Cutting-Edge Applications of Nanomaterials in Biomedical Sciences

Pranav Kumar Prabhakar
Lovely Professional University, India

Ajit Prakash
University of North Carolina, USA

IGI Global
PUBLISHER of TIMELY KNOWLEDGE

A volume in the Advances in Medical Diagnosis, Treatment, and Care (AMDTC) Book Series

Published in the United States of America by
IGI Global
Medical Information Science Reference (an imprint of IGI Global)
701 E. Chocolate Avenue
Hershey PA, USA 17033
Tel: 717-533-8845
Fax: 717-533-8661
E-mail: cust@igi-global.com
Web site: http://www.igi-global.com

Library of Congress Cataloging-in-Publication Data

Names: Kumar Prabhakar, Pranav editor. | Prakash, Ajit, 1986- editor.
Title: Cutting-edge applications of nanomaterials in biomedical sciences / edited by Pranav Prabhakar, Ajit Prakash.
Description: Hershey, PA : Medical Information Science Reference, [2024] | Includes bibliographical references and index. | Summary: "The book provides a comprehensive overview of challenges, opportunities, and potential impact of nanotechnology-based substances in drug delivery, precision medicine, diagnostics, and therapeutics"-- Provided by publisher.
Identifiers: LCCN 2023037093 (print) | LCCN 2023037094 (ebook) | ISBN 9798369304488 (hardcover) | ISBN 9798369304495 (paperback) | ISBN 9798369304501 (ebook)
Subjects: MESH: Nanostructures--therapeutic use | Nanotechnology--methods
Classification: LCC R857.M3 (print) | LCC R857.M3 (ebook) | NLM QT 36.5 | DDC 610.28/4--dc23/eng/20230901
LC record available at https://lccn.loc.gov/2023037093
LC ebook record available at https://lccn.loc.gov/2023037094

This book is published in the IGI Global book series Advances in Medical Diagnosis, Treatment, and Care (AMDTC) (ISSN: 2475-6628; eISSN: 2475-6636)

British Cataloguing in Publication Data
A Cataloguing in Publication record for this book is available from the British Library.

For electronic access to this publication, please contact: eresources@igi-global.com.

Advances in Medical Diagnosis, Treatment, and Care (AMDTC) Book Series

ISSN:2475-6628
EISSN:2475-6636

Mission

Advancements in medicine have prolonged the life expectancy of individuals all over the world. Once life-threatening conditions have become significantly easier to treat and even cure in many cases. Continued research in the medical field will further improve the quality of life, longevity, and wellbeing of individuals.

The **Advances in Medical Diagnosis, Treatment, and Care (AMDTC)** book series seeks to highlight publications on innovative treatment methodologies, diagnosis tools and techniques, and best practices for patient care. Comprised of comprehensive resources aimed to assist professionals in the medical field apply the latest innovations in the identification and management of medical conditions as well as patient care and interaction, the books within the AMDTC series are relevant to the research and practical needs of medical practitioners, researchers, students, and hospital administrators.

Coverage

- Disease Management
- Chronic Conditions
- Experimental Medicine
- Internal Medicine
- Diagnostic Medicine
- Emergency Medicine
- Patient-Centered Care
- Disease prevention
- Alternative Medicine
- Cancer Treatment

IGI Global is currently accepting manuscripts for publication within this series. To submit a proposal for a volume in this series, please contact our Acquisition Editors at Acquisitions@igi-global.com or visit: http://www.igi-global.com/publish/.

The Advances in Medical Diagnosis, Treatment, and Care (AMDTC) Book Series (ISSN 2475-6628) is published by IGI Global, 701 E. Chocolate Avenue, Hershey, PA 17033-1240, USA, www.igi-global.com. This series is composed of titles available for purchase individually; each title is edited to be contextually exclusive from any other title within the series. For pricing and ordering information please visit http://www.igi-global.com/book-series/advances-medical-diagnosis-treatment-care/129618. Postmaster: Send all address changes to above address.

Titles in this Series

For a list of additional titles in this series, please visit: www.igi-global.com/book-series/advances-medical-diagnosis-treatment-care/129618

Geriatric Dentistry in the Age of Digital Technology
Dachel Martínez Asanza (University of Medical Sciences of Havana, Cuba)
Medical Information Science Reference • copyright 2024 • 347pp • H/C (ISBN: 9798369302606) • US $360.00 (our price)

Clinical Practice and Post-Infection Care for COVID-19 Patients
Gunda Varaprasad Rao (NMH Heart Care Center, Nashik, India) and Sangeeta Dhamdhere-Rao (Modern College of Arts, Science, and Commerce, Pune, India)
Medical Information Science Reference • copyright 2024 • 262pp • H/C (ISBN: 9781668468555) • US $435.00 (our price)

Exploring Complementary and Alternative Medicinal Products in Disease Therapy
Etetor Roland Eshiet (Sustainable Energy Environmental and Educational Development (SEEED), USA)
Medical Information Science Reference • copyright 2023 • 348pp • H/C (ISBN: 9781799841203) • US $325.00 (our price)

Natural Products as Cancer Therapeutics
Narayanaswamy Radhakrishnan (Saveetha Medical College and Hospital (SIMATS), India) Srinivasan Vasantha (Saveetha Medical College and Hospital (SIMATS), India) and Ashok Kumar Pandurangan (B.S. Abdur Rahman Crescent Institute of Science and Technology, India)
Medical Information Science Reference • copyright 2023 • 388pp • H/C (ISBN: 9798369307038) • US $325.00 (our price)

Experimental and Clinical Evidence of the Neuropathology of Parkinson's Disease
Ahmed Draoui (Cadi Ayyad University, Morocco) Omar El Hiba (Chouaib Doukkali University, Morocco) and Arumugam R. Jayakumar (Miami Veterans Affairs Medical Center, USA)
Medical Information Science Reference • copyright 2023 • 447pp • H/C (ISBN: 9781668451564) • US $325.00 (our price)

Pharmacological Benefits of Natural Agents
Narayanaswamy Radhakrishnan (Saveetha Medical College and Hospital (SIMATS), India) Srinivasan Vasantha (Saveetha Medical College and Hospital (SIMATS), India) and Ashok Kumar Pandurangan (B.S. Abdur Rahman Crescent Institute of Science and Technology, India)

IGI Global
PUBLISHER of TIMELY KNOWLEDGE

701 East Chocolate Avenue, Hershey, PA 17033, USA
Tel: 717-533-8845 x100 • Fax: 717-533-8661
E-Mail: cust@igi-global.com • www.igi-global.com

Table of Contents

Detailed Table of Contents

The advancements in the molecular sciences have been a driving force for the search of unconventional nanomaterials to be used in Biomedical applications. Nanobiotechnology has proved its potential for the development of specialized materials for targeted drug and gene delivery, diagnosis, regenerative medicine, bioimaging, biosensing, tissue engineering, and implants. Nanomaterials are capable of integrating well into biomedical devices since the majority of the biological systems are also nanosized. The integration of nanotechnology and medical sciences offers a range of properties that offer nanomaterials as a robust, highly sensitive, cost-effective approach for further exploration in various fields. The present chapter offers a basic understanding of emerging nano-structured materials in biomedical sciences eliciting the possible usage and further avenues in research.

This chapter provides a comprehensive review of recent advances in nanomaterials for drug delivery, focusing on the design and preparation of nanocarriers. It also dissects the intricate mechanisms underpinning drug loading and release, and delves into the strategic planning inherent in achieving target delivery. It further outlines the potential applications of these nanomaterials in treating various diseases, including cancer, infectious diseases, and neurological disorders. A distinct case study is incorporated into the chapter, elucidating the promising utility of electrospun nanofibers in drug delivery paradigms. In its concluding remarks, the chapter engages in a thoughtful discourse about the persistent challenges within this rapidly evolving field. It also forecasts the potential trajectories for future exploration and innovation in the captivating domain of nanomaterials for drug delivery.

The use of nanotechnology products in biomedicine has led to the emergence of a hybrid science known as nano-biotechnology. Due to the nanoscale nature of most biological systems, nanoscale materials integrate well into biomedical devices. In response to certain stimuli, highly ordered bottom-up nano-structured materials exhibit specific behaviours. Nanomaterial applications are tuned by surface chemistry and physics. This chapter provides an overview of the use of metallic, metal oxide, and carbon nanoparticles for specific biomedical applications. It also discusses liposomes and nano-patterned flat surfaces. A challenge is determining the effects of nanomaterials on biological systems. However, a detailed understanding of nanomaterial potential toxicity is needed to take advantage of their potential applications in medicine. To minimize false results, it is important to interpret the relationship between toxicity and physicochemical properties cautiously.

Cancer is one of the most abundant lethal diseases globally threatening public health. There is considerable research effort on the prevention, diagnosis, and treatment of cancer. The current practices for cancer treatment are usage of synthetic chemicals (i.e. chemotherapy), radiotherapy, and surgery. Besides these conventional therapies, there are contemporary, innovative approaches, e.g., targeting of the drugs to the cancerous tissues, synergetic enhancement via simultaneous usage of conventional methods, and contemporary methods. Therefore, the process of drug research and development in the field of cancer is increasingly challenging, due to the limited success of current therapies and the constant need to find safer and more effective novel approaches. The utilization of nanotechnology may present new opportunities in cancer treatment. Metal nanoparticles prepared via "bottom-up" approach may be used for triggering the selective cell apoptosis mechanisms for cancerous cells, while sparing healthy cells considerably.

Polymeric nanoparticles (PNPs) are tiny particles with a size between 1 and 1000 nm that can include active substances that have been surface-adsorbed over onto polymeric core or are entrapped inside of them. Both nanospheres and nanocapsules fall under the umbrella of "nanoparticles," which are characterized by their morphological structure. This material is anticipated to be extensively used in various sectors, including drug delivery systems, catalysts, biosensors, nanocomposites, agriculture, and the environment because of its extremely small size and large surface area. Particle size, geometry, material selection, and processing methods are all study topics of interest to establish the optimal nanosystem for more efficient and focused delivery of therapeutic applications. Drug delivery methods such as drug conjugation and drug entrapment, prodrugs, stimuli-responsive systems, imaging modalities, and theranostics all use PNPs. The goal of the technique of using polymeric nanoparticles for drug delivery is to maximize therapeutic effectiveness while reducing side effects.

Diabetes mellitus is a chronic metabolic disorder characterized by impaired glucose regulation, which leads to various complications affecting multiple organs and systems. This chapter discusses various types of nanomaterials, such as liposomes, polymeric nanoparticles, dendrimers, and carbon-based nanomaterials, and their potential for encapsulating and delivering therapeutic agents to specific sites affected by diabetic complications. The advantages of nanomaterial-based drug delivery, including enhanced drug stability, prolonged circulation time, and improved targeting efficiency, are highlighted. The challenges and considerations associated with targeted nanotherapy development, including biocompatibility, toxicity, and regulatory aspects, are also discussed. The chapter serves as a valuable resource for researchers, clinicians, and healthcare professionals involved in the development and translation of targeted nano therapies, ultimately contributing to the advancement of diabetic complication management.

Infectious diseases are a major global burden according to the latest WHO reports. The problems of drug resistance, emergence, and reemergence cases are rising when treatment is given by conventional therapy. These therapeutic insufficiencies lead to treatment failure. Nanomaterials are a class of carrier systems that offer some desirable properties to combat the aforementioned problems related to the treatment of infectious diseases. They offer better targetability and better bioavailability than conventional systems. Thus, they are being explored to their full potential in the treatment of infectious diseases. The use of metallic nanoparticles, carbon dots, are a major area where research is being carried out to mark them as effective carriers. This book chapter gives an insight to various nanomaterials which are widely used and explored for the treatment of various diseases along with the safety and regulatory aspects of nanomaterials.

Nanotechnology has been applied in healthcare to cure diseases, especially cancer. Cancer is one of the heterogenous diseases which lacks symptoms in the early stage thus has made it difficult to cure at a

cancer, cardiovascular diseases, and renal failure, which can improve patient's lifestyle. Nanomaterials offer properties like enhanced diagnostic specificity, increased blood circulation time, and organ specific delivery just with the help of functionalization and conjugation with desired materials. Nanomaterials like dendrimer, silica nanoparticles, and some magnetic nanoparticles are used as contrast agents in imaging technology such as magnetic resonance imaging (MRI), computed tomography (CT) and radiopharmaceuticals. This chapter covers nanomaterials (NPs) as a biomedical tool for imaging and diagnosis of various diseases.

Materials with 10-9m dimensions are considered nanomaterials, which exhibit beneficial aspects against health-related complications and thus have received much attention. Modern knowledge of the various functions of nanomaterials has advanced it to a new level of revolution. Several chemical, physical, and biological techniques can be used to create nanomaterials. A variety of methods are available for figuring out their physical characteristics and chemical makeup. Their unique physical and chemical properties, due to nanoscale size, enhance their utilization and applications in the field of medicine and biomedical sciences. However, glimpse of certain harmful paradigms offered by nanoparticles forces us to rethink the negative impacts against the human health. This chapter reviews an introductory overview covering the current concepts related to the properties and application of various sorts of nanomaterials used in the field of medical science, with special reference to their metabolic and physiological influence in many types of pathophysiological disorders.

A new era in healthcare has been ushered in by the development of nanotechnology. Materials with exceptional properties at the nanoscale are being used to enhance the accuracy and efficacy of diagnostic methods. In particular, nanoparticles have become potent tools with a variety of applications in medical imaging. They can be employed as contrast agents in a number of imaging techniques, such as ultrasounds, computed tomography, and magnetic resonance imaging (MRI), to increase tissue visibility and help diagnose diseases. Increased sensitivity and specificity are two benefits of using nanomaterials in medical diagnostics. They allow for the creation of novel biosensors and diagnostic platforms that can identify biomarkers at lower concentrations, enabling the early identification and monitoring of illnesses. Precision healthcare benefits from the use of drug delivery systems based on nanomaterials because they enable customised therapy, lessen side effects, and enhance patient outcomes.

Recognizing and promoting contributions relevant to public health is crucial as the range of nanotechnology uses in medicine expands. Nanomedical advances promise to have far-reaching effects across the medical spectrum, revealing exciting new approaches to enhance health and lengthen life that can be quantified on both an individual and a societal scale. In the United States, for instance, cardiovascular disease and cancer account for over half of all deaths each year, yet there is promising evidence that improvements in nanomedicine can help cut these numbers. Nanomedicine's public health uses, like quicker and more portable diagnostics and more potent immunizations, could radically alter the state of global health. Diverse innovators from engineering, biology, medicine, and public health should collaborate to maximize the impact of their research on human health.

Drug delivery research aims to deliver exact doses of anti-tumor drugs to tumors. Recent nanoparticle engineering trials have improved drug targeting, but results need to be better. Nanoparticles, like traditional medicine, target their target via blood circulation. The enhanced permeability and retention (EPR) effect helps most nanoparticles, PEGylated or not, reach their target. Nanoparticles with targeting moieties like antibodies or ligands do not deliver drugs to tumors, according to research. Targeted medicine delivery tumors created complicated biological, mechanical, chemical, and transport systems with changing properties. However, most research has focused on making and modifying drug-carrying nanoparticle surfaces. Bioactive substances delivered utilizing stimuli-responsive controlled-release nanomedicine may reduce side effects and boost effectiveness.

Bacteria that secrete exopolysaccharides (EPS) when colonised on living and non-living surfaces also protect from stressors in a variety of environments. EPS is considered a complex carbohydrate, which is part of their extracellular matrix. EPS play magnificent roles in microbial biofilm formation, providing structural integrity and protection for microbial communities. Chemically synthesised nanomaterials are not ideal for use as antimicrobial agents because they are harmful to environments and also ineffective. An alternative, sustainable approach is needed to control biofilm-related infections. Therefore, in this chapter, the authors discuss the techniques of optimisation and characterization of bacterial exopolysaccharide-mediated nanoparticles and nanomaterials for targeting oral biofilm-forming pathogens. It will be essential for the use of exopolysaccharide-mediated nanoparticles in biomedical applications to prevent biofilm-associated infections such as urinary catheter devices and biofilm-related chronic wounds.

Researchers have directed their attention to the application of nanotechnology in the biomedical sciences owing to their promising effects. In light of this, the present chapter is a concerted effort to highlight the emerging application of nanotechnology in the field of biomedical sciences. The first part of the chapter describes the introduction to biomedical science, followed by an introduction to the development of nanotechnology, the types and characteristics of nanosized materials, and their potential therapeutic properties. Next, the present chapter describes the application of nanotechnology in biomedical sciences. It also highlights the current issues regarding the usage of nanotechnology in biomedical science, especially safety, regulation, and toxicity. This chapter aims to provide new insights into the extraordinary application of nanotechnology in the biomedical science field for researchers, policymakers, regulators, healthcare professionals, and others involved in the nano biomedical application field.

Understanding how nanomaterials (NMs) and biological systems interact at the interface is of great research interest. Nanoparticles (NPs) such as carbon nanotubes, graphene oxides, carbon dots, graphite nanopowders, and others are included in NMs. Through organic layers, medicinal compounds, proteins, DNA, and cellular matrices, these NPs exhibit a range of interactions with biological interfaces. The morphological surface of bio-nanoconjugates is influenced by a variety of biophysical and colloidal factors that control their biological responses, giving the NMs unique physical characteristics. Future-generation nano-tool design is essentially focused on the fundamental characteristics of NMs, such as shape, size, composition, functionality, etc., and substantial research has been done in this area. Understanding their characteristics encourages study in the biological and medical fields and enhances their relevance in the field of health management.

Nanomaterials' unique physicochemical features make them suitable for biological applications such medication delivery, imaging, and tissue engineering. However, there is growing concern regarding their safety and toxicity due to their small size and high surface area, which can result in unanticipated interactions with biological systems. Studies have demonstrated that cationic nanoparticles exhibit a propensity to interact with cellular membranes and elicit oxidative stress, while anionic nanoparticles have a tendency to accumulate within lysosomes and trigger inflammatory responses. Numerous methods have been developed to evaluate the safety and toxicity of nanomaterials, such as in-vitro, in-vivo assays, computational modeling, etc. Nanomaterials in medical sciences are subject to regulatory scaffolds that give guidelines/ policies for safety assessment and risk management, nonetheless more research is required to entirely comprehend the possible long-term effects or interactions of nanoparticles with other environmental elements.

This chapter focuses on the viscometric, volumetric, and spectroscopic techniques to investigate the thermo-acoustic parameters and nature of molecular interactions. This in-depth analysis of the literature focuses on the properties and uses of benzoate-based combinations in aqueous solutions. Studies examining the density and volumetric properties, excess parameters, molecular interactions, and thermal properties of benzoate-based compounds like sodium benzoate, ethyl benzoate, and methyl benzoate are the main subject of interest. The current review presents research and studies on acoustic and thermodynamic investigations as well as molecular interactions of the mixtures. This review aims not only to consolidate the existing knowledge but also to inspire future investigations that contribute to the development of novel materials used in many applications of ultrasonic sound in the disciplines of medical, pharmacology, agricultural practices, etc.

Phosphate-based mixtures are widely used in various industries, and understanding their thermodynamic properties is crucial for optimizing their applications in medicine, pharmaceuticals, leather manufacturing, textiles, etc. This comprehensive review explores the literature on the thermodynamic characteristics and applications of phosphate-based mixtures in aqueous solutions. The focus is on studies investigating density and volumetric properties, phase equilibrium, molecular interactions, and thermal properties of phosphate compounds such as Disodium dihydrogen pyrophosphate and DiPotassium hydrogen phosphate. The chapter provides a comprehensive summary of the extensive research conducted on the thermodynamics of mixtures, specifically in aqueous solutions. The focus of these investigations has been on exploring the thermodynamic properties of various compounds containing phosphates. The findings presented in this review contribute to the existing knowledge base and provide a foundation for further research and optimization of phosphate-based mixtures in aqueous solutions.

Utilizing the ultrasonic speed of sound and density of ternary mixture of butoxyethanol (BE), phenoxyethanol(PE) in aqueous solution of biotin (Vitamin B7) at concentrations (0.0012, 0.0017, 0.0022) mol•⟦kg⟧^(-1)and varying temperature from (288.15 to 303.15 K) for constant frequency (3 MHz), various thermoacoustic parameters, such as acoustic impedance (Z), adiabatic compressibility (β), Wada's constant (W), Rao's constant (R), intermolecular free length (LF), and Vander Waal's constant (b) have been determined. The experimental work was carried out by using Anton Paar DSA 5000 M at constant pressure 0.1 MPa. The calculated values obtained from experimental values provided the understanding of intermolecular interaction between solute and solvent in liquid mixture. Variation in these parameters describes the understanding of behavior and interaction between the components in solution. Decrease in ultrasonic velocity depicts the weak interaction between molecules.

In order to examine the non-ideal behaviour of a liquid, it is crucial to conduct investigations. To determine excess properties, a range of measurable properties can be utilized in experimental calculations. Major characteristics to consider in binary and ternary mixtures include density and apparent molar volume. From a thermodynamic standpoint, several combination characteristics, various thermodynamic features, such as partial molar volumes, at infinite dilution, hold great significance. The purpose of this review is to provide a summary of recent research on the acoustics and thermodynamics of sugar alcohols in various mixtures and temperatures. Sugar alcohols are widely used in the nutrition and pharmacological industries, and many medical applications. They function as low-calorie sweeteners, providing a sweet flavour without rapidly raising blood sugar levels. Specific sugar alcohols, like xylitol, support dental health. Furthermore, acoustics can be employed as a tool for particle sizing, as well as for revealing information about the microstructure of the dispersed system.

Preface

In the ever-evolving landscape of biomedical sciences, the pursuit of knowledge is not merely a noble endeavor—it's a necessity. *Cutting-Edge Applications of Nanomaterials in Biomedical Sciences* seeks to underscore the paramount importance of research, innovation, and the transformative power of nanomaterials in addressing critical challenges facing healthcare today.

The complexities of modern medicine demand innovative solutions, and it is research that stands as the beacon, guiding us towards these solutions. Our book, edited by *Pranav Kumar Prabhakar* and *Ajit Prakash*, acts as a testament to the significance of research in revolutionizing healthcare by harnessing the potential of nanotechnology-based substances.

RESEARCH AS THE CATALYST FOR CHANGE

a) **Comprehensive Overview:** At the core of our book lies the belief in the power of comprehensive research. It is through this research that we can understand, harness, and implement the latest advancements in nanomaterials for medical applications. This knowledge empowers us to unlock new frontiers in medicine.

b) **Challenges and Opportunities:** Our exploration of challenges and opportunities is a call to action. Research enables us to confront these challenges head-on, and it illuminates the path to seizing the opportunities that nanotechnology offers. By conducting rigorous investigations, we can craft innovative solutions for drug delivery, precision medicine, diagnostics, and therapeutics, thus shaping the future of healthcare.

c) **Regulatory and Commercial Aspects:** As we delve into the regulatory and commercialization aspects, it becomes clear that research plays a pivotal role in bridging the gap between discovery and implementation. Robust research is essential for developing safe, effective, and ethical approaches to the use of nanomaterials in medicine. Furthermore, it fuels the commercialization engine, making these innovations accessible to patients.

TRANSFORMING CHALLENGES INTO SOLUTIONS

(a) Our book, filled with the latest research findings, equips researchers, clinicians, and students with the knowledge they need to drive progress in biomedical sciences. It offers a solid foundation upon which they can build their own research endeavors, thereby advancing our collective understanding of nanomaterials in medicine.

(b) Through research, we can overcome obstacles and turn them into opportunities. By engaging in rigorous investigation, we can navigate the intricate terrain of drug delivery, precision medicine, diagnostics, and therapeutics, and develop cutting-edge solutions that will redefine healthcare.

(c) Policymakers and regulators will discover in-depth insights to help them make informed decisions, based on solid research, about the safety and ethical implications of nanomaterials in medicine. In doing so, they can safeguard public health and ensure the responsible use of these groundbreaking technologies.

THE PROMISE OF RESEARCH

As we embark on this journey through the pages of *Cutting-Edge Applications of Nanomaterials in Biomedical Sciences*, let us remember that it is research that propels us forward. Research is the key to addressing the challenges, seizing the opportunities, and realizing the immense potential of nanomaterials in medicine.

Through research, we transform problems into solutions, questions into answers, and possibilities into realities. It is our hope that this book will not only inform but also inspire you to embark on your own research adventures in this exciting and dynamic field. Together, we can shape the future of healthcare and improve the lives of countless individuals through the power of nanomaterials and research-driven innovation.

CHAPTER OVERVIEW

Chapter 1: An Insight into the Application of Nanotechnology in Biomedical Sciences: Exploration of Biomedical Sciences with Relation to Nanotechnology

In this opening chapter, the authors provide a foundational understanding of the application of nanotechnology in biomedical sciences. They explore the pivotal role nanotechnology plays in fields like targeted drug delivery, gene therapy, regenerative medicine, and more. This chapter serves as a bridge, connecting the realm of nanotechnology with the vast opportunities it offers in biomedical applications.

Chapter 2: Advances in Nanomaterials for Drug Delivery

Chapter 2 delves into the cutting-edge advancements in nanomaterials for drug delivery. It not only reviews the recent progress in designing and preparing nanocarriers but also discusses the mechanisms underlying drug loading and release. The chapter further explores the potential applications of these nanomaterials in treating diseases, including cancer, infectious diseases, and neurological disorders, providing a glimpse into the future of drug delivery.

Chapter 3: Nanotechnology and its Applications in Biomedical Sciences

The third chapter focuses on the integration of nanotechnology and biomedicine, forming the intriguing field of nano-biotechnology. It covers a wide range of nanomaterials, such as metallic, metal oxide, and carbon nanoparticles, and their applications in various biomedical contexts. Surface chemistry and physics are highlighted as key factors in tuning nanomaterial applications. The chapter also discusses the challenges and safety concerns associated with nanomaterial use in medicine.

Chapter 4: Metal Nanoparticles via Green Synthesis: A New Cancer Treatment Approach

Cancer treatment is a major concern globally, and this chapter sheds light on an innovative approach involving metal nanoparticles synthesized through green methods. It explores how metal nanoparticles can selectively induce apoptosis in cancer cells while sparing healthy cells. This novel approach to cancer therapy is presented as a beacon of hope in the fight against this deadly disease.

Chapter 5: Polymeric Nanoparticles in Drug Delivery

Chapter 5 takes a closer look at polymeric nanoparticles and their applications in drug delivery systems. It explains the versatility of polymeric nanoparticles, which can carry active substances, and discusses the key parameters for optimizing their use, including particle size, geometry, material selection, and processing methods. The goal is to maximize therapeutic effectiveness while minimizing side effects.

Chapter 6: Targeted Nanotherapies for Diabetic Complications

This chapter focuses on the challenges posed by diabetes mellitus, a chronic metabolic disorder. It discusses how nanomaterials, such as liposomes, polymeric nanoparticles, dendrimers, and carbon-based nanomaterials, can be harnessed to encapsulate and deliver therapeutic agents to specific sites affected by diabetic complications. The advantages and considerations of targeted nanotherapies are highlighted, offering valuable insights for researchers and healthcare professionals in this field.

Chapter 7: Nanomaterials in Treatment of Infectious Diseases: Treatment and Regulatory Aspect

Infectious diseases remain a global challenge, and conventional therapies face issues like drug resistance. This chapter explores how nanomaterials are being investigated as carriers to combat these issues. It delves into the use of metallic nanoparticles and carbon dots and also discusses safety and regulatory aspects, shedding light on the potential for nanomaterials in treating various diseases.

Chapter 8: Nanomaterials in Cancer Therapy

Chapter 8 introduces the role of nanotechnology in cancer therapy. Cancer, often diagnosed at later stages, presents a significant challenge for effective treatment. This chapter explores the diverse applications of various types of nanoparticles in cancer therapy, emphasizing hybrid nanoparticles' effectiveness in treating this heterogeneous disease. The combination of multiple therapies is also discussed, representing the forefront of cancer treatment.

Chapter 9: Quantum Nanoscience in Targeted Drug Delivery: Understanding Mechanism of Bio-Nano Interactions in Targeting and Drug Delivery

The ninth chapter delves into the intricate world of targeted drug delivery (TDD) using quantum nanoscience. It highlights the various aspects of TDD, such as drug loading, transport, and unloading at precise locations in the body. It emphasizes the need for interdisciplinary collaboration in fields like polymer science, pharmacology, and biology to unlock the full potential of TDD and advance clinical applications.

Chapter 10: Nanomaterials in Imaging and Diagnostics

Chapter 10 uncovers the application of nanomaterials in medical imaging and diagnostics. These materials offer enhanced diagnostic specificity, increased circulation time, and organ-specific delivery. The chapter reviews the use of nanomaterials as contrast agents in imaging techniques such as MRI, CT, and radiopharmaceuticals. The enhanced sensitivity and specificity of these nanomaterials hold immense promise for early disease diagnosis and monitoring.

Chapter 11: Nanotechnology and its Application in Medical Sciences

This chapter provides an introductory overview of the properties and applications of various nanomaterials in medical science. It emphasizes the unique characteristics of nanomaterials, stemming from their nanoscale size, and their significance in addressing various pathophysiological disorders. The chapter provides an essential foundation for researchers, policymakers, regulators, healthcare professionals, and others interested in the field of nanobiomedical applications.

Chapter 12: The Significance of Nanomaterials in Medical Imaging and Diagnostics

Chapter 12 explores the profound significance of nanomaterials in enhancing medical imaging and diagnostics. Nanoparticles serve as potent tools to improve the accuracy and efficacy of diagnostic methods. The chapter reviews the applications of nanomaterials as contrast agents and their role in developing novel biosensors and diagnostic platforms. These innovations enable early disease detection and monitoring, contributing to the field of precision healthcare.

Chapter 14: The Importance of Nanomedicine and its Prospects for the Public Health and Research Field in the Present and Future

This chapter highlights the crucial role of nanomedicine in public health and research. It discusses how nanomedicine can revolutionize healthcare by providing new ways to enhance health and extend life. Various applications of nanomedicine, from quicker and more portable diagnostics to more potent immunizations, are explored. The chapter emphasizes the potential of nanomedicine to address global health challenges.

Chapter 15: The Development of Nanomaterials for the Regulated and Sustained Delivery of Medications for Future Health and Research

Chapter 15 focuses on the development of nanomaterials for controlled drug delivery. It explores the challenges and innovations in this field, aiming to improve therapeutic effectiveness while minimizing side effects. The chapter discusses various techniques, such as stimuli-responsive controlled-release systems, and emphasizes the importance of sustainable, regulated drug delivery for future healthcare and research.

Chapter 16: Bacterial Exopolysaccharides Based Nanomaterials for Targeting Biofilm-Associated Infections: Bacterial Nanomaterials

This chapter delves into a sustainable approach to combating biofilm-associated infections, using bacterial exopolysaccharides to create nanomaterials. It explores the potential of these nanomaterials in preventing infections in applications like urinary catheter devices and chronic wound management. The chapter also addresses the optimization and characterization of bacterial exopolysaccharide-mediated nanoparticles for targeted therapies.

Chapter 17: Emerging Application of Nanomaterial with Less Toxicity and More Efficacy in Modern Biomedical Engineering

Chapter 17 explores the interface between nanomaterials and biological systems, highlighting the interactions that occur at this juncture. It delves into the effects of various nanoparticles on biological interfaces, offering insights into the unique physical characteristics of nan omaterials. The chapter emphasizes the role of nanomaterials in advancing healthcare and enhancing patient outcomes.

Chapter 18: Safety and Toxicity of Nanomaterials in Medicine

This chapter addresses the safety and toxicity concerns associated with nanomaterials used in medicine. It explores the unique physicochemical features of nanomaterials that may lead to unanticipated interactions with biological systems. The chapter discusses various methods for evaluating the safety and toxicity of nanomaterials, from in-vitro and in-vivo assays to computational modeling. It also considers regulatory frameworks for nanomaterials in medical sciences.

Chapter 19: Thermo-Acoustic Investigations on Benzoate-Based Mixtures Using Ultrasonic Technique: A Review

This chapter reviews the research on benzoate-based mixtures using thermo-acoustic investigations. It covers various parameters, such as acoustic impedance, adiabatic compressibility, and more. These investigations aim to understand the interactions between different components in the mixtures, providing insights into the behavior and properties of these compounds.

Chapter 20: Thermo-Acoustic Investigations on Phosphate-Based Mixtures in Aqueous Solutions: A Review

Chapter 20 focuses on the thermo-acoustic investigations of phosphate-based mixtures in aqueous solutions. These mixtures are essential in various industries, including medicine and pharmaceuticals. The chapter reviews the studies examining density, phase equilibrium, molecular interactions, and thermal properties, offering valuable insights for optimizing their applications.

Chapter 21: Thermodynamic Investigations of Vitamin B7 with Glycol Ethers as the Function of Temperature

Chapter 21 explores the ultrasonic investigations of vitamin B7 in glycol ethers, observing changes in ultrasonic velocity with varying temperatures and concentrations. This research helps to understand the intermolecular interactions within these mixtures and their effects.

Chapter 22: A Review on Acoustic and Thermodynamic Properties of Sugar Alcohols

This chapter presents a comprehensive review of the acoustic and thermodynamic properties of sugar alcohols in various mixtures and temperatures. Sugar alcohol is widely used in several industries, including medical applications. The review covers various aspects of their behavior, making it a valuable resource for understanding their applications in diverse fields.

IN SUMMARY

In bringing together this comprehensive edited reference book on *"Nanomaterials in Biomedical Sciences and Beyond,"* we have embarked on a remarkable journey through the intersection of nanotechnology and the vast domains of biomedical research, healthcare, and beyond. The collection of 22 meticulously crafted chapters, contributed by experts in their respective fields, has shed light on the innovative and dynamic landscape that is reshaping the future of medicine, healthcare, and several other disciplines.

This reference book has unfolded the immense potential of nanomaterials in addressing some of the most challenging problems in healthcare and beyond. Each chapter serves as a window into the exciting world of nanotechnology, where remarkable progress is made every day. The authors have provided insights into the latest advancements, focusing on their applications in drug delivery, imaging, disease treatment, and more.

From targeted Nanotherapies for diabetic complications to the use of metal nanoparticles for new cancer treatment approaches, from the significance of nanomedicine in public health to investigations of thermodynamic properties in various mixtures, this book reflects the breadth and depth of nanomaterial research. We've explored the role of nanotechnology in improving the diagnosis, treatment, and monitoring of diseases, emphasizing its potential to revolutionize the healthcare landscape.

However, this journey also highlights the importance of safety, regulation, and thorough evaluation of the potential toxicity of nanomaterials. While the promise of nanotechnology is undeniable, the ethical, safety, and environmental implications of this evolving field must not be overlooked.

As we conclude this preface, we would like to express our gratitude to the dedicated authors who contributed their expertise to this project, as well as to the readers who embark on their own journey into the world of nanomaterials. We hope that this edited reference book will serve as a valuable resource for researchers, clinicians, policymakers, and healthcare professionals and inspire the next wave of breakthroughs in this rapidly evolving field.

Our journey through the pages of this book has been both enlightening and inspiring, and it is our sincere hope that it serves as a catalyst for further exploration, innovation, and collaboration in the dynamic world of nanomaterials in biomedical sciences and beyond.

Thank you for joining us on this journey.

With warm regards,

Pranav Kumar Prabhakar
Lovely Professional University, Punjab India

Ajit Prakash
University of North Carolina at Chapel Hill, United States

Chapter 1
An Insight Into the Application of Nanotechnology in Biomedical Sciences:
Exploration of Biomedical Sciences With Relation to Nanotechnology

Mayank Bahuguna
https://orcid.org/0000-0003-1344-5511
Swami Rama Himalayan University, India

Charu Sharma
https://orcid.org/0009-0001-4206-4905
Swami Rama Himalayan University, India

Geeta Bhandari
https://orcid.org/0000-0003-0617-3714
Swami Rama Himalayan University, India

Sanjay Gupta
Swami Rama Himalayan University, India

ABSTRACT

The advancements in the molecular sciences have been a driving force for the search of unconventional nanomaterials to be used in Biomedical applications. Nanobiotechnology has proved its potential for the development of specialized materials for targeted drug and gene delivery, diagnosis, regenerative medicine, bioimaging, biosensing, tissue engineering, and implants. Nanomaterials are capable of integrating well into biomedical devices since the majority of the biological systems are also nanosized. The integration of nanotechnology and medical sciences offers a range of properties that offer nanomaterials as a robust, highly sensitive, cost-effective approach for further exploration in various fields. The present chapter offers a basic understanding of emerging nano-structured materials in biomedical sciences eliciting the possible usage and further avenues in research.

DOI: 10.4018/979-8-3693-0448-8.ch001

INTRODUCTION

Nanobiotechnology is an amalgamation realm of biotechnology and nanotechnology with the potential to revolutionize fields, like medicine, energy, biosensors, and electronics. The knowledge acquired from the field of Nanotechnology involves the designing, fabrication, modification, and implementation of materials, devices, and systems at the nanoscale (0.1-100 nm) level. Therefore, with properties of being nanoscaled, with a high surface area to volume ratio, nanomaterials display unique characteristics distinguishing them from bulk particles including; physical strength, durability, optical, electrical, magnetic characteristics, reactivity, and conductivity (Bhandari et al., 2023). An avenue of possible modifications in consideration of size, shape, and composition, proves them to be ideal for a wide range of applications, including medicine, electronics, and energy. Several significant properties including surface composition, topographical features, roughness, wettability, free energy, electronic, magnetic, and optical features, along with their toxicological impact specificies their application in different areas. A vast range of possibilities also aligns with the usage of nanoparticles in the biomedical sector for diagnostics, therapies, and disease prevention such as novel diagnostic technologies, imaging, targeted pharmaceuticals delivery, biomedical implants, disease monitoring, regenerative medicine, and tissue engineering. Furthermore, nanoprobes, hybrid sensory nano-electronic devices, and multifunctional chemical compounds for pharmaceutical delivery and disease targeting are future applications in nanotechnology. Additionally, Nanomedicine consists of science and technology which employs molecular methods and information about the human body for:

1. Production of novel therapeutically active agents for disease treatment and tissue repair
2. Development of diagnostics methods for fast monitoring such as; high throughput analysis, imaging instruments, nanoparticle labels, highly sensitivity detectors, and nano-sensors
3. Development of bio-pharmaceutics for target-specific drug and gene delivery, improvement of cell-material interactions for tissue regeneration and repair
4. Development of surgical tools and aids

Moreover, Nanomaterials possess the ability to integrate specifically into biomedical instruments due to the nanosizing of biological systems. For the following reason, Inorganic and metal nanomaterials, carbon nanotubes, liposomes, and metallic surfaces are generally employed for developing medically important materials (H. Liu et al., 2016). Particularly, biomolecules can be conjugated with nanomaterials using physicochemical techniques in consideration of antibody-antigen, receptor-ligand, and DNA-DNA interactions. The major contributing factors for the following process involve conjugation, encapsulation, or adsorption for the agents used in drug delivery systems, therapeutics, biomolecules, and imaging. Several reports on the use of nanomaterials for different biomedical applications are available in the literature. Discussing further, Nanobots are employed for targeting tissue-specific cancerous cells with the usage of smart tablets, which enables the data scientists for suggesting the correct diagnosis and treatment for patients to the medicos. *In-vitro* diagnostics by replacing current methods with nano-biosensors for a more cost-effective and easy-to-use alternative is a recent trend among researchers of the age. Nanoparticles may also contribute to the innovation of molecular imaging devices with reference to cancer-related genetic modifications and tumor cell functional characters (Haleem et al., 2023). In general, the functional nanomaterial-based coating for the possible intervention includes TiO_2, SiO_2, carbon black, Fe_3O_4, ZnO, and AgO (Keskinbora & Jameel, 2018). Such possible, devices and methods entail the improvement in terms of physicochemical determination, safety, and effective use of nanomaterial and nano-surfaces in the field of nano-medicine. On another note, the Anti-microbial/viral effects of nanoparticles in integration with treatment methods are also employed for treating drug-resistant microbial infections, immunization, and vaccine development in the latest reportings at a lab scale design. Liposomal nano-materials consisting of PGE-1 has been reported by using fabricated design for the treatment of thrombosis, peripheral arterial diseases and myocardial infarction which enables the decrease in PGE-1 degradation and enhancing the results of drug actions (Chandarana et al., 2018). Likewise, the nanoparticles can be used for controlling the circulation of tumorous cells related to progenitor of metastatic stages in different type of cancers (Haleem et al., 2023). Thus, nanobiotechnology has established a new perspectives in the biomedical sciences and the current chapter will help in providing a detailed insight into wide biomedical applications of different nanomaterials.

APPLICATIONS OF NANOPARTICLES IN INFECTIOUS DISEASES AND TREATMENT

The reach of nanoparticles for infectious diseases majorly depends on the ability of biocompatibility and biosorption on the integral membrane channels, along with chemical stability, mechanical properties, and high-end photocatalytic capacity for regulating antibacterial properties (Fang et al., 2018). Based on recent advancements in anti-inflammatory approaches, electroporation-enhanced nanoparticles have been reported for their highly specific binding ability to the pathogenic bacteria at the infectious sites in the case of bone disease "Osteoporosis". The local treatment in the in vivo system has reported a decrease of S. aureus, Escherichia coli (E. coli), and multi-drug-resistance bacteria via electroporating coated nanoparticles, with a good efficacy of antimicrobial effects (Shi et al., 2021). For the detection of certain diseases including Keratosis, rapid disease detection is required which is achievable through different theranostic agents, made up of vancomycin (Van)-modified fluorescent silicon nanoparticles (SiNPs-Van). The simultaneous diagnosis and therapy of Gram-positive bacteria in cases of keratitis are proven to be effective against majorly S. aureus (L. Zhang et al., 2021). Another prime infectious disease, Tuberculosis (TB) has been a research area in the present scenario, which still poses a serious global public health threat. In contrast to conventional treatment regimens, CpG oligodeoxynucleotides (CpG ODNs) synthesized nanoparticles are made in use which are capable of inducing Th1-type immune response via (TLRs). The metallic–organic framework based on zirconium ions and porphyrin ligands, displays an advantage of high drug loading capacity, but also as an action of photosensitizer, allowing the avenue for photodynamic therapy (PDT). These PDT-combined immunotherapy approaches are found to be associated with macrophage-targeted killing of latent Mtb (Tian et al., 2023). Therefore, the potential of nanoparticles is highly explored in the present scenario. Metal oxide nanoparticles, quantum, carbon dots, and graphene oxides endure the capability to impact the viability of viral particles on surfaces when linked with polymers and textiles. These nanomaterials generate reactive oxygen species on exposure to illumination and inhibit viral particles in three steps. In the initial stage, nanoparticle attaches to the viral particles and blocks its penetration into the cell. Thereafter, generation of reactive oxygen species occurs with subsequent destruction of structure and functionality of virus proteins and genetic material. Lastly, it is presumed that nucleus enhances the immune response of the host cell and reduces the budding and spread of the viral genome (Zhou et al., 2020). Photothermal materials including carbon dots, graphene, and Ag nanoparticles have been fabricated for designing for facemasks to prevent antibacterial and antiviral infections. Nano-porous membranes made up of carbon dots and polymers exhibit a hydrophobic surface that inhibits moisture accumulation in the face masks. Furthermore, a compact nanopore film enables both breathability and efficient particle (>100nm) filtration (Singh et al., 2021).

APPLICATION IN DIAGNOSTIC AND DRUG DELIVERY THERAPY

The current diagnostic methods available for different diseases rely on observable parameters for the identification of distinct kinds of diseases. Various electrochemical and enzymatic sensors are being fabricated for disease diagnosis. Early disease detection enables timely treatment and prevention. Nano-biotechnology can expand the possibilities that were previously available, as diagnosis methods rely on response analysis and the efficacy of the detection system. Nanotechnology-empowered instruments may be capable of non-invasive, fast, inexpensive, accurate, and ultrasensitive in vitro and in vivo diagnostics of cellular and sub-cellular features (Qamar et al., 2019). Nanoparticles allow accurate and rapid DNA sequencing, *in vivo* staining, and targeted imaging of cancerous cells and tissues thus reducing the requirement of biopsy. Furthermore, small nanotechnology-based quasi-robot devices enable defect correction. These remarkably significant inventions may also assist in designing DNA molecules for medical and computer scientists, such as nano-biosensors, nano-electronics and bio-electronic instruments, and DNA computational devices (Zahid et al., 2013). The nano-wires also allow the determination of pathological alterations in distinct and non-accessible tissues, including CNS, small blood vessels, and nerve fibers which are difficult to assess by employing current procedures. Magnetic and luminescent nanomaterials assist in non-invasive, sensitive, and specific *in vivo* imaging without the risk of renal toxicity. Nano-imaging has immensely advanced in recent times for the betterment of biomedical sciences. Intercellular imaging can be easily performed in the current times by employing chromophores or quantum dots labeled target agents (Mongin et al., 2016). Currently, the sparse autoencoder is being employed for the effective determination of the nucleus on histopathological high-resolution images for detecting breast cancer (J. Xu et al., 2016).

The major drawback in disease treatment is the transfer of therapeutical agents to the targeted tissues. The deficiency in selective, effective, and poorly biodistributed conventional drugs limits their efficacy. Drug transport to the target site of action by controlling the drug delivery system and its side effects are some of the possibilities to overcome the usage hurdles (Qamar et al., 2019). Drug delivery methods also prevent drug clearance or fast degradation and therefore improve the active amount of drug in relevant sites (Chamundeeswari et al., 2018). For resolving the challenges, nanosized drug encapsulation (e.g. nano-shells, hollow capsules, and organic dendrimers), can assist in controlled and targeted drug release. Functional inorganic nanocarriers and robust nano-scaffold have also been employed in gene therapy. For the following reason, surface modification is the major contributing factor responsible for the functionality and specificity of drug action. In the case of nanoparticles bearing magnetic properties, a biocompatible layer is coated to functionalize the conjugation/ encapsulation property of the drug. The magnetic field is further used to guide the complex and release of enzyme activity by various factors involved such as pH, temperature, or osmolality (Patel et al., 2019). In relation to morbidity and mortality factors, available agents for cancerous treatment have severe systemic side effects, and gradually lose their therapeutic effects (Bahrami et al., 2017). For a prognostic approach, platinum nanoparticles (PtNPs) possess some intrinsic anticancer activity, leading to slowing tumor growth. The targeted ligands are attached to these functionalized metal PtNPs enabling a controlled release of drugs, to improve the

Figure 1. Illustration of nano-carrier composite use for targeted drug delivery for breast cancer cells

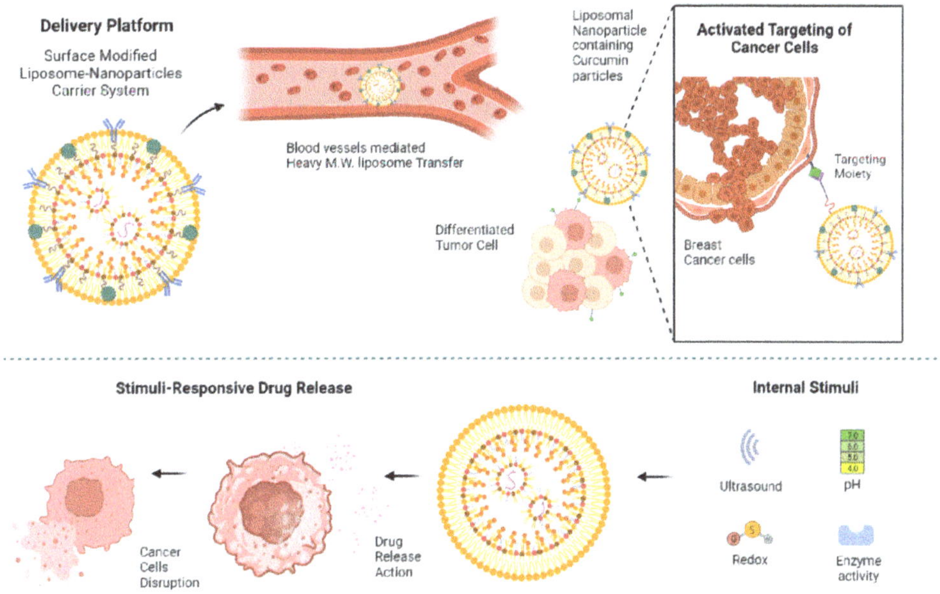

efficiency and simultaneously reduce the side effects of cancer therapy (Abed et al., 2022). Furthermore, another study has displayed a glioma cell targeted therapy via the treatment of conjugated nanoparticles. The anti-glioma efficacy is evident in both 2D and 3D-spheroid models supported with novel organic cation/ carnitine transporters (Kou et al., 2018).

Liposome-based therapy via nanoparticles is also known for its potential for anti-cancerous effects as a Nano-carrier composite, which requires surface modification for its proper functioning without the limitations of drug instability or leakages. The thin film hydration method has been reported for the construction of 3 different nano-capsules, encapsulating curcumin into the core of the liposome (Othman et al., 2022).

APPLICATIONS OF NANOPARTICLES IN IMPLANTS AND PROSTHESES

Nanotechnology has various applications in tissue and implant engineering. In the case of tissue implants, the biological responses of osteogenic cells and the mechanical contact between tissue and implant can be improved by regulating surface area and coarseness of the materials at the nanoscale (Rack & Qazi, 2006). By altering the metallic surfaces, a stronger bone-implant interface can be obtained which leads to better osteointegration of the implant (Jalota et al., 2007). Another approach used to improve the tissue-implant interaction is the addition of bioactive substances thus modifying the coarseness of the surfaces at the nano scale. These strategies have influenced the prospects of nanotechnology in biomedicine (Puleo & Nanci, 1999). The treated surface of the implants impacts the anchorage, morphology, and performance of the living tissue at the tissue-implant interface. These interactions are influenced by the features, charge, chemical constitution, and adhesion ability of the interacting surfaces. Many researchers have demonstrated significant differences in the in vivo and in vitro response of the optimized implant surfaces, thus supporting the role of modifying the topography of the implant surfaces in enhancing bone formation (Chen et al., 2014; Healy et al., 2000). Nanoengineering involves refining the interacting surface by regulating these properties. At times, the metallic surface of the implants is modified by the addition of certain bioactive substances (Biomimetics) which helps in defining chemical and physical features at the nanoscale (Shkodra-Pula et al., 2020; Surmenev et al., 2014).

Several research have extended the use of silver nanoparticles as a coating material in cardiovascular implants, as well as central nervous and neurosurgical stents (Chaloupka et al., 2010). Further, metal implants have been lately used as bone and tooth replacements during commonly practiced surgical procedures. One of the most sought-after materials for bone grafting applications is Titanium and its alloys. Numerous studies have indicated that roughening or treating the implant surfaces at the nanoscale supports cell differentiation and adhesion (Kunzler et al., 2007). As in the case of dental implants, various coatings like thin ceramic layers are used to facilitate the binding of a prosthesis and osseous tissue, which improves long-term incorporation. The most used bioactive coating substances are calcium phosphate (hydroxyapatite, tricalcium phosphate) and bioactive glasses. These materials improve cell adhesion, differentiation, and bone development. Though one can vouch for the advantages of using ceramic coatings such as faster healing, better bone remodeling, stronger implant-tissue attachment, etc., still there is a lot of scope for research in the field to further improve the efficacy and reliability on a specific coating material (Tomsia et al., 2011). Modifying the implant surfaces to improve implant-tissue interaction is critical in the case of dental implants where successful and steady osteointegration is crucial for its functionality and durability (Healy et al., 2000).

With new developments in the field of nanotechnology, researchers have been trying to make the most of it in the development of prosthetic limbs and aids to help the disabled. Nanomaterials exhibit different electrical, magnetic, thermal, and mechanical characteristics which can be harnessed for the manufacturing of better and more efficient prosthetics (Inamuddin, 2018). Lately, various nanocomposite materials have been investigated for the development of prosthetics like cellular electronic skin (e-skin), intelligent robotic skin, prosthetic bones, biosensors, etc. Nanomaterials have shown promising results in the designing of electronic skin exhibiting neuro tactile functions. Mostly carbon-based, metal, metal-polymer composite materials, and hydrogels are used for studying the development of prosthetic neural sensors (Zarrintaj et al., 2018). Studies have shown that prosthetic nerve sensors can monitor physiological indexes, sense the body's actions, conduct electrophysiological signals, etc. Bionic neural sensors can be used in wearable devices to monitor and regulate temperature, respiration, blood pressure, pulse, and so on. These prosthetic nerve sensors can be used as neurotransmitters and can be implanted subcutaneously (Cao et al., 2021; Leal-Junior & Frizera-Neto, n.d.). Carbon nanotube polyester thread can be used for studying neurotransmission in the epidermal layer of the skin, whereas 3D graphene-based pressure sensors have been used in the e-skin (Cao et al., 2021; Liao et al., 2021). Hydrogel nanomaterial is yet another material that can be used for manufacturing neural sensors because of its compatibility with biological material, antimicrobial properties, thermal stability, and bio-degradable nature (Khalid & Chang, 2022; Rahmani & Shojaei, 2021). Many studies have demonstrated the manufacturing of prosthetic skin using Crosslinked gold nanoparticles, carbon nanotube films, and Polyacrylonitrile. Laser-induced graphene is being employed for the development of cellular electronic skin and vertical graphene array has been promising in recognizing multifunctional tactility when incorporated in e-skin (Fastier-Wooller et al., 2021; Yao et al., 2022).

Researchers have used composite materials like ionic tactile sensors to mimic human skin (Scaffaro et al., 2021), and HCl-doped poly (o-toluidine) (POMANI)-Mn3O4 film nanocomposite material for developing amenable thermal sensors for prosthetic limbs and gloves (Kumar et al., 2019). Various studies have established the use of Polydimethylsiloxane -zinc oxide nanorods for developing intelligent artificial limbs which can act as feedback systems translating fingertip responses to electronic signals and thus helping in the advancement of rehabilitation of the disabled (Demolder et al., 2021; Liao et al., 2019). Commonly used nanomaterials for constructing skeletal tissue in prosthetic limbs are fiber materials, composite metal mixtures, and other composite materials. Carbon fiber, Kevlar fiber, and glass fiber, commonly called reinforced fibers are used in developing prosthetic sockets, which are crucial for the connection of prosthetic limbs at the sites (Khare et al., 2021).

Many researchers have used agave fibers and strengthened polyester resin, such as carbon, jute, glass, and perlon in the artificial sockets (Oleiwi et al., 2022). One of the metallic materials, commonly a Ti-Ta composite, has shown good prospects in orthopedic applications owing to its properties such as better ductility, low elasticity, and compatibility with biological materials (Qianli Huang et al., 2021). Considering all the recent advancements and ongoing research one can appropriately articulate that manufacturing an intelligent prosthetic limb is unfathomable without the use of nanomaterials. The amalgamation of biomedicine and material medicine has paved the way for the development of nano-materials that can improve the present quality and functionality of prosthetic limbs, thus improving the lives of the disabled (Tan et al., 2022).

APPLICATION OF NANOPARTICLES FOR MAGNETIC HYPERTHERMIA TREATMENT

Iron Oxide is an extensively utilized and researched nanoparticle for biological purposes. Its chemically stable nature along with non-toxicity, high magnetization, high magnetic vulnerability, and compatibility with various biological materials has made it popular (Chen et al., 2008; Karimi et al., 2013; McNamara & Tofail, 2016). The highest biocompatibility among iron oxides is demonstrated by maghemite (γ-Fe_2O_3) and magnetite (Fe_3O_4), though has seen the widest application in the field of biomedicine (McNamara & Tofail, 2013). For instance, iron oxide had been researched for treating magnetic hyperthermia as well as its use as a contrast agent in imaging (Magnetic Resonance Imaging) (Liao et al., 2015; Liu & Fan, 2014a, 2014b; Sharma et al., 2014; Wabler et al., 2014). Magnetic hyperthermia treatment is used

Figure 2. Representational illustration of magnetic hyperthermia

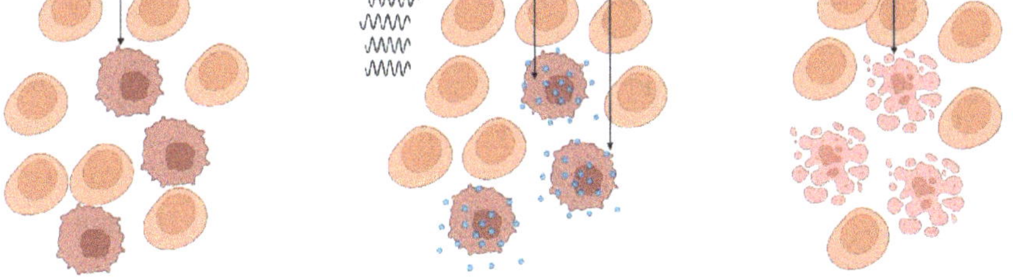

to selectively kill cancerous cells by subjecting them to moderately high temperatures. The temperature used is generally above 43 °C, causing the death of cancerous cells which are more heat sensitive than the normal cells. This treatment method induces localized heating with external alternating electromagnetic radiation through energy absorbed by the metallic magnetic nanoparticles such as Fe, Co, Ni, and their oxides (Fatima et al., 2021).

Magnetic hyperthermia treatment is preferred over chemotherapy for being site-specific, though sometimes it is used in combination with chemotherapy and radiotherapy. Magnetic Iron oxide (Fe3O4) nanoparticles can be delivered to the cancerous site by arterial injections or by using hydrogels to form in situ implants. Sometimes, another approach is used which involves injecting magnetic nanoparticles coated with tumor-specific antibodies into the circulatory system (Chatterjee et al., 2014; McNamara & Tofail, 2016). Various types of magnetic nanoparticles are being developed to treat specific cancerous sites with explicit coating materials of varying shapes and surface charges (Kong et al., 2012). One of the most important characteristics of magnetic nanoparticles is that they can cross the blood-brain barrier which can be used to treat brain tumors (Pankhurst et al., 2003). The efficacy of magnetic nanoparticles in magnetic hyperthermia is based on various factors like heating efficiency, selectivity, clearance, and accumulation/distribution in vivo. Uniform dispersion of magnetic nanoparticles enhances their heating performance in comparison with amassed nanoparticles (Fatima et al., 2021).

APPLICATIONS OF NANOPARTICLES IN IMAGING

In the last few years, a lot of research has been done with nanomaterials which has helped in the designing of nanoparticles with specific characteristics, which can be employed in the field of diagnostics and therapeutics (Baetke et al., 2015). In today's world, molecular imaging is considered one of the important branches of medical research, which helps in advancing the current techniques used for the diagnosis and prognosis of diseases. Thus, enabling the designing and personalization of treatment for the patients (Chen et al., 2014; Weissleder & Pittet, 2008). There are various imaging techniques like magnetic resonance imaging, computed tomography, positron emission tomography, and ultrasound for the diagnosis of ailments. For the advancement of several imaging methods by enhancing biocompatibility and imaging time, several nanomaterials have been researched for their use as contrast agents (Chatterjee et al., 2014; Rümenapp et al., 2012).

Due to features like as absorption and refraction in the visible and near-infrared spectrums, metallic nanomaterials comprising gold, silver, or platinum and magnetic properties can be employed as a contrast agent for different bio-sensing and imaging methods (Bhattacharya & Mukherjee, 2008). The powerful optical absorption exhibited by the inert elements makes them appropriate to develop molecular contrast imaging techniques (Liao et al., 2006). For instance, the magnetic characteristics of iron oxide enabled its use for magnetic resonance imaging, magnetic particle imaging, magneto-motive ultrasound, photoacoustic imaging techniques as well as magnetic hyperthermia treatment (Liu et al., 2016; Oh et al., 2006). Mostly transition and lanthanide elements, as well as iron oxide-containing mixtures, have been used clinically to achieve improved accuracy with imaging (Das et al., 2019). Nanomaterials containing gold and bismuth sulphide have shown promising results as an alternative to iodine-based contrast agents used in CT imaging techniques (Rosen et al., 2011). Intrinsic fluorescence of Zinc oxide particles is also being used for imaging tumor cells (Hong et al., 2011). Studies have also demonstrated gold nanoparticles employed for the in vivo monitoring of blood circulation along with photoacoustic imaging (Wang et al., 2005).

Particularly, properties such as dimensions in nanomaterials influence the bioavailability, half-life, cellular absorption, site-specific action, and rapid cellular clearance through the renal system (for the size ≤ 10nm) (Hoshyar et al., 2016; Longmire et al., 2008; Scott & Quaggin, 2015). One of the approaches used for site-specific targeting is labeling the surface of nanomaterials with different ligands and receptors which enhance the contrast agent's concentration at the cancerous sites during imaging. For example, during imaging of prostate cancer, gold nanoparticles labeled with specific RNA aptamer antigens have demonstrated higher density at the affected site. Also, superparamagnetic iron oxide nanoparticles labeled with anti-EGFR antibodies have exhibited site-specific localization at affected lung tissues during MRI (Kim et al., 2010; Wang et al., 2017). In another study, involving a mouse model, gold nanocages coupled with α-melanocyte-stimulating hormone (α-MSH) peptide and Cu radio labeled melanocortin 1 receptor-(MC1R) have been employed for diagnosis of cancer using PET imaging (Zhao et al., 2018).

Comfortably one can say that, in contrast to conventional imaging agents, nanomaterials can be optimized by labeling the surfaces with different biomolecules, providing enhanced imaging efficiency. A study concerning breast cancer patients demonstrated the successful detection of sentinel lymph nodes using SPIO nanoparticles as a suitable substitute for general nuclear imaging techniques (Karakatsanis et al., 2016; Taruno et al., 2019). Another study involving the identification of human breast cancer cells in blood serum and tissue employed liposome-encapsulated gold particles activated with Her2 antibody (Tao et al., 2017). Several similar studies have reinforced the use of nanoparticles for the detection of specific cancer biomarkers (Coutinho & Somoza, 2019; Li et al., 2017). Improved half-life and bioavailability of nanomaterials enhance the contrast signal as against the signal obtained with conventional agents. As discussed earlier, modification of the surface chemistry of nanoparticles is crucial for augmenting imaging results. Studies have shown enhanced solubility and half-life of nanoparticles encapsulated in polyethylene glycol covering (Han et al., 2019). Another important and astonishing nanomaterial-based imaging device is fluorescent quantum dots, commonly called QDs which enable the simultaneous detection of multiple biological molecules. These quantum dots are tolerant to photobleaching and have narrow emission bandwidth (Y. Xu et al., 2018). Because of exceptional properties like enhanced stability and optimizable emission bandwidth, quantum dots can be employed in fluorescence-based imaging techniques (Zhao & Zeng, 2015). One strategy for high throughput, fast and parallel identification of multiple biological entities employs quantum dots with multiple "noses" (sites) with each "nose" (site) labeled with a different receptor for the detection of a target molecule. Currently, researchers are trying to construct microfluidic chips that would enable us to identify several biomolecules as a vigorous and bedside diagnostic technique (Bharathala & Sharma, 2019). Other nanoparticles that need a mention are carbon dots and nanodiamonds which are being investigated for their suitability in the field of fluorescence imaging. These nano assemblies exhibit characteristics like small size, photostability, optimizable topography and non-toxic nature (Montalti et al., 2015). Current research is focussed on "Smart fluorophores" that can tune their emission characteristics according to the changes in the microenvironment like temperature, pH, etc and corelate these changes with the progression or diagnosis of a disease (Freidus et al., 2018).

Exploring further, nanoparticles do contributes to the diagnosis and prognosis of the disease in vivo as well ex vivo, in the body fluids like serum, urine, saliva, etc (Qinqin Huang et al., 2018). For example, CdSe/ZnS QDs stimulated with dopamine or oxidized cytochrome C has demonstrated the ability to detect changes in intracellular pH (Medintz et al., 2010) or reactive oxygen species (Li et al., 2011).

Table 1. Application of nanomaterials in detection and sensory devices by employing nanotechnology and biomedical sciences

S. No	Nanomaterial	Applications	Reference
1	Graphene	**Piezoresistive sensors:**Electronic Skin	M. Cao, J. Su, S. Fan, H. Qiu, D. Su, and L. Li, "Wearable piezoresistive pressure sensors based on 3D graphene," Chemical Engineering Journal, vol. 406, article 126777, 2021.
2	Carbon-based	**Wearable healthcare devices:**Monitoring pulse, respiration, blood pressure, movements	Z. Lou, L. Wang, K. Jiang, Z. Wei, and G. Shen, "Reviews of wearable healthcare systems: materials, devices and system integration," Materials Science and Engineering: R: Reports, vol. 140, article 100523, 2020. (Lou et al., 2020)
3	Carbon nanotube polyester wire	**Bionic electronic neural sensors:**Human-computer communication	X. Liao, W. Wang, L. Wang et al., "A highly stretchable and deformation-insensitive bionic electronic exteroceptive neural sensor for human-machine interfaces," Nano Energy, vol. 80, article 105548, 2021. (X. Liao et al., 2021)
4	Metal-carbon polymer combination	**Implantation Devices:** Prosthetic limbs, Nerve prosthesis	P. Zarrintaj, M. R. Saeb, S. Ramakrishna, and M. Mozafari, "Biomaterials selection for neuroprosthetics," Current Opinion in Biomedical Engineering, vol. 6, pp. 99–109, 2018.
5	Hydrogel	**Simulation Detection:**Limbs, and human body movement	P. Rahmani and A. Shojaei, "A review on the features, performance and potential applications of hydrogel-based wearable strain/pressure sensors," Advances in Colloid and Interface Science, vol. 298, article 102553, 2021.
6	Proanthocyanidins/reduced graphene oxide (PC/ rGO), glycerol-plasticized polyvinyl alcohol-borax hydrogel	**Imitation & Detection:**Epidermal movement, Simulation of skin tactility	X. Pan, Q. Wang, P. He et al.,"A bionic tactile plastic hydrogelbased electronic skin constructed by a nerve-like nanonetwork combining stretchable, compliant, and self-healing properties," Chemical Engineering Journal, vol. 379, article 122271, 2020. (Pan et al., 2020)
7	Nickel cobalt nanoparticles	**Automatic Sensor Controls**	K. Arikan, H. Burhan, R. Bayat, and F. Sen, "Glucose nano biosensor with non-enzymatic excellent sensitivity prepared with nickel–cobalt nanocomposites on f-MWCNT," Chemosphere, vol. 291, Part 3, article 132720, 2022.(Arikan et al., 2022)
8	Cross-linked gold nanoparticles	**Prosthetic skin**	D. Alvares, L. Wieczorek, B. Raguse, F. Ladouceur, and N. H. Lovell, "Development of nanoparticle film-based multi-axial tactile sensors for biomedical applications," Sensors and Actuators A: Physical, vol. 196, pp. 38–47, 2013.(Alvares et al., 2013)
9	Polydimethylsiloxane- zinc nanorods	**Tactile sensors:**e-skin, wearable devices, biological robotic skin	M.-S. Suen, Y.-C. Lin, and R. Chen, "A flexible multifunctional tactile sensor using interlocked ZnO nanorod arrays for artificial electronic skin," Procedia Engineering, vol. 168, pp. 1044– 1047, 2016.(Suen et al., 2018)
10	Silver nanowire-polyurethane scaffold-Carbon fiber composite material	**Virtual Translation:**Potential for translating fingertip responses into auditory and visual feedback	X. Liao, W. Song, X. Zhang et al., "Hetero-contact microstructure to program discerning tactile interactions for virtual reality," Nano Energy, vol. 60, pp. 127–136, 2019.(X. Liao et al., 2019)
11	Carbon nanotubes and polyacrylonitrile	**Sensors:**Development of sensing ability in artificial robotic skin	J. W. Fastier-Wooller, V. T. Dau, T. Dinh, C. D. Tran, and D. V. Dao, "Pressure and temperature sensitive e-skin for in situ robotic applications," Materials & Design, vol. 208, article 109886, 2021.
12	Carbon black, carbon nanotubes, carbon fibers, graphene sheets, and graphene oxide	**Detection Devices:** Human movement detection, soft robots	M. A. U. Khalid and S. H. Chang, "Flexible strain sensors for wearable applications fabricated using novel functional nanocomposites: a review," Composite Structures, vol. 284, article 115214, 2022.
13	Vertical graphene array	**Prosthetics and e-Skin:**Wearable devices, prosthetic limbs	D. Yao, L. Wu, S. A et al., "Stretchable vertical graphene arrays for electronic skin with multifunctional sensing capabilities," Chemical Engineering Journal, vol. 431, article 134038, 2022.
14	Derivatives of Silane and keratin	**Mimicking Approach:**For human nails	S. Sakuri, E. Surojo, D. Ariawan, and A. R. Prabowo, "Investigation of Agave cantala-based composite fibers as prosthetic socket materials accounting for a variety of alkali and microcrystalline cellulose treatments," Theoretical and Applied Mechanics Letters, vol. 10, no. 6, pp. 405 –411, 2020.(Sakuri et al., 2020)
15	Composite Agave fibres	**Prosthetic Sockets**	
16	Fiber-reinforced polyester resin (Carbon, jute, glass, and perlon)	**Prosthetic Sockets**	J. K. Oleiwi, Q. A. Hamad, and S. A. Abdulrahman, Flexural, impact and max. shear stress properties of fibers composite for prosthetic socket, Materials Today: Proceedings, Amsterdam, Netherlands, 2022.(Oleiwi et al., 2022)
17	Ti-Ta based nanomaterial	**Orthopaedic Applications:**	Q. Huang, S. Xu, Z. Ouyang, Y. Yang, and Y. Liu, "Multi-scale nacre-inspired lamella-structured Ti-Ta composites with high strength and low modulus for load-bearing orthopedic and dental applications, " Materials Science and Engineering: C, vol. 118, article 111458, 2021.
18	MWCNT–(polydimethylsiloxane) PDMS	**Development & Casting Ability:**For Tensile Sensory Devices, and Prosthetic Liners	B. Oldfrey, A. Tchorzewska, R. Jackson et al., "Additive manufacturing techniques for smart prosthetic liners, " Medical Engineering & Physics, vol. 87, pp. 45–55, 2021. (Oldfrey et al., 2021)

Studies have also demonstrated the use of carbon-based quantum dots for detecting intracellular pH and metal ions (Du et al., 2013; Jiang et al., 2016). Scientists have elaborated on fluorophores embedded in the silica nanoparticles to detect intracellular variations in pH, oxygen, and metal ion concentrations as well (Koo et al., 2004; Park et al., 2003; Wu et al., 2011). Taking the use of nanomaterials as a step forward, scientists have employed nanoparticles as biosensors for measuring drug metabolites related to diseased cells and toxic ion concentrations (Guerrini et al., 2014; Sanles-Sobrido et al., 2009). Ever-increasing evidence supports the role of nanoparticles as a tumor contrast agent to enhance the sensitivity and specificity in disease diagnosis and prognosis.

APPLICATIONS OF NANOPARTICLES FOR CANCER TREATMENT

Cancer correlates with a wide range of diseases that consists of abnormally growing cells, and these cells may spread and affect other distinct cells and tissues. Current treatments consist of chemotherapy, radiation, and surgery, and generally, these methods destruct not only the tumor but also normal cells. The prime challenge in cancer diagnostics are evaluating the inter-relationship between cancer biomarkers and clinical pathology; localized drug delivery against tumor in infancy to maximize the treatment effectiveness. Nanoparticles are being used in cancer diagnostics to collect cancer biomarkers such as cancer-associated proteins, circulating tumor DNA, circulating tumor cells, and exosomes. (Jia et al., 2017). The increased surface area to volume ratio of nanoparticles in comparison to bulk materials is a critical benefit for cancer detection. Because of this feature, antibodies, small molecules, peptides, aptamers, and other moieties can be thickly coated on nanoparticle surfaces. These compounds bear the capability to attach and identify certain cancer molecules. Multivalent effects can also be obtained by introducing multiple binding ligands to cancer cells, which can increase the specificity and sensitivity of an experiment (Y. Zhang et al., 2019).

Quantum dots, gold nanoparticles, and polymer dots are three common nanoparticle probes used in diagnosing cancer. A sandwich immunoassay based on zinc oxide quantum dots was developed for ZnO nanowire substrates, which provided a wide surface area with many binding sites for detection. CEA, the most extensively used cancer biomarker, has been used to monitor anticancer therapy as well as to predict tumor recurrence following surgical resection in late-stage cancer patients, making it widely investigated (Y. Zhang et al., 2019). In relation to a latest reported study, lung cancer metastases can be detected by creating immunological superparamagnetic iron oxide nanoparticles (SPIONs) that can be used in MRI imaging with cancer cell lines as the SPIONs' targets (Wan et al., 2016). Furthermore, the high specificity of SPIONs has been reported without any significant side effects has been reported enabling them to be a suitable approach for aerosol detection via MRI imaging in lung cancer patients. Carbon nanotubes assist in delivering proteins and immunotherapy components for cancer treatment. Additionally, they are capable of natural cancer treatment by usage of photo-thermal therapy. Fluorescent nanoprobes allow the detection of fibroblast-activated protein-a on the cell membrane of tumor-associated fibroblasts (Ji et al., 2013). In a recent paper, adriamycin-conjugated nanoparticles were effectively used to treat several types of malignancies, but they also had many adverse effects, such as toxicity and cardiac difficulties, restricting their application. Doxil (a liposomal version of doxorubicin), which is less related to cardiotoxicity in patients and hence may give a safer nanomaterial synthetic technique for researchers in the future, can further address these difficulties (Jin et al., 2020). Quantum dots can co-aggregate in certain areas of the body and transport the medications. The capacity of QDs to concentrate in a single internal organ gives them a unique ability as an alternative to untargeted medication delivery, as well as a possible way to prevent chemotherapy side effects. Highly sensitive quantum dot-based probes for multi-color fluorescence in vivo imaging of cancer cells have been produced and reported for their utilization to detect the ovarian cancer marker antigen 125 (CA125) in different types of specimens (Jin et al., 2020).

LIMITATIONS

Nanoparticles' distinctive qualities, such as optical, fluorescent, and magnetic properties, allow unprecedented possibilities for illness detection and therapy. With the emergence of nanotechnology and its ramifications in medicine and theranostics, assessing its negative impact and toxicities has become increasingly important. Different types of nanomaterials can result in the generation of oxidative stress and inflammation in different cells and tissues. Nanoparticles may also result in a toxic impact on the liver, respiratory, excretory, immune, and reproductive tissue of the body (Chakravarty & Vora, 2020). Furthermore, gold nanoparticles have been found to go through cyanidation and oxidation in the body, which results in the production of toxic by-products. These by-products are readily absorbed by kidneys with subsequent nephrotoxic impact (Ray & Bandyopadhyay, 2021). Thus, a detailed evaluation of probable hazards of nanoparticle materials is much needed for the advancement of Nanobiotechnology. However, a major setback in toxicity studies is to develop efficient procedures and instruments for the assessment of exposure of nanoparticles with water and air. Furthermore, *in vivo,* case studies consisting of animal models for the determination of nanomaterial toxicities in the environment and humans can be an inevitable problem. The commercialization of nanotechnology, consisting of effective, scalable, patient, funding, innovative, and scarce resources is another challenge.

CONCLUSION AND FUTURE PROSPECTS

Nanobiotechnology has revolutionized how biocompatible nanomaterials may be synthesized enabling the incorporation of different chemotherapeutic agents, imaging probes as well as targeting molecules, thus improving the results of treatment and reducing the overall cost. Nanobiotechnology offers a diverse range of applications in the biomedical sectors such as; drug, tissue, and gene engineering, targeted delivery, diagnostics devices, imaging, therapy, and antiviral/microbial agents. Nonetheless, the efficacy of these applications needs to be evaluated through clinical studies with compliance to the standard procedures or demonstration of remarkable equivalence with an already available product. The potential of nanomaterial-based devices/products is projected to drive the market with immense capabilities of growth. The occurrence of approximately 40% of the nanotechnology-based products in phase II of clinical trials can result in a huge amount of potential commercialized opportunities in the coming decade. Additionally, this application in diagnostics and therapies still requires proper evaluation for safety and risk factors related to nanotechnology.

REFERENCES

Abed, A., Derakhshan, M., Karimi, M., Shirazinia, M., Mahjoubin-Tehran, M., Homayonfal, M., Hamblin, M. R., Mirzaei, S. A., Soleimanpour, H., Dehghani, S., Dehkordi, F. F., & Mirzaei, H. (2022). Platinum Nanoparticles in Biomedicine: Preparation, Anti-Cancer Activity, and Drug Delivery Vehicles. *Frontiers in Pharmacology*, *13*, 797804. doi:10.3389/fphar.2022.797804 PMID:35281900

Alvares, D., Wieczorek, L., Raguse, B., Ladouceur, F., & Lovell, N. H. (2013). Development of nanoparticle film-based multi-axial tactile sensors for biomedical applications. *Sensors and Actuators. A, Physical*, *196*, 38–47. doi:10.1016/j.sna.2013.03.021

Arikan, K., Burhan, H., Bayat, R., & Sen, F. (2022). Glucose nano biosensor with non-enzymatic excellent sensitivity prepared with nickel–cobalt nanocomposites on f-MWCNT. *Chemosphere*, *291*, 132720. doi:10.1016/j.chemosphere.2021.132720 PMID:34743867

Baetke, S. C., Lammers, T., & Kiessling, F. (2015). Applications of nanoparticles for diagnosis and therapy of cancer. *The British Journal of Radiology*, *88*(1054), 20150207. doi:10.1259/bjr.20150207 PMID:25969868

Bahrami, B., Hojjat-Farsangi, M., Mohammadi, H., Anvari, E., Ghalamfarsa, G., Yousefi, M., & Jadidi-Niaragh, F. (2017). Nanoparticles and targeted drug delivery in cancer therapy. *Immunology Letters*, *190*, 64–83. doi:10.1016/j.imlet.2017.07.015 PMID:28760499

Bhandari, G., Dhasmana, A., Chaudhary, P., Gupta, S., Gangola, S., Gupta, A., Rustagi, S., Shende, S. S., Rajput, V. D., Minkina, T., Malik, S., & Slama, P. (2023). A Perspective Review on Green Nanotechnology in Agro-Ecosystems: Opportunities for Sustainable Agricultural Practices & Environmental Remediation. *Agriculture*, *13*(3), 668. doi:10.3390/agriculture13030668

Bharathala, S., & Sharma, P. (2019). Biomedical applications of nanoparticles. In *Nanotechnology in Modern Animal Biotechnology: Concepts and Applications*. Elsevier. doi:10.1016/B978-0-12-818823-1.00008-9

Bhattacharya, R., & Mukherjee, P. (2008). Biological properties of "naked" metal nanoparticles. *Advanced Drug Delivery Reviews*, *60*(11), 1289–1306. doi:10.1016/j.addr.2008.03.013 PMID:18501989

Cao, M., Su, J., Fan, S., Qiu, H., Su, D., & Li, L. (2021). Wearable piezoresistive pressure sensors based on 3D graphene. *Chemical Engineering Journal*, *406*, 126777. doi:10.1016/j.cej.2020.126777

Chakravarty, M., & Vora, A. (2020). Nanotechnology-based antiviral therapeutics. *Drug Delivery and Translational Research 2020 11:3*, *11*(3), 748–787. doi:10.1007/s13346-020-00818-0

Chaloupka, K., Malam, Y., & Seifalian, A. M. (2010). Nanosilver as a new generation of nanoproduct in biomedical applications. *Trends in Biotechnology*, *28*(11), 580–588. doi:10.1016/j.tibtech.2010.07.006 PMID:20724010

Chamundeeswari, M., Jeslin, J., & Verma, M. L. (2018). Nanocarriers for drug delivery applications. *Environmental Chemistry Letters 2018 17:2*, *17*(2), 849–865. doi:10.1007/s10311-018-00841-1

Chandarana, M., Curtis, A., & Hoskins, C. (2018). The use of nanotechnology in cardiovascular disease. *Applied Nanoscience 2018 8:7*, *8*(7), 1607–1619. doi:10.1007/s13204-018-0856-z

Chatterjee, K., Sarkar, S., Jagajjanani Rao, K., & Paria, S. (2014). Core/shell nanoparticles in biomedical applications. *Advances in Colloid and Interface Science*, *209*, 8–39. doi:10.1016/j.cis.2013.12.008 PMID:24491963

Chen, Z., Kang, L., Wang, Z., Xu, F., Gu, G., Cui, F., & Guo, Z. (2014). Recent progress in the research of biomaterials regulating cell behavior. *RSC Advances*, *4*(109), 63807–63816. doi:10.1039/C4RA05534A

Chen, Z. P., Zhang, Y., Zhang, S., Xia, J. G., Liu, J. W., Xu, K., & Gu, N. (2008). Preparation and characterization of water-soluble monodisperse magnetic iron oxide nanoparticles via surface double-exchange with DMSA. *Colloids and Surfaces. A, Physicochemical and Engineering Aspects*, *316*(1–3), 210–216. doi:10.1016/j.colsurfa.2007.09.017

Chen, Z. Y., Wang, Y. X., Lin, Y., Zhang, J. S., Yang, F., Zhou, Q. L., & Liao, Y. Y. (2014). Advance of molecular imaging technology and targeted imaging agent in imaging and therapy. *BioMed Research International*, *2014*, 1–12. doi:10.1155/2014/819324 PMID:24689058

Coutinho, C., & Somoza, Á. (2019). MicroRNA sensors based on gold nanoparticles. *Analytical and Bioanalytical Chemistry*, *411*(9), 1807–1824. doi:10.100700216-018-1450-7 PMID:30390112

Das, S., Kotcherlakota, R., & Patra, C. R. (2019). Noninvasive imaging techniques of metal nanoparticles and their future diagnostic applications. *Medical Imaging Methods: Recent Trends*, 119–141. https://doi.org/ doi:10.1007/978-981-13-9121-7_5/COVER

Demolder, C., Molina, A., Hammond, F. L. III, & Yeo, W. H. (2021). Recent advances in wearable biosensing gloves and sensory feedback biosystems for enhancing rehabilitation, prostheses, healthcare, and virtual reality. *Biosensors & Bioelectronics*, *190*, 113443. doi:10.1016/j.bios.2021.113443 PMID:34171820

Du, F., Ming, Y., Zeng, F., Yu, C., & Wu, S. (2013). A low cytotoxic and ratiometric fluorescent nanosensor based on carbon-dots for intracellular pH sensing and mapping. *Nanotechnology*, *24*(36), 365101. doi:10.1088/0957-4484/24/36/365101 PMID:23942146

Fang, R. H., Kroll, A. V., Gao, W., & Zhang, L. (2018). Cell Membrane Coating Nanotechnology. *Advanced Materials*, *30*(23), 1706759. doi:10.1002/adma.201706759 PMID:29582476

Fastier-Wooller, J. W., Dau, V. T., Dinh, T., Tran, C. D., & Dao, D. V. (2021). Pressure and Temperature Sensitive e-Skin for in situ Robotic Applications. *Materials & Design*, *208*, 109886. doi:10.1016/j.matdes.2021.109886

Fatima, H., Charinpanitkul, T., & Kim, K. S. (2021). Fundamentals to Apply Magnetic Nanoparticles for Hyperthermia Therapy. *Nanomaterials, 11*(5), 1203. doi:10.3390/nano11051203

Freidus, L. G., Pradeep, P., Kumar, P., Choonara, Y. E., & Pillay, V. (2018). Alternative fluorophores designed for advanced molecular imaging. *Drug Discovery Today*, *23*(1), 115–133. doi:10.1016/j.drudis.2017.09.008 PMID:29111179

Guerrini, L., Rodriguez-Loureiro, I., Correa-Duarte, M. A., Lee, Y. H., Ling, X. Y., García De Abajo, F. J., & Alvarez-Puebla, R. A. (2014). Chemical speciation of heavy metals by surface-enhanced Raman scattering spectroscopy: Identification and quantification of inorganic- and methyl-mercury in water. *Nanoscale*, *6*(14), 8368–8375. doi:10.1039/C4NR01464B PMID:24938410

Haleem, A., Javaid, M., Singh, R. P., Rab, S., & Suman, R. (2023). Applications of nanotechnology in medical field: A brief review. *Global Health Journal (Amsterdam, Netherlands)*, *7*(2), 70–77. doi:10.1016/j.glohj.2023.02.008

Han, X., Xu, K., Taratula, O., & Farsad, K. (2019). Applications of nanoparticles in biomedical imaging. *Nanoscale*, *11*(3), 799–819. doi:10.1039/C8NR07769J PMID:30603750

Healy, K. E., Harbers, G. M., Barber, T. A., & Sumner, D. R. (2000). Osteoblast Interactions with Engineered Surfaces. In J. E. Davies (Ed.), Bone engineering. em squared.

Hong, H., Shi, J., Yang, Y., Zhang, Y., Engle, J. W., Nickles, R. J., Wang, X., & Cai, W. (2011). Cancer-targeted optical imaging with fluorescent zinc oxide nanowires. *Nano Letters*, *11*(9), 3744–3750. doi:10.1021/nl201782m PMID:21823599

Hoshyar, N., Gray, S., Han, H., & Bao, G. (2016). The effect of nanoparticle size on in vivo pharmacokinetics and cellular interaction. *Nanomedicine (London)*, *11*(6), 673–692. doi:10.2217/nnm.16.5 PMID:27003448

Huang, Q., Wang, Y., Chen, X., Wang, Y., Li, Z., Du, S., Wang, L., & Chen, S. (2018). Nanotechnology-Based Strategies for Early Cancer Diagnosis Using Circulating Tumor Cells as a Liquid Biopsy. *Nanotheranostics*, *2*(1), 21–41. doi:10.7150/ntno.22091 PMID:29291161

Huang, Q., Xu, S., Ouyang, Z., Yang, Y., & Liu, Y. (2021). Multi-scale nacre-inspired lamella-structured Ti-Ta composites with high strength and low modulus for load-bearing orthopedic and dental applications. *Materials Science and Engineering C*, *118*, 111458. doi:10.1016/j.msec.2020.111458 PMID:33255043

Inamuddin. (2018). Applications of Nanocomposite Materials in Orthopedics. *Applications of Nanocomposite Materials in Orthopedics*, 1–328. doi:10.1016/C2016-0-05076-3

Jalota, S., Bhaduri, S. B., & Tas, A. C. (2007). Osteoblast proliferation on neat and apatite-like calcium phosphate-coated titanium foam scaffolds. *Materials Science and Engineering C*, *27*(3), 432–440. doi:10.1016/j.msec.2006.05.052

Ji, T., Zhao, Y., Wang, J., Zheng, X., Tian, Y., Zhao, Y., & Nie, G. (2013). Tumor Fibroblast Specific Activation of a Hybrid Ferritin Nanocage-Based Optical Probe for Tumor Microenvironment Imaging. *Small*, *9*(14), 2427–2431. doi:10.1002mll.201300600 PMID:23853124

Jia, S., Zhang, R., Li, Z., Li, J., Jia, S., Zhang, R., Li, Z., & Li, J. (2017). Clinical and biological significance of circulating tumor cells, circulating tumor DNA, and exosomes as biomarkers in colorectal cancer. *Oncotarget*, *8*(33), 55632–55645. doi:10.18632/oncotarget.17184 PMID:28903450

Jiang, Y., Wang, Z., & Dai, Z. (2016). Preparation of Silicon-Carbon-Based Dots@Dopamine and Its Application in Intracellular Ag+ Detection and Cell Imaging. *ACS Applied Materials & Interfaces*, *8*(6), 3644–3650. doi:10.1021/acsami.5b08089 PMID:26502274

Jin, C., Wang, K., Oppong-Gyebi, A., & Hu, J. (2020). Application of Nanotechnology in Cancer Diagnosis and Therapy - A Mini-Review. *International Journal of Medical Sciences*, *17*(18), 2964–2973. doi:10.7150/ijms.49801 PMID:33173417

Karakatsanis, A., Christiansen, P. M., Fischer, L., Hedin, C., Pistioli, L., Sund, M., Rasmussen, N. R., Jørnsgård, H., Tegnelius, D., Eriksson, S., Daskalakis, K., Wärnberg, F., Markopoulos, C. J., & Bergkvist, L. (2016). The Nordic SentiMag trial: A comparison of super paramagnetic iron oxide (SPIO) nanoparticles versus Tc(99) and patent blue in the detection of sentinel node (SN) in patients with breast cancer and a meta-analysis of earlier studies. *Breast Cancer Research and Treatment*, *157*(2), 281–294. doi:10.100710549-016-3809-9 PMID:27117158

Karimi, Z., Karimi, L., & Shokrollahi, H. (2013). Nano-magnetic particles used in biomedicine: Core and coating materials. *Materials Science and Engineering C*, *33*(5), 2465–2475. doi:10.1016/j.msec.2013.01.045 PMID:23623057

Keskinbora, K. H., & Jameel, M. A. (2018). Nanotechnology Applications and Approaches in Medicine: A Review. *J Nanosci Nanotechnol Res*, *2*(2), 6. www.imedpub.com

Khalid, M. A. U., & Chang, S. H. (2022). Flexible strain sensors for wearable applications fabricated using novel functional nanocomposites: A review. *Composite Structures*, *284*, 115214. doi:10.1016/j.compstruct.2022.115214

Khare, J. M., Dahiya, S., Gangil, B., & Ranakoti, L. (2021). Influence of different resins on Physico-Mechanical properties of hybrid fiber reinforced polymer composites used in human prosthetics. *Materials Today: Proceedings*, *38*, 345–349. doi:10.1016/j.matpr.2020.07.420

Kim, D., Jeong, Y. Y., & Jon, S. (2010). A drug-loaded aptamer - Gold nanoparticle bioconjugate for combined ct imaging and therapy of prostate cancer. *ACS Nano*, *4*(7), 3689–3696. doi:10.1021/nn901877h PMID:20550178

Kong, S. D., Lee, J., Ramachandran, S., Eliceiri, B. P., Shubayev, V. I., Lal, R., & Jin, S. (2012). Magnetic targeting of nanoparticles across the intact blood–brain barrier. *Journal of Controlled Release*, *164*(1), 49–57. doi:10.1016/j.jconrel.2012.09.021 PMID:23063548

Koo, Y. E. L., Cao, Y., Kopelman, R., Koo, S. M., Brasuel, M., & Philbert, M. A. (2004). Real-Time Measurements of Dissolved Oxygen Inside Live Cells by Organically Modified Silicate Fluorescent Nanosensors. *Analytical Chemistry*, *76*(9), 2498–2505. doi:10.1021/ac035493f PMID:15117189

Kou, L., Hou, Y., Yao, Q., Guo, W., Wang, G., Wang, M., Fu, Q., He, Z., Ganapathy, V., & Sun, J. (2018). L-Carnitine-conjugated nanoparticles to promote permeation across blood–brain barrier and to target glioma cells for drug delivery via the novel organic cation/carnitine transporter OCTN2. *Artificial Cells, Nanomedicine, and Biotechnology*, *46*(8), 1605–1616. doi:10.1080/21691401.2017.1384385/SUPPL_FILE/IANB_A_1384385_SM9430.DOC PMID:28974108

Kumar, A., Singla, M. L., Kumar, A., & Rajput, J. K. (2019). Fabrication and linearisation of conformable POMANI-Mn3O4 nanocomposite based thermistor for temperature monitoring applications in prosthetic gloves. *Sensors and Actuators. A, Physical*, *285*, 588–598. doi:10.1016/j.sna.2018.11.036

Kunzler, T. P., Drobek, T., Schuler, M., & Spencer, N. D. (2007). Systematic study of osteoblast and fibroblast response to roughness by means of surface-morphology gradients. *Biomaterials*, *28*(13), 2175–2182. doi:10.1016/j.biomaterials.2007.01.019 PMID:17275082

Leal-Junior, A., & Frizera-Neto, A. (n.d.). *Optical Fiber Sensors for the Next Generation of Rehabilitation Robotics*. Science Direct. http://www.sciencedirect.com:5070/book/9780323859523/optical-fiber-sensors-for-the-next-generation-of-rehabilitation-robotics

Li, D. W., Qin, L. X., Li, Y., Nia, R. P., Long, Y. T., & Chen, H. Y. (2011). CdSe/ZnS quantum dot–Cytochrome c bioconjugates for selective intracellular O2˙− sensing. *Chemical Communications*, *47*(30), 8539–8541. doi:10.1039/c1cc13160e PMID:21709927

Li, R., Liu, B., & Gao, J. (2017). The application of nanoparticles in diagnosis and theranostics of gastric cancer. *Cancer Letters*, *386*, 123–130. doi:10.1016/j.canlet.2016.10.032 PMID:27845158

Liao, H., Nehl, C. L., & Hafner, J. H. (2006). Biomedical applications of plasmon resonant metal nanoparticles. *Nanomedicine (London)*, *1*(2), 201–208. doi:10.2217/17435889.1.2.201 PMID:17716109

Liao, S. H., Liu, C. H., Bastakoti, B. P., Suzuki, N., Chang, Y., Yamauchi, Y., Lin, F. H., & Wu, K. C. W. (2015). Functionalized magnetic iron oxide/alginate core-shell nanoparticles for targeting hyperthermia. *International Journal of Nanomedicine*, *10*, 3315. doi:10.2147/IJN.S68719 PMID:26005343

Liao, X., Song, W., Zhang, X., Zhan, H., Liu, Y., Wang, Y., & Zheng, Y. (2019). Hetero-contact microstructure to program discerning tactile interactions for virtual reality. *Nano Energy*, *60*, 127–136. doi:10.1016/j.nanoen.2019.03.048

Liao, X., Wang, W., Wang, L., Jin, H., Shu, L., Xu, X., & Zheng, Y. (2021). A highly stretchable and deformation-insensitive bionic electronic exteroceptive neural sensor for human-machine interfaces. *Nano Energy*, *80*, 105548. doi:10.1016/j.nanoen.2020.105548

Liu, H., Zhang, J., Chen, X., Du, X. S., Zhang, J. L., Liu, G., & Zhang, W. G. (2016). Application of iron oxide nanoparticles in glioma imaging and therapy: From bench to bedside. *Nanoscale*, *8*(15), 7808–7826. doi:10.1039/C6NR00147E PMID:27029509

Liu, X. L., & Fan, H. M. (2014). Innovative magnetic nanoparticle platform for magnetic resonance imaging and magnetic fluid hyperthermia applications. *Current Opinion in Chemical Engineering*, *4*, 38–46. doi:10.1016/j.coche.2013.12.010

Longmire, M., Choyke, P. L., & Kobayashi, H. (2008). Clearance properties of nano-sized particles and molecules as imaging agents: Considerations and caveats. *Nanomedicine (London)*, *3*(5), 703–717. doi:10.2217/17435889.3.5.703 PMID:18817471

Lou, Z., Wang, L., Jiang, K., Wei, Z., & Shen, G. (2020). Reviews of wearable healthcare systems: Materials, devices and system integration. *Materials Science and Engineering R Reports*, *140*, 100523. doi:10.1016/j.mser.2019.100523

McNamara, K., & Tofail, S. A. M. (2013). Biomedical applications of nanoalloys. *Nanoalloys: From Fundamentals to Emergent Applications*, 345–371. doi:10.1016/B978-0-12-394401-6.00010-2

McNamara, K., & Tofail, S. A. M. (2016). Nanoparticles in biomedical applications. *Advances in Physics: X*, *2*(1), 54–88. doi:10.1080/23746149.2016.1254570

Medintz, I. L., Stewart, M. H., Trammell, S. A., Susumu, K., Delehanty, J. B., Mei, B. C., Melinger, J. S., Blanco-Canosa, J. B., Dawson, P. E., & Mattoussi, H. (2010). Quantum-dot/dopamine bioconjugates function as redox coupled assemblies for in vitro and intracellular pH sensing. *Nature Materials, 9*(8), 676–684. doi:10.1038/nmat2811

Mongin, C., Garakyaraghi, S., Razgoniaeva, N., Zamkov, M., & Castellano, F. N. (2016). Direct observation of triplet energy transfer from semiconductor nanocrystals. *Science*, *351*(6271), 369–372. doi:10.1126cience.aad6378 PMID:26798011

Montalti, M., Cantelli, A., & Battistelli, G. (2015). Nanodiamonds and silicon quantum dots: Ultrastable and biocompatible luminescent nanoprobes for long-term bioimaging. *Chemical Society Reviews*, *44*(14), 4853–4921. doi:10.1039/C4CS00486H PMID:26051500

Oh, J., Feldman, M. D., Kim, J., Condit, C., Emelianov, S., & Milner, T. E. (2006). Detection of magnetic nanoparticles in tissue using magneto-motive ultrasound. *Nanotechnology*, *17*(16), 4183–4190. doi:10.1088/0957-4484/17/16/031 PMID:21727557

Oldfrey, B., Tchorzewska, A., Jackson, R., Croysdale, M., Loureiro, R., Holloway, C., & Miodownik, M. (2021). Additive manufacturing techniques for smart prosthetic liners. *Medical Engineering & Physics*, *87*, 45–55. doi:10.1016/j.medengphy.2020.11.006 PMID:33461673

Oleiwi, J. K., Hamad, Q. A., & Abdulrahman, S. A. (2022). Flexural, impact and max. shear stress properties of fibers composite for prosthetic socket. *Materials Today: Proceedings*, *56*, 3121–3128. doi:10.1016/j.matpr.2021.12.368

Othman, A. K., El Kurdi, R., Badran, A., Mesmar, J., Baydoun, E., & Patra, D. (2022). Liposome-based nanocapsules for the controlled release of dietary curcumin: PDDA and silica nanoparticle-coated DMPC liposomes enhance the fluorescence efficiency and anticancer activity of curcumin. *RSC Advances*, *12*(18), 11282–11292. doi:10.1039/D2RA00071G PMID:35425076

Pan, X., Wang, Q., He, P., Liu, K., Ni, Y., Chen, L., Ouyang, X., Huang, L., Wang, H., & Xu, S. (2020). A bionic tactile plastic hydrogel-based electronic skin constructed by a nerve-like nanonetwork combining stretchable, compliant, and self-healing properties. *Chemical Engineering Journal*, *379*, 122271. doi:10.1016/j.cej.2019.122271

Pankhurst, Q. A., Connolly, J., Jones, S. K., & Dobson, J. (2003). Applications of magnetic nanoparticles in biomedicine. *Journal of Physics. D, Applied Physics*, *36*(13), R167–R181. doi:10.1088/0022-3727/36/13/201

Park, E. J., Brasuel, M., Behrend, C., Philbert, M. A., & Kopelman, R. (2003). Ratiometric optical PEBBLE nanosensors for real-time magnesium ion concentrations inside viable cells. *Analytical Chemistry*, *75*(15), 3784–3791. doi:10.1021/ac0342323 PMID:14572044

Patel, P., Hanini, A., Shah, A., Patel, D., Patel, S., Bhatt, P., & Pathak, Y. V. (2019). Surface Modification of Nanoparticles for Targeted Drug Delivery. In *Surface Modification of Nanoparticles for Targeted Drug Delivery* (pp. 19–31). Springer International Publishing. doi:10.1007/978-3-030-06115-9_2

Puleo, D. A., & Nanci, A. (1999). Understanding and controlling the bone-implant interface. *Biomaterials*, *20*(23–24), 2311–2321. doi:10.1016/S0142-9612(99)00160-X PMID:10614937

Qamar, S. A., Asgher, M., Khalid, N., & Sadaf, M. (2019). Nanobiotechnology in health sciences: Current applications and future perspectives. *Biocatalysis and Agricultural Biotechnology*, *22*, 101388. doi:10.1016/j.bcab.2019.101388

Rack, H. J., & Qazi, J. I. (2006). Titanium alloys for biomedical applications. *Materials Science and Engineering C*, *26*(8), 1269–1277. doi:10.1016/j.msec.2005.08.032

Rahmani, P., & Shojaei, A. (2021). A review on the features, performance and potential applications of hydrogel-based wearable strain/pressure sensors. *Advances in Colloid and Interface Science*, *298*, 102553. doi:10.1016/j.cis.2021.102553 PMID:34768136

Ray, S. S., & Bandyopadhyay, J. (2021). Nanotechnology-enabled biomedical engineering: Current trends, future scopes, and perspectives. *Nanotechnology Reviews*, *10*(1), 728–743. doi:10.1515/ntrev-2021-0052

Rosen, J. E., Yoffe, S., Meerasa, A., Verma, M., & Gu, F. X. (2011). Nanotechnology and Diagnostic Imaging: New Advances in Contrast Agent Technology. *Journal of Nanomedicine & Nanotechnology*, *2*(5). doi:10.4172/2157-7439.1000115

Rümenapp, C., Gleich, B., & Haase, A. (2012). Magnetic nanoparticles in magnetic resonance imaging and diagnostics. *Pharmaceutical Research*, *29*(5), 1165–1179. doi:10.100711095-012-0711-y PMID:22392330

Sakuri, S., Surojo, E., Ariawan, D., & Prabowo, A. R. (2020). Investigation of Agave cantala-based composite fibers as prosthetic socket materials accounting for a variety of alkali and microcrystalline cellulose treatments. *Theoretical & Applied Mechanics Letters*, *10*(6), 405–411. doi:10.1016/j.taml.2020.01.052

Sanles-Sobrido, M., Rodríguez-Lorenzo, L., Lorenzo-Abalde, S., González-Fernández, Á., Correa-Duarte, M. A., Alvarez-Puebla, R. A., & Liz-Marzán, L. M. (2009). Label-free SERS detection of relevant bioanalytes on silver-coated carbon nanotubes: The case of cocaine. *Nanoscale*, *1*(1), 153–158. doi:10.1039/b9nr00059c PMID:20644874

Scaffaro, R., Maio, A., & Citarrella, M. C. (2021). Ionic tactile sensors as promising biomaterials for artificial skin: Review of latest advances and future perspectives. *European Polymer Journal*, *151*, 110421. doi:10.1016/j.eurpolymj.2021.110421

Scott, R. P., & Quaggin, S. E. (2015). The cell biology of renal filtration. *The Journal of Cell Biology*, *209*(2), 199–210. doi:10.1083/jcb.201410017 PMID:25918223

Sharma, P., Rana, S., Barick, K. C., Kumar, C., Salunke, H. G., & Hassan, P. A. (2014). Biocompatible phosphate anchored Fe3O4 nanocarriers for drug delivery and hyperthermia. *New Journal of Chemistry*, *38*(11), 5500–5508. doi:10.1039/C4NJ01431F

Shi, M., Shen, K., Yang, B., Zhang, P., Lv, K., Qi, H., Wang, Y., Li, M., Yuan, Q., & Zhang, Y. (2021). An electroporation strategy to synthesize the membrane-coated nanoparticles for enhanced anti-inflammation therapy in bone infection. *Theranostics*, *11*(5), 2349–2363. doi:10.7150/thno.48407 PMID:33500729

Shkodra-Pula, B., Vollrath, A., Schubert, U. S., & Schubert, S. (2020). Polymer-based nanoparticles for biomedical applications. *Frontiers of Nanoscience*, *16*, 233–252. doi:10.1016/B978-0-08-102828-5.00009-7

Singh, S., Shauloff, N., Sharma, C. P., Shimoni, R., Arnusch, C. J., & Jelinek, R. (2021). Carbon dot-polymer nanoporous membrane for recyclable sunlight-sterilized facemasks. *Journal of Colloid and Interface Science*, *592*, 342–348. doi:10.1016/j.jcis.2021.02.049 PMID:33677194

Suen, M. S., Lin, Y. C., & Chen, R. (2018). A flexible multifunctional tactile sensor using interlocked zinc oxide nanorod arrays for artificial electronic skin. *Sensors and Actuators. A, Physical*, *269*, 574–584. doi:10.1016/j.sna.2017.11.053

Surmenev, R. A., Surmeneva, M. A., & Ivanova, A. A. (2014). Significance of calcium phosphate coatings for the enhancement of new bone osteogenesis—A review. *Acta Biomaterialia*, *10*(2), 557–579. doi:10.1016/j.actbio.2013.10.036 PMID:24211734

Tan, Q., Wu, C., Li, L., Shao, W., & Luo, M. (2022). Nanomaterial-Based Prosthetic Limbs for Disability Mobility Assistance: A Review of Recent Advances. *Journal of Nanomaterials*, *2022*, 1–10. doi:10.1155/2022/3425297

Tao, Y., Li, M., Kim, B., & Auguste, D. T. (2017). Incorporating gold nanoclusters and target-directed liposomes as a synergistic amplified colorimetric sensor for HER2-positive breast cancer cell detection. *Theranostics*, *7*(4), 899–911. doi:10.7150/thno.17927 PMID:28382162

Taruno, K., Kurita, T., Kuwahata, A., Yanagihara, K., Enokido, K., Katayose, Y., Nakamura, S., Takei, H., Sekino, M., & Kusakabe, M. (2019). Multicenter clinical trial on sentinel lymph node biopsy using superparamagnetic iron oxide nanoparticles and a novel handheld magnetic probe. *Journal of Surgical Oncology*, *120*(8), 1391–1396. doi:10.1002/jso.25747 PMID:31667855

Tian, N., Duan, H., Cao, T., Dai, G., Sheng, G., Chu, H., & Sun, Z. (2023). Macrophage-targeted nanoparticles mediate synergistic photodynamic therapy and immunotherapy of tuberculosis. *RSC Advances*, *13*(3), 1727–1737. doi:10.1039/D2RA06334D PMID:36712647

Tomsia, A. P., Launey, M. E., Lee, J. S., Mankani, M. H., Wegst, U. G. K., & Saiz, E. (2011). Nanotechnology Approaches for Better Dental Implants. *The International Journal of Oral & Maxillofacial Implants, 26*(Suppl), 25. /pmc/articles/PMC3087979/

Wabler, M., Zhu, W., Hedayati, M., Attaluri, A., Zhou, H., Mihalic, J., Geyh, A., Deweese, T. L., Ivkov, R., & Artemov, D. (2014). Magnetic resonance imaging contrast of iron oxide nanoparticles developed for hyperthermia is dominated by iron content. *International Journal of Hyperthermia*, *30*(3), 192–200. doi:10.3109/02656736.2014.913321 PMID:24773041

Wan, X., Song, Y., Song, N., Li, J., Yang, L., Li, Y., & Tan, H. (2016). The preliminary study of immune superparamagnetic iron oxide nanoparticles for the detection of lung cancer in magnetic resonance imaging. *Carbohydrate Research*, *419*, 33–40. doi:10.1016/j.carres.2015.11.003 PMID:26649917

Wang, H., Huff, T. B., Zweifel, D. A., He, W., Low, P. S., Wei, A., & Cheng, J. X. (2005). In vitro and in vivo two-photon luminescence imaging of single gold nanorods. *Proceedings of the National Academy of Sciences of the United States of America*, *102*(44), 15752–15756. doi:10.1073/pnas.0504892102 PMID:16239346

Wang, Z., Qiao, R., Tang, N., Lu, Z., Wang, H., Zhang, Z., Xue, X., Huang, Z., Zhang, S., Zhang, G., & Li, Y. (2017). Active targeting theranostic iron oxide nanoparticles for MRI and magnetic resonance-guided focused ultrasound ablation of lung cancer. *Biomaterials*, *127*, 25–35. doi:10.1016/j.biomaterials.2017.02.037 PMID:28279919

Weissleder, R., & Pittet, M. J. (2008). Imaging in the era of molecular oncology. *Nature 2008 452:7187*, *452*(7187), 580–589. doi:10.1038/nature06917

Wu, S., Li, Z., Han, J., & Han, S. (2011). Dual colored mesoporous silica nanoparticles with pH activable rhodamine-lactam for ratiometric sensing of lysosomal acidity. *Chemical Communications*, *47*(40), 11276–11278. doi:10.1039/c1cc14627k PMID:21931895

Xu, J., Xiang, L., Liu, Q., Gilmore, H., Wu, J., Tang, J., & Madabhushi, A. (2016). Stacked sparse autoencoder (SSAE) for nuclei detection on breast cancer histopathology images. *IEEE Transactions on Medical Imaging*, *35*(1), 119–130. doi:10.1109/TMI.2015.2458702 PMID:26208307

Xu, Y., Wang, X., Zhang, W. L., Lv, F., & Guo, S. (2018). Recent progress in two-dimensional inorganic quantum dots. *Chemical Society Reviews*, *47*(2), 586–625. doi:10.1039/C7CS00500H PMID:29115355

Yao, D., Wu, L. A. S., Zhang, M., Fang, H., Li, D., Sun, Y., Gao, X., & Lu, C. (2022). Stretchable vertical graphene arrays for electronic skin with multifunctional sensing capabilities. *Chemical Engineering Journal*, *431*, 134038. doi:10.1016/j.cej.2021.134038

Zahid, M., Kim, B., Hussain, R., Amin, R., & Park, S. H. (2013). DNA nanotechnology: A future perspective. *Nanoscale Research Letters*, *8*(1), 1–13. doi:10.1186/1556-276X-8-119 PMID:23497147

Zarrintaj, P., Saeb, M. R., Ramakrishna, S., & Mozafari, M. (2018). Biomaterials selection for neuroprosthetics. *Current Opinion in Biomedical Engineering*, *6*, 99–109. doi:10.1016/j.cobme.2018.05.003

Zhang, L., Ji, X., Su, Y., Zhai, X., Xu, H., Song, B., Jiang, A., Guo, D., & He, Y. (2021). Fluorescent silicon nanoparticles-based nanotheranostic agents for rapid diagnosis and treatment of bacteria-induced keratitis. *Nano Research*, *14*(1), 52–58. doi:10.100712274-020-3039-7

Zhang, Y., Li, M., Gao, X., Chen, Y., & Liu, T. (2019). Nanotechnology in cancer diagnosis: Progress, challenges and opportunities. *Journal of Hematology & Oncology*, *12*(1), 1–13. doi:10.118613045-019-0833-3 PMID:31847897

Zhao, M. X., & Zeng, E. Z. (2015). Application of functional quantum dot nanoparticles as fluorescence probes in cell labeling and tumor diagnostic imaging. *Nanoscale Research Letters*, *10*(1), 1–9. doi:10.118611671-015-0873-8 PMID:25897311

Zhao, Y., Pang, B., Detering, L., Luehmann, H., Yang, M., Black, K., Sultan, D., Xia, Y., & Liu, Y. (2018). Melanocortin 1 Receptor Targeted Imaging of Melanoma With Gold Nanocages and Positron Emission Tomography. *Molecular Imaging*, *17*. Advance online publication. doi:10.1177/1536012118775827 PMID:29873290

Zhou, J., Hu, Z., Zabihi, F., Chen, Z., & Zhu, M. (2020). Progress and Perspective of Antiviral Protective Material. *Advanced Fiber Materials*, *2*(3), 123–139. doi:10.100742765-020-00047-7

Chapter 2
Advances in Nanomaterials for Drug Delivery

Bancha Yingngam
https://orcid.org/0000-0001-7215-9123
Faculty of Pharmaceutical Sciences, Ubon Ratchathani University, Thailand

ABSTRACT

This chapter provides a comprehensive review of recent advances in nanomaterials for drug delivery, focusing on the design and preparation of nanocarriers. It also dissects the intricate mechanisms underpinning drug loading and release, and delves into the strategic planning inherent in achieving target delivery. It further outlines the potential applications of these nanomaterials in treating various diseases, including cancer, infectious diseases, and neurological disorders. A distinct case study is incorporated into the chapter, elucidating the promising utility of electrospun nanofibers in drug delivery paradigms. In its concluding remarks, the chapter engages in a thoughtful discourse about the persistent challenges within this rapidly evolving field. It also forecasts the potential trajectories for future exploration and innovation in the captivating domain of nanomaterials for drug delivery.

INTRODUCTION

The emergence of nanomaterials signifies a pivotal transformation in drug delivery systems, largely attributable to their unique physicochemical attributes. These include an elevated surface-to-volume ratio, superior biocompatibility, and the ability to encapsulate a variety of drugs—both hydrophilic and hydrophobic (Dutt et al., 2023). The employment of nanomaterial properties for drug delivery has instigated a transformative shift in the medical sciences, enabling the precise delivery of therapeutics to targeted cells, tissues, and organs while minimizing off-target effects (H. Zhu et al., 2024). Recent strides in nanotechnology have resulted in the inception of innovative nanomaterials that are characterized by improved drug-loading capacity, controlled release kinetics, and enhanced targeting precision (Al-Awsi et al., 2024). Among the diverse types of nanomaterials, lipid-based nanocarriers, polymer-based nanoparticles, inorganic nanomaterials, carbon-based nanomaterials, and nanofibers have undergone extensive study for their potential applicability in drug delivery systems (Gautam et al., 2023; Prajapati

DOI: 10.4018/979-8-3693-0448-8.ch002

et al., 2023; Xu & Chow, 2023). These nanomaterials' strengths lie in their capacity to facilitate targeted drug delivery, modulate release rates, and optimize pharmacokinetics. Conceptualizing and fabricating nanomaterials for drug delivery requires a comprehensive understanding of their physicochemical characteristics, including size, shape, surface charge, and biocompatibility (Mokhtar et al., 2023). To develop nanomaterials that are both safe and effective for drug delivery, a nuanced understanding of the interactions between these materials and biological systems is essential, along with an awareness of potential toxicological implications (Dutt et al., 2023).

This chapter aims to provide an overview of recent advances in nanomaterials for drug delivery. It scrutinizes the design and synthesis processes of nanomaterials, considers biocompatibility and toxicity, and explores applications of these materials within the domain of drug delivery. An illustrative case study on the use of electrospun nanofibers for drug delivery is also presented, underscoring the potential of this technique for the sustained release of therapeutic agents. To achieve a comprehensive analysis of the advances in nanomaterials for drug delivery, a search was performed across the Scopus database. As a premier abstract and citation database encompassing peer-reviewed research literature, Scopus offers a treasure trove of information that can be tapped to enrich one's understanding of this specialized domain (Yingngam, 2023a).

This chapter is structured as follows: Section 2, "Bibliometric Analysis of Nanomaterials for Drug Delivery", focuses on evaluating the research output, citation analysis, and research trends in the field of nanomaterials for delivery. Section 3, titled "Types of Nanomaterials for Drug Delivery", provides an overview of various types of nanocarriers in the field of drug delivery. Section 4, "Designs and Synthesis of Nanomaterials", explores innovative techniques and factors to consider when creating pharmaceutical nanomaterials. It includes an analysis of various strategies used to modify their size, shape, and surface charge and how these factors affect the encapsulation and release of drugs. Section 5, "Biocompatibility and Toxicity of Nanomaterials", addresses the vital aspect of safety in the application of nanomaterials for drug delivery. This section emphasizes the importance of biocompatibility and offers an examination of potential toxicity issues, citing recent research on how to minimize these risks while maximizing efficacy. Section 6, "Application of Nanomaterials in Drug Delivery", presents a range of potential and current uses of nanomaterials within the field of drug delivery. This section details how lipid-based nanocarriers, polymer-based nanoparticles, and nanofibers are being employed. It specifically highlights their significant roles in delivering drugs to precise targets and managing controlled releases. Section 7, "Case Study: Electrospun Nanofibers for Drug Delivery", presents an in-depth examination of electrospun nanofibers. This section details the electrospinning process, discusses its potential benefits for sustained drug release, and examines a practical application through a case study. Section 8, "Strategies for Developing Novel Nanomaterials for Drug Delivery", discusses innovative methods and procedures that have the potential to revolutionize the production and use of nanomaterials in drug delivery. Section 9, "Future Directions", casts a forward-looking gaze over the landscape of this field. It identifies key trends, potential challenges, and promising areas for future research, aiming to shape the discourse and guide future innovation in the development of nanomaterials for drug delivery. The chapter concludes with Section 10, "Conclusion".

BIBLIOMETRIC ANALYSIS OF NANOMATERIALS FOR DRUG DELIVERY

A comprehensive bibliometric analysis was conducted to examine the advancements and research trends in the field of nanomaterials for drug delivery. This analysis was accomplished by using Scopus, one of the most comprehensive and credible databases for scientific literature, which incorporates a broad spectrum of disciplines (Yingngam, 2023a).

Methodology

Search Strategy

The search strategy was designed to be as comprehensive as possible. The author utilized the advanced search feature in the Scopus database to identify articles related to nanomaterials for drug delivery. The search terms employed in this study were ("nanomaterials" OR "nanoparticles" OR "nanostructures" OR "nanocarriers" OR "nanofibers") AND ("drug delivery" OR "therapeutic delivery"). To focus on the advancements in the field, the time frame for the search was set from 2000 (1 January 2000) to the present (31 July 2023). The search was limited to articles written in English due to the author's capacity to review and analyze these sources. Both open access and subscription-based articles were included in the search to avoid any potential publication bias.

Data Extraction and Management

The search results were exported from Scopus in research information system (RIS) format, including details such as title, authors, year of publication, journal, keywords, affiliations, abstracts, and citations. The CSV files were then imported into a bibliometric analysis tool (VOSviewer version 1.6.16) for further evaluation (van Eck & Waltman, 2010).

Inclusion and Exclusion Criteria

The initial results were screened for relevance. Studies were included if they met the following criteria: (1) original research articles; (2) articles focusing on the synthesis, properties, or applications of nanomaterials in drug delivery; and (3) articles that presented novel findings or trends in the field. On the other hand, papers were excluded if they (1) were not written in English, (2) did not focus on the use of nanomaterials for drug delivery, (3) were review articles, opinion pieces, editorials, letters, or commentaries, or (4) were conference abstracts without full text availability.

Bibliometric Analysis

The extracted data were analyzed to identify trends over time, such as the number of publications per year, the most cited papers, the journals with the most publications, and the countries contributing the most to this field of research. Keywords were analyzed to understand the main themes and trends in the research, while authorship and institutional data provided insight into the leading researchers and institutions in the field.

Results and Discussion

This section will discuss the results obtained from the systematic search and bibliometric analysis based on the methodology described in the previous section.

Publication Output and Trend

The analysis of publication output and trends within the realm of nanomaterials for drug delivery furnishes critical insights into the velocity of scholarly progress and innovation in this domain. Furthermore, it serves to delineate principal areas of emphasis and nascent themes, thereby bestowing indispensable perspectives on the evolution of the field and charting the course for forthcoming investigations. Figure 1 shows the PRISMA flowchart of the literature search and selection process. This figure illustrates the steps taken during the search strategy, from the initial search in the Scopus database to the application of inclusion and exclusion criteria and the final number of included articles. The literature search strategy yielded a total of 101,662 documents. This comprehensive collection comprised a variety of document types, including 69,049 research articles, 22,114 review articles, 4,849 book chapters, 3,064 conference papers, 1,015 editorials, 457 notes, 375 short survey articles, 310 books, 122 conference papers, 115 errata, 109 letters, 65 retracted papers, 15 data papers, and 3 undefined document types. These documents were mainly written in English, accounting for 99,893 papers, followed by 1,297 in Chinese, 155 in Japanese, 58 in Russian, and 40 in French, among other languages. Following initial curation, the author narrowed down the corpus to 67,850 research articles, which were subsequently subjected to systematic analyses. In the context of investigating the advances in nanomaterials for drug delivery, focusing on research articles rather than other types of documents, such as review articles, book chapters, or conference papers, can be more beneficial for several reasons. First, research articles typically contain original data and new findings, offering the most current and precise details about advances in the field. These papers present specific methodologies, results, and interpretations from unique studies, giving you access to primary, firsthand research information. Second, research articles usually undergo rigorous peer-review processes, which ensure that the data are credible and that the conclusions are well supported. This quality assurance is critical when analyzing advances in a scientific field. On the other hand, review articles, while valuable for obtaining a broad overview of a field, summarize and synthesize existing research. They might not delve into the precise details of a study or offer new, original data. Similarly, book chapters and conference papers can vary widely in their depth of detail, scope, and peer-review rigor. Therefore, to gain the most reliable, detailed, and current information about the advances in nanomaterials for drug delivery, it is prudent to focus primarily on research articles for analysis.

The annual publication count in the field of nanomaterials for drug delivery is depicted in Figure 2. This figure illustrates the growth and progression of research in this field over time. A consistent increase in the number of annual publications indicates a rising interest in this area of research. In particular, a notable surge is observed post-2010, with peak publication counts recorded in 2021 (7,215 documents) and 2022 (7,345 documents). Up to the end of July 2023, a total of 4,398 documents had already been published. Assuming a consistent publishing pace throughout the year, it can be inferred that approximately 628 articles are being published each month, as calculated by dividing the total number of articles (4,398) published in the first 7 months of the year. Projecting this monthly publication rate onto the remaining 5 months of 2023, it is possible to anticipate that approximately 3,140 additional articles (628 articles/month × 5 months) will be published by year-end. This would bring the total for 2023 to an

Figure 1. PRISMA flowchart of the literature search and selection process

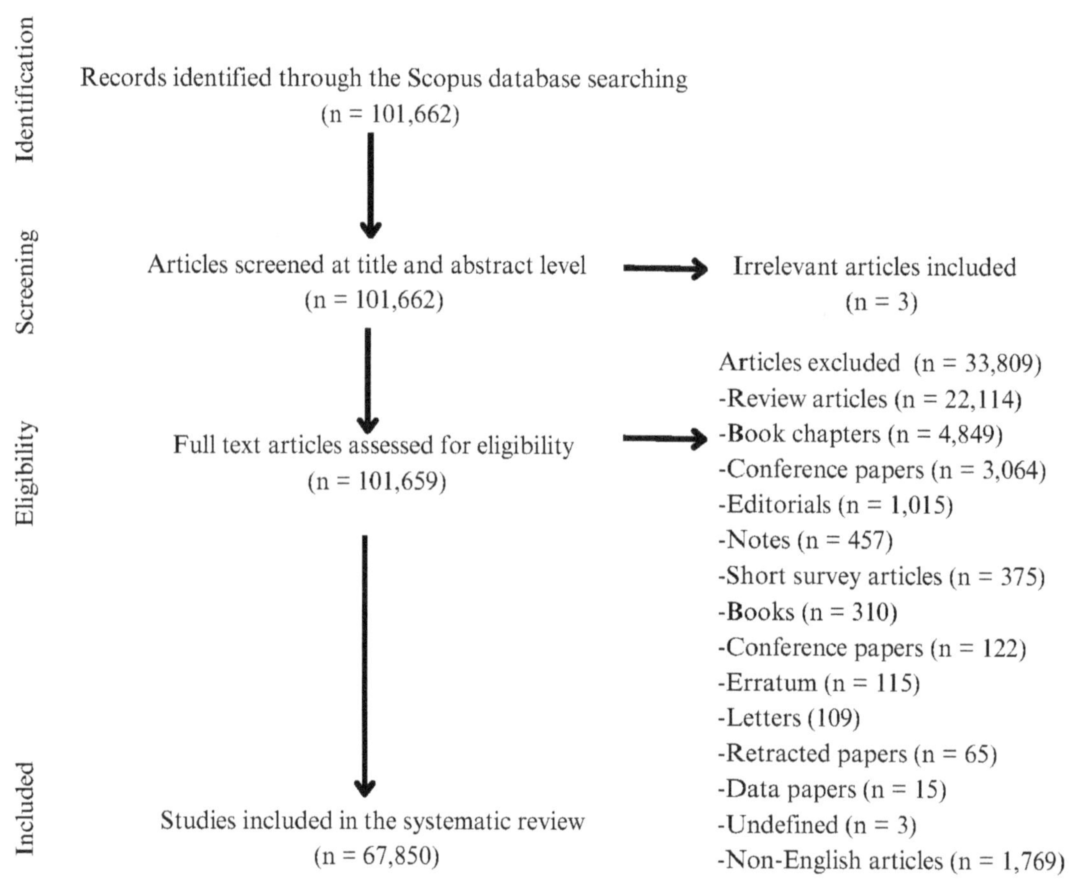

estimated 7,538 documents, signaling a continued upward trend in publication numbers. However, the publication rate may vary throughout the year due to factors such as academic calendars, conferences, and other events. Furthermore, the ongoing impact of global events or changes in funding trends could influence the final count. Hence, while the projection indicates a continuing upward trend, the actual total at the end of 2023 may be slightly higher or lower.

This upward trend reflects the maturation of the field and the increasing recognition of the potential of nanomaterials in drug delivery applications. The consistent upsurge in publication output is a testament to the maturation of the field. This indicates that researchers worldwide have recognized the potential of nanomaterials to revolutionize drug delivery systems, leading to more effective, safer, and personalized therapeutic strategies. This continuous growth trajectory suggests that the field is expected to maintain its momentum in the coming years. However, while the increasing publication output demonstrates the vibrancy of the field, it also suggests a rapidly growing body of knowledge that can be challenging to navigate. This highlights the importance of regular bibliometric analyses, such as the one conducted in this study, to monitor the progression of the field, identify key trends, and highlight the most impactful research directions. Moreover, the rising trend should also prompt ongoing discussion about the quality

Figure 2. Annual publication count in the field of nanomaterials for drug delivery from 2000 (1 January 2000) to 2023 (31 July 2023)

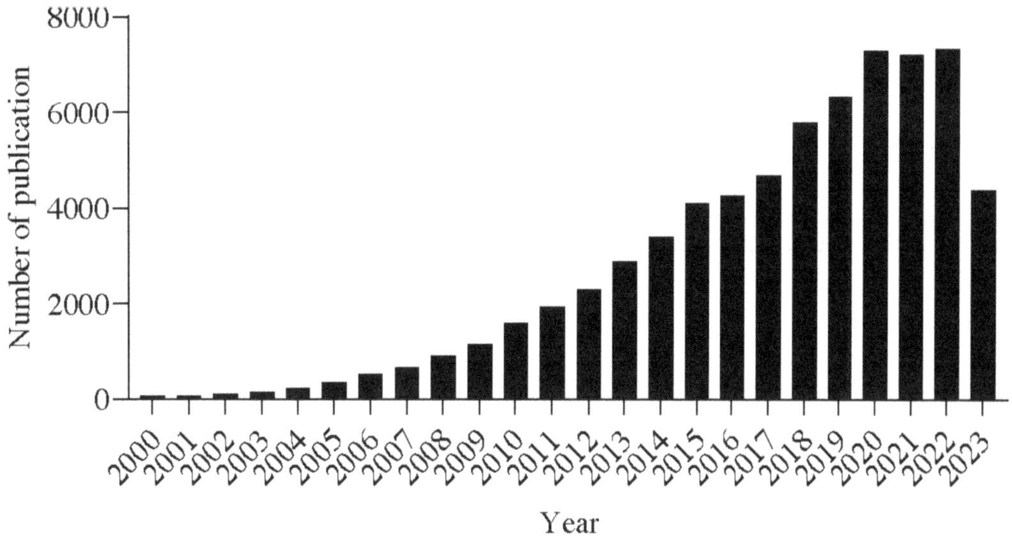

of the research being produced, emphasizing the need for rigorous peer review, replication of findings, and translational research to ensure that these advancements in nanomaterials for drug delivery contribute meaningfully to healthcare improvements.

Most-Cited Papers and Journals

The examination of the most cited papers provides an understanding of the seminal works that have had substantial influence in shaping the field of nanomaterials for drug delivery. The top 10 most cited papers in the field of nanomaterials for drug delivery are summarized in Table 1. This figure highlights the most influential publications in the field based on the number of citations. The most cited paper, with over 5,600 citations, was titled "Magnetic Iron Oxide Nanoparticles: Synthesis, Stabilization, Vectorization, Physicochemical Characterizations and Biological Applications" and was published in "Chemical Reviews" in 2008. This underscores the long-standing interest in targeted drug delivery using nanomaterials. This finding underscores the consistent interest in targeted drug delivery as a key application area of nanomaterials, which has driven a great deal of research innovation over the years.

Analyzing the distribution of publications across various scientific journals, as shown in Figure 3, offers further insights into the outlets that play a crucial role in disseminating research findings in this field. The International Journal of Pharmaceutics stands out as the journal with the most publications on the topic, contributing approximately 3.27% of the total output (2,222 documents). This indicates its status as a leading platform for sharing advances in nanomedicine and, more specifically, in the use of nanomaterials for drug delivery. The dominance of this journal could be attributed to its multidisciplinary nature, which aligns well with the cross-disciplinary character of nanomaterials research in drug delivery, and its open-access model, which ensures a broad reach for its published work. It is worth noting that the concentration of articles in this journal reflects the focused dedication toward nanomedicine, but

Table 1. The top 10 most cited papers in the field of nanomaterials for drug delivery as of July 31, 2023

No.	Article	Author	Source	Year	Citation
1	Magnetic iron oxide nanoparticles: Synthesis, stabilization, vectorization, physicochemical characterizations, and biological applications	Laurent, S., Forge, D., Port, M., Roch, A., Robic, C., Vander Elst, L., Muller, R. N.	Chemical Reviews, 108(6), pp. 2064–2110	2008	5,622
2	*In vivo* cancer targeting and imaging with semiconductor quantum dots	Gao, X., Cui, Y., Levenson, R. M., Chung, L. W.K., Nie, S.	Nature Biotechnology, 22(8), pp. 969–976	2004	4,421
3	PEGylated nanographene oxide for delivery of water-insoluble cancer drugs	Liu, Z., Robinson, J.T., Sun, X., Dai, H.	Journal of the American Chemical Society, 130(33), pp. 10876–10877	2008	3,263
4	Impact of nanotechnology	Farokhzad, O.C., Langer, R.	ACS Nano, 3(1), pp. 16 – 20	2009	2,563
5	Chitosan chemistry and pharmaceutical perspectives	Kumar, M.N.V.R., Muzzarelli, R.A.A., Muzzarelli, C., Sashiwa, H., Domb, A.J.	Chemical Reviews, 104(12), pp. 6017–6084	2004	2,496
6	Mesoporous silica nanoparticles: Synthesis, biocompatibility, and drug delivery	Tang, F., Li, L., Chen, D.	Advanced Materials, 24(12), pp. 1504–1534	2012	2,220
7	Shape effects of filaments versus spherical particles in flow and drug delivery	Geng, Y., Dalhaimer, P., Cai, S., Tsai, R., Tewari, M., Minko, T., Discher, D.E.	Nature Nanotechnology, 2(4), pp. 249–255	2007	2,158
8	Evidence of RNAi in humans from systematically administered siRNA via targeted nanoparticles	Davis, M.E., Zucker, J.E., Choi, C.H.J.,David, S., Tolcher, A., Alabi, C.A., Yen, Y., Heidel, J.D., Ribas, A.	Nature, 464(7291), pp. 1067–1070	2010	2,113
9	Carbon nanotubes as multifunctional biological transporters and near-infrared agents for selective cancer cell destruction	Kam, N.W.S., O'Connell, M., Wisdom, J.A., Dai, H.	Proceedings of the National Academy of Sciences of the United States of America, 102(33), pp. 11600–11605	2005	2,085
10	*In vivo* tumor targeting and spectroscopic detection with surface-enhanced Raman nanoparticle tags	Qian, X., Peng, X.-H., Ansari, D.O., Yin-Goen, Q., Chen, G.Z., Shin, M., Yang, L., Yong, A.N., Wang, M.D., Nie, S.	Nature Biotechnology, 26(1), pp. 83–90	2008	2,074

it also emphasizes the importance of other journals that, although contributing fewer articles, provide outlets for niche research areas and promote diversity in the field.

Taken together, the analysis of the most cited papers and journals reveals not only the impactful research and key outlets in the field of nanomaterials for drug delivery but also provides insight into the research trends and the evolving interests of the research community. It is clear that the field is flourishing, with impactful contributions and strong publishing outlets. This growth, coupled with the focus on targeted drug delivery, indicates a promising future for nanomaterials in the field of drug delivery.

Figure 3. Distribution of publications across ten scientific journals

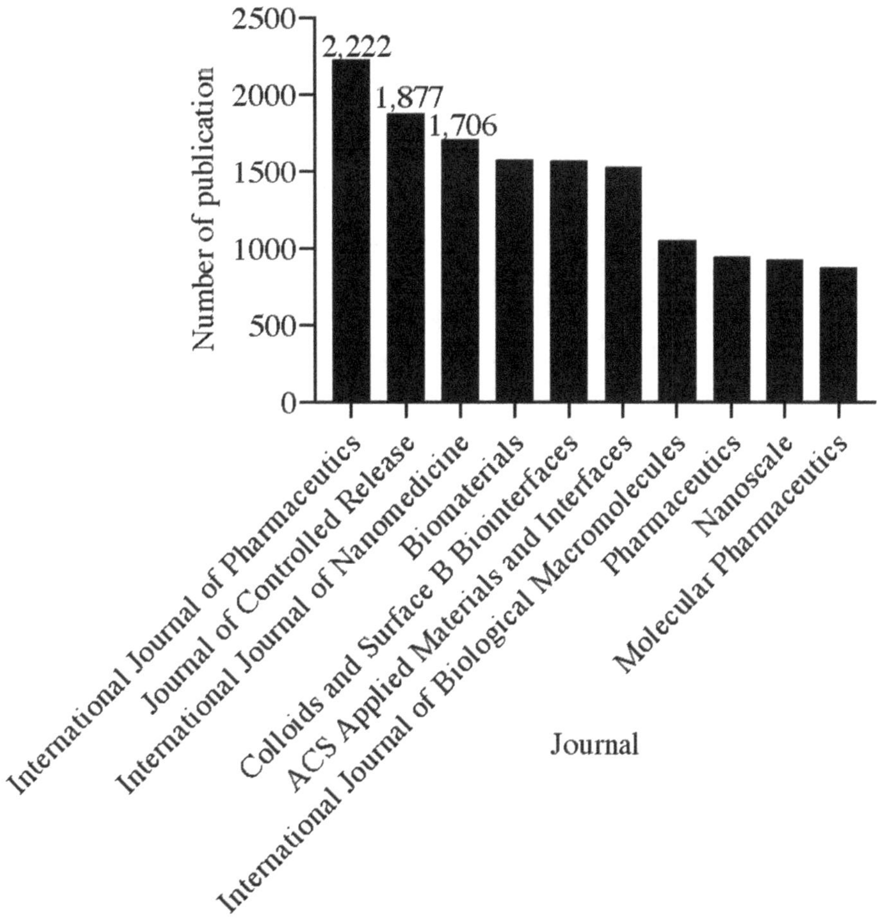

Country and Institution Analysis

The geographical distribution of publications in the field of nanomaterials for drug delivery is demonstrated in Figure 4. This analysis of the publications revealed that China was the leading contributor to the field, followed by the United States, India, Iran, South Korea, Germany, the United Kingdom, Italy, Spain, and France. This result offers an intriguing perspective on the global landscape of this research domain. China's leading contribution signifies the country's robust scientific and technological capabilities as well as a high level of investment in nanotechnology and drug delivery research. Following China, the United States, India, Iran, South Korea, and Germany are significant contributors, reflecting their growing prominence in nanomaterial research, driven by strategic investment in nanoscience and nanotechnology. Interestingly, the substantial contributions from both developed and developing nations suggest a global recognition of the importance of nanomaterials in advancing drug delivery systems. The investment of these diverse countries also indicates the potential for international collaboration in this research area.

Figure 4. Geographical distribution of publications in the field of nanomaterials for drug delivery

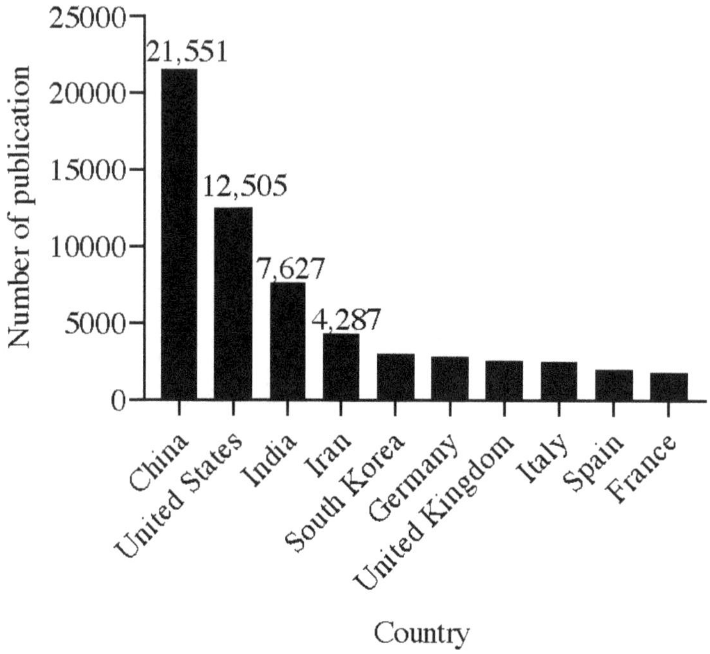

The institutional analysis, depicted in Figure 5, provides additional insights into the entities driving these research advancements. Among institutions, the Ministry of Education China had the highest number of publications (3,508 documents), followed by the Chinese Academy of Sciences (2,478 documents) and Sichuan University (1,015 documents). This leadership position of the Ministry of Education China could be attributed to the institute's emphasis on interdisciplinary research and its world-renowned programs in nanotechnology, material science, and biomedical engineering. The Chinese Academy of Sciences, another leading contributor, is known for its research strength in the biomedical field, which likely contributes to the productivity of nanomaterials for drug delivery. Sichuan University, one of China's most prestigious institutions, follows closely, reflecting China's significant advancements in the field of nanotechnology. It is noteworthy that these institutions are not only well known for their contributions to science and technology but also for their commitment to innovation and collaboration. Their prominence in the field of nanomaterials for drug delivery suggests that they serve as important nodes in the global research network, driving innovation and fostering collaborations. It is important to note, however, that while this analysis highlights the leading contributors, it does not diminish the vital contributions from other institutions and countries worldwide. These findings should further stimulate international and interinstitutional collaborations, promote knowledge exchange, and accelerate advancements in the field of nanomaterials for drug delivery.

The examination of publication output in the realm of nanomaterials for drug delivery systems, as cataloged in Scopus, elucidates the five most prominent scholars in this domain. Prof. Qiang Zhang, affiliated with Peking University Health Science Center in China, holds a seminal position with a corpus of 120 documents, closely trailed by Assoc. Prof. Bruno Sarmento from Universidade do Porto, Portugal, with a body of 119 documents. Prof. Rassoul Dinarvand of the Tehran University of Medical Science,

Figure 5. Top contributing institutions to the research of nanomaterials for drug delivery

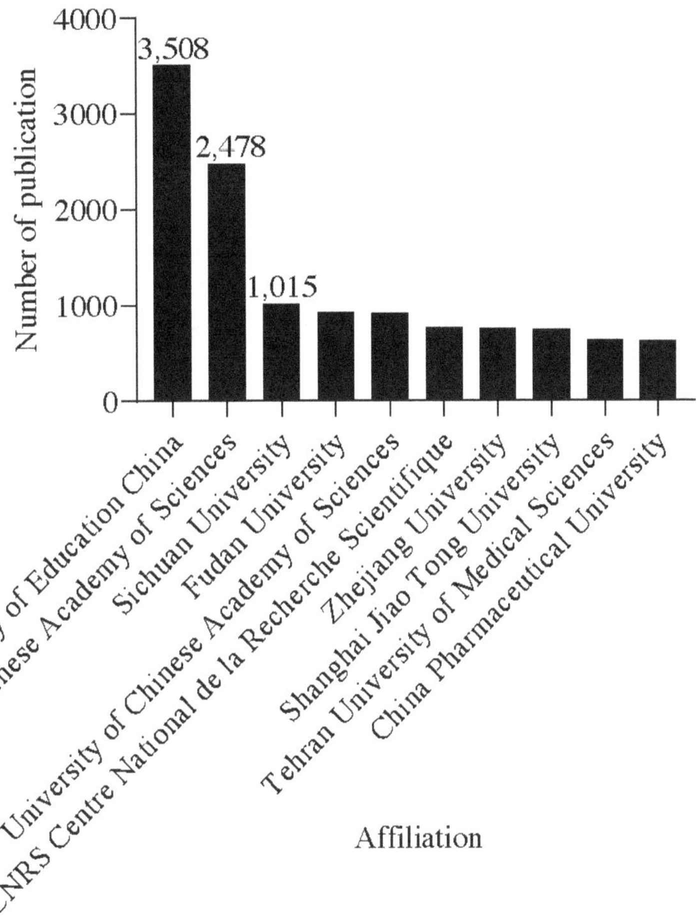

Iran, occupies second place with 113 published documents. Prof. Xuesi Chen of the Chinese Academy of Science, China, and Prof. Hélder A. Santos from Helsingin Yliopisto, Finland, follow with 112 and 111 documents, respectively. The substantial contributions made by these scholars underscore their notable influence on the field of nanomaterials for drug delivery systems. Their exhaustive research endeavors enhance our comprehension of the field and catalyze innovation, consistently expanding the frontiers of knowledge and application in this sphere.

Keyword Analysis

A network visualization analysis was conducted, setting the minimum number of occurrences for a keyword at 5. Out of the 139,284 keywords identified, 24,024 met this threshold. For each of these 24,024 keywords, we calculated the total strength of co-occurrence links with other keywords. The keywords with the greatest total link strength were then selected. For this section, we limited our selection to the top 1,000 keywords. The network diagram in Figure 6 represents the most commonly used keywords in the articles, their frequency, and the connections between them. Keyword analysis revealed terms such as "drug delivery system", "controlled release", "nanoparticles", "human", "nonhuman", and "animals" as the most prevalent.

Research themes could be classified into five clusters. Each of the five clusters identified reflects a unique research theme in the field of nanomaterials, offering diverse and valuable contributions to the development and understanding of this area. Cluster 1 (red), comprising 364 items, focused on the development and characterization of drug delivery systems. This theme recognizes the critical role that nanomaterials can play in delivering drugs to targeted areas within the body. It involves investigating and designing various delivery systems at the nanoscale, assessing their physicochemical properties, and evaluating their biocompatibility. By defining these properties, researchers can ensure that these nanomaterial-based drug delivery systems are safe, effective, and can be optimally utilized in various medical applications. and the characterization of their physicochemical and biocompatibility properties. Cluster 2 (green), consisting of 228 items, centers on the application of smart nanomaterials for cancer therapies. These smart nanomaterials often have properties that allow for targeted drug delivery or controlled drug release, which can improve the efficacy and safety of cancer treatment. This could involve nanomaterials that respond to specific triggers in the body (such as pH or temperature changes), allowing for the direct targeting of cancer cells, thereby minimizing damage to healthy cells. Cluster 3 (blue), with 214 items, involves the application of nanomaterials in immunotherapy and gene therapy. This cluster indicates a growing interest in leveraging the unique properties of nanomaterials to stimulate immune responses or deliver gene-editing tools to specific cells. This can result in more effective treatments for a range of diseases, from cancer to genetic disorders. Cluster 4 (yellow), including 192 items, covered studies of drug delivery using nanocarriers. This theme focuses on the practical aspects of using nanocarriers for drug delivery, including the investigation of different administration routes, studying the pharmacokinetic profiles in animal models, and evaluating pharmacological responses. This information is essential for understanding how these nanocarriers behave in a biological system and how they can be best used in clinical settings. Last, cluster 5 (purple), represented by 1 item, is a specific study of the potential toxicity of nanocarriers, particularly their effects on hemolysis, which is the breakdown of red blood cells. As the use of nanocarriers in medicine expands, it is vital to understand their potential impacts on human health, including possible adverse effects. Even though this cluster is smaller than the others, its importance should not be underestimated, as ensuring the safety of nanomaterials is crucial for their broader acceptance and usage in healthcare.

The timeline illustrated in Figure 7 maps the progression and emerging trends in nanomaterial research based on keyword analysis. This highlights the field's significant focus on improving drug delivery efficiency, particularly in cancer treatment, immunotherapy, and gene therapy, with considerable interest in polymeric nanoparticles due to their biocompatibility and ease of functionalization. "Immunotherapy" and "gene therapy" keywords indicate the increasing trend of leveraging nanomaterials to enhance the immune response or deliver therapeutic genes, promising strategies that could potentially revolutionize disease treatment. The focus on "targeted delivery" and "bioavailability" suggests that current challenges and research efforts aim to enhance drug delivery system efficiency and improve the bioavailability of therapeutics. This aligns with one of the main advantages of nanomaterials in drug delivery—their potential to increase the solubility and stability of drugs, improving bioavailability. It also mirrors ongoing efforts to design nanomaterials for delivering therapeutics to specific target sites, which can minimize side effects and increase treatment efficacy. The frequent appearance of "cancer therapy" as a keyword underscores the significant application of nanomaterials for drug delivery in oncology. Nanomaterials promise to revolutionize cancer treatment due to their potential for targeted delivery, which can address

Figure 6. Keyword co-occurrence network in the field of nanomaterials for drug delivery (VOSviewer 1.6.16)

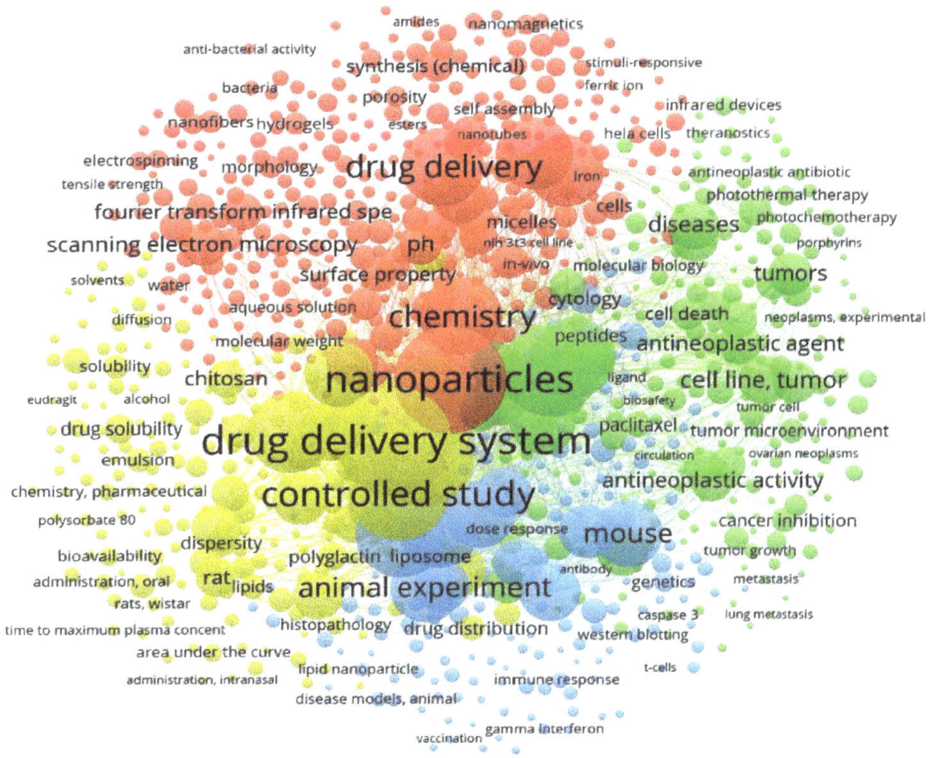

the challenges of conventional cancer therapy, such as systemic toxicity and nonspecific distribution. The dominance of "polymeric nanoparticles" as a keyword suggests a major trend in the type of nanomaterials being investigated for drug delivery applications. Polymeric nanoparticles are increasingly valued for their biocompatibility, tunable physical and chemical properties, and potential for functionalization, allowing a wide range of applications in drug delivery. The evolution of these themes over time shows the dynamic nature of this research field, reflecting continuous innovation and adaptation to address changing needs and challenges in drug discovery. However, it also underscores the consistent focus on improving therapeutic efficacy and precision, particularly in cancer therapy. This keyword analysis, while providing an understanding of the dominant themes and trends, should be interpreted in conjunction with other bibliometric findings. The prevalence of these keywords does not negate the importance of other, less frequent but potentially emerging themes in nanomaterials for drug delivery. Future research may delve deeper into these emergent themes, potentially revealing the next frontier in this fast-evolving field.

In conclusion, the results of this bibliometric analysis provide a comprehensive overview of the research landscape in the field of nanomaterials for drug delivery. The consistent increase in publications over the years demonstrates the ongoing advancement and evolution of this field. The focus on targeted drug delivery and cancer therapy implies the critical role of nanomaterials in revolutionizing therapeutic strategies. Additionally, the leading roles of China, the United States, India, Iran, South Korea, and Germany indicate the significant contributions these entities are making toward the development of this research

Figure 7. Evolution of key themes in nanomaterials for drug delivery research from 2020 to 2023 (VOSviewer 1.6.16)

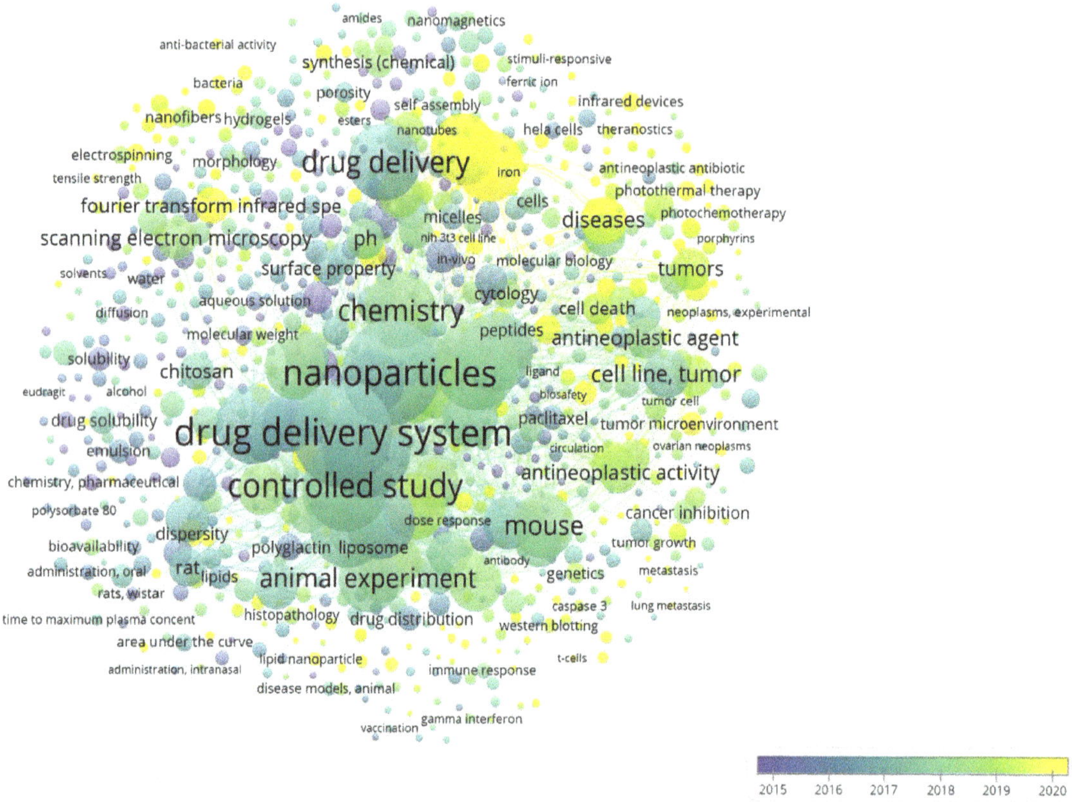

area. These data, however, should be interpreted considering the database's inherent limitations and the fact that a single database (Scopus) was used for the analysis. Future studies may expand this analysis to include other databases and use additional bibliometric and scientometric tools for a more detailed examination of the research trends and advancements in the field of nanomaterials for drug delivery.

TYPES OF NANOMATERIALS FOR DRUG DELIVERY

The use of nanomaterials in drug delivery has drastically transformed the landscape of therapeutic approaches. They have proven crucial in increasing drug bioavailability, prolonging drug release, and targeting precise delivery sites. Among the broad spectrum of nanomaterials, lipid-based nanocarriers, polymer-based nanoparticles, inorganic nanomaterials, carbon-based nanomaterials, and nanofibers have gained significant attention for their potential applications (Husni et al., 2023; T. Liu et al., 2023). In this section, the author explains the wide range of nanomaterials currently employed or being explored for the application of drug delivery. Readers will gain comprehensive insights into the role and significance of various nanocarriers, including lipid-based nanocarriers, polymer-based nanoparticles, nanofibers, and other innovative forms of nanomaterials. Each type of nanomaterial is carefully discussed, revealing

Figure 8. Chemical structures of selected drugs discussed in this chapter, which are delivered via nano-carrier systems
(ChemDraw 20.1.1)

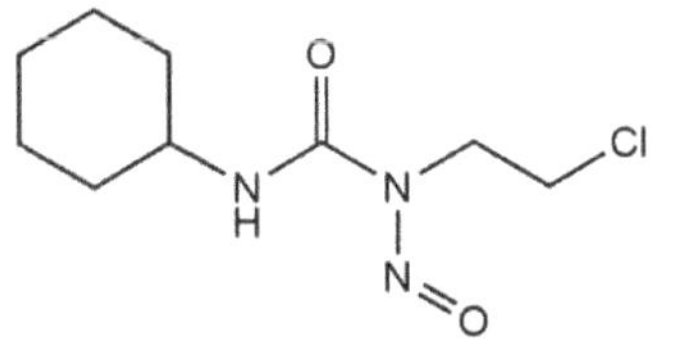

Lomustine

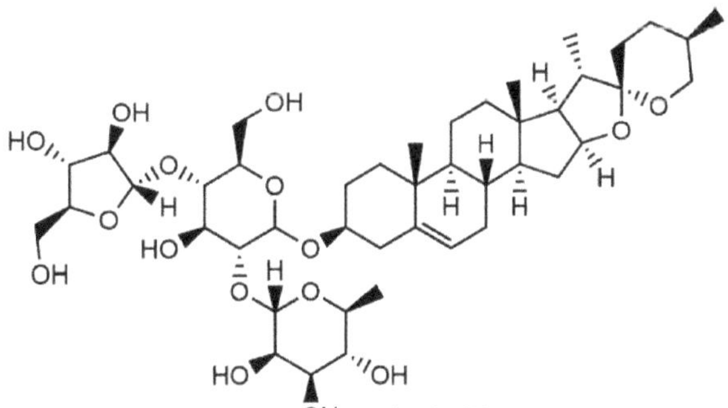

Polyphyllin D

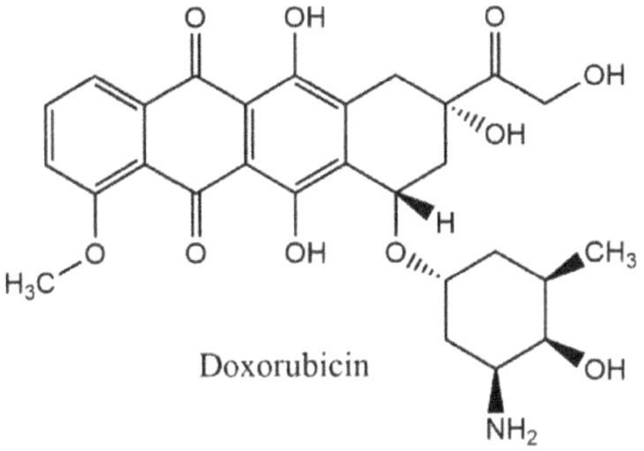

Doxorubicin

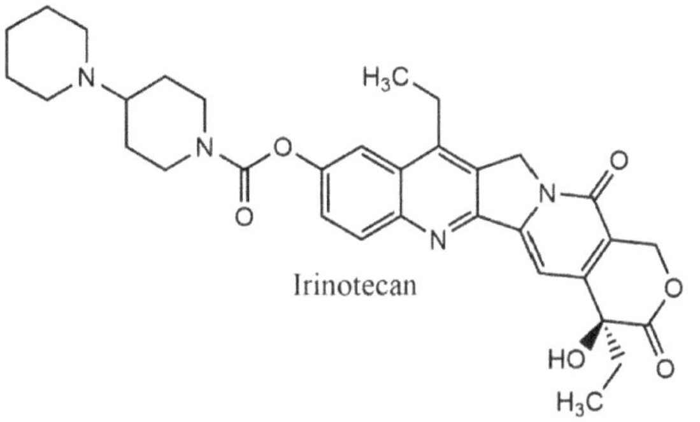

Irinotecan

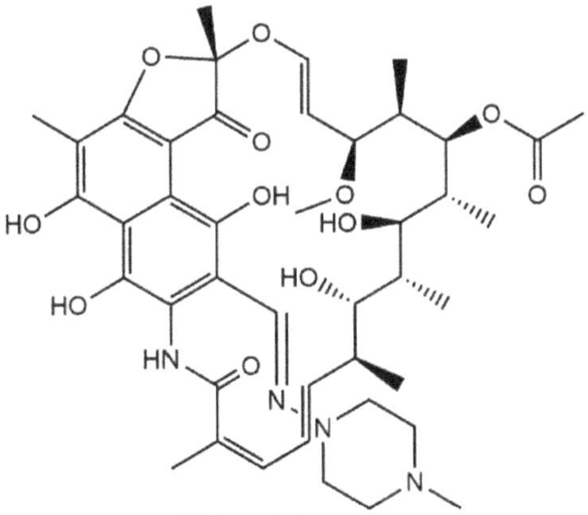

Rifampicin

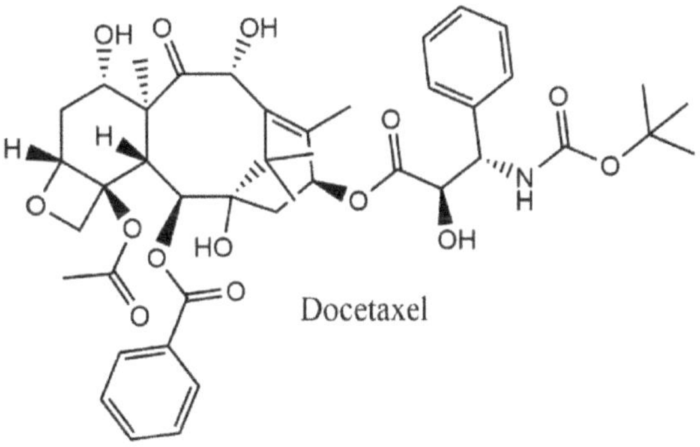

Docetaxel

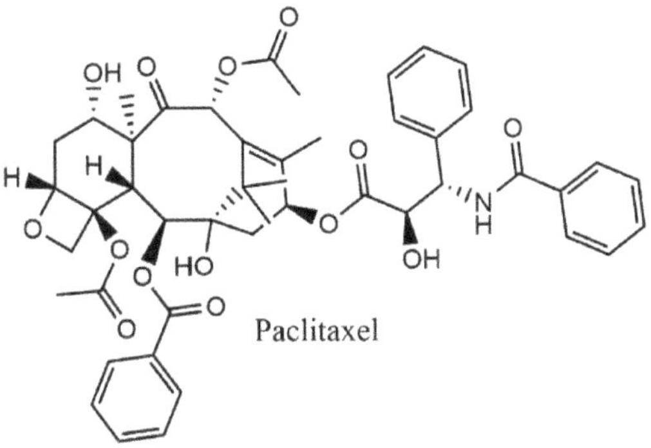

Paclitaxel

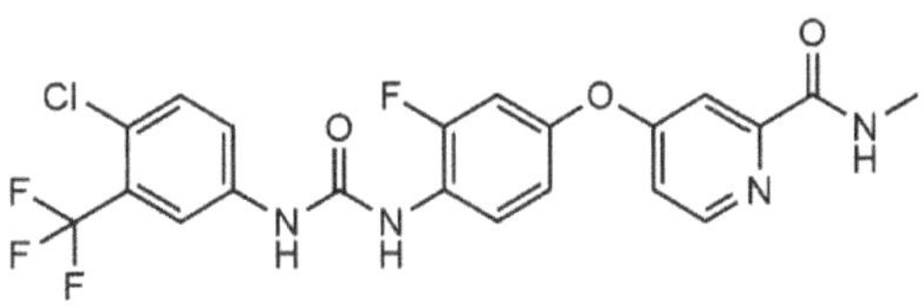

Regorafenib

their unique properties, mechanisms of action, and respective advantages for facilitating the delivery of drugs. Figure 8 displays the chemical structures of specific drugs that are discussed in this chapter. These drugs are unique in that they are delivered to their target locations in the body via nanocarrier systems. Moreover, this section sheds light on how these nanomaterials overcome challenges associated with conventional drug delivery systems. For instance, it outlines how certain nanocarriers enhance the solubility and stability of therapeutics and can also allow for targeted drug delivery, thereby improving the therapeutic index and reducing side effects. Readers will also discover how these nanomaterials contribute to controlling drug release, thus ensuring that therapeutic agents can be delivered at the right time and at the optimal dosage.

Lipid-Based Nanomaterials

Lipid-based nanocarriers are gaining substantial recognition in the realm of drug delivery due to their unique attributes. Structurally, they are composed of biocompatible and biodegradable lipids, which encapsulate drug molecules and facilitate their transport through biological systems. The lipidic nature of these nanocarriers enables them to accommodate both hydrophilic and hydrophobic drugs, thereby amplifying their applicability in delivering a diverse range of therapeutics (Das et al., 2022). One illustrative success story of lipid-based drug delivery systems in recent times is the mRNA-based COVID-19 vaccines developed by Moderna and Pfizer, known by their commercial names as mRNA-1273 and Comirnaty, respectively. These vaccines utilize lipid nanoparticles to transport mRNA, which encodes the spike protein of the SARS-CoV-2 virus – the culprit behind COVID-19. By doing so, the lipid nanoparticles shield the mRNA from degradation while also boosting its absorption into cells. This initiates an immune response that provides defense against COVID-19 (Husni et al., 2023). On the other hand, patisiran or Onpattro serves as a further testament to the effectiveness of lipid-based drug delivery systems. This therapeutic was developed by Alnylam Pharmaceuticals and uses RNA interference (RNAi) for treating hereditary transthyretin-mediated amyloidosis, a relatively uncommon genetic disorder (Maurer et al., 2023). Like vaccines, lipid components provide a protective layer for small interfering RNA (siRNA) against degradation and amplify its cellular uptake. This allows the siRNA to target and trigger the gene responsible for generating the transthyretin protein, which accumulates in peripheral nerves and contributes to the disease (Schmidt et al., 2022). Several types of lipid-based nanocarriers exist, each offering distinctive characteristics that determine their suitability for specific applications. Key examples, including lipid-based drug delivery systems (lipid nanoparticles, liposomes, and other vesicular delivery systems) and lipid drug conjugates, are provided in the following details.

Lipid Nanoparticles

Lipid nanoparticles are emerging as powerful platforms for drug delivery due to their remarkable characteristics, including biocompatibility, biodegradability, and the ability to encapsulate both hydrophilic and hydrophobic drugs (Navabhatra et al., 2022). This subsection will cover three primary types of lipid nanoparticles utilized in drug delivery: nanoemulsions, solid lipid nanoparticles (SLNs), and nanostructured lipid carriers (NLCs).

1) Nanoemulsions

Nanoemulsions are colloidal dispersions comprised of two immiscible liquids, typically oil and water, stabilized by surfactants. With a size ranging from 20 to 200 nm, they can solubilize lipophilic drugs within their oil phase, enabling their systemic delivery. The small droplet size of nanoemulsions provides a large surface area for drug absorption and allows the drug to bypass first-pass metabolism, thereby improving bioavailability (X. Shen et al., 2023). Additionally, nanoemulsions can be tuned to control the drug release rate, which is beneficial for prolonged or targeted therapeutic delivery (Attama et al., 2023). For example, glioblastoma multiforme is a highly aggressive type of cancer with a five-year survival rate of less than 5%. It can occur at any age but is most commonly found in elderly individuals. The disease is marked by significant angiogenesis, rampant cell proliferation, and extensive tissue infiltration (Vojdani et al., 2021). Currently, chemotherapeutic strategies, including oral or parenteral methods, only marginally improve the survival rate. As such, novel strategies that increase the localization of chemotherapeutic agents to the brain tumor are required to reduce fatality rates. One such agent, lomustine (refer to Figure 8), an alkylating chemotherapy drug, is often employed to treat this cancer. However, it indiscriminately affects rapidly dividing cells, resulting in potential side effects and toxicity. The need to balance dosage reduction to minimize adverse effects with the requirement for a sufficiently high dose to kill cancer cells presents a significant challenge. Lomustine is lipophilic and can be absorbed orally and passed through lipophilic membranes. After absorption, it is metabolized extensively in the liver with a half-life of approximately 94 minutes (Khan et al., 2022; Lombardi et al., 2021). Recently, a study by Al-Awsi et al. (2024) explored the use of nanoemulsions to deliver lomustine directly to the brain via nasal administration, bypassing the blood–brain barrier and minimizing systemic side effects. They chose nanoemulsions for their simplicity of production and good solubilizing abilities. This is particularly beneficial given lomustine's poor oral bioavailability and severe side effects. The researchers created eighteen different nanoemulsion formulations after examining lomustine's solubility in various substances. These formulations were then assessed for their characteristics, such as droplet size, entrapment efficiency, and stability. The most promising formulation showed efficient drug entrapment efficiency, stability, and complete lomustine release within 15 minutes. This suggests that nanoemulsions could rapidly and directly deliver the drug to the brain, offering a potentially safer and more effective alternative to oral delivery.

2) Solid lipid nanoparticles

SLNs are submicron colloidal carriers, typically ranging in size from 10 to 1000 nanometers. They are composed predominantly of lipids that remain solid at both room temperature and body temperature. These lipids can be either natural or synthetic, such as triglycerides, fatty acids, or waxes (Dhanya et al., 2023). The core advantages of SLNs as drug delivery systems revolve around their high stability, controlled drug release capabilities, biocompatibility, and capacity for large-scale production. Additionally, SLNs can be formulated to enhance the solubility of lipophilic drugs, protect sensitive drugs from degradation, and deliver drugs to specific target sites in the body (Elkateb et al., 2023). The solid core allows for a high drug loading capacity and protects the encapsulated drug from degradation. Furthermore, SLNs can control drug release, enhance stability, and improve bioavailability. They are particularly useful for the delivery of lipophilic drugs and provide a potential platform for targeted drug delivery (Harish et al., 2023). The preparation of SLNs involves the emulsification of a melted lipid, in which the drug is dissolved or dispersed, followed by a rapid cooling process that leads to the solidification of the lipid, entrapping the drug within. There are several methods for producing SLNs, including high-pressure homogenization, microemulsion, and solvent evaporation. Each of these methods has unique advantages and can be chosen based on the specific properties of the drug to be loaded and the intended application (Almawash, 2023). The incorporation of drugs into SLNs can be achieved either by dispersing the drug in the lipid matrix (homogeneous matrix model) or by creating a drug-enriched shell or core (drug-enriched model). These techniques allow for versatile drug delivery mechanisms, such as immediate, delayed, or sustained release, depending on the distribution of the drug within the SLNs (Aguilera-Garrido et al., 2023). Despite their numerous advantages, SLNs also face some challenges. For instance, the limited drug loading capacity due to the crystalline structure of the lipid matrix and the potential for drug expulsion during storage are significant considerations. However, innovative approaches are being developed to mitigate these issues, such as the development of nanostructured lipid carriers, which blend solid lipids with liquid lipids to disrupt the crystalline structure and increase the drug loading capacity.

Several drugs have been delivered via SLNs, including polyphyllin D (Emami, Ghafouri, & Sariri, 2023), tofacitinib citrate (Roy et al., 2023), and maslinic acid (Aguilera-Garrido et al., 2023). For instance, in the 2023 study, Emai and colleagues examined the potential of an SLN formulation containing polyphyllin D (refer to Figure 8) to treat breast cancer. Polyphyllin D is a steroidal saponin found in *Paris polyphylla* and is known to initiate apoptosis in various cancer types. However, its application has been limited due to hemolysis and cytotoxicity related to its structure. To overcome these limitations, the researchers optimized a polyphyllin D-loaded SLN formulation and evaluated its impact on breast cancer cells. They identified cell death through apoptosis via Annexin V/propidium iodide staining and western blot analysis. Subsequent in vivo studies on 4T1-implanted BALB/c mice compared the tumor inhibitory effectiveness of various doses of polyphyllin D-loaded SLNs. The researchers calculated the half-maximal inhibitory concentration (IC_{50}) of PD-loaded SLN to be 33.25 and 35.74 μg/mL for MCF7 and MDA-MB-231 cells, respectively. There was a noticeable increase in apoptosis in cells treated with PD-loaded SLN, as evidenced by flow cytometry analysis. Western blot analysis revealed that treatment with PD-loaded SLN downregulated Bcl2 and HSP70 protein levels while upregulating Bax, Bad, P53, Apaf-1, p-p53, and Noxa protein levels in both cell lines. These results were further corroborated by *in vivo* tests on BALB/c mice (Emami et al., 2023).

3) Nanostructured lipid carriers

NLCs represent the second generation of lipid nanoparticles, aiming to overcome the limitations of SLNs, such as their low drug loading capacity and expulsion of the drug during storage. They are formulated using a blend of solid and liquid lipids, leading to an imperfect matrix structure. This disordered, nonhomogeneous structure provides better encapsulation of the drug, reduces drug expulsion during storage, and allows the controlled release of the drug. The fabrication process of NLCs typically involves high-pressure homogenization, ultrasonication, or microemulsion techniques (Navabhatra et al., 2022). The selection of solid and liquid lipids is contingent upon factors such as the nature of the drug to be delivered, its compatibility with the lipids, the desired release profiles, and the intended route of administration. A key advantage of NLCs is their ability to enhance the solubility of lipophilic drugs. Their high lipid content also contributes to their biocompatibility, making them suitable for various administration routes, including oral, topical, intravenous, ocular, and nasal (Agrawal et al., 2022). Moreover, NLCs have the potential to bypass biological barriers, facilitating targeted delivery of drugs and reducing off-target effects (Şen et al., 2021). Another essential feature of NLCs is their capability to offer controlled and sustained drug release. By manipulating the lipid matrix's composition, one can effectively adjust the drug release rate to maintain therapeutic levels of the drug over extended periods (Navabhatra et al., 2022). NLCs have also shown significant potential for the delivery of fragile biomolecules such as proteins, peptides, and genes. The lipid matrix offers protection against enzymatic degradation and enhances stability during storage (Nguyen et al., 2022). Recently, Z. Zhang et al. (2023) reported the potential of *Artemisia argyi* essential oil-loaded NLCs for hepatitis B treatment. This essential oil was found to inhibit the replication of hepatitis B virus DNA, and its effects were enhanced when delivered via NLCs. This treatment led to a substantial reduction in viral DNA levels, and the beneficial effects were sustained even after stopping the treatment. Furthermore, the developed NLCs improved essential oil oral bioavailability and liver exposure. Network pharmacology and molecular docking revealed that the studied essential oil impacts immune-related signaling pathways and has strong binding interactions with prostaglandin-endoperoxide synthase-2, suggesting that the developed NLCs could be a potential therapeutic strategy for hepatitis B virus infection.

Liposomes and Other Vesicular Delivery Systems

Liposomes and other vesicular delivery systems have been at the forefront of pharmaceutical research due to their potential to revolutionize drug delivery. These vesicular systems, which include liposomes, niosomes, ethosomes, and transfersomes, are unique because they can encapsulate both lipophilic and hydrophilic drugs, improving their stability, solubility, and bioavailability (A. Liu et al., 2023). Notably, liposomes, which are lipid-based vesicles with more or less phospholipid bilayers, have been extensively researched for their versatile applicability in targeted drug delivery, gene therapy, and vaccine development (Yong Wang et al., 2023). These systems can protect the entrapped active pharmaceutical ingredients from degradation, control their release, and enhance their distribution in the body (L. Cheng et al., 2021). Additionally, they can be manipulated to target specific cells or tissues, thereby improving therapeutic efficacy while minimizing side effects (J. Li et al., 2023). The following sections will highlight liposomes and other vesicular delivery systems, highlighting their structure, mechanisms, and applications in drug delivery and beyond.

Liposomes are spherical, self-assembling structures composed of one or more concentric lipid bilayers enclosing an aqueous core. Figure 9 represents a liposomal structure, a spherical vesicle consisting of one or more phospholipid bilayers. The outer layer is hydrophilic (attracted to water), and the inner space is hydrophobic (repels water). This unique structure allows liposomes to encapsulate both hydrophilic drugs within the aqueous core and hydrophobic drugs within the lipid bilayer, making them highly versatile for various drug delivery applications. The biological characteristics of liposomes can be fine-tuned by altering their physicochemical and biophysical attributes, such as their lipid composition, dimensions, volume, and surface charge (Kansız & Elçin, 2023). Deploying liposomes in drug delivery systems has substantially enhanced the pharmacokinetic profiles of numerous bioactive compounds in pharmaceuticals (Kim et al., 2023). Nevertheless, the broad utilization of liposomes faces certain constraints, predominantly due to issues associated with their thermodynamic instability (Michlewska et al., 2023). This instability can limit their effectiveness and, consequently, their potential applications in various therapeutic settings.

Liposomal drug delivery systems have been widely used in oncology due to their ability to improve the therapeutic index of chemotherapeutic agents. For example, Doxil®, a liposomal formulation of the chemotherapeutic agent doxorubicin, has been approved by the United States Food and Drug Administration for the treatment of ovarian cancer and multiple myeloma. Liposomal encapsulation enhances the delivery of doxorubicin (refer to Figure 8) to the tumor site, thereby improving therapeutic effectiveness and reducing systemic toxicity (Taher et al., 2023). Similarly, Onivyde®, a liposomal formulation of irinotecan (refer to Figure 8), is used for the treatment of metastatic pancreatic cancer (Zhang et al., 2022). Liposomal encapsulation allows prolonged circulation and improved accumulation at the tumor site, enhancing therapeutic efficiency and reducing side effects. A recent study by M. Mishra et al. (2023) investigated a novel approach to tackling tuberculosis, a disease caused by the intracellular pathogen *Mycobacterium tuberculosis*. The researchers focused on the potential of liposomes, lipid-based structures that were developed using immunostimulatory lipids obtained from tuberculosis-causing bacteria. These liposomes are found to moderate the immune response of the host and aid in the effective eradication of the pathogen when combined with sustained drug delivery. The study extensively evaluated the intracellular and *in vitro* release of the antituberculosis drug rifampicin (refer to Figure 8) from these liposomes, its impact on cell viability, its long-term stability, and its antimicrobial efficiency. The researchers noted a higher intracellular drug concentration following treatment with these liposome-encapsulated drugs compared to the free drug. This indicates a sustained release of the drug. The encapsulated drug within the liposomes was internalized by cells via clathrin-mediated endocytosis and was found to trigger a strong proinflammatory immune response. Interestingly, the drug-loaded liposomes and the pathogen were found in the same cellular compartments (recycling and late endosomes), suggesting localized intracellular targeting. The results also suggest that these liposomal drug formulations might have lipid-centric and species-specific selectivity.

Beyond liposomes, other vesicular systems, such as niosomes and ethosomes, have also been explored for drug delivery. Niosomes are small vesicular systems that have gained significant attention for their potential use in drug delivery. Composed of nonionic surfactants and cholesterol, they are similar to liposomes but have key advantages that make them an attractive alternative, such as cost-effectiveness, better storage stability, and a wider choice of materials (Bashkeran et al., 2023). Ethosomes, which are composed of phospholipids and a high concentration of ethanol (typically ranging from 20% to 45%), have been used for the transdermal delivery of drugs, as ethanol enhances the permeability of the skin (Aljohani et al., 2023). In addition, transfersomes, menthosomes, flexosomes, and phytosomes represent innovative vesicular systems in the domain of drug delivery, each offering unique advantages. Transfersomes, as ultraflexible vesicles, can penetrate the skin deeply, carrying both hydrophilic and lipophilic drugs for transdermal administration (Sun et al., 2023). Menthosomes loaded with menthol enhance skin permeability and provide a soothing effect, demonstrating potential for topical and transdermal drug delivery (Nayak & Tippavajhala, 2021). Flexosomes incorporate an edge activator to induce elasticity, enabling their penetration through pores smaller than their own diameter, thus optimizing transdermal delivery (Hongda Zhu et al., 2022). Finally, phytosomes form a complex of natural products from herbal compounds (Gaikwad et al., 2023). Vesicular delivery systems, with versatile encapsulation capabilities and potential for targeted drug delivery, continue to revolutionize the field of drug delivery. Ongoing research and development of these systems promise the advent of more precise, efficient, and safer therapeutic strategies.

Lipid-Drug Conjugates

Lipid-drug conjugates (LDCs) have emerged as a potent tool in the field of drug delivery, leveraging the natural compatibility of lipids within the body to potentially improve the delivery, efficacy, and safety of therapeutics. These systems utilize lipids as carriers to enhance the solubility of hydrophobic drugs,

Figure 9. Illustration of a liposomal structure

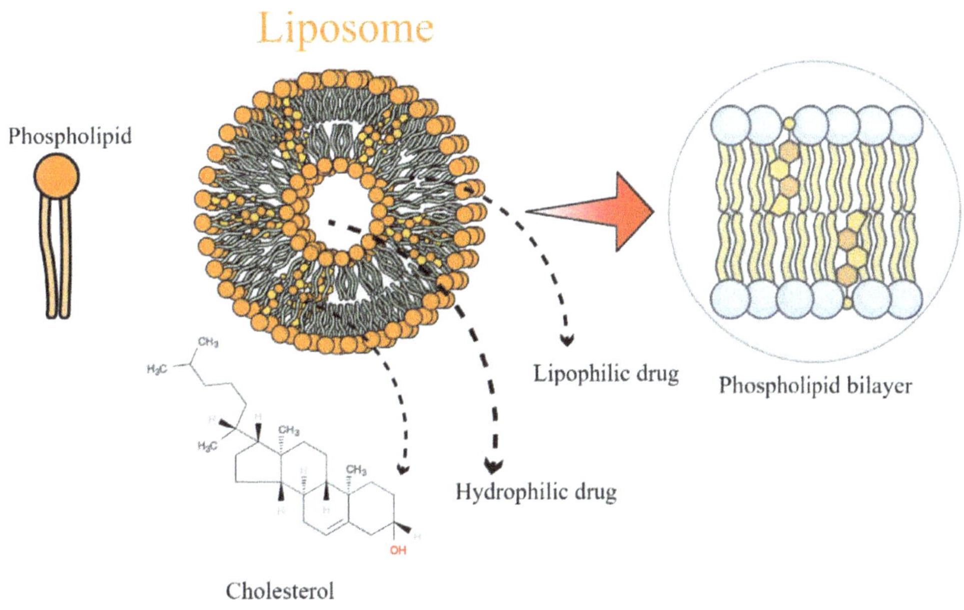

protect them from biological degradation, and facilitate cellular membrane crossing (Husni et al., 2023). A crucial aspect in the design of LDCs is the linkage between the drug and lipid. The bond must be resilient enough to endure systemic circulation while maintaining the ability to dissociate at the target site. This chemical design, although challenging, is a fundamental step in ensuring efficient drug delivery. For instance, disulfide linkages are often employed due to their sensitivity to the reducing environment in cells, ensuring efficient intracellular drug release (Y. Pan et al., 2023). However, realizing the full potential of LDCs is not without challenges. High drug loading, which is often desirable for improving therapeutic outcomes, may destabilize LDCs, affecting their overall performance. In fact, these instabilities could potentially lead to premature drug release or a reduction in half-life in the body (Dissanayake et al., 2022). Moreover, the immune system could potentially recognize and eliminate LDCs before the drug reaches its intended target. Strategies such as PEGylation - the addition of polyethylene glycol (PEG) to the lipid - are often employed to reduce this risk and prolong the circulation time (Srivastav et al., 2023). Finally, the scalability and cost-effectiveness of producing LDCs are formidable challenges. These complexities underscore the need for innovative manufacturing strategies and stringent quality control processes to ensure the robustness, safety, and efficacy of the final product. Overall, while LDCs present promising opportunities for improving drug delivery, it is essential to address these challenges through continued research and innovation. This will aid in realizing the full potential of LDCs in clinical applications and improving patient outcomes.

Polymer-Based Nanomaterials

Polymer-based nanomaterials, characterized by their unique properties and applications, have emerged as potent tools in drug discovery. This technology encompasses polymeric nanoparticles, micelles, dendrimers, and nanohydrogels, each offering specific advantages for various therapeutic applications.

Polymeric Nanoparticles

Polymeric nanoparticles, typically ranging in size from 10 to 1,000 nm, have positioned themselves as promising carriers for drug delivery. These nanoparticles are typically made up of synthetic or natural polymers, the choice of which largely hinges on the required characteristics of the nanoparticles, such as size, surface charge, and the type of drug to be encapsulated. Table 2 summarizes the key types of polymeric nanoparticles, their core compositions, and some common applications they have in the field of drug delivery. Polylactic-co-glycolic acid (PLGA), a copolymer of lactic acid and glycolic acid, is commonly used due to its biocompatibility, biodegradability, and ability to provide a slow and controlled release of drugs (Manhas et al., 2023). Polylactic acid (PLA) is another frequently used polymer; it is a biodegradable and bioresorbable polyester derived from renewable resources such as corn starch, marking it as an environmentally friendly choice (Bakr et al., 2023). Poly(ε-caprolactone) (PCL), a biodegradable polyester, is often used for the extended controlled release of drugs due to its slow degradation rate (Yingngam et al., 2019). Polyethylene glycol (PEG), commonly used as a coating for nanoparticles, offers "stealth" features, helping to evade the immune system and extend the circulation time of the nanoparticles in the body (Korake et al., 2023). Chitosan, a linear polysaccharide derived from chitin, has found extensive use in drug delivery due to its biocompatibility, biodegradability, and ability to open tight junctions, improving drug permeability (Jalal et al., 2023). Finally, polyethylenimine (PEI), a cationic polymer, is particularly beneficial in gene delivery applications due to its ability to condense DNA into nanoparticles and facilitate cellular uptake (T. T. Nguyen et al., 2023). These polymers are used to fabricate polymeric nanoparticles through various methods, such as emulsion, coacervation, and nanoprecipitation. The choice of method depends on the type of polymer, the drug to be encapsulated, and the desired characteristics of the nanoparticles.

Polymeric nanoparticles offer distinct advantages due to their nanoscale size, which ensures stability, optimized biodistribution, and extended circulation times in the bloodstream. They can encapsulate therapeutic agents in their core, protecting them from premature enzymatic degradation and unwanted interactions with biological components, thus improving bioavailability. Alternatively, drugs can be conjugated onto the nanoparticle surface for targeted release and enhanced pharmacological activity. Polymeric nanoparticles have been employed across a broad range of therapeutic applications. For instance, PLGA nanoparticles can deliver chemotherapy drugs such as doxorubicin effectively to tumor sites, minimizing toxicity to healthy tissues (Panda & Jain, 2023). Significant progress has also been made in the delivery of genetic material in gene therapy using polymeric nanoparticles. PEGylated polyethylenimine nanoparticles, for example, have been used to deliver DNA and RNA molecules to specific cells for the treatment of genetic diseases. These nanoparticles protect the genetic material from degradation and facilitate efficient uptake by target cells, showcasing their potential in gene therapy (Sands et al., 2023). In the context of neurodegenerative disorders such as Alzheimer's and Parkinson's disease, polymeric nanoparticles such as those made from PLGA have shown promise by crossing the blood–brain barrier—a major challenge in neurotherapeutics—and delivering drugs directly to the brain

Table 2. Summary of various types of polymeric nanoparticles, their compositions, and applications in drug delivery

Polymeric nanoparticle	Composition	Drug delivery application	Reference
Polylactic-co-glycolic acid nanoparticles	Biodegradable and biocompatible copolymer of lactic acid and glycolic acid	Used to encapsulate and deliver chemotherapy drugs like doxorubicin to tumor sites due to its slow and controlled release properties	Manhas et al. (2023)
Polylactic acid nanoparticles	Biodegradable and bioresorbable resources such as corn starch	Utilized in various drug delivery systems due to its eco-friendly nature and biocompatibility	Bakr et al. (2023)
Poly(ε-caprolactone) nanoparticles	Biodegradable polyester with a slow degradation rate	Used for long-term drug delivery due to its slow degradable rate	Chen Xu et al. (2023); Yingngam et al. (2019)
Polyethylene glycol-coated nanoparticles	Polyethylene glycol coating provides "stealth" characteristics	Increases the circulation time of the nanoparticles in the body, avoiding rapid clearance by the immune system	Korake et al. (2023)
Chitosan nanoparticles	Linear polysaccharide derived from chitin	Frequently used in drug delivery due to its biocompatibility, biodegradability, and ability to enhance drug permeability	Jalal et al. (2023)
Polyethylenimine nanoparticles	Cationic polymer	Often used in gene delivery applications due to its ability to condense DNA into nanoparticles and facilitate cellular uptake	T. T. Nguyen et al. (2023)

(Chacko & Jose, 2023). Furthermore, they have been employed in antimicrobial therapy, with chitosan nanoparticles used for the delivery of various antibiotics, enhancing antimicrobial activity due to the increased concentration of the drug at the infection site (Elmehbad et al., 2023).

Polymeric Micelles

Polymeric micelles are another class of polymeric nanomaterials. These are self-assembling nanoparticles formed by amphiphilic block copolymers, meaning they have both hydrophobic (water-repelling) and hydrophilic (water-attracting) segments. In an aqueous environment, the hydrophobic segments cluster together to form the core of the micelle, while the hydrophilic segments form the shell. The core of the micelle is capable of encapsulating hydrophobic drugs, while the shell stabilizes the micelle in the aqueous environment and can prevent the rapid clearance of the encapsulated drug by the immune system. The hydrophilic shell can also be modified with targeting moieties for targeted drug delivery (B. Huang et al., 2023). Table 3 provides a comparative analysis of various polymers used in micelle formation and highlights their advantages in drug delivery applications. Some examples of polymers used to form polymeric micelles include the following:

1) Poly(ethylene glycol)-b-poly(caprolactone) (PEG-b-PCL): PEG forms the hydrophilic shell, while PCL forms the hydrophobic core. PCL can encapsulate a variety of hydrophobic drugs.
2) Poly(ethylene glycol)-b-poly(D,L-lactide) (PEG-b-PDLLA): PDLLA forms the core and can encapsulate hydrophobic drugs, while PEG forms the shell.
3) Poly(ethylene glycol)-b-poly(L-glutamic acid) (PEG-b-PGA): PGA forms the core and can encapsulate cationic drugs or proteins, while PEG forms the shell.

Polymeric micelles can be prepared using several methods. Here are a few common ones:

1) Direct dissolution method: The amphiphilic block copolymer and the drug are dissolved in an organic solvent, and then the solution is poured into water. The solvent is then evaporated, leaving behind micelles.
2) Film hydration method: The copolymer and drug are dissolved in a volatile organic solvent, and then the solvent is evaporated to form a thin film. This film is then hydrated in an aqueous solution to form micelles.
3) Solvent evaporation method (oil/water emulsion method): The drug and copolymer are dissolved in an organic solvent and emulsified in water with or without a surfactant. The solvent is then evaporated to form micelles.
4) Dialysis method: The drug and copolymer are dissolved in a solvent, and then the solution is placed into a dialysis tube and dialyzed against water. The solvent molecules diffuse out of the tube, and micelles form.

Each method has its own advantages and disadvantages in terms of control over size and drug loading efficiency, stability of the micelles, and simplicity of the procedure, among other factors. The choice of method depends on the specific requirements of the drug delivery system being developed.

Polymeric micelles have found extensive applications across a range of therapeutic domains. Chemotherapeutics, for example, have been used to improve the delivery of poorly water-soluble chemotherapeutic agents. One such example is the use of pteroyl-γ-l-glutamate/Pluronic® F68 (poly(ethylene oxide)-b-poly(propylene oxide)-b-poly(ethylene oxide)) modified polymeric micelles for the encapsulation and delivery of docetaxel (refer to Figure 8). This system not only enhances the solubility of docetaxel but also allows for its preferential accumulation at the tumor site due to the enhanced permeability and retention effect, improving therapeutic outcomes (Rarokar et al., 2023). Another example includes the use of PEG-b-PCL micelles for the delivery of paclitaxel and regorafenib (refer to Figure 8), a chemotherapeutic agent used for the treatment of various cancers. The micelles increase the solubility of both drugs, provide stability in the bloodstream, and allow for passive targeting of the tumor site, thus maximizing therapeutic efficacy while minimizing toxicity (Nezhadi et al., 2023). In gene therapy, polymeric micelles have been used for the delivery of genetic material. For instance, poly(ethylene glycol)-block-polyethylenimine (PEG-b-PEI) micelles have been used for the encapsulation and delivery of plasmid DNA, demonstrating efficient gene transfection (Karayianni et al., 2023). In the field of cancer therapy, polymeric micelles have been used to enhance the delivery of anticancer agents. An example of this includes the use of Pluronic® micelles for the delivery of curcumin, leading to improved anticancer activity (Patel et al., 2022).

Dendrimers

Dendrimers are highly branched, tree-like, symmetrical molecules with a well-defined, three-dimensional structure. They consist of a central core, a branching interior layer (generation), and exterior surface groups. Dendrimers can encapsulate small drug molecules in their internal cavities or bind larger molecules to numerous surface functional groups, making them highly useful for drug delivery (Kannan et al., 2023). The nature of the drug, the intended use, and the route of administration dictate the type of dendrimer used. Here are a few examples of dendrimers used for drug delivery.

Table 3. Comparison of different polymers used in micelle formation and their advantages in drug delivery applications

Polymer type	Advantages in drug delivery applications	Reference
Poly(ethylene glycol)-b-poly(caprolactone) (PEG-b-PCL)	PEG provides the hydrophilic shell for the micelle, making it water-soluble and biocompatible, while PCL forms the hydrophobic core, which is excellent for encapsulating a variety of hydrophobic drugs and enhancing their solubility and bioavailability.	Di Trani et al. (2021)
Poly(ethylene glycol)-b-poly(D,L-lactide) (PEG-b-PDLLA)	PEG forms the hydrophilic shell of the micelle, enhancing its water solubility, while PDLLA forms the hydrophobic core, which is ideal for encapsulating hydrophobic drugs. PDLLA is biodegradable and safe for use in the body, enabling the controlled release of the encapsulated drug.	Tao Liu et al. (2023)
Poly(ethylene glycol)-b-poly(L-glutamic acid) (PEG-b-PGA)	PEG forms the hydrophilic shell, providing water solubility to the micelle, while PGA forms the hydrophobic core. PGA is capable of encapsulating cationic drugs or proteins, enabling targeted and controlled delivery of these substances.	H. Yuan et al. (2022)
Triblock copolymers poly(2-phenoxyethyl methacrylate)-b-poly(2-oxopropyl methacrylate)-b-poly[poly(ethylene glycol) methyl ether methacrylate] (PPOEMA-b-POPMA-b-PPEGMA)	Triblock copolymers, equipped with both hydrophobic and hydrophilic segments, offer an effective method for encapsulating a range of drugs, from hydrophilic to hydrophobic. These copolymers provide a platform for controlled and sustained drug release, facilitated by the variation in hydrophobicity across their different blocks. Notably, the POPMA block can undergo hydrolysis, which triggers structural changes, leading to a controlled drug release. Furthermore, these copolymers exhibit sensitivity to both temperature and pH. These characteristics can be harnessed for targeted drug delivery, allowing for a more precise approach. This enables the delivery of drugs to specific areas in the body where temperature or pH may vary, such as tumor tissues, thus enhancing the efficiency of the treatment.	B. Huang et al. (2023)

1) Poly(amidoamine) (PAMAM) dendrimers: These are the most extensively studied dendrimers due to their ease of synthesis and wide range of available surface groups. The primary amines on the dendrimer surface can be readily modified for drug conjugation, and the internal cavities can encapsulate small molecules.
2) Poly(propylenimine) (PPI) dendrimers: These are also frequently studied and offer similar opportunities for drug encapsulation and conjugation as PAMAM dendrimers.
3) Poly(L-lysine) (PLL) dendrimers: PLL dendrimers are biodegradable and have been used to deliver a variety of drugs, including anticancer agents, antivirals, and gene therapy agents.
4) Triazine dendrimers: These dendrimers offer a highly flexible structure that can be customized for specific drug delivery applications.

Two main methods for the synthesis of dendrimers are divergent and convergent. For drug delivery applications, drugs can be incorporated into dendrimers by encapsulation in the internal cavities or by covalent attachment to the surface groups.

1) Divergent method: In this method, synthesis starts from the core, and branches (generations) are added step by step, moving outward. Each step involves two stages: the addition of a branching unit and then the addition of a functional group that can react with the next branching unit. However, the problem with this method is that as the size of the dendrimer increases, it becomes more dif-

ficult to fully react with all the functional groups on the surface, leading to defects in the dendrimer structure.

2) Convergent method: In this method, synthesis starts from the surface and moves inward toward the core. The advantage of this method is better control over the size and shape of the dendrimer and fewer structural defects. However, it can be challenging to link the final surface groups to the core.

Dendrimers have found diverse applications across the spectrum of therapeutics due to their unique structural features and tunability. In oncology, dendrimers have been explored as carriers for chemotherapeutic drugs. For example, poly(amidoamine) (PAMAM) dendrimers have been employed to encapsulate and deliver methotrexate, enhancing its solubility and allowing for targeted delivery to an intra-articular joint arthritic rat model (Essien et al., 2023). In the field of gene therapy, dendrimers serve as effective vectors for DNA and siRNA delivery. The cationic nature of certain dendrimers, such as PAMAM and poly(propylenimine) (PPI) dendrimers, allows for effective complexation with negatively charged nucleic acids. For instance, PAMAM dendrimers have been used to deliver plasmid DNA and siRNA, demonstrating efficient gene transfection and gene silencing, respectively (Joubert et al., 2023). In the context of drug delivery across the blood–brain barrier (BBB), dendrimers have shown promising results. PAMAM dendrimers have been exploited to deliver drugs, such as doxorubicin, to the brain, demonstrating the potential of dendrimers to enhance drug delivery across the BBB (Kurawattimath et al., 2023). Michlewska et al. (2023) compared two established methods for creating liposomal locked-in dendrimers. These systems incorporate a carbosilane ruthenium metallodendrimer and an anticancer drug (doxorubicin) within a liposomal structure. The results showed that the lipid-coated dendrimers improved the transfer of genetic material and reduced toxicity toward blood cells and other cell types. These complexes, with their nanoscale size, low variability in size, and decreased positive charge, show potential for future use in drug delivery. However, systems prepared via the hydrophobic locking protocol were ineffective, while those formed using the hydrophilic loading method demonstrated promising outcomes, exhibiting enhanced effectiveness of the anticancer drug doxorubicin against cancer cells compared to normal cells.

Nanohydrogels

Nanohydrogels are nanoparticulate, hydrophilic, three-dimensional polymeric networks capable of absorbing large quantities of water or biological fluids. They can contain over 90% water. These systems can encapsulate and deliver various types of therapeutic agents and have been widely studied due to their high water content, biocompatibility, nontoxicity, and ability to carry both hydrophilic and hydrophobic drugs (Yu Wang et al., 2023). The composition of nanohydrogels includes the following components.

1) Polymer backbone: Nanohydrogels are typically composed of natural, synthetic, or semisynthetic polymers. The choice of polymer depends on the desired properties, including biocompatibility, biodegradability, and mechanical strength. Natural polymers include proteins (e.g., gelatin or albumin) and polysaccharides (e.g., chitosan, alginate, and hyaluronic acid), while synthetic polymers include poly(ethylene glycol) (PEG), poly(vinyl alcohol) (PVA), and poly(acrylic acid) (PAA).
2) Cross-linker: The cross-linker is essential to the formation of the three-dimensional network of the nanohydrogel. It can be a chemical cross-linker that forms covalent bonds (e.g., glutaraldehyde,

genipin) or a physical cross-linker that forms noncovalent bonds (e.g., temperature, pH, ionic interactions).

3) Drug: The therapeutic agent to be delivered is incorporated into the nanohydrogel. The drug can be physically entrapped in the network of the hydrogel, chemically bound to the polymer backbone, or a combination of both.

Several methods can be used to prepare nanohydrogels.

1) Inverse emulsion polymerization: In this method, an aqueous phase containing the monomer, cross-linker, and drug is emulsified in an organic phase to create an inverse emulsion. Polymerization is then initiated, forming nanohydrogels.
2) Precipitation polymerization: Similar to nanogels, nanohydrogels can also be synthesized by precipitation polymerization. Monomers are polymerized in a solvent where they are soluble, but the resulting polymer is not, leading to precipitation of the formed polymer.
3) Self-assembly: Certain polymers can self-assemble into nanohydrogels. For example, amphiphilic block copolymers can self-assemble in water to form a core-shell structure, where the hydrophobic core can entrap hydrophobic drugs, and the hydrophilic shell can stabilize the nanoparticles in an aqueous environment.
4) Electrostatic assembly: In this method, oppositely charged polymers are mixed in an aqueous solution to form nanohydrogels. This method is particularly useful when working with polyelectrolytes.

The drug can be incorporated into the nanohydrogel during the preparation process or after the nanohydrogel is formed by swelling it in a solution containing the drug. There are several types of nanohydrogels that are classified by their stimulus-responsive behaviors (Table 4). This means that they can change their structure or properties in response to changes in their environment. The choice of method depends on the nature of the drug and the polymer, as well as the desired release characteristics. Nanohydrogels have been employed in numerous applications across the therapeutic spectrum, showing their versatility as drug delivery systems. In oncology, nanohydrogels have been used to encapsulate anticancer agents for targeted cancer therapy. For instance, folic acid/resveratrol-loaded poly(N-isopropylacrylamide) (PNIPAM) nanohydrogels have been developed, which demonstrated temperature-responsive drug release and enhanced cytotoxicity against cancer cells (Metawea et al., 2023). Nanohydrogels have also been explored for the delivery of biotherapeutics such as proteins and peptides, which are typically prone to degradation and have poor bioavailability. An example includes the encapsulation of insulin in *O*-carboxymethyl chitosan/sodium alginate nanohydrogels, providing a pH-responsive and sustained release of insulin, which has potential applications in diabetes management (Haibin Zhang et al., 2022).

Inorganic Nanomaterials

Inorganic nanomaterials, distinguished by their physical stability, biocompatibility, and unique optical, magnetic, and electrical properties, have emerged as potential platforms for innovative drug delivery systems (Asad et al., 2022). Some common types of inorganic nanomaterials used for drug delivery are detailed in the following subsections. Each has been explored for its potential in drug delivery, and each brings its own unique properties to this field.

Table 4. Properties of various types of nanohydrogels, their stimuli-responsive behaviors, and their uses in drug delivery

Type of nanohydrogel	Stimuli-responsive behavior	Use in drug delivery	Reference
Thermosensitive nanohydrogels	Changes in volume or sol-gel transition upon variations in temperature	Effective for controlled drug release, often used for cancer therapy where localized temperature increases can trigger drug release	B. Wu et al. (2022)
pH-sensitive nanohydrogels	Swell or shrink based on pH changes	Useful for targeting drug delivery to specific parts of the body (e.g., stomach, intestine, or tumor environments) where pH levels are distinct	Haibin Zhang et al. (2022)
Magnetic nanohydrogels	Affected by external magnetic fields	Used to enhance drug targeting and release, they can be directed to specific locations using magnets	Kheiri et al. (2022)
Light-sensitive nanohydrogels	React to specific wavelengths of light	Can be used for site-specific drug delivery, often used in cancer treatment for controlled release upon exposure to a specific light wavelength	Omrani et al. (2022)
Enzyme-responsive nanohydrogels	Respond to specific enzymes	Used for drug delivery in specific diseases where certain enzymes are overexpressed (e.g., cancer, inflammatory diseases)	Omrani et al. (2022)
Redox-responsive nanohydrogels	Sensitive to changes in redox potential	Suitable for targeted delivery of drugs to cells or organelles with different redox states, such as tumor cells	Metawea et al. (2023)

1) Gold nanoparticles (AuNPs): These nanoparticles are biocompatible and can be synthesized in different shapes and sizes. They have strong light absorption and scattering properties, making them useful in imaging and photothermal therapies.
2) Silver Nanoparticles (AgNPs): These nanocarriers have strong antimicrobial properties and can be used in wound healing and infection control. They can also be used as carriers for drug delivery.
3) Iron oxide nanoparticles: Iron oxide nanoparticles, especially magnetite (Fe_3O_4) and maghemite (γ-Fe_2O_3), are extensively used for magnetic drug targeting and hyperthermia treatment in cancer.
4) Silica nanoparticles (SiNPs): These nanoparticles are used for drug delivery due to their large surface area and pore volume, which allows for a high drug loading capacity. They are also biocompatible and degrade into harmless silicic acid in the body.
5) Quantum dots: Quantum dots are semiconducting nanoparticles that exhibit size-dependent fluorescence. They can be used in imaging and as carriers for drug delivery.
6) Calcium phosphate nanoparticles: Calcium phosphate nanoparticles are biocompatible and biodegradable. They can be used for the delivery of various therapeutic agents, including small molecule drugs, proteins, and nucleic acids.

The drug can be loaded onto inorganic nanoparticles by various methods, including adsorption, covalent conjugation, or encapsulation, depending on the nature of the drug and the nanoparticles.

1) Chemical reduction: This is the most common method used for the synthesis of metallic nanoparticles such as gold and silver nanoparticles. The metal salt is reduced by a reducing agent, leading to the formation of nanoparticles.
2) Coprecipitation: This method is often used for the synthesis of iron oxide nanoparticles. Iron salts are coprecipitated in a basic solution, forming iron oxide nanoparticles.

Figure 10. Different types of carbon-based nanomaterials for drug delivery: graphene oxide (a two-dimensional monolayer of carbon atoms in a honeycomb lattice); carbon nanotubes (cylindrical structures composed of rolled sheets of single-layer carbon atoms); nanorods (elongated carbon-based structures that offer superior cellular uptake and controlled drug release in response to external stimuli); and graphene quantum dots (diminutive fragments of graphene that enable targeted drug delivery and offer inherent fluorescence for real-time tracking and imaging)

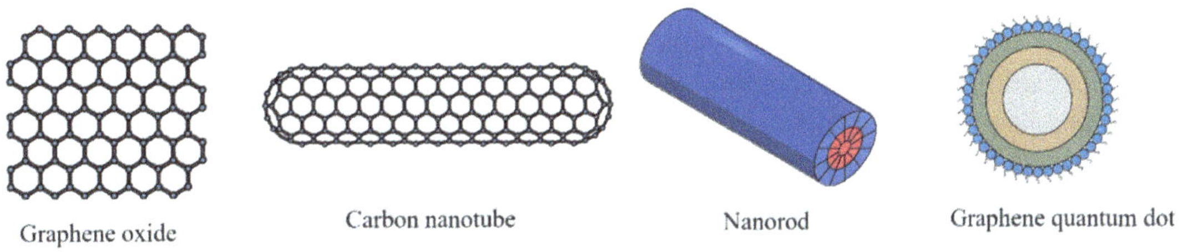

3) Sol-gel method: This method is commonly used for the synthesis of silica nanoparticles. Silica precursors are hydrolyzed and condensed in a solvent, forming a gel that can then be aged, dried, and calcined to obtain silica nanoparticles.
4) Thermal decomposition: This method can be used for the synthesis of quantum dots. Precursors are thermally decomposed in a high-boiling solvent, leading to the formation of quantum dots.
5) Wet chemical method: This method is often used for the synthesis of calcium phosphate nanoparticles. Calcium and phosphate salts are mixed in a solution, leading to the precipitation of calcium phosphate nanoparticles.

Carbon-Based Nanomaterials

The scientific community has recently focused on carbon-based nanomaterials, such as graphene oxide, carbon nanotubes, nanorods, nanowires, and graphene quantum dots. Figure 10 illustrates the variety of carbon-based nanomaterials being utilized for drug delivery applications. The fascination with these materials arises from their exceptional physicochemical properties, inherent tunability, and remarkable biocompatibility. Coupled with their unique interactions within biological systems, these nanomaterials hold tremendous potential as vehicles in the field of drug delivery (Brindhadevi et al., 2023).

Graphene Oxide

Derived from graphene, graphene oxide presents as a monolayer of carbon atoms densely aggregated into a two-dimensional honeycomb lattice. The enormity of its surface area offers a considerable advantage by facilitating high drug loading capacities. The availability of oxygen-containing functional groups on the graphene oxide surface provides a robust platform for interactions with various therapeutics, thus permitting controlled and targeted drug release. For example, Matiyani et al. (2023) demonstrated how multifunctional graphene oxide can deliver curcumin and quercetin to cancer cells, leveraging the pH sensitivity of graphene oxide-based nanocarriers for controlled release in acidic tumor environments. Its innate ability to penetrate cell membranes establishes graphene oxide as an ideal candidate for intracellular drug delivery. It has found applicability in diverse fields, extending from oncology, where it has facilitated direct chemotherapy drug delivery to cancer cells, to antimicrobial therapeutics, where it serves as a transport medium for antibiotics to target specific pathogens. Moreover, S. Wu et al. (2022) utilized a graphene oxide/alginate-based antisense hydrogel for antibiotic properties, demonstrating a marked increase in the antimicrobial activity against *Staphylococcus aureus* infection.

Carbon Nanotubes

Carbon nanotubes, characterized by their distinctive cylindrical structures, are composed of rolled sheets of single-layer carbon atoms. This morphology offers a shield-like protective role, enabling the encapsulation of therapeutic agents and protection against *in vivo* degradation. Moreover, the external surface of carbon nanotubes can undergo functionalization with biological markers, enhancing targeted drug delivery. In cancer therapy, for instance, Yasmin Begum (2023) illustrated how folic acid-functionalized carbon nanotubes carrying doxorubicin and gemcitabine, a chemotherapeutic agent, effectively inhibit tumor growth in mice due to the enhanced permeability and retention effect.

Nanorods and Nanowires

Owing to their elongated shapes, nanorods and nanowires constitute yet another class of carbon-based nanomaterials. Their shape affords a distinct advantage by facilitating superior cellular uptake, thereby making them ideal for drug delivery applications. In a study by Lihuang et al. (2021), gold nanorods were used to deliver YAP-siRNA into glioblastoma cells, resulting in gene silencing and cell death. These materials can be tailored to carry a diverse array of therapeutics and release them in response to external stimuli, such as changes in light intensity or pH. This unique property paves the way toward targeted and controlled drug delivery.

Graphene Quantum Dots

Graphene quantum dots, small fragments of graphene less than 10 nanometers in size, exhibit unique properties owing to quantum confinement and edge effects. These characteristics make them particularly desirable for drug delivery applications. Graphene quantum dots possess the ability to conjugate with therapeutic agents, allowing for targeted drug delivery. Moasses Ghafary et al. (2022) demonstrated how these quantum dots, conjugated with the anticancer drug doxorubicin/curcumin, effectively targeted cancer cells. Additionally, their intrinsic fluorescence can be exploited for real-time tracking and imaging, thereby improving therapeutic efficiency and monitoring. This amalgamation of drug delivery and bioimaging capabilities positions graphene quantum dots at the forefront of theranostics—a promising field that seamlessly integrates therapy and diagnostics (Sengupta et al., 2023).

Nanodiamonds

Nanodiamonds (a class of carbon nanocarriers) are tiny particles on the scale of a few nanometers that are composed of diamond. These particles have unique properties that make them promising for targeted drug delivery applications (F. Pan et al., 2023). Nanodiamonds have a high surface area-to-volume ratio and can be functionalized or modified to carry a variety of drug molecules. The outer shell of a nanodiamond can be chemically altered to attach different types of molecules, including anticancer drugs, antibiotics, or other therapeutic agents. They can be engineered to release the drugs they carry in a controlled manner (Wu et al., 2023). This means that drugs can be delivered directly to a specific location (such as a tumor) over an extended period of time, improving the efficacy of the treatment and reducing side effects (Xu & Chow, 2023). In addition to their drug delivery capabilities, nanodiamonds have unique optical properties that allow them to be used in imaging. They can fluoresce under certain conditions, making them useful for tracking the delivery of drugs within the body (San-Martin et al., 2023). In addition, nanodiamonds are resistant to degradation within the body, which allows for sustained release of the drug over time (Wu et al., 2023).

Chemotherapy for cancer often results in harmful side effects that compromise quality of life and can reduce adherence to treatment. These negative effects could be diminished by selectively delivering cytotoxic drugs directly to cancer cells, thus reducing the dosage, side effects, and cost. For example, Sharoyko et al. (2023) presented the preparation of nanodiamond covalent conjugates with doxorubicin and 1,3,5-triazine class cytostatic drugs, which were confirmed via various physicochemical methods. The conjugates demonstrated good hemocompatibility and did not impact plasma coagulation, platelet activity, or the erythrocyte membrane. Additionally, the developed conjugates could bind to human serum albumin with a greater cytostatic effect than individual cytostatic effects. In tests on the T98G glioblastoma cell line, these conjugates showed more significant cytotoxicity at lower drug concentrations compared to individual drugs. The developed conjugates mainly entered HeLa cells through a nonspecific action-dependent mechanism. These results suggest that these nanodiamonds hold promise as intertumoral administration agents.

In addition, a dual-function folate-modified nanodiamond drug delivery system has been developed for doxorubicin. This system features activated fluorescence and cytotoxicity. When doxorubicin is covalently attached to the nanodiamond, both its toxicity and fluorescence are suppressed. Cancer cells that overexpress the folate receptor preferentially uptake the developed nanodiamonds. Within these cells, the chemotherapy drug is released due to the levels of glutathione, which breaks a disulfide link to release the drug. Intriguingly, once the drug is on the nanodiamond, it can bypass resistance mechanisms that typically expel drugs from the cell. In a live model, this nanodrug effectively hindered tumor growth with fewer side effects than direct injection of free doxorubicin when locally injected (Wu et al., 2023). This result indicates its potential as an enhanced platform for improving therapeutic outcomes.

DESIGNS AND SYNTHESIS OF NANOMATERIALS

Designing and synthesizing nanomaterials for drug delivery systems is a multidisciplinary endeavor that has seen significant strides over the past few decades. The primary goal is to fabricate nanomaterials that protect the therapeutic agent during transit, precisely guide it to the desired site of action, and control its release to maximize therapeutic efficacy and minimize adverse effects (Navabhatra et al., 2022; C.-H. Nguyen et al., 2023).

Nanocarrier Types and Materials

The type of nanocarrier is one of the first considerations in the design and synthesis of nanocarriers for a particular application. There are several types of nanocarriers, each with unique characteristics that make them suitable for specific uses. Common types include liposomes and derivatives, polymeric nanoparticles, dendrimers, micelles, lipid-based nanoparticles, and nanotubes, among others. For example, liposomes are often used for drug delivery due to their ability to encapsulate both hydrophilic and lipophilic substances (M. Mishra et al., 2023). Dendrimers, with their well-defined, branched structures, can provide precise control over size and functionality. The selection of nanocarrier type is influenced by factors such as the natural profile, biocompatibility, and target specificity. In addition, the choice of material for constructing the nanocarrier is critically important and is dictated by the type of nanocarrier, the intended application, and the need for biocompatibility and biodegradability. Lipid-based materials, such as phospholipids, are used in the synthesis of liposomes, while polymers (both natural and synthetic) form the basis for polymeric nanoparticles and dendrimers. Other materials, such as surfactants, are utilized in the construction of micelles. In recent years, materials such as metal-organic frameworks, carbon-based materials, and silica have been increasingly used due to their unique properties. For instance, metal-organic frameworks have high porosity and can be chemically modified for desired functionality, making them suitable for applications such as drug delivery and catalysis (Molaei, 2023).

Synthesis of Nanomaterials

The synthesis of nanocarriers for drug delivery systems is contingent on the type of material and the desired properties. The specific synthesis approach can significantly influence the size, shape, surface properties, and internal architecture of the nanocarriers and thus their overall performance in drug delivery (Navabhatra et al., 2022). Various methods are used to synthesize nanocarriers, often categorized as either top-down or bottom-up approaches. Top-down methods, such as milling and high-pressure homogenization, involve reducing larger structures to the nanoscale. These methods are straightforward and widely used, particularly in the synthesis of lipid-based nanocarriers, such as liposomes, SLNs, and NLCs. For instance, NLCs can be synthesized through methods such as hot-melted homogenization followed by extrusion or sonication, which enable control over their size and uniformity (Navabhatra et al., 2022). Bottom-up methods, on the other hand, involve the assembly of smaller units into larger structures. These include methods such as nanoprecipitation, emulsification, and self-assembly. Nanoprecipitation, for example, is often used for synthesizing polymeric nanoparticles. It involves the addition of a polymer solution to a nonsolvent, leading to the formation of nanoparticles due to differences in solubility (Yingngam et al., 2019). Both methods have advantages and drawbacks. Top-down methods, while straightforward, often result in larger size distributions and potential damage to sensitive molecules during the synthesis process. On the other hand, bottom-up methods allow for more precise control over the size and shape of the nanocarriers but may involve more complex and time-consuming processes. Recent advancements in synthesis technologies aim to overcome these challenges, offering improved control over nanocarrier properties and broadening the scope for the design of innovative drug delivery systems. For example, inorganic nanoparticles such as gold nanoparticles can be synthesized via chemical reduction methods, with the size and shape of the nanoparticles modifiable by the concentration of the reducing agent, temperature, and reaction time (X. Cheng et al., 2023).

Surface Modifications

Surface modification is a key design element in the synthesis of nanomaterials for drug delivery systems. By altering the surface characteristics of nanocarriers, researchers can significantly enhance their biocompatibility, stability, and drug loading efficiency. Additionally, surface modifications can introduce target specificity and modulate drug release kinetics, allowing for greater control over the delivery of therapeutic agents within the body (Freis et al., 2023). Surface modifications can be performed using hydrophilic polymers such as polyethylene glycol (PEG), often referred to as PEGylation, which enhances biocompatibility and stability. PEGylated nanocarriers display increased stability in biological environments and prolonged systemic circulation. This is achieved by reducing protein adsorption on the nanocarrier surface, thereby preventing rapid clearance by the reticuloendothelial system (Digiacomo et al., 2023). Targeted drug delivery is another advantage conferred by surface modifications, particularly through the attachment of specific ligands. These ligands can bind to receptors overexpressed on target cells, ensuring that drugs are delivered precisely where they are needed (Freis et al., 2023). For instance, liposomes conjugated with folate have been designed for the targeted delivery of chemotherapeutic drugs to cancer cells, which often overexpress folate receptors (Dinakar et al., 2023). Furthermore, nanocarriers can be surface-modified with stimuli-responsive molecules that respond to specific triggers, such as pH, temperature, or the presence of particular enzymes. This responsiveness can result in the controlled release of drugs at the target site, improving therapeutic efficacy while minimizing potential side effects. An example of this approach is seen in polymersomes coated with hyaluronic acid-b-poly (β-amino ester), which exhibit pH-responsive behavior, releasing loaded doxorubicin within the acidic environment of tumors (Borhaninia et al., 2023).

Intelligent Design for Controlled Drug Release

Advancements in nanotechnology and machine learning algorithms have provided new avenues for designing intelligent drug delivery systems capable of controlled release. The fusion of these technologies facilitates the creation of nanocarriers capable of releasing drugs based on specific stimuli at precise locations and times, enhancing therapeutic efficacy and reducing side effects. Machine learning algorithms can aid in predicting, analyzing, and controlling drug release from nanocarriers. They do this by leveraging patterns and dependencies found in the existing biomedical data. Various machine learning algorithms, such as decision trees, support vector machines, random forests, and deep learning networks, have been employed for this purpose (Navabhatra et al., 2022). In a study conducted by Ijaz et al. (2023), a machine learning model was developed with the goal of predicting and controlling the release of the chemotherapeutic drug doxorubicin from zinc oxide nanoflowers. The model considered various features, such as improved stability and maximized anticancer activity, as well as factors related to time-dependent drug release patterns. This approach enabled more precise control of drug efficacy and helped minimize toxicity. Another approach is the use of deep learning for designing nanocarriers for tumor targeting. For instance, deep learning networks can be trained on datasets incorporating various physicochemical conditions and their corresponding pharmacokinetic profiles. The trained model can then predict the response of the nanocarrier under new conditions. This approach guides the design of more efficient and responsive drug delivery systems (Chou et al., 2023). The integration of machine learning into nanomedicine opens new doors for personalized medicine. However, it is worth noting that these methods often require large, high-quality datasets for training, and the generated models may need experimental validation. Nonetheless, the combination of nanotechnology and machine learning offers significant potential to revolutionize drug delivery systems, paving the way for more effective and tailored therapies.

BIOCOMPATIBILITY AND TOXICITY OF NANOMATERIALS

In the field of nanomedicine, biocompatibility and toxicity are paramount considerations in nanomaterial design, especially as capabilities progress toward more complex and targeted nanocarriers for drug delivery. Acquiring a comprehensive understanding of the safety profiles associated with this engineered nanomaterial has become an absolute necessity.

Biocompatibility of Nanomaterials

Biocompatibility, defined as the ability of a material to perform its designated function in a living system without inducing harmful reactions, is central to the application of nanomaterials in drug delivery (Vaudagna et al., 2023). This concept implies that while nanomaterials aid in the delivery of therapeutic agents, they should not trigger unwanted physiological responses. Various factors contribute to the biocompatibility of nanomaterials, with their physicochemical properties—such as size, shape, charge, and chemical composition—having a significant role in how they interact with biological systems (Elansary et al., 2023). For example, smaller nanoparticles may cross cellular barriers more easily, but the increased reactivity attributable to their high surface area-to-volume ratio could lead to potential cytotoxicity (Mertdinç-Ülküseven et al., 2023). Surface modification methods, such as PEGylation (attachment of polyethylene glycol), have been utilized to enhance nanomaterial biocompatibility (Korake et al., 2023). PEGylated nanoparticles exhibit an extended circulation time, decreased immunogenicity, and minimal nonspecific protein binding, which collectively make them more suitable for *in vivo* applications (X. Wang et al., 2023).

Toxicity of Nanomaterials

While nanomaterials hold great promise for drug delivery, their potential toxicity remains a critical issue that necessitates thorough investigation (Y. Liu et al., 2023). Because of their nanoscale size, nanomaterials may display unique bioactive properties, leading to distinct cellular responses compared to their larger counterparts (Mahamuni-Badiger & Dhanavade, 2023). The toxicity of nanomaterials often arises from several mechanisms, including the generation of reactive oxygen species (ROS), interactions with cellular proteins, disruption of cellular processes, or accumulation due to nonbiodegradability (Li et al., 2022). For instance, certain metal-based nanoparticles, such as gold and silver, can catalyze ROS generation, triggering oxidative stress and inflammation and potentially leading to cell death (Y. Huang et al., 2022). The physicochemical properties of nanoparticles, including their shape and size, can also influence their biodistribution, accumulation, and excretion, thereby impacting their toxicity profile. Nanocarriers with high aspect ratios or elongated morphologies may not be readily cleared from the body, leading to prolonged exposure and potential toxicity (Darbasizadeh et al., 2022).

Mitigating Toxicity and Enhancing Efficacy

Recent research on nanomaterials for drug delivery strives to engineer nanocarriers that minimize toxicity while ensuring optimal drug delivery (Oladipo et al., 2023). Various strategies are being employed, such as surface modifications, utilizing biocompatible and biodegradable materials, and smart nanocarrier design. Surface modifications, including the coating of nanoparticles with biomimetic materials, can help camouflage their foreign nature, thereby mitigating immune responses (Teixeira et al., 2023). Coatings can also be designed to emit specific signaling molecules to actively suppress immune reactions, which further diminishes the potential for adverse reactions (Büyükbayraktar et al., 2023). An alternate approach is to use naturally derived or biodegradable materials to synthesize nanoparticles. Polymer-based nanoparticles and lipid-based nanoparticles, for instance, are not only biocompatible but also offer versatile platforms for drug encapsulation and targeted delivery (Yingngam et al., 2019). Furthermore, the intelligent design of nanocarriers, harnessing principles from biology and materials science, is an effective strategy. For instance, the development of stimulus-responsive release mechanisms has been demonstrated to significantly decrease off-target effects and increase therapeutic efficiency (H.-S. Kim et al., 2023). These mechanisms respond to changes in the tumor microenvironment, such as pH or temperature variations, ensuring targeted and timely drug release, thereby enhancing the therapeutic outcome while reducing systemic side effects.

APPLICATIONS OF NANOMATERIALS FOR DRUG DELIVERY

The most recent wave of nanomaterial research for drug delivery focuses on the design of nanocarriers with minimal toxicity and optimized drug delivery. Strategies encompass surface modifications, the utilization of biocompatible and biodegradable materials, and smart nanocarrier design. For instance, surface modifications such as coating nanoparticles with biomimetic materials can help mask their foreignness, thus reducing immune responses. These coatings can also be tailored to release specific signaling molecules that actively suppress immune reactions, thereby reducing potential adverse reactions. Another approach employs naturally derived or biodegradable materials to construct nanoparticles. Not only are polymer- and lipid-based nanoparticles biocompatible, but they also offer versatile platforms for drug encapsulation and targeted delivery. Moreover, the intelligent design of nanocarriers using insights from biology and materials science—such as stimuli-responsive release mechanisms—significantly reduces off-target effects and enhances therapeutic efficacy. This amalgamation of disciplines and strategies underlines the promise and ongoing evolution of nanomaterials in drug delivery.

Cancer Therapy

The integration of nanomaterials into drug delivery systems has instigated significant progress in cancer therapy by facilitating personalized interventions, amplifying therapeutic efficacy, and attenuating adverse side effects. Nanomaterials, distinguished by their payload versatility and singular physicochemical traits, are pioneering a promising frontier in circumventing the limitations inherent in conventional cancer treatment approaches. An exemplary application of nanomaterials in cancer therapy is their role in targeted drug delivery. Leveraging the tumor-specific enhanced permeability and retention effect, nanoparticle-mediated drug delivery systems can preferentially accumulate within the tumor milieu, thereby mitigating collateral damage to healthy tissues. This principle is exemplified by Doxil®, a liposomal formulation of doxorubicin that exploits the enhanced permeability and retention effect to amplify drug concentration within the tumor and attenuate systemic toxicity (Taher et al., 2023). In the case of theragnostics – an integrative strategy that combines therapy and diagnostics – nanomaterials have made pivotal contributions. For instance, nanoparticles such as gold nanoparticles and quantum dots can be engineered to simultaneously carry therapeutic agents and imaging probes. This permits synchronous treatment and surveillance of disease progression. Gold AuroShell Nanoshells® Therapy, a platform utilizing gold-silica nanoshells, embodies this concept, allowing both hyperthermal treatment and real-time imaging of solid tumors (Sung et al., 2023).

Furthermore, the delivery of genetic material for gene therapies in cancer has been made possible through nanomaterials. They can be tailored to deliver small interfering RNAs (siRNAs) or plasmid DNAs to manipulate the expression of oncogenes or tumor suppressor genes, thereby offering a novel dimension to cancer treatment. A prime example is ONPATTRO® (patisiran), an RNAi therapeutic encapsulated within a lipid nanoparticle, highlighting the capabilities of such therapies (Rouge, 2023). Finally, nanomaterials have played a crucial role in bolstering the effectiveness of immunotherapies, such as cancer vaccines and CAR-T-cell therapies. For instance, they can be deployed to deliver tumor-specific antigens to antigen-presenting cells, thereby augmenting the patient's immune response against cancer cells. Moreover, nanocarriers can encapsulate immune checkpoint inhibitors, fortifying their stability and facilitating their delivery to the tumor microenvironment. Current clinical trials of mRNA-based cancer vaccines encapsulated within lipid nanoparticles underscore these advancements in immunotherapy (Snow et al., 2022; Z. Wang et al., 2023).

Immunotherapy

Immunotherapy marks a significant leap forward in contemporary healthcare, opening new avenues for combating diseases, especially cancer (Han et al., 2023). However, this innovative therapeutic strategy is not without hurdles, such as off-target effects and complex *in vivo* environments, that can constrain the effectiveness of the therapeutic agents. Herein, nanomaterials, with their unique properties, have emerged as a promising tool to navigate these challenges, thereby enhancing the precision and efficiency of immunotherapies. Nanomaterials find utility across multiple types of immunotherapies, including immune checkpoint inhibitors, cancer vaccines, and CAR-T-cell therapies. Immune checkpoint inhibitors function by blocking proteins that hinder immune responses against cancer cells. Their encapsulation within nanocarriers, such as the chitosan nanoparticles used for PD-L1 checkpoint blockade, enhances their stability and delivery to the tumor microenvironment and diminishes off-target effects (Song et al., 2023). Nanocarriers also play a critical role in cancer vaccines by delivering tumor-specific antigens and adjuvants to antigen-presenting cells, thus stimulating an immune response against cancer cells. For instance, the nanoparticle-based NeoVax vaccine, which triggers a robust T-cell response against neoantigens, is currently in clinical trials (Yu et al., 2022). In the context of CAR-T-cell therapy, nanomaterials can be utilized to ferry genetic material into T cells to express specific chimeric antigen receptors (CARs), thereby amplifying their ability to destroy tumors. CRISPR–Cas9 gene editing, assisted by nanoparticle delivery systems, is a notable example of this approach (Hajifathali et al., 2023). Moreover, nanomaterials can assist in modulating the tumor microenvironment to enhance the efficacy of immunotherapies. Tumors often establish an immunosuppressive microenvironment to elude the immune system. Nanomaterials can be designed to deliver immunostimulatory agents to the tumor site, reversing this immunosuppression and rendering the tumors more susceptible to immune attacks. An example of this is the use of STING agonist-loaded nanoparticles that activate innate immune responses within tumors (Cheng Xu et al., 2023). In addition, nanomaterials can deliver drugs designed to inhibit the proliferation of tumor-associated blood vessels, thus cutting off the nutrient supply to the tumor cells, as demonstrated by angiogenesis inhibitor-loaded nanoparticles (Mabrouk et al., 2023).

Gene Therapy

Gene therapy, with its immense potential, stands as a promising frontier in the field of medicine. Its success, however, is contingent on the efficient delivery of genetic material into target cells. To address this challenge, nanomaterials, with their unique physicochemical properties, have emerged as pivotal players. They serve not only to protect the genetic materials but also to augment their stability and negotiate biological barriers, thereby delivering the payload to targeted cells (Pardridge, 2023). Two broad categories of nanocarriers—viral and nonviral—have been the subject of extensive research, each presenting unique advantages. Viral nanocarriers, owing to their inherent aptitude for gene delivery, exhibit high efficiency across a diverse range of cells and tissues (Lundstrom, 2023). The utilization of viral vectors such as lentiviruses in therapies such as Luxturna™, a treatment for an inherited form of blindness, is a notable example (Kumar et al., 2023). Nonviral nanocarriers, encompassing entities such as liposomes and nanoparticles, are less efficient but compensate for a considerable gene carrying capacity, lower immunogenicity, and diminished risk of insertional mutagenesis. The development of lipid nanoparticles for the delivery of mRNA in the Pfizer-BioNTech and Moderna COVID-19 vaccines underscores their potential (Neamatallah, 2023).

The field of targeted gene delivery has witnessed remarkable advancements with the advent of nanomaterials. Nanocarriers can be engineered with targeting ligands that bind to specific receptors overexpressed in target cells. The attachment of transferrin ligands to liposomal nanocarriers for target delivery of genes to cancer cells illustrates this strategy's efficacy (Ying et al., 2022). Nanomaterials have proven invaluable in negotiating biological barriers to gene delivery. Their role extends from shielding genetic material against nuclease degradation, thus extending stability in the bloodstream, to facilitating the cellular uptake of genetic material through endocytosis. Moreover, they assist in the subsequent endosomal escape, securing the payload's transportation to its intended destination within the cell. Certain nanocarriers, for instance, gold nanoparticles, have shown potential for facilitating the entry of DNA into the nucleus, thereby enabling its transcription and subsequent translation into therapeutic proteins (Salesa et al., 2023).

Infectious Disease Treatment

The treatment of infectious diseases often presents significant challenges, including drug resistance, inadequate bioavailability, and off-target side effects. Nanomaterials, due to their unique properties, are increasingly being utilized as potential solutions to these issues. By virtue of their small size and large surface area, nanomaterials can effectively encapsulate antimicrobial drugs, enhancing their stability and bioavailability. They can also be engineered to target specific pathogens, thereby increasing therapeutic efficacy and minimizing systemic side effects (Thankappan et al., 2023). Significant advancements have been made in employing nanomaterials for the treatment of various infectious diseases. For instance, in the fight against bacterial infections, silver nanoparticles have shown excellent antimicrobial properties and, when combined with antibiotics, can effectively combat antibiotic-resistant bacteria (Caballero Gómez et al., 2023). Similarly, gold nanoparticles have been used as carriers for antiretroviral drugs in the treatment of HIV, enabling targeted drug delivery and reducing drug toxicity (Rawat & Gupta, 2021; Soundararajan et al., 2022). Nanocarriers such as liposomes and polymeric nanoparticles have been instrumental in delivering antifungal drugs for fungal infections, improving drug penetration and retention in infected tissues (Abd El- Salam et al., 2023). In the field of viral infections, nanomaterials have also been successfully used in the delivery of antiviral drugs and vaccines. For instance, lipid nanoparticles played a crucial role in the formulation of mRNA-based vaccines for COVID-19, protecting the mRNA from degradation and facilitating its delivery into host cells (Bernard et al., 2023). This approach marked a significant milestone in nanotechnology, demonstrating its potential for responding to global health emergencies.

Neurological Disorders

Effective treatment of neurological disorders is a persistent challenge owing to the inherent complexities associated with the brain's physiology, such as the presence of the BBB and the specificity required for drug targeting. Nanomaterials have emerged as a potential solution to these challenges due to their unique properties. They can be engineered to traverse the BBB, specifically target neuronal cells, and encapsulate therapeutic agents to enhance their bioavailability, thereby improving the efficacy of drug delivery systems. Notable applications of nanomaterials in treating neurological disorders include the delivery of therapeutic agents for Alzheimer's disease, Parkinson's disease, and brain tumors (Attia et al., 2023). Transferrin-functionalized NLCs have shown promise in carrying Alzheimer's drugs such as resveratrol and rivastigmine across the BBB, enhancing their therapeutic potential (Jain et al., 2023). In the case of Parkinson's disease, lipid-based nanoparticles and polymeric nanoparticles have been employed to deliver levodopa directly to the brain, thereby improving the therapeutic outcome and reducing systemic side effects (van Vliet et al., 2023). For brain tumors, a variety of nanomaterials, including gold nanoparticles, superparamagnetic iron oxide nanoparticles, and carbon nanotubes, have been investigated for their potential to deliver chemotherapy drugs while minimizing harm to healthy tissues (L. Yuan et al., 2023). Despite these advancements, there are still several challenges to be overcome before nanomaterials can be fully integrated into clinical practice. Potential issues include nanotoxicity, control over drug release, and long-term effects on the human body. Future research needs to address these challenges while also optimizing nanomaterials in terms of size, surface properties, and targeting capabilities to improve their efficacy and safety. Overall, the application of nanomaterials holds immense promise in developing drug delivery systems for neurological disorders, but a considerable amount of research is required to harness their full potential.

Wound Healing

The application of nanocarriers in the field of wound healing has shown promising results, primarily due to their ability to deliver therapeutic agents directly to the wound site. Nanocarriers can carry a range of bioactive substances, including growth factors, anti-inflammatory agents, antimicrobial agents, and even genetic materials, all of which can play a role in the healing process (Dutt et al., 2023). The delivery of growth factors is an important way nanocarriers contribute to wound healing. Growth factors are proteins that play crucial roles in wound healing by promoting cell proliferation and migration, angiogenesis (the formation of new blood vessels), and the synthesis of the extracellular matrix. However, the topical application of growth factors can be challenging due to their instability and short half-life. Nanocarriers can protect growth factors from degradation, prolong their release, and increase their local concentration at the wound site, enhancing their efficacy (Maatouk et al., 2021). Inflammation is an essential part of the wound healing process, but chronic inflammation can impede healing and result in chronic wound inflammation that can impede healing and result in wound chronicity. Nanocarriers can be used to deliver anti-inflammatory agents directly to the wound site, controlling inflammation and promoting the healing process (Tran et al., 2023).

Infection is a common complication in wound healing that can delay the process and even lead to life-threatening conditions such as sepsis. Nanocarriers can deliver antimicrobial agents (including antibiotics and antiseptics) directly to the wound, combating infection. Moreover, some nanomaterials have intrinsic antimicrobial properties. For example, silver nanoparticles and *Centella asiatica* have been widely used for their broad-spectrum antimicrobial activity and wound healing properties, respectively. Bozkaya et al. (2023) synthesized and examined silver nanoparticles coated with *Centella asiatica* extract for their biocompatibility, antimicrobial, and analgesic properties, with potential applications in wound dressings. The produced nanoparticles were biocompatible according to an MTT (3-(4,5-dimethylthiazol-2-yl)-2,5-diphenyl-2H-tetrazolium bromide) cytotoxicity assay, showing that fibroblasts could tolerate the prepared nanoparticles at concentrations of 1 mM or less. Furthermore, the antimicrobial effectiveness of the prepared nanoparticles was demonstrated through significant inhibition of two bacterial types: *Staphylococcus aureus* and *Escherichia coli*. These bacteria served as gram-positive and gram-negative bacteria, respectively. The analgesic properties of the formulated nanoparticles were also studied. Using tail-flick and hot plate methods, the nanoparticles demonstrated statistically significant analgesic effects. The findings of this study suggest that the synthesized nanoparticles have potential for use as an effective antibacterial and pain-relieving agent in the coating of wound dressings.

Nanocarriers can deliver genetic material to cells at the wound site, allowing the cells to produce therapeutic proteins locally. For example, they can deliver plasmid DNA or mRNA encoding growth factors, enhancing the wound healing process. Research explores a potential treatment for diabetic ulcers, which often heal slowly due to poor angiogenesis (the process of new blood vessel formation). One suggested treatment is to increase promoters of angiogenesis and decrease suppressors using RNA interference. Small RNA molecules, such as microRNAs (miRNAs) and small interfering RNAs (siRNAs), can be utilized for this purpose. This research involves the development of various antagonists for miRNAs and siRNAs that target multiple genes to promote angiogenesis and wound healing. For example, Beheshtizadeh et al. (2023) reported *in silico* engineering of RNA nanocarriers to promote diabetic wound healing. The process began with gene ontology analysis across several datasets, followed by systems biology approach analysis. The next step was to investigate the potential of incorporating the proposed siRNAs and miRNA antagomirs into polymeric bioresponsive nanocarriers for wound delivery. This was done using a technique known as molecular dynamics simulation. The study evaluated three nanocarriers: PLGA, PEI, and chitosan. The simulations showed that the PLGA/hsa-mir-422a complex was the most stable for gene delivery. In contrast, the siRNA/chitosan complex showed the least favorable results. The findings suggest that the proposed RNA molecules could be delivered via bioresponsive nanocarriers to accelerate wound healing by enhancing angiogenesis. Nanocarriers can control the release rate of therapeutic agents, ensuring sustained delivery over an extended period. This is beneficial for wound healing, as it reduces the frequency of dressing changes, enhances patient compliance, and provides a prolonged therapeutic effect (Younas et al., 2023). Another aspect of nanocarriers is their targeted delivery properties. Nanocarriers can be engineered to deliver their payload specifically to target cells in the wound, such as fibroblasts, keratinocytes or immune cells. This can be achieved by attaching specific ligands to the surface of the nanocarriers that bind to receptors overexpressed on the target cells. This targeted delivery enhances the efficacy of the therapeutic agents and reduces potential side effects (Yang et al., 2023).

CASE STUDY: ELECTROSPUN IBUPROFEN-LOADED NANOFIBERS

Electrospun nanofibers have recently garnered significant interest, especially within the realm of drug delivery systems, thanks to their unique properties. This discussion provides a comprehensive examination of electrospun nanofibers, covering their manufacturing process, characteristics, and potential drug delivery applications, as evidenced by a case study from the author's research. Electrospinning, a cost-efficient and versatile method, employs electrostatic forces to produce fibers with diameters ranging from a few nanometers to several micrometers. This technique allows manipulation of the nanofiber morphology, structure, and properties by adjusting variables such as the solution characteristics, operational conditions, and choice of polymer. Electrospun nanofibers, with their high surface area-to-volume ratio, significant porosity, and adaptable surface morphology, prove highly beneficial for drug delivery applications. Furthermore, their physicochemical properties can be effortlessly modified, bolstering their suitability for drug delivery.

Figure 11 illustrates the electrospinning process, which employs an electric field to form nanofibers from a polymer solution or melt. The process initiates with the preparation of a polymer solution or melt, either by dissolving a polymer in an appropriate solvent or heating it until it melts. This solution or melt is placed in a syringe fitted with a metallic needle, or spinneret, connected to a high-voltage power supply, with the other end grounded. When the electric field between the spinneret and the ground intensifies enough (approximately 15–50 kV), it overcomes the droplet's surface tension at the spinneret tip, morphing it into what is known as a Taylor cone. A sufficiently strong electric field ejects a jet of the polymer solution or melts it from the tip of the Taylor cone. As this jet traverses through air or another gaseous medium, the solvent (in the case of a solution) evaporates, leaving behind a solid fiber. In the case of a melt, the jet cools and solidifies into a fiber. Under the electric field's influence, the jet undergoes a process called "instability", wherein it stretches and whips in the air, reducing the jet's diameter and leading to nanofiber formation. The fibers are collected on a grounded collector, which could range from a flat plate to a rotating drum, depending on the desired fiber alignment and structure. The resulting nanofibers create a nonwoven mat on the collector, which can be dried to remove any residual solvent and subsequently peeled off for future use.

In this section, the author details a case study (unpublished study) conducted by the author, which demonstrates the potential of electrospun nanofibers in drug delivery via the creation of an ibuprofen controlled-release system. Initially, ibuprofen (see Figure 8) and a 12% *w/w* solution of polymers (PCL and polyvinyl alcohol) were dissolved in a mixture of dimethylformamide and chloroform (3:1, *v/v*). The author fixed the ibuprofen concentration at 10% by polymer weight. The polymer not only helped form the nanofibers but also served as a carrier for the drug. The author stirred the solution until it became a homogeneous mixture and then loaded it into a syringe equipped with a spinneret. After placing the syringe in a syringe pump to control the feed rate of the solution, the author connected a high-voltage power supply to the spinneret and positioned a grounded collector 10 cm away (Figure 12a). As the polymer solution flowed through the needle, the high voltage triggered the formation of a jet directed toward the collector. As the solvent evaporated during this process, it left fibers on the collector. Once the electrospinning process was completed, the author dried the fibrous mat in a vacuum to remove any residual solvent. The author then collected and characterized the fibers using various techniques, such as scanning electron microscopy (SEM) for fiber morphology analysis and Fourier transform infrared spectroscopy, to confirm the presence of ibuprofen. The author submerged the ibuprofen-loaded fibers in a medium (phosphate-buffered saline) to simulate physiological conditions and studied the release of

Figure 11. Schematic illustration of the electrospinning processes: (a) preparation of polymer solution or melt; (b) creation of the Taylor cone; (c) jet ejection and solvent evaporation; (d) formation of nanofibers; and (e) collection and drying

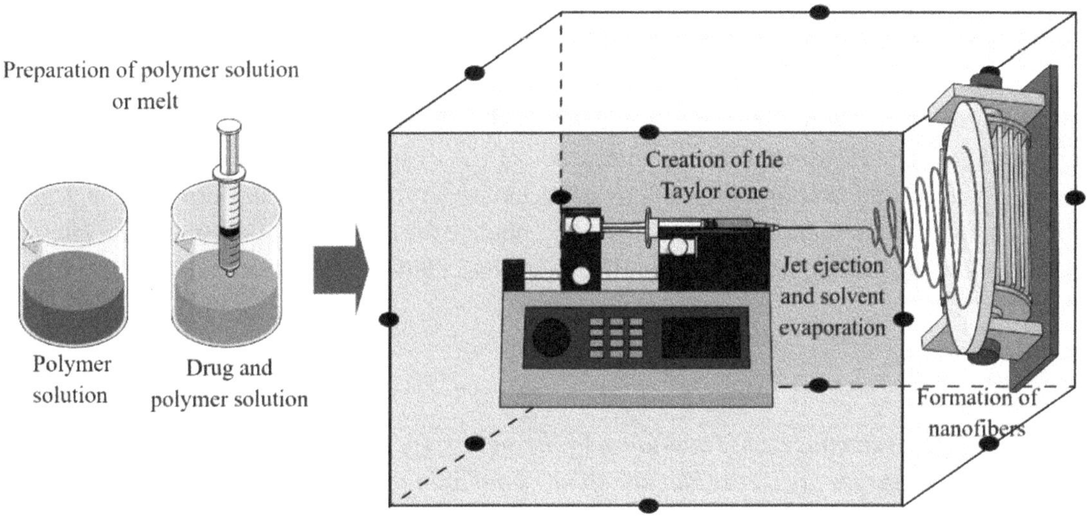

ibuprofen over time (24 hours). The author periodically sampled the medium and used high-performance liquid chromatography to determine the amount of ibuprofen released.

SEM analysis helped the author inspect the morphological characteristics of the ibuprofen-loaded nanofibers. The SEM images revealed well-formed nanofibers with a predominantly smooth surface. The fibers had an approximate diameter in the range of 300–600 nm, indicative of a successful electrospinning process (Figure 12b). However, the author sporadically observed small defects in the form of bead formations along the length of the fibers (Figures 12c and d). These bead-like structures varied in size but were generally larger than the fiber diameter, potentially indicating inconsistencies in the electrospinning process. The formation of beads in electrospun nanofibers is generally attributed to an imbalance between the solution's viscosity and the electric field strength during the electrospinning process. In this case, bead formation might have resulted from the relatively low viscosity of the polymer solution. A low-viscosity solution might not have sufficient chain entanglement, causing it to break up into droplets under the electrostatic field, which could lead to bead formation. As the solvent evaporated during electrospinning, ibuprofen, which cannot evaporate, might concentrate and form these bead-like structures.

The *in vitro* release study of ibuprofen from the electrospun nanofibers employed a phosphate-buffered saline (PBS, pH 7.4) medium to mimic physiological conditions. The release profile exhibited a biphasic pattern, with an initial rapid release of ibuprofen during the first 2 hours, during which approximately 30% of the total loaded ibuprofen was released. This burst release was followed by a slower, more controlled release phase. By the end of the 24-hour study period, approximately 85% of the total ibuprofen had been released from the nanofibers. The initial burst release can be attributed to ibuprofen molecules located near the nanofiber surface or embedded in areas with thinner polymer matrices. These molecules can easily diffuse out of the nanofibers upon contact with the release medium. The subsequent sustained release is likely due to ibuprofen being more deeply embedded within the polymer matrix. The release of these molecules is governed by the diffusion of ibuprofen through the polymer matrix and potentially by the slow degradation of the polymer itself. The results suggest that the electrospun ibuprofen-loaded nanofibers could offer immediate pain relief due to burst release, followed by sustained analgesia over a 24-hour period. This release profile positions them as potential candidates for postoperative pain management, where both immediate and prolonged pain relief are desirable.

Overall, ibuprofen was successfully incorporated into polymeric nanofibers via the electrospinning process, creating an efficient, controlled-release drug delivery system that could potentially enhance transdermal drug permeation. These results underscore the potential of electrospun nanofibers for transforming drug delivery. However, further optimization of electrospinning parameters, including solution concentration, feed rate, and applied voltage, is necessary to minimize bead formation and improve nanofiber quality. Future studies should also aim to modulate the release profile to meet specific clinical needs and assess the biocompatibility and efficacy of ibuprofen-loaded nanofibers in relevant *in vitro* and *in vivo* models.

Figure 12. (a) Electrospinning device developed by the author's research group and (b) scanning electron microscopy (SEM) images of electrospun nanofibers containing ibuprofen, observed at ×1000 magnification, (c) SEM image of bead formation observed at ×10,000 magnification, and (d) SEM image of bead formation of the fibers, observed at ×20,000 magnification

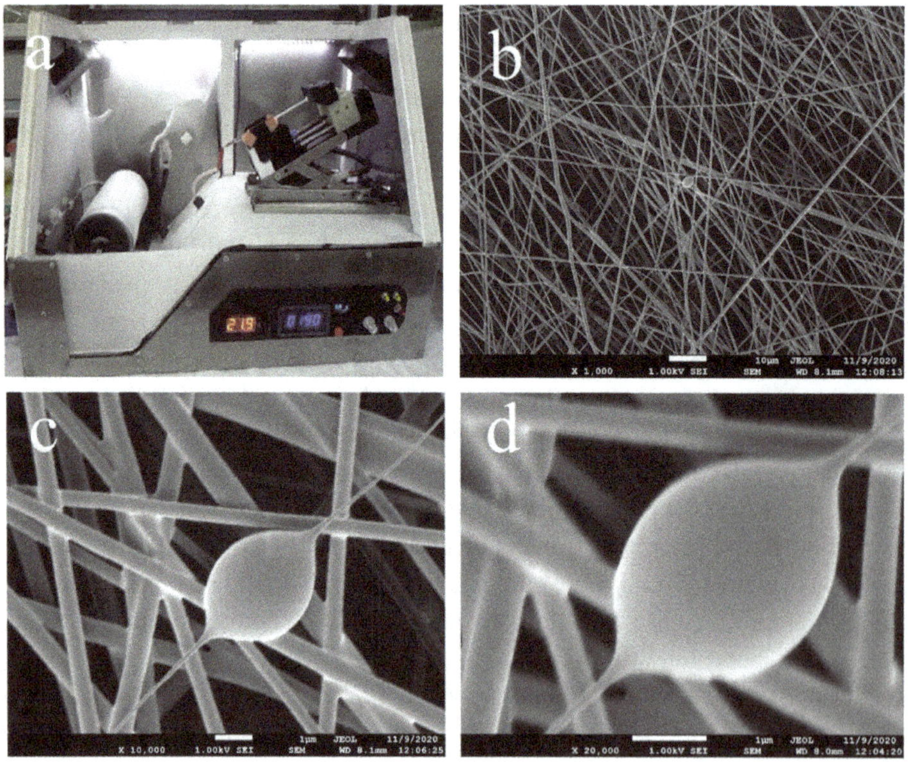

STRATEGIES FOR DEVELOPING NOVEL NANOMATERIALS FOR DRUG DELIVERY

The domain of nanomaterials possesses tremendous potential to revolutionize drug delivery by introducing innovative solutions that surpass the limitations inherent to traditional pharmaceutical formulations. Essential attributes of nanomaterials, such as their minuscule size, extensive surface area, and capability for functionalization, offer distinctive advantages. These include enhanced solubility, improved pharmacokinetics, targeted drug delivery and controlled release of therapeutic agents. However, the development of novel nanomaterials for drug delivery requires an understanding of their physicochemical properties, biological interactions, and potential therapeutic and adverse effects. This section presents the strategic approach toward the development of these novel nanomaterials for drug delivery. Key factors influencing the design and development of these materials are explored, from grasping essential physicochemical properties to incorporating biological functionality and stimuli-responsive systems. The strategies further delve into the creation of smart nanomaterials, for instance, stimuli-responsive drug delivery systems, self-assembling nanomaterials, and multifunctional nanomaterials that integrate biological functionality. Approaches to enhance biocompatibility and minimize toxicity are considered, along with strategies to circumvent biological barriers. An interdisciplinary approach, harnessing advanced computational techniques and machine learning algorithms, is underscored as a necessity for progress. These strategies are graphically illustrated in Figure 13, with detailed discussions following in subsequent sections.

Stimuli-Responsive Drug Delivery Systems

The development of "smart" or stimuli-responsive nanomaterials has become a focal point in the field of drug delivery. Such systems are engineered to respond to specific physiological or environmental stimuli, including pH changes, temperature variations, magnetic fields, or enzymatic activity, result-

Figure 13. A comprehensive overview of strategies for developing novel nanomaterials for drug delivery

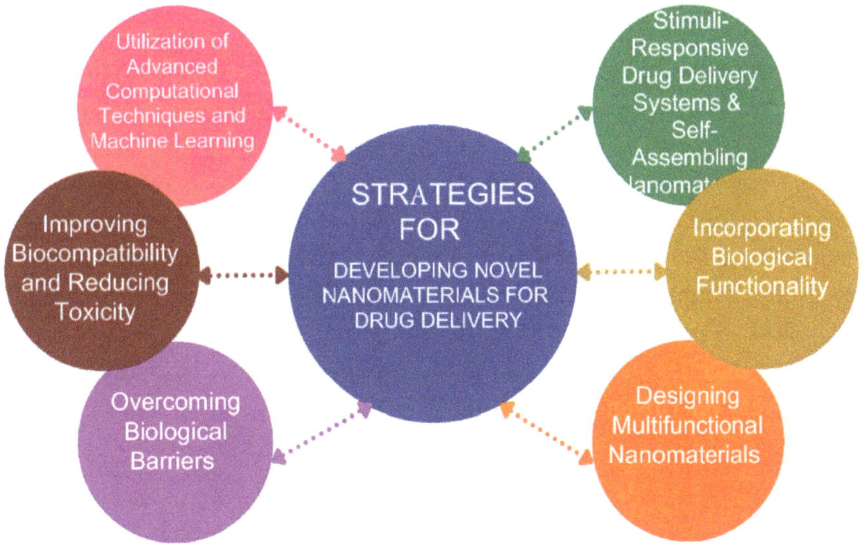

ing in targeted and timely drug release. This presents a significant advancement over traditional drug delivery methods, optimizing therapeutic efficacy and reducing adverse side effects. An emblematic example of this strategy is the development of pH-responsive nanocarriers. These carriers are designed to exploit the acidic microenvironment of tumorous tissues, which typically present a lower pH than healthy tissues. Upon reaching such a milieu, the nanocarrier undergoes a conformational change or disassembly, triggering the release of its therapeutic payload. For instance, hydrazone bonds are commonly used in the design of pH-responsive nanocarriers due to their ability to hydrolyze under acidic conditions. A prominent example includes the work of Rahmani et al. (2023), wherein pH-responsive aldehyde-modified polycaprolactone and hydrazine-modified polyvinyl alcohol-drug (curcumin and methotrexate) polymersomes exhibited enhanced anticancer efficacy in MCF-7 human breast cancer cells. Another innovative approach involves the utilization of thermoresponsive nanomaterials for drug delivery. These systems undergo a phase transition at a specific temperature (often near the physiological temperature), allowing for the controlled release of drugs. Poly(*N*-isopropylacrylamide) (PNIPAM) is a frequently used thermoresponsive polymer that exhibits a lower critical solution temperature around body temperature, making it ideal for biomedical applications. For instance, studies by Metawea et al. (2023) demonstrated that PNIPAM-based nanohydrogels could effectively deliver anticancer drugs to tumor sites, with drug release triggered by a slight increase in local temperature.

Self-Assembling Nanomaterials

Research on self-assembling nanomaterials has become a dynamic frontier in the field of drug delivery. Such nanomaterials are typically composed of building blocks, including lipids, peptides, or polymers, that can spontaneously assemble into complex, higher-order structures under appropriate conditions. This self-assembly process, governed by various noncovalent interactions such as hydrophobic interactions, electrostatic interactions, or hydrogen bonding, often leads to the formation of well-defined nanostructures such as micelles, vesicles, or nanofibers. These nanostructures offer potential benefits as drug carriers, including high loading capacity, enhanced stability, and the capability for controlled drug release. A notable example of self-assembling nanomaterials is liposomes, which are lipid-based vesicles that can encapsulate both hydrophilic and hydrophobic drugs. Liposomes, such as Doxil®, a liposomal formulation of doxorubicin, have already gained FDA approval for use in cancer therapy due to their ability to enhance the bioavailability of drugs and reduce systemic toxicity (X. Zhang et al., 2023). Another instance involves peptide-based self-assembling nanomaterials. These structures can be designed to form a variety of nanostructures, including nanofibers, nanotubes, or hydrogels, under physiological conditions. A pioneering work by Lu et al. (2023) reported the use of a self-assembling peptide nanofiber as a carrier for the anticancer drug paclitaxel. This peptide-based carrier demonstrated increased drug solubility, enhanced tumor targeting, and improved therapeutic efficacy in a breast cancer model. Similarly, self-assembling polymers, such as block copolymers, can form micelles or vesicles that are valuable in drug delivery applications. An example includes Pluronic® block copolymers, which can self-assemble into micelles in aqueous solutions and have been extensively investigated for their potential in drug delivery (Garibyan et al., 2023).

Incorporating Biological Functionality

The incorporation of biological functionality into novel nanomaterials for drug delivery signifies an innovative field of study intended to amplify the effectiveness, safety, and individualization of therapeutic interventions. This undertaking encompasses several strategies. First, surface functionalization involves the modification of nanomaterial surfaces with biological molecules, such as antibodies, proteins, peptides, or small molecules, which can interact with specific biological targets. A notable example of this can be observed in targeted cancer therapy, where the surfaces of nanoparticles are functionalized with antibodies specific to cancer cells. This modification allows the precise delivery of anticancer drugs to the intended site, thus minimizing collateral damage to healthy cells. This strategy has been employed in therapies such as antibody–drug conjugates, which consist of an antibody linked to a cytotoxic drug. The antibody binds to a specific antigen on the cancer cells, allowing precise drug delivery (Yeom et al., 2023). Second, the integration of bioactive compounds within the nanomaterial matrix constitutes another approach. Such embedded compounds can enhance the therapeutic performance of the drug or introduce additional functionalities to the nanomaterial. For instance, nanomaterials loaded with anti-inflammatory agents can mitigate localized inflammation upon drug delivery (Deepika et al., 2023). Finally, in certain sophisticated designs, nanomaterials facilitate the delivery of genetic material, a method employed in gene therapy. A notable example is the utilization of lipid nanoparticles to deliver mRNA in novel mRNA vaccines developed for COVID-19 (Zamani et al., 2023).

Designing Multifunctional Nanomaterials

The design of multifunctional nanomaterials that can perform several functions simultaneously is another promising strategy. These multifunctional nanomaterials can perform several functions concurrently, extending far beyond merely serving as drug carriers. They can enhance the efficacy of therapeutics, reduce side effects, and provide real-time monitoring of treatment progress. One approach to multifunctionality is the design of nanomaterials capable of carrying multiple drugs simultaneously, an approach referred to as combined therapy. This strategy holds significant promise for complex diseases such as cancer, where different drugs can target different cellular mechanisms to exert a synergistic therapeutic effect. For example, the delivery of doxorubicin and paclitaxel using niosomes has been explored for its potential to improve cancer treatment. The biocompatibility and biodegradability of niosomes, coupled with their ability to encapsulate both hydrophilic and hydrophobic drugs, make them an effective delivery system for combination therapy (Rezaei et al., 2023).

A further dimension of multifunctionality involves incorporating diagnostic capabilities into therapeutic nanomaterials, thus creating "theragnostic" nanocarriers. These can provide simultaneous therapy and diagnostic functions, enabling real-time monitoring of drug distribution, pharmacokinetics, and therapeutic responses. One notable example is the use of iron oxide nanoparticles that can be simultaneously loaded with a chemotherapeutic drug for cancer therapy and a contrast agent for magnetic resonance imaging. This allows for both therapeutic intervention and monitoring of the tumor's response to therapy in real time (Turrina et al., 2023). Another noteworthy application of multifunctional nanomaterials is in the field of phototherapy. Nanoparticles such as gold nanorods can be designed to carry a chemotherapeutic drug and have inherent optical properties that allow them to convert absorbed light into heat. This dual functionality can be used for combination chemotherapy and photothermal therapy, where the heat generated by the nanorods enhances the efficacy of the chemotherapy and can also be used for imaging purposes (M. Wang et al., 2023).

Overcoming Biological Barriers

Nanomaterials for drug delivery must effectively traverse biological barriers to deliver their therapeutic payloads to target sites. These barriers, which include the BBB, cellular membranes, and the nuclear envelope, have evolved to protect the body and maintain homeostasis, presenting challenges for drug delivery. However, advances in nanotechnology have led to innovative strategies to circumvent these barriers. The BBB, for example, is a tightly regulated structure that controls the entry of substances into the brain, thus protecting it from potential harm. However, this also limits the delivery of therapeutic agents for neurological disorders. Nanomaterials, when designed appropriately, can facilitate delivery across the BBB. For instance, nanoparticles coated with polysorbate 80 have demonstrated enhanced transport across the BBB, presumably via adsorption-mediated transcytosis (Fateh Basharzad et al., 2022). Similarly, nanoparticles functionalized with ligands that target BBB-specific receptors, such as transferrin or LDL receptor-related proteins, can exploit receptor-mediated transcytosis to cross the BBB (A. Mishra et al., 2023). The cellular membrane also poses a barrier to drug delivery. To cross this barrier, nanoparticles can be engineered with cationic surface charges to enhance interaction with negatively charged cell membranes, thereby facilitating cellular uptake (C. Shen et al., 2023). Moreover, nanoparticles can be functionalized with specific ligands (such as antibodies or peptides) that bind to receptors on target cells, promoting receptor-mediated endocytosis (Choi et al., 2023). The nuclear envelope is a barrier for therapeutic agents targeting DNA or nuclear proteins. To reach these targets, nanomaterials can be designed to leverage the nuclear import machinery of the cell. For example, nanoparticles conjugated with nuclear localization signals, sequences that are recognized by the cell's nuclear import machinery, can be transported into the nucleus (Wei et al., 2023). External stimuli can also facilitate the penetration of biological barriers. For instance, ultrasound can temporarily increase the permeability of the BBB, allowing for the enhanced delivery of nanomaterials to the brain (Q. Li et al., 2023). Similarly, magnetically responsive nanoparticles can be directed to specific target sites using external magnetic fields (García-García et al., 2023).

Improving Biocompatibility and Reducing Toxicity

Assuring biocompatibility and addressing the potential toxicity of nanomaterials are fundamental considerations in the pursuit of effective drug delivery systems. Biocompatibility indicates the capability of the material to function with an appropriate host response in a specific application, while toxicity refers to the adverse effects that a material can have on biological systems. Therefore, the design and development strategies for nanomaterials should aim to enhance biocompatibility and mitigate toxicity. The use of biodegradable materials is a significant approach to enhancing the biocompatibility of nanomaterials. Biodegradable materials can breakdown into biocompatible byproducts within the body, thus reducing the risk of long-term toxicity. For instance, PLGA is an FDA-approved, biodegradable polymer commonly used in nanomaterial design for drug delivery that safely degrades into lactic and glycolic acids in the body (Razavi et al., 2023). The size of nanomaterials plays a pivotal role in their interaction with biological systems and can be manipulated to reduce their potential toxicity. Smaller nanoparticles can enhance cellular uptake and permeability across biological barriers but may also lead to increased accumulation in nontarget tissues, possibly leading to toxicity (Windell et al., 2023). Thus, careful tuning of the nanoparticle size based on the intended application is essential. Surface modification of nanomaterials offers another promising approach to improving biocompatibility and minimizing toxicity. This could involve the attachment of hydrophilic polymers, such as PEG, to the surface of nanoparticles, a process known as PEGylation. PEGylated nanoparticles exhibit reduced protein adsorption, immune recognition, and clearance by the mononuclear phagocyte system, thereby prolonging circulation time in the body and reducing potential toxicity (Tenchov et al., 2023). Furthermore, coating nanoparticles with cell membrane-derived materials (e.g., cancer cell membranes and red blood cell membranes) has emerged as a novel strategy to enhance biocompatibility and reduce immune recognition (Yuqi Liu et al., 2023). This approach also offers the advantage of potentially enabling targeted drug delivery, as shown in several preclinical studies. The choice of strategy for improving biocompatibility and reducing toxicity will largely depend on the specific requirements of the intended drug delivery application, highlighting the importance of an integrative and versatile approach to the design and development of nanomaterials for drug delivery.

Utilization of Advanced Computational Techniques and Machine Learning

The utilization of advanced computational techniques and machine learning can expedite the design and development process (Navabhatra et al., 2022; Yingngam, 2023b). For instance, computational modeling, encompassing techniques such as molecular dynamics simulations and quantum mechanical calculations, allows a thorough exploration of the interactions between drugs and nanomaterials at the atomic level. This can lead to optimized drug encapsulation, release kinetics, and targeted delivery with a specific nanocarrier design. For example, molecular dynamics simulations have been used to explore the structural view of insulin adsorption on Cu nanoparticles of multiple sizes (Jomhori Baloch et al., 2022). Additionally, machine learning algorithms, when trained on robust datasets, can serve as potent predictive tools. Machine learning can analyze vast datasets composed of the physicochemical properties and biological activities of successful and unsuccessful nanomaterials, potentially identifying new patterns or trends that can inform the design of novel, effective nanomaterials for drug delivery. An example is the work of the author and colleagues (Maharjan et al., 2023; Navabhatra et al., 2022), where a machine learning model was trained to predict the optimal formulation of nanoparticles based on their physicochemical properties. Moreover, the interdisciplinary field of materials informatics can assist in the high-throughput screening of nanomaterials, leading to the accelerated and cost-effective design of novel nanomaterials. For instance, the application of materials informatics in the analysis of physical properties for carbon nanotubes was exemplified by Vivanco-Benavides's group at Instituto Politécnico Nacional, Mexico (Vivanco-Benavides et al., 2022). These examples illustrate the vital role of advanced computational techniques and machine learning in the design and development of novel nanomaterials for drug delivery, emphasizing the need for their wider adoption in the field.

FUTURE DIRECTIONS

In the field of nanomaterials for drug delivery, a new epoch in medical therapeutics appears to be within grasp. Nevertheless, it remains of paramount importance to anticipate and speculate on the future directions of this dynamic domain. There exists an array of intriguing possibilities for research and implementation that hold the potential to fundamentally recalibrate the conceptualization of drug delivery systems.

Figure 14 presents a conceptual roadmap detailing potential future perspectives in the field of nanomaterials for drug delivery. It encapsulates novel nanomaterial design and synthesis, integration with genetic medicine and biomedical imaging, the development of patient-specific nanodrug delivery systems, and the convergence of nanotechnology with artificial intelligence (AI). First, a promising pathway for future exploration involves the design and synthesis of novel nanomaterials that are purposefully crafted to enhance drug delivery. The diversity of nanomaterials remains largely untapped, and their exploitation could yield highly specialized delivery systems capable of addressing a wide spectrum of therapeutic needs. As the domain of genetic medicine expands, the use of nanomaterials for the delivery of genetic material offers a promising direction. Furthermore, the integration of nanomaterials with biomedical imaging could initiate a dual-functionality system that serves as both a therapeutic carrier and a diagnostic tool. Such a convergence has the potential to facilitate real-time monitoring of drug distribution and release within the body. This property provides crucial data on treatment efficacy.

However, even as the exploration of this captivating frontier progresses, it is imperative to remain aware of potential challenges. The biocompatibility and prospective toxicity of nanomaterials remain significant concerns, necessitating dedicated research efforts to mitigate potential health and environmental impacts. The development of patient-specific nanodrug delivery systems presents a valuable opportunity to align with the broader trend toward personalized medicine. These systems, tailored to the unique genetic and disease profiles of individual patients, have the potential to optimize treatment efficacy and minimize adverse effects.

Finally, the confluence of nanotechnology and AI offers substantial promise. Utilizing AI and machine learning techniques to expedite the design of nanomaterials for drug delivery could provoke a paradigm

Figure 14. Schematic overview of future directions in nanomaterials for drug delivery

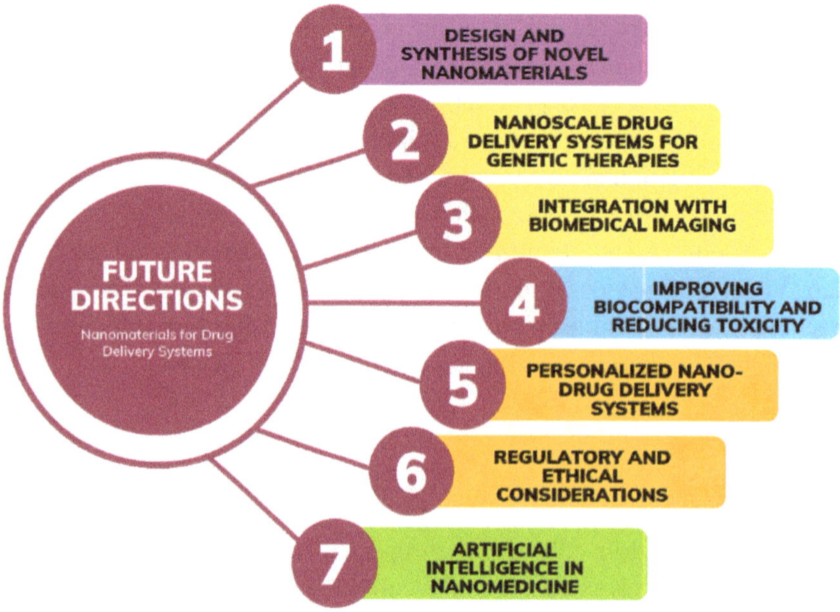

shift, providing a swift, cost-effective route to optimal nanoparticle design (Yingngam, 2023b). However, as with any transformative technology, the ethical and regulatory implications of nanomaterials require careful deliberation. A concerted effort from both policymakers and researchers is necessary to ensure the safe and responsible implementation of these powerful technologies. The future of nanomaterials for drug delivery is both exhilarating and challenging, promising a multitude of advancements and opportunities that could irrefutably revolutionize healthcare.

CONCLUSION

The rapidly evolving field of nanotechnology is reshaping various disciplines, including pharmaceutical sciences. In this chapter, the author has detailed how advances in nanomaterials have revolutionized the pharmaceutical sector, introducing new perspectives for drug delivery systems and treatments. Nanomaterials offer a promising approach to overcoming some traditional drug delivery challenges. Their unique attributes, such as a high surface-to-volume ratio, tunable size, and adaptable surface functionalities, allow them to transport therapeutic agents efficiently and target specific sites. This significantly reduces side effects and enhances therapeutic outcomes. The extensive study of lipid-based nanoparticles, polymeric nanoparticles, inorganic nanoparticles, carbon-based nanoparticles, and other nanocarriers has resulted in innovative, more effective methods of drug administration. This exploration is merely the beginning, and the field stands on the threshold of groundbreaking advancements that could redefine healthcare. While optimism is warranted, it is crucial to remember that the creation of new nanomaterial-based therapies should also address potential challenges and ethical considerations, such as biocompatibility, toxicity, environmental impact, and regulatory aspects.

The convergence of nanotechnology and drug delivery has enormous potential. One exciting prospect is the integration of AI with nanomedicine. AI could be employed to create nanoparticles with optimal properties and predict their behavior in biological environments. This could fast-track the design of effective nanomaterials for drug delivery and reduce the costs of trial-and-error experimental procedures. Additionally, integrating nanotechnology with bioengineering offers vast potential for personalized medicine. Customizable, patient-specific nanodrug delivery systems could be developed to align with the unique genetic makeup and disease profiles of individual patients, significantly increasing treatment efficacy and reducing side effects. Furthermore, advances in stimulus-responsive nanomaterials that react to specific biological signals or external triggers provide a new aspect of controlled and targeted drug delivery. Imagine a future where drugs are released in the body only when and where they are needed, significantly minimizing side effects and maximizing efficacy.

In conclusion, the advances in nanomaterials for drug delivery signify a new context in healthcare and therapeutics. The potential of nanotechnology to transform the field of drug delivery is immense, but it requires continued research, interdisciplinary collaboration, and careful consideration of ethical implications. Both researchers and practitioners must navigate this promising yet intricate terrain with care and diligence. The forthcoming years will undoubtedly witness even greater strides in this dynamic, rapidly evolving field. The author eagerly awaits the next phase of these revolutionary advancements.

REFERENCES

Abd El- Salam, A. M., Tahoun, A., & Hanafy, N. A. N. (2023). Evaluation of liposomal hydrocolloidal NPs loaded by tea tree oil as antifungal agent in vitro and in vivo investigations: Preclinical studies. *Food Hydrocolloids for Health*, *3*, 100136. doi:10.1016/j.fhfh.2023.100136

Agrawal, Y. O., Patil, K. D., More, K. R., Mohd Siddique, M. U., Alkahtani, S., Aljarba, N. H., & Hasnain, M. S. (2022). Amelioration of bioavailability through formulating and optimizing Azilsartan Entrapped nanostructured lipid carriers and its pharmacokinetic assessment. *Journal of Drug Delivery Science and Technology*, *77*, 103894. doi:10.1016/j.jddst.2022.103894

Aguilera-Garrido, A., Graván, P., Navarro-Marchal, S. A., Medina-O'Donnell, M., Parra, A., Gálvez-Ruiz, M. J., Marchal, J. A., & Galisteo-González, F. (2023). Maslinic acid solid lipid nanoparticles as hydrophobic anticancer drug carriers: Formulation, in vitro activity and in vivo biodistribution. *Biomedicine and Pharmacotherapy*, *163*, 114828. doi:10.1016/j.biopha.2023.114828 PMID:37163783

Al-Awsi, G. R. L., Alameri, A. A., Al-Dhalimy, A. M. B., Gabr, G. A., & Kianfar, E. (2024). Application of nano-antibiotics in the diagnosis and treatment of infectious diseases. *Brazilian Journal of Biology*, *84*, e114828. doi:10.1590/1519-6984.264946 PMID:36722677

Aljohani, A. A., Alanazi, M. A., Munahhi, L. A., Hamroon, J. D., Mortagi, Y., Qushawy, M., & Soliman, G. M. (2023). Binary ethosomes for the enhanced topical delivery and antifungal efficacy of ketoconazole. *OpenNano*, *11*, 100145. doi:10.1016/j.onano.2023.100145

Almawash, S. (2023). Solid lipid nanoparticles, an effective carrier for classical antifungal drugs. *Saudi Pharmaceutical Journal*, *31*(7), 1167–1180. doi:10.1016/j.jsps.2023.05.011 PMID:37273269

Asad, S., Jacobsen, A.-C., & Teleki, A. (2022). Inorganic nanoparticles for oral drug delivery: Opportunities, barriers, and future perspectives. *Current Opinion in Chemical Engineering*, *38*, 100869. doi:10.1016/j.coche.2022.100869

Attama, A. A., Agbo, C. P., Onokala, O. B., Kenechukwu, F. C., Ugwueze, M. E., Mbah, C. C., Umeryor, C. E., Uronnachi, E. M., & Nnamani, P. O. (2023). Applications of nanoemulsions as drug delivery vehicle for phytoconstituents. In S. Thomas, A. O. Oyedeji, O. S. Oluwafemi, & R. Jaquilin Pj (Eds.), *Nanotechnology in Herbal Medicine* (pp. 119–194). Woodhead Publishing. doi:10.1016/B978-0-323-99527-6.00017-3

Attia, M. S., Yahya, A., Monaem, N. A., & Sabry, S. A. (2023). Mesoporous silica nanoparticles: Their potential as drug delivery carriers and nanoscavengers in Alzheimer's and Parkinson's diseases. *Saudi Pharmaceutical Journal*, *31*(3), 417–432. doi:10.1016/j.jsps.2023.01.009 PMID:37026045

Bakr, E. A., Gaber, M., Saad, D. R., & Salahuddin, N. (2023). Comparative study between two different morphological structures based on polylactic acid, nanocellulose and magnetite for co-delivery of fluro-uracil and curcumin. *International Journal of Biological Macromolecules*, *230*, 123315. doi:10.1016/j.ijbiomac.2023.123315 PMID:36708892

Bashkeran, T., Kamaruddin, A. H., Ngo, T. X., Suda, K., Umakoshi, H., Watanabe, N., & Nadzir, M. M. (2023). Niosomes in cancer treatment: A focus on curcumin encapsulation. *Heliyon*, *18710*(8), e18710. Advance online publication. doi:10.1016/j.heliyon.2023.e18710 PMID:37593605

Beheshtizadeh, N., Salimi, A., Golmohammadi, M., Ansari, J. M., & Azami, M. (2023). In-silico engineering of RNA nanoplatforms to promote the diabetic wound healing. *BMC Chemistry*, *17*(1), 52. doi:10.118613065-023-00969-4 PMID:37291669

Bernard, M.-C., Bazin, E., Petiot, N., Lemdani, K., Commandeur, S., Verdelet, C., Margot, S., Perkov, V., Ripoll, M., Garinot, M., Ruiz, S., Boudet, F., Rokbi, B., & Haensler, J. (2023). The impact of nucleoside base modification in mRNA vaccine is influenced by the chemistry of its lipid nanoparticle delivery system. *Molecular Therapy. Nucleic Acids*, *32*, 794–806. doi:10.1016/j.omtn.2023.05.004 PMID:37346973

Borhaninia, M., Zahiri, M., Abnous, K., Taghdisi, S. M., Ramezani, M., & Alibolandi, M. (2023). Self-targeted hyaluronic acid-b-poly (β-amino ester) pH-switchable polymersome for guided doxorubicin delivery to metastatic breast cancer. *International Journal of Biological Macromolecules*, *248*, 125882. doi:10.1016/j.ijbiomac.2023.125882 PMID:37473882

Bozkaya, O., Ekici, H., Gün Gök, Z., Arat, E., Ekici, S., Yiğitoğlu, M., & Vargel, İ. (2023). Investigation of the in vitro antibacterial, cytotoxic and in vivo analgesic effects of silver nanoparticles coated with Centella asiatica plant extract. *Ankara Üniversitesi Veteriner Fakültesi Dergisi*, *70*(1), 87–96. doi:10.33988/auvfd.1014802

Brindhadevi, K., Garalleh, H. A. L., Alalawi, A., Al-Sarayreh, E., & Pugazhendhi, A. (2023). Carbon nanomaterials: Types, synthesis strategies and their application as drug delivery system for cancer therapy. *Biochemical Engineering Journal*, *192*, 108828. doi:10.1016/j.bej.2023.108828

Büyükbayraktar, H. K., Pelit Arayıcı, P., Ihlamur, M., Gökkaya, D., Karahan, M., Abamor, E. Ş., & Topuzoğulları, M. (2023). Effect of polycation coating on the long-term pulsatile release of antigenic ESAT-61–20 peptide from PLGA nanoparticles. *Colloids and Surfaces. B, Biointerfaces*, *228*, 113421. doi:10.1016/j.colsurfb.2023.113421 PMID:37356137

Caballero Gómez, N., Manetsberger, J., Benomar, N., & Abriouel, H. (2023). Novel combination of nanoparticles and metallo-β-lactamase inhibitor/antimicrobial-based formulation to combat antibiotic resistant Enterococcus sp. and Pseudomonas sp. strains. *International Journal of Biological Macromolecules*, *248*, 125982. doi:10.1016/j.ijbiomac.2023.125982 PMID:37499723

Chacko, J. B., & Jose, S. (2023). PLGA-based nanoparticles for treatment of cerebral diseases. In P. Kesharwani (Ed.), *Poly(lactic-co-glycolic acid) (PLGA) Nanoparticles for Drug Delivery* (pp. 235–266). Elsevier. doi:10.1016/B978-0-323-91215-0.00018-2

Cheng, L., Zhang, X., Tang, J., Lv, Q., & Liu, J. (2021). Gene-engineered exosomes-thermosensitive liposomes hybrid nanovesicles by the blockade of CD47 signal for combined photothermal therapy and cancer immunotherapy. *Biomaterials*, *275*, 120964. doi:10.1016/j.biomaterials.2021.120964 PMID:34147721

Cheng, X., Li, D., & Cui, R. (2023). Introducing a novel therapeutic supplement for osteoporosis: Remedial, cytotoxicity and antioxidant effects of plant extract green-formulated gold nanoparticles. *Journal of Engineering Research*, *100151*. doi:10.1016/j.jer.2023.100151

Choi, Y., Cho, B. K., Seok, S. H., Kim, C., Ryu, J. H., & Kwon, I. C. (2023). Controlled spatial characteristics of ligands on nanoparticles: Determinant of cellular functions. *Journal of Controlled Release*, *360*, 672–686. doi:10.1016/j.jconrel.2023.07.020 PMID:37437847

Chou, W.-C., Chen, Q., Yuan, L., Cheng, Y.-H., He, C., Monteiro-Riviere, N. A., Riviere, J. E., & Lin, Z. (2023). An artificial intelligence-assisted physiologically-based pharmacokinetic model to predict nanoparticle delivery to tumors in mice. *Journal of Controlled Release, 361*, 53–63. doi:10.1016/j.jconrel.2023.07.040 PMID:37499908

Darbasizadeh, B., Feyzi-barnaji, B., & Naderi, N. (2022). Chapter 19 - Toxicity and biocompatibility of nanomaterials: In vivo studies. In M. Saravanan, H. Barabadi, E. Mostafavi, & T. Webster (Eds.), Emerging Nanomaterials and Nano-Based Drug Delivery Approaches to Combat Antimicrobial Resistance (pp. 701-732): Elsevier. doi:10.1016/B978-0-323-90792-7.00014-2

Das, B., Nayak, A. K., & Mallick, S. (2022). Lipid-based nanocarriers for ocular drug delivery: An updated review. *Journal of Drug Delivery Science and Technology*, *76*, 103780. doi:10.1016/j.jddst.2022.103780

Deepika, G., Suresh, V., Rupula, K., Bantal, V., & Rb, S. (2023). Synthesis and evaluation of anti-inflammatory and anti-nociceptive potentials of biopolymer based curcumin nanoparticle construct: In silico, in vitro and in vivo studies. *Bioactive Carbohydrates and Dietary Fibre*, *30*, 100381. doi:10.1016/j.bcdf.2023.100381

Dhanya, C. S., Paul, W., Rekha, M. R., & Joseph, R. (2023). Solid lipid nanoparticles of lauric Acid: A prospective drug carrier for oral drug delivery. *Journal of Molecular Liquids*, *380*, 121738. doi:10.1016/j.molliq.2023.121738

Di Trani, N., Liu, H.-C., Qi, R., Viswanath, D. I., Liu, X., Chua, C. Y. X., & Grattoni, A. (2021). Long-acting tunable release of amlodipine loaded PEG-PCL micelles for tailored treatment of chronic hypertension. *Nanomedicine; Nanotechnology, Biology, and Medicine*, *37*, 102417. doi:10.1016/j.nano.2021.102417 PMID:34171469

Digiacomo, L., Renzi, S., Quagliarini, E., Pozzi, D., Amenitsch, H., Ferri, G., Pesce, L., Lorenzi, V. D., Matteoli, G., Cardarelli, F., & Caracciolo, G. (2023). Investigating the mechanism of action of DNA-loaded PEGylated lipid nanoparticles. *Nanomedicine; Nanotechnology, Biology, and Medicine*, *102697*, 102697. doi:10.1016/j.nano.2023.102697 PMID:37507061

Dinakar, Y. H., Karole, A., Parvez, S., Jain, V., & Mudavath, S. L. (2023). Folate receptor targeted NIR cleavable liposomal delivery system augment penetration and therapeutic efficacy in breast cancer. *Biochimica et Biophysica Acta (BBA) -. Biochimica et Biophysica Acta. G, General Subjects*, *1867*(9), 130396. doi:10.1016/j.bbagen.2023.130396 PMID:37271407

Dissanayake, T., Sun, X., Abbey, L., & Bandara, N. (2022). Recent advances in lipid-protein conjugate-based delivery systems in nutraceutical, drug, and gene delivery. *Food Hydrocolloids for Health*, *2*, 100054. doi:10.1016/j.fhfh.2022.100054

Dutt, Y., Pandey, R. P., Dutt, M., Gupta, A., Vibhuti, A., Vidic, J., Raj, V. S., Chang, C.-M., & Priyadarshini, A. (2023). Therapeutic applications of nanobiotechnology. *Journal of Nanobiotechnology*, *21*(1), 148. doi:10.118612951-023-01909-z PMID:37149615

Elansary, M., Belaiche, M., Mouhib, Y., Lemine, O. M., Bentarhlia, N., & Bsoul, I. (2023). Novel biocompatible nanomaterial for biomedical application: Structural, morphological, magnetic, and in vivo toxicity investigations. *Ceramics International*, *49*(3), 4551–4570. doi:10.1016/j.ceramint.2022.09.341

Elkateb, H., Cauldbeck, H., Niezabitowska, E., Hogarth, C., Arnold, K., Rannard, S., & McDonald, T. O. (2023). High drug loading solid lipid nanoparticles, nanostructured lipid carriers and nanoemulsions for the dual drug delivery of the HIV drugs darunavir and ritonavir. *JCIS Open*, *11*, 100087. doi:10.1016/j.jciso.2023.100087

Elmehbad, N. Y., Mohamed, N. A., Abd El-Ghany, N. A., & Abdel-Aziz, M. M. (2023). Reinforcement of the antimicrobial activity and biofilm inhibition of novel chitosan-based hydrogels utilizing zinc oxide nanoparticles. *International Journal of Biological Macromolecules*, *246*, 125582. doi:10.1016/j.ijbiomac.2023.125582 PMID:37379952

Emami, A., Ghafouri, H., & Sariri, R. (2023). Polyphyllin D-loaded solid lipid nanoparticles for breast cancer: Synthesis, characterization, in vitro, and in vivo studies. *International Journal of Pharmaceutics*, *639*, 122976. doi:10.1016/j.ijpharm.2023.122976 PMID:37088118

Essien, E. N., Revi, N., Khatri, V., Liu, S., Van Thiel, G., & Bijukumar, D. (2023). Methotrexate and sulforaphane loaded PBA-G5-PAMAM dendrimers as a combination therapy for anti-inflammatory response in an intra-articular joint arthritic animal model. *International Journal of Pharmaceutics*, *642*, 123150. doi:10.1016/j.ijpharm.2023.123150 PMID:37336302

Fateh Basharzad, S., Hamidi, M., Maleki, A., Karami, Z., Mohamadpour, H., & Reza Saghatchi Zanjani, M. (2022). Polysorbate-coated mesoporous silica nanoparticles as an efficient carrier for improved rivastigmine brain delivery. *Brain Research*, *1781*, 147786. doi:10.1016/j.brainres.2022.147786 PMID:35041841

Freis, B., Ramírez, M. D. L. Á., Furgiuele, S., Journe, F., Cheignon, C., Charbonnière, L. J., Henoumont, C., Kiefer, C., Mertz, D., Affolter-Zbaraszczuk, C., Meyer, F., Saussez, S., Laurent, S., Tasso, M., & Bégin-Colin, S. (2023). Bioconjugation studies of an EGF-R targeting ligand on dendronized iron oxide nanoparticles to target head and neck cancer cells. *International Journal of Pharmaceutics*, *635*, 122654. doi:10.1016/j.ijpharm.2023.122654 PMID:36720449

Gaikwad, S. S., Morade, Y. Y., Kothule, A. M., Kshirsagar, S. J., Laddha, U. D., & Salunkhe, K. S. (2023). Overview of phytosomes in treating cancer: Advancement, challenges, and future outlook. *Heliyon*, *9*(6), e16561. doi:10.1016/j.heliyon.2023.e16561 PMID:37260890

García-García, G., Caro, C., Fernández-Álvarez, F., García-Martín, M. L., & Arias, J. L. (2023). Multi-stimuli-responsive chitosan-functionalized magnetite/poly(ε-caprolactone) nanoparticles as theranostic platforms for combined tumor magnetic resonance imaging and chemotherapy. *Nanomedicine; Nanotechnology, Biology, and Medicine*, *52*, 102695. doi:10.1016/j.nano.2023.102695 PMID:37394106

Garibyan, A., Delyagina, E., & Terekhova, I. (2023). Improving properties of baricitinib due to interaction with Pluronic micelles. *Journal of Molecular Liquids*, *382*, 121968. doi:10.1016/j.molliq.2023.121968

Gautam, S., Das, D. K., Kaur, J., Kumar, A., Ubaidullah, M., Hasan, M., Yadav, K. K., & Gupta, R. K. (2023). Transition metal-based nanoparticles as potential antimicrobial agents: Recent advancements, mechanistic, challenges, and future prospects. *Discover Nano*, *18*(1), 84. Advance online publication. doi:10.118611671-023-03861-1 PMID:37382784

Hajifathali, A., Lasemi, M. V., Mehravar, M., Moshari, M. R., Alizadeh, A. M., & Roshandel, E. (2023). Novelty in improvement of CAR T cell-based immunotherapy with the aid of CRISPR system. *Hematology, Transfusion and Cell Therapy*. doi:10.1016/j.htct.2023.05.009 PMID:37451978

Han, G., Noh, D., Lee, H., Lee, S., Kim, S., Yoon, H. Y., & Lee, S. H. (2023). Advances in mRNA therapeutics for cancer immunotherapy: From modification to delivery. *Advanced Drug Delivery Reviews*, *199*, 114973. doi:10.1016/j.addr.2023.114973 PMID:37369262

Harish, V., Mohd, S., Tewari, D., Pandey, N. K., Vishwas, S., Babu, M. R., Salkini, M. A., Rehman, Z., Alotaibi, J. T., Alotaibi, R. F., Alrashed, F. A., Prasher, P., Sharma, N., Gupta, G., Jakhmola, V., Singh, Y., Pinto, T. J. A., Paudel, K. R., Mittal, N., & Singh, S. K. (2023). Unravelling the role of solid lipid nanoparticles in drug delivery: Journey from laboratory to clinical trial. *Journal of Drug Delivery Science and Technology*, *85*, 104616. doi:10.1016/j.jddst.2023.104616

Huang, B., Zhang, F., Cai, C., & Zhang, L. (2023). Toward understanding polymeric micelle stability regulated by diverse physico-chemical strategies and their stabilized mechanism. *Colloids and Surfaces. A, Physicochemical and Engineering Aspects*, *674*, 131880. doi:10.1016/j.colsurfa.2023.131880

Huang, Y., Li, X., Cao, J., Wei, X., Li, Y., Wang, Z., Cai, X., Li, R., & Chen, J. (2022). Use of dissociation degree in lysosomes to predict metal oxide nanoparticle toxicity in immune cells: Machine learning boosts nano-safety assessment. *Environment International*, *164*, 107258. doi:10.1016/j.envint.2022.107258 PMID:35483183

Husni, P., Lim, C., & Oh, K. T. (2023). Tumor microenvironment stimuli-responsive lipid-drug conjugates for cancer treatment. *International Journal of Pharmaceutics*, *639*, 122942. doi:10.1016/j.ijpharm.2023.122942 PMID:37037397

Ijaz, S., Sultana, M., Shamim, R., & Bukhari, N. I. (2023). Development and DoE-ANN based optimization of novel swellable matrix-diffusible doxorubicin loaded zinc oxide nanoflowers using sonochemical-precipitation method. *International Journal of Pharmaceutics*, *633*, 122584. doi:10.1016/j.ijpharm.2023.122584 PMID:36621704

Jain, D., Hasan, N., Zafar, S., Thakur, J., Haider, K., Parvez, S., & Ahmad, F. J. (2023). Transferrin functionalized nanostructured lipid carriers for targeting Rivastigmine and Resveratrol to Alzheimer's disease: Synthesis, in vitro characterization and brain uptake analysis. *Journal of Drug Delivery Science and Technology*, *86*, 104555. doi:10.1016/j.jddst.2023.104555

Jalal, R. R., Ways, T. M. M., Abu Elella, M. H., Hassan, D. A., & Khutoryanskiy, V. V. (2023). Preparation of mucoadhesive methacrylated chitosan nanoparticles for delivery of ciprofloxacin. *International Journal of Biological Macromolecules*, *242*, 124980. doi:10.1016/j.ijbiomac.2023.124980 PMID:37236558

Jomhori Baloch, M., Mosaddeghi, H., & Jamshidian-Mojaver, M. (2022). Structural view of insulin adsorption on the multiple sizes of Cu nanoparticles; molecular dynamics simulation study. *Archives of Biochemistry and Biophysics*, *722*, 109219. doi:10.1016/j.abb.2022.109219 PMID:35427577

Joubert, F., Munson, M. J., Sabirsh, A., England, R. M., Hemmerling, M., Alexander, C., & Ashford, M. B. (2023). Precise and systematic end group chemistry modifications on PAMAM and poly(l-lysine) dendrimers to improve cytosolic delivery of mRNA. *Journal of Controlled Release*, *356*, 580–594. doi:10.1016/j.jconrel.2023.03.011 PMID:36918085

Kannan, R. M., Pitha, I., & Parikh, K. S. (2023). A new era in posterior segment ocular drug delivery: Translation of systemic, cell-targeted, dendrimer-based therapies. *Advanced Drug Delivery Reviews*, *200*, 115005. doi:10.1016/j.addr.2023.115005 PMID:37419213

Kansız, S., & Elçin, Y. M. (2023). Advanced liposome and polymersome-based drug delivery systems: Considerations for physicochemical properties, targeting strategies and stimuli-sensitive approaches. *Advances in Colloid and Interface Science*, *317*, 102930. doi:10.1016/j.cis.2023.102930 PMID:37290380

Karayianni, M., Chroni, A., Chrysostomou, V., Giaouzi, D., Kafetzi, M., Selianitis, D., Sentoukas, T., & Pispas, S. (2023). Polymeric micelles for therapeutics and diagnosis. In M. S. Hasnain, A. K. Nayak, & T. M. Aminabhavi (Eds.), *Advanced Nanoformulations* (pp. 97–157). Academic Press. doi:10.1016/B978-0-323-85785-7.00019-X

Khan, I., Pandit, J., Ahmed, S., Zameer, S., Nikita, Ahmad, S., Bano, S., Ansari, M. D., Solanki, P., Jahan, R. N., Waheed, A., Aqil, M., & Sultana, Y. (2022). Development and evaluation of biodegradable polymeric lomustine nanofibres for the efficient tumor targeting: In vitro characterization, ex vivo permeation and degradation study. *Journal of Drug Delivery Science and Technology*, *75*, 103685. doi:10.1016/j.jddst.2022.103685

Kheiri, K., Sohrabi, N., Mohammadi, R., & Amini-Fazl, M. S. (2022). Preparation and characterization of magnetic nanohydrogel based on chitosan for 5-fluorouracil drug delivery and kinetic study. *International Journal of Biological Macromolecules*, *202*, 191–198. doi:10.1016/j.ijbiomac.2022.01.028 PMID:35033524

Kim, H.-S., Kang, J.-H., Jang, J., Lee, E.-J., Kim, J. H., Byun, J., & Shin, U. S. (2023). Dual stimuli-responsive mesoporous silica nanoparticles for efficient loading and smart delivery of doxorubicin to cancer with RGD-integrin targeting. *European Journal of Pharmaceutical Sciences*, *188*, 106525. doi:10.1016/j.ejps.2023.106525 PMID:37437854

Kim, M., Kim, S.-B., Kim, J., Kim, K.-S., & Kim, D.-E. (2023). Co-delivery of curcumin and PTTG1 siRNA by galactose receptor-targeted liposomes for enhanced anti-tumor effects in hepatocellular carcinoma. *Journal of Drug Delivery Science and Technology*, *86*, 104692. doi:10.1016/j.jddst.2023.104692

Korake, S., Bothiraja, C., & Pawar, A. (2023). Design, development, and in-vitro/in-vivo evaluation of docetaxel-loaded PEGylated solid lipid nanoparticles in prostate cancer therapy. *European Journal of Pharmaceutics and Biopharmaceutics*, *189*, 15–27. doi:10.1016/j.ejpb.2023.05.020 PMID:37270157

Kumar, S., Fry, L. E., Wang, J.-H., Martin, K. R., Hewitt, A. W., Chen, F. K., & Liu, G.-S. (2023). RNA-targeting strategies as a platform for ocular gene therapy. *Progress in Retinal and Eye Research*, *92*, 101110. doi:10.1016/j.preteyeres.2022.101110 PMID:35840489

Kurawattimath, V., Wilson, B., & Geetha, K. M. (2023). Nanoparticle-based drug delivery across the blood-brain barrier for treating malignant brain glioma. *OpenNano*, *10*, 100128. doi:10.1016/j.onano.2023.100128

Li, B., Zhang, T., & Tang, M. (2022). Toxicity mechanism of nanomaterials: Focus on endoplasmic reticulum stress. *The Science of the Total Environment*, *834*, 155417. doi:10.1016/j.scitotenv.2022.155417 PMID:35472346

Li, J., Zhang, L., Tao, Y., Sun, Z., Ge, Y., & Hu, S. (2023). Combination of transcatheter arterial chemoembolization and anti-PD-L1 liposomes therapy suppressed hepatocellular carcinoma progression in mice. *European Journal of Pharmaceutical Sciences*, *106549*, 106549. doi:10.1016/j.ejps.2023.106549 PMID:37524271

Li, L., Guo, Q., Liu, Y., Lu, M., Yang, J., Ge, Y., Zhang, Q., Sun, B., Wang, X., Liang-cheng, L., & Ren, L. (2021). Targeted combination therapy for glioblastoma by co-delivery of doxorubicin, YAP-siRNA and gold nanorods. *Journal of Materials Science and Technology*, *63*, 81–90. doi:10.1016/j.jmst.2020.03.009

Li, Q., Tang, Z., Zhang, Y., Yuan, T., Yuan, B., Du, L., & Jin, Y. (2023). Application of low-intensity ultrasound by opening blood–brain barrier for enhanced brain-targeted drug delivery. *International Journal of Pharmaceutics*, *642*, 123191. doi:10.1016/j.ijpharm.2023.123191 PMID:37391108

Liu, A., Chai, X., Zhu, S., Chin, P., He, M., Xu, Y.-J., & Liu, Y. (2023). Effects of N-succinyl-chitosan coating on properties of astaxanthin-loaded PEG-liposomes: Environmental stability, antioxidant/antibacterial activities, and in vitro release. *International Journal of Biological Macromolecules*, *244*, 125311. doi:10.1016/j.ijbiomac.2023.125311 PMID:37302627

Liu, T., Lu, Y., Zhan, R., Qian, W., & Luo, G. (2023). Nanomaterials and nanomaterials-based drug delivery to promote cutaneous wound healing. *Advanced Drug Delivery Reviews*, *193*, 114670. doi:10.1016/j.addr.2022.114670 PMID:36538990

Liu, T., Zou, H., Mu, J., Zhang, X., Liu, G., Yu, N., Yuan, B., Yuan, X., Liang, X., & Guo, S. (2023). PDLLA length on anti-breast cancer efficacy of acid-responsive self-assembling mPEG-PDLLA–docetaxel conjugates. *Chinese Chemical Letters*, *34*(9), 108135. doi:10.1016/j.cclet.2023.108135

Liu, Y., Li, S., Ding, C., Ge, Z., Aierken, A., Li, J., Qin, L., Liu, J., Guo, X., Wang, Y., Xing, Z., Yuan, F., & Zhou, P. (2023). Dual-responsive and controlled-release paclitaxel-loaded mesoporous silicon nanoparticles with cell membrane coating for homologous targeted therapy of tongue squamous cell carcinoma. *Materials & Design*, *229*, 111886. doi:10.1016/j.matdes.2023.111886

Liu, Y., Zhu, S., Gu, Z., & Chen, C. (2023). Toxicology of nanomaterials: From toxicokinetics to toxicity mechanisms. In Y. Yin, Y. Lu, & Y. Xia (Eds.), *Encyclopedia of Nanomaterials* (1st ed., pp. 718–732). Elsevier. doi:10.1016/B978-0-12-822425-0.00025-7

Lombardi, G., Del Bianco, P., Brandes, A. A., Eoli, M., Rudà, R., Ibrahim, T., Lolli, I., Rizzato, S., Daniele, B., Pace, A., Pasqualetti, F., Caccesse, M., Bergo, E., Magni, G., Salvo, G. L. D., & Zagonel, V. (2021). Patient-reported outcomes in a phase II randomised study of regorafenib compared with lomustine in patients with relapsed glioblastoma (the REGOMA trial). *European Journal of Cancer*, *155*, 179–190. doi:10.1016/j.ejca.2021.06.055 PMID:34388515

Lu, S., Hao, D., Xiang, X., Pei, Q., & Xie, Z. (2023). Carboxylated paclitaxel prodrug nanofibers for enhanced chemotherapy. *Journal of Controlled Release*, *355*, 528–537. doi:10.1016/j.jconrel.2023.02.013 PMID:36787820

Lundstrom, K. (2023). Viral vectors engineered for gene therapy. In *International Review of Cell and Molecular Biology*. Academic Press.

Maatouk, B., Jaffa, M. A., Karam, M., Fahs, D., Nour-Eldine, W., Hasan, A., Jaffa, A. A., & Mhanna, R. (2021). Sulfated alginate/polycaprolactone double-emulsion nanoparticles for enhanced delivery of heparin-binding growth factors in wound healing applications. *Colloids and Surfaces. B, Biointerfaces*, *208*, 112105. doi:10.1016/j.colsurfb.2021.112105 PMID:34536674

Mabrouk, A. A., El-Mezayen, N. S., Awaad, A. K., Tadros, M. I., El-Gazayerly, O. N., & El-Refaie, W. M. (2023). Novel celecoxib-loaded chitosan-fucoidan nanoparticles as potential immunotherapy for oral squamous cell carcinoma: Mechanistic insights. *Journal of Drug Delivery Science and Technology*, *81*, 104228. doi:10.1016/j.jddst.2023.104228

Mahamuni-Badiger, P., & Dhanavade, M. J. (2023). Challenges and toxicity assessment of inorganic nanomaterials in biomedical applications: Current status and future roadmaps. *Journal of Drug Delivery Science and Technology*, *104806*, 104806. doi:10.1016/j.jddst.2023.104806

Maharjan, R., Hada, S., Lee, J. E., Han, H.-K., Kim, K. H., Seo, H. J., Foged, C., & Jeong, S. H. (2023). Comparative study of lipid nanoparticle-based mRNA vaccine bioprocess with machine learning and combinatorial artificial neural network-design of experiment approach. *International Journal of Pharmaceutics*, *640*, 123012. doi:10.1016/j.ijpharm.2023.123012 PMID:37142140

Manhas, P., Sharma, R., Wangoo, N., Saini, R., Saima, Agrewala, J. N., & Sharma, R. K. (2023). Dox-loaded TPU-PLGA nanoparticles embedded chitosan hydrogel formulation as an effective anti-cancer therapy. *Journal of Molecular Liquids*, *383*, 122170. doi:10.1016/j.molliq.2023.122170

Matiyani, M., Rana, A., Karki, N., Garwal, K., Pal, M., & Sahoo, N. G. (2023). Development of multi-functionalized graphene oxide based nanocarrier for the delivery of poorly water soluble anticancer drugs. *Journal of Drug Delivery Science and Technology*, *83*, 104412. doi:10.1016/j.jddst.2023.104412

Maurer, M. S., Fontana, M., Berk, J., Gustafsson, F., Simoes, M., Grogan, M., Fernandes, F., Gottlieb, R. L., Kubanek, M., Poulsen, S., Damy, T., Diemberger, I., Tahara, N., Yu, W.-C., Tang, W. H. W., Obic, L., Gonzalez-Duarte, A., Sekijima, Y., White, M. T., & Gillmore, J. D. (2023). Primary results from apollo-B, a phase 3 study of patisiran in patients with transthyretin-mediated amyloidosis with cardiomyopathy. *Journal of Cardiac Failure*, *29*(4), 550. doi:10.1016/j.cardfail.2022.10.013

Mertdinç-Ülküseven, S., Khakzad, F., Aslan, C., Onbasli, K., Çevik, Ç., İşçi, S., Balcı-Çağıran, Ö., Acar, H. Y., Öveçoğlu, M. L., & Ağaoğulları, D. (2023). Fe_2B magnetic nanoparticles: Synthesis, optimization and cytotoxicity for potential biomedical applications. *Journal of Science. Advanced Materials and Devices*, *8*(3), 100602. doi:10.1016/j.jsamd.2023.100602

Metawea, O. R. M., Teleb, M., Haiba, N. S., Elzoghby, A. O., Khafaga, A. F., Noreldin, A. E., Khattab, S. N., & Khalil, H. H. (2023). Folic acid-poly(N-isopropylacrylamide-maltodextrin) nanohydrogels as novel thermo-/pH-responsive polymer for resveratrol breast cancer targeted therapy. *European Polymer Journal*, *182*, 111721. doi:10.1016/j.eurpolymj.2022.111721

Michlewska, S., Garaiova, Z., Šubjakova, V., Hołota, M., Kubczak, M., Grodzicka, M., Okła, E., Naziris, N., Balcerzak, Ł., Ortega, P., de la Mata, F. J., Hianik, T., Waczulikova, I., Bryszewska, M., & Ionov, M. (2023). Lipid-coated ruthenium dendrimer conjugated with doxorubicin in anti-cancer drug delivery: Introducing protocols. *Colloids and Surfaces. B, Biointerfaces*, *227*, 113371. doi:10.1016/j.colsurfb.2023.113371 PMID:37244201

Mishra, A., Kumar, R., Mishra, J., Dutta, K., Ahlawat, P., Kumar, A., Dhanasekaran, S., Gupta, A. K., Sinha, S., Bishi, D. K., Gupta, P. K., & Nayak, S. (2023). Strategies facilitating the permeation of nanoparticles through blood-brain barrier: An insight towards the development of brain-targeted drug delivery system. *Journal of Drug Delivery Science and Technology*, *86*, 104694. doi:10.1016/j.jddst.2023.104694

Mishra, M., Gupta, A. D., Dadhich, R., Ahmad, M. N., Dasgupta, A., Chopra, S., & Kapoor, S. (2023). Mycobacterial lipid-derived immunomodulatory drug- liposome conjugate eradicates endosome-localized mycobacteria. *Journal of Controlled Release*, *360*, 578–590. doi:10.1016/j.jconrel.2023.07.013 PMID:37442202

Moasses Ghafary, S., Rahimjazi, E., Hamzehil, H., Modarres Mousavi, S. M., Nikkhah, M., & Hosseinkhani, S. (2022). Design and preparation of a theranostic peptideticle for targeted cancer therapy: Peptide-based codelivery of doxorubicin/curcumin and graphene quantum dots. *Nanomedicine; Nanotechnology, Biology, and Medicine*, *42*, 102544. doi:10.1016/j.nano.2022.102544 PMID:35192939

Mokhtar, N., Fouda, F., Zaazaa, A. M., & Mahmoud, M. H. (2023). Nano-Encapsulation of Doxorubicin Using Pectin: Safety an Activity on Chemotherapy-Induced Cardiotoxicity in Carcinoma Mice. *Letters in Applied NanoBioScience*, *12*(4), 107. doi:10.33263/LIANBS124.107

Molaei, M. J. (2023). Carbon quantum dots-based fluorescent layered double hydroxide for targeted drug delivery application. *Diamond and Related Materials*, *137*, 110135. doi:10.1016/j.diamond.2023.110135

Navabhatra, A., Brantner, A., & Yingngam, B. (2022). Artificial neural network modeling of nanostructured lipid carriers containing 5-*O*-caffeoylquinic acid-rich *Cratoxylum formosum* leaf extract for skin application. *Advanced Pharmaceutical Bulletin*, *12*(4), 801–817. doi:10.34172/apb.2022.082 PMID:36415630

Nayak, D., & Tippavajhala, V. K. (2021). A comprehensive review on preparation, evaluation and applications of deformable liposomes. *Iranian Journal of Pharmaceutical Research*, *20*(1), 186–205. doi:10.22037/ijpr.2020.112878.13997 PMID:34400952

Neamatallah, T. (2023). Delayed inflammatory reaction to hyaluronic acid lip filler after the Pfizer-BioNTech COVID-19 vaccine: A case report. *Heliyon*, *9*(7), e18274. doi:10.1016/j.heliyon.2023.e18274 PMID:37539264

Nezhadi, S., Norouzi, P., Rasouli, A., Akbari Javar, H., Ostad, S. N., & Dorkoosh, F. (2023). Co-delivery of paclitaxel and regorafenib by F127/TPGS mixed micelles for triple negative breast cancer treatment. *Journal of Drug Delivery Science and Technology*, *86*, 104673. doi:10.1016/j.jddst.2023.104673

Nguyen, C.-H., Banh, K.-S., An, T. N. M., Anh, N. T. H., Dang, C.-H., Doan, V.-D., Chi, T. T. K., Vu-Quang, H., & Nguyen, T.-D. (2023). Cyclodextrin modified with different groups to enhance the drug delivery efficiency of gold nanoparticles to treat cancer. *Arabian Journal of Chemistry*, *16*(9), 105079. doi:10.1016/j.arabjc.2023.105079

Nguyen, T. T., Chuang, E.-Y., Chen, Y.-P., Tseng, P.-C., Jhan, M.-K., Lai, C.-Y., Wang, Y.-T., Hung, Y.-P., Changou, C. A., Lee, C.-M., Chen, C.-L., & Lin, C.-F. (2023). Anticancer polypyrrole-polyethylenimine drug-free nanozyme for precise B-cell lymphoma therapy. *Biomedicine and Pharmacotherapy*, *160*, 114397. doi:10.1016/j.biopha.2023.114397 PMID:36796279

Nguyen, V. H., Thuy, V. N., Van, T. V., Dao, A. H., & Lee, B.-J. (2022). Nanostructured lipid carriers and their potential applications for versatile drug delivery via oral administration. *OpenNano*, *8*, 100064. doi:10.1016/j.onano.2022.100064

Oladipo, A. O., Lebelo, S. L., & Msagati, T. A. M. (2023). Nanocarrier design–function relationship: The prodigious role of properties in regulating biocompatibility for drug delivery applications. *Chemico-Biological Interactions*, *377*, 110466. doi:10.1016/j.cbi.2023.110466 PMID:37004951

Omrani, M., Naimi-Jamal, M. R., & Far, B. F. (2022). The design of multi-responsive nanohydrogel networks of chitosan for controlled drug delivery. *Carbohydrate Polymers*, *298*, 120143. doi:10.1016/j.carbpol.2022.120143 PMID:36241333

Pan, F., Khan, M., Ragab, A. H., Javed, E., Alsalmah, H. A., Khan, I., Lei, T., Hussain, A., Mohamed, A., Zada, A., & Ansari, M. Z. (2023). Recent advances in the structure and biomedical applications of nanodiamonds and their future perspectives. *Materials & Design*, *233*, 112179. doi:10.1016/j.matdes.2023.112179

Pan, Y., Guan, J., Gao, Y., Zhu, Y., Li, H., Guo, H., He, Q., Guan, Z., & Yang, Z. (2023). Modified ASO conjugates encapsulated with cytidinyl/cationic lipids exhibit more potent and longer-lasting anti-HCC effects. *Molecular Therapy. Nucleic Acids*, *32*, 807–821. doi:10.1016/j.omtn.2023.04.028 PMID:37251692

Panda, P. K., & Jain, S. K. (2023). Doxorubicin bearing peptide anchored PEGylated PLGA nanoparticles for the effective delivery to prostate cancer cells. *Journal of Drug Delivery Science and Technology*, *86*, 104667. doi:10.1016/j.jddst.2023.104667

Pardridge, W. M. (2023). Brain gene therapy with Trojan horse lipid nanoparticles. *Trends in Molecular Medicine*, *29*(5), 343–353. doi:10.1016/j.molmed.2023.02.004 PMID:36907687

Patel, H. S., Shaikh, S. J., Ray, D., Aswal, V. K., Vaidya, F., Pathak, C., Varade, D., Rahdar, A., & Sharma, R. K. (2022). Structural transitions in mixed Phosphatidylcholine/Pluronic micellar systems and their in vitro therapeutic evaluation for poorly water-soluble drug. *Journal of Molecular Liquids*, *364*, 120003. doi:10.1016/j.molliq.2022.120003

Prajapati, B. G., Prajapati, B., & Khunt, D. (2023). In-vivo pharmacokinetics study of exemestane hydrochloride self-nanoemulsifying drug delivery systems via oral route. *Letters in Applied NanoBioScience*, *12*(4), 98. doi:10.33263/LIANBS124.098

Rahmani, D., Torbat, N. A., & Boddohi, S. (2023). Synthesis and characterization of pH-responsive PCL-PVA polymersome for dual delivery to breast cancer cells. *European Polymer Journal, 191*, 112032. doi:10.1016/j.eurpolymj.2023.112032

Rarokar, N., Agrawal, R., Yadav, S., Khedekar, P., Ravikumar, C., Telange, D., & Gurav, S. (2023). Pteroyl-γ-l-glutamate/Pluronic® F68 modified polymeric micelles loaded with docetaxel for targeted delivery and reduced toxicity. *Journal of Molecular Liquids, 369*, 120842. doi:10.1016/j.molliq.2022.120842

Rawat, P., & Gupta, S. (2021). Dual engineered gold nanoparticle based synergistic prophylaxis delivery system for HIV/AIDS. *Medical Hypotheses, 150*, 110576. doi:10.1016/j.mehy.2021.110576 PMID:33799160

Razavi, M. S., Abdollahi, A., Malek-Khatabi, A., Ejarestaghi, N. M., Atashi, A., Yousefi, N., Ebrahimnejad, P., Elsawy, M. A., & Dinarvand, R. (2023). Recent advances in PLGA-based nanofibers as anticancer drug delivery systems. *Journal of Drug Delivery Science and Technology, 85*, 104587. doi:10.1016/j.jddst.2023.104587

Rezaei, N., Kazem Arki, M., Miri-Lavasani, Z., Solhi, R., Khoramipour, M., Rashedi, H., Aghdaei, H. A., Hossein-Khannazer, N., Mostafavi, E., & Vosough, M. (2023). Co-delivery of doxorubicin and paclitaxel via niosome nanocarriers attenuates cancerous phenotypes in gastric cancer cells. *European Journal of Pharmaceutics and Biopharmaceutics, 188*, 33–47. doi:10.1016/j.ejpb.2023.04.016 PMID:37105361

Rouge, J. (2023). RNA and nanocarriers: Next generation drug and delivery platform take center stage. *Trends in Biotechnology, 41*(3), 281–282. doi:10.1016/j.tibtech.2022.12.019 PMID:36609034

Roy, H., Panda, S. P., Panda, S. K., Tripathi, A. K., Srivastava, S. K., Nayak, B. S., Singh, P. K., & Singh, G. D. (2023). N-trimethyl chitosan and tripalmitin loaded solid lipid nanoparticles of tofacitinib citrate: Characterization and in-vivo anti-inflammatory assessment. *Journal of Drug Delivery Science and Technology, 87*, 104789. doi:10.1016/j.jddst.2023.104789

Salesa, B., Ferrús-Manzano, P., Tuñón-Molina, A., Cano-Vicent, A., Assis, M., Andrés, J., & Serrano-Aroca, Á. (2023). Study of biological properties of gold nanoparticles: Low toxicity, no proliferative activity, no ability to induce cell gene expression and no antiviral activity. *Chemico-Biological Interactions, 382*, 110646. doi:10.1016/j.cbi.2023.110646 PMID:37506996

San-Martin, C. R., Zhang, Y., Hamoh, T., Berendse, L., Klijn, C., Li, R., Sigaeva, A., Kawałko, J., Li, H. T., Tehrani, J., Mzyk, A., & Schirhagl, R. (2023). Fluorescent nanodiamond labels: Size and concentration matters for sperm cell viability. *Materials Today. Bio, 20*, 100629. doi:10.1016/j.mtbio.2023.100629 PMID:37441134

Sands, I., Lee, J., & Chen, Y. (2023). Nanotechnology for DNA and RNA delivery. In T. J. Webster (Ed.), *Nanomedicine* (2nd ed., pp. 81–111). Woodhead Publishing. doi:10.1016/B978-0-12-818627-5.00008-7

Schmidt, H. H., Wixner, J., Planté-Bordeneuve, V., Muñoz-Beamud, F., Lladó, L., Gillmore, J. D., Mazzeo, A., Li, X., Arum, S., Jay, P. Y., & Adams, D. (2022). Patisiran treatment in patients with hereditary transthyretin-mediated amyloidosis with polyneuropathy after liver transplantation. *American Journal of Transplantation, 22*(6), 1646–1657. doi:10.1111/ajt.17009 PMID:35213769

Şen, Ö., Emanet, M., Marino, A., Belenli Gümüş, M., Bartolucci, M., Doccini, S., Catalano, F., Genchi, G. G., Santorelli, F. M., Petretto, A., & Ciofani, G. (2021). Evaluation of the therapeutic potential of resveratrol-loaded nanostructured lipid carriers on autosomal recessive spastic ataxia of Charlevoix-Sagucnay patient-derived fibroblasts. *Materials & Design*, *209*, 110012. doi:10.1016/j.matdes.2021.110012

Sengupta, S., Pal, S., Pal, A., Maity, S., Sarkar, K., & Das, M. (2023). A review on synthesis, toxicity profile and biomedical applications of graphene quantum dots (GQDs). *Inorganica Chimica Acta*, *557*, 121677. doi:10.1016/j.ica.2023.121677

Sharoyko, V. V., Berdichevsky, G. M., Vasina, L. V., Shemchuk, O. S., Maystrenko, D. N., Molchanov, O. E., Abdelhalim, A. O. E., Nashchekin, A. V., Nerukh, D. A., Tochilnikov, G. V., Murin, I. V., & Semenov, K. N. (2023). Covalent conjugates based on nanodiamonds with doxorubicin and a cytostatic drug from the group of 1,3,5-triazines: Synthesis, biocompatibility and biological activity. *Biochimica et Biophysica Acta (BBA) -. Biochimica et Biophysica Acta. G, General Subjects*, *1867*(9), 130384. doi:10.1016/j.bbagen.2023.130384 PMID:37209777

Shen, C., Xue, Y., Li, Y., Wei, M., Wen, M., Zhang, L., & Shang, L. (2023). Kinetically regulated one-pot synthesis of cationic gold nanoparticles and their size-dependent antibacterial mechanism. *Journal of Materials Science and Technology*, *162*, 145–156. doi:10.1016/j.jmst.2023.03.061

Shen, X., Cui, Z., Wei, Y., Huo, Y., Yu, D., Zhang, X., & Mao, S. (2023). Exploring the potential to enhance drug distribution in the brain subregion via intranasal delivery of nanoemulsion in combination with borneol as a guider. *Asian Journal of Pharmaceutical Sciences*, *100778*(6), 100778. Advance online publication. doi:10.1016/j.ajps.2023.100778 PMID:38089837

Snow, A., Lin, L., Hunsucker, S. A., Wang, Y., Liu, R., & Armistead, P. M. (2022). Development of a mRNA lipid nanoparticle (mRNA-LNP) cancer vaccine to prevent leukemia relapse after stem cell transplant. *Blood*, *140*(Supplement 1), 7382–7383. doi:10.1182/blood-2022-160218

Song, S., Shim, M. K., Yang, S., Lee, J., Yun, W. S., Cho, H., Moon, Y., Min, J. Y., Han, E. H., Yoon, H. Y., & Kim, K. (2023). All-in-one glycol chitosan nanoparticles for co-delivery of doxorubicin and anti-PD-L1 peptide in cancer immunotherapy. *Bioactive Materials*, *28*, 358–375. doi:10.1016/j.bioactmat.2023.05.016 PMID:37334068

Soundararajan, D., Ramana, L. N., Shankaran, P., & Krishnan, U. M. (2022). Nanoparticle-based strategies to target HIV-infected cells. *Colloids and Surfaces. B, Biointerfaces*, *213*, 112405. doi:10.1016/j.colsurfb.2022.112405 PMID:35255375

Srivastav, A. K., Karpathak, S., Rai, M. K., Kumar, D., Misra, D. P., & Agarwal, V. (2023). Lipid based drug delivery systems for oral, transdermal and parenteral delivery: Recent strategies for targeted delivery consistent with different clinical application. *Journal of Drug Delivery Science and Technology*, *85*, 104526. doi:10.1016/j.jddst.2023.104526

Sun, Y., Zhang, Y., Liu, X., Tingting, Y., Shen, L., Ye, D., Kong, X., Su, Y., & Tian, Q. (2023). The preparation of high minoxidil loaded transfersomes and its gel for effective topical treatment of alopecia. *Journal of Drug Delivery Science and Technology*, *84*, 104458. doi:10.1016/j.jddst.2023.104458

Sung, D., Sanchez, A., & Tward, J. D. (2023). Successful salvage brachytherapy after infusion of gold auroshell nanoshells for localized prostate cancer in a human patient. *Advances in Radiation Oncology*, *8*(4), 101202. doi:10.1016/j.adro.2023.101202 PMID:37082724

Taher, M., Susanti, D., Haris, M. S., Rushdan, A. A., Widodo, R. T., Syukri, Y., & Khotib, J. (2023). PEGylated liposomes enhance the effect of cytotoxic drug: A review. *Heliyon*, *9*(3), e13823. doi:10.1016/j.heliyon.2023.e13823 PMID:36873538

Teixeira, M. I., Lopes, C. M., Amaral, M. H., & Costa, P. C. (2023). Surface-modified lipid nanocarriers for crossing the blood-brain barrier (BBB): A current overview of active targeting in brain diseases. *Colloids and Surfaces. B, Biointerfaces*, *221*, 112999. doi:10.1016/j.colsurfb.2022.112999 PMID:36368148

Tenchov, R., Sasso, J. M., & Zhou, Q. A. (2023). PEGylated Lipid Nanoparticle Formulations: Immunological Safety and Efficiency Perspective. *Bioconjugate Chemistry*, *34*(6), 941–960. doi:10.1021/acs.bioconjchem.3c00174 PMID:37162501

Thankappan, B., Thomas, A., Sakthivadivel, A., Shanmuganathan, N., & Angayarkanni, J. (2023). In vitro and in vivo antimicrobial activity of self-assembled melittin nanoparticles: A comparative study with melittin peptide. *Colloids and Surfaces. B, Biointerfaces*, *226*, 113331. doi:10.1016/j.colsurfb.2023.113331 PMID:37150105

Tran, V. N., Strnad, O., Šuman, J., Veverková, T., Sukupová, A., Cejnar, P., Hynek, R., Kronusová, O., Šach, J., Kaštánek, P., & Viktorová, J. (2023). Cannabidiol nanoemulsion for eye treatment – Anti-inflammatory, wound healing activity and its bioavailability using in vitro human corneal substitute. *International Journal of Pharmaceutics*, *643*, 123202. doi:10.1016/j.ijpharm.2023.123202 PMID:37406946

Turrina, C., Schoenen, M., Milani, D., Klassen, A., Rojas Gonzaléz, D. M., Cvirn, G., Mela, P., Berensmeier, S., Slabu, I., & Schwaminger, S. P. (2023). Application of magnetic iron oxide nanoparticles: Thrombotic activity, imaging and cytocompatibility of silica-coated and carboxymethyl dextrane-coated particles. *Colloids and Surfaces. B, Biointerfaces*, *228*, 113428. doi:10.1016/j.colsurfb.2023.113428 PMID:37379701

van Eck, N. J., & Waltman, L. (2010). Software survey: VOSviewer, a computer program for bibliometric mapping. *Scientometrics*, *84*(2), 523–538. doi:10.100711192-009-0146-3 PMID:20585380

van Vliet, E. F., Knol, M. J., Schiffelers, R. M., Caiazzo, M., & Fens, M. H. A. M. (2023). Levodopa-loaded nanoparticles for the treatment of Parkinson's disease. *Journal of Controlled Release*, *360*, 212–224. doi:10.1016/j.jconrel.2023.06.026 PMID:37343725

Vaudagna, M. V., Aiassa, V., Marcotti, A., Pince Beti, M. F., Constantín, M. F., & Pérez, M. F., & Silvero C., M. J. (2023). Titanium Dioxide Nanoparticles in sunscreens and skin photo-damage. Development, synthesis and characterization of a novel biocompatible alternative based on their in vitro and in vivo study. *Journal of Photochemistry and Photobiology*, *15*, 100173. doi:10.1016/j.jpap.2023.100173

Vivanco-Benavides, L. E., Martínez-González, C. L., Mercado-Zúñiga, C., & Torres-Torres, C. (2022). Machine learning and materials informatics approaches in the analysis of physical properties of carbon nanotubes: A review. *Computational Materials Science*, *201*, 110939. doi:10.1016/j.commatsci.2021.110939

Vojdani, S., Ghaderian, S. M. H., Zali, A., Rakhshan, A., Oraee Yazdani, S., Poursheikhani, A., Zerehpoush, F. B., & Sharifi, G. (2021). Altered expression of EGFR and miR-34a derived from serum and tumoral tissue was associated with glioblastoma multiform. *Experimental and Molecular Pathology*, *121*, 104655. doi:10.1016/j.yexmp.2021.104655 PMID:34062187

Wang, M., Zhang, M., Hu, X., Wang, W., Zhang, Y., Zhang, L., & Wang, J. (2023). Lipid-functionalized gold nanorods with plug-to-direct mitochondria targeting ligand for synergetic photothermal-chemotherapy of tumor therapy. *European Journal of Pharmaceutics and Biopharmaceutics*, *185*, 71–81. doi:10.1016/j.ejpb.2023.02.010 PMID:36828240

Wang, X., Meng, X., Mao, K., Chen, H., Cong, X., Liu, F., Wang, J., Liu, S., Xin, Y., Zhu, G., Tan, H., Yang, Y.-G., & Sun, T. (2023). Maleimide as the PEG end-group promotes macrophage-targeted drug delivery of PEGylated nanoparticles in vivo by enhancing interaction with circulating erythrocytes. *Biomaterials*, *300*, 122187. doi:10.1016/j.biomaterials.2023.122187 PMID:37302279

Wang, Y., Ji, J.-Y., Guo, K., Zhang, T., Zhong, X.-C., Zhuang, Z.-M., Zhong, Y.-F., Lin, X.-F., Du, Y.-Z., Chen, J., & Tan, W.-Q. (2023). Gene liposome nanocomplex-loaded dermal substitute promotes diabetic chronic wound healing and angiogenesis in rat. *Biomedicine and Pharmacotherapy*, *163*, 114794. doi:10.1016/j.biopha.2023.114794 PMID:37121150

Wang, Y., Yuan, K., Shang, Z., Tan, G., Zhong, Q., He, Y., Miao, G., Lai, K., Li, Y., & Wang, X. (2023). Construction of nanohydrogels for enhanced delivery of hydrophilic and hydrophobic drugs and improving chemotherapy efficacy. *European Polymer Journal*, *186*, 111838. doi:10.1016/j.eurpolymj.2023.111838

Wang, Z., Ma, W., Fu, X., Qi, Y., Zhao, Y., & Zhang, S. (2023). Development and applications of mRNA treatment based on lipid nanoparticles. *Biotechnology Advances*, *65*, 108130. doi:10.1016/j.biotechadv.2023.108130 PMID:36933868

Wei, C., Xu, Y., Shen, Q., Li, R., Xiao, X., Saw, P. E., & Xu, X. (2023). Role of long non-coding RNAs (lncRNAs) in cancer: From subcellular localization to nanoparticles (NPs)-mediated targeted regulation. *Molecular Therapy. Nucleic Acids*, *33*, 774–793. doi:10.1016/j.omtn.2023.07.009 PMID:37655045

Windell, D. L., Mourabit, S., Moger, J., Owen, S. F., Winter, M. J., & Tyler, C. R. (2023). The influence of size and surface chemistry on the bioavailability, tissue distribution and toxicity of gold nanoparticles in zebrafish (*Danio rerio*). *Ecotoxicology and Environmental Safety*, *260*, 115019. doi:10.1016/j.ecoenv.2023.115019 PMID:37269610

Wu, B., Feng, J., Zeng, T., Guo, Q., Zhang, Z., Ding, C., Tian, B., & Sai, S. (2022). Flurbiprofen loaded thermosensitive nanohydrogel for ophthalmic anti-inflammatory therapy. *Journal of Drug Delivery Science and Technology*, *70*, 103253. doi:10.1016/j.jddst.2022.103253

Wu, J., Du, X., Zhang, D., Cui, J., Zhang, X., Duan, X., Trant, J. F., & Li, Y. (2023). A nanodiamond chemotherapeutic folate receptor-targeting prodrug with triggerable drug release. *International Journal of Pharmaceutics*, *630*, 122432. doi:10.1016/j.ijpharm.2022.122432 PMID:36435503

Wu, S., Gan, T., Xie, L., Deng, S., Liu, Y., Zhang, H., Hu, X., & Lei, L. (2022). Antibacterial performance of graphene oxide/alginate-based antisense hydrogel for potential therapeutic application in *Staphylococcus aureus* infection. *Biomaterials Advances*, *141*, 213121. doi:10.1016/j.bioadv.2022.213121 PMID:36162343

Xu, C., Dobson, H. E., Yu, M., Gong, W., Sun, X., Park, K. S., Kennedy, A., Zhou, X., Xu, J., Xu, Y., Tai, A. W., Lei, Y. L., & Moon, J. J. (2023). STING agonist-loaded mesoporous manganese-silica nanoparticles for vaccine applications. *Journal of Controlled Release*, *357*, 84–93. doi:10.1016/j.jconrel.2023.03.036 PMID:36948420

Xu, C., Li, S., Chen, J., Wang, H., Li, Z., Deng, Q., Li, J., Wang, X., Xiong, Y., Zhang, Z., Yang, X., & Li, Z. (2023). Doxorubicin and erastin co-loaded hydroxyethyl starch-polycaprolactone nanoparticles for synergistic cancer therapy. *Journal of Controlled Release*, *356*, 256–271. doi:10.1016/j.jconrel.2023.03.001 PMID:36871643

Xu, J., & Chow, E. K.-H. (2023). Biomedical applications of nanodiamonds: From drug-delivery to diagnostics. *SLAS Technology*, *28*(4), 214–222. doi:10.1016/j.slast.2023.03.007 PMID:37004790

Yang, X., Mo, W., Shi, Y., Fang, X., Xu, Y., He, X., & Xu, Y. (2023). Fumaria officinalis-loaded chitosan nanoparticles dispersed in an alginate hydrogel promote diabetic wounds healing by upregulating VEGF, TGF-β, and b-FGF genes: A preclinical investigation. *Heliyon*, *9*(7), e17704. doi:10.1016/j.heliyon.2023.e17704 PMID:37519642

Yasmin Begum, M. (2023). Co-loading of doxorubicin and gemcitabine on folic acid functionalized carbon nanotubes; a molecular dynamics simulation study. *Journal of Molecular Liquids*, *384*, 122244. doi:10.1016/j.molliq.2023.122244

Yeom, J.-H., Shin, E., Jin, H., Liu, H., Luo, Y., Nam, Y., Ryu, M., Song, W., Chi, H., Kim, J., Lee, K., & Bae, J. (2023). Aptamer-conjugated gold nanoparticles platform as the intracellular delivery of antibodies for cancer therapy. *Journal of Industrial and Engineering Chemistry*, *126*, 480–491. doi:10.1016/j.jiec.2023.06.036

Ying, N., Lin, X., Xie, M., & Zeng, D. (2022). Effect of surface ligand modification on the properties of anti-tumor nanocarrier. *Colloids and Surfaces. B, Biointerfaces*, *220*, 112944. doi:10.1016/j.colsurfb.2022.112944 PMID:36274398

Yingngam, B. (2023a). Chapter 11 - Modern solvent-free microwave extraction with essential oil optimization and structure-activity relationships. In R. Atta ur (Ed.), Studies in Natural Products Chemistry (Vol. 77, pp. 365-420): Elsevier. doi:10.1016/B978-0-323-91294-5.00011-7

Yingngam, B. (2023b). New Drug Discovery. In M. S. Aslam & M. A. Ahmad (Eds.), *Multidisciplinary Applications of Natural Science for Drug Discovery and Integrative Medicine* (pp. 134–184). IGI Global. doi:10.4018/978-1-6684-9463-9.ch005

Yingngam, B., Chiangsom, A., Pharikarn, P., Vonganakasame, K., Kanoknitthiran, V., Rungseevijitprapa, W., & Prasitpuriprecha, C. (2019). Optimization of menthol-loaded nanocapsules for skin application using the response surface methodology. *Journal of Drug Delivery Science and Technology*, *53*, 101138. doi:10.1016/j.jddst.2019.101138

Younas, A., Dong, Z., Hou, Z., Asad, M., Li, M., & Zhang, N. (2023). A chitosan/fucoidan nanoparticle-loaded pullulan microneedle patch for differential drug release to promote wound healing. *Carbohydrate Polymers*, *306*, 120593. doi:10.1016/j.carbpol.2023.120593 PMID:36746584

Yu, G., He, X., Li, X., & Wu, Y. (2022). Driving neoantigen-based cancer vaccines for personalized immunotherapy into clinic: A burdensome journey to promising land. *Biomedicine and Pharmacotherapy*, *153*, 113464. doi:10.1016/j.biopha.2022.113464 PMID:36076493

Yuan, H., Zhou, L., Qi, Z., Zhang, C., & Wang, C. (2022). Preparation of pH-responsive solanesol-based poly (glutamic acid) micellar carrier for doxorubicin delivery. *Materials Today. Communications*, *33*, 104800. doi:10.1016/j.mtcomm.2022.104800

Yuan, L., Chen, Q., Riviere, J. E., & Lin, Z. (2023). Pharmacokinetics and tumor delivery of nanoparticles. *Journal of Drug Delivery Science and Technology*, *83*, 104404. doi:10.1016/j.jddst.2023.104404 PMID:38037664

Zamani, P., Mashreghi, M., Rezazade Bazaz, M., Zargari, S., Alizadeh, F., Dorrigiv, M., Abdoli, A., Aminianfar, H., Hatamipour, M., Zarqui, J., Behboodiar, S., Samsami, Y., Sokhangouy, S. K., Sefidbakht, Y., Uskoković, V., Rezayat, S. M., Jaafari, M. R., & Mozaffari-Jovin, S. (2023). Characterization of stability, safety and immunogenicity of the mRNA lipid nanoparticle vaccine Iribovax® against COVID-19 in nonhuman primates. *Journal of Controlled Release*, *360*, 316–334. doi:10.1016/j.jconrel.2023.06.025 PMID:37355212

Zhang, H., Gu, Z., Li, W., Guo, L., Wang, L., Guo, L., Wang, L., Guo, L., Ma, S., Han, B., & Chang, J. (2022). pH-sensitive O-carboxymethyl chitosan/sodium alginate nanohydrogel for enhanced oral delivery of insulin. *International Journal of Biological Macromolecules*, *223*, 433–445. doi:10.1016/j.ijbiomac.2022.10.274 PMID:36347366

Zhang, H., Wang, T., He, W., Wang, J., & Li, X. (2022). Irinotecan-loaded ROS-responsive liposomes containing thioether phosphatidylcholine for improving anticancer activity. *Journal of Drug Delivery Science and Technology*, *71*, 103321. doi:10.1016/j.jddst.2022.103321

Zhang, X., Wei, Z., Ding, Z., Lv, W., Li, J., Li, X., Liu, H., Yu, P., Yang, X., & Gan, L. (2023). Boosting doxil-based chemoimmunotherapy via reprogramming tumor-associated macrophages. *Chemical Engineering Journal*, *451*, 138971. doi:10.1016/j.cej.2022.138971

Zhang, Z., Fu, X., Wang, Y., Wang, J., Feng, S., Zhao, Z., Zheng, L., Zhang, J., Zhang, X., & Peng, Y. (2023). In vivo anti-hepatitis B activity of Artemisia argyi essential oil-loaded nanostructured lipid carriers. Study of its mechanism of action by network pharmacology and molecular docking. *Phytomedicine*, *116*, 154848. doi:10.1016/j.phymed.2023.154848 PMID:37163901

Zhu, H., Yang, C., & Ma, K. (2022). Nanovesicles for transdermal drug delivery. In A. K. Nayak, M. S. Hasnain, T. M. Aminabhavi, & V. P. Torchilin (Eds.), *Applications of Nanovesicular Drug Delivery* (pp. 103–114). Academic Press., doi:10.1016/B978-0-323-91865-7.00012-2

Zhu, H., Zhang, L., Kou, F., Zhao, J., Lei, J., & He, J. (2024). Targeted therapeutic effects of oral magnetically driven pectin nanoparticles containing chlorogenic acid on colon cancer. *Particuology*, *84*, 53–59. doi:10.1016/j.partic.2023.02.021

Chapter 3
Nanotechnology and Its Applications in Biomedical Sciences

Niteshkumar Agrawal
Pillai College of Engineering (Autonomous), Navi Mumbai, India

Moutusi De
Pillai College of Engineering (Autonomous), Navi Mumbai, India

Shreedevi Avinash Kulkarni
Pillai College of Engineering (Autonomous), Navi Mumbai, India

Lokendra Singh
Koneru Lakshmaiah Educational Foundation, Vaddeswaram, India

S. K. Tripathy
National Institute of Technology, Silchar, India

ABSTRACT

The use of nanotechnology products in biomedicine has led to the emergence of a hybrid science known as nano-biotechnology. Due to the nanoscale nature of most biological systems, nanoscale materials integrate well into biomedical devices. In response to certain stimuli, highly ordered bottom-up nano-structured materials exhibit specific behaviours. Nanomaterial applications are tuned by surface chemistry and physics. This chapter provides an overview of the use of metallic, metal oxide, and carbon nanoparticles for specific biomedical applications. It also discusses liposomes and nano-patterned flat surfaces. A challenge is determining the effects of nanomaterials on biological systems. However, a detailed understanding of nanomaterial potential toxicity is needed to take advantage of their potential applications in medicine. To minimize false results, it is important to interpret the relationship between toxicity and physicochemical properties cautiously.

DOI: 10.4018/979-8-3693-0448-8.ch003

INTRODUCTION

Nanotechnology is gaining wider application in the biomedical sciences, and it has resulted in the development of two new cross-disciplinary fields, nano-biology, and nano-biomedicine. In Biomedical Nanotechnology and Its Applications, the authors provide a brief overview of the research that has been conducted so far (Ramos et al. 2017). A hybrid science known as nano-biotechnology has developed out of the use of nanotechnology products in biomedicine. Nanoscale materials integrate well into biomedical devices due to their nanoscale nature. Highly ordered nanostructures (NSs) exhibit specific behaviors when exposed to certain stimuli (Zhao et al. 2002). Surface chemistry and physics have a significant influence on nanomaterials (NMs) applications. Materials with different biological properties and functions can be produced by modifying NMs surfaces in different ways (Gulumian et al. 2021). Physiological conditions facilitate the solubility of these materials. By applying novel materials to Nanobiotechnology, new opportunities have been created (Jeevanandam et al. 2018). Implantable technologies, drug delivery, and diagnosis all rely on these materials. Due to their chemical and physical properties, they are used in diagnostic devices, biosensors, bioimaging devices, and drug delivery systems (Zhou et al. 2015, Cicha et al. 2022). The field of nanotoxicology is also discussed, which examines how nanostructured materials affect their surfaces as well as the toxicology of these particles (Wu et al. 2023). Nanoparticles (NPs) and nano-patterned flat surfaces for diagnostics, biosensing, bioimaging devices, medication delivery, immunosensing, and bone substitutes are explored here using inorganic (metal, metal oxide, and carbon nanotube) and organic (carbon nanotube, liposome) NPs (Joseph et al. 2023). In recent years, NMs have had various advantages in the bioimaging arena. Due to near-infrared (NIR) excitation, visible emission lines with high signal-to-background ratio, and long fluorescence lifetimes, non-invasive and deep tissue penetration are preferred (Kashyap et al. 2023, Gholami et al. 2020). These imaging modalities are summarized in Figure 1.

Biomedical applications of metal, metal oxide, and carbon NPs are explored in this chapter. It also discusses liposomes and nano-patterned flat surfaces. NMs affect biological systems. To benefit from NMs potential application in medicine, however, an in-depth knowledge of toxicity is required. To minimize false results, it is important to interpret Physicochemical properties and toxicity carefully (Zielińska et al. 2020, Zhang et al. 2012). Nanotechnology is used in biomedical sciences for various reasons, primarily due to its unique properties and potential applications at

the nanoscale (Khan, Saeed, and Khan 2019). The properties and behaviors of materials at this scale are distinct from those of bulk materials (Guisbiers, Mejía-Rosales, and Leonard Deepak 2012). Nanotechnology aims to understand and utilize these properties to design and create new materials, devices, and systems with enhanced functionalities (Haleem et al. 2023). Key features and concepts of nanotechnology include viz. (i) NMs: Nanotechnology involves the synthesis, characterization, and manipulation of nanoscale materials. These materials have precise properties and functions, such as improved strength, conductivity, reactivity, or optical properties. Examples of NMs include NPs, nanotubes, nanowires, and thin films (Chausali, Saxena, and Prasad 2023), (ii) Nanotechnology employs both bottom-up and top-down approaches. Bottom-up tactics involve building structures atom by atom to create nanoscale materials with desired properties. Top-down approaches involve scaling down larger structures or materials to the nanoscale using techniques like lithography or etching (Jitendra Pal et al. 2020), (iii) Size-dependent Properties: At the nanoscale, materials exhibit unique properties. These properties can include enhanced mechanical strength, altered optical properties, different electrical conductivity, and modified chemical reactivity (Joseph Adeyemi et al. 2018), (iv) Characterization Techniques: Advanced

Figure 1. An overview of the main imaging modalities used in biomedical applications of NMs (Chen et al. 2013)

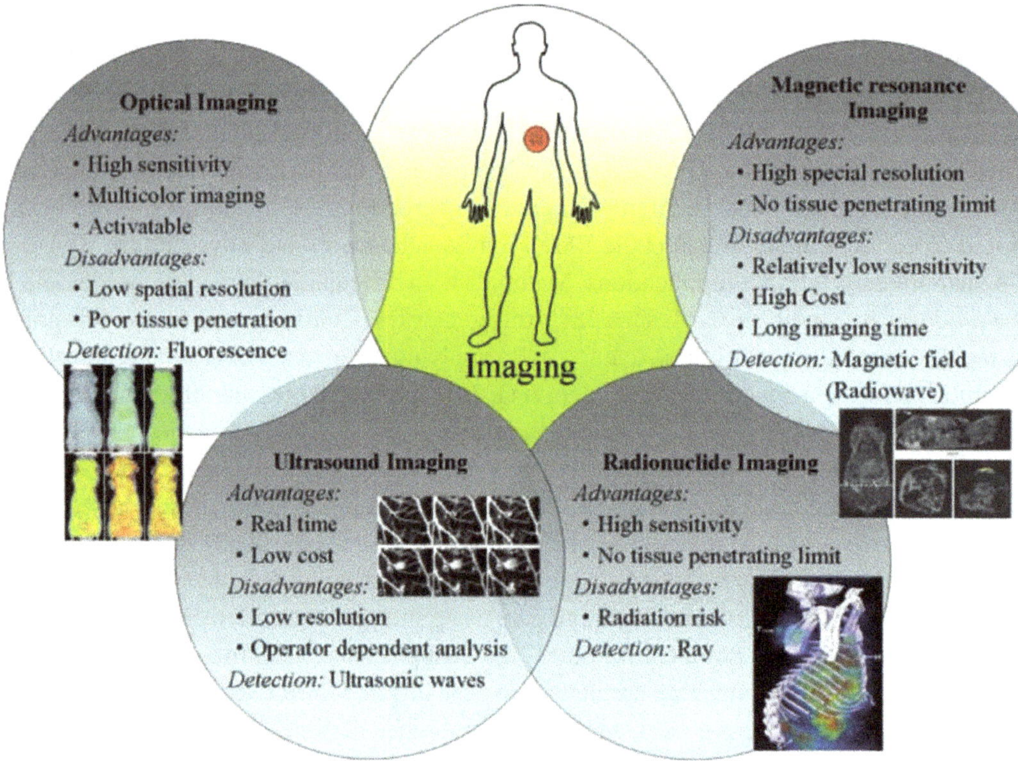

characterization techniques are crucial for understanding and analyzing nanoscale materials and structures. Techniques such as scanning electron microscopy (SEM), transmission EM (TEM), atomic force microscopy (AFM), and spectroscopic methods provide insights into the structure, composition, and behavior of NMs (Venkateshaiah et al. 2020), (v) Interdisciplinary Nature: Nanotechnology combines knowledge and expertise from various scientific disciplines. This interdisciplinary approach allows for innovation and collaboration across fields to address complex challenges and develop novel applications, (vi) Applications: Nanotechnology has diverse applications across numerous sectors. In electronics, it enables the development of smaller, faster, and more energy-efficient devices. In medicine, nanotechnology contributes to targeted drug delivery, imaging agents, biosensors, and regenerative medicine. Other areas of application include energy, environmental remediation, agriculture, information technology, and more (Zhu et al. 2020), and (vii) Ethical and Safety Considerations: As nanotechnology advances, ethical considerations, and safety concerns arise. The potential impact on health, atmosphere, and ethical aspects of nanotechnology research and applications requires careful evaluation and regulation to ensure responsible and safe practices (Agrawal, Saha, Kumar, Singh, Zhang, Jha, et al. 2020). The diverse sensors used in biosensing are shown in Fig. 2. Nanotechnology holds immense promise for advancing technology, improving healthcare, and addressing global challenges. It continues to drive innovation and contribute to various fields, concrete the way for groundbreaking discoveries and future applications (Agrawal, Zhang, Saha, Kumar, Pu, et al. 2020). Here are some key reasons why nanotechnology is employed in the biomedical field:

Drug Delivery: Nanotechnology offers opportunities for targeted drug delivery. NPs can be engineered to encapsulate drugs and deliver them directly to specific cells or tissues in the body. This targeted delivery approach enhances therapeutic efficacy, reduces side effects, and improves patient compliance (Kumar et al., 2022).

Disease Treatment and Therapeutics: Nanotechnology offers new avenues for the development of innovative therapeutics. NPs can be designed to bypass biological barriers, deliver drugs to specific disease sites, or penetrate cells more efficiently (Sim and Wong 2021). Additionally, nanotechnology-based approaches, such as photothermal therapy and magnetic hyperthermia, utilize NPs to selectively heat and destroy cancer cells while minimizing damage to healthy tissues (Patra et al. 2018).

Imaging and Diagnostics: NPs can be used as contrast agents in medical imaging techniques viz. MRI, CT scan, and PET. These NPs can enhance the imaging quality, enable early disease detection, and facilitate the monitoring of disease progression or treatment response (Estelrich, Sánchez-Martín, and Busquets 2015).

Tissue Engineering: Nanotechnology plays an important role in tissue engineering and regenerative medicine. Nanoscale scaffolds and matrices are designed to mimic the structure and function of native tissues, differentiation, and tissue regeneration (Shi et al. 2010). NMs also offer the potential to stimulate specific cellular behaviors and promote tissue healing (Chun et al. 2013).

Biosensors and Diagnostics: Nano-sensors and nanodevices can detect and measure specific molecules or biomarkers in biological samples. These devices can enable rapid and sensitive disease diagnosis viz. cancer or infectious diseases, by detecting disease-specific biomarkers in body fluids (Bohunicky and Mousa 2010).

Therapeutics and Theranostics: NPs can be engineered to possess therapeutic properties themselves or carry therapeutic agents such as drugs or genes (Mundekkad and Cho 2022). These NPs can selectively target diseased cells, deliver therapeutic payloads, and monitor treatment

response simultaneously, combining diagnostics and therapeutics into a single system known as theranostics (Yetisgin et al. 2020).

Disease Monitoring: Nanotechnology-based sensors can continuously monitor physiological parameters, biomarkers, or drug levels within the body. These sensors provide real-time data, enabling personalized medicine, remote patient monitoring, and early detection of disease progression or complications (Lokendra et al. 2021).

Nanoscale Imaging and Manipulation: Nanotechnology tools and techniques, such as AFM and nanomanipulation, allow researchers to study biological structures, cells, and molecules at the nanoscale. This capability aids in understanding fundamental biological processes and enables the development of novel therapeutic interventions (Kiio and Park 2020).

Biosensors and Point-of-Care Devices: Nanotechnology enables the development of the biosensor for rapid and accurate biomarkers detection, pathogens, and disease-related molecules. NMs, such as quantum dots or nanowires, enable real-time monitoring and personalized healthcare (Agrawal, Zhang, Saha, Kumar, Kaushik, et al. 2020).

Biomaterials and Implants: NMs are used to develop advanced biomaterials for medical implants and devices. Nanostructured coatings improve the biocompatibility and durability of implants, reducing the risk of rejection or infection (Zhang and Liu 2019). Nanotechnology also enables the integration of sensors and drug delivery systems into implants, enhancing their functionality and patient outcomes (Salhi et al. 2016).

Figure 2. Different types of sensors used in biomedical sensing
(Naresh and Lee 2021a)

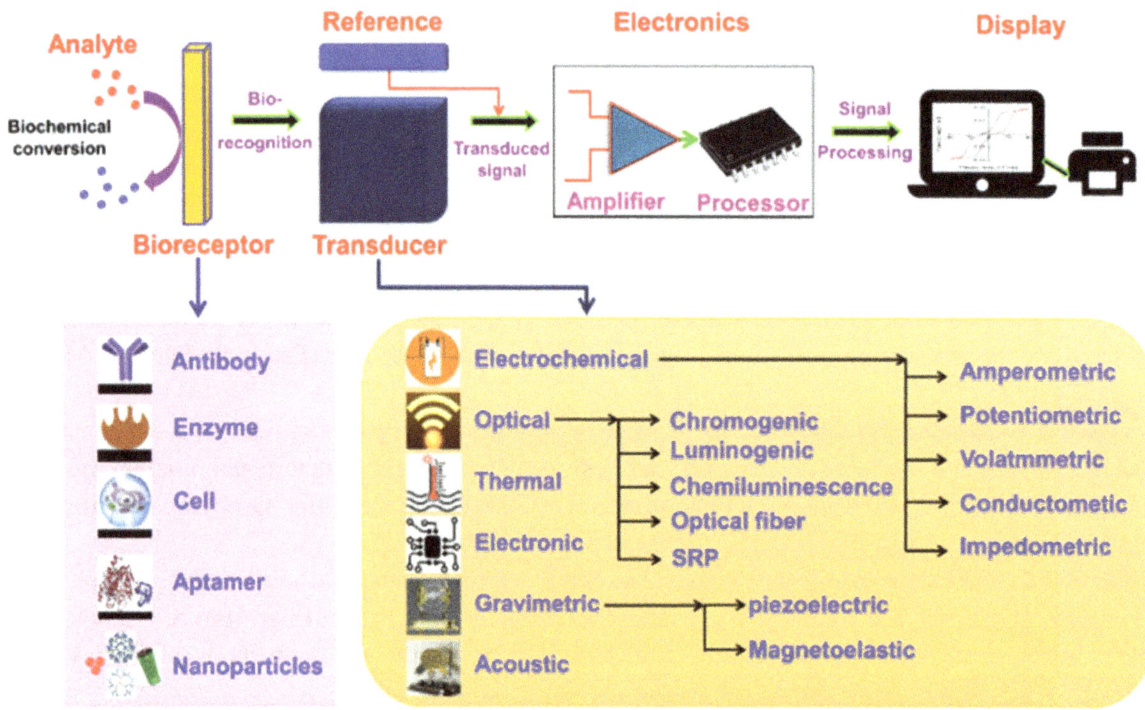

NanoBodies (NBs): It has many unique properties, such as small size, excellent solubility, superior stability, quick clearance from the blood, and deep tissue penetration. This has led to the development of NBs as promising diagnostic and therapeutic tools for diseases. The use of NBs with biosensors offers different advantages to the conventionally used antibodies (Jin et al. 2023). Although these antibodies can be used for the diagnosis. Thus, NBs can eliminate these disadvantages and make them attractive to be used with biosensors. Other than the methods of detection mentioned above, the nanobodies can be tagged with fluorescence material or radioactive materials, and based on the fluorescence or the radioactivity the imaging process is done for disease imaging, biomarker detection, and disease progression monitoring (Mirón-Barroso, Domènech, and Trigueros 2021).

Gene Therapy and Gene Editing

With the latest advancements in molecular genetics have created a better understanding of the genetic basis of many pathologies and thereby led to the development of new therapies. Gene therapy repairs or rebuilds defective genetic material in cells to treat disease. By correcting defective genes responsible for disease development by delivering repaired genes or by replacing incorrect ones, gene therapy is used for treating or preventing genetic disorders. To replace nonfunctional genes, normal genes are usually inserted into a nonspecific location within the genome to correct faulty genes. The goal of gene therapy is to alter gene expression instead of administering drugs. The goal of genome editing, or gene editing, is to understand gene function and develop ways to treat genetic diseases and acquired illnesses by editing genes in living organisms. Following observations that yeast can perform homologous recombination naturally, scientists developed this technique in the late 1970s (Jin et al. 2023). Genomic sequences corresponding to the portion of the genome that will be edited must be synthesized and isolated to perform homologous recombination in a laboratory (Mirón-Barroso, Domènech, and Trigueros 2021). By injecting the fragments or using chemicals, these isolated fragments can be taken up by individual cells. As soon as these fragments are inside a cell, they can recombine with the cell's DNA to replace the target (Soleimani et al. 2016).

Gene Augmentation

An alternative method involves delivering the correct gene via a delivery vector to replace the mutant gene that doesn't function. There are several kinds of therapeutic nucleic acids, including DNA, mRNA, mRNA analogy, and oligonucleotides. Because RNA does not need to be delivered into the nucleus, it has a low risk of insertion into the host genome (Mirón-Barroso, Domènech, and Trigueros 2021). In contrast, it is both unstable and immunogenic, which are major disadvantages. In recent years, plasmid DNA has become the most popular method of introducing genes due to its highly stable nature. Once in the nucleus, plasmid genes remain episomal because plasmids rapidly chromaticism once internalized (Jin et al. 2023).

Overall, nanotechnology offers unprecedented opportunities to revolutionize biomedical sciences by providing precise control and manipulation at the nanoscale, thereby addressing key challenges in drug delivery, diagnostics, tissue engineering, and therapeutics.

ROLE OF NANOMATERIALS IN NANOTECHNOLOGY

Nanotechnology focuses on designing, structures, and systems that are fabricated from atoms and molecules at a nanoscale, i.e., with dimensions of 100 nm or less. It is the design, manipulation, and manufacture of materials at the nanoscale that constitutes nanotechnology (Agrawal, Saha, Kumar, Singh, Zhang, and Kumar 2020). NMs are materials manufactured using nanotechnology. NMs (typically between 1-100 nm) are the building blocks of nanotechnology (Singh, Agrawal, Saha, Singh, et al. 2022). NMs play a critical role in nanotechnology because they are used to make new devices, and systems with unprecedented properties and functions such as improved sensing, imaging, and energy conversion, to name a few. They are used in electronics, medicine, energy, and environmental sustainability field (Surana et al. 2019). Additionally, the development of NMs is crucial for addressing some of the world's most pressing challenges, such as energy and water shortages, pollution, and disease outbreaks. There are several types of NMs used in nanotechnology. Here are a few examples:

Nanoparticles- These are typically spherical particles with a diameter ranging from 1-100 nm. They are used in drug delivery, imaging, and energy storage (Agrawal et al. 2022).

Nanotubes- These are cylindrical structures with a diameter of a few nm to hundreds of nm and a length of several μm to a few mm. They are used in electronics, sensors, and energy storage.

Nanowires- These are ultra-thin wires with diameters of 1-100 nm. They are used in electronics, solar cells, and biosensors (Ha et al. 2022).

Figure 3. Classification of NMs according to their dimensionality
(Naresh and Lee 2021b)

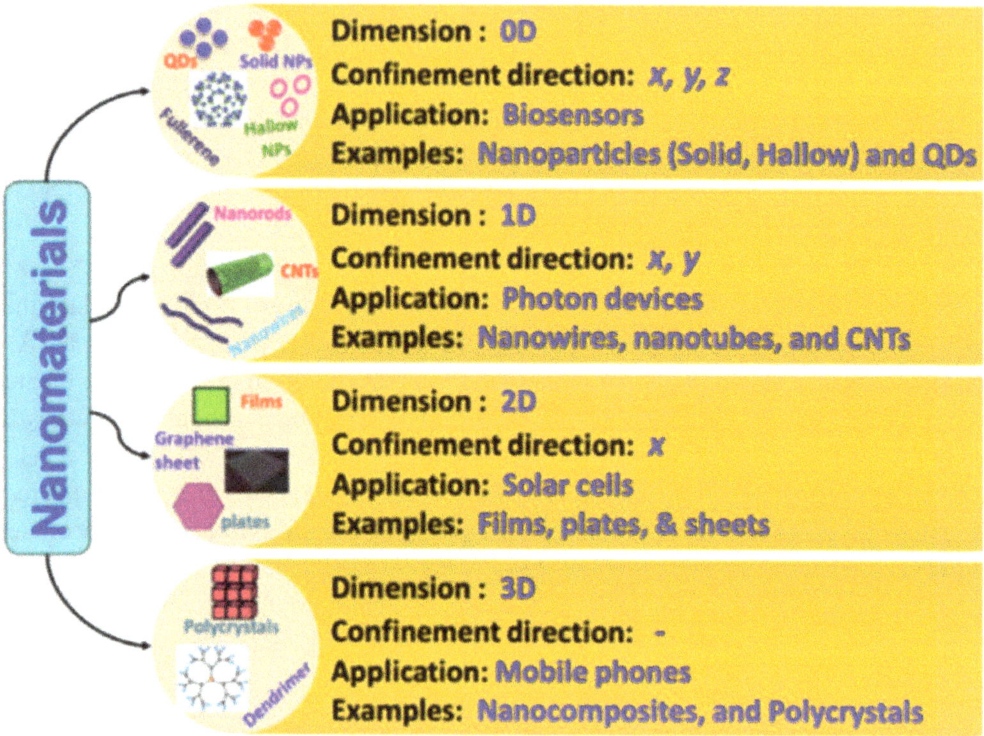

Quantum Dots- These are semiconductor nanocrystals with a diameter of a few nm. They have unique optical properties, making them useful for imaging, lighting, and solar energy (Singh, Iadicicco, et al. 2022).

Nanocomposites- They consist of two or more different NMs. They can have superior mechanical, and electrical properties and are used in applications such as catalysis, energy storage, and coatings (Chack et al. 2013). The classification of NMs according to their dimensionality is shown in Figure 4. These are just a few examples of the types of NMs used in nanotechnology. There are many more, each with its unique properties and potential applications. NMs have unique properties at the nanoscale due to their high surface area-to-volume ratio. Some of the potential applications of NMs in nanotechnology include:

Nano-sensors: NMs can be used in the development of various nano-sensors due to their high sensitivity and selectivity. For example, carbon nanotubes can be used to detect changes in pH levels, while metal nanowires can be used to detect temperature changes (Cash and Clark 2010).

Drug Delivery: NMs can be used to deliver drugs to specific parts of the body. NPs made of biocompatible materials can be used to increase the bioavailability of drugs and improve drug efficacy (Patra et al. 2018).

Energy Storage: NMs can be used in energy storage devices viz. batteries and supercapacitors. This is because NPs can store more electrical charge than larger particles (Adedoja, Sadiku, and Hamam 2023).

Catalysis: NMs can be used as catalysts in various chemical reactions. This is because they have a large surface area for reacting with other compounds (Huang et al. 2020).

Figure 4. Characterization of NPs based on dimensions, morphology, composition, aggregation state, and charge
(McClements and Xiao 2017)

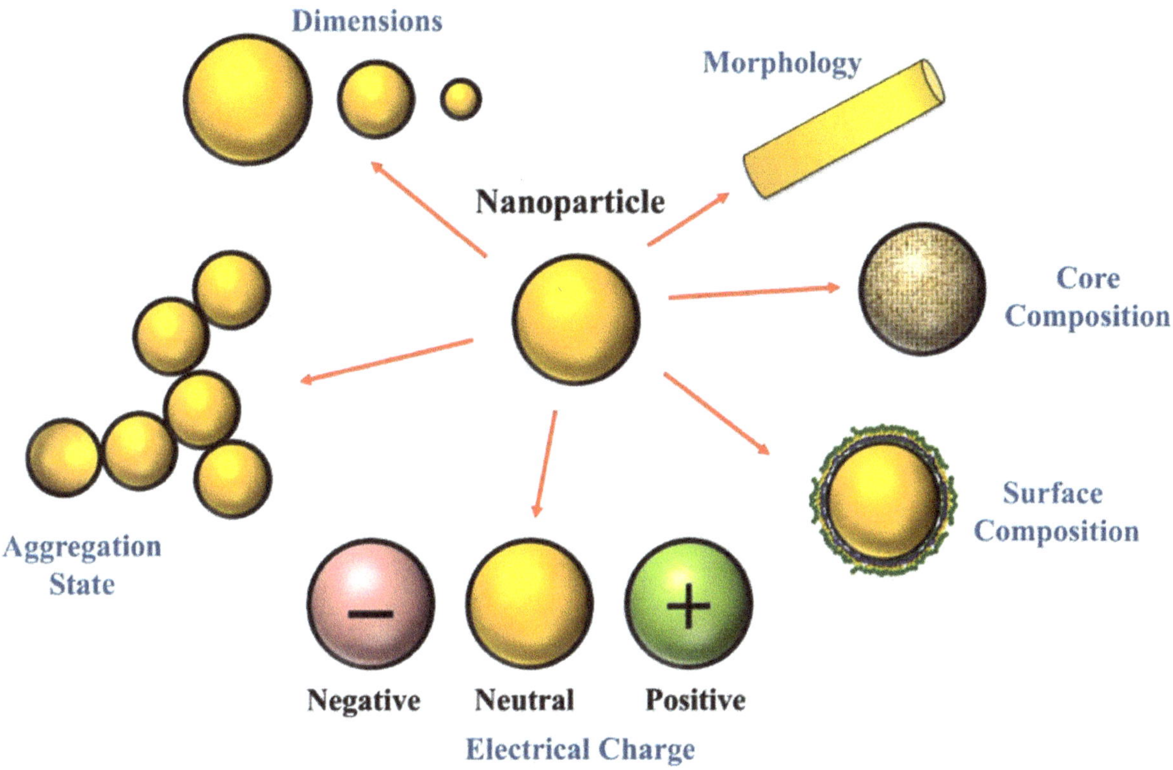

Water Purification: NMs can be used to purify water by removing impurities such as heavy metals and bacteria. NPs made of materials such as graphene oxide and silver are effective in removing contaminants from water (Ethaib et al. 2022).

A wide range of nanotechnology applications can benefit from NMs' unique properties.

APPLICATION OF NANOTECHNOLOGY IN BIOMEDICAL SCIENCE

Nanotechnology finds numerous applications in biomedical science, leading to advancements in diagnostics, therapeutics, regenerative medicine, and more. Here are some specific applications of nanotechnology in biomedical science:

NPs-based Drug Delivery: NPs can be engineered to carry and deliver drugs to specific targets. Functionalization of NPs with targeting ligands to selectively deliver drugs to diseased cells or tissues, and reduce side effects (Singh, Agrawal, and Saha 2021).

Nanoscale Imaging Agents: NPs enable the improved visualization of biological structures (Nune et al. 2009). QDs, iron oxide NPs, and AuNPs are examples of NMs used as imaging agents for fluorescence imaging, MRI, and CT imaging, respectively. These NPs provide enhanced sensitivity, resolution, and multiplexing capabilities for diagnostic imaging (Han et al. 2019).

Biosensors and Diagnostics: Nanotechnology-based biosensors offer highly sensitive and specific detection of biomarkers and disease-related molecules. NMs, such as carbon nanotubes, graphene, or metallic NPs, can be used to construct biosensors that detect minute quantities of analytes. These biosensors find applications in early disease detection, monitoring treatment responses, and point-of-care diagnostics (Kumar et al. 2020).

Tissue Engineering and Regenerative Medicine: Nanotechnology plays a significant role in tissue engineering and regenerative medicine. Nanoscale scaffolds made of biocompatible materials provide a framework for cells to grow and regenerate damaged tissues (Funda et al. 2020, Saxena et al. 2023).

Nanomedicine and Cancer Therapy: Nanotechnology offers innovative approaches to cancer diagnosis and treatment (Singh 2019). Additionally, NMs can be used for photothermal therapy, where NPs convert light energy into heat to selectively destroy cancer cells. NPs-based systems also enable image-guided surgery, improving precision and outcomes in cancer treatment (Mundekkad and Cho 2022).

Antimicrobial Applications: NMs possess unique antimicrobial properties. Silver NPs, for example, exhibit potent antimicrobial activity against bacteria and fungi. These NPs can be incorporated into wound dressings, medical implants, or coatings to prevent infections. Nanotechnology-based approaches also offer new strategies for combating antibiotic-resistant bacteria by developing targeted therapies or drug delivery systems (Bruna et al. 2021).

Nanotechnology-Based Sensors for Biosensing Application

Nanotechnology-based sensors have revolutionized biosensing applications by offering high sensitivity, selectivity, and miniaturization. These sensors utilize NMs and nanoscale structures to detect and analyze biomolecules, pathogens, and other biological entities (Singh, Agrawal, Gola, et al. 2022). The different types of NMs-based nano-biosensors are presented in Fig. 5. Here are some examples of nanotechnology-based sensors for biosensing applications:

Nanoparticle-Based Biosensors

Metallic NPs, such as Au or AgNPs, are commonly used in biosensors. They can be functionalized with biomolecules viz. anti-bodies or DNA probes, to selectively bind. Changes in the NPs' optical properties, such as color or fluorescence, indicate the presence of the target, enabling sensitive detection. There are many uses for NMs, including the use of biomolecules as immobilizers, the use of bioactive species as amplifiers, and the detection of biomarkers using nanoprobes. NMs are used in biosensors according to their transduction mechanisms including electrochemical, optical, thermoelectric, etc.

Primary NPs (Gold and Silver) Based Biosensors

AuNPs are commonly used in biosensing applications owing to their unique optical and surface properties. They offer several advantages for biosensing, including high stability, biocompatibility, and ease of functionalization. Here are some key aspects and applications of AuNPs-based biosensors:

Surface Plasmon Resonance (SPR) Sensing: AuNPs exhibit a phenomenon called SPR, where the collective oscillation of electrons on the NPs surface interacts with incident light, resulting in enhanced absorption and scattering at specific wavelengths (Hong et al. 2012). The localized SPR (LSPR) of AuNPs can be tailored by controlling their size, shape, and surface chemistry. Changes in the LSPR are

Figure 5. Types of NMs-based biosensors (nano-biosensors)
(Naresh and Lee 2021b)

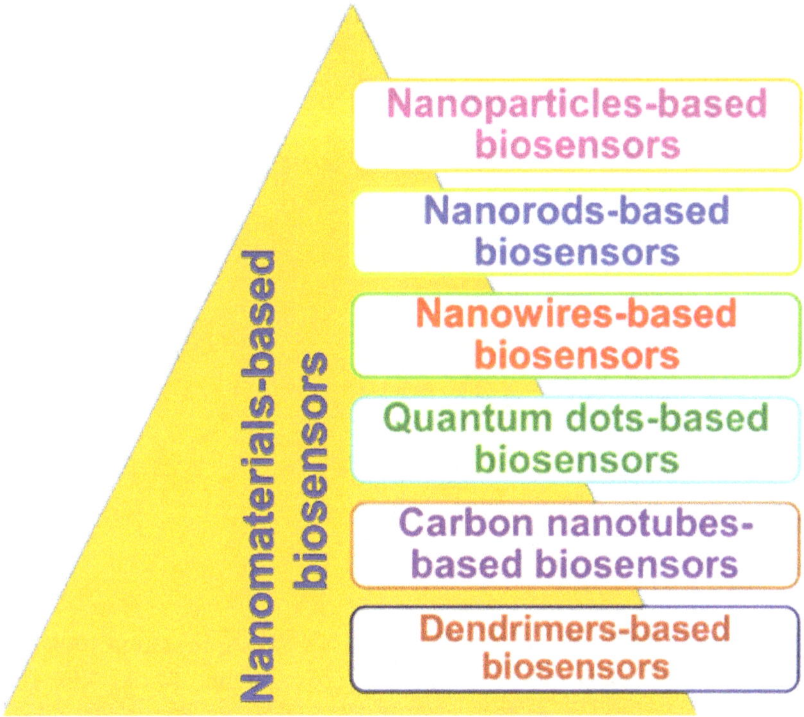

due to binding events or changes in the local environment (Kang et al. 2020, Akouibaa et al. 2022). The sensor chip on the prism is mounted on the SPR immunoassay as shown in schematic Fig. 6.

Colorimetric Assays: AuNPs can produce distinct color changes based on their size, shape, and aggregation state. Functionalizing gold NPs with precise recognition elements, viz. antibodies or DNA probes, allows them to bind to target analytes. The binding event induces aggregation or disassembly of the NPs, leading to a visible color change that can be observed with the naked eye or measured using spectrophotometric techniques. These colorimetric assays provide simple and rapid detection methods for various biomolecules, pathogens, and environmental analytes (López-Lorente 2021).

Lateral Flow Assays: AuNPs are commonly used in lateral flow assay platforms, also known as immunochromatographic assays or rapid diagnostic tests. In these assays, AuNPs are functionalized with capture probes, such as antibodies or aptamers, and immobilized on a test strip. The target analyte in the sample binds to the capture probes, forming a colored line on the strip, indicating a positive result. Lateral flow assays are widely used for PoC diagnostics and on-site testing due to their simplicity, and rapid results (Wang et al. 2021).

SERS-based Sensing: Surface-enhanced Raman scattering (SERS) can detect and characterize molecules based on their vibrational spectra. AuNPs can serve as excellent SERS substrates due

to their strong EM enhancement properties. By functionalizing AuNPs with Raman reporters and specific recognition elements, they can be used to detect and identify trace amounts of target analytes, including biomarkers, drugs, and environmental contaminants (Aldosari 2022).

Figure 6. The sensor chip on the prism is mounted on the SPR immunoassay schematic (Chen et al. 2023)

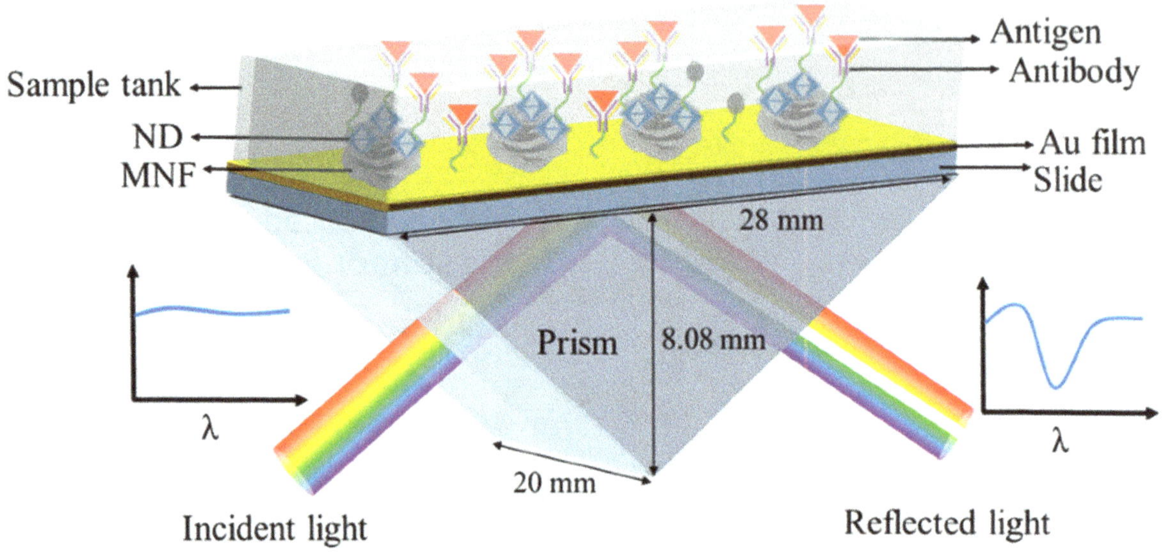

Biosensing Amplification Strategies: AuNPs also serve as amplification tools in biosensing. The presence of the target DNA induces the aggregation or crosslinking of gold NPs, resulting in a color change or enhanced signal amplification. This amplification strategy improves the sensitivity and detection limit of the biosensor (Israelsen, Hanson, and Vargis 2015).

AuNPs-based biosensors find applications in the medical, environmental, and bioanalytical research fields (Singh, Agrawal, Saha, and Kaushik 2022). Their unique properties, ease of functionalization, and compatibility with existing detection methods make them valuable tools for the sensitive and selective target detection of analytes in complex samples (Sapsford et al. 2006).

Carbon Nanotube-Based Biosensors

Carbon nanotubes (CNTs) have novel electrical properties, making them appropriate for biosensing applications. Functionalized CNTs can interact with target biomolecules, causing changes in their electrical conductivity. These changes can be measured by the presence of specific analytes, including proteins, DNA, or viruses.

Sensors functionalized with multiwalled CNTs and GO for histamine detection are reported by Zhang et al. 2023 in their recent study. Using LSPR to detect varying histamine concentrations, authors have developed an optical fiber biosensor that is humanoid-shaped and tapered in shape (HTOF) (Zhang et al. 2023, Chack, Agrawal, and Raghuwanshi 2014).

QDs-Based Biosensors

QDs are semiconductor nanocrystals with excellent fluorescence properties. QDs can be engineered to bind to target biomolecules, generating fluorescence signals upon binding. This fluorescence can be detected and quantified, enabling sensitive and multiplexed detection of various analytes simultaneously (Shao, Gao, and Yan 2011, Rizvi et al. 2010).

1.3.5. ***Nanowire-Based Biosensors***: Nanowires, typically made of silicon or metal oxides, offer high sensitivity and can be functionalized for biosensing applications. When target molecules bind to the nanowire surface, it induces changes in electrical conductivity or optical properties, allowing for their detection (Unser et al. 2015).

1.3.6. ***2D Material-Based Biosensors***: 2D materials, viz. graphene and GO, have excellent electrical and mechanical properties. Functionalized 2D materials can interact with biomolecules, leading to changes in their electrical conductivity or surface properties (Mayer and Hafner 2011).

1.3.7. ***Plasmonic Biosensors***: Plasmonic sensors utilize the unique properties of plasmons, which are a collective oscillation of electrons in metallic NSs. Plasmonic sensors can detect changes in the RI caused by the binding of biomolecules, leading to shifts in the plasmon resonance, which can be measured to determine the presence and concentration of analytes (Hill 2015, Sriram et al. 2015).

These are just a few examples of nanotechnology-based sensors for biosensing applications. These sensors offer advantages viz. high sensitivity, rapid response, and the potential for miniaturization, making them invaluable tools for biomedical research, diagnostics, environmental monitoring, and food safety. Continued advancements in nanotechnology will likely lead to even more sensitive and versatile biosensors in the future.

NANOPARTICLES-BASED IMMUNOSENSOR

Immunosensor is a biosensing device embedded with transducers, antibodies and that convert biochemical changes into measurable signals due to precise bio interaction. In an immunosensor specific immuno-reaction takes place between an antibody and its target antigen, as a result a stable immunocomplex is formed (Figure 7). Tremendous improvisation took place in immune-sensing technology when transducers were combined with NMs, like MNPs, metal-oxide NPs, QDs, CNTs, graphene, semiconductor NMs *etc.(de la Escosura-Muñiz, Parolo, and Merkoçi 2010)*. NPs incorporating immunosensors are showing superior sensitivity, resolution, selectivity, and rapid response for protein detection over conventional diagnostic systems. For their high sensitivity and specificity, these immunosensors have gained a lot of interest in rapid disease detection, clinical diagnosis, antibiotic detection, and industrial as well as environmental monitoring. Even label-free immunosensors have already proven themselves suitable for *PoC* analysis (Li et al. 2020). Due to the high electron transfer ability electroactive NPs are extremely useful in fabricating immunosensors. The sensing response of different transducers can be enhanced multiple times by coating them with a thin layer of electroactive NPs. Electroactive NPs are crucial for the transduction of quantifiable electrical signals thanks to their large surface area, high electron density, tunable electrical properties, high absorbance in the visible range, large power density,

high bandwidth, *etc. (de la Escosura-Muñiz, Parolo, and Merkoçi 2010, Hasanzadeh et al. 2017)*. IgG structured antibody is commonly used in immune-sensing assays. Antibody and antigen interaction takes place in an immunosensor (Figure 8) (de la Escosura-Muñiz, Parolo, and Merkoçi 2010). This kind of antibody-antigen interaction is too specific and able to identify antigens at the ppb level (Halkare et al. 2019, Chandra, Bharadwaj, and Mukherji 2017). Different immune-sensing technologies are discussed in the following section which are empowered by NMs. AuNPs characterization results are presented in Fig. 9.

Figure 7. Immunosensor and its field of applications

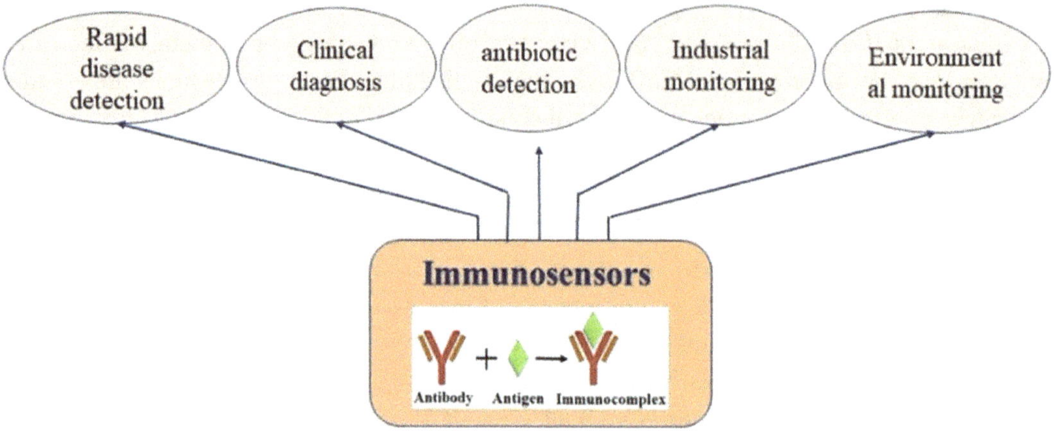

Figure 8. Immunosensor and functionalization of NP (I–V) functionalized NP preparation and (VI–X) biochemical treatment of Au-disk
(Domínguez-Aragón et al. 2023)

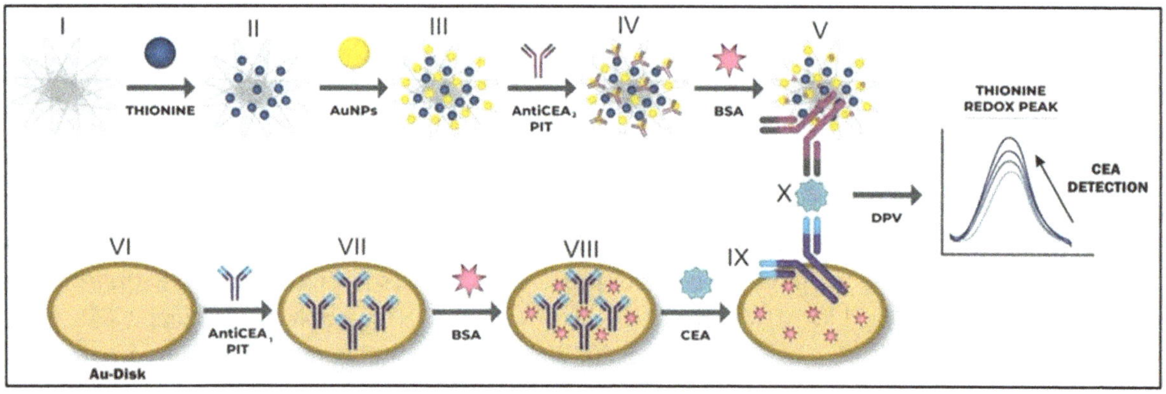

Figure 9. (i) TEM image of functionalized AuNPs and (ii) image of treated Au-disk
(Domínguez-Aragón et al. 2023)

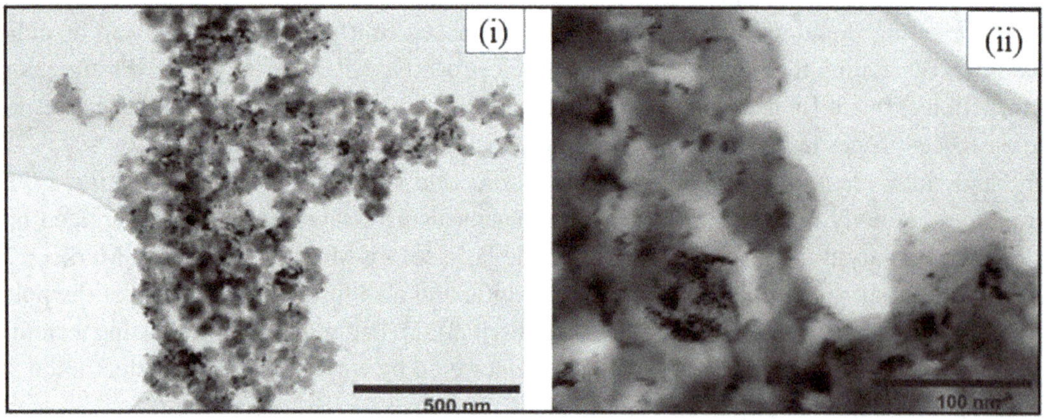

Figure 10. Colorimetric immunosensor based on the colloidal solution of functionalized gold nanoparticles and antibody
(Acunzo et al. 2022)

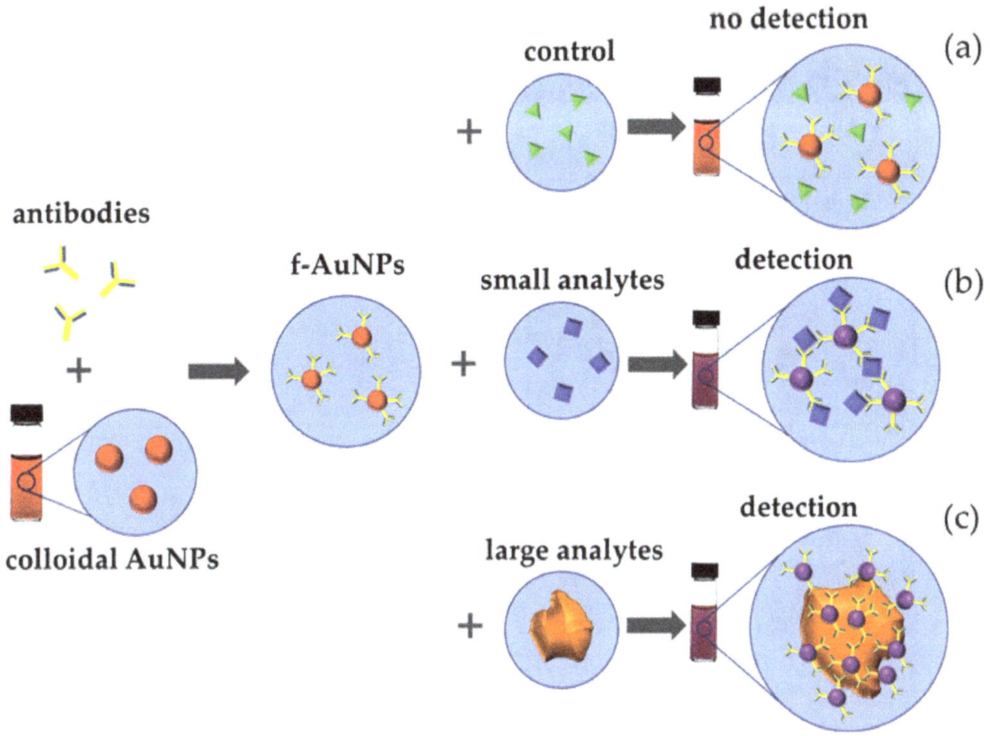

1.4.1 Colorimetric detection: AuNPs are the most useful element for colorimetric immunosensing. These NPs have extremely high extinction coefficient and their optical properties dependent on interatomic spacing. Due to the aggregation color of suspended AuNPs shifts from red to purple. These sensors are designed during immunological reactions due to the binding of an analyte with an antibody (present on the surface of AuNPs), NPs got disaggregated, or vice versa (Acunzo et al. 2022). As a result, distinguishable color shifts of the solution take place which can be observed by the naked eye (Figure 10). Not only AuNPs but also AgNPs can be used to suit this purpose.

1.4.2 Fluorescence detection: QDs, semiconductors, and polystyrene NPs which are exhibiting particle diameter-dependent emission bands are popular as fluorescent markers (Figure 11) (Tsai et al. 2022). These sensors show high sensitivity as well as selectivity. These immunoassays are useful for clinical human hepatitis B surface antigen detection, prostate-specific antigen, interleukin-6, etc.

1.4.3 Optical or surface plasmon resonance-based detection: Prism and optical fiber are the two most popular transducers in this domain. These transducers are combined with plasmonic NPs and electronic coupling interaction takes place between these NPs and the transducer-guided wave. The resonance associated with this phenomenon is known as LSPR. Plasmonic immunosensors can measure extremely small changes in RI in situ of the NPs surface. Generally, for the immunosensing study, an antibody is immobilized on the metal surface and the target antigen from the solution docks to the antibody which will cause a RI change around the metal surfaces. These changes are detectable with LSPR by tracking

Figure 11. Schematic diagram of a fluorescence-based immunoassay
(Tsai et al. 2022)

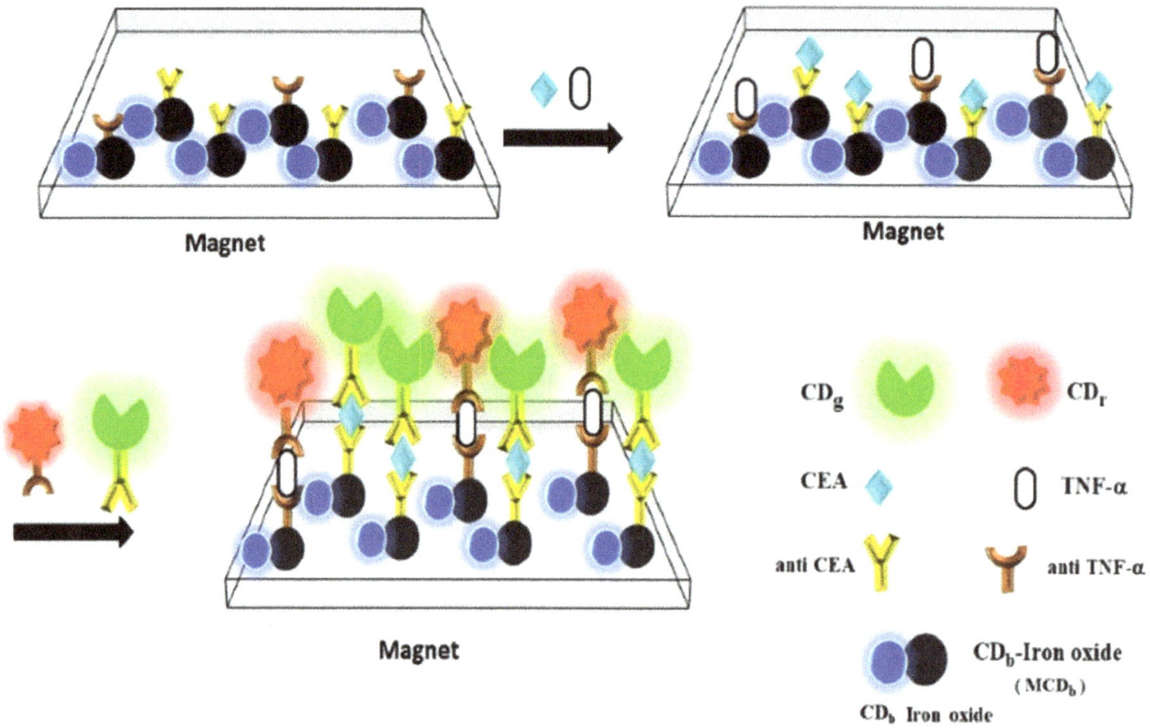

Figure 12. Schematic illustration of a plasmonic immunosensor for melamine detection
(Oh et al. 2019)

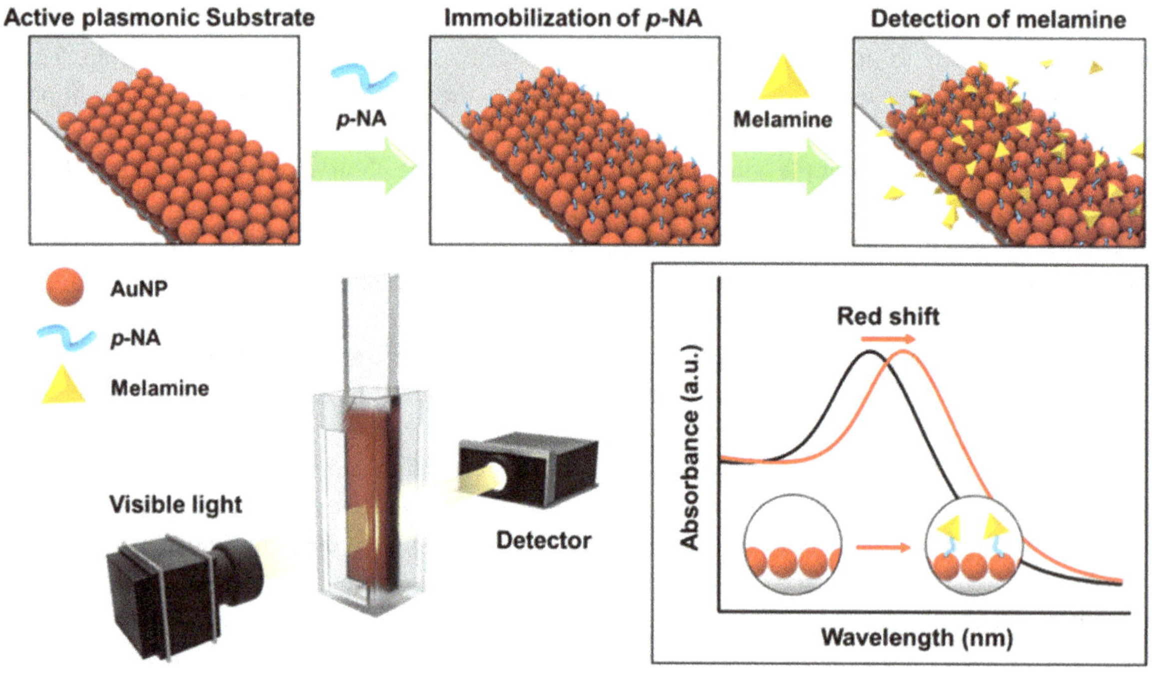

the change in resonance wavelength or resonance amplitude or resonance angle (Figure 12) (Oh et al. 2019). SERS is another sensitive immunosensing technology that works based on the SPR principle. SERS is extremely sensitive and selectivity toward the bioanalytical changes around the metal surface in comparison to the conventional Raman scattering. Also, it is a label-free detection system.

Direct Electrical Detection

AuNPs and heavy metal (like, CdS, ZnS, PbS, etc.) based QDs show excellent electroactivity which makes them suitable for the fabrication of electrical or electrochemical immunosensor. Direct

detection of NPs is possible due to their proactive property. For this detection, electrode surface and metal direct contact is necessary. But in this phenomenon, there is a chance of less sensitivity due to the large no. of non-touching particles. However rapid response, the acceptable limit of detection, and compact structure are key features of this immunosensor.

1.4.5 Indirect electrical detections: Indirect electrochemical detection is the most popular bioassay in the immunosensing domain. Here, also electroactive NMs are in use. In this assay, NPs are loaded with other NPs and with enzymes to obtain labels as well as signal enhancement. They show a low detection limit in the order of pM. Even multi-detection of different proteins is possible by using different inorganic quantum dots as electroactive labels on the same immunoassay.

1.4.6 NPs as modifiers of electro-transducing surfaces: Electroactive NPs coating on the electro-transducer enhances its sensitivity multiple times. NPs are immobilized on the transducer surface based on their absorbance over the conventional electrode. These NPs provide congenial microenvironments for more bioactivity as well as freedom for the protein molecules. Electroactive polymers, Au, and platinum NPs are mostly used to suit this application. A graphical representation of direct, indirect, and NPs-modified immunosensor is shown in Figure 13 (Iglesias-Mayor et al. 2019).

1.4.7 Electromechanical detection: Microcantilevers and quartz crystal microbalances have been demonstrated as a high sensitive and label-free biosensors (Zhao and Sun 2018). For these assays, the antibody-antigen reaction rises a change in the impedance as well as the resonance frequency. Even AuNPs combined microcantilever can detect prostate-specific antigen at a pg/ml level (Figure 14).

1.4.8 Lateral flow and lab-on-a-chip: Lateral flow immunoassay (LFIA) is a carrier material coated rectangular strip-shaped biosensor as shown in Fig. 15. LFIA is activated when some liquid sample is poured into the sample pad. Then sample flows are driven by capillary force and the antibody-antigen interaction takes place (Bernabeu et al. 2020). For this sensor, sensitivity is dependent on the density of a sample. It is mainly a colorimetric and qualitative analysis. LFIA is fast responding, chip, and suitable for *PoC* testing. The first LFIA was made for a pregnancy test (Serafinelli et al. 2023). These chips are made of polymer or silica and modified with NPs and antibodies. A low sample volume is needed for this bioassay and they can detect various cancer biomarkers.

CONCLUSION AND FUTURE PERSPECTIVE

In conclusion, nanotechnology plays a crucial role in various fields and offers significant contributions to science, technology, and society. Here are some key conclusive points on the role of nanotechnology: (i) Advancing Technology: Nanotechnology enables the development of smaller, faster, and more efficient electronic devices, leading to advancements in computing power, energy storage, and communication

Figure 13. Mechanism of direct, indirect, and nanoparticle-modified immunosensor
(Iglesias-Mayor et al. 2019)

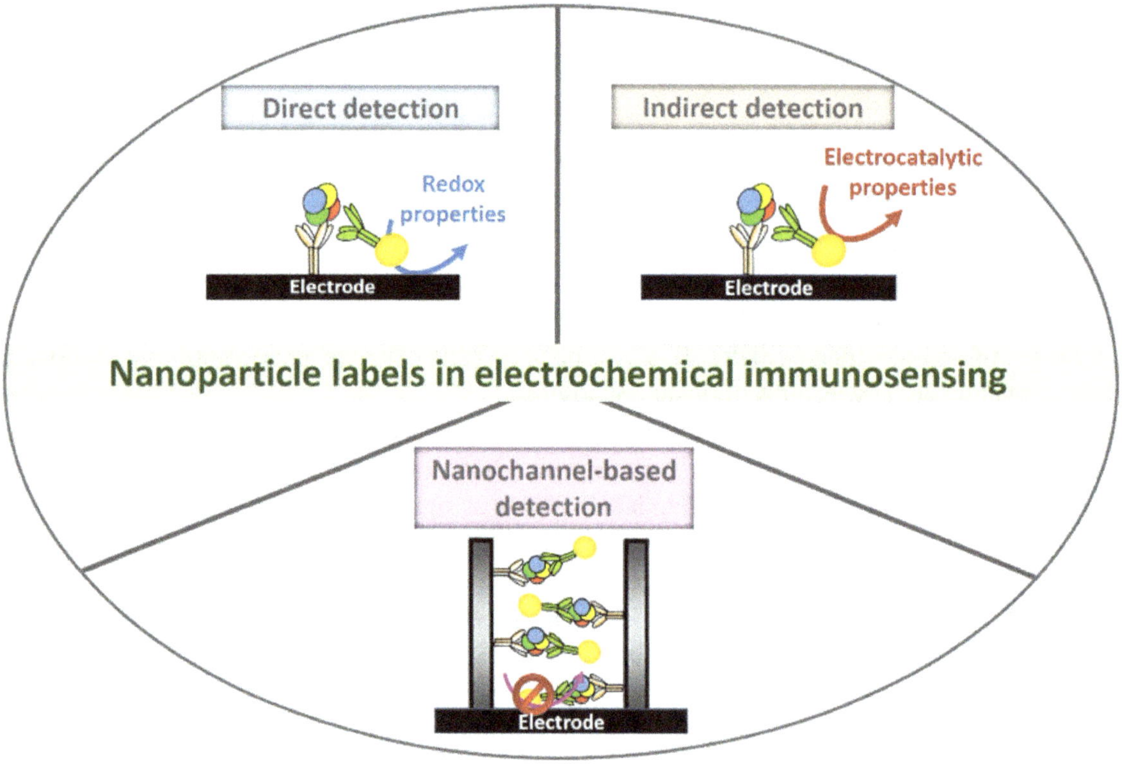

Figure 14. Schematic diagram of a microcantilever
(Zhao and Sun 2018)

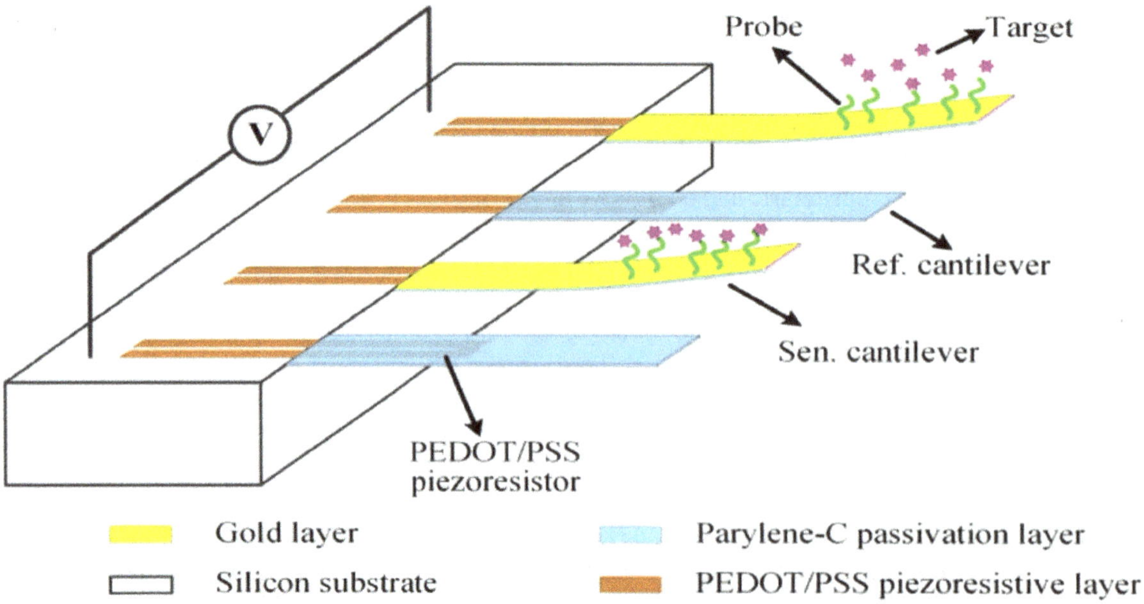

Figure 15. Principle of the LFIA
(Bernabeu et al. 2020)

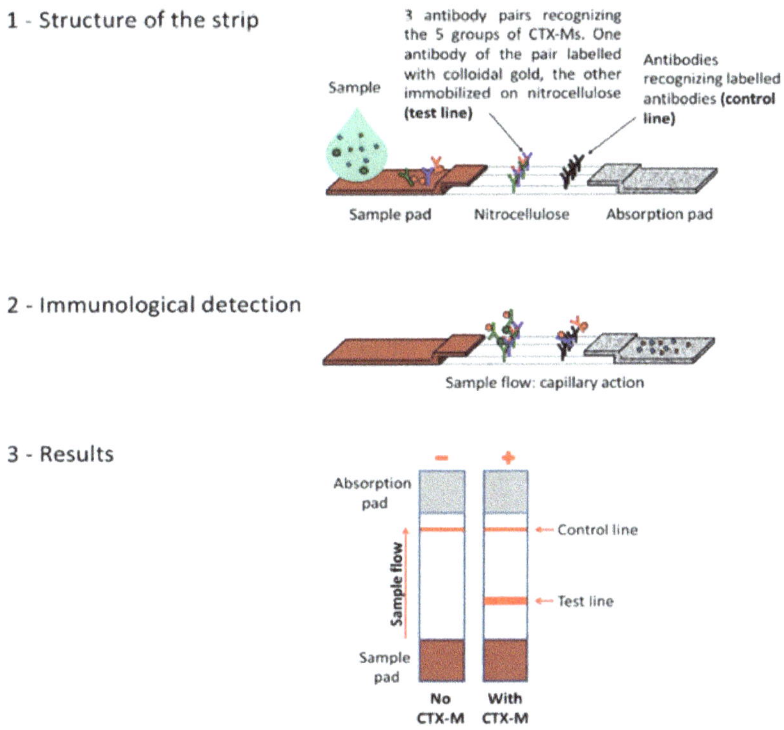

technologies, (ii) Healthcare Revolution: Nanotechnology revolutionizes healthcare by providing targeted drug delivery systems, sensitive diagnostics, regenerative medicine solutions, and innovative cancer therapies. It enhances treatment efficacy, reduces side effects, and improves patient outcomes, (iii) Environmental Solutions: Nanotechnology offers potential solutions to environmental challenges by enabling efficient water purification, air filtration, pollution detection, and remediation. NMs and nano-sensors contribute to sustainable energy production and storage, (iv) Enhanced Materials: Nanotechnology allows the engineering of materials with improved properties such as strength, conductivity, and reactivity. This leads to the development of lightweight and high-performance materials for aerospace, automotive, and construction industries, (v) Sustainable Agriculture: Nanotechnology offers opportunities for sustainable agriculture through targeted delivery of fertilizers and pesticides, soil remediation, and efficient water management. It promotes precision farming and reduces environmental impact, (vi) Sensor and Detection Systems: Nanotechnology-based sensors enable highly sensitive detection of biomarkers, toxins, and pollutants. These sensors find healthcare, environmental monitoring, and security applications, and (vii) Ethical and Safety Considerations: As nanotechnology advances, it is essential to address ethical concerns and ensure the safe use of NMs. Research on potential health and environmental impacts, ethical implications, and responsible regulations are necessary for the responsible development and application of nanotechnology. Overall, nanotechnology's role is multidimensional and far-reaching, impacting various sectors and offering solutions to global challenges. With ongoing research and development, nanotechnology holds great potential for transformative advancements in biomedical science and other fields, benefiting society as a whole.

In the future, a number of global challenges can be addressed through nanotechnology, including healthcare improvements and the advancement of technology. In many fields, it continues to drive innovation, paving the way for groundbreaking discoveries and applications in the future. These areas are Drug Delivery, Disease Treatment and Therapeutics, Imaging and Diagnostics, Tissue Engineering, Biosensors and Diagnostics, Therapeutics and Theragnostic, Disease Monitoring, Nanoscale Imaging and Manipulation, Biosensors and Point-of-Care Devices, and Biomaterials and Implants.

A major challenge in developing biosensing diagnostic devices for the next generation is their integration into electronic health systems. Wirelessly operated *PoC* devices are now able to connect with health experts and hospitals through technological developments in the Internet of Medical Things (IoMT). Data analytics and machine learning (ML) algorithms, such as AI, are integrated with POC platforms to create an innovative model for making decisions based on data. First, portable instruments that automatically digitize biomarker concentrations are used by AI sensors to analyze the sample. Through algorithms such as classification, clustering, and patterning, we can predict the disease spectrum based on the acquired data. With AI, medical practitioners can provide patients with more personalized care and observation in this context. By using IoMT and AI, health analytics contribute to the proactive management and prevention of disease, which serves to improve the health of the patients.

REFERENCES

Acunzo, A., Scardapane, E., De Luca, M., Marra, D., Velotta, R., & Minopoli, A. (2022). Plasmonic Nanomaterials for Colorimetric Biosensing: A Review. *Chemosensors (Basel, Switzerland)*, *10*(4), 136. doi:10.3390/chemosensors10040136

Adedoja, O. S., Sadiku, E. R., & Hamam, Y. (2023). An Overview of the Emerging Technologies and Composite Materials for Supercapacitors in Energy Storage Applications. *Polymers*, *15*(10), 2272. doi:10.3390/polym15102272 PMID:37242851

Adeyemi, J., Adekoya, O. K. O., Oluwasegun, S. T., Olugbenga, D. E., & Neerish, R. (2018). Band Structure, Morphology, Functionality, and Size- Dependent Properties of Metal Nanoparticles. In S. M. Singh & D. Bristow Alan (Eds.), *Noble and Precious Metals*. IntechOpen.

Agrawal, N., Saha, C., Kumar, C., Singh, R., Zhang, B., Jha, R., & Kumar, S. (2020). Detection of L-Cysteine Using Silver Nanoparticles and Graphene Oxide Immobilized Tapered SMS Optical Fiber Structure. *IEEE Sensors Journal*, *20*(19), 11372–11379. doi:10.1109/JSEN.2020.2997690

Agrawal, N., Saha, C., Kumar, C., Singh, R., Zhang, B., & Kumar, S. (2020). Development of Uric Acid Sensor Using Copper Oxide and Silver Nanoparticles Immobilized SMSMS Fiber Structure-Based Probe. *IEEE Transactions on Instrumentation and Measurement*, *69*(11), 9097–9104. doi:10.1109/TIM.2020.2998876

Agrawal, N., Saxena, R., Singh, L., Saha, C., & Kumar, S. (2022). Recent advancements in plasmonic optical biosensors: A review. *ISSS Journal of Micro and Smart Systems*, *11*(1), 31–42. doi:10.100741683-021-00079-0

Agrawal, N., Zhang, B., Saha, C., Kumar, C., Kaushik, B. K., & Kumar, S. (2020). Development of Dopamine Sensor Using Silver Nanoparticles and PEG-Functionalized Tapered Optical Fiber Structure. *IEEE Transactions on Biomedical Engineering*, *67*(6), 1542–1547. doi:10.1109/TBME.2019.2939560 PMID:31494542

Agrawal, N., Zhang, B., Saha, C., Kumar, C., Pu, X., & Kumar, S. (2020). Ultra-Sensitive Cholesterol Sensor Using Gold and Zinc-Oxide Nanoparticles Immobilized Core Mismatch MPM/SPS Probe. *Journal of Lightwave Technology*, *38*(8), 2523–2529. doi:10.1109/JLT.2020.2974818

Akouibaa, A., Masrour, R., Jabar, A., Benhamou, M., Ouarch, M., & Derouiche, A. (2022). Study of the Optical and Thermoplasmonics Properties of Gold Nanoparticle Embedded in Al(2)O(3) Matrix. *Plasmonics*, *17*(3), 1157–1169. doi:10.100711468-022-01607-w PMID:35228839

Aldosari, F. M. M. (2022). Characterization of Labeled Gold Nanoparticles for Surface-Enhanced Raman Scattering. *Molecules (Basel, Switzerland)*, *27*(3), 892. doi:10.3390/molecules27030892 PMID:35164155

Bernabeu, S., Ratnam, K. C., Boutal, H., Gonzalez, C., Vogel, A., Devilliers, K., Plaisance, M., Oueslati, S., Malhotra-Kumar, S., Dortet, L., Fortineau, N., Simon, S., Volland, H., & Naas, T. (2020). A Lateral Flow Immunoassay for the Rapid Identification of CTX-M-Producing Enterobacterales from Culture Plates and Positive Blood Cultures. *Diagnostics (Basel)*, *10*(10), 764. doi:10.3390/diagnostics10100764 PMID:32998433

Bohunicky, B., & Mousa, S. A. (2010). Biosensors: The new wave in cancer diagnosis. *Nanotechnology, Science and Applications*, *4*, 1–10. doi:10.2147/NSA.S13465 PMID:24198482

Bruna, T., Maldonado-Bravo, F., Jara, P., & Caro, N. (2021). Silver Nanoparticles and Their Antibacterial Applications. *International Journal of Molecular Sciences*, *22*(13), 7202. doi:10.3390/ijms22137202 PMID:34281254

Cash, K. J., & Clark, H. A. (2010). Nanosensors and nanomaterials for monitoring glucose in diabetes. *Trends in Molecular Medicine*, *16*(12), 584–593. doi:10.1016/j.molmed.2010.08.002 PMID:20869318

Chack, D., Agrawal, N., & Raghuwanshi, S. K. (2014). To analyse the performance of tapered and MMI assisted splitter on the basis of geographical parameters. *Optik (Stuttgart)*, *125*(11), 2568–2571. doi:10.1016/j.ijleo.2013.11.019

Chack, D., Raghuwanshi, S. K., Kumar, V., & Agrawal, N. (2013). Analyzing the Optimum Parameter of an 1x2 MMI Splitter. *2013 International Conference on Communication Systems and Network Technologies*. IEEE. 10.1109/CSNT.2013.41

Chandra, S., Bharadwaj, R., & Mukherji, S. (2017). Label free ultrasensitive optical sensor decorated with polyaniline nanofibers: Characterization and immunosensing application. *Sensors and Actuators. B, Chemical*, *240*, 443–450. doi:10.1016/j.snb.2016.08.103

Chausali, N., Saxena, J., & Prasad, R. (2023). Nanotechnology as a sustainable approach for combating the environmental effects of climate change. *Journal of Agriculture and Food Research*, *12*, 100541. doi:10.1016/j.jafr.2023.100541

Chen, S., Zhang, Q., Hou, Y., Zhang, J., & Liang, X. (2013). Nanomaterials in medicine and pharmaceuticals: nanoscale materials developed with less toxicity and more efficacy. *EJNM, 5*(2), 61-79. doi: . doi:10.1515/ejnm-2013-0003

Chen, Y., Xiong, X., Chen, Y., Chen, L., Liu, G., Xiao, W., Shi, J., Chen, Z., & Luo, Y. (2023). MoS2-Nanoflower and Nanodiamond Co-Engineered Surface Plasmon Resonance for Biosensing. *Biosensors (Basel), 13*(5), 506. doi:10.3390/bios13050506 PMID:37232867

Chun, Y. W., Crowder, S. W., Mehl, S. C., Wang, X., Bae, H., & Sung, H.-J. (2013). THERAPEUTIC APPLICATION OF NANOTECHNOLOGY IN CARDIOVASCULAR AND PULMONARY REGENERATION. *Computational and Structural Biotechnology Journal, 7*(8), e201304005. doi:10.5936/csbj.201304005 PMID:24688735

Cicha, I., Priefer, R., Severino, P., Souto, E. B., & Jain, S. (2022). Biosensor-Integrated Drug Delivery Systems as New Materials for Biomedical Applications. *Biomolecules, 12*(9), 1198. doi:10.3390/biom12091198 PMID:36139035

de la Escosura-Muñiz, A., Parolo, C., & Merkoçi, A. (2010). Immunosensing using nanoparticles. *Materials Today, 13*(7), 24–34. doi:10.1016/S1369-7021(10)70125-5

Domínguez-Aragón, A., Zaragoza-Contreras, E. A., Figueroa-Miranda, G., Offenhäusser, A., & Mayer, D. (2023). Electrochemical Immunosensor Using Electroactive Carbon Nanohorns for Signal Amplification for the Rapid Detection of Carcinoembryonic Antigen. *Biosensors (Basel), 13*(1), 63. doi:10.3390/bios13010063 PMID:36671898

Estelrich, J., Sánchez-Martín, M. J., & Busquets, M. A. (2015). Nanoparticles in magnetic resonance imaging: From simple to dual contrast agents. *International Journal of Nanomedicine, 10*, 1727–1741. doi:10.2147/IJN.S76501 PMID:25834422

Ethaib, S., Al-Qutaifia, S., Al-Ansari, N., & Zubaidi, S. L. (2022). Function of Nanomaterials in Removing Heavy Metals for Water and Wastewater Remediation: A Review. *Environments (Basel, Switzerland), 9*(10), 123. doi:10.3390/environments9100123

Funda, G., Taschieri, S., Bruno, G. A., Grecchi, E., Paolo, S., Girolamo, D., & Del Fabbro, M. (2020). Nanotechnology Scaffolds for Alveolar Bone Regeneration. *Materials (Basel), 13*(1), 201. doi:10.3390/ma13010201 PMID:31947750

Gholami, A., Hashemi, S. A., Yousefi, K., Mousavi, S. M., Chiang, W.-H., Ramakrishna, S., Mazraedoost, S., Alizadeh, A., Omidifar, N., Behbudi, G., & Babapoor, A. (2020). 3D Nanostructures for Tissue Engineering, Cancer Therapy, and Gene Delivery. *Journal of Nanomaterials, 1852946*, 1–24. doi:10.1155/2020/1852946

Guisbiers, G., Mejía-Rosales, S., & Deepak, F. L. (2012). Nanomaterial Properties: Size and Shape Dependencies. *Journal of Nanomaterials, 180976*, 1–2. doi:10.1155/2012/180976

Gulumian, M., Andraos, C., Afantitis, A., Puzyn, T., & Coville, N. J. (2021). Importance of Surface Topography in Both Biological Activity and Catalysis of Nanomaterials: Can Catalysis by Design Guide Safe by Design? *International Journal of Molecular Sciences, 22*(15), 8347. doi:10.3390/ijms22158347 PMID:34361117

Ha, H., Amicucci, C., Matteini, P., & Hwang, B. (2022). Mini review of synthesis strategies of silver nanowires and their applications. *Colloid and Interface Science Communications*, *50*, 100663. doi:10.1016/j.colcom.2022.100663

Haleem, A., Javaid, M., Singh, R. P., Rab, S., & Suman, R. (2023). Applications of nanotechnology in medical field: A brief review. *Global Health Journal (Amsterdam, Netherlands)*, *7*(2), 70–77. doi:10.1016/j.glohj.2023.02.008

Halkare, P., Punjabi, N., Wangchuk, J., Nair, A., Kondabagil, K., & Mukherji, S. (2019). Bacteria functionalized gold nanoparticle matrix based fiber-optic sensor for monitoring heavy metal pollution in water. *Sensors and Actuators. B, Chemical*, *281*, 643–651. doi:10.1016/j.snb.2018.10.119

Han, X., Xu, K., Taratula, O., & Farsad, K. (2019). Applications of nanoparticles in biomedical imaging. *Nanoscale*, *11*(3), 799–819. doi:10.1039/C8NR07769J PMID:30603750

Hasanzadeh, M., Shadjou, N., Lin, Y., & de la Guardia, M. (2017). Nanomaterials for use in immunosensing of carcinoembryonic antigen (CEA): Recent advances. *Trends in Analytical Chemistry*, *86*, 185–205. doi:10.1016/j.trac.2016.11.003

Hill, R. T. (2015). Plasmonic biosensors. *Wiley Interdisciplinary Reviews. Nanomedicine and Nanobiotechnology*, *7*(2), 152–168. doi:10.1002/wnan.1314 PMID:25377594

Hong, Y., Huh, Y.-M., Yoon, D. S., & Yang, J. (2012). Nanobiosensors Based on Localized Surface Plasmon Resonance for Biomarker Detection. *Journal of Nanomaterials*, *759830*, 1–13. doi:10.1155/2012/759830

Huang, Y., Yu, D., Qiu, Y., Chu, L., & Lin, Y. (2020). The Role of Nanomaterials in Modulating the Structure and Function of Biomimetic Catalysts. *Frontiers in Chemistry*, *8*, 764. doi:10.3389/fchem.2020.00764 PMID:33134257

Iglesias-Mayor, A., Amor-Gutiérrez, O., Costa-García, A., & de la Escosura-Muñiz, A. (2019). Nanoparticles as Emerging Labels in Electrochemical Immunosensors. *Sensors (Basel)*, *19*(23), 5137. doi:10.339019235137 PMID:31771201

Israelsen, N. D., Hanson, C., & Vargis, E. (2015). Nanoparticle properties and synthesis effects on surface-enhanced Raman scattering enhancement factor: An introduction. *TheScientificWorldJournal*, *124582*, 1–12. doi:10.1155/2015/124582 PMID:25884017

Jeevanandam, J., Barhoum, A., Chan, Y. S., Dufresne, A., & Danquah, M. K. (2018). Review on nanoparticles and nanostructured materials: History, sources, toxicity and regulations. *Beilstein Journal of Nanotechnology*, *9*, 1050–1074. doi:10.3762/bjnano.9.98 PMID:29719757

Jin, B., Odongo, S., Radwanska, M., & Magez, S. (2023). Nanobodies: A Review of Generation, Diagnostics and Therapeutics. *International Journal of Molecular Sciences, 24*(6). . doi:10.3390/ijms24065994

Joseph, T. M., Mahapatra, D. K., Esmaeili, A., Piszczyk, Ł., Hasanin, M. S., Kattali, M., Haponiuk, J., & Thomas, S. (2023). Nanoparticles: Taking a Unique Position in Medicine. *Nanomaterials (Basel, Switzerland)*, *13*(3), 574. doi:10.3390/nano13030574 PMID:36770535

Kang, M. S., Lee, S. Y., Kim, K. S., & Han, D. W. (2020). State of the Art Biocompatible Gold Nanoparticles for Cancer Theragnosis. *Pharmaceutics, 12*(8), 701. doi:10.3390/pharmaceutics12080701 PMID:32722426

Kashyap, B. K., Singh, V. V., Solanki, M. K., Kumar, A., Ruokolainen, J., & Kesari, K. K. (2023). Smart Nanomaterials in Cancer Theranostics: Challenges and Opportunities. *ACS Omega, 8*(16), 14290–14320. doi:10.1021/acsomega.2c07840 PMID:37125102

Khan, I., Saeed, K., & Khan, I. (2019). Nanoparticles: Properties, applications and toxicities. *Arabian Journal of Chemistry, 12*(7), 908–931. doi:10.1016/j.arabjc.2017.05.011

Kiio, T. M., & Park, S. (2020). Nano-scientific Application of Atomic Force Microscopy in Pathology: From Molecules to Tissues. *International Journal of Medical Sciences, 17*(7), 844–858. doi:10.7150/ijms.41805 PMID:32308537

Kumar, H., Kuča, K., Bhatia, S. K., Saini, K., Kaushal, A., Verma, R., Bhalla, T. C., & Kumar, D. (2020). Applications of Nanotechnology in Sensor-Based Detection of Foodborne Pathogens. *Sensors (Basel), 20*(7), 1966. doi:10.339020071966 PMID:32244581

Kumar, S., Agrawal, N., Saha, C., & Jha, R. (2022). *Optical Fiber-Based Plasmonic Biosensors: Trends, Techniques, and Applications*. CRC Press. doi:10.3389/978-2-88974-680-4

Kumar, S., Agrawal, N., Saha, C., & Jha, R. (2020). Optical Fiber-based Plasmonic Biosensors: Trends, Techniques and Applications.

Li, F., You, M., Li, S., Hu, J., Liu, C., Gong, Y., Yang, H., & Xu, F. (2020). Paper-based point-of-care immunoassays: Recent advances and emerging trends. *Biotechnology Advances, 39*, 107442. doi:10.1016/j.biotechadv.2019.107442 PMID:31470046

Lokendra, S., Niteshkumar, A., Himnashu, B., Bhupal, A., & Taresh, S. (2021). Application of Fiber Optics in Bio-Sensing. In H.-C. Guillermo (Ed.), *Fiber Optics*. IntechOpen.

López-Lorente, Á. I. (2021). Recent developments on gold nanostructures for surface enhanced Raman spectroscopy: Particle shape, substrates and analytical applications. A review. *Analytica Chimica Acta, 1168*, 338474. doi:10.1016/j.aca.2021.338474 PMID:34051992

Mayer, K. M., & Hafner, J. H. (2011). Localized Surface Plasmon Resonance Sensors. *Chemical Reviews, 111*(6), 3828–3857. doi:10.1021/cr100313v PMID:21648956

McClements, D., & Xiao, H. (2017). Is nano safe in foods? Establishing the factors impacting the gastrointestinal fate and toxicity of organic and inorganic food-grade nanoparticles. *npj Science of Food, 1*(1), 6. . doi:10.1038/s41538-017-0005-1

Mirón-Barroso, S., Domènech, E. B., & Trigueros, S. (2021). Nanotechnology-Based Strategies to Overcome Current Barriers in Gene Delivery. *International Journal of Molecular Sciences, 22*(16), 8537. doi:10.3390/ijms22168537 PMID:34445243

Mundekkad, D., & Cho, W. C. (2022). Nanoparticles in Clinical Translation for Cancer Therapy. *International Journal of Molecular Sciences, 23*(3), 1685. doi:10.3390/ijms23031685 PMID:35163607

Naresh, V., & Lee, N. (2021a). A Review on Biosensors and Recent Development of Nanostructured Materials-Enabled Biosensors. *Sensors (Basel), 21*(4), 1109. doi:10.339021041109 PMID:33562639

Naresh, V., & Lee, N. (2021b). A Review on Biosensors and Recent Development of Nanostructured Materials-Enabled Biosensors. *Sensors (Basel), 21*(4), 1109. doi:10.339021041109 PMID:33562639

Nune, S. K., Gunda, P., Thallapally, P. K., Lin, Y. Y., Forrest, M. L., & Berkland, C. J. (2009). Nanoparticles for biomedical imaging. *Expert Opinion on Drug Delivery, 6*(11), 1175–1194. doi:10.1517/17425240903229031 PMID:19743894

Oh, S. Y., Lee, M. J., Heo, N. S., Kim, S., Oh, J. S., Lee, Y., Jeon, E. J., Moon, H., Kim, H. S., Park, T. J., Moon, G., Chun, H. S., & Huh, Y. S. (2019). Cuvette-Type LSPR Sensor for Highly Sensitive Detection of Melamine in Infant Formulas. *Sensors (Basel), 19*(18), 3839. doi:10.339019183839 PMID:31491964

Pal, J., Singh, K. M., Aditya, S., Ganesh, P., Hwa, C. K., & Sangsul, L. (2020). Bottom-Up and Top-Down Approaches for MgO. In K. Selcan (Ed.), *Sonochemical Reactions*. IntechOpen.

Patra, J. K., Das, G., Fraceto, L. F., Estefania, V. R. C., Maria del Pilar, R.-T., Acosta-Torres, L. S., Diaz-Torres, L. A., Grillo, R., Swamy, M. K., Sharma, S., Habtemariam, S., & Shin, H.-S. (2018). Nano based drug delivery systems: Recent developments and future prospects. *Journal of Nanobiotechnology, 16*(1), 71. doi:10.118612951-018-0392-8 PMID:30231877

Ramos, A. P., Cruz, M. A. E., Tovani, C. B., & Ciancaglini, P. (2017). Biomedical applications of nanotechnology. *Biophysical Reviews, 9*(2), 79–89. doi:10.100712551-016-0246-2 PMID:28510082

Rizvi, S. B., Ghaderi, S., Keshtgar, M., & Seifalian, A. M. (2010). Semiconductor quantum dots as fluorescent probes for in vitro and in vivo bio-molecular and cellular imaging. *Nano Reviews, 1*(1), 5161. doi:10.3402/nano.v1i0.5161 PMID:22110865

Salhi, B., Hossain, M. K., Mukhaimer, A. W., & Al-Sulaiman, F. A. (2016). Nanowires: A new pathway to nanotechnology-based applications. *Journal of Electroceramics, 37*(1), 34–49. doi:10.100710832-016-0037-y PMID:32214875

Sapsford, K. E., Pons, T., Medintz, I. L., & Mattoussi, H. (2006). Biosensing with Luminescent Semiconductor Quantum Dots. *Sensors (Basel), 6*(8), 925–953. doi:10.33906080925

Saxena, R., Sharma, P., Kumar, S., Agrawal, N., Sharma, S. K., & Awasthi, A. (2023). Modulation of mitochondria by viral proteins. *Life Sciences, 313*, 121271. doi:10.1016/j.lfs.2022.121271 PMID:36526048

Serafinelli, C., Fantoni, A., Alegria, E. C. B. A., & Vieira, M. (2023). Recent Progresses in Plasmonic Biosensors for Point-of-Care (POC) Devices: A Critical Review. *Chemosensors (Basel, Switzerland), 11*(5), 303. doi:10.3390/chemosensors11050303

Shao, L., Gao, Y., & Yan, F. (2011). Semiconductor quantum dots for biomedicial applications. *Sensors (Basel), 11*(12), 11736–11751. doi:10.3390111211736 PMID:22247690

Shi, J., Votruba, A. R., Farokhzad, O. C., & Langer, R. (2010). Nanotechnology in drug delivery and tissue engineering: From discovery to applications. *Nano Letters, 10*(9), 3223–3230. doi:10.1021/nl102184c PMID:20726522

Sim, S., & Wong, N. K. (2021). Nanotechnology and its use in imaging and drug delivery (Review). *Biomedical Reports*, *14*(5), 42. doi:10.3892/br.2021.1418 PMID:33728048

Singh, L., Agrawal, N., Gola, K. K., Saha, C., & Pareek, P. (2022). Numerical investigation of all optical SR flip-flop using plasmonic metal–insulator-metal (MIM) waveguides. *Optical and Quantum Electronics*, *54*(6), 381. doi:10.100711082-022-03666-z

Singh, L., Agrawal, N., & Saha, C. (2021). Investigation of Glucose Sensor by using Plasmonic MIM Waveguide Based M. *2021 IEEE MTT-S International Microwave and RF Conference (IMARC)*. IEEE. 10.1109/IMaRC49196.2021.9714533

Singh, L., Agrawal, N., Saha, C., & Kaushik, B. K. (2022). A Plus Shaped Cavity in Optical Fiber Based Refractive Index Sensor. *IEEE Transactions on Nanobioscience*, *21*(2), 199–205. doi:10.1109/TNB.2021.3121779 PMID:34673494

Singh, L., Agrawal, N., Saha, C., Singh, B. M., & Singh, T. (2022). Highly Sensitive Plus Shaped Cavity in Silicon Fiber for RI Detection of Water Samples. *Silicon*, *14*(13), 7819–7828. doi:10.100712633-021-01519-0

Singh, L., Iadicicco, A., Agrawal, N., Saha, C., & Chauhan, R. (2022). A compact formulation of all optical signal router by using plasmonic waveguides. *Optical and Quantum Electronics*, *54*(8), 478. doi:10.100711082-022-03878-3

Singh, R. (2019). Nanotechnology based therapeutic application in cancer diagnosis and therapy. *3 Biotech* *9*(11), 415. . doi:10.1007/s13205-019-1940-0

Soleimani, M., Zaabi, A., Merheb, M., & Matar, R. (2016). Nanoparticles in Gene Therapy. *International Journal of Integrative Biology*, *17*, 7–16.

Sriram, M., Zong, K., Vivekchand, S., & Gooding, J. (2015). Single Nanoparticle Plasmonic Sensors. *Sensors (Basel)*, *15*(10), 25774–25792. doi:10.3390151025774 PMID:26473866

Surana, H., Agarwal, N., Udaykumar, A., & Darekar, R. (2019). *Blackbox-Based Night Vision Camouflage Robot for Defence Applications*. Computing, Communication and Signal Processing. doi:10.1007/978-981-13-1513-8_64

Tsai, H., Chang, K., Lee, W., & Fuh, C. B. (2022). Rapid Preparation of Fluorescent Carbon Dots from Pine Needles for Chemical Analysis. *Nanomaterials (Basel, Switzerland)*, *12*(1), 66. doi:10.3390/nano12010066 PMID:35010016

Unser, S., Bruzas, I., He, J., & Sagle, L. (2015). Localized Surface Plasmon Resonance Biosensing: Current Challenges and Approaches. *Sensors (Basel)*, *15*(7), 15684–15716. doi:10.3390150715684 PMID:26147727

Venkateshaiah, A., Padil, V. V. T., Nagalakshmaiah, M., Waclawek, S., Černík, M., & Varma, R. S. (2020). Microscopic Techniques for the Analysis of Micro and Nanostructures of Biopolymers and Their Derivatives. *Polymers*, *12*(3), 512. doi:10.3390/polym12030512 PMID:32120773

Wang, S.-Y., Shi, X.-C., Zhu, G.-Y., Zhang, Y.-J., Jin, D.-Y., Zhou, Y.-D., Liu, F.-Q., & Laborda, P. (2021). Application of surface-enhanced Raman spectroscopy using silver and gold nanoparticles for the detection of pesticides in fruit and fruit juice. *Trends in Food Science & Technology*, *116*, 583–602. doi:10.1016/j.tifs.2021.08.006

Wu, J., Liu, H., Chen, W., Ma, B., & Ju, H. (2023). Device integration of electrochemical biosensors. *Nature Reviews Bioengineering*, *1*(5), 346–360. doi:10.103844222-023-00032-w PMID:37168735

Yetisgin, A. A., Cetinel, S., Zuvin, M., Kosar, A., & Kutlu, O. (2020). Therapeutic Nanoparticles and Their Targeted Delivery Applications. *Molecules (Basel, Switzerland)*, *25*(9), 2193. doi:10.3390/molecules25092193 PMID:32397080

Zhang, W., Singh, R., Wang, Z., Li, G., Xie, Y., Jha, R., Marques, C., Zhang, B., & Kumar, S. (2023). Humanoid shaped optical fiber plasmon biosensor functionalized with graphene oxide/multi-walled carbon nanotubes for histamine detection. *Optics Express*, *31*(7), 11788–11803. doi:10.1364/OE.486844 PMID:37155805

Zhang, X. Q., Xu, X., Bertrand, N., Pridgen, E., Swami, A., & Farokhzad, O. C. (2012). Interactions of nanomaterials and biological systems: Implications to personalized nanomedicine. *Advanced Drug Delivery Reviews*, *64*(13), 1363–1384. doi:10.1016/j.addr.2012.08.005 PMID:22917779

Zhang, Y., & Liu, H. (2019). Nanowires for High-Efficiency, Low-Cost Solar Photovoltaics. *Crystals*, *9*(2), 87. doi:10.3390/cryst9020087

Zhao, R., & Sun, Y. (2018). Polymeric Flexible Immunosensor Based on Piezoresistive Micro-Cantilever with PEDOT/PSS Conductive Layer. *Sensors (Basel)*, *18*(2), 451. doi:10.339018020451 PMID:29401669

Zhao, W., Cao, H., Wan, C. S., & Zhang, W. B. (2002). Application of nanotechnology in biomedical sciences. *Di Yi Jun Yi Da Xue Xue Bao*, *22*(5), 461–463. PMID:12390718

Zhou, H., Hernandez, C., Goss, M., Gawlik, A., & Exner, A. A. (2015). Biomedical Imaging in Implantable Drug Delivery Systems. *Current Drug Targets*, *16*(6), 672–682. doi:10.2174/1389450115666141122211920 PMID:25418857

Zhu, G., Agrawal, N., Singh, R., Kumar, S., Zhang, B., Saha, C., & Kumar, C. (2020). A novel periodically tapered structure-based gold nanoparticles and graphene oxide – Immobilized optical fiber sensor to detect ascorbic acid. *Optics & Laser Technology*, *127*, 106156. doi:10.1016/j.optlastec.2020.106156

Zielińska, A., Costa, B., Ferreira, M. V., Miguéis, D., Louros, J. M. S., Durazzo, A., Lucarini, M., Eder, P., Chaud, M. V., Morsink, M., Willemen, N., Severino, P., Santini, A., & Souto, E. B. (2020). Nanotoxicology and Nanosafety: Safety-By-Design and Testing at a Glance. *International Journal of Environmental Research and Public Health*, *17*(13). doi:10.3390/ijerph17134657 PMID:32605255

Chapter 4
Metal Nanoparticles via Green Synthesis: A New Cancer Treatment Approach

Demet Saylan
https://orcid.org/0000-0002-1969-428X
Abdullah Gul University, Turkey

İlker Erdem
https://orcid.org/0000-0001-5743-0835
Abdullah Gul University, Turkey

ABSTRACT

Cancer is one of the most abundant lethal diseases globally threatening public health. There is considerable research effort on the prevention, diagnosis, and treatment of cancer. The current practices for cancer treatment are usage of synthetic chemicals (i.e. chemotherapy), radiotherapy, and surgery. Besides these conventional therapies, there are contemporary, innovative approaches, e.g., targeting of the drugs to the cancerous tissues, synergetic enhancement via simultaneous usage of conventional methods, and contemporary methods. Therefore, the process of drug research and development in the field of cancer is increasingly challenging, due to the limited success of current therapies and the constant need to find safer and more effective novel approaches. The utilization of nanotechnology may present new opportunities in cancer treatment. Metal nanoparticles prepared via "bottom-up" approach may be used for triggering the selective cell apoptosis mechanisms for cancerous cells, while sparing healthy cells considerably.

NANOPARTICLES: SYNTHESIS AND CHARACTERIZATION

Nanoparticles (NPs) are formed by agglomeration of atoms and/or molecules with a size around or less than 100 nanometers (nm) at least in two dimensions (Klaine, *et al.* 2008; Vaid, *et al.*, 2020). The NPs are appreciated for their relatively higher surface areas compared to the same amount of bulk material.

DOI: 10.4018/979-8-3693-0448-8.ch004

The high surface area and small size of the NPs make them promising versatile applications. The high surface area increases their interaction with the surrounding media and makes them more interactive / reactive. The smaller size enables approaching / penetration of material to the fine microstructures / micropores. The NPs may be of different material types e.g., metals (e.g., silver (Ag), gold (Au), copper (Cu), platinum (Pt), ceramics (metal-oxides (e.g., iron oxide (FeO), zinc oxide (ZnO), magnesium oxide (MgO), metal-hydroxides (e.g., magnesium hydroxide ($Mg(OH)_2$)), or various organics / polymers and composites composed of inorganic and polymer structures.

The synthesis of NPs may be performed by two main approaches: "top-down" and "bottom-up". The former approach consists of size reduction of bulk material to have smaller pieces of it. The size reduction may be performed with some mechanical / physical methods like grinding, milling, etc. "Top-down" approach may end-up with a very wide particle size range, decreasing the efficiency (i.e., the product may be composed of relatively coarse, micro, and nano particles). The later approach ("bottom-up") is performed by atomic or molecular level precursors. The precursors are treated / reacted under controlled conditions to form / synthesize agglomerates with desired size. The methods following "bottom-up" approach may be exemplified as chemical precipitation, vapor deposition, sol-gel (Erdem & Çakır, 2022). The synthesis methods of NPs may further be classified as biological, physical (e.g., ball milling) and chemical methods (Vijayaram *et al.*, 2023). The NPs with their superior properties like being antimicrobial, antifungal, catalytic, having high adsorption capability, may be used in various applications (e.g., chemical processes, biomedical applications, environmental applications).

The characterization of NPs is crucial to assure their quality for utilization in different applications. The first concern may be about the particle size distribution and the average particle size. The size of the NPs may be monitored by appropriate methods considering the sample properties. Mainly some microscopic techniques are preferred to determine the microstructure and particle size of NPs. Scanning electron microscopy (SEM) and transmission electron microscopy (TEM) are the most common methods to determine the particle size and shape of NPs. The energy dispersive X-ray (EDX) accessory for the electron microscopes (e.g., SEM) enables monitoring the elemental distribution of the sample and may be helpful in controlling the purity of the NPs. The electron microscopes are very helpful tools to visualize the shape and size of the NPs. But the micrographs captured are showing only a small portion of the NPs in the batch. The researchers may prefer to increase the number of micrographs by focusing on different points of the sample and use some image processing software to report the average particle size of NPs more precisely. The particle size distribution and average particle size of NPs may also be determined via light scattering methods. The NPs suspended in liquid phase (e.g., water) are used in the dynamic light scattering (DLS) methods. The NPs making random diffusional movements (Brownian motion) in the liquid media are aimed by a light beam (e.g., laser light). The scattered portion of the laser beam is determined in time by a detector. The NPs with smaller size (mass) will be diffusing faster and they will scatter light with a more fluctuating frequency while NPs with bigger size (mass) will be diffusing more slowly and will be passing through the laser beam (and scatter the laser beam) with a lower frequency. Iterative comparisons of scattered beam in time will be used to calculate the average particle size using the Einstein-Stokes and Schmoluchowsky equations. The advantage of DLS methods is the number of NPs used in the analysis may be higher than the ones in electron microscopy methods, which will be more representative. The disadvantage of the DLS methods is that the NPs may tend to form agglomerates and the determined particle size and distribution may be of the agglomerates instead of singular NPs. The utilization of both electron microscopy methods and DLS methods may present more accurate characterization about the size and size distribution of NPs. The Fourier Transform Infrared (FT-IR) spectroscopy may be used to monitor the chemical bondings and how they alter with varying synthesis conditions. The IR radiation sent to the sample will be either absorbed by the bondings vibrating in the same frequency with the IR radiation or will be transmitted in the absence of certain chemical bonding. UV-vis spectrophotometry may also be used to monitor the evolution of chemicals in the reaction media which utilizes ultraviolet (UV) and visible (vis) light. Again, the distinctive absorption of radiation at certain wavelengths will supply information about the material to be analysed. X-ray diffraction (XRD) analysis may be used for determining the crystallinity of NPs. The X-ray radiation sent on the material with varying angles will be constructively interfere while being scattered from the well-organized crystalline layers of the NPs. The scattering will be forming destructive interference of X-ray radiation, and no radiation will be detected by the detector, if the material is not crystalline (i.e., amorphous).

GREEN SYNTHESIS

Green synthesis is aiming at the optimization of current processes and proposes new methodologies which are more economical, more sustainable, more environmentally friendly, and less hazardous to human health (Anastas & Kirchoff, 2002). Natural resources like plants and microorganisms are used as a replacement for the synthetic chemicals/processes in green synthesis, which makes it more sustainable and environmentally friendly. Green synthesis in general may be considered as a more beneficial choice than the conventional methods, because of decreasing cost and pollution. It is also less threating the environment and human health. Metal nanoparticles (NPs) may propose enhanced chemical, physical, optical, electronic properties compared to the bulk form of metals (Nakkala, *et al.* 2017). Preparation of metal NPs (e.g., Ag, Au) via green synthesis has been possible by using metal salts and several organic materials to reduce the ionic metal (e.g., Ag^{+}) to neutral metallic element (e.g., Ag^{0}) (Erdem & Çakır, 2022). The organic materials to be used in green synthesis may be versatile. Microorganisms (bacteria, yeast, fungi) or different parts of various plants may be used. The utilization of plant tissues instead of microorganisms is reported to be more advantageous in terms of efficiency (Dong *et al.*, 2017, Nakkala *et al.* 2018, Beyene *et al.*, 2017). Preparation of metal NPs by using different parts of the plants (e.g., leaves, shells, roots, etc.) may be considered as "green synthesis" because the phytochemicals are used in synthesis of NPs instead of harsh, synthetic chemicals and the reaction may be performed in aqueous environment instead of environmentally less friendly organic solvents. The phytochemicals may be varying with respect to the source plant. They may be in the form of phenolic compounds, organic acids, amino acids, polysaccharides, etc. (Chopra *et al.*, 2022). Some of these organic compounds (phytochemicals) may contribute to the dispersion of forming metal NPs. They will attach to the surface of metal NPs and form a barrier of same surface charge / characteristics to prevent the agglomeration of metal NPs. That hindrance on agglomeration will help better suspension of metal NPs and keep them "nano". Different metal NPs were synthesized successfully via green synthesis (e.g., copper (Cu), silver, (Ag), gold (Au)) (Makarov *et al.* 2014). Metal salt type and concentration, organic materials (e.g., phytochemicals from plant parts) type and concentration may be effective on the formation of metal NPs and their particle sizes. The temperature and pH of the aqueous media may also be effective on green synthesis of metal NPs. The reduction reaction of metal ions can be enhanced by increasing the temperature (e.g., from room temperature to 60°C). Elevated temperatures (beyond 60°C) may result in degradation of some organic structures and adversely affect the metal NP formation. This will shorten the reaction time and the neutral metal NPs will be formed faster. During the green synthesis of metal NPs via green synthesis the average particle size / particle size distribution should be controlled by setting the parameters of synthesis. In the case of using plant extracts as the source of reducing organic material, for example, the amount of plant component used in extraction, the extraction solvent and temperature should be chosen appropriately. Then the ratio of plant extract / metal salt solution, the concentration of metal salt solution, the temperature (and maybe the pH) of the reaction mixture will be important parameters in order to end up with metal NPs with desired size, shape and characteristics. Especially silver (Ag) NPs may be prepared extremely small, consisting of silver atoms, and typically range in size from 1 to 100 nms. They are excellent for a variety of biomedical applications because of their small size, which enables them to interact with biological molecules and cellular structures. Silver nanoparticles have been used by researchers for their potential as an antimicrobial (Chahar, *et al.*, 2018; Erdem & Çakır, 2022) and antifungal (Ediz *et al.*, 2021) agent. There is an increasing research interest on the utilization of metal NPs (like Ag-NPs) prepared via green chemistry for their utilization in cancer therapy (Vaid *et al.*, 2020, Nakkala *et al.*, 2017, Nayak *et al.*, 2016, Palaniapan *et al.*, 2015). The green synthesized metal NPs (like Ag-NPs) are found to be more reliable thanks to the lack of synthetic chemicals during their preparation. The natural phytochemicals in the extract of the plant parts may have beneficial properties in biomedical applications like cancer therapy. The possible side effects of synthetic chemicals during cancer therapy may be eliminated with the utilization of green synthesis method for preparation of metal NPs (like Ag-NPs) for cancer therapy (Vaid *et al.*, 2020).

Some examples of research activities on green synthesis of Ag-NPs and their anticancer potential are listed on Table 1 (Jain *et al.*, 2021). Considering the particle sizes reported for Ag-NPs prepared via different plants, the NPs prepared are mostly in a size range (e.g., 5 – 15, 20 – 100 nm) in 1 – 100 nm size range. The particle size analysis was mostly performed via SEM or TEM. A number of particles and / or micrographs were investigated to give the size range and / or report the average particle size. Some researchers also used DLS for particle size determination (Huo *et al.*, 2018, Zhang *et al.*, 2019, Pei *et al.* 2019, Kuppusamy *et al.* 2016). The values determined via DLS method were all higher than the average particle size values determined via electron microscopy (SEM, TEM) (e.g., 5 – 15 nm via electron microscopy and 247.6 nm via DLS method (Huo *et al.*, 2018)). This may be explained by the possible agglomeration of NPs in the aqueous suspension used as sample for particle size distribution (PSD) analysis via DLS method. Some researchers did not use the XRD analysis for characterizing the crystallinity of Ag-NPs but they also used it for calculating the crystallite size using the Scherrer Equation and compared the crystalline size with average particle size values determined via electron microscopy (or DLS method). The crystalline size values were mostly smaller or similar to the particle size values determined via electron microscopy, and they were smaller than the particle size values determined via DLS method.

Nanoparticle applications on cancer cells cause oxidative stress by increased reactive oxygen species (ROS) production and eventually DNA damage. These nanoparticles make the mitochondrial membrane more permeable and decreasing ATP synthesis, causes mitochondrial death. Additionally, nanoparticles stop the cell cycle at the G2/M phase. By activating pro-apoptotic proteins, which is important for initiating the apoptosis process. Intracellular pro-apoptotic proteins are released after DNA damage, activating caspases and resulting in cell death. Adopted from Jain *et al.*, 2021. Created by BioRender.

Figure 1. Synthesis of nanoparticles through green synthesis method and effects on cancer cells

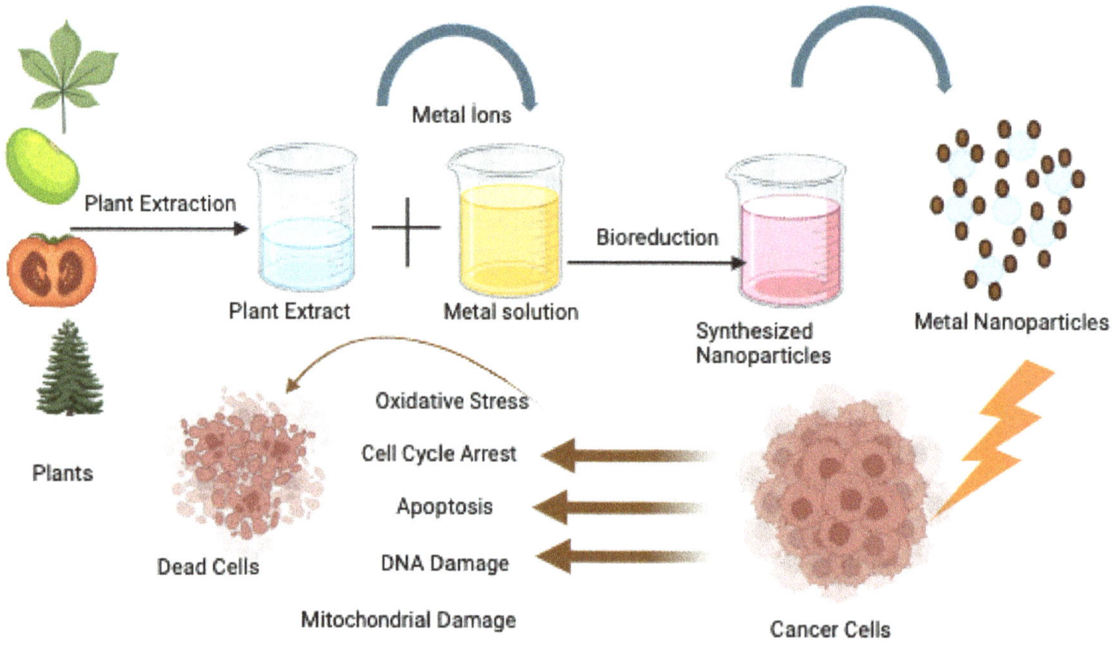

ANTICANCER BEHAVIOUR OF METAL NPs

According to the majority of studies (Miethling-Graff *et al.*, 2014; Raja *et al.*, 2020; Chairuangkitti *et al.*, 2013), the generation of reactive oxygen species (ROS) is linked to the anti-cancer effects. It has been demonstrated that exposure to silver nanoparticles (Ag-NPs) raises ROS levels, which causes cellular toxicity, lowers the rate of cell division, damages biological molecules and cell structures, and finally causes cell death (Figure 1) (Miranda *et al.*, 2022). Ag-NPs also interfere with the antioxidant molecules that are present in cells. For instance, Miranda and colleagues conducted a study using human hepatocarcinoma cells (HepG2) and 10 nm citrate-coated Ag-NPs, which revealed a decrease in proteins linked to glutathione metabolism in cancer cells but not in normal cells exposed to the same nanoparticles (Rank Miranda *et al.*, 2020).

Similar results were found in a study by Barcińska and collagues, who found that after treatment with Ag NPs, pancreatic tumour cells had higher ROS levels and lower antioxidant levels (Barcińska *et al.*, 2018). In addition, the authors observed that smaller Ag-NPs (2.6 nm) were more harmful than bigger ones (18 nm). Additionally, Ag-NPs have an impact on a number of cancer-related characteristics, including drug resistance, mitochondrial function, and respiratory chain (Plackal Adimuriyil George *et al.*, 2018; Lee *et al.*, 2015; Miranda *et al.*, 2018; Kovács *et al.*, 2016). This disruption causes the release of electrons and the creation of ROS, causing oxidative stress that interferes with other molecular pathways and ultimately causes the death of cancer cells (Sofi *et al.*, 2022).

The activation of p53, Caspase-3, LC3-II, ATG7, beclin-1, ATG5, and p-Er K1/2 as well as the deactivation of AKT, P62, and p-AKT autophagic indicators are only a few of the signalling pathways that Ag-NPs disrupt in tumour cells (Buttacavoli *et al.*, 2018; Sofi *et al.*, 2022). This ultimately leads to programmed cell death in cancer cells.

Table 1. Green synthesised silver nanoparticles and their anticancer activities

Type of cancer	Plant	Cell model	NP size (nm)	IC 50 (µg/mL) @24 h	Mechanism of Action	References
Human breast cancer	Artocarpus integer	MCF-7, MG-63 cells	5.76 - 19.1	90 – 70 (110 for healthy cells)	Interfere with DNA, cell damage, cytotoxicity	Majeed *et al.*, 2019
	Annona squamosa	MCF-7 cells	20 - 100	50 (30 for healthy cells)	Induction of apoptosis	Vivek *et al.*, 2012
	Cynara scolymus	MCF7 cells	98.47		Mitochondrial apoptosis	Erdogan *et al.*, 2019
	Camellia Sinensis Green tea	MCF-7 cells	50		Decrease O-GlcNAc Transferase (OGT) and cytotoxicity	Rasheed *et al.*, 2019
	Couroupita guianensis	MCF-7 Cell Line	28.4	20	Cytotoxicity	Deveraj *et al.*, 2013
	Glycyrrhiza uralensis	MCF7cells	5 – 15 (247.6 nm via DLS)		Cytotoxicity	Huo *et al.*, 2018
	Juglans regia (Walnuts)	MCF-7 cell	31.4		Disturb the signaling pathway, increase ROS	Khorrami *et al.*, 2018
	Lonicera hypoglauca	MCF-7 cells	10 – 50		Increases in expressions of pro-apoptotic Bax, caspase-3 & caspase-9	Jang *et al.*, 2016
	Sesbania grandiflora	MCF-7	22		Apoptosis, oxidative stress, interfere cell membrane integrity, decrease cell proliferation, DNA damage	Jeyaraj *et al.*, 2013
	Melia dubia	KB cell line	5 – 35	31.2	Cell toxicity	Kathiravan *et al.*, 2014
	Nostoc linckia	MCF-7			Inhibits growth of tumor	El-Naggar *et al.*, 2017
Prostate cancer cells	Alternanthera sessili	PC3	30 – 50		Antiproliferative, cell toxicity	Firdhouse & Lalitha, 2013
	Salvia miltiorrhiza	LNCaP cell lines	12 – 80, (128 nm via DLS)	50 – 75	Apoptosis and cytotoxicity by bax, Bcl2 intrinsic pathway	Zhang *et al.*, 2019
Lung carcinoma	Bauhinia tomentosa Linn	A-549	11.6 - 33	28.125	Inhibits proliferation	Mukundan *et al.*, 2015
	Capparis zeylanicu	A549 cell line	28		Induce apoptosis	Nilavukkarasi *et al.*, 2020
	Coptis chinensis	A549-cell	6 – 45 (135.8 nm via DLS)	15 – 20	Induce intrinsic pathway apoptosis	Pei *et al.*, 2019
	Indigofera tinctoria	A549	9 – 26	59.33	Increase ROS and leads to cell death	Vijayan *et al.*, 2018
	Zanthoxylum rhetsa	A549	10 – 68	65.17	Ag+ ion interact with cell membrane, protein, DNA, RNA leads to cell death	Nayaka *et al.*, 2020
Hepatic cancer	Asafoetida	HepG2 cell line	90 – 100		Antiproliferative	Satsangi, 2020

continued on following page

Table 1. Continued

Type of cancer	Plant	Cell model	NP size (nm)	IC 50 (µg/mL) @24 h	Mechanism of Action	References
	Myrtus communis	HepG2	20 – 30		down regulation of Pl3k/Akt, ERK and NF-kB pathways and inhibit cell proliferation	Ali Abuderman *et al.*, 2019
	Nigella sativa	HepG2 cell lines	10 - 20		Apoptosis & increase ROS production	Usmani *et al.*, 2019
	Phyllanthus emblica	HeLa cells, HUH-7			Cytotoxicity	Singh *et al.*, 2019
Cervical cancer	Iresine herbstii	HeLa	44 – 64	51	Cytotoxic activity	Dipankar & Murugan, 2012
	Moringa oleifera	HeLa	40		reactive oxygen species (ROS)	Vasanth *et al.*, 2014
	Nepeta deflersiana	HeLA	33		Increase oxidative stress, apoptosis and necrosis	Al-Sheddi *et al.*, 2018
	Nothapodytes nimmonian	HeLA cell	44 – 64	87.32	Inhibits proliferations	Mahendran & Kumari, 2016
	Punica granatum Pomegranate	HeLa cell line	41.69 - 69.61	100	Apoptosis	Sarkar & Kotteeswaran, 2018
	Prunus domestica	HeLa	5 – 30	3.45	Cytotoxic	Islam *et al.*, 2017
Colon Cancer	Commelina nudiflora	HCT-116	24 – 80 (280 via DLS)	100	Upregulate apoptotic genes, apoptosis	Kuppusamy *et al.*, 2016
	Flavonoids	HCT116	2 – 10	4 – 6	Mitochondrial impairment, DNA damage	Gurunathan *et al.*, 2018
	Vitex negundo	HCT15	5 - 47	> 100	Cell cycle arrest at G0/G1-phase, DNA damage, apoptosis	Prabhu *et al.*, 2013
Breast cancer, liver cancer	Cucumis prophetarum	A549, MDA-MB-231, HepG2, and MCF-7	–	105.8	Apoptosis, cytotoxicity	Hemlata *et al.*, 2020
Breast and prostate cancer	Hyptis suaveolens	MDA-MB-231 and PC-3 Cells	12 – 25	74.66 (for MDA-MB-231), 173.21 (for PC-3)	Interfere with protein, nitrogen base, DNA and cause apoptosis	Botcha & Prattipati, 2020
Prostate & Breast adeno-carcinoma	Momordica cymbalaria	PC-3 & MDA-MB 231 cells	10 – 50	81.1	Damage genetic material, cell organelle- leads to cell death	Hemlata *et al.*, 2020
	Momordica cymbalaria	PC-3 & MDA-MB 231 cells	10 – 50	81.1	Damage genetic material, cell organelle- leads to cell death	Hemlata *et al.*, 2020

Effects of Metal Nanoparticles on Cancer

The results of the research reports about the anticancer potential of green synthesized Ag-NPs are tabulated on Table 1 for various cancer types. The plants used were very versatile and synthesized Ag-NPs have varying average particle sizes. The IC50 values showing the concentration of the AgNPs to result in death for 50% of the cells are also changing in a wide range (e.g., 4 to >100 μg/mL). The Ag-NPs were reported to be more lethal to the cancer cells than to the regular healthy cells in general. The IC50 values 70 – 90 μg/mL for the cancer cells while it was a higher value (110 μg/mL) for healthy cells (Majeed *et al.*, 2019). There was an exceptional case where the IC50 value for the healthy cells (30 μg/mL) was lower than the value for cancer cells (50 μg/mL) reported by Vivek *et al.* (2012) for Ag-NPs tested with breast cancer cells.

Since the Ag-NPs were prepared via various plants and tested against various cancer types the reported research activities may be further investigated by classifying them with respect to the type of cancer for which the green synthesized Ag-NPs were tested.

NPs Affecting Breast Cancer

Recent years have seen a notable movement in the direction of creative and environmentally friendly methods for synthesising NPs with potential applications in cancer treatment. One noteworthy method involves using reducing agents generated from plants to produce NPs using green synthesis techniques. This not only allays worries about the negative environmental effects of conventional synthesis methods, but also bears potential results for battling breast cancer—a major worldwide health issue.

Particularly in the context of breast cancer, silver nanoparticles (Ag-NPs) have shown promising inhibitory effects against cancer cells. Chemotherapy is less successful because having the multidrug resistance transporters that cause drug resistance in breast cancer cells and these NPs interfere with the multidrug resistance transporters (Gopisetty *et al.*, 2019; Goebel *et al.*, 2021). Breast cancer cells quickly absorb Ag-NPs because they overexpress folate receptors, which makes cancer cells more hazardous than healthy cells (Frigerio *et al.*, 2019). Additionally, some Ag-NPs, such as those conjugated to soybean agglutinin, are more toxic to breast cancer cell lines due to altered surface glycosylation patterns (Pimentel *et al.*, 2016).

Cell-penetrating peptides are frequently employed to enhance the intracellular transport of Ag-NPs within cancer cells (Åmand *et al.*, 2012). Studies have demonstrated that Ag-NPs functionalized peptides improve the internalisation and cell toxicity against breast cancer cells (Mussa Farkhani *et al.*, 2017). Additionally, it has been discovered that Ag-NPs can overcome multidrug resistance by causing endoplasmic reticulum stress and autophagy induction in breast cancer cells (Gopisetty *et al.*, 2019).

Ag-NPs have been shown to cause apoptosis, which is an important mechanism that controls cell survival and death, often known as programmed cell death, in human breast cancer cells by ROS production, mitochondrial damage, and DNA damage in a dose-dependent way in certain studies that have investigated novel approaches to AgNP synthesis, such as using tamarind fruit shells (Gomathi *et al.*, 2020).

Ag-NPs have also demonstrated the capacity to increase the expression of vascular endothelial growth factor-A (VEGF) and restrict the transcription of hypoxia-inducible factor-1 (HIF-1), both of which have an effect on angiogenesis and tumour progression (Jabeen *et al.*, 2021). The development of blood vessels was shown to be decreased and the harmful effects on tumour cells to be increased by Ag-NPs made from red amaranth (Yang *et al.*, 2016).

Adenium obesum's aqueous leaf extract was used to synthesize Ag-NPs (10–30 nm), and reactive oxygen species (ROS) and DNA damage were the first two things that happened after being exposed to these NPs, which set off a series of events in human breast cancer cells, which led to the induction of apoptosis and autophagy in the MCF-7 cell lines (Farah *et al.* 2016). Another research also uncovered an intriguing link between autophagy, a cellular recycling process, and the anti-cancer properties of the Ag-NPs, suggesting a complex mechanism obtained by Jeyarah and colleagues found that NPs made from Sesbania grandiflora aqueous leaf extract killed breast cancer cells by inducing apoptosis (Jeyaraj *et al.* 2013). The ability of the NPs to induce apoptosis in breast cancer cells was later demonstrated through experimentation, correlating with the findings of Farah and colleagues. The success of the researchers in synthesizing Ag-NPs with a size of 22 nm using this Sesbania grandiflora aqueous leaf extract is evidenced by the subsequent demonstration of the NPs' anti-cancer effects on breast cancer.

One study concentrated on that production of Ag-NPs with oak fruit hull (Jaft) extract and their possible cytotoxic effects on breast cancer cells. On MCF-7 breast cancer cells, the cytotoxicity of the Ag-NPs was assessed, and it was discovered that the extract had more cytotoxic activity than the isolated Ag-NPs. These results imply that the Jaft extract containing Ag-NPs might be a possible substitute agent for the treatment of breast cancer. Overall, the study offers insightful information about biosynthesis and possible uses of Ag-NPs in the treatment of cancer. On cancer cell lines (MCF-7), results indicate that the presence of Jaft extract increased the cytotoxic effects of Ag-NPs were investigated (Heydari & Rashidipour; 2015). The outcomes demonstrated that the biosynthesized Ag-NPs exhibited cytotoxic activity, indicating their potential as a substitute agent for the treatment of human breast cancer.

Diethyldithiocarbamate (DE) is a potent Cancer Stem Cell (CSC) inhibitor that works by targeting a detoxifying enzyme (ALDH1A) (Deitrich and Erwin, 1971; Kitson, 1975; Vallari and Pietruszko, 1982; Kitson, 1983; Lipsky *et al.*, 2001). Nanoformulating DE with copper oxide (Cu4O3) and zinc oxide NPs enhances its effects. The resulting nanocomplexes, CD NPs and ZD NPs, demonstrate superior apoptotic and anti-migration potential in MDA-MB 231 cells. These nanocomplexes selectively elevate reactive oxygen species and deplete glutathione in tumour tissues, unlike fluorouracil. CD NPs, with higher uptake and oxidant activity, induce apoptosis, suppress hypoxia-inducing factor genes, and eliminate CD44+CSCs (metastasis initiating cells), reducing tumour size and metastasis to the liver.

With respect to breast cancer cells, Ag-NPs exhibit a variety of anti-cancer properties, including the ability to undermine drug resistance pathways, exhibit cancer cell-specific toxicity, enhance intracellular trafficking via cell-penetrating peptides, activate autophagy, induce ROS-dependent stress and influence angiogenesis. These results suggest the therapeutic potential of Ag-NPs for breast cancer, but further studies are required to determine their clinical efficacy and safety.

These studies demonstrate an amazing blending of green synthesis techniques with breast cancer treatment. Through DNA damage, ROS production and induction of programmed cell death, NPs specifically designed in size and properties for efficient contact with cancer cells have a significant impact on a variety of cancer cell survival pathways. A comprehensive study of NP-cellular process interactions is enabled by the simultaneous induction of autophagy.

In conclusion, the combination of green synthesis methods with NP-based breast cancer treatment represents a promising development in the fight against cancer. These results demonstrate the ability of plant-derived NPs to selectively target and destroy breast cancer cells, providing hope for future effective and green therapeutic approaches.

NPs Affecting Lung Cancer

The battle against lung cancer is ferocious and scientists are working to find new ways to treat this fatal condition. NPs have become viable options for targeted cancer therapy in recent years. Among them, silver NPs have drawn a lot of interest because of their distinctive characteristics and prospective uses in the treatment of cancer.

A study on the anti-cancer capabilities of silver NPs produced with Artemisia princeps leaf extract was published in 2015 by Gurunathan and his colleagues. The potential of these NPs to fight lung cancer was demonstrated. More particular, they were discovered to kill lung cancer A549 cells in a dose-dependent manner while sparing healthy L132 lung cell lines. In order to effectively treat cancer, cancer therapy must be selective to minimize harm to healthy tissues. Artemisia princeps leaf extract is used in a novel and environmentally friendly way to create these silver NPs (Gurunathan *et al.* 2015). This method's attraction is increased using Artemisia princeps, a plant renowned for its numerous medical benefits. In addition to highlighting the potential of silver NPs, it also emphasizes how crucial it is to use natural resources to create novel medicines.

In 2018, Padinjarathil and his team made another big advancement when they investigated the usage of silver NPs coated with galactomannan, a polysaccharide produced from the pomegranate's (Punica granatum) fruit peel. These 30 nm-sized NPs were examined for their potential to inhibit the growth of the A549 lung cancer cell line. The explanation of the fundamental mechanism underlying the reported anti-cancer effects was what made this study unique. The apoptotic pathways in the A549 lung cancer cells were shown to be activated by the galactomannan-coated silver NPs (Padinjarathil *et al.* 2018). In this case, the cancer cells underwent apoptosis due to the silver NPs, which ultimately caused their death. The potential of silver NPs in the treatment of lung cancer is a testament to how rapidly cancer research is developing. The research carried out by Gurunathan, Padinjarathil, and their individual teams has created promising new opportunities for the treatment of cancer. Silver NPs' capacity to specifically target and eradicate cancer cells while leaving healthy ones unharmed raises the prospect of more effective and non-toxic treatments.

Lung cancer treatment using silver NPs (Ag-NPs) made from diverse plant extracts has showed encouraging outcomes. These Ag-NPs predominantly use the apoptotic route to cause cytotoxicity. Key discoveries and mechanisms consist of:

Ag-NPs cause lung cancer cells to undergo apoptosis as its mode of action. Bax and Bak proteins help with the release of cytochrome c from mitochondria during this phase. A critical stage occurs when the mitochondrial membrane becomes more permeable during pro-apoptotic processes.

Gene and Protein Regulation: In tumour cells, Ag-NPs reduce the expression of the anti-apoptotic Bcl-2 genes while increasing the expression of pro-apoptotic proteins such CASP3 and CASP9. Cell death is facilitated by this change in the ratio of pro- to anti-apoptotic molecules.

MiR-192 regulation: The RB1 gene's expression is decreased by miR-192, which is probably activated by Ag-NPs. This decrease intensifies the apoptotic process in tumour cells even more.

Ag-NPs show dose-dependent cytotoxicity, with lung cancer cells (the A549 cell line) showing more toxicity than healthy cells. The increased activity of mitochondria in tumour cells is thought to be the cause of this selectivity (Fard *et al.*, 2018; Scatena, 2012).

Interference with DNA and Proteins: Silver ions produced from Ag-NPs can bind to DNA and proteins inside cancer cells, potentially preventing their normal function and limiting the cancer cells' survival and proliferative ability (Othman & Nagoor, 2014).

In conclusion, the future looks bright as scientists continue to learn more about NPs and how they may be used to treat cancer. The development of silver NPs with natural extracts like Artemisia princeps and coatings like galactomannan is a prime example of the creative thinking needed to fight a difficult and deadly disease like lung cancer. Ag-NPs created from plant extracts have proven to have significant potential as a lung cancer treatment strategy. They offer a promising route for additional study and advancement in the field of cancer treatment because of their capacity to trigger apoptosis, control essential genes and proteins, and demonstrate specific cytotoxicity towards cancer cells. However, in order to confirm their efficacy and safety for potential therapeutic usage, more thorough research and clinical trials are required. Although there is still more to be done before these medicines can be extensively used in clinical settings, the journey has unquestionably started, and the future looks more promising than ever.

NPs Affecting Colon Cancer

Studies have shown that NPs are effective in preventing the spread of malignant cells and triggering their death in the case of colon cancer. This innovation in cancer research represents a big step forward in the fight against this fatal condition and gives sufferers new hope.

In 2015 a study by Mata *et al.* provides one convincing example of the anticancer activities of silver NPs. Using the aqueous leaf extract of Abutilon indicum, silver NPs with sizes ranging from 5 to 25 nms were created in this study. Subsequently, the COLO 205 cell line was used to test these NPs against colon cancer cells (Mata *et al.* 2015). The findings were startling, showing that the silver NPs were harmful to colon cancer cells. This toxicity most likely results from the capacity of NPs to interact with the cellular structures and processes of cancer cells, causing disruption of those processes and cell death.

Another study examined the possibility of silver NPs in colon cancer treatment using a different strategy and was carried out by Padinjarathil *et al.* in 2018. In this instance, galactomannan from the fruit rind of Punica granatum was used to produce silver NPs with a size of about 30 nms. These NPs, specifically the HCT116 cell line, caused a series of events that ultimately resulted in cell death when they were administered to colon cancer cells (Padinjarathil *et al.* 2018). The result, according to the researchers, was brought on by the activation of apoptotic pathways. In this situation, caspase-2, 3, 8, and 9-mediated pathways were critical in inducing the death of colon cancer cells. This finding is particularly important because it sheds light on how silver NPs work to effectively fight colon cancer.

There are various benefits to using NPs in cancer treatment, such as silver NPs in the circumstances listed above. They can target cancer cells more precisely due to their microscopic size, which enables them to delve deeply into tumour tissues. The possibility of injuring healthy surrounding tissues, a typical worry in conventional cancer treatments like chemotherapy and radiation therapy, is decreased by this tailored approach.

Additionally, therapeutic compounds such as medications or genetic material can be delivered directly to cancer cells through nanoparticle engineering. As a result, negative effects on the rest of the body are reduced when medications are delivered precisely to the tumour location.

In conclusion, many studies have indicated that the use of NPs in the treatment of colon cancer has produced positive outcomes. They have made tremendous progress towards the creation of more potent and minimally invasive cancer treatments by being able to cause cell death in colon cancer cells either through toxicity or by activating apoptotic pathways. Although additional investigation is required to fully comprehend the mechanisms at play and to evaluate long-term safety and efficacy, these discoveries have a significant impact on the lives of colon cancer patients and raise the possibility of future, more focused, less toxic treatment approaches.

NPs Affecting Cervical Cancer

NPs have attracted a lot of attention in recent years due to their special qualities and prospective uses in treating a variety of cancer types. Against cervical cancer cells like HeLa cells, NPs have shown potential anticancer effects. Their capacity to cause DNA damage and start apoptotic cell death in cancer cells is credited with this discovery.

The utilization of materials originating from plants is one significant method used in the manufacture of NPs with anticancer characteristics. The therapeutic potential of plants, particularly their ability to treat cancer, has long been acknowledged. This method boosts the efficiency of plants against cervical cancer by combining their natural anticancer capabilities with the positive aspects of silver NPs.

In a 2014 study by Vasanth *et al.*, a unique formulation was made using Styrax benzoin gum powder and silver nanoparticles. Styrax benzoin, sometimes referred to as benzoin resin, is a substance that is traditionally used in herbal medicine and is derived from the bark of specific plants. It contributed to the creation of NPs with improved anticancer activity when it was added into the synthesis of silver NPs. In cervical cancer cells, these silver nanoparticles demonstrated the ability to cause DNA damage, which compromises the integrity of the cells' genetic code.

The potential of plant-based materials in the manufacture of silver NPs for the treatment of cervical cancer was further investigated in a study done by Du *et al.* in 2016. The drumstick tree's Moringa oleifera stem bark extract was used in this experiment together with silver NPs. The nutritional advantages and wide range of medical benefits of Moringa oleifera are well known. Silver NPs were combined with this plant extract to create NPs that had a stronger anticancer effect. An essential component in eliminating cancer cells, known as apoptosis, was discovered to be the mechanism of action in HeLa cells.

In summary, the utilization of silver NPs in the treatment of cervical cancer has been significantly enhanced by incorporating plant-derived materials, such as Styrax benzoin gum powder and Moringa oleifera stem bark extract, into the synthesis process. These studies have demonstrated that these plant-based additives can augment the anticancer properties of silver NPs, leading to DNA damage and the induction of apoptotic cell death in cervical cancer cells. This research represents an innovative and promising avenue in the development of targeted therapies for cervical cancer, potentially offering improved outcomes for patients in the future. Further research in this field may uncover additional plant-derived compounds that can enhance the efficacy of silver NPs in cervical cancer treatment.

NPs Affecting Prostate Cancer

In the field of cancer therapy, NPs have shown promise as tools, with possible application to the treatment of prostate cancer. Finding novel methods for treating prostate cancer, one of the most prevalent malignancies in males, is essential. Particularly those made from natural extracts, NPs have demonstrated tremendous potential for locating and killing prostate cancer cells.

During the work has been done using silver NPs (9–32 nm) made with D. longan Lour. extract, it was discovered that these nanoparticles had cytotoxic effects only on the PC3 prostate cancer cell line (He *et al.*, 2016a,b). Because PC3 cells are an aggressive and advanced stage of prostate cancer and are therefore a difficult target for traditional therapies, this discovery is particularly important.

Apoptosis, or programmed cell death, is one of the primary processes by which these silver NPs exercise their anticancer effects. A natural mechanism called apoptosis serves to maintain tissue homeostasis by removing damaged or unneeded cells. Apoptosis is frequently compromised in the context of cancer, allowing cancer cells to avoid cell death and continue to proliferate. However, prostate cancer cells can undergo apoptosis when exposed to silver NPs.

As seen in the study, a critical stage in the apoptotic cascade is the activation of caspase-3. By cleaving different cellular proteins, the enzyme caspase-3 is essential for carrying out apoptosis, which results in cell death. The fact that caspase-3 is activated suggests that silver NPs cause prostate cancer cells to undergo a controlled and orderly process of cell death. The study also found that the expression of numerous proteins linked to cancer cell survival and resistance to apoptosis decreased. These proteins include Bcl-2 (Bcl-2: The Bcl-2 protein family controls apoptosis by either encouraging it or suppressing it. Cancer cells frequently overexpress Bcl-2 proteins that prevent apoptosis. Silver NPs may be able to tip the scales in favour of apoptosis in prostate cancer cells based on the reduced expression of Bcl-2), Stat-3, and survivin. As seen in the study, a critical stage in the apoptotic cascade is the activation of caspase-3. By cleaving different cellular proteins, the enzyme caspase-3 is essential for carrying out apoptosis, which results in cell death. The fact that caspase-3 is activated suggests that silver NPs cause prostate cancer cells to undergo a controlled and orderly process of cell death.

Green technologies used to synthesise Ag-NPs have demonstrated promising anticancer activity against prostate cancer cells. Numerous studies have emphasised their ability to suppress tumour growth and trigger apoptosis via a variety of mechanisms:

Caspase Pathway Activation: According to one study, Ag-NPs produced through green synthesis caused prostate cancer cells to undergo apoptosis (Eid *et al.*, 2002). The programmed cell death pathway is essential.

Activation of the AMPK-mTOR Pathway: According to another study, Ag-NPs activated the protein Hypoxia-Inducible Factor 1-alpha (HIF-1), which in turn triggered the AMPK-mTOR pathway and caused prostate cancer cells to die (Chen *et al.*, 2020). Cell growth and survival are regulated by this mechanism.

ROS-Independent Autophagy: In a separate work, Ag-NPs activated the same AMPK-mTOR pathway to induce autophagy in prostate cancer cells without the creation of reactive oxygen species (ROS) (Chen *et al.*, 2018). Cellular processes like autophagy can result in cell death.

Ag-NPs made from Pinus roxburghii have been demonstrated to trigger apoptosis through the intrinsic mechanism by resulting in mitochondrial depolarization and DNA damage (Kumari *et al.*, 2020).

Ag-NPs created from a variety of plant extracts, such as Salvia miltiorrhiza, Alternanthera sessilis, Dimocarpus longan lor, Elderberry, Acai berry, and Azadirachta indica, have also demonstrated anticancer action against prostate cancer cells. These investigations have repeatedly demonstrated that Ag-NPs can affect critical proteins such PARP-1, Bcl2, Bclxl, Bax, and Caspase-3 to cause cell toxicity, produce ROS, and increase apoptosis in prostate cancer cells (Kumari *et al.*, 2020; Zhang *et al.*, 2019). Importantly, there is frequently an up-regulation of Caspase-3 and a down-regulation of proteins such Stat-3, Survivin, and Bcl2, which together contribute to the inhibition of tumour growth (he *et al.*, 2016). It's noteworthy that these impacts seem to spare healthy cells.

Green-synthesized Ag-NPs have shown substantial promise as a therapeutic choice for the treatment of prostate cancer. They may be a useful addition to the arsenal of anticancer treatments due to their capacity to cause apoptosis, prevent cell growth, and modify essential proteins in cancer cells. But before they can be taken into consideration for therapeutic usage, more study, including preclinical and clinical studies, is required to fully understand their safety and effectiveness in humans.

Overall, the results of this work point to the possibility of using silver NPs produced with D. longan Lour. extract to treat prostate cancer by triggering apoptosis and concentrating on key molecular actors involved in cancer cell survival and development. This study is a critical step towards the development of innovative prostate cancer medicines based on NPs that may be more effective and have fewer side effects than current medications. To validate these results and establish the safety and effectiveness of silver NPs as a prostate cancer treatment option, more research and clinical investigations are nonetheless required.

NPs Affecting Liver Cancer

Due to its potential to provide focused and efficient therapies with few side effects, the use of nanoparticles (NPs) in the treatment of liver cancer has attracted considerable attention in recent years. The studies you've described, which used synthesised silver nanoparticles from various sources, emphasise the positive effects of NPs on liver cancer.

In the study by Padinjarathil *et al.* (2018), galactomannan from the fruit rind of Punica granatum (pomegranate) was used to create silver nanoparticles with a size of 30 nm. When compared to conventional approaches, this novel approach to NP synthesis may offer a number of benefits, including cost effectiveness and lower environmental impact.

When exposed to these silver nanoparticles, the HepG2 liver cancer cell line underwent caspase-2, 3, 8, and 9-mediated programmed cell death (apoptosis). This is a critical discovery since apoptosis naturally kills off damaged or malignant cells. The fact that caspases are activated suggests that these NPs can cause liver cancer cells to go through a tightly controlled and regulated cell death process.

The research on silver nanoparticles (20–47 nm) generated from Balanites aegyptiaca's aqueous fruit extract revealed that these NPs had cytotoxicity towards liver cancer cells. The possibility that the NPs can precisely target and harm cancer cells while sparing healthy ones raises tremendous interest in this cytotoxic impact.

According to Yassin *et al.*'s (2017) study, these silver nanoparticles have the ability to control the expression of numerous crucial genes in liver cancer cells. Notably, the downregulation of Bcl-2, TGF (transforming growth factor), survivin, and MMP-7 raises the possibility that these NPs might prevent cancer cells from growing, invasive, and surviving. Additionally, the modulation of nuclear factor-kappa B (NF-B), a crucial transcription factor implicated in inflammation and cancer, may be linked to the overexpression of IK (perhaps alluding to IB kinase).

The combined results of these research indicate that silver nanoparticles have a great deal of potential as liver cancer therapeutics. They have the ability to particularly affect cancer cells by inducing apoptosis, blocking the production of genes that promote survival and growth, and cytotoxic effects. To assess the safety and effectiveness of these effects in preclinical and clinical contexts, as well as to better understand the mechanisms underlying them, more research is nonetheless required. Future liver cancer treatments may provide patients with more specialised and non-toxic options thanks to nanoparticle-based medicines, which show promise in the fight against the disease.

CONCLUSION

In conclusion, the combination of green synthesised metal NPs (like Ag-NPs) represents a new strategy for transforming cancer treatment. Green synthesis of metal NPs promotes sustainability and environmental responsibility, in addition to exploiting the inherent qualities of natural resources. This green strategy is in line with international initiatives to improve medical research without harming the environment.

Being more cost-effective and environmentally friendly the green synthesis offers a promising alternative method for the preparation of metal NPs, which may be used in versatile applications. The scale-up of green synthesis of metal NPs is relatively more practical than the conventional methods, which is another advantage of using green synthesis for metal NP preparations.

In addition, by addressing different aspects of the treatment pathway, green-synthesised metal NPs offer a ray of hope for people suffering from cancer. These metal NPs have exceptional selectivity in drug delivery, reducing the dreaded off-target side effects associated with conventional therapy. As a result, patients can enjoy a better quality of life during treatment without experiencing negative side effects.

In addition to their delivery capabilities, green-synthesised metal NPs have become stand-alone therapeutic agents. They have the potential to improve the stability and bioavailability of substances such as curcumin, making it a potent anticancer agent. In addition to overcoming formulation difficulties, this improves the effectiveness of targeting cancer cells. The utilization of metal NPs may be a promising alternative for the conventional cancer treatments. Considering the research results reporting that the metal NPs are relatively more lethal for cancer cells than normal cells, metal NPs may be utilized as an alternative cancer therapy. This will be possible only if the average size / size distribution and surface characteristics of the metal NPs are optimized. The metal NPs should be prepared at certain size and with certain surface characteristics to enhance their uptake to the cell efficiently.

The diagnostic capabilities of green-synthesised NPs open up new avenues for the accurate and early detection of cancer. Using cancer-specific proteins, these NPs enable non-invasive imaging methods that identify tumours with unparalleled precision. This early detection significantly improves the prospects and outcomes of treatment.

In addition, the ability of these NPs to be functionalised with targeting ligands ensures that therapeutic drugs reach their intended site, sparing healthy tissue and minimising side effects. Better outcomes for cancer patients are expected thanks to the controlled release of chemotherapeutic drugs coupled with these NPs.

The green synthesis enabling utilization of plants (natural phytochemicals) for preparation of metal NPs may present some synergistic effect of metal NPs and some phytochemicals for cancer treatment. The phytochemicals in green synthesis act as reducing agent in the formation of metal NPs. Some phytochemicals act as capping (i.e., stabilizing) agent to keep the metal NPs suspended away from each other (i.e., preventing agglomeration and keeping the NPs "nano"). Besides these important roles of them, the phytochemicals may alter the surface charge / characteristics of the metal NPs and enhance the intake mechanism of the metal NPs by the cell (i.e., enhanced bioactivity). The phytochemicals should not be washed away after the metal NP formation to use their contribution as capping / stabilizing agent and possible assistance in enhanced bioactivity during intake of the metal NPs to the cell.

Green synthesis and nanotechnology working together to solve complex medical problems is an example of how interdisciplinary approaches can be used. The future holds the promise of more efficient, targeted and long-lasting therapeutic approaches in the fight against cancer, as research in this field continues to grow. In the fight against this terrible disease, we can pave the way for a better and healthier future by combining innovation and environmental awareness.

REFERENCES

Al-Sheddi, E. S., Farshori, N. N., Al-Oqail, M. M., Al-Massarani, S. M., Saquib, Q., Wahab, R., Musarrat, J., Al-Khedhairy, A. A., & Siddiqui, M. A. (2018). Anticancer Potential of Green Synthesized Silver Nanoparticles Using Extract of Nepeta deflersiana against Human Cervical Cancer Cells (HeLA). *Bioinorganic Chemistry and Applications*, *9390784*, 1–12. doi:10.1155/2018/9390784 PMID:30515193

Ali Abuderman, A., Syed, R., & Alyousef, A., A., S. Alqahtani, M., Shamsul Ola, M., & Malik, A. (2019). Green synthesized silver Nanoparticles of Myrtus communis L (AgMC) extract inhibits cancer hallmarks via targeting aldose reductase (AR) and associated signaling network. *Processes (Basel, Switzerland)*, *7*(11), 860. doi:10.3390/pr7110860

Åmand, H. L., Rydberg, H. A., Fornander, L. H., Lincoln, P., Nordén, B., & Esbjörner, E. K. (2012). Cell surface binding and uptake of arginine- and lysine-rich penetratin peptides in absence and presence of proteoglycans. *Biochimica et Biophysica Acta. Biomembranes*, *1818*(11), 2669–2678. doi:10.1016/j.bbamem.2012.06.006 PMID:22705501

Barcińska, E., Wierzbicka, J., Zauszkiewicz-Pawlak, A., Jacewicz, D., Dabrowska, A., & Inkielewicz-Stepniak, I. (2018). Role of oxidative and nitro-oxidative damage in silver nanoparticles cytotoxic effect against human pancreatic ductal adenocarcinoma cells. *Oxidative Medicine and Cellular Longevity*, *2018*, 1–15. doi:10.1155/2018/8251961 PMID:30186549

Beyene, H. D., Werkneh, A. A., Bezabh, H. K., & Ambaye, T. G. (2017). Synthesis paradigm and applications of silver nanoparticles (AgNPs), a review. *Sustainable materials and technologies*, *13*, 18-23.

Botcha, S., & Prattipati, S. D. (2020). Callus extract mediated green synthesis of silver nanoparticles, their characterization and cytotoxicity evaluation against MDA-MB-231 and PC-3 cells. *BioNanoScience*, *10*(1), 11–22. doi:10.100712668-019-00683-3

Buttacavoli, M., Albanese, N. N., Di Cara, G., Alduina, R., Faleri, C., Gallo, M., Pizzolanti, G., Gallo, G., Feo, S., Baldi, F., & Cancemi, P. (2018). Anticancer activity of biogenerated silver nanoparticles: An integrated proteomic investigation. *Oncotarget*, *9*(11), 9685–9705. doi:10.18632/oncotarget.23859 PMID:29515763

Chahar, V., Sharma, B., Shukla, G., Srivastava, A., & Bhatnagar, A. (2018). Study of antimicrobial activity of silver nanoparticles synthesized using green and chemical approach. *Colloids and Surfaces. A, Physicochemical and Engineering Aspects*, *554*, 149–155. doi:10.1016/j.colsurfa.2018.06.012

Chairuangkitti, P., Lawanprasert, S., Roytrakul, S., Aueviriyavit, S., Phummiratch, D., Kulthong, K., Chanvorachote, P., & Maniratanachote, R. (2013). Silver nanoparticles induce toxicity in A549 cells via ROS-dependent and ROS-independent pathways. *Toxicology In Vitro*, *27*(1), 330–338. doi:10.1016/j.tiv.2012.08.021 PMID:22940466

Chen, Y., Wang, M., Zhang, T., Du, E., Liu, Y., Qi, S., Xu, Y., & Zhang, Z. (2018). Autophagic effects and mechanisms of silver nanoparticles in renal cells under low dose exposure. *Ecotoxicology and Environmental Safety*, *166*, 71–77. doi:10.1016/j.ecoenv.2018.09.070 PMID:30248563

Chen, Y., Yang, T., Chen, S., Qi, S., Zhang, Z., & Xu, Y. (2020). Silver nanoparticles regulate autophagy through lysosome injury and cell hypoxia in prostate cancer cells. *Journal of Biochemical and Molecular Toxicology*, *34*(5), e22474. doi:10.1002/jbt.22474 PMID:32043710

Chopra, H., Bibi, S., Singh, I., Hasan, M. M., Khan, M. S., Yousafi, Q., Baig, A. A., Rahman, M. M., Islam, F., Emran, T. B., & Cavalu, S. (2022). Green Metallic Nanoparticles: Biosynthesis to Applications. *Frontiers in Bioengineering and Biotechnology*, *10*, 874742. doi:10.3389/fbioe.2022.874742 PMID:35464722

Dadashpour, M., Firouzi-Amandi, A., Pourhassan-Moghaddam, M., Maleki, M. J., Soozangar, N., Jeddi, F., Nouri, M., Zarghami, N., & Pilehvar-Soltanahmadi, Y. (2018). Biomimetic synthesis of silver nanoparticles using Matricaria chamomilla extract and their potential anticancer activity against human lung cancer cells. *Materials Science and Engineering C*, *92*, 902–912. doi:10.1016/j.msec.2018.07.053 PMID:30184820

Deitrich, R. A., & Erwin, V. G. (1971). Mechanism of the inhibition of aldehyde dehydrogenase in vivo by disulfiram and diethyldithiocarbamate. *Molecular Pharmacology*, *7*(3), 301–307. PMID:4328422

Devaraj, P., Kumari, P., Aarti, C., & Renganathan, A. (2013). Synthesis and characterization of silver nanoparticles using cannonball leaves and their cytotoxic activity against MCF-7 cell line. *Journal of Nanotechnology*, *2013*, 2013. doi:10.1155/2013/598328

Dipankar, C., & Murugan, S. (2012). The green synthesis, characterization and evaluation of the biological activities of silver nanoparticles synthesized from Iresine herbstii leaf aqueous extracts. *Colloids and Surfaces. B, Biointerfaces*, *98*, 112–119. doi:10.1016/j.colsurfb.2012.04.006 PMID:22705935

Dong, C., Cao, C., Zhang, X., Zhan, Y., Wang, X., Yang, X., Zhou, K., Xiao, X., & Yuan, B. (2017). Wolfberry fruit (Lycium barbarum) extract mediated novel route for the green synthesis of silver nanoparticles. *Optik (Stuttgart)*, *130*, 162–170. doi:10.1016/j.ijleo.2016.11.010

Ediz, E., Kurtay, G., Karaca, B., Büyük, İ., Gökdemir, F. Ş., & Aras, S. (2021). Green synthesis of silver nanoparticles from Phaseolus vulgaris L. extracts and investigation of their antifungal activities. *Hacettepe Journal of Biology and Chemistry*, *49*(1), 11–23. doi:10.15671/hjbc.680371

Eid, M. A., Lewis, R. W., Abdel-Mageed, A. B., & Kumar, M. V. (2002). Reduced response of prostate cancer cells to TRAIL is modulated by NFkappaB-mediated inhibition of caspases and bid activation. *International Journal of Oncology*. doi:10.3892/ijo.21.1.111 PMID:12063557

El-Naggar, N. E., Hussein, M. H., & El-Sawah, A. A. (2017). Bio-fabrication of silver nanoparticles by phycocyanin, characterization, in vitro anticancer activity against breast cancer cell line and in vivo cytotxicity. *Scientific Reports*, *7*(1), 10844. doi:10.103841598-017-11121-3 PMID:28883419

Erdem, İ., & Çakır, Ş. (2022). Green synthesis of silver nanoparticles using walnut shell powder and cynara sp. and their antibacterial activities. *Hacettepe Journal of Biology and Chemistry*, *50*(4), 335–347. doi:10.15671/hjbc.984727

Erdogan, O., Abbak, M., Demirbolat, G. M., Birtekocak, F., Aksel, M., Pasa, S., & Cevik, O. (2019). Green synthesis of silver nanoparticles via Cynara scolymus leaf extracts: The characterization, anti-cancer potential with photodynamic therapy in MCF7 cells. *PLoS One*, *14*(6), e0216496. doi:10.1371/journal.pone.0216496 PMID:31220110

Farah, M., Ali, M. A., Chen, S. M., Li, Y., Al-Hemaid, F. M., & Abou-Tarboush, F. M. (2016). Silver nanoparticle synthesized from Adenium obesum leaf extract: Anticancer, antimicrobial, antioxidant and catalytic activities. *Arabian Journal of Chemistry*, *9*(6), 970–975.

Fard, N. N., Noorbazargan, H., Mirzaie, A., Hedayati, Ch. M., Moghimiyan, Z., & Rahimi, A. (2018). Biogenic synthesis of Ag-NPs using Artemisia oliveriana extract and their biological activities for an effective treatment of lung cancer. *Artificial Cells, Nanomedicine, and Biotechnology*, *46*(sup3), 1047–1058. doi:10.1080/21691401.2018.1528983 PMID:30479160

Firdhouse, M. J., & Lalitha, P. (2013). Biosynthesis of silver nanoparticles using the extract of Alternanthera sessilis-antiproliferative effect against prostate cancer cells. *Cancer Nanotechnology*, *4*(6), 137–143. doi:10.100712645-013-0045-4 PMID:26069509

Frigerio, B., Bizzoni, C., Jansen, G., Leamon, C. P., Peters, G. J., Low, P. S., Matherly, L. H., & Figini, M. (2019). Folate receptors and transporters: Biological role and diagnostic/therapeutic targets in cancer and other diseases. *Journal of Experimental & Clinical Cancer Research: Cr.* . doi:10.1186/s13046-019-1123-1

Goebel, J., Chmielewski, J., & Hrycyna, C. A. (2021). The roles of the human ATP-binding cassette transporters P-glycoprotein and ABCG2 in multidrug resistance in cancer and at endogenous sites: Future opportunities for structure-based drug design of inhibitors. *Cancer Drug Resistance (Alhambra, Calif.).* doi:10.20517/cdr.2021.19 PMID:34993424

Gomathi, A. C., Xavier Rajarathinam, S. R., Mohammed Sadiq, A., & Rajeshkumar, S. (2020). Anticancer activity of silver nanoparticles synthesized using aqueous fruit shell extract of Tamarindus indica on MCF-7 human breast cancer cell line. *Journal of Drug Delivery Science and Technology*, *55*, 101376. doi:10.1016/j.jddst.2019.101376

Gopisetty, M. K., Kovács, D., Igaz, N., Rónavári, A., Bélteky, P., Rázga, Z., Venglovecz, V., Csoboz, B., Boros, I. M., Kónya, Z., & Kiricsi, M. (2019). Endoplasmic reticulum stress: Major player in size-dependent inhibition of P-glycoprotein by silver nanoparticles in multidrug-resistant breast cancer cells. *Journal of Nanobiotechnology*, *17*(1), 1–15. doi:10.118612951-019-0448-4 PMID:30670028

Gurunathan, S., Jeong, J. K., Han, J. W., Zhang, X. F., Park, J. H., & Kim, J. H. (2015). Multidimensional effects of biologically synthesized silver NPs in Helicobacter pylori, Helicobacter felis, and human lung (L132) and lung carcinoma A549 cells. *Nanoscale Research Letters*, *10*(1), 35. doi:10.118611671-015-0747-0 PMID:25852332

Gurunathan, S., Qasim, M., Park, C., Yoo, H., Kim, J. H., & Hong, K. (2018). Cytotoxic Potential and Molecular Pathway Analysis of Silver Nanoparticles in Human Colon Cancer Cells HCT116. *International Journal of Molecular Sciences*, *19*(8), 2269. doi:10.3390/ijms19082269 PMID:30072642

He, Y., Du, Z., Ma, S., Cheng, S., Jiang, S., Liu, Y., Li, D., Huang, H., Zhang, K., & Zheng, X. (2016). Biosynthesis, Antibacterial Activity and Anticancer Effects against prostate Cancer (PC-3) cells of silver nanoparticles using Dimocarpus Longan Lour. Peel Extract. *Nanoscale Research Letters*, *11*(1), 300. doi:10.118611671-016-1511-9 PMID:27316741

He, Y., Du, Z., Ma, S., Cheng, S., Jiang, S., Liu, Y., Li, D., Huang, H., Zhang, K., & Zheng, X. (2016a). Biosynthesis, antibacterial activity and anticancer effects against prostate cancer (PC-3) cells of silver NPs using Dimocarpus Longan Lour. peel extract. *Nanoscale Research Letters*, *11*(1), 300. doi:10.118611671-016-1511-9 PMID:27316741

He, Y., Du, Z., Ma, S., Liu, Y., Li, D., Huang, H., Jiang, S., Cheng, S., Wu, W., Zhang, K., & Zheng, X. (2016b). Effects of green-synthesized silver NPs on lung cancer cells in vitro and grown as xenograft tumors in vivo. *International Journal of Nanomedicine*, *11*, 1879. doi:10.2147/IJN.S103695 PMID:27217750

Hemlata, M., Meena, P. R., Singh, A. P., & Tejavath, K. K. (2020). Biosynthesis of Silver Nanoparticles Using Cucumis prophetarum Aqueous Leaf Extract and Their Antibacterial and Antiproliferative Activity Against Cancer Cell Lines. *ACS Omega*, *5*(10), 5520–5528. doi:10.1021/acsomega.0c00155 PMID:32201844

Heydari, R., & Rashidipour, M. (2015). Green synthesis of silver nanoparticles using extract of oak fruit hull (jaft): Synthesis and in vitro cytotoxic effect on mcf-7 cells. *International Journal of Breast Cancer*, *846743*, 1–6. doi:10.1155/2015/846743 PMID:25685560

Huo, Y., Singh, P., Kim, Y. J., Soshnikova, V., Kang, J., Markus, J., Ahn, S., Castro-Aceituno, V., Mathiyalagan, R., Chokkalingam, M., Bae, K. S., & Yang, D. C. (2018). Biological synthesis of gold and silver chloride nanoparticles by Glycyrrhiza uralensis and in vitro applications. *Artificial Cells, Nanomedicine, and Biotechnology*, *46*(2), 303–312. doi:10.1080/21691401.2017.1307213 PMID:28375686

Islam, N. U., Amin, R., Shahid, M., Amin, M., Zaib, S., & Iqbal, J. (2017). A multi-target therapeutic potential of Prunus domestica gum stabilized nanoparticles exhibited prospective anticancer, antibacterial, urease-inhibition, anti-inflammatory and analgesic properties. *BMC Complementary and Alternative Medicine*, *17*(1), 276. doi:10.118612906-017-1791-3 PMID:28535789

Jabeen, S., Qureshi, R., Munazir, M., Maqsood, M., Munir, M., Shah, S. S. H., & Rahim, B. Z. (2021). Application of green synthesized silver nanoparticles in cancer treatment - A critical review. *Materials Research Express*, *8*(9), 092001. doi:10.1088/2053-1591/ac1de3

Jain, N., Jain, P., Rajput, D., & Patil, U. K. (2021). Green synthesized plant-based silver nanoparticles: Therapeutic prospective for anticancer and antiviral activity. *Micro and Nano Systems Letters*, *9*(1), 5. doi:10.118640486-021-00131-6

Jang, S. J., Yang, I. J., Tettey, C. O., Kim, K. M., & Shin, H. M. (2016). In-vitro anticancer activity of green synthesized silver nanoparticles on MCF-7 human breast cancer cells. *Materials Science and Engineering C*, *68*, 430–435. doi:10.1016/j.msec.2016.03.101 PMID:27524038

Jeyaraj, M., Sathishkumar, G., Sivanandhan, G., MubarakAli, D., Rajesh, M., Arun, R., Kapildev, G., Manickavasagam, M., Thajuddin, N., Premkumar, K., & Ganapathi, A. (2013). Biogenic silver nanoparticles for cancer treatment: An experimental report. *Colloids and Surfaces. B, Biointerfaces*, *106*, 86–92. doi:10.1016/j.colsurfb.2013.01.027 PMID:23434696

Kathiravan, V., Ravi, S., & Ashokkumar, S. (2014). Synthesis of silver nanoparticles from Melia dubia leaf extract and their in vitro anticancer activity. *Spectrochimica Acta. Part A: Molecular and Biomolecular Spectroscopy*, *130*, 116–121. doi:10.1016/j.saa.2014.03.107 PMID:24769382

Khorrami, S., Zarrabi, A., Khaleghi, M., Danaei, M., & Mozafari, M. R. (2018). Selective cytotoxicity of green synthesized silver nanoparticles against the MCF-7 tumor cell line and their enhanced antioxidant and antimicrobial properties. *International Journal of Nanomedicine*, *13*, 8013–8024. doi:10.2147/IJN.S189295 PMID:30568442

Kitson, T. M. (1975). The effect of disulfiram on the aldehyde dehydrogenases of sheep liver. *The Biochemical Journal*, *151*(2), 407–412. doi:10.1042/bj1510407 PMID:3167

Kitson, T. M. (1983). Mechanism of inactivation of sheep liver cytoplasmic aldehyde dehydrogenase by disulfiram. *The Biochemical Journal*, *213*(2), 551–554. doi:10.1042/bj2130551 PMID:6615449

Klaine, S. J., Alvarez, P. J., Batley, G. E., Fernandes, T. F., Handy, R. D., Lyon, D. Y., Mahendra, S., McLaughlin, M. J., & Lead, J. R. (2008). Nanomaterials in the environment: Behavior, fate, bioavailability, and effects. *Environmental Toxicology and Chemistry*, *27*(9), 1825–1851. doi:10.1897/08-090.1 PMID:19086204

Kovács, D., Szoke, K., Igaz, N., Spengler, G., Molnár, J., Tóth, T., Madarász, D., Rázga, Z., Kónya, Z., Boros, I. M., & Kiricsi, M. (2016). Silver nanoparticles modulate ABC transporter activity and enhance chemotherapy in multidrug resistant cancer. *Nanomedicine; Nanotechnology, Biology, and Medicine*, *12*(3), 601–610. doi:10.1016/j.nano.2015.10.015 PMID:26656631

Kumari, R., Saini, A. K., Kumar, A., & Saini, R. V. (2020). Apoptosis induction in lung and prostate cancer cells through silver nanoparticles synthesized from Pinus roxburghii bioactive fraction. *Journal of Biological Inorganic Chemistry*, *25*(1), 23–37. doi:10.100700775-019-01729-3 PMID:31641851

Kuppusamy, P., Ichwan, S. J., Al-Zikri, P. N., Suriyah, W. H., Soundharrajan, I., Govindan, N., Maniam, G. P., & Yusoff, M. M. (2016). In Vitro Anticancer Activity of Au, Ag Nanoparticles Synthesized Using Commelina nudiflora L. Aqueous Extract Against HCT-116 Colon Cancer Cells. *Biological Trace Element Research*, *173*(2), 297–305. doi:10.100712011-016-0666-7 PMID:26961292

Lee, M. J., Lee, S. J., Yun, S. J., Jang, J. Y., Kang, H., Kim, K., Choi, I. H., & Park, S. (2015). Silver nanoparticles affect glucose metabolism in hepatoma cells through production of reactive oxygen species. *International Journal of Nanomedicine*, 55. doi:10.2147/IJN.S94907 PMID:26730190

Lipsky, J. J., Shen, M. L., & Naylor, S. (2001). In vivo inhibition of aldehyde dehydrogenase by disulfiram. *Chemico-Biological Interactions*, *130-132*(1-3), 93–102. doi:10.1016/S0009-2797(00)00225-8 PMID:11306034

Mahendran, G., & Kumari, B. R. (2016). Biological activities of silver nanoparticles from Nothapodytes nimmoniana (Graham) Mabb. fruit extracts. *Food Science and Human Wellness*, *5*(4), 207–218. doi:10.1016/j.fshw.2016.10.001

Majeed, S., Bakhtiar, N. F. B., Danish, M., Ibrahim, M. M., & Hashim, R. (2019). Green approach for the biosynthesis of silver nanoparticles and its antibacterial and antitumor effect against osteoblast MG-63 and breast MCF-7 cancer cell lines. *Sustainable Chemistry and Pharmacy*, *12*, 100138. doi:10.1016/j.scp.2019.100138

Makarov, V. V., Love, A. J., Sinitsyna, O. V., Makarova, S. S., Yaminsky, I. V., Taliansky, M. E., & Kalinina, N. O. (2014). "Green" nanotechnologies: Synthesis of metal nanoparticles using plants. [англоязычная версия]. *Acta Naturae (English Ed.)*, *6*(1 (20)), 35–44. doi:10.32607/20758251-2014-6-1-35-44 PMID:24772325

Mata, R., Nakkala, J. R., & Sadras, S. R. (2015). Biogenic silver NPs from Abutilon indicum: Their antioxidant, antibacterial and cytotoxic effects in vitro. *Colloids and Surfaces. B, Biointerfaces*, *128*, 76–86. doi:10.1016/j.colsurfb.2015.01.052 PMID:25701118

Miethling-Graff, R., Rumpker, R., Richter, M., Verano-Braga, T., Kjeldsen, F., Brewer, J., Hoyland, J., Rubahn, H. G., & Erdmann, H. (2014). Exposure to silver nanoparticles induces size- and dose-dependent oxidative stress and cytotoxicity in human colon carcinoma cells. *Toxicology In Vitro*, *28*(7), 1280–1289. doi:10.1016/j.tiv.2014.06.005 PMID:24997297

Miranda, R. R., Gorshkov, V., Korzeniowska, B., Kempf, S. J., Neto, F. F., & Kjeldsen, F. (2018). Co-exposure to silver nanoparticles and cadmium induce metabolic adaptation in HepG2 cells. *Nanotoxicology*, *12*(7), 781–795. doi:10.1080/17435390.2018.1489987 PMID:29996704

Miranda, R. R., Sampaio, I., & Zucolotto, V. (2022). Exploring silver nanoparticles for cancer therapy and diagnosis. *Colloids and Surfaces. B, Biointerfaces*, *210*, 112254. doi:10.1016/j.colsurfb.2021.112254 PMID:34896692

Mukundan, D., Mohankumar, R., & Vasanthakumari, R. (2015). Green synthesis of silver nanoparticles using leaves extract of Bauhinia tomentosa linn and its invitro anticancer potential. *Materials Today: Proceedings*, *2*(9), 4309–4316. doi:10.1016/j.matpr.2015.10.014

Mussa Farkhani, S., Asoudeh Fard, A., Zakeri-Milani, P., Shahbazi Mojarrad, J., & Valizadeh, H. (2017). Enhancing antitumor activity of silver nanoparticles by modification with cell-penetrating peptides. *Artificial Cells, Nanomedicine, and Biotechnology*, *45*(5), 1029–1035. doi:10.1080/21691401.2016.1200059 PMID:27357085

Nakkala, J. R., Mata, R., Raja, K., Khub Chandra, V., & Sadras, S. R. (2018). Green synthesized silver nanoparticles: Catalytic dye degradation, in vitro anticancer activity and in vivo toxicity in rats. *Materials Science and Engineering C*, *91*, 372–381. doi:10.1016/j.msec.2018.05.048 PMID:30033267

Nakkala, J. R., Mata, R., & Sadras, S. R. (2017). Green synthesized nano silver: Synthesis, physicochemical profiling, antibacterial, anticancer activities and biological in vivo toxicity. *Journal of Colloid and Interface Science*, *499*, 33–45. doi:10.1016/j.jcis.2017.03.090 PMID:28363102

Nayak, D., Ashe, S., Rauta, P. R., Kumari, M., & Nayak, B. (2016). Bark extract mediated green synthesis of silver nanoparticles: Evaluation of antimicrobial activity and antiproliferative response against osteosarcoma. *Materials Science and Engineering C*, *58*, 44–52. doi:10.1016/j.msec.2015.08.022 PMID:26478285

Nayaka, S., Chakraborty, B., Pallavi, S. S., Bhat, M. P., Shashiraj, K. N., & Ghasti, B. (2020). Synthesis of biogenic silver nanoparticles using Zanthoxylum rhetsa (Roxb.) DC seed coat extract as reducing agent and in-vitro assessment of anticancer effect on A549 lung cancer cell line. *International Journal of Pharmaceutical Research*, *12*(3), 302–314.

Nilavukkarasi, M., Vijayakumar, S., & Kumar, S. P. (2020). Biological synthesis and characterization of silver nanoparticles with Capparis zeylanica L. leaf extract for potent antimicrobial and anti proliferation efficiency. *Materials Science for Energy Technologies*, *3*, 371–376. doi:10.1016/j.mset.2020.02.008

Padinjarathil, H., Joseph, M. M., Unnikrishnan, B. S., Preethi, G. U., Shiji, R., Archana, M. G., Maya, S., Syama, H. P., & Sreelekha, T. T. (2018). Galactomannan endowed biogenic silver NPs exposed enhanced cancer cytotoxicity with excellent biocompatibility. *International Journal of Biological Macromolecules*, *118*, 1174–1182. doi:10.1016/j.ijbiomac.2018.06.194 PMID:30001604

Palaniappan, P., Sathishkumar, G., & Sankar, R. (2015). Fabrication of nano-silver particles using Cymodocea serrulata and its cytotoxicity effect against human lung cancer A549 cells line. *Spectrochimica Acta. Part A: Molecular and Biomolecular Spectroscopy*, *138*, 885–890. doi:10.1016/j.saa.2014.10.072 PMID:25467657

Pei, J., Fu, B., Jiang, L., & Sun, T. (2019). Biosynthesis, characterization, and anticancer effect of plant-mediated silver nanoparticles using Coptis chinensis. *International Journal of Nanomedicine*, *14*, 1969–1978. doi:10.2147/IJN.S188235 PMID:30936697

Pimentel, R. G. C., Robles Botero, V., Martínez, E. S. M., Gómez García, C., & Hinestroza, J. P. (2016). Soybean agglutinin-conjugated silver nanoparticles nanocarriers in the treatment of breast cancer cells. *Journal of Biomaterials Science. Polymer Edition*, *27*(3), 218–234. doi:10.1080/09205063.2015.1116892 PMID:26540350

Plackal Adimuriyil George, B., Kumar, N., Abrahamse, H., & Ray, S. S. (2018). Apoptotic efficacy of multifaceted biosynthesized silver nanoparticles on human adenocarcinoma cells. *Scientific Reports*, *8*(1), 14368. doi:10.103841598-018-32480-5 PMID:30254325

Prabhu, D., Arulvasu, C., Babu, G., Manikandan, R., & Srinivasan, P. (2013). Biologically synthesized green silver nanoparticles from leaf extract of Vitex negundo L. induce growth-inhibitory effect on human colon cancer cell line HCT15. *Process Biochemistry (Barking, London, England)*, *48*(2), 317–324. doi:10.1016/j.procbio.2012.12.013

Raja, G., Jang, Y. K., Suh, J. S., Kim, H. S., Ahn, S. H., & Kim, T. J. (2020). Microcellular environmental regulation of silver nanoparticles in cancer therapy: *A critical review, cancers (Basel).* . doi:10.3390/cancers12030664

Rank Miranda, R., Pereira da Fonseca, M., Korzeniowska, B., Skytte, L., Lund Rasmussen, K., & Kjeldsen, F. (2020). Elucidating the cellular response of silver nanoparticles as a potential combinatorial agent for cisplatin chemotherapy. *Journal of Nanobiotechnology*, *18*(1), 164. doi:10.118612951-020-00719-x PMID:33168016

Rasheed, M., Ali, A., Kanwal, S., Ismail, M., Sabir, N., & Amin, F. (2019). Synergy of green tea reduced tamoxifen-loaded silver nanoparticles exhibit OGT downregulation in breast cancer cell line. *Digest Journal of Nanomaterials and Biostructures*, *14*(3), 695–704.

Sarkar, S., & Kotteeswaran, V. (2018). Green synthesis of silver nanoparticles from aqueous leaf extract of Pomegranate (Punica granatum) and their anticancer activity on human cervical cancer cells. *Advances in Natural Sciences: Nanoscience and Nanotechnology*, *9*(2), 025014. doi:10.1088/2043-6254/aac590

Satsangi, N. (2020). Synthesis and characterization of biocompatible silver nanoparticles for anticancer application. *Journal of Inorganic and Organometallic Polymers and Materials*, *30*(6), 1907–1914. doi:10.100710904-019-01372-0

Scatena, R. (2012). Mitochondria and cancer: A growing role in apoptosis, Cancer cell metabolism and dedifferentiation. *Advances in Experimental Medicine and Biology*, *942*, 287–308. doi:10.1007/978-94-007-2869-1_13 PMID:22399428

Shedrack, R. K., Peter, K., Judith, S., Dominic, O., Peter, M., & Naomi, M. (2022). Biogenic synthesis of silver nanoparticles using Azadirachta indica methanolic bark extract and their anti-proliferative activities against DU-145 human prostate cancer cells. *African Journal of Biotechnology*, *21*, 64–72.

Sibuyi, N. R. S., Thipe, V. C., Panjtan-Amiri, K., Meyer, M., & Katti, K. V. (2021). Green synthesis of gold nanoparticles using Acai berry and elderberry extracts and investigation of their effect on prostate and pancreatic Cancer cells. *BJGP Open*, *8*. doi:10.1177/1849543521995310 PMID:33643450

Singh, D., Yadav, E., Falls, N., Kumar, V., Singh, M., & Verma, A. (2019). RETRACTED ARTICLE: Phytofabricated silver nanoparticles of Phyllanthus emblica attenuated diethylnitrosamine-induced hepatic cancer via knock-down oxidative stress and inflammation. *Inflammopharmacology*, *27*(5), 1037–1054. doi:10.100710787-018-0525-6 PMID:30219979

Sofi, M. A., Sunitha, S., Sofi, M. A., Pasha, S. K., & Choi, D. (2022). An overview of antimicrobial and anticancer potential of silver nanoparticles. *Journal of King Saud University. Science*, *34*(2), 101791. doi:10.1016/j.jksus.2021.101791

Usmani, A., Mishra, A., Jafri, A., Arshad, M., & Siddiqui, M. A. (2019). Green synthesis of silver nanocomposites of Nigella sativa seeds extract for hepatocellular carcinoma. *Current Nanomaterials*, *4*(3), 191–200. doi:10.2174/2468187309666190906130115

Vaid, P., Raizada, P., Saini, A. K., & Saini, R. V. (2020). Biogenic silver, gold and copper nanoparticles-A sustainable green chemistry approach for cancer therapy. *Sustainable Chemistry and Pharmacy*, *16*, 100247. doi:10.1016/j.scp.2020.100247

Vallari, R. C., & Pietruszko, R. (1982). Human aldehyde dehydrogenase: Mechanism of inhibition of disulfiram. *Science*, *216*(4546), 637–639. doi:10.1126cience.7071604 PMID:7071604

Vasanth, K., Ilango, K., MohanKumar, R., Agrawal, A., & Dubey, G. P. (2014). Anticancer activity of Moringa oleifera mediated silver nanoparticles on human cervical carcinoma cells by apoptosis induction. *Colloids and Surfaces. B, Biointerfaces*, *117*, 354–359. doi:10.1016/j.colsurfb.2014.02.052 PMID:24681047

Vijayan, R., Joseph, S., & Mathew, B. (2018). Indigofera tinctoria leaf extract mediated green synthesis of silver and gold nanoparticles and assessment of their anticancer, antimicrobial, antioxidant and catalytic properties. *Artificial Cells, Nanomedicine, and Biotechnology*, *46*(4), 861–871. doi:10.1080/21691401.2017.1345930 PMID:28681622

Vijayaram, S., Razafindralambo, H., Sun, Y.-Z., Vasantharaj, S., Ghafarifarsani, H., Hoseinifar, S. H., & Raeeszadeh, M. (2023). Applications of green synthesized metal nanoparticles – a review. *Biological Trace Element Research*. doi:10.100712011-023-03645-9 PMID:37046039

Vivek, R., Thangam, R., Muthuchelian, K., Gunasekaran, P., Kaveri, K., & Kannan, S. (2012). Green biosynthesis of silver nanoparticles from Annona squamosa leaf extract and its in vitro cytotoxic effect on MCF-7 cells. *Process Biochemistry (Barking, London, England)*, *47*(12), 2405–2410. doi:10.1016/j.procbio.2012.09.025

Yang, T., Yao, Q., Cao, F., Liu, Q., Liu, B., & Wang, X. H. (2016). Silver nanoparticles inhibit the function of hypoxia-inducible factor-1 and target genes: Insight into the cytotoxicity and antiangiogenesis. *International Journal of Nanomedicine*, *11*, 6679–6692. doi:10.2147/IJN.S109695 PMID:27994464

Zhang, K., Liu, X., Samuel Ravi, S. O. A., Ramachandran, A., Aziz Ibrahim, I. A., Nassir, A. M., & Yao, J. (2019). Synthesis of silver nanoparticles (Ag-NPs) from leaf extract of Salvia miltiorrhiza and its anticancer potential in human prostate cancer LNCaP cell lines. *Artificial Cells, Nanomedicine, and Biotechnology*. doi:10.1080/21691401.2019.1638792 PMID:31299869

KEY TERMS AND DEFINITIONS

Apoptosis: A type of programmed cell death that is important for maintaining tissue homeostasis and is often targeted in cancer treatments.

Biocompatibility: The ability of a substance to interact safely with biological systems.

Bio-Reduction: Bio-reduction is the conversion of metal ions into nanoparticles using biological agents such as bacteria or enzymes.

Bottom-Up Synthesis: The construction of nanoparticles from smaller components or starting molecules.

Cancer Therapy: The treatment of cancer using various methods and approaches to prevent or eliminate malignant cells.

Chemotherapy: The process of treating cancer by either destroying or slowing the growth of cancer cells using chemicals, often drugs.

Clinical Trials: Research projects involving human subjects to evaluate the efficacy and safety of new medical therapies.

Cytotoxicity: Cell death or damage caused by a chemical.

Drug Delivery: The technique of delivering drugs to specific sites in the body to improve the effectiveness of treatment.

Drug Resistance: A major obstacle in cancer treatment because it allows cancer cells to evolve and become resistant to therapy.

Green Capping Agents: Green capping agents are natural compounds or polymers that can stabilise metal nanoparticles and protect them from aggregation and oxidation.

Green Synthesis: An environmentally friendly process that uses natural resources or environmentally safe reducing agents to create nanoparticles.

Metal Nanoparticles: Nanoparticles made of metals such as gold, silver etc.

Nanoparticle Characterization: Analytical methods for determining the dimensions, content and surface properties of nanoparticles are known as nanoparticle characterisation.

Phytochemicals: Phytochemicals are organic substances that occur naturally in plants and can be used as stabilising and reducing agents in green synthesis.

ROS (Reactive Oxygen Species): Highly reactive chemicals, such as free radicals, that cause oxidative stress and damage to cancer cells.

Sustainability: The process of producing and using metal nanoparticles to treat cancer, considering the impact on the environment and the conservation of resources.

Synergistic Therapy: Combining different treatment techniques, such as chemotherapy and nanoparticle-based therapy, to increase the effectiveness of treatment is known as synergistic therapy.

Targeted Therapy: A medical strategy that selectively kills cancer cells while minimising damage to healthy cells.

Chapter 5
Polymeric Nanoparticles in Drug Delivery

Kajal Parashar
https://orcid.org/0009-0007-0627-0844
Lovely Professional University, India

Minhaj Ahmad Khan
Lovely Professional University, India

ABSTRACT

Polymeric nanoparticles (PNPs) are tiny particles with a size between 1 and 1000 nm that can include active substances that have been surface-adsorbed over onto polymeric core or are entrapped inside of them. Both nanospheres and nanocapsules fall under the umbrella of "nanoparticles," which are characterized by their morphological structure. This material is anticipated to be extensively used in various sectors, including drug delivery systems, catalysts, biosensors, nanocomposites, agriculture, and the environment because of its extremely small size and large surface area. Particle size, geometry, material selection, and processing methods are all study topics of interest to establish the optimal nanosystem for more efficient and focused delivery of therapeutic applications. Drug delivery methods such as drug conjugation and drug entrapment, prodrugs, stimuli-responsive systems, imaging modalities, and theranostics all use PNPs. The goal of the technique of using polymeric nanoparticles for drug delivery is to maximize therapeutic effectiveness while reducing side effects.

INTRODUCTION: POLYMERIC NANOPARTICLES (PNPs)

For decades, polymeric nanoparticles having active medicinal components embedded inside or adsorbing on macromolecules have been created as drug delivery methods (DDS). As DDS, they have a variety of benefits including site-specific targeting of particular organs or tissues, general biocompatibility, biodegradability, ease of production, non-toxicity, and non-immunogenicity. Liposomes and drug-bound albumin are two examples of polymeric nanoparticles that the U.S. Food & Drug Administration (FDA) has licensed for use in nanomedicines (Wang et al., 2022). Polymeric substrates are now being studied

DOI: 10.4018/979-8-3693-0448-8.ch005

Figure 1. Polymeric nanoparticles in drug delivery

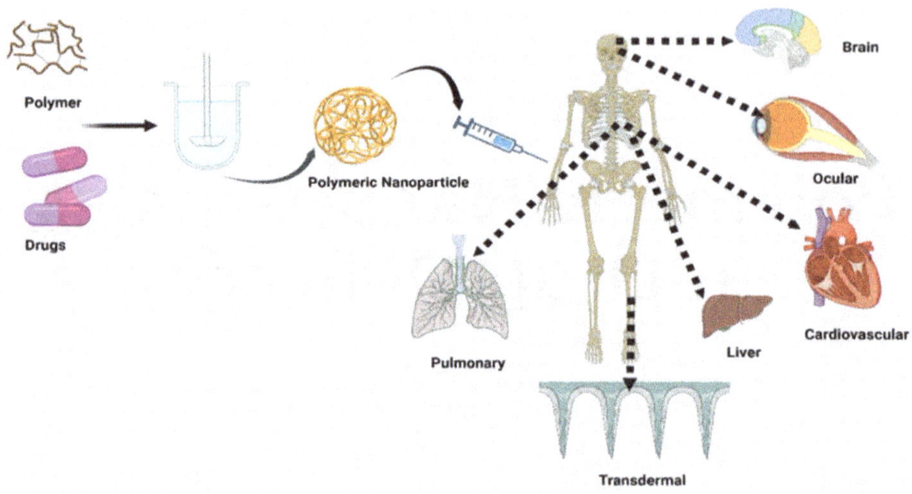

for drug delivery and, specifically, in cancer therapy. Polymeric nanoparticles are used in pharmaceutical sciences to increase drug solubility and bioavailability while minimizing toxicity and negative effects (Shelma et al., 2022).

Smart polymers quickly and irreversibly transition from a hydrophilic to a hydrophobic state in their microstructure. These modifications are brought about by minute alterations in the environment, yet they become visible at the macroscopic scales as precipitate formation from a solution or orders-of-magnitude modifications in the size and water content of polymers. These macroscopic modifications are likewise

Figure 2. Diagrammatic representation of fundamental components of PNPs (Nanocapsule and Nanosphere)

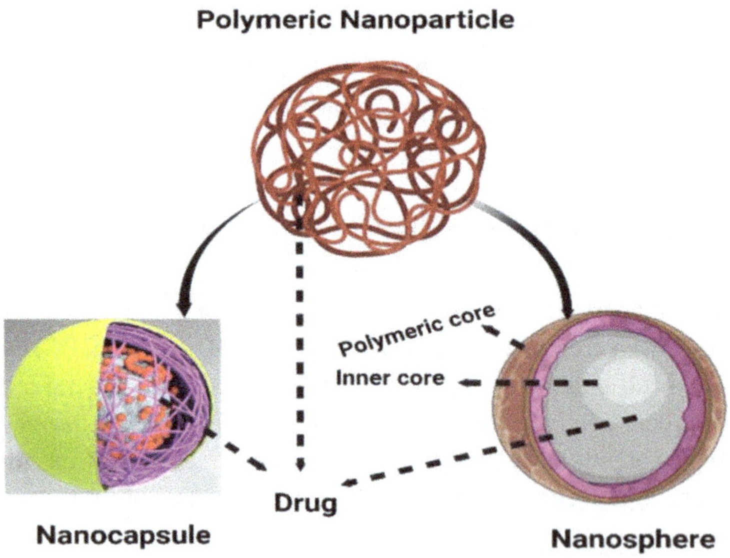

reversible, with the removal of the trigger causing the system to revert to its original condition. Common stimuli for these transitions include the neutralization of charged groups by a pH change or the addition of a polymer with an opposite charge, changes in hydrogen bonding efficiency brought on by an increase in temperature as well as ionic strength, and the dissolution of polymers & interpenetrating polymer networks (Malviya et al., 2022).

The significant consistency of PNPs in biofluids along with the abundance of different polymers, the ability created to serve their surfaces and control polymer degradation, and the spillages of the apprehended compound(s) as a function of particular stimuli are additional peculiarities of polymeric nanoparticles (Gagliardi et al., 2021). The features of polymeric nanoparticles (PNPs), which result from their small size, have generated a great deal of interest in recent years (Zielinska et al., 2020). One of the most cutting-edge non-invasive methods for medication delivery applications is polymer nanoparticles (PNPs). The primary goal of NPs is to deliver the therapeutic material, whether it be a medication, protein, or nucleic acid, directly to the organ or tissue of interest (Calzoni et al., 2019).

The benefits of using polymeric NPs as drug carriers include their capacity for controlled release, ability to shield drugs and other molecules from the environment, and ability to increase bioavailability and therapeutic efficacy (Shoppimath et al., 2001). Both nanocapsules & nanospheres, which have different morphologies, are included in the term "nanoparticle." Nanocapsules consist of an oily core, in which the medicine is typically dissolved, and a polymeric shell, which regulates the drug's release profile from the core. The medicine can be kept inside of or adsorbed onto the surface of nanospheres thanks to their continuous polymeric network (Gutteres et al., 2007). These two varieties of polymeric nanoparticles (NPs) are known as a matrix system and a reservoir system.

Due to their superior benefits, such as effective cargo dissolving, entanglement, encapsulation, or ground attachment, the ability to form antimicrobial groups for selective recognition and destruction, biodegradability and biocompatibility low toxicity, and synergistic therapy, nanostructured antimicrobial polymers have attracted more attention in recent years (Spirecue et al., 2021). Ursula Scheffel's initial experimental work served as the foundation for Paul Ehrlich's historical analysis of PNPs. At ETH Zürich, the Peter Speiser group carried out extensive research in the 1960s and early 1970s. PNPs are a rapidly expanding sector with significant applications in a wide range of fields, including photonics, electronics, sensing, medicine, pollution control, & environmental technology. PNPs have been a staple in well-known, common coatings, paints, and adhesives for a very long time. They have more recently found use in biomedical disciplines like medication delivery, diagnostics, and bioimaging. PNP-based materials with distinct physical and chemical properties could eventually serve as guidelines for the development of novel nanomaterials (Mallakpour et al., 2016).

Due to its better efficacy in delivering therapeutic substances directly to the targeted site of action, the polymer has played a crucial role in the area of smart drug delivery. To successfully design a nanoparticulate delivery system and achieve the target & specific activity at a set rate and time, it is ideal to effectively control the particle size, and surface character, and enhance permeation, flexibility, solubility, and relieve therapeutically active agents. The development of smart medication delivery systems in the realm of bio-nanotechnology is made possible by advancements in polymer science. These developments have recently been discovered in numerous medicinal applications for smart medication delivery using nano-scale structures. Smart drug administration systems should include features like pre-scheduled rates, self-control, targeting, predetermined times, and delivery monitoring. The polymer nanoparticle therapeutic regimen is improved by the smart medication delivery system (Bennet et al., 2014).

They are nano- to micro-scale drug delivery systems made of natural, semi-synthetic, & synthetic polymeric materials. Spheres and capsules are the aggregate names for polymeric particles. The majority of polymeric nanoparticles containing surfactants provide stability of several active drug forms and have beneficial smart release features. Many biological uses for nanoscale to microscale-sized particles have been discovered, including site-targeted, regulated, and improved bioavailability of hydrophobic medicines. Additionally, polymeric particles demonstrated their efficiency in maintaining and shielding medicinal compounds like proteins and peptides from environmental degradation (Brigger et al., 2012). There are many ways to create nanoparticles; it all relies on the chemical and physical properties of the polymer and the active components. The majority of formulation procedures include a variety of mechanisms that can degrade the pharmaceutically active components, including the use of organic solvents, heat, ultrasonication, and mechanical agitation. To ensure that the formulation approach does not harm the active medicinal ingredients, a nanoparticulate system can be designed. To create smart nanoparticles, a variety of biocompatible and biodegradable polymers with various physicochemical properties are available; these polymeric nanocarriers may be natural, semi-natural, or manufactured (Panyam et al., 2003).

The most recent developments in self-regulating devices, micro, and nanofabricated carriers enable sustained and focused distribution: micro-needles for transdermal drug delivery using biodetectable devices have demonstrated the flexibility and improved permeability of such polymeric materials. The development of a micro- and nano-fabricated therapeutic medication release device with the ability to retain and release a variety of active agents on demand is the ultimate objective of smart drug delivery (Kasagana et al., 2011).

The four main modes of controlled drug delivery are as follows:

(1) Rate-programmed delivery of drugs, where drug dispersion from the system follows a particular release rate profile.
(2) Activation-modulated delivery of drugs, where the release of drugs is induced by numerous factors like physical, chemical, electrical, or biochemical modules.
(3) Feedback-regulated drug development, where the release rate is determined by biochemical substances.
(4) The rate of drug release is controlled by the active targeting moiety, solubilizer, and drug moiety in site-targeted drug delivery systems, which is a complicated process with numerous steps of diffusion rate and partitioning (Cao et al., 2001).

Over the past ten years, researchers have recognized the expansion of bio nanotechnology's prospective applications as delivering significant improvements in new drug delivery & targeting. The most beneficial effects are delivered to clinical levels by the innovative drug delivery platform, which reduces toxicity and improves therapeutic efficacy. The administration route is one of the most important components of drug targeting in strategies for drug delivery systems. To reach the therapeutic target and increase efficacy, drug delivery systems concentrate on breaking down various membrane obstacles, such as the blood-brain barrier and tight junction barrier (Cui et al., 2002). In this chapter, recent revolutionary nanofabrication techniques for unique drug delivery systems will be briefly discussed. A few of these novel technologies are also highlighted, and their potential for ongoing clinical use is considered. Following this chapter, a more in-depth examination of the creation of innovative drug delivery systems from the perspective of polymeric nanoparticles and their many bio-applications will be presented without attempting to cover all the studies that have been conducted in this area.

POLYMERS USED IN THE PREPARATION OF NANOPARTICLES (NPs)

The following polymers are used to make nanoparticles (Vyas et al., 2004):

1. Natural Polymers
2. Synthetic Polymers

Natural Polymers

Natural polymers are produced by bacteria, fungi, plants, and mammals. Polysaccharides & protein-based polymers are the two primary categories. Both have undergone in-depth research on drug delivery. Both are capable of forming scaffolds as functional extracellular matrix (ECM). This will result in tailored medicine administration with great loading efficiency and little intrusive behaviour (Wong et al., 2020). Due to some distinct and relatively safe characteristics, such as biocompatibility, biodegradability, abundance in nature, and affordability compared to bioresorbable synthetic polymers, interest has been generated in producing nanoparticles that use natural polymers intending to encourage their use in drug delivery for examining more advanced pharmaceutical applications against various indications. Alginate, chitosan, gelatine, albumin, and collagen are among the most often utilized natural polymers in the delivery of drugs. Natural polymer-based nanodevices are created using a variety of methods. The type of active ingredient, the polymer, and the characteristics of the nanoparticles—such as size, zeta potential, and encapsulation effectiveness—are taken into consideration when choosing a procedure. The most often utilized methods include ionotropic gelation, coacervation, and emulsion-cross linking (Barratt et al., 2000).

A). Natural Polysaccharides

The carbohydrate-based polymers known as polysaccharides are made up of several sugar molecules bound together by glycosidic linkages. A variety of physical characteristics that result from the fact that polysaccharides can have straight or branching structures affect their suitability as a material for tissue engineering and drug delivery applications. Numerous reviews of polysaccharide-based Nanoparticles have been published (Jarai et al., 2020). Among the most popular polysaccharide-based polymers utilized in biomedical applications are chitosan, cellulose, & hyaluronic acid (HA).

A1). Hyaluronic acid

HA is a repeating D-glucuronic acid & N-acetyl-D-glucosamine unit-based linear chain polysaccharide. HA is an extracellular matrix polymer that occurs naturally in many human tissues. It is non-toxic and biodegradable. HA has been widely used for both increasing targeted medication delivery and regulating API release because of its widespread presence in the human body (Ulery et al., 2011). Interestingly, tumor cells frequently overexpress the human receptor CD44, which is specific for HA, leading several researchers to use HA in NP-based compositions to improve delivery to tumors (Alaniz et al., 2002).

A2). Cellulose

The linear chain polysaccharide known as cellulose is composed of glucose units joined together by b(1 / 4) glycosidic linkages. The most prevalent polysaccharide in the natural world, cellulose is innately biocompatible with human tissue. The two categories of cellulose-based nanoparticles are cellulose crystals and nano-fibrillated cellulose (Sequiera et l., 2010). To conjugate APIs to the interface of the crystals, cellulose nanocrystals have an extremely high surface area & a net negative charge. Doxorubicin (DOX), for instance, has been successfully attached to the surfaces of cellulose nanocrystals, demonstrating the viability of using cellulose-based NPs for the delivery of anticancer drugs. Additionally, the steroidal small molecule beclomethasone dipropionate has been released in a regulated manner using nanofibrillated cellulose (Jackson et al., 2011).

B). Natural Proteins

One or more amino acid chains make up proteins, which are macromolecules that resemble natural polymers in that the amino acid chains can complexly self-assemble to form macromolecular structures. Because they may be easily modified and are biodegradable, proteins are employed in the creation of NP. Additionally, when included in an NP, proteins' capacity to recognize compounds can be used to enhance targeted medication delivery. The most popular protein polymers utilized in the biomedical field are albumin, elastin, collagen, and silk (Seib et al., 2013). Notably, a variety of protein-based NP therapies have received FDA approval, including Abraxane, an intravenous NP albumin-bound chemotherapy used to treat various malignancies (Hawkins et al., 2018).

Synthetic Polymers

The most common processes used to create and produce polymeric particles are emulsion techniques, solvent exchange, salting out, emulsion freeze-dry or spray drying, and supercritical fluid technologies. Significantly faster, more reproducible, and readily scaled-up, the multiple emulsion spray-drying methods has potential advantages over the freeze-drying method. To encapsulate hydrophilic or hydrophobic medicines into specific polymeric nanoparticles, these approaches can be adjusted. Because they may change functional groups and offer a variety of preparation options, the application of synthetic polymers is advocated. Polymeric nanoparticles' increased reactivity to various stimuli has also been a huge plus for targeted delivery methods (Ghosh et al., 2004).

The term "nanoparticle" refers to both nanospheres and nanocapsules that are composed of solid carriers comprised of either synthetic or natural polymers but are either biodegradable or not. These solid carriers may encapsulate the drug or gene by absorbing onto the surface of the nanoparticles or embedding them into the matrix. Liposomes haven't garnered as much attention as nanoparticles have due to liposomes' lack of therapeutic potential and nanoparticles' higher durability in bodily fluids and during storage (Reis et al., 2006). Nanoparticles can be made using a variety of techniques, however, the ones that are suitable for use in the industry employ safe solvents. Although many insoluble medications tend to dissolve in solvents like DMSO and DMF, their cost and toxicity prevent their use for any therapeutic purpose, especially whenever the process of creating nanoparticles is carried out on an industrial scale. Nowadays, it is widely acceptable to make nanoparticles from pre-formed polymers or by polymerizing a monomer (Nafee et l., 2009).

A). Polyesters

Polymeric polymers used in drug delivery applications must meet important criteria such as biodegradability and low immunogenicity. Excellent biocompatibility and biodegradability have been demonstrated for polyesters, and the by-products of degradation are often metabolites that are absorbed by natural routes. Because of this, polyesters—particularly PLGA—have been widely used in biomedical applications (Allen et al., 2018).

B). Poly (glycolic acid)

One of the earliest biodegradable synthetic polymers to be employed in biological applications was poly (glycolic acid, or PGA). Glycolic acid is most frequently used to create PGA through polycondensation or ring-opening polymerization. In the 1960s, PGA was utilized in the first biodegradable suture that the US Food & Drug Administration (FDA) approved (Pillai et al., 2010). Due to its high crystallinity & low solubility in the majority of organic solvents, PGA is stiff and difficult to dissolve. The biggest disadvantage of employing PGA as a drug administration method is that it degrades quickly and loses mechanical strength quickly after use. In order to enhance mechanical qualities and degradability, PGA is combined with other polymers like poly(-caprolactone) (PCL) & poly (lactic acid) (PLA) (Lee et al., 2003).

C). Polyanhydrides

Due to their biocompatibility, polyanhydrides, a group of biodegradable synthetic polymers, have found extensive usage in biomedical applications, particularly in the delivery of drugs. Compared to bulk-eroding polyesters, polyanhydride-based materials have stronger control over persistent API release due to their surface erosion (Petersen et al., 2010). Dicarboxylic acid units are produced during the breakdown of polyanhydrides by cleaving the anhydride link. 90 In the production of NP, poly (sebacic acid)91 and poly(1,6-bis(p-carboxyphenoxy) hexane) are two examples of polyanhydrides (Kipper et al., 2002).

D). Polyamines

One of the most often utilized polymers for genome delivery is poly (ethylenimine, or PEI). Because PEI has a positive charge, it can form polyplexes, which are complexes containing negatively charged DNA. PEI is a cationic polyamine. The degree of polyplex formation is influenced by both the degree of branching and the proportion of DNA to PEI, which can be found in both linear & branched forms of PEI (Lungwitz et al., 2005). Despite showing promise in gene transfer applications, PEI/DNA complexes have a severe lethal effect in vivo because PEI impairs cell activity. Due to this, numerous attempts have been made to increase the biocompatibility of PEI-based complexes by covering them with biocompatible polymers, particularly PEG (Tang et al., 2003).

PNPs IN NANOMEDICINE

Due to the fusion of nanotechnology with biomedicine, a new field known as nanomedicine has emerged (Molinero et al., 2023). The field of medicine known as nanomedicine uses nanotechnology to cure and prevent disease. By enhancing drug solubility, modifying biodistribution, and managing the release, nanotechnology is one of the most efficient methods for increasing a medicine's therapeutic efficacy and lowering toxicity. The advancement of nanotechnology and new materials has sparked a dramatic revolution in medicine that has had a big impact on how many serious diseases, including cancer, injection-related diseases, and cardiovascular diseases, are treated. The field of nanomedicine has grown rapidly in recent years (Jia et al., 2023).

One of the organic approaches to nanomedicine that has received the most research is polymeric nanoparticles (PNPs). The polymer nano-revolution in medicine is an exciting promise because it has the ability to turn existing therapeutic, diagnostic, preventive, and biological issues' plausible answers into alternatives that are more dependable and effective. The difficulties come from the numerous interactions of complicated physiological systems, as well as the weighty feature considerations and accompanying impacts, which result in a complex system that is difficult to understand and analyze. At the nanoscale level, cellular responses are drastically different (Banik et al., 2016).

Polymeric nanoparticles have completely changed the way that medicine is thought of and practiced. Block copolymer micelles, polymer protein conjugates, medicines, and aptamers, polymeric pharmaceuticals, and multicomponent nonviral carriers with covalent links are all included in Duncan and Vicent's definition of "polymer therapies." Due to their design flexibility based on functionalization, macromolecular manufacturing techniques, and polymer variety, polymers are attractive for use in therapeutic applications (Delplace et al., 2014). Nanostructures that range in size from one to a thousand nanometres are denoted by the prefix "nano." Enhancing cell permeability, enhancing therapeutic delivery, reducing dosage levels and frequency, and improving the efficacy of medicines employed in nanomedicine are all possible with nanoscale characteristics (Kobayashi et al., 2014).

Through the examination of physicochemical structure qualities and the biological interface, current research concentrates on the search for the "perfect nanosystem." In general, the layout of the structure, the treatment of the carrier, & the material selected for the device are comparable considerations made for each studying target in the fields of nanomedicine. These characteristics have a significant impact on cell signaling and particle uptake. The initial surface contacts of the cell receptors, which can involve cell membrane elongation or compression, and protein interactions, among other things, determine the cellular responses & ultimately changes in phenotype. All of these responses are dependent on the chemical makeup, geometry, and functionalization of the NP as well as the microenvironment of the cell, which consists of the cell membrane and any subsequent transmembrane proteins, the surrounding extracellular matrix, & the geometry of the target cells (for example, spindle-shaped endothelial cells developing on a basement membrane are a very different target than surrounding connective tissue formed of fibroblasts around them) (Su et al., 2015).

The first generation of NPs focused on the biocompatibility & toxicity of nanomaterials via material design; the second generation examined surface chemistry optimization with a focus on the stability, stealth, and targeting capabilities of the NPs; and the third generation of NPs started to raise the possibility of dynamic "smart nanomedicine" with environment-responsive systems to enhance the targeting mechanisms and theranostics abilities (Kamaly et al., 2012).

A large number of publications and commercially available products (approximately 90 authorized nanomedicines) show that nanomedicine has made great progress. Given that more than 90 nanomedicines were recently made available for purchase, the transition percentage is still small in comparison to the enormous volume of publications. Between 2018 and 2022, there were over 50,000 studies on nanomedicine, but only nine items were released (Lammers et al., 2020).

Because there are no reliable methods for examining metabolism, the in vivo destiny of nanomedicine is not well understood. Fortunately, attention is being paid to the in vivo outcome. Nanoparticle destiny exploration is being done using an increasing number of innovative approaches, such as fluorescence bioimaging and radioactive tracing. Based on aggregation-caused quenching, aggregation-induced emission, and Forster resonance transfer of energy-responsive fluorescent probes (Cai et al., 2022). It is anticipated that nanotechnology will continue to have a significant impact on the development of biopharmaceuticals and that more nanomedicine related to biologics will be commercialized in the future.

FABRICATION METHODS OF PNPs

The utilization of surfactants may be necessary while creating polymeric nanoparticles. Amphiphilic chemical compounds known as surfactants have the capacity to self-assemble in solutions. The majority of commonly used surfactants are made up of a hydrocarbon chain (hydrophobic portion) attached to an

Figure 3. Fabrication methods of polymeric nanoparticles

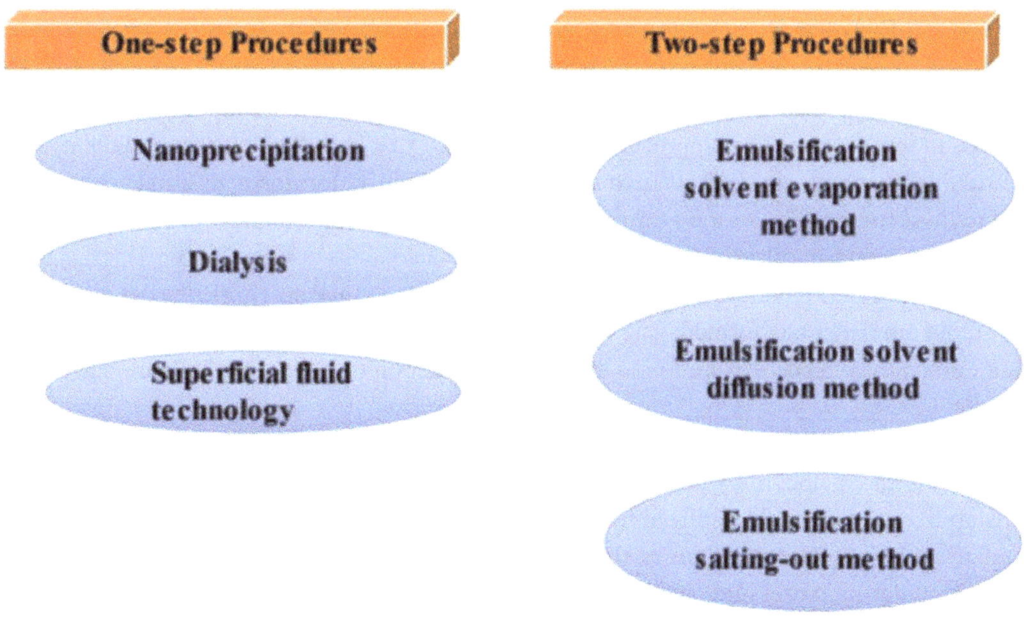

ionic functional group, creating so-called cationic surfactants like benzalkonium chloride hydroxide or anionic surfactants like docusate or sodium laurate.

There are other non-ionic surfactants that combine hydrophobic and hydrophilic molecules to provide an amphiphilic property (e.g., ethoxylated amines, & nonyl-phenol ethoxylates) (Begines et al., 2020). Various techniques have been used to create polymeric nanoparticles depending on their intended use and the physicochemical properties of the medication. To get PNPs with the appropriate qualities for a specific application, the most effective technique selection is crucial (Crucho et al., 2017). Numerous preparation techniques have been created, and they can be split into two categories: those that use premade polymers and those that rely on the synthesis of monomers. These techniques can be further divided into two groups: one-step procedures where nanoparticle formation does not require emulsification, and two-step procedures comprising the formation of an emulsification environment followed by nanoparticle formation in the second stage of the process (Allouche et al., 2013).

Two-Step Procedures

The food and pharmaceutical sectors frequently use emulsion-based colloidal delivery methods to enclose, safeguard, and administer bioactive ingredients. The basic definition of an emulsion is a mixture of two liquid phases that are either entirely or partially incompatible. To ensure stability, amphiphilic surface-active particles (surfactants) are used to lower the interfacial strain between the two liquids. Emulsions can likewise be categorized according to their morphology or content (oil, water, surfactants). According to whether the oil is disseminated as droplets in the water or not, emulsions can either be of either oil-in-water (o/w) or water-in-oil (w/o) varieties. Also possible are more advanced systems like (water-in-oil)-in-water (w/o/w). The emulsion created can be divided into three groups based on the size of the droplets: There are three types of emulsions: nano, micro, and macro (Mason et al., 2006).

Emulsification Solvent Evaporation Method

One of the most popular techniques for creating nanoparticles is the solvent evaporation technique. There are two steps in this process. This approach relies on the fact that both the polymer and the hydrophobic drug are soluble in an organic solvent (such as dichloromethane, chloroform, or ethyl acetate), which is also used to dissolve the. The resulting mixture of a medication solution and a polymer is next emulsified in water. To create an oil-in-water (o/w) emulsion, this aqueous solution comprises a surfactant or emulsifying agent. The organic solvent is vaporized either by continual stirring or by decreasing pressure after the stable emulsion has formed. The types and concentrations of stabilizers, polymer concentrations, and homogenizer speeds were found to have an impact on the size range of nanoparticles (Kwon et al., 2001).

To create small particle sizes, high-speed homogenization or ultrasonication may frequently be used. The nanoparticles are gathered by ultracentrifugation, cleaned with purified water to get rid of any free drugs or stabilizers, and then lyophilized for storage. Solvent evaporation procedure and highly pressurized emulsification are two variations of this technique. With this technique, an emulsion is prepared, homogenized under high pressure, and then thoroughly stirred to eliminate organic solvent (Jaiswal et al., 2004). The viscosity of the organic and aqueous phases, temperature, kind, and amount of the dispersion agent can all be changed to alter the size. However, this approach can be used with liposoluble medications, and the scale-up issue places restrictions on its use. The polymers PLGA, cellulose acetate phthalate, PLA EC, Poly (-hydroxybutyrate) (PHB), and Poly (-caprolactone) (PCL) are employed in this process (Lemarchand et al., 2006).

Due to the technological advancement of emulsification devices during the past ten years, methods for preparing nanoscale emulsions have undergone significant development. This has led to the creation of the solvent evaporation approach. Although this procedure is straightforward and adaptable, it can only be used for medications that are liposoluble, it takes a lot of time, and there is a chance that nanoparticles will agglomerate during evaporation. Additionally, other techniques with minimal energy requirements for homogenization, including the phase inversion compositional (PIC) technique, are favored for scale-up production (Fornaguera et al., 2015).

Emulsification Solvent Diffusion Method

Leroux was the one who first proposed the emulsification-solvent diffusion technique. It involves creating a typical oil-in-water emulsion between a partially water-soluble solvent containing the medication and polymer and an aqueous solution containing a surfactant (Leroux et al., 1995). The polymer solvent and water must be mutually saturated at ambient temperature for this approach to work. This maintains the two liquids' initial thermodynamic equilibrium. As a result of the following dilution with a large volume of water, solvent diffusion from the emulsion droplets into the exterior phase causes the development of colloidal particles. Indirect evaporation of the solvent system from the nanodroplets is more severe than the diffusion process. Unlike techniques based on the evaporation of the solvent, this technique's droplet size falls abruptly in a millisecond timeframe during solvent diffusion (Moniard et al., 2008). Typically, this process yields nanospheres, but nanocapsules can be made simply by introducing a tiny amount of oil, like miglyol, into the organic phase. Finally, the solvent can be removed by evaporation relying on its boiling point. The size of the PNPs produced by solvent diffusion can be influenced by a number of formulation parameters. For instance, it has been demonstrated that the emulsification stage determines the majority of the features of nanocapsules.

It has been demonstrated that higher polymer concentrations result in larger particle sizes and a higher polydispersity index. In contrast hand, it was discovered that a moderate reduction in PNP size was caused by an increase in stirring pace and surfactant content (Trimaille et al., 2003). The water-miscible solvent and a little proportion of the organic solvent (which is water-immiscible) are employed as the oil phase in this procedure. Solvents spontaneously diffuse between the two phases, creating interfacial turbulence that may ultimately result in the creation of tiny particles. Increasing the concentration of a water-miscible solvent will result in a smaller particle size. Both hydrophilic and hydrophobic medicines can be processed using this approach. When dealing with hydrophilic medications, a multiple w/o/w emulsion must be created with the medication dissolved in the inner aqueous phase (Niwa et al., 1993). The solvent diffusion step's experimental conditions don't appear to have an impact on particle size. As long as the solubility of the organic solvent criterion is met, free solvent diffusion is assured (Song et al., 2006). It was demonstrated that the size of the particle reduced as the dilution water's temperature rose. In this instance, lowering the exterior phase's viscosity encouraged solvent diffusion, which led to a reduction in particle size (Kwon et al., 2001).

With regards to batch-to-batch repeatability, high yields, ease of scaling up, lack of requirement for ultrasonication, and usually good encapsulation efficiencies, the emulsification-diffusion approach offers evident advantages. There are, however, drawbacks as well. Examples include the need to remove large amounts of water from the suspension as well as the potential leaking of medications that are water soluble into the external phase during the emulsification step (Quintanar et al., 1997).

Emulsification Salting-Out Method

A salting-out action is used in the method to separate water-miscible solvents from an aqueous solution. It is based on the salting-out action, which separates a water-miscible solvent from an aqueous solution. The salting-out agents & colloidal stabilizers are added to an aqueous gel after the initial step in which the medication and polymer are dissolved into a solvent. There are many different kinds of salting-out agents (electrolytes, like magnesium chloride and calcium chloride, or non-electrolytes, like sucrose) and colloidal stabilizers, including polyvinylpyrrolidone or hydroxyethyl cellulose. As a result, an oil/water emulsion is created, which is then further diluted with enough water to improve the solvent's ability to diffuse into the aqueous medium and, ultimately, trigger the production of nanospheres. Variables in this process include the rate of stirring, the internal/external phase ratio, the concentration of polymeric materials in the organic phase, the kind of electrolyte concentration, and the type of stabilizer in the aqueous phase (Couvreur et al., 1995). It does not need a rise in temperature, making it potentially beneficial when processing heat-sensitive materials. Its main drawback is the limited use of lipophilic drugs and lengthy nanoparticle cleaning procedures.

Emulsification Reverse Salting-Out Method

Considered a variant of the emulsification-reverse salting-out technique is the previously described emulsification solvent diffusion approach. The structure of the emulsion, which is made from an aqueous gel including the salting-out agent & a colloidal stabilizer, and an acetone-like water-miscible polymer solvent, is where the main distinction is found (Ibrahim et al., 1992). Electrolytes like magnesium chloride, calcium chloride, or magnesium acetate are examples of acceptable salting-out agents, as are non-electrolytes like sucrose. Without using any strong shear pressures, an Ouzo effect causes the emulsion to form (Ganachaud et al., 2005). By saturation of the aqueous solution, acetone and water's miscibility is decreased, allowing the two normally miscible phases to form an o/w emulsion. By diluting the created o/w emulsion with too much water, one might induce the reverse salting-out effect. This occurs when acetone diffuses into the aqueous phase, precipitating the polymer that was absorbed in the emulsified nanodroplets. Crossflow filtering is used to remove any leftover polymer solvent & salting-out agent (Konan et al., 2002).

The emulsification-reverse salting-out approach has been used to successfully manufacture PNPs using a variety of polymers, solvents, and salting-out agents. The existence of the salting-out product requires a two-phase system, which is the only prerequisite that needs to be satisfied (Allemann et al., 1992). First, acetone with magnesium chloride was used as the solvent & salting-out agent, respectively, to create Eudragit® S PNPs. As a rheological agent & emulsion stabilizer, PVA was additionally included in the aqueous phase. The size of the PNPs may be regulated within a wide range by altering the molecular weight & PVA's concentration in the external phase (186–1130 nm). A modest reduction in particle size was additionally made possible by accelerating the stirring rate. The polymer content or the internal or external phase ratio was changed to produce PNPs with a size range of 200 to 500 nm (Zweers et al., 2003).

Avoiding chlorinated solvents, which seem to be harmful to the environment and the body's physiological systems, is one of the salting-out method's key benefits. The two main drawbacks of using salts are the fact that they can only be used to encapsulate pharmaceuticals that are lipophilic and the necessity of extensive purifying procedures. The latter may be to blame for the limited number of studies that have been released in recent years that mention the salting-out procedure (Song et al., 2008).

One-Step Procedures

Nanoprecipitation Method

This technique's fundamental concept is founded on the interface coating of a polymer when the organic solvent is displaced from a lipophilic mixture to the aqueous phase. A water-miscible solvent with intermediate polarity is used to dissolve the polymer, and this solution is then added to an agitated aqueous solution either all at once, in steps, as drops, or at a regulated addition rate (Fessi et al., 1989). The nanoparticles develop right away in an effort to stay away from the water molecules because of the quick spontaneous diffusion of the polymer solution into the aqueous phase. This procedure seems to be controlled by the Marangoni effect, which is characterized by a reduction in the interfacial tension that exists between the phases, an increase in the surface area brought on by rapid diffusion, and the production of tiny droplets of organic solvent (Sternling et al., 1959).

The polymer precipitates as nanocapsules or nanospheres as the solvent diffuses from the nanodroplets. Normally, the organic layer is introduced to the aqueous phase, however, the procedure might alternatively be reversed without endangering the creation of nanoparticles. Acetone is the most often used organic solvent because it is easily removed by evaporation and is miscible with water. Although it is also possible to utilize mixtures of ethanol and binary solvents, such as acetone plus a small amount of water, ethanol, or methanol (Chang et al., 2009). Surfactants are frequently used in the procedure to ensure colloidal suspension stability, but their availability is not necessary to assure the creation of nanoparticles. The resulting nanoparticles often exhibit a well-defined size and a limited size distribution, which is preferable to those made using emulsification solvent evaporation. The essential parameters relating to the experimental design are those that influence the final nanoparticle properties. The PNP physicochemical parameters can be carefully adjusted by carefully altering the composition, the ratio of the organic phase to the aqueous phase, the rate at which the organic phase is injected, the fluid dynamics, and the mixing speed. For instance, a general increase in particle size is produced by increasing the concentration of polymer or polymer molecular weight. The larger nanodroplets produced by the greater organic phase viscosity, which prevents solvent diffusion, are the cause of these results (Chorny et al., 2002).

This technique has been modified to work with hydrophilic medications as well as hydrophobic ones; it is typically used to entrap hydrophobic pharmaceuticals. A polar, water-miscible solvent like acetone, acetonitrile, methanol, or ethanol, is used to dissolve medicines and polymers. The then is added gradually, drop by drop, to an aqueous phase containing a surfactant. Rapid solvent diffusion results in the instantaneous formation of nanoparticles. The solvent is then eliminated at reduced pressure (Govender et al., 1999). Finding an appropriate drug/polymer/solvent/non-solvent system that enables successful nanoparticle formation and drug encapsulation is the problem in nanoprecipitation, in general. However, because of its ease of use, speed, and reproducibility, this method is commonly utilized. The mixing procedure during nanoprecipitation is one of the challenges. For the nanoparticles synthesized of PNPs, a microfluidic platform may hold promise because the hydrodynamic circulation ensures quick and adaptable mixing of the solvent and non-solvent in the microchannels (Xie et al., 2010).

The automated approach to nanoprecipitation with high-throughput sequencing experimentation is another new breakthrough (pipetting robot & inkjet printing). Because the medication might diffuse to the aqueous solution during polymer precipitation, hydrophilic medicines have poor encapsulation efficacy, which is another disadvantage. Other ways to increase encapsulation effectiveness include altering the drug's solubility by changing the pH or the solvent makeup (Leo et al., 2004).

Dialysis

The creation of tiny PNPs with a restricted size distribution has been accomplished with success using the dialysis approach (Jeon et al., 2004). Similar to the nanoprecipitation approach, it is controlled by a similar process with a bit distinct experimental setup. This approach uses semipermeable membranes or dialysis tubes as a physical border for the polymer with an appropriate molecular weight cut-off (MWCO). Typically, the polymer is dialyzed against a non-solvent after being mixed in an organic solvent and deposited into the dialysis membrane (Rao et al., 2011). The miscibility of the solvents as well as the presence of diluted polymer solutions is fundamental conditions. The mixture's capacity to decompose the polymer decreases over time due to the displacement of the solvent within the membrane. Additionally, a rise in interfacial tension causes the polymer to aggregate and creates a colloidal dispersion of nanoparticles. Dialysis is a straightforward and widely used operation, but because it takes so long, the huge number of counter-dialyzing media can cause the nanoparticle payload to escape too soon. Numerous experimental factors, including the solvent/non-solvent pair, the dialysis MWCO, the temperatures at which the procedure is conducted, the polymer concentration, and the rate of solvent mixing, might affect the morphology & particle size distribution of the produced PNPs (Akagi et al., 2005).

A linear relationship between polymer content and nanosphere size was found for poly (methyl methacrylate) (PMMA) nanoparticles. Nanospheres made of poly(phenylacetylene) (PPA) displayed the same behavior. Additionally, PPA nanoparticles having smaller diameters were produced at low temperatures than at room temperature at low concentrations. It also investigated how the MWCO affected this synthetic polymer. It was demonstrated that lowering the membrane's MWCO causes the average particle size to decrease. The investigated biopolymers likewise exhibited a similar pattern. This is caused by a reduction in the solvent mixing rate, which prioritizes thermodynamic over kinetic variables as seen for hyaluronic acid-based nanostructures. This is accomplished by altering the chemical characteristics of the solvent/nonsolvent pair (Jeong et al., 2001).

Superficial Fluid Technology

The use of organic solvents, which pose risks to the environment and the body, is required by conventional techniques such as solvent extraction by evaporation, solvent diffusion, and organic phase separation. As a result, because higher viscosity is benign for the environment, they have been researched as a substitute for creating biodegradable micro- and nanoparticles (Jung et al., 2001). In general, a supercritical fluid is a solvent that has reached its critical temperature and that, regardless of pressure, maintains a single phase. Due to its moderate severe situations ($T_c = 31.1$ °C & $P_c = 73.8$ bars), nontoxicity, nonflammability, and inexpensive cost, supercritical CO2 (SC CO2) is the most often employed supercritical fluid. Supercritical anti-solvent (SAS) and fast inflation of supercritical solution (RESS) are the two most often used processing methods employing supercritical fluids.

In the supercritical solvent removal approach, both the medicine and the polymer are dissolved in the appropriate organic solvent before being atomized through a nozzle into supercritical CO_2. Since CO_2 is only miscible with the solvent, the scattered organic solvent stage and antisolvent CO_2 stage diffuse into one another. As the solvent is extracted, the solid that is insoluble in supercritical fluid precipitates as nanoparticles because CO_2 is only miscible with the solvent (Subramaniam et al., 1997). The solute is mixed in supercritical CO2 and this mixture is ionized through a nozzle into a collection chamber under atmospheric conditions in the massive development of the supercritical solutions technique. When the solute is expanded, CO2 instantly evaporates, and a coprecipitate of the medication embedded in the polymer matrix forms. Despite being environmentally friendly and ideal for mass manufacturing, supercritical fluid technology is more costly and necessitates specialized equipment (Dadwal et al., 2014).

TYPES OF PNPs IN THE DRUG DELIVERY SYSTEM

Most medications, notably those used to treat cancer, are extremely lipophilic, polar, and unstable in aqueous environments and degrade more slowly through hydrolysis. Since these tiny medications can diffuse through a cellular membrane that isn't the drug's target when administered systemically, they may have negative side effects. Therefore, in order to safeguard the drug during circulation & release it under specified circumstances, researchers have been concentrating on the synthesis of polymer composites that would aid in improving their solubility and serving as carriers (Ventura et al., 2015).

Polymeric drug carriers should have the following properties:

- The ability to encapsulate lipophilic drug molecules inside of their core.
- A desirable surface area to achieve trying to target through the EPR effect.
- The ability to stably incorporate the molecules to avoid sudden release.
- The ability to release their components in response to a particular stimulus provoked by the target cell environment.
- An easily modified surface for the complexation of targeting ligands.
- Demonstrate minimal intrinsic toxicity.
- Use synthetic techniques that are repeatable (Ventura et al., 2015).

Redox Responsive PNPs

Reducing agents in high concentrations, such as reduced glutathione (GSH) with thioredoxin, can cause nanoscopic redox-responsive nanoparticles to cleave, which makes them particularly appealing (Gao et al., 2009). Human plasma has micromolar levels of GSH, whereas cell cytosol contains roughly 10 mM of GSH. It's interesting to note that cancer cells have a seven-fold greater GSH concentration in their cytoplasm than healthy cells do. Consequently, the creation of delivery methods that are sensitive to the disulfide functionality caused by the action of GSH can promote the intracellular release of medication molecules that have been encapsulated (Ge et al., 2011). The drug compound can be enclosed in the polymeric carriers or covalently joined to them by the disulfide functionality, which can be found in the side groups or backbone of the polymeric carriers. The disulfide bond may also be found at the point where two polymer blocks are joined. For the creation of self-assembled micelles, an approach that is frequently used is the employment of amphiphilic polymers having disulfide activity inside their hydrophobic backbone (Geisow et al., 1984).

The micelles will break down when confronted with GSH because they lose their amphiphilic nature, allowing the cargo to be released. A polymer micelle system was made with sheddable polyethyleneimine (PEI) coatings that become unshielded when the disulfide links separating the micelle core are broken. The medication, in this instance doxorubicin, is then discharged into the cell's cytoplasm. The creation of micellar clumps from the self-assembly of an amphiphilic polymer made of triethylene glycol as well as an alkyl strand as the hydrophobic component attached to the polymer's backbone by a disulfide bond has also been documented by our research (Ghosh et al., 2007).

pH-Responsive PNPs

Controlled medication release in particular organs, intracellular elements, or surroundings linked to pathology has been examined through the exploration of the pH gradient there in human organism's intra and extracellular settings (Castro et al., 2022). These nanosystems are typically created utilizing polymers (polyacids or polybases) containing ionizable groups that vary in conformation and/or solubility in response to changes in the pH of the environment, releasing the cargo they were carrying (Lu et al., 2018). Polymeric Nanoparticles (NPs) practical use as chemotherapeutic devices for drug delivery is frequently limited by problems including low circulation stability and ineffective targeting. Here, we've used a straightforward method to create pH-responsive hybrid NPs that are both biocompatible and biodegradable, which solves these problems. The NPs are made of a drug-loaded PLGA (polylactic-co-glycolic acid) core that is covalently "wrapped" around a crosslinked BSA (bovine serum albumin) shell to reduce interactions with macrophages and serum proteins that impair target identification (Palanikumar et al., 2020).

It has also been used to cause changes in the characteristics of polymeric materials in response to environmental cues like pH gradient. For instance, delivery methods have been created to react to variations in the gastrointestinal tract's pH at the organ level. The pH of the gastric lumen for digestion ranges between 1-3, while that of the duodenum, jejunum, and ileum is between 6.6 and 7.5. The use of polymers with an acrylic base is a typical strategy for achieving medication release in the gastrointestinal system. These polymers continue to be in their collapsed condition at low pH. The hydrogenation of the carboxylic groups with loss of hydrogen bonds caused by an increase in pH causes the nanoparticle to swell. Because of the build-up of lactic acid, solid tumors' extracellular environment is more acidic (pH 6.5) at the tissue level than the extracellular environment for normal cells (pH 7.4) (Gonzalez et al., 2012).

Utilizing these pH changes to trigger hydrophobic-hydrophilic transitions in the polymer is one tactic used. The loss of the hydrophobic-hydrophilic equilibrium results in the breakdown of the nanoparticles at the end of this transition. Since the protonation of the amine changes the polymer from hydrophilic to hydrophobic at pH values below 6.5, -amino ester-containing polymers are frequently used (Gu et al., 2011). Targeting acid response at the cellular level can be accomplished by lowering the pH of certain compartments, such as the early endosome and the lysosome, to 5.0 or below. Endosomal escape has frequently been enhanced by amine-containing polymers, such as polyethyleneimine, poly(amidoamine), and imidazole-containing polymers which moderate the pH of intracellular compartments (Guo et al., 2014).

Temperature-Responsive PNPs

Since studies have shown that tumors and other inflammatory disorders exhibit aberrant temperatures due to high metabolic activity and high rates of cell growth in sick tissues, thermo-responsive nanoparticles have gained popularity (Danheir et al., 2010). Due to the fact that heat-responsive polymers alter their chemical and physical properties in reaction to heat, medications are released when nanocarriers experience a slight temperature change. In response to temperature variations brought on by sick tissue, external factors may also affect the temperature at particular locations (Banik et al., 2016).

When exposed to a range of temperatures, polymers can experience conformational changes that alter their solubility or hydrophobicity. Below a particular temperature, they are hydrophilic, and once it rises, they become hydrophobic (Kamaly et al., 2016). The upper critical solution temperature (UCST), which denotes the temperature at which a mixture's components are miscible in all proportions, is another characteristic that is used to produce thermoresponsive materials. The most typical materials exhibiting UCST and utilized as temperature-responsive materials are polyoxazolines and polysulfobetaines.

Light Responsive PNPs

Another stimulus used to cause phase transition and subsequent carrier collapse in polymers is light. The polymeric nanoparticles' structure includes photochromic moieties to make them light-sensitive. These molecules, or chromophores, go through photo-induced structural changes that cause the block to become more polar and water-soluble. When exposed to radiation at a specific wavelength, certain molecules undergo transformations such as cyclization, structural isomerization, or ring opening. Azobenzene is a chromophore that is frequently used due to its quick conversion to cis photoisomerization when exposed to light. The lower critical solubility (LCST) of the molecule and the dipole moment of the molecule both rise as a result of this isomerization (Hamilton et al., 2009).

When exposed to UV light, another molecule, salicylideneaniline, isomerizes from the enol towards the trans-keto form (Heredia et al., 2005). Due to the fact that the cargo is really only released when it is radiated from an external source, these drug-delivery systems offer spatiotemporal control over the triggering event. Light- and radiation-sensitive functional groups in the polymers used to create these nanocapsules are necessary for their proper release because they cause structural changes in the polymeric structure (Crucho et al., 2015).

Magnetic Field Responsive PNPs

Materials that are magnetic, super magnetic, or paramagnetic can generate magnetic field-responsive nanoparticles. Nanosystems are often composed of a core-shell structure, in which a magnetic center is encased in polymers with great biocompatibility (Fleige et al., 2012). Depending on the application, these nanosystems can be exposed to permanent as well as alternating magnetic fields. Controlling the amount of charge discharged over time and repeatedly by these nanoparticles is made possible by alternating magnetic fields (Mura et al., 2013). Performing the magnetic resonance of the nanocarriers and, consequently, combining diagnoses and treatments in a single system, is an important component (Yang et al., 2011).

Using a temperature-sensitive hydrogel, fluorescein (negatively charged) or daunorubicin (positively charged) charged polypyrrole (conductive polymer) nanoparticles were created and applied subcutaneously in vivo (PLGA-PEG PLGA). The electrochemical reduction/oxidation process that the release mechanisms involved were triggered by the application of a weak external direct current electric field. As the surface charge of the polypyrrole nanoparticles varies, the nanoparticles shrink and non-covalently attached drug molecules are attracted to them, which results in the liberation of the nanoparticle active principle, which is directly related to the total net energy within the nanoparticles. The system has shown promise because applications with good biological findings and little invasiveness have been documented (Deckers et al., 2010).

CHARACTERIZATION METHODS OF PNPs

A new age of disease detection and therapy has begun thanks to the use of PNPs in pharmacological and biological applications. Comprehensive characterization of nanomaterials is a crucial prerequisite for preclinical development and is at the heart of any substantial advancements in applications based on them. There are currently no FDA regulatory guidelines or established methodologies for the characterization of nanoparticles (Lin et al., 2014).

However, it is widely known that the physicochemical characteristics of the particles influence physiological interactions. Understanding and forecasting how the system within the body will behave require developing a pretty precise image of the PNPs. Physicochemical characterization, chastity, and pyrogenicity evaluation, biodistribution & toxicity characterization are all parts of a tiered preclinical characterization process for nanomedicines (Hall et al., 2007).

Figure 4. Characterization parameters of polymeric nanoparticles

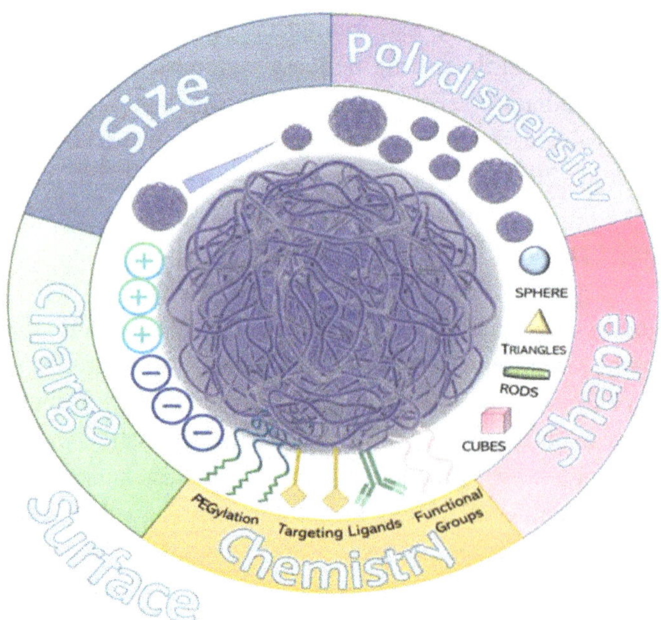

In this chapter, nanoparticles are typically described in terms of their size distribution, shape, surface characteristics, stability, pH, zeta potential, and interactions with drugs and polymers

Morphology, Size, Surface Properties, and Stability

The size and shape of polymeric NPs have been extensively studied using scanning & transmission electron microscopy (TEM and SEM). To undertake the NPs morphology analysis, they are typically paired with cryofracture techniques. The commonly used TEM can measure the thickness of the wall of a nanocapsule and can distinguish between nanospheres and nanocapsules (Bhorey et al., 2016). Nanocapsules are created by wrapping an oily core in a thin (5 nm) polymeric envelope, as opposed to nanospheres, which have a spherical shape and a solid polymeric structure. Atomic force microscopy is a different method that has been applied to describe the morphologies of polymeric NPs (AFM) (Andreani et al., 2015). It can discern surface details down to the atomic level and gives information with great resolution in three dimensions and on a nanometric scale. By using this technique, a complex topology on the nanoparticles' surfaces has been seen, and by examining sample slices, the presence of tiny cavities & pores has also been seen (Mathurin et al., 2018).

The distribution of particle sizes and shapes is the primary criterion used to assess nanoparticle characteristics. The morphology and size of nanoparticles can now be determined with the help of electron microscopy. It is simple to assess how nanoparticles are used in drug delivery and targeting by using a variety of methods. The impact of nanoparticle particle size on medication release has already been well-documented. Faster drug release is achieved by smaller nanoparticles with a bigger surface area. When a loaded drug is exposed to a particle's surface area, a considerable amount of the drug is released. In contrast, medicines' slower diffusion of bigger particles takes place inside the nanoparticles. Therefore, during the storage and transit of nanoparticle dispersion, smaller particles tend to agglomerate. Consequently, there is a mutual trade-off between maximal stability and small nanoparticle size (Redhead et al., 2001). Additionally, particle size can have an impact on how well a polymer degrades. For example, in vitro research has shown that degradation of poly (lactic-co-glycolic acid) increases with increasing particle size (Betancor et al., 2008).

The most important variables used to assess the physical characteristics of polymer nanoparticles are particle size & size distribution. For measuring the size and the size distribution of polymer nanoparticles, methods including photon correlation spectroscopy (PCS), commonly referred to as dynamic light scattering (DLS), light diffraction (LD), and colter counter are frequently utilized. The size & size distribution of submicron particles floating in liquid media are frequently determined using PCS/DLS. The most often measured metric for this technique is the mean particle size with a size distribution, which is represented by the polydispersity index (PDI). A tight size distribution is denoted by a PDI value range of 0.1 to 0.25 whereas a broad distribution is denoted by a PDI value range of more than 0.5. The size of dry polymer nanoparticle powders cannot be determined using this method (Cun et al., 2011).

The stability of drug-loaded particles in vitro shows how well they hold up to storage over time. Typically, polymer nanoparticles are kept at 4 C or room temperature for 6 or 12 months before stability parameters are assessed and compared to those of samples kept at room temperature. The technique of manufacture, particle size & distribution, shape, and effectiveness of drug loading and drug encapsulation all have a significant impact on the durability of polymer nanoparticles. The in vitro stabilization capabilities can also be influenced by the dosage form, delivery method, and drug type (small molecules vs. big macromolecules). For the creation of drug carriers, the sustainability of drug-loaded polymer nanoparticles continues a particularly difficult problem. The most popular and recommended method for improving the stability of polymer nanoparticle suspensions is the inclusion of a stabilizer or combination of stabilizers. With the ongoing advancements in the field of polymer particle engineering, the production of self-stabilized polymer nanoparticle suspensions is anticipated to increase (Catarina et al., 2006).

Drug Polymer Interactions

The nature of the polymer-drug interactions in addition to the type of polymer and its physical and chemical properties should be taken into consideration in order to increase drug loading capacity and prolong drug release. Due to their increased internal energy, which promotes improved solubility and bioavailability, the amorphous form of pharmacologically active compounds has drawn a lot of interest (Yu et al., 2001). Both the unstructured state as well as the crystalline form are possible, however because of physical instability, a drug's amorphous form frequently transforms into a crystalline form on its own. Fortunately, the medication can be incorporated into an amorphous polymer with the simultaneous production of an amorphous solid mixture to accomplish structural stabilization. The solubility of these substances in each other is controlled by interactions among the two types of molecules, which are mediated by hydrogen bonds and van der Walls forces. The drug material can be solubilized by the polymeric component and significant amounts of the drug can be included in the polymer matrices without drug crystallization when the drug-polymer intermolecular interaction is comparable to drug-drug and polymer-polymer interactions. On the other hand, drug crystallization happens when the contacts between the drug & the polymer are weaker because the drug and also the polymer prefer to associate with molecules of the same kind (Raula et al., 2007).

In order to investigate the physicochemical state and potential interactions of the drug-loaded in PNPs, differential scanning calorimetry (DSC) is frequently performed. Phase transitions like melting, crystallization, and glass transition can be found via DSC. The reversible change from a hard, brittle state to a molten or rubber-like state in amorphous materials or in amorphous areas of semi-crystalline materials is known as the glass transition temperature (Tg). In their glassy form, polymers can give PNPs mechanical strength and prevent particle aggregation (Kerc et al., 1995). The thermal properties of PLGA nanoparticles loaded with ketoprofen were investigated in a study. The drug was represented in a non-crystalline state, as shown by the DSC scanned image of the loaded nanoparticles, which did not show a melting peak. Due to their propensity to bind, glycosylated nanoparticles may find innovative uses in targeted medication delivery mediated by carbohydrates. Today, it is understood that polysaccharides have great promise for the creation of long-circulating systems. Sugars also have very appealing biocompatibility, biodegradability, and non-toxicity properties (Corrigan et al., 2009).

Crystal Structure and Chemical Composition

Chemical composition can be determined using an ensemble or single-particle compositional analysis approach and refers to the atomic elements that make up a nanoparticle as well as compounds' natural or manufactured functional groups. Atomic absorption spectroscopy, one of the most widely used ensemble techniques, is based on the concept of atomic absorption, whereby ground-state electrons of the atoms leap to an active state by absorbing a given amount of energy from light at a particular wavelength (Mourdikaudis et al., 2018). The mass concentration of the sample can be determined by correlating the signal to calibration curves at known concentrations since the quantity of energy absorbed is dependent on the type and number of atoms in the light path. Time-of-flight mass spectrometry (TOFMS), which involves ionizing small to large organic solutes into the gas phase with minimal separation and their subsequent separation/detection using a time-of-flight mass analyzer, is one method used to determine the chemical structure of a single particle (Lu et al., 2007). A nanoparticle's arrangement of constituent atoms can either be amorphous or structured into a crystal form. Typically, powder X-ray diffraction or chosen area energy dispersive using transmission electron microscopy (TEM is used to identify the crystal structure. Approximately one gram of material must be supplied for X-ray diffraction, whereas electron diffraction can be performed on single particles (Yang et al., 2007).

Zeta Potential

The zeta potential (ζ) represents the surface energy of the particles and is affected by changes at the particle-dispersing medium interface, changes brought on by the dissociation of ligands on the particle's surface or by the adsorption of ionic species existing in the aqueous dispersion medium, as well as the solvation effect (Honary et al., 2013). The surface charge can be measured indirectly using the zeta potential. It can be discovered by assessing the potential discrepancy between the surface of the shear and the outer Helmholtz plane. Thus, the zeta potential of dispersion based on colloidal particles aids in determining its storage stability. In order to guarantee stability and prevent particle aggregation, high zeta potential values—either positive or negative—are attained. Zeta potential measurements can be used to assess the nature of the material contained within nanocapsules or deposited on a surface, as well as its surface hydrophobicity (Otsuka et al., 2003). A PNP colloidal suspension's stability and surface charge, or how much aggregation will happen over time, are typically assessed using -potential analysis. Additionally, it has a significant role in how PNP behaves in vivo, such as when interacting with cell membranes. The well-known electrophoresis method is typically used to measure the ζ potential of a suspension in order to calculate the particle surface charge. The fundamental idea is to measure the carrier concentration of charged particles when an electrical potential is applied (Tantra et al., 2010).

The major elements of polymeric NPs are phospholipids, poloxamers, and polymers, and when included in formulations, they have the power to alter the zeta potential. For the colloidal solution to be physiochemically stable, an elevated zeta potential value, defined as $|30\ mV|$, is necessary because strong repulsive forces tend to prevent aggregation due to sporadic collisions with nearby nanoparticles. Zeta potential measurements are helpful in clarifying the mechanism of drug interaction with nanoparticles (Zielinska et al., 2019).

pH of the Suspension

Monitoring pH as a time-varying variable allows for the collection of pertinent data regarding the stability of microparticle suspensions. For instance, a pH shift may signal the degradation of a polymer since it suggests a change in the protonation of a particle's surface. After six months of storage, molar mass was confirmed in suspensions of nanocapsules and nanospheres, according to a study, which led to a drop in the pH of these formulations (Guterres et al., 2007). However, depending on how hydrophobic the polymer is, the rapid reduction in pH values of suspensions can be due to the ionization of carboxylic groups present in the polymer, which releases protons into the surrounding media. Additionally, the zeta potential and the electrostatic persistence of the formulation may be influenced by the medium's pH, making it extremely important to monitor.

CONTROLLED DRUG RELEASE BY PNPs

Rate Programmed Drug Delivery Systems

Recent improvements in rate-programmed drug administration systems and smart drug carriers have been made possible by functionalizing rate-controlling surfaces. A new pace of pre-programmed medication delivery has been made possible by transdermal patches, which transfer a specific concentration of pharmaceuticals to the bloodstream through the skin and provide therapeutic benefits at clinical levels. The discharge of drug molecules from the rate-controlling membrane system has already been pre-programmed to occur at a specific rate kinetics in rate-programmed drug delivery systems. The rate-controlling membranes demonstrate their ability to be used as rate-controlling membranes in any dose form, including nano- to microscale level particle-contained matrixes or transdermal patches. They are manufactured from natural & semi-synthetic polymeric materials. It must be easy to use, affordable, and flexible enough to bend or stretch without splitting or cracking. Recently, novel rate-controlling reinforced membranes have been created as rate-controlling barriers for transdermal application. These membranes have flexible and smooth surfaces with embedded scaffolds that could lower the risk of wounding or being rubbed off during dressing, which is an improvement over conventional dressings and can lead to higher patient compliance (Bennet et al., 2013).

This is accomplished by system design optimization, which establishes how easily active agents diffuse across membranes. Different regulating relationships, like membrane permeation-controlled, permeability, membrane hybrid type, and reservoir partition-controlled systems, can be used to categorize this rate-programmed drug delivery system. The polymer and their scaffolds play crucial roles in the recent advancement in smart frequency programmed drug delivery systems, such as improved drug-loaded nano/microparticle encapsulation ability, overcoming pre-systemic metabolism, increased bioavailability, and environmentally sensitive properties for different applications. Consider certain crucial elements when choosing polymers for medicinal applications, like reduced tensile strength, anti-infective, and biocompatibility (Zhang et al., 2002).

Feedback -Regulated Drug Delivery

Various controlled delivery systems, including bio-erosion regulated, bio-responsive regulated, and self-regulating drug delivery systems, have been developed using the feedback-regulated drug delivery idea. One of the ideas in this has to do with intelligent controlled delivery systems. For this reason, numerous research projects are also ongoing to create such drug-containing nanoparticles with feedback-modulated drug release, (Zhao et al., 2013). A triggering factor, such as a biological substance, triggers the release of the drug through some feedback systems in the body. The concentration of the triggering chemical has been used to calculate the release rate. The release is initiated when the activating agent rises above a specific threshold. This can start and halt the release of the medication. A system that identified the specific warning signal brought on by the disease-affected component evaluated the signal's magnitude ratio, and then took action to release the precise number of active medications in response would have a significant potential for advantages. This type of medication delivery device needed a feedback mechanism to satisfy the physiological necessity. For the rate-control release, the self-regulated drug-delivery systems employ a number of techniques, including pH-responsive polymers, enzyme-substrate reactions, enzyme-mediated, pH-dependent drug-dissolving nature, competitive binding mechanism, and metal concentration-dependent hydrolysis. In an aquatic environment, a hydrogel can swell while maintaining its structure (Zhou et al., 2013).

The sensor implanted in the delivery mechanism can enable the simulation of the recognition function of different bio-chemicals like enzymes, cell-mediated receptors, and different proteins in humans for maintaining control and equilibrium. This method is used for drug-incorporated polymeric performance appraisal-controlled delivery methods, and it is based on the understanding that alters in control mechanisms, such as pH, ionic strength, or temperatures, can affect significant changes in drug solubility, which can be the primary determinant of release rate control.

The pH within the polymeric system can be changed by the outside trigger molecule with the polymer-bound enzyme. If the pH of the polymer system changes, this may affect the drug's solubility and cause diffusion, dissolution, or disintegration, changing the rate of release in accordance. The rumen has been bypassed by a membrane that several researchers have constructed, but it still permits the polymeric framework to release the medicine in the stomach via the gastric retention mechanism (Singh et al., 2000). It is impermeable to the rumen's pH 7 due to the polymer membrane, but it expands and releases at pH 4, which is the level of the fourth stomach. Various polymers carrying slightly basic or acidic functional groups in the polymer membrane have been the subject of numerous studies. By altering the pH of the surroundings, this polymeric framework can swell or shrink-swell. In this manner, a matrix or device formed by pH-dependent polymers will release the medicine, and this method can offer controlled release rates.

Site-Targeting Drug Delivery System

The most recent developments in site-targeting medication release and smart delivery devices. A site-targeted drug delivery system is intricate and involves many partitioning and diffusion processes. Today's site-targeted drug delivery systems are the subject of extensive research since scientists are so keen to outperform current medicinal applications. Recent reports describe a well-designed faceted polymeric transporter for site-targeted drug carriers in the treatment of a variety of disorders, including genitourinary, kidney, and colon ailments (Kumar et al., 2008). For biomedical purposes, a number of water-soluble polymers, both natural and synthetic, have been utilized. Because they are so excellent at regulating drug release, these polymers have been utilized frequently in biopharmaceutics. Traditional compositions are not very effective in targeting molecules, thus novel and clever drug delivery techniques are being researched as a solution. Smart drug delivery systems are designed to enable localized medication delivery while also ensuring that healthy tissues are unaffected and that there are no adverse effects. The medications are made up of micro- or nano-sized particle systems, which can pass through arteries, veins, capillaries, and other body organs as well as membrane barriers. They can also travel via systemic circulation (Patel et al., 2010).

The molecular communication paradigm has been used to view communications and transportation because the movement of nanoparticles and their targeting of tissue are complex processes. It has been observed how drug-loaded nanoparticles move throughout the human body, and a signaling molecule carries the message to the area where the nanoparticle travels. The relevance of developing a smart granular delivery system is demonstrated by the communication system's clear reading of particulate diffusion, distribution, and disintegration across time all through the biological system. The communication system was initially solved through computer simulation using the kinetic Monte Carlo approach (Heaton et al., 2012).

Recently, scientists created a method of analysis based on the separation of systems for delivering targeted particulates as a kind of communication. Intracellular & intercellular signaling are used to transmit this information from sender to receiver. Up to this point, various molecular communication types that require either passive or active molecule transport have been studied. When distributing active medication particles from the point of ingestion to the systemic circulation to a desired target, the smart site-tailored delivery system makes use of the systemic circulation. In essence, the delivery systems have been designed with the objective to control the release rate from the systems, but greater control is still needed over the transport of nanoparticles to the target site. The administration route and nanoparticle mobility should ideally be well controlled as well (Pierobon et al., 2012).

TOXICITY AND BIOCOMPATIBILITY CONCERNS

Biocompatibility

PNPs have the ability to cross cell membranes, spread throughout blood arteries, and accumulate in particular cell types. PNPs that have a high ability to penetrate membranes boost the efficiency of medications but can create a number of possible dangers. The significant differences between live tissue & non-living polymeric biomaterials give rise to the biocompatibility issue. Polymeric nanoparticles interact with live tissues when they enter the body, which can have both positive and negative consequences. According to a popular definition, biocompatibility is “the attribute of being consistent with living cells or a living body by not being toxic or harmful and not triggering immunological rejection.” Williams expanded the meaning of biocompatibility in 2008. According to him, “biocompatibility” refers to a biomaterial’s capacity to carry out its intended function in relation to a medical therapy without causing any unfavorable systemic or local effects in the recipient and otherwise beneficiary of that therapy, while simultaneously generating the most beneficial cellular or tissue reactions in that particular circumstance and optimizing the clinically relevant ones. Blood compatibility and histocompatibility are two terms used to describe how polymers interact with tissues and cells, respectively (cytocompatibility) (Saini et al., 2018).

Histocompatibility

The contact between PNPs and tissues is referred to as histocompatibility. The choice of biomaterial is typically based on its tissue biocompatibility for applications that do not involve blood contact (such as dental procedures). The biocompatibility of a polymer biomaterial varies from one site to another, and a biological material may be biocompatible for one application but bioincompatible for another. In contrast to the intense acute inflammations, they generate in the loose connective tissue surrounding the nerves, poly (lactic-co-glycolic acid) based nano- & microparticles exhibit modest tissue reactivity (He et al., 2010).

Hemocompatibility

In applications where there is direct contact with blood, such as drug delivery, gene transfer, or as biosensors, NPs are utilized as vectors. Biocompatibility for blood interaction applications is mostly governed by the measure that shows with blood and its constituents. Numerous scientists studied PNPs regarding their blood compatibility characteristics, and the results of their studies revealed that the surface qualities of the material had an impact on blood compatibility. Surface area, surface charge, hydrophobicity/hydrophilicity, and other physicochemical characteristics all affect how blood reacts when it comes into touch with a substance. For NPs, these reactions are determined by the size effect, structure, and surface (Chouhan et al., 2010).

Nanotoxicity

Toxic side effects must be thoroughly tested for in all pharmaceutical drugs authorized for use in both humans and animals. The preclinical and ultimate clinical assessment and evaluation are complicated by the use of novel materials in the formulation of nanocarriers that have not yet been well characterized. Before the clinical efficacy of the system can be evaluated, the toxicity profile of the different components must be identified. After incubation with nanoparticles, tissues from cell cultures can be examined histologically to get a preliminary estimate of the toxicity. In vitro cytotoxicity, however, is typically significantly greater than in vivo cytotoxicity. This could be explicated by the fact that the hazardous breakdown products are continuously removed from the application site in vivo. PNPs can vary in size, shape, and chemical architecture depending on how they are made. These variables fundamentally influence how PNPs interact with living tissues or cells. PNPs can influence the operation of the immune function by interacting with a variety of immune system cells (Grabowski et al., 2015).

They can be harmful or benign depending on how they interact. When polymeric material interfaces with live tissue, two different sorts of responses may take place. A systemic response affects sections of the body outside the local part, whereas a local reaction only affects the part of the body that is in immediate contact with the substance. Unless it is specifically created for such needs, such as PNPs that target and kill cancer cells, a biomaterial should generally be harmless. The study of the possible harm caused by interactions between nanoparticles and biological systems is known as nanotoxicology (Hussain et al., 2012).

APPLICATIONS OF PNPs

For Cancer Therapy

PNPs targeted delivery can overcome issues with traditional anticancer treatments, such as their poor water solubility, rapid elimination, and lack of selectivity, which result in a wide range of side effects for healthy tissues and a reduction in the anticancer concentration that reaches cancer tissues. The use of PNPs for the oral administration of anticancer medications has grown significantly. PNPs' ability to capture anticancer medications protects them from efflux transporters, and their range of nanoscale PNPs speeds up an entry through biological membranes. Additionally, the polymer coating protects the medication from bodily enzymes. On the other hand, hydrolysis, diffusion, and enzymatic degradation are potential routes for the release of anticancer properties from PNPs. PNPs also demonstrated the ability to improve medication stability, prolong the results of remediation, modify cellular uptake, and reduce deterioration as well as metabolism (Khalid et al., 2017).

Figure 5. Applications of polymeric nanoparticles

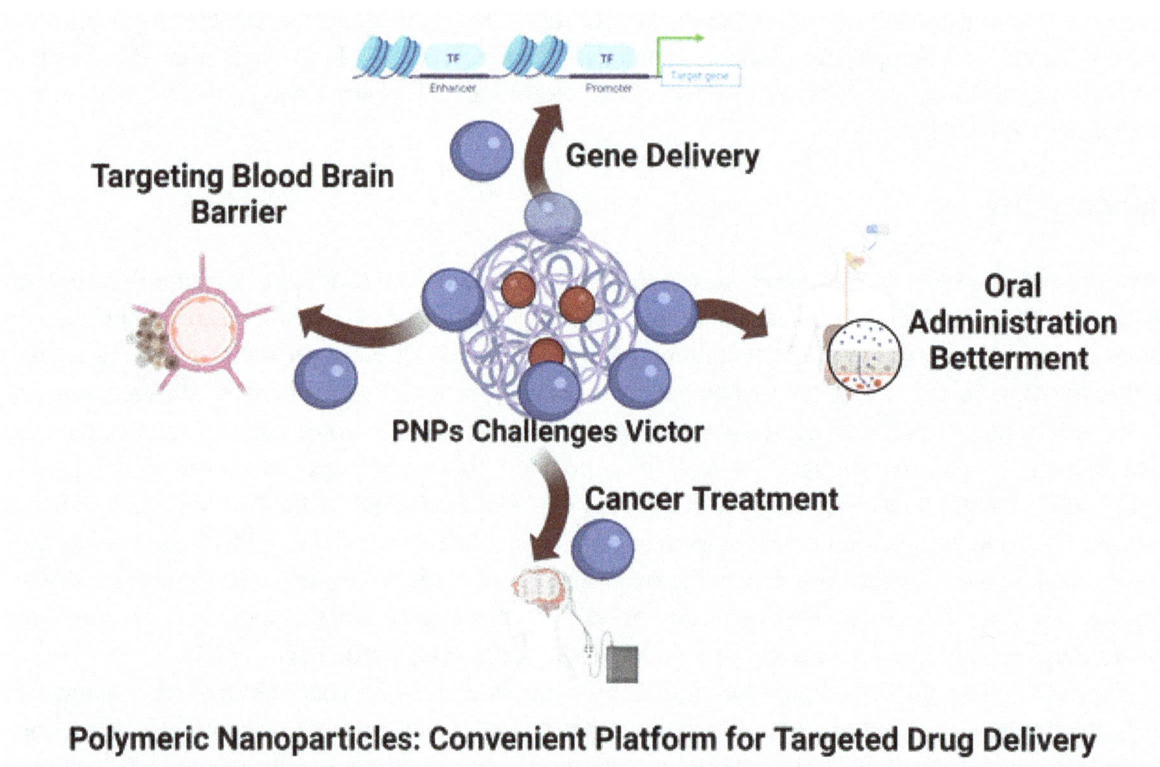

The PNPs intended for targeted delivery (TDDS) can increase the tissue particular anticancer active ingredients receive and send through either active or passive targeting tumors devoid of affecting non-cancerous regions. Recent advances in nanotechnology have revealed many different targeting strategies for supplementing drug accumulation into the tumor while limiting the undesirable toxicity to normal cells. PNPs only have an effect on tumors during the targeted delivery of tumors because of the damaged lymphatic network and the dysfunctional porous assembly of tumor vasculature. The drug-PNPs will consequently build up in the cellular interstices of the tumor as a result of what is known as an increased permeability & retention (EPR) effect. On the other hand, in active tumor targeting, ternary-constructed particles enter the tissues and/or vasculature of the tumor by receptor-intermediated endocytosis. An anticancer moiety, a polymer acting as an importer, and a ligand serving as a targeting element make up this assemblage (Khalid et al., 2017).

Long-circulating PNPs, a new class of PNPs for more precise and targeted distribution, are created by PNPs assembled with surface modification using polymers with good water solubility including poly-ethylene oxide (PEO) & PEG. The hydrophilic surface modifiers were thought to be the ones that reduce the interactions between PNPs and plasma proteins, resulting in a lower absorption by the reticuloendo-thelial system (RES). The main result of adaptation employing PEG, poly (propylene oxide) (PPO), or other hydrophilic flexible polymers is a significant increase in circulation time, ensuring maintenance of the optimal drug blood concentration, the better chance of extravasation, and PNPs' retention ability in areas of dispersed endothelium (Kommareddy et al., 2006).

Natural diterpene oridonin has shown the ability to block nuclear factor-KB (NF-KB), bottom the Bcl-2 family of proteins, and trigger apoptosis in lymphoid malignancies cells. Although this potential medication has several clinical uses, oridonin suffers from a number of drawbacks, including a limited therapeutic index & poor water solubility. By adopting the emulsion solvent diffusion approach, oridonin-loaded PLA-PNPs were created. The results of pharmacokinetic tests showed that oridonin incorporated in PLA-PNPs was incredibly effective at extending blood circulation time. After the administration of oridonin-PLA-PNPs, the amount of oridonin in the spleen, liver, and lung is reported to be steady and highly concentrated, whereas the amounts in the kidney and heart have significantly decreased (Ikezoe et al., 2005).

These challenges may be overcome by the potent, extremely adaptable carrier systems known as polymeric nanoparticles (PNPs). According to several studies, properly made polymeric NPs can pass the blood-brain barrier, improve medication bioavailability, lessen systemic toxicity, and target cancer cells in the central nervous system. Although there are no clinical trials for research involving their use in curing brain cancer, there are growing preclinical indications that polymeric NPs may be helpful for treating brain tumors. This review examines several polymeric NPs and also how their associated compositions, surface changes, and delivery techniques affect their ability to enhance the treatment of brain tumors (Caraway et al., 2022).

For Immune Engineering

It is well known that vaccine distribution within PNPs has great promise. However, in order to transport the plasmid DNA, researchers have relied on polymeric microparticle (PMP) or PNP systems. Both chitosan and PLGA, which are natural and artificial polymers, have become important factors in oral DNA delivery. Through persistent release, antigen encapsulation inside PNPs may actually lengthen the antigen exhibition. When PLGA PNPs were employed to transport the BCG antigen 85B from Mycobacterium TB, this is what happened. When PNPs are used to transport antigens, the absorption efficiency into dendritic cells is significantly increased in comparison to the free antigen. For the delivery of PNPs antigens, PLGA, a biodegradable polymer, is also being scientifically enhanced. Comparatively, to free, unentrapped core Hepatitis B antigen, PLGA PNPs loaded with the antigen elicited a stronger cellular immune response. It is clear from much prior research that PNPs have the ability to increase antigen absorption and influence the type and extent of antigen performance. These PNPs' strengths are seen as being critical in coordinating the necessary immune response against a wide range of infectious diseases (Bolhassani et al., 2014).

For Infectious Disease

To establish an infection site, both viruses and bacteria infiltrate bodily tissue and cells, multiply, and produce proteins and cell signaling chemicals. Antimicrobial or virulence-suppressing APIs, which typically target mitochondrial systems, cell wall integrity, or proliferation pathways, are used to treat infections. There are pathogens that are quiescent and can escape the APIs which can eventually cause resistance in some illnesses. The poor water solubility and stability of many antibiotic APIs further reduce their bioavailability & biodistribution. As a result, PNPs have been thought of as potential beneficial carriers to enhance medicinal formulations (Zhu et al., 2014). Polymer NPs provide greater design flexibility than lipid nanoparticles or metallic NPs, allowing for the creation of copolymers with a variety of functionalities. To localize the release of antibiotics to the infection site, a polymeric NP was made, for instance, using a copolymer of poly(L-histidine) and PEG for bioinert contacts and hydrogenation in an acidic environment (Radovic et al., 2012).

This further illustrates a polymer NP's stimulus-responsive nature. A variety of APIs can be used with polymer NP systems due to the design's adaptability, which increases the API's solubility and stability in vivo. For instance, antiviral nucleoside analog azidothymidine, which is poorly soluble in water, was loaded onto poly (hexyl cyanoacrylate) particles, and these particles demonstrated potential as a treatment for preventing human immunodeficiency virus. In the creation of nanoparticles (NPs), certain natural polymers, such as chitosan, can engage with bacteria to trigger cell death, which has inherent antibacterial characteristics. When release kinetics, durability, retention, and stimulus-response are controlled in polymer NPs, antibiotic efficacy is 120 times more than it is for free antibiotics (Turos et al., 2007).

For Cardiovascular Diseases

Cardiovascular disease is the primary cause of death in all developed nations, and atherosclerotic is one of the main causes. An inflammatory response to cardiovascular disease, atherosclerosis is characterized by constricted arteries brought on by the build-up of fatty plaque formation along vessel walls and upregulates immune response in infected locations. Destabilization of the plaque and possible thrombosis can result from the aggravation of inflected endothelium brought on by macrophage recruitment in the atherosclerotic vasculature. These deposits have the potential to rupture during thrombosis and result in deadly obstructions in the veins that are typical of stroke or myocardial infarction (Choi et al., 2010).

Current therapies for atherosclerosis often try to lower cholesterol levels with statins or suppress immunological response with anticoagulants, barring surgical intervention to remove actual plaque plaques. While both statin & anticoagulant medication has limited absorption, with the delivery of higher dosages approaching toxicity, statin therapy treating atherosclerosis may be clouded with muscle-related myopathy and other unwanted side effects. Because of the flexibility in adjusting the size and surface charge characteristics for enhanced bioavailability, PNPs can be used for sustained distribution over time for the long-term therapy of a high-potency API. For instance, PLGA NPs have been created to replicate the high-density lipoprotein's size, shape, & surface charge in order to target atherosclerotic tissue (Sanchez et al., 2015).

SAFETY ISSUES AND CHALLENGES OF PNPs

A variety of polymers, including biodegradable and non-biodegradable polymers, can be utilized to create polymeric nanoparticles. Comparatively speaking, biodegradable polymers are safer than non-biodegradable polymers. Preferably, the polymer should be both biocompatible and biodegradable. Safety issues may arise if the polymer builds up inside the body. Currently, the FDA has only approved and guaranteed the safety of a small number of polymers. The FDA has not yet authorized PACA, the most often used polymer in the CNS, raising serious concerns about its safety. However, polymers like PLGA, PLA, and others have been shown to be free from toxic usage. Additionally, to be biocompatible and biodegradable, they have US FDA approval (Marcowicz et al., 2015).

Since natural polymers are made from natural materials and are biocompatible and biodegradable, they are typically favored over synthetic polymers. Synthetic polymer emerged as a solution to issues like inconsistent sourcing, production challenges, seasonal polymer procurement, easy microorganism contamination, etc. Before using polymers in the manufacture of nanoparticles, it is important to properly investigate their properties. Before creating a specific nanoparticle, one should confirm its safety and non-toxicity. The production of polymeric nanoparticles also carries a significant danger. The primary danger is present in the production of dry, powdery polymeric nanoparticles. Such powders are challenging to handle and expose employees to high exposure levels by ingestion through the GI system, through skin absorption, and inhalation into the lungs. By maintaining proper personal hygiene, adhering to fundamental safety guidelines, and using personal protection equipment, these work dangers can be avoided (Othman et al., 2018).

In addition to the concern indicated above, polymeric nanoparticles also present some environmental risks. Some nanoparticles have the potential to harm both the environment and living things. For instance, a polymeric nanoparticle poses a serious threat to the ecosystem and can be extremely dangerous to microorganisms, contaminating groundwater in the process. Additionally, the nanoparticle has the potential to penetrate the food chain and harm the environment. For instance, the implantation of polymeric nanoparticles in fish, plants, or other living things may have a negative impact on the environment and food chain. Specific regulations should be established to prevent environmental pollution in order to avert such environmental concerns. Additionally, waste from the facility that produces polymeric nanoparticles needs to be disposed of properly (Gatti et al., 2018).

CONCLUSION

A clever drug delivery technology is the polymeric nanoparticle that has been functionalized. Numerous variations of the polymers have been investigated for their safety and efficiency in delivering drugs to a particular spot. The synthesized polymeric nanoparticle has many different applications, including the delivery of drugs to the brain, the treatment of cancer, gene therapy, and the vagina. There have been many developments in the functionalized nanoparticle sector over the past few decades, including the release of drugs in reaction to external stimuli, goal drug release, magnetic nanocapsules, ligand-based polymeric nanoparticles, nanogels, and many others. While many synthesized polymeric nanoparticles are still in various stages of clinical testing, many have already hit the market. These nanoparticles successfully load the medication and target the desired spot, reducing adverse effects.

Future advances in nanomedicine, particularly in functionalized polymeric nanoparticles, will help treat severe diseases like cancer with fewer side effects. The procedures for illness diagnosis, therapy, and prevention will be improved by the ongoing study on functionalized nanoparticles. A new approach to research is needed to create an easy scaling-up method and a plain, simple, efficient production method. To increase the safety of the nanoparticles for people and the ecology, some regulatory requirements should be established.

The numerous current shortcomings of some technological solutions can be addressed by fusion technologies, which have a high potential for synergistic improvement in the safest nanoparticle-based drug delivery. A promising and mostly unexplored field of research is the consideration of combining and incorporating two or more appropriate technologies to produce a high-throughput technology. The evaluation of smart medication delivery and the development of novel polymeric-based nanoparticles must now consider this new understanding. Additionally, the effectiveness and side effects of the next wave of polymeric nanoparticle-based delivery systems for pharmaceuticals including growth factors, hormones, autoantibodies, genes, peptides, etc. should be improved.

The assessment, treatment, and prevention of illnesses will be substantially altered and improved by ongoing research on PNPs in both preclinical and clinical investigations. With newly found disease site-specific medications and current poorly soluble pharmaceuticals, polymeric nanoparticles provide a novel way to achieve delivery of drug and therapeutic targeting. Polymeric nanoparticles are expected to improve application and effective medication delivery by overcoming the limitations of current drug delivery technologies, which would eventually improve patient compliance and treatment.

In conclusion, toxicity, immune system recognition and authorization, stability and repeatability, and regulatory approval are some of the difficulties that polymeric nanoparticles in biomedicine face. The successful application of polymeric nanoparticle-based technologies in clinical settings will depend on how well these issues are resolved.

REFERENCES

Akagi, T., Kaneko, T., Kida, T., & Akashi, M. (2005). Preparation and characterization of biodegradable nanoparticles based on poly (γ-glutamic acid) with L-phenylalanine as a protein carrier. *Journal of Controlled Release*, *108*(2-3), 226–236. doi:10.1016/j.jconrel.2005.08.003 PMID:16125267

Alaniz, L., Cabrera, P. V., Blanco, G., Ernst, G., Rimoldi, G., Alvarez, E., & Hajos, S. E. (2002). Interaction of CD44 with different forms of hyaluronic acid. Its role in adhesion and migration of tumor cells. *Cell Communication & Adhesion*, *9*(3), 117–130. doi:10.1080/15419060214522 PMID:12521133

Allémann, E., Gurny, R., & Doelker, E. (1992). Preparation of aqueous polymeric nanodispersions by a reversible salting-out process: Influence of process parameters on particle size. *International Journal of Pharmaceutics*, *87*(1-3), 247–253. doi:10.1016/0378-5173(92)90249-2

Allen, R. P., Bolandparvaz, A., Ma, J. A., Manickam, V. A., & Lewis, J. S. (2018). Latent, Immunosuppressive Nature of Poly (lactic-co-glycolic acid) Microparticles. *ACS Biomaterials Science & Engineering*, *4*(3), 900–918. doi:10.1021/acsbiomaterials.7b00831 PMID:30555893

Allouche, J. (2013). Synthesis of organic and bioorganic nanoparticles: an overview of the preparation methods. *Nanomaterials: a danger or a promise?* 27-74.

Andreani, T., Kiill, C. P., de Souza, A. L. R., Fangueiro, J. F., Doktorovová, S., Garcia, M. L., Gramião, M. P. D., Silva, A. M., & Souto, E. B. (2015). Effect of cryoprotectants on the reconstitution of silica nanoparticles produced by sol–gel technology. *Journal of Thermal Analysis and Calorimetry*, *120*(1), 1001–1007. doi:10.100710973-014-4275-4

Banik, B. L., Fattahi, P., & Brown, J. L. (2016). Polymeric nanoparticles: The future of nanomedicine. *Wiley Interdisciplinary Reviews. Nanomedicine and Nanobiotechnology*, *8*(2), 271–299. doi:10.1002/wnan.1364 PMID:26314803

Barratt, G. M. (2000). Therapeutic applications of colloidal drug carriers. *Pharmaceutical Science & Technology Today*, *3*(5), 163–171. doi:10.1016/S1461-5347(00)00255-8 PMID:10785658

Begines, B., Ortiz, T., Pérez-Aranda, M., Martínez, G., Merinero, M., Argüelles-Arias, F., & Alcudia, A. (2020). Polymeric nanoparticles for drug delivery: Recent developments and future prospects. *Nanomaterials (Basel, Switzerland)*, *10*(7), 1403. doi:10.3390/nano10071403 PMID:32707641

Bennet, D., & Kim, S. (2013). A transdermal delivery system to enhance quercetin nanoparticle permeability. *Journal of Biomaterials Science. Polymer Edition*, *24*(2), 185–209. doi:10.1163/156856212X630258 PMID:23565597

Bennet, D., & Kim, S. (2014). *Polymer nanoparticles for smart drug delivery* (*Vol. 8*).

Betancor, L., & Luckarift, H. R. (2008). Bioinspired enzyme encapsulation for biocatalysis. *Trends in Biotechnology*, *26*(10), 566–572. doi:10.1016/j.tibtech.2008.06.009 PMID:18757108

Bohrey, S., Chourasiya, V., & Pandey, A. (2016). Polymeric nanoparticles containing diazepam: Preparation, optimization, characterization, in-vitro drug release and release kinetic study. *Nano Convergence*, *3*(1), 1–7. doi:10.118640580-016-0061-2 PMID:28191413

Bolhassani, A., Javanzad, S., Saleh, T., Hashemi, M., Aghasadeghi, M. R., & Sadat, S. M. (2014). Polymeric nanoparticles: Potent vectors for vaccine delivery targeting cancer and infectious diseases. *Human Vaccines & Immunotherapeutics*, *10*(2), 321–332. doi:10.4161/hv.26796 PMID:24128651

Brigger, I., Dubernet, C., & Couvreur, P. (2012). Nanoparticles in cancer therapy and diagnosis. *Advanced Drug Delivery Reviews*, *64*, 24–36. doi:10.1016/j.addr.2012.09.006 PMID:12204596

Cai, Y., Qi, J., Lu, Y., He, H., & Wu, W. (2022). The in vivo fate of polymeric micelles. *Advanced Drug Delivery Reviews*, *188*, 114463. doi:10.1016/j.addr.2022.114463 PMID:35905947

Calzoni, E., Cesaretti, A., Polchi, A., Di Michele, A., Tancini, B., & Emiliani, C. (2019). Biocompatible polymer nanoparticles for drug delivery applications in cancer and neurodegenerative disorder therapies. *Journal of Functional Biomaterials*, *10*(1), 4. doi:10.3390/jfb10010004 PMID:30626094

Cao, X., Lai, S., & James Lee, L. (2001). Design of a self-regulated drug delivery device. *Biomedical Microdevices*, *3*(2), 109–118. doi:10.1023/A:1011494008729

Caraway, C. A., Gaitsch, H., Wicks, E. E., Kalluri, A., Kunadi, N., & Tyler, B. M. (2022). Polymeric nanoparticles in brain cancer therapy: A review of current approaches. *Polymers*, *14*(14), 2963. doi:10.3390/polym14142963 PMID:35890738

Castro, K. C. D., Costa, J. M., & Campos, M. G. N. (2022). Drug-loaded polymeric nanoparticles: A review. *International Journal of Polymeric Materials*, *71*(1), 1–13. doi:10.1080/00914037.2020.1798436

Catarina Pinto, R., Neufeld, R. J., Ribeiro, A. J., Francisco, V., & Nanoencapsulation, I. (2006). Methods for preparation of drug-loaded polymeric nanoparticles Nanomedicine. *Nanotechnol Biol Med*, *2*, 8–21. doi:10.1016/j.nano.2005.12.003

Chang, J., Jallouli, Y., Kroubi, M., Yuan, X. B., Feng, W., Kang, C. S., Pu, P., & Betbeder, D. (2009). Characterization of endocytosis of transferrin-coated PLGA nanoparticles by the blood–brain barrier. *International Journal of Pharmaceutics*, *379*(2), 285–292. doi:10.1016/j.ijpharm.2009.04.035 PMID:19416749

Choi, H. S., Ashitate, Y., Lee, J. H., Kim, S. H., Matsui, A., Insin, N., Bawendi, M. G., Semmler-Behnke, M., Frangioni, J. V., & Tsuda, A. (2010). Rapid translocation of nanoparticles from the lung airspaces to the body. *Nature Biotechnology*, *28*(12), 1300–1303. doi:10.1038/nbt.1696 PMID:21057497

Chorny, M., Fishbein, I., Danenberg, H. D., & Golomb, G. (2002). Lipophilic drug loaded nanospheres prepared by nanoprecipitation: Effect of formulation variables on size, drug recovery and release kinetics. *Journal of Controlled Release*, *83*(3), 389–400. doi:10.1016/S0168-3659(02)00211-0 PMID:12387947

Chouhan, R., & Bajpai, A. K. (2010). Release dynamics of ciprofloxacin from swellable nanocarriers of poly (2-hydroxyethyl methacrylate): An in vitro study. *Nanomedicine; Nanotechnology, Biology, and Medicine*, *6*(3), 453–462. doi:10.1016/j.nano.2009.11.006 PMID:20044034

Corrigan, O. I., & Li, X. (2009). Quantifying drug release from PLGA nanoparticulates. *European Journal of Pharmaceutical Sciences*, *37*(3-4), 477–485. doi:10.1016/j.ejps.2009.04.004 PMID:19379812

Couvreur, P., Dubernet, C., & Puisieux, F. (1995). Controlled drug delivery with nanoparticles: Current possibilities and future trends. *European Journal of Pharmaceutics and Biopharmaceutics*, *41*(1), 2–13.

Crucho, C. I. (2015). Stimuli-responsive polymeric nanoparticles for nanomedicine. *ChemMedChem*, *10*(1), 24–38. doi:10.1002/cmdc.201402290 PMID:25319803

Crucho, C. I., & Barros, M. T. (2017). Polymeric nanoparticles: A study on the preparation variables and characterization methods. *Materials Science and Engineering C*, *80*, 771–784. doi:10.1016/j.msec.2017.06.004 PMID:28866227

Cui, Z., & Mumper, R. J. (2002). Plasmid DNA-entrapped nanoparticles engineered from microemulsion precursors: In vitro and in vivo evaluation. *Bioconjugate Chemistry*, *13*(6), 1319–1327. doi:10.1021/bc0255586 PMID:12440869

Cun, D., Jensen, D. K., Maltesen, M. J., Bunker, M., Whiteside, P., Scurr, D., Foged, C., & Nielsen, H. M. (2011). High loading efficiency and sustained release of siRNA encapsulated in PLGA nanoparticles: Quality by design optimization and characterization. *European Journal of Pharmaceutics and Biopharmaceutics*, *77*(1), 26–35. doi:10.1016/j.ejpb.2010.11.008 PMID:21093589

Dadwal, M., Solan, D., & Pradesh, H. (2014). Polymeric nanoparticles as promising novel carriers for drug delivery: An overview. *Journal of Advanced Pharmacy Education & Research Jan-Mar*, *4*(1).

Danhier, F., Feron, O., & Préat, V. (2010). To exploit the tumor microenvironment: Passive and active tumor targeting of nanocarriers for anti-cancer drug delivery. *Journal of Controlled Release*, *148*(2), 135–146. doi:10.1016/j.jconrel.2010.08.027 PMID:20797419

Deckers, R., & Moonen, C. T. (2010). Ultrasound triggered, image guided, local drug delivery. *Journal of Controlled Release*, *148*(1), 25–33. doi:10.1016/j.jconrel.2010.07.117 PMID:20709123

Delplace, V., Couvreur, P., & Nicolas, J. (2014). Recent trends in the design of anticancer polymer prodrug nanocarriers. *Polymer Chemistry*, *5*(5), 1529–1544. doi:10.1039/C3PY01384G

Fessi, H. P. F. D., Puisieux, F., Devissaguet, J. P., Ammoury, N., & Benita, S. (1989). Nanocapsule formation by interfacial polymer deposition following solvent displacement. *International Journal of Pharmaceutics*, *55*(1), R1–R4. doi:10.1016/0378-5173(89)90281-0

Fleige, E., Quadir, M. A., & Haag, R. (2012). Stimuli-responsive polymeric nanocarriers for the controlled transport of active compounds: Concepts and applications. *Advanced Drug Delivery Reviews*, *64*(9), 866–884. doi:10.1016/j.addr.2012.01.020 PMID:22349241

Fornaguera, C., Feiner-Gracia, N., Calderó, G., García-Celma, M. J., & Solans, C. (2015). Galantamine-loaded PLGA nanoparticles, from nano-emulsion templating, as novel advanced drug delivery systems to treat neurodegenerative diseases. *Nanoscale*, *7*(28), 12076–12084. doi:10.1039/C5NR03474D PMID:26118655

Gagliardi, A., Giuliano, E., Venkateswararao, E., Fresta, M., Bulotta, S., Awasthi, V., & Cosco, D. (2021). Biodegradable polymeric nanoparticles for drug delivery to solid tumors. *Frontiers in Pharmacology*, *12*, 601626. doi:10.3389/fphar.2021.601626 PMID:33613290

Ganachaud, F., & Katz, J. L. (2005). Nanoparticles and nanocapsules created using the ouzo effect: Spontaneous emulsification as an alternative to ultrasonic and high-shear devices. *ChemPhysChem*, *6*(2), 209–216. doi:10.1002/cphc.200400527 PMID:15751338

Gao, J., Gu, H., & Xu, B. (2009). Multifunctional magnetic nanoparticles: Design, synthesis, and biomedical applications. *Accounts of Chemical Research*, *42*(8), 1097–1107. doi:10.1021/ar9000026 PMID:19476332

Gatti, T. H. H., Eloy, J. O., Ferreira, L. M. B., Silva, I. C. D., Pavan, F. R., Gremião, M. P. D., & Chorilli, M. (2018). Insulin-loaded polymeric mucoadhesive nanoparticles: Development, characterization and cytotoxicity evaluation. *Brazilian Journal of Pharmaceutical Sciences*, *54*(1), 54. doi:10.15902175-97902018000117314

Ge, J., Lei, J., & Zare, R. N. (2011). Bovine serum albumin–poly (methyl methacrylate) nanoparticles: An example of frustrated phase separation. *Nano Letters*, *11*(6), 2551–2554. doi:10.1021/nl201303q PMID:21553851

Geisow, M. J., & Evans, W. H. (1984). pH in the endosome: Measurements during pinocytosis and receptor-mediated endocytosis. *Experimental Cell Research*, *150*(1), 36–46. doi:10.1016/0014-4827(84)90699-2 PMID:6198190

Ghosh, S. (2004). Recent research and development in synthetic polymer-based drug delivery systems. *Journal of Chemical Research*, *2004*(4), 241–246. doi:10.3184/0308234041209158

Ghosh, S., Irvin, K., & Thayumanavan, S. (2007). Tunable disassembly of micelles using a redox trigger. *Langmuir*, *23*(15), 7916–7919. doi:10.1021/la700981z PMID:17567057

González-Toro, D. C., Ryu, J. H., Chacko, R. T., Zhuang, J., & Thayumanavan, S. (2012). Concurrent binding and delivery of proteins and lipophilic small molecules using polymeric nanogels. *Journal of the American Chemical Society*, *134*(16), 6964–6967. doi:10.1021/ja3019143 PMID:22480205

Govender, T., Stolnik, S., Garnett, M. C., Illum, L., & Davis, S. S. (1999). PLGA nanoparticles prepared by nanoprecipitation: Drug loading and release studies of a water soluble drug. *Journal of Controlled Release*, *57*(2), 171–185. doi:10.1016/S0168-3659(98)00116-3 PMID:9971898

Grabowski, N., Hillaireau, H., Vergnaud, J., Tsapis, N., Pallardy, M., Kerdine-Römer, S., & Fattal, E. (2015). Surface coating mediates the toxicity of polymeric nanoparticles towards human-like macrophages. *International Journal of Pharmaceutics*, *482*(1-2), 75–83. doi:10.1016/j.ijpharm.2014.11.042 PMID:25448553

Gu, Z., Biswas, A., Zhao, M., & Tang, Y. (2011). Tailoring nanocarriers for intracellular protein delivery. *Chemical Society Reviews*, *40*(7), 3638–3655. doi:10.1039/c0cs00227e PMID:21566806

Guo, X., Shi, C., Yang, G., Wang, J., Cai, Z., & Zhou, S. (2014). Dual-responsive polymer micelles for target-cell-specific anticancer drug delivery. *Chemistry of Materials*, *26*(15), 4405–4418. doi:10.1021/cm5012718

Guterres, S. S., Alves, M. P., & Pohlmann, A. R. (2007). Polymeric nanoparticles, nanospheres and nanocapsules, for cutaneous applications. *Drug Target Insights*, *2*, 117739280700200002. doi:10.1177/117739280700200002 PMID:21901071

Guterres, S. S., Alves, M. P., & Pohlmann, A. R. (2007). Polymeric nanoparticles, nanospheres and nanocapsules, for cutaneous applications. *Drug Target Insights*, *2*, 117739280700200002. doi:10.1177/117739280700200002 PMID:21901071

Hall, J. B., Dobrovolskaia, M. A., Patri, A. K., & McNeil, S. E. (2007). *Characterization of nanoparticles for therapeutics.*

Hamilton, S. K., & Harth, E. (2009). Molecular dendritic transporter nanoparticle vectors provide efficient intracellular delivery of peptides. *ACS Nano*, *3*(2), 402–410. doi:10.1021/nn800679z PMID:19236078

Hawkins, M. J., Soon-Shiong, P., & Desai, N. (2008). Protein nanoparticles as drug carriers in clinical medicine. *Advanced Drug Delivery Reviews*, *60*(8), 876–885. doi:10.1016/j.addr.2007.08.044 PMID:18423779

He, Q., Zhang, J., Chen, F., Guo, L., Zhu, Z., & Shi, J. (2010). An anti-ROS/hepatic fibrosis drug delivery system based on salvianolic acid B loaded mesoporous silica nanoparticles. *Biomaterials*, *31*(30), 7785–7796. doi:10.1016/j.biomaterials.2010.07.008 PMID:20674009

Heaton, L. L., López, E., Maini, P. K., Fricker, M. D., & Jones, N. S. (2012). Advection, diffusion, and delivery over a network. *Physical Review. E*, *86*(2), 021905. doi:10.1103/PhysRevE.86.021905 PMID:23005783

Heredia, K. L., Bontempo, D., Ly, T., Byers, J. T., Halstenberg, S., & Maynard, H. D. (2005). In situ preparation of protein–"smart" polymer conjugates with retention of bioactivity. *Journal of the American Chemical Society*, *127*(48), 16955–16960. doi:10.1021/ja054482w PMID:16316241

Honary, S., & Zahir, F. (2013). Effect of zeta potential on the properties of nano-drug delivery systems-a review (Part 2). *Tropical Journal of Pharmaceutical Research*, *12*(2), 265–273.

Hussain, S., Vanoirbeek, J. A., & Hoet, P. H. (2012). Interactions of nanomaterials with the immune system. *Wiley Interdisciplinary Reviews. Nanomedicine and Nanobiotechnology*, *4*(2), 169–183. doi:10.1002/wnan.166 PMID:22144008

Ibrahim, H., Bindschaedler, C., Doelker, E., Buri, P., & Gurny, R. (1992). Aqueous nanodispersions prepared by a salting-out process. *International Journal of Pharmaceutics*, *87*(1-3), 239–246. doi:10.1016/0378-5173(92)90248-Z

Ikezoe, T., Yang, Y., Bandobashi, K., Saito, T., Takemoto, S., Machida, H., Togitani, K., Koeffler, H. P., & Taguchi, H. (2005). Oridonin, a diterpenoid purified from Rabdosia rubescens, inhibits the proliferation of cells from lymphoid malignancies in association with blockade of the NF-κB signal pathways. *Molecular Cancer Therapeutics*, *4*(4), 578–586. doi:10.1158/1535-7163.MCT-04-0277 PMID:15827331

Jackson, J. K., Letchford, K., Wasserman, B. Z., Ye, L., Hamad, W. Y., & Burt, H. M. (2011). The use of nanocrystalline cellulose for the binding and controlled release of drugs. *International Journal of Nanomedicine*, *6*, 321. PMID:21383857

Jaiswal, J., Gupta, S. K., & Kreuter, J. (2004). Preparation of biodegradable cyclosporine nanoparticles by high-pressure emulsification-solvent evaporation process. *Journal of Controlled Release*, *96*(1), 169–178. doi:10.1016/j.jconrel.2004.01.017 PMID:15063039

Jarai, B. M., Kolewe, E. L., Stillman, Z. S., Raman, N., & Fromen, C. A. (2020). Polymeric nanoparticles. In *Nanoparticles for biomedical applications* (pp. 303–324). Elsevier. doi:10.1016/B978-0-12-816662-8.00018-7

Jeon, H. J., Jeong, Y. I., Jang, M. K., Park, Y. H., & Nah, J. W. (2000). Effect of solvent on the preparation of surfactant-free poly (DL-lactide-co-glycolide) nanoparticles and norfloxacin release characteristics. *International Journal of Pharmaceutics*, *207*(1-2), 99–108. doi:10.1016/S0378-5173(00)00537-8 PMID:11036235

Jeong, Y. I., Cho, C. S., Kim, S. H., Ko, K. S., Kim, S. I., Shim, Y. H., & Nah, J. W. (2001). Preparation of poly (DL-lactide-co-glycolide) nanoparticles without surfactant. *Journal of Applied Polymer Science*, *80*(12), 2228–2236. doi:10.1002/app.1326

Jia, Y., Jiang, Y., He, Y., Zhang, W., Zou, J., Magar, K. T., Boucetta, H., Teng, C., & He, W. (2023). Approved Nanomedicine against Diseases. *Pharmaceutics*, *15*(3), 774. doi:10.3390/pharmaceutics15030774 PMID:36986635

Jung, J., & Perrut, M. (2001). Particle design using supercritical fluids: Literature and patent survey. *The Journal of Supercritical Fluids*, *20*(3), 179–219. doi:10.1016/S0896-8446(01)00064-X

Kamaly, N., Xiao, Z., Valencia, P. M., Radovic-Moreno, A. F., & Farokhzad, O. C. (2012). Targeted polymeric therapeutic nanoparticles: Design, development and clinical translation. *Chemical Society Reviews*, *41*(7), 2971–3010. doi:10.1039/c2cs15344k PMID:22388185

Kamaly, N., Yameen, B., Wu, J., & Farokhzad, O. C. (2016). Degradable controlled-release polymers and polymeric nanoparticles: Mechanisms of controlling drug release. *Chemical Reviews*, *116*(4), 2602–2663. doi:10.1021/acs.chemrev.5b00346 PMID:26854975

Kasagana, V., Karumuri, S. S., & Margesan, M. T. (2011). Recent advances in smart drug delivery systems. *Int J Nov Drug Deliv Tech*, *1*(3), 201–207.

Kerc, J., & Srcic, S. (1995). Thermal analysis of glassy pharmaceuticals. *Thermochimica Acta, 248*, 81–95. doi:10.1016/0040-6031(94)01949-H

Khalid, M., & El-Sawy, H. S. (2017). Polymeric nanoparticles: Promising platform for drug delivery. International journal of pharmaceutics, 528(1-2), 675-691.

Kipper, M. J., Shen, E., Determan, A., & Narasimhan, B. (2002). Design of an injectable system based on bioerodible polyanhydride microspheres for sustained drug delivery. *Biomaterials*, *23*(22), 4405–4412. doi:10.1016/S0142-9612(02)00181-3 PMID:12219831

Kobayashi, H., Watanabe, R., & Choyke, P. L. (2014). Improving conventional enhanced permeability and retention (EPR) effects; what is the appropriate target? *Theranostics*, *4*(1), 81–89. doi:10.7150/thno.7193 PMID:24396516

Konan, Y. N., Gurny, R., & Allémann, E. (2002). Preparation and characterization of sterile and freeze-dried sub-200 nm nanoparticles. *International Journal of Pharmaceutics*, *233*(1-2), 239–252. doi:10.1016/S0378-5173(01)00944-9 PMID:11897428

Kumar, M. R. (Ed.). (2008). *Handbook of particulate drug delivery*. American Scientific Publishers.

Kwon, H. Y., Lee, J. Y., Choi, S. W., Jang, Y., & Kim, J. H. (2001). Preparation of PLGA nanoparticles containing estrogen by emulsification–diffusion method. *Colloids and Surfaces. A, Physicochemical and Engineering Aspects*, *182*(1-3), 123–130. doi:10.1016/S0927-7757(00)00825-6

Kwon, H. Y., Lee, J. Y., Choi, S. W., Jang, Y., & Kim, J. H. (2001). Preparation of PLGA nanoparticles containing estrogen by emulsification–diffusion method. *Colloids and Surfaces. A, Physicochemical and Engineering Aspects*, *182*(1-3), 123–130. doi:10.1016/S0927-7757(00)00825-6

Lammers, T., & Ferrari, M. (2020). The success of nanomedicine. *Nano Today*, *31*, 100853. doi:10.1016/j.nantod.2020.100853 PMID:34707725

Lee, S. H., Kim, B. S., Kim, S. H., Choi, S. W., Jeong, S. I., Kwon, I. K., Kang, S. W., Nikolovski, J., Mooney, D. J., Han, Y.-K., & Kim, Y. H. (2003). Elastic biodegradable poly (glycolide-co-caprolactone) scaffold for tissue engineering. *Journal of Biomedical Materials Research. Part A*, *66*(1), 29–37. doi:10.1002/jbm.a.10497 PMID:12833428

Lemarchand, C., Gref, R., Passirani, C., Garcion, E., Petri, B., Müller, R., Costantini, D., & Couvreur, P. (2006). Influence of polysaccharide coating on the interactions of nanoparticles with biological systems. *Biomaterials*, *27*(1), 108–118. doi:10.1016/j.biomaterials.2005.04.041 PMID:16118015

Leo, E., Brina, B., Forni, F., & Vandelli, M. A. (2004). In vitro evaluation of PLA nanoparticles containing a lipophilic drug in water-soluble or insoluble form. *International Journal of Pharmaceutics*, *278*(1), 133–141. doi:10.1016/j.ijpharm.2004.03.002 PMID:15158956

Leroux, J. C., Allemann, E., Doelker, E., & Gurny, R. (1995). New approach for the preparation of nanoparticles by an emulsification-diffusion method. *European Journal of Pharmaceutics and Biopharmaceutics*, *41*(1), 14–18.

Lin, P. C., Lin, S., Wang, P. C., & Sridhar, R. (2014). Techniques for physicochemical characterization of nanomaterials. *Biotechnology advances, 32*(4), 711-726.99.

Lu, C., & Urban, M. W. (2018). Stimuli-responsive polymer nano-science: Shape anisotropy, responsiveness, applications. *Progress in Polymer Science*, *78*, 24–46. doi:10.1016/j.progpolymsci.2017.07.005

Lu, M., Yang, X., Yang, Y., Qin, P., Wu, X., & Cai, Z. (2017). Nanomaterials as assisted matrix of laser desorption/ionization time-of-flight mass spectrometry for the analysis of small molecules. *Nanomaterials (Basel, Switzerland)*, *7*(4), 87. doi:10.3390/nano7040087 PMID:28430138

Lungwitz, U., Breunig, M., Blunk, T., & Göpferich, A. (2005). Polyethylenimine-based non-viral gene delivery systems. *European Journal of Pharmaceutics and Biopharmaceutics*, *60*(2), 247–266. doi:10.1016/j.ejpb.2004.11.011 PMID:15939236

Mallakpour, S., & Behranvand, V. (2016). Polymeric nanoparticles: Recent development in synthesis and application. *Express Polymer Letters*, *10*(11), 895–913. doi:10.3144/expresspolymlett.2016.84

Malviya, N., Malviya, S., Saxena, R., Chauhan, V., & Dhere, M. (2022). Smart Biodegradable Polymeric Nanoparticles: Synthesis, Characterization, and Applications. In Advancements in Controlled Drug Delivery Systems (pp. 257-280). IGI Global.

Markowicz-Piasecka, M., Sikora, J., Szymański, P., Kozak, O., Studniarek, M., & Mikiciuk-Olasik, E. (2015). PAMAM dendrimers as potential carriers of gadolinium complexes of iminodiacetic acid derivatives for magnetic resonance imaging. *Journal of Nanomaterials*, *2015*, 2015. doi:10.1155/2015/394827

Mason, T. G., Wilking, J. N., Meleson, K., Chang, C. B., & Graves, S. M. (2006). Nanoemulsions: Formation, structure, and physical properties. *Journal of Physics Condensed Matter*, *18*(41), R635–R666. doi:10.1088/0953-8984/18/41/R01

Mathurin, J., Pancani, E., Deniset-Besseau, A., Kjoller, K., Prater, C. B., Gref, R., & Dazzi, A. (2018). How to unravel the chemical structure and component localization of individual drug-loaded polymeric nanoparticles by using tapping AFM-IR. *Analyst*, *143*(24), 5940–5949. doi:10.1039/C8AN01239C PMID:30345433

Moinard-Chécot, D., Chevalier, Y., Briançon, S., Beney, L., & Fessi, H. (2008). Mechanism of nanocapsules formation by the emulsion–diffusion process. *Journal of Colloid and Interface Science*, *317*(2), 458–468. doi:10.1016/j.jcis.2007.09.081 PMID:17936772

Mourdikoudis, S., Pallares, R. M., & Thanh, N. T. (2018). Characterization techniques for nanoparticles: Comparison and complementarity upon studying nanoparticle properties. *Nanoscale*, *10*(27), 12871–12934. doi:10.1039/C8NR02278J PMID:29926865

Mura, S., Nicolas, J., & Couvreur, P. (2013). Stimuli-responsive nanocarriers for drug delivery. *Nature Materials*, *12*(11), 991–1003. doi:10.1038/nmat3776 PMID:24150417

Nafee, N., Schneider, M., Schaefer, U. F., & Lehr, C. M. (2009). Relevance of the colloidal stability of chitosan/PLGA nanoparticles on their cytotoxicity profile. *International Journal of Pharmaceutics*, *381*(2), 130–139. doi:10.1016/j.ijpharm.2009.04.049 PMID:19450671

Niwa, T., Takeuchi, H., Hino, T., Kunou, N., & Kawashima, Y. (1993). Preparations of biodegradable nanospheres of water-soluble and insoluble drugs with D, L-lactide/glycolide copolymer by a novel spontaneous emulsification solvent diffusion method, and the drug release behavior. *Journal of Controlled Release*, *25*(1-2), 89–98. doi:10.1016/0168-3659(93)90097-O

Othman, N., Masarudin, M. J., Kuen, C. Y., Dasuan, N. A., Abdullah, L. C., & Md. Jamil, S. N. A. (2018). Synthesis and optimization of chitosan nanoparticles loaded with L-ascorbic acid and thymoquinone. *Nanomaterials (Basel, Switzerland)*, *8*(11), 920. doi:10.3390/nano8110920 PMID:30405074

Otsuka, H., Nagasaki, Y., & Kataoka, K. (2003). PEGylated nanoparticles for biological and pharmaceutical applications. *Advanced Drug Delivery Reviews*, *55*(3), 403–419. doi:10.1016/S0169-409X(02)00226-0 PMID:12628324

Palanikumar, L., Al-Hosani, S., Kalmouni, M., Nguyen, V. P., Ali, L., Pasricha, R., Barrera, F. N., & Magzoub, M. (2020). pH-responsive high stability polymeric nanoparticles for targeted delivery of anticancer therapeutics. *Communications Biology*, *3*(1), 1–17. doi:10.103842003-020-0817-4 PMID:32127636

Panyam, J., & Labhasetwar, V. (2003). Biodegradable nanoparticles for drug and gene delivery to cells and tissue. *Advanced Drug Delivery Reviews*, *55*(3), 329–347. doi:10.1016/S0169-409X(02)00228-4 PMID:12628320

Patel, M. P., Patel, R. R., & Patel, J. K. (2010). Chitosan mediated targeted drug delivery system: A review. *Journal of Pharmacy & Pharmaceutical Sciences*, *13*(4), 536–557. doi:10.18433/J3JC7C PMID:21486530

Petersen, L. K., Sackett, C. K., & Narasimhan, B. (2010). High-throughput analysis of protein stability in polyanhydride nanoparticles. *Acta Biomaterialia*, *6*(10), 3873–3881. doi:10.1016/j.actbio.2010.04.004 PMID:20388561

Pierobon, M., & Akyildiz, I. F. (2012). Capacity of a diffusion-based molecular communication system with channel memory and molecular noise. *IEEE Transactions on Information Theory*, *59*(2), 942–954. doi:10.1109/TIT.2012.2219496

Pillai, C. K. S., & Sharma, C. P. (2010). Absorbable polymeric surgical sutures: Chemistry, production, properties, biodegradability, and performance. *Journal of Biomaterials Applications*, *25*(4), 291–366. doi:10.1177/0885328210384890 PMID:20971780

Quintanar-Guerrero, D., Allémann, E., Doelker, E., & Fessi, H. (1997). A mechanistic study of the formation of polymer nanoparticles by the emulsification-diffusion technique. *Colloid & Polymer Science*, *275*(7), 640–647. doi:10.1007003960050130

Radovic-Moreno, A. F., Lu, T. K., Puscasu, V. A., Yoon, C. J., Langer, R., & Farokhzad, O. C. (2012). Surface charge-switching polymeric nanoparticles for bacterial cell wall-targeted delivery of antibiotics. *ACS Nano*, *6*(5), 4279–4287. doi:10.1021/nn3008383 PMID:22471841

Rao, J. P., & Geckeler, K. E. (2011). Polymer nanoparticles: Preparation techniques and size-control parameters. *Progress in Polymer Science*, *36*(7), 887–913. doi:10.1016/j.progpolymsci.2011.01.001

Raula, J., Eerikäinen, H., Lähde, A., & Kauppinen, E. I. (2007). Aerosol flow reactor method for the synthesis of multicomponent drug nano-and microparticles. In *Nanoparticulate Drug Delivery Systems* (pp. 111–128). CRC Press.

Redhead, H. M., Davis, S. S., & Illum, L. (2001). Drug delivery in poly (lactide-co-glycolide) nanoparticles surface modified with poloxamer 407 and poloxamine 908: In vitro characterisation and in vivo evaluation. *Journal of Controlled Release*, *70*(3), 353–363. doi:10.1016/S0168-3659(00)00367-9 PMID:11182205

Reis, C. P., Neufeld, R. J., Ribeiro, A. J., & Veiga, F. (2006). Nanoencapsulation II. Biomedical applications and current status of peptide and protein nanoparticulate delivery systems. *Nanomedicine; Nanotechnology, Biology, and Medicine*, *2*(2), 53–65. doi:10.1016/j.nano.2006.04.009 PMID:17292116

Saini, R. K., Bagri, L. P., Bajpai, A. K., & Mishra, A. (2018). Responsive polymer nanoparticles for drug delivery applications. In *Stimuli Responsive Polymeric Nanocarriers for Drug Delivery Applications* (Vol. 1, pp. 289–320). Woodhead Publishing. doi:10.1016/B978-0-08-101997-9.00015-1

Sanchez-Gaytan, B. L., Fay, F., Lobatto, M. E., Tang, J., Ouimet, M., Kim, Y., van der Staay, S. E. M., van Rijs, S. M., Priem, B., Zhang, L., Fisher, E. A., Moore, K. J., Langer, R., Fayad, Z. A., & Mulder, W. J. (2015). HDL-mimetic PLGA nanoparticle to target atherosclerosis plaque macrophages. *Bioconjugate Chemistry*, *26*(3), 443–451. doi:10.1021/bc500517k PMID:25650634

Seib, F. P., Jones, G. T., Rnjak-Kovacina, J., Lin, Y., & Kaplan, D. L. (2013). pH-dependent anticancer drug release from silk nanoparticles. *Advanced Healthcare Materials*, *2*(12), 1606–1611. doi:10.1002/adhm.201300034 PMID:23625825

Shelma, R. (2022). Polymeric Nanoparticles for Drug Delivery. In *A Holistic and Integrated Approach to Lifestyle Diseases* (pp. 319–332). Apple Academic Press.

Singh, B. N., & Kim, K. H. (2000). Floating drug delivery systems: An approach to oral controlled drug delivery via gastric retention. *Journal of Controlled Release*, *63*(3), 235–259. doi:10.1016/S0168-3659(99)00204-7 PMID:10601721

Siqueira, G., Bras, J., & Dufresne, A. (2010). Cellulosic bionanocomposites: A review of preparation, properties and applications. *Polymers*, *2*(4), 728–765. doi:10.3390/polym2040728

Song, K. C., Lee, H. S., Choung, I. Y., Cho, K. I., Ahn, Y., & Choi, E. J. (2006). The effect of type of organic phase solvents on the particle size of poly (d, l-lactide-co-glycolide) nanoparticles. *Colloids and Surfaces. A, Physicochemical and Engineering Aspects*, *276*(1-3), 162–167. doi:10.1016/j.colsurfa.2005.10.064

Song, X., Zhao, Y., Wu, W., Bi, Y., Cai, Z., Chen, Q., Li, Y., & Hou, S. (2008). PLGA nanoparticles simultaneously loaded with vincristine sulfate and verapamil hydrochloride: Systematic study of particle size and drug entrapment efficiency. *International Journal of Pharmaceutics*, *350*(1-2), 320–329. doi:10.1016/j.ijpharm.2007.08.034 PMID:17913411

Soppimath, K. S., Aminabhavi, T. M., Kulkarni, A. R., & Rudzinski, W. E. (2001). Biodegradable polymeric nanoparticles as drug delivery devices. *Journal of Controlled Release*, *70*(1-2), 1–20. doi:10.1016/S0168-3659(00)00339-4 PMID:11166403

Spirescu, V. A., Chircov, C., Grumezescu, A. M., & Andronescu, E. (2021). Polymeric nanoparticles for antimicrobial therapies: An up-to-date overview. *Polymers*, *13*(5), 724. doi:10.3390/polym13050724 PMID:33673451

Sternling, C. A., & Scriven, L. E. (1959). Interfacial turbulence: Hydrodynamic instability and the Marangoni effect. *AIChE Journal. American Institute of Chemical Engineers*, *5*(4), 514–523. doi:10.1002/aic.690050421

Su, Y., Xie, Z., Kim, G. B., Dong, C., & Yang, J. (2015). Design strategies and applications of circulating cell-mediated drug delivery systems. *ACS Biomaterials Science & Engineering*, *1*(4), 201–217. doi:10.1021/ab500179h PMID:25984572

Subramaniam, B., Rajewski, R. A., & Snavely, K. (1997). Pharmaceutical processing with supercritical carbon dioxide. *Journal of Pharmaceutical Sciences*, *86*(8), 885–890. doi:10.1021/js9700661 PMID:9269864

Tang, G. P., Zeng, J. M., Gao, S. J., Ma, Y. X., Shi, L., Li, Y., Too, H.-P., & Wang, S. (2003). Polyethylene glycol modified polyethylenimine for improved CNS gene transfer: Effects of PEGylation extent. *Biomaterials*, *24*(13), 2351–2362. doi:10.1016/S0142-9612(03)00029-2 PMID:12699673

Tantra, R., Schulze, P., & Quincey, P. (2010). Effect of nanoparticle concentration on zeta-potential measurement results and reproducibility. *Particuology*, *8*(3), 279–285. doi:10.1016/j.partic.2010.01.003

Trimaille, T., Pichot, C., Elaissari, A., Fessi, H., Briançon, S., & Delair, T. (2003). Poly (D, L-lactic acid) nanoparticle preparation and colloidal characterization. *Colloid & Polymer Science*, *281*(12), 1184–1190. doi:10.100700396-003-0894-1

Turos, E., Reddy, G. S. K., Greenhalgh, K., Ramaraju, P., Abeylath, S. C., Jang, S., Dickey, S., & Lim, D. V. (2007). Penicillin-bound polyacrylate nanoparticles: Restoring the activity of β-lactam antibiotics against MRSA. *Bioorganic & Medicinal Chemistry Letters*, *17*(12), 3468–3472. doi:10.1016/j.bmcl.2007.03.077 PMID:17420125

Ulery, B. D., Nair, L. S., & Laurencin, C. T. (2011). Biomedical applications of biodegradable polymers. *Journal of Polymer Science. Part B, Polymer Physics*, *49*(12), 832–864. doi:10.1002/polb.22259 PMID:21769165

Vargas-Molinero, H. Y., Serrano-Medina, A., Palomino-Vizcaino, K., López-Maldonado, E. A., Villarreal-Gómez, L. J., Pérez-González, G. L., & Cornejo-Bravo, J. M. (2023). Hybrid Systems of Nanofibers and Polymeric Nanoparticles for Biological Application and Delivery Systems. *Micromachines*, *14*(1), 208. doi:10.3390/mi14010208 PMID:36677269

Ventura, J. A. (2015). Design and Synthesis of Polymeric Nanoparticles for Drug and Protein Delivery.

Vyas, S. P., & Khar, R. K. (2004). *Targeted & controlled drug delivery: novel carrier systems*. CBS publishers & distributors.

Wang, X., Fan, Y., Yan, J., & Yang, M. (2022). Engineering polyphenol-based polymeric nanoparticles for drug delivery and bioimaging. *Chemical Engineering Journal*, *439*, 135661. doi:10.1016/j.cej.2022.135661

Wong, K. H., Lu, A., Chen, X., & Yang, Z. (2020). Natural ingredient-based polymeric nanoparticles for cancer treatment. *Molecules (Basel, Switzerland)*, *25*(16), 3620. doi:10.3390/molecules25163620 PMID:32784890

Xie, H., & Smith, J. W. (2010). Fabrication of PLGA nanoparticles with a fluidic nanoprecipitation system. *Journal of Nanobiotechnology*, *8*(1), 1–7. doi:10.1186/1477-3155-8-18 PMID:20707919

Yang, H. W., Hua, M. Y., Liu, H. L., Huang, C. Y., Tsai, R. Y., Lu, Y. J., Chen, J.-Y., Tang, H.-J., Hsien, H.-Y., Chang, Y.-S., Yen, T.-C., Chen, P.-Y., & Wei, K. C. (2011). Self-protecting core-shell magnetic nanoparticles for targeted, traceable, long half-life delivery of BCNU to gliomas. *Biomaterials*, *32*(27), 6523–6532. doi:10.1016/j.biomaterials.2011.05.047 PMID:21645920

Yang, Y., Jiang, Y., Xu, J., & Yu, J. (2007). Conducting polymeric nanoparticles synthesized in reverse micelles and their gas sensitivity based on quartz crystal microbalance. *Polymer*, *48*(15), 4459–4465. doi:10.1016/j.polymer.2007.06.005

Yu, L. (2001). Amorphous pharmaceutical solids: Preparation, characterization and stabilization. *Advanced Drug Delivery Reviews*, *48*(1), 27–42. doi:10.1016/S0169-409X(01)00098-9 PMID:11325475

Zhang, M., Li, X. H., Gong, Y. D., Zhao, N. M., & Zhang, X. F. (2002). Properties and biocompatibility of chitosan films modified by blending with PEG. *Biomaterials*, *23*(13), 2641–2648. doi:10.1016/S0142-9612(01)00403-3 PMID:12059013

Zhao, L., Xiao, C., Ding, J., He, P., Tang, Z., Pang, X., Zhuang, X., & Chen, X. (2013). Facile one-pot synthesis of glucose-sensitive nanogel via thiol-ene click chemistry for self-regulated drug delivery. *Acta Biomaterialia*, *9*(5), 6535–6543. doi:10.1016/j.actbio.2013.01.040 PMID:23403168

Zhou, G., Lu, Y., Zhang, H., Chen, Y., Yu, Y., Gao, J., & Zhong, Y. (2013). A novel pulsed drug-delivery system: Polyelectrolyte layer-by-layer coating of chitosan–alginate microgels. *International Journal of Nanomedicine*, *8*, 877. PMID:23486565

Zhu, X., Radovic-Moreno, A. F., Wu, J., Langer, R., & Shi, J. (2014). Nanomedicine in the management of microbial infection–overview and perspectives. *Nano Today*, *9*(4), 478–498. doi:10.1016/j.nantod.2014.06.003 PMID:25267927

Zielińska, A., Carreiró, F., Oliveira, A. M., Neves, A., Pires, B., Venkatesh, D. N., Durazzo, A., Lucarini, M., Eder, P., Silva, A. M., Santini, A., & Souto, E. B. (2020). Polymeric nanoparticles: Production, characterization, toxicology and ecotoxicology. *Molecules (Basel, Switzerland)*, *25*(16), 3731. doi:10.3390/molecules25163731 PMID:32824172

Zielińska, A., Ferreira, N. R., Durazzo, A., Lucarini, M., Cicero, N., Mamouni, S. E., Silva, A. M., Nowak, I., Santini, A., & Souto, E. B. (2019). Development and optimization of alpha-pinene-loaded solid lipid nanoparticles (SLN) using experimental factorial design and dispersion analysis. *Molecules (Basel, Switzerland)*, *24*(15), 2683. doi:10.3390/molecules24152683 PMID:31344802

Zweers, M. L., Grijpma, D. W., Engbers, G. H., & Feijen, J. (2003). The preparation of monodisperse biodegradable polyester nanoparticles with a controlled size. *Journal of Biomedical Materials Research. Part B, Applied Biomaterials*, *66*(2), 559–566. doi:10.1002/jbm.b.10046 PMID:12861608

Chapter 6
Targeted Nanotherapies for Diabetic Complications

Pranav Kumar Prabhakar
https://orcid.org/0000-0001-8130-1822
Lovely Professional University, India

ABSTRACT

Diabetes mellitus is a chronic metabolic disorder characterized by impaired glucose regulation, which leads to various complications affecting multiple organs and systems. This chapter discusses various types of nanomaterials, such as liposomes, polymeric nanoparticles, dendrimers, and carbon-based nanomaterials, and their potential for encapsulating and delivering therapeutic agents to specific sites affected by diabetic complications. The advantages of nanomaterial-based drug delivery, including enhanced drug stability, prolonged circulation time, and improved targeting efficiency, are highlighted. The challenges and considerations associated with targeted nanotherapy development, including biocompatibility, toxicity, and regulatory aspects, are also discussed. The chapter serves as a valuable resource for researchers, clinicians, and healthcare professionals involved in the development and translation of targeted nano therapies, ultimately contributing to the advancement of diabetic complication management.

INTRODUCTION

Overview of Diabetes Mellitus

Diabetes mellitus is a chronic metabolic disorder characterized by high blood glucose levels, known as hyperglycemia. It occurs when the body is unable to properly regulate insulin, a hormone produced by the pancreas that helps control blood sugar levels. Insulin allows glucose to enter cells, where it is used as a source of energy. There are three main types of diabetes mellitus: type 1, type 2, and gestational diabetes (Prabhakar et al., 2019).

i. **Type 1 Diabetes:** Type 1 diabetes, also known as insulin-dependent diabetes or juvenile-onset diabetes, is an autoimmune condition where the immune system mistakenly attacks and destroys

DOI: 10.4018/979-8-3693-0448-8.ch006

the insulin-producing beta cells in the pancreas. As a result, the pancreas is unable to produce insulin, leading to a complete deficiency. People with type 1 diabetes require lifelong insulin therapy through injections or insulin pump to regulate their blood sugar levels (Nankar et al., 2017).

ii. **Type 2 Diabetes:** Type 2 diabetes, also referred to as non-insulin dependent diabetes or adult-onset diabetes, is the most common form of diabetes, accounting for approximately 90-95% of all cases. It occurs when the body becomes resistant to the effects of insulin or when the pancreas fails to produce enough insulin to meet the body's needs. Type 2 diabetes is strongly associated with lifestyle factors such as obesity, sedentary lifestyle, poor diet, and genetics. Initially, it can often be managed through lifestyle modifications, such as healthy eating, regular physical activity, and weight loss (Prabhakar et al., 2016). However, over time, medication or insulin therapy may be required to manage blood sugar levels effectively.

iii. **Gestational Diabetes:** Gestational diabetes develops during pregnancy and affects approximately 2-10% of pregnant women. It occurs when hormonal changes during pregnancy lead to insulin resistance, resulting in elevated blood sugar levels. While gestational diabetes usually resolves after childbirth, it increases the risk of developing type 2 diabetes later in life for both the mother and the child. Pregnant women with gestational diabetes require careful monitoring of their blood sugar levels and may need dietary changes, physical activity, and in some cases, medication or insulin therapy (Prabhakar et al., 2016).

Diabetic Complications

In recent times, as people's living standards and quality of life have steadily improved, there have been significant shifts in people's eating habits and daily routines. These changes have contributed to a notable rise in the prevalence of diabetes. The global incidence of diabetes has been consistently increasing over the past years, with a worldwide prevalence rate of 9.3% in 2019 (Prabhakar et al., 2016). Diabetes is a metabolic disorder characterized by persistent and chronic high blood sugar levels resulting from various factors. Once developed, the disease is challenging to completely cure. Numerous clinical studies have demonstrated that prolonged elevated blood sugar levels can lead to the emergence of several concurrent ailments. Diabetes exerts substantial stress on vital organs such as the heart, brain, liver, and kidneys, resulting in organ damage (Prabhakar et al., 2016). The subsequent complications that arise are also profoundly severe, potentially impacting the overall quality of life for patients.

Poorly controlled diabetes over a prolonged period can lead to various complications that affect multiple organ systems in the body. These complications include:

a) **Diabetic Cardiovascular Disease (DCM):** Diabetes significantly increases the risk of developing cardiovascular diseases such as coronary artery disease, heart attack, stroke, and peripheral arterial disease. High blood sugar levels can damage the blood vessels, leading to atherosclerosis (hardening and narrowing of the arteries) and an increased risk of cardiovascular events (Prabhakar, 2016).

Some studies suggest that oxidative stress-induced damage to myocardial cells caused by diabetes plays a pivotal role in triggering various complications, including DCM, ultimately leading to impairments in myocardial contractility and relaxation (Liu et al., 2014). DCM commonly manifests with myocardial fibrosis and apoptosis, key pathological traits contributing to subsequent cardiac functional deterioration (Cao et al., 2023). Another critical facet of DCM is microvascular disease. Diabetes-related microvascular changes in the heart are closely tied to the decline in left ventricular function (Jia et al., 2018). In the realm of nanotechnology applied to DCM, poly(lactic-co-glycolic acid) (PLGA)-based nanoparticles loaded with pexelizumab (PSS) were formulated, employing a modified double emulsion solvent evaporation method. Yu et al. investigated the effects of PSS-loaded nanoparticles on vascular endothelial function in DCM-afflicted rats. The outcomes demonstrated that these nanoparticles significantly enhanced ventricular wall movement and cardiac systolic and diastolic functions in DCM rats. They exhibited the capacity to modulate the ultrastructure of myocardial microvascular endothelial cells within DCM rat hearts, thereby decelerating the progression of vascular endothelial dysfunction. Notably, there was a significant increase in the concentrations of nitric oxide synthase (eNOS) and vascular endothelial growth factor A (VEGFA) in the serum, contributing to the mitigation of vascular endothelial injury in DCM rats (Jia et al., 2018). Furthermore, investigations delved into the therapeutic potential of acidic fibroblast growth factor-1 (FGFl) nanoliposomes combined with ultrasound-targeted microbubble disruption (UTMD) for DCM. The impact of this combination was assessed through cardiac function measurements. Results exhibited that left ventricular systolic pressure (LVESP), left ventricular end-diastolic pressure (LVEDP), and the maximum rate of left ventricular development pressure (LV ± DP/dtmax) were markedly improved in the FGFl-combined treatment group, surpassing other treatment groups and the DCM group. This highlights the potential of FGFl to ameliorate both systolic and diastolic functions in DCM rats. Further assessments of collagen volume fraction (CVF) and the apoptotic index of cardiomyocytes reinforced these findings, revealing significantly lower CVF and apoptosis rates in the FGFl-combined treatment group compared to other groups. It suggests that the DCM combined with fluorescence light microscopy (FLM) can enhance cardiac function in rats. Intriguingly, the microvessel density (MVD) of rats in the FGFl-combined treatment group was notably higher than that in the DCM group and other treatment groups, suggesting that this combined approach has the potential to alleviate myocardial microvascular abnormalities in DCM rats, potentially enhancing myocardial blood flow and reducing oxidative stress injury. Consequently, the combination of FGFl nanoliposomes and UTMD offers promise in ameliorating both pathological and functional alterations triggered by diabetes (Xiong et al., 2021). It's apparent that nanotechnology has demonstrated promise in animal studies targeting DCM treatment. Nonetheless, it's essential to ponder whether these interventions will translate into efficacious clinical outcomes as in animal experiments, and to consider the biocompatibility, biodegradability, and controlled drug release properties of the aforementioned nanodrugs.

b) **Diabetic Retinopathy (DR):** Diabetic retinopathy is a complication that affects the eyes and is a leading cause of blindness in adults. It occurs due to damage to the blood vessels in the retina, the light-sensitive tissue at the back of the eye. Persistent high blood sugar levels can cause the blood vessels to leak or become blocked, leading to vision problems and potential vision loss if left untreated (Prabhakar, 2016).

With the rising number of individuals afflicted by diabetes, diabetic retinopathy has emerged as the leading cause of blindness among those aged 16 to 64 (Prabhakar, 2016). The factors contributing to the development of DR are intricate and encompass hypertension, genetic predisposition, and the duration of diabetes. Pathological transformations commonly involve damage to retinal capillary endothelial cells, thickening of the basement membrane, microvascular blockages, and impairment of the blood-retinal barrier function, leading to retinal swelling and the emergence of new blood vessels (Mrugacz et al., 2021). Nanotechnology has gained substantial traction in DR treatment, marking a new chapter and practical applications in clinical settings. Researchers have engineered silicate (SI) nanoparticles, assessing their capacity to counteract retinal neovascularization. Microscopic examination affirmed the benign impact of silicon nanoparticles on retinal tissue, alongside their capability to hinder retinal neovascularization formation. Consequently, silicon nanoparticles show promise in effectively managing neovascularization driven by vascular endothelial growth factor (Veith et al., 2019). Another study by Kim and colleagues focused on gold nanoparticles, demonstrating their potential to suppress retinal neovascularization. Their findings underscored the capacity of gold nanoparticles to effectively impede the proliferation and migration of retinal microvascular endothelial cells, as well as the formation of capillary-like networks induced by vascular endothelial growth factor. Importantly, these gold nanoparticles exhibited no adverse influence on the activity of microvascular endothelial cells and posed no retinal toxicity concerns (Mandal et al., 2023). In a separate line of investigation, Jo et al. explored the application of titanium dioxide (TiO2) nanoparticles, which exhibited noteworthy in vitro anti-angiogenic effects without inducing retinal toxicity. Intravitreal injection of these particles also demonstrated neovascularization inhibition. This study lends support to the potential utilization of TiO2 nanoparticles in treating retinopathy in mouse models at specific concentrations (Mandal et al., 2023). Gurunathan and colleagues conducted a study highlighting silver nanoparticles as capable of thwarting VEGF-induced angiogenesis in mice (Mandal et al., 2023).

c) **Diabetic Nephropathy (DN):** Diabetic nephropathy refers to kidney damage caused by diabetes. Over time, high blood sugar levels can damage the small blood vessels in the kidneys, impairing their ability to filter waste products and excess fluids from the blood. This can result in chronic kidney disease and, in severe cases, end-stage renal disease requiring dialysis or kidney transplantation (Dable, 2010).

Currently, there is a lack of effective methods to prevent or halt the progression of DN, resulting in unsatisfactory outcomes in its prevention and treatment. In recent times, the integration of nanotechnology into DN treatment has emerged, holding potential to enhance drug effectiveness and prognosis for diabetic patients, consequently alleviating patient suffering and financial burden. The underlying causes of DN are intricate and encompass genetic factors mutation, disrupted glucose metabolism leading to the activation of multiple endocrine pathways, heightened production of endothelial nitric oxide synthase and advanced glycation end products (AGEs), and inhibited nitric oxide formation. Contributing factors also include insulin resistance, inflammatory responses, and alterations in renal hemodynamics, all culminating in the development of DN (Imig and Ryan, 2013). Research indicates that advanced glycation end products (RAGE) and their interactions with various binding ligands play a pivotal role in DN (Imig and Ryan, 2013). Poly(lactic-co-glycolic acid) (PLGA), a synthetic polymer material, has been employed in novel ways. Yang devised and refined a nanoscale formulation of crocin (CT-PLGA-NP), a therapeutic agent for streptozotocin (STZ)-induced diabetic nephropathy. Experimental results revealed that CT-PLGA-NPs accumulated in the kidneys and livers of diabetic rats, providing anti-inflammatory and antifibrotic effects. The administration of CT-PLGA-NPs notably reduced the production and expression of renal fibrosis markers (TGF-β1 and fibronectin) as well as inflammatory cytokines like MCP-1 and TNF-α, concurrently diminishing the activation of NF-κB expression and PKC activity. It can be deduced from existing research that CT-PLGA-NPs exert their effects through antifibrotic and anti-inflammatory mechanisms, thus ameliorating diabetic nephropathy (Karthikeyan et al., 2020). Ahangarpour et al. assessed the impact of myricetin solid lipid nanoparticles (SLN) on streptozotocin-nicotinamide (STZ-

NA)-induced diabetic nephropathy in mice. The administration of myricetin and its SLN counterpart ameliorated diabetic nephropathy-related changes by curbing oxidative stress and elevating antioxidant enzyme levels, with the SLN formulation demonstrating more pronounced effects (Ahangarpour et al., 2019). Additionally, nanoliposomes containing Eprosartan mesylate were formulated by Ahad et al. and tested in Wistar rats with STZ-induced diabetic nephropathy. Substantial reductions in serum creatinine, urea, lactate dehydrogenase, total albumin, and malondialdehyde levels were observed, signifying the renal protective potential of Eprosartan mesylate-loaded nanoliposomes.

d) **Diabetic Peripheral Neuropathy (DNP):** Diabetic peripheral neuropathy is a condition characterized by nerve damage caused by high blood sugar levels. It can affect various types of nerves, including those involved in sensation, movement, and organ function. Symptoms may include numbness, tingling, pain, or weakness, typically starting in the feet and gradually progressing to other areas of the body. Diabetic neuropathy can also affect the nerves that control the digestive system, leading to problems such as gastroparesis (delayed stomach emptying), constipation, and diarrhea. Additionally, it can affect the nerves responsible for sexual function, causing sexual dysfunction in both men and women. Statistical data highlight that, for a significant number of diabetic patients, DNP frequently coincides with other complications. Ongoing clinical inquiries underscore a multitude of factors contributing to DNP, encompassing microvascular damage, disrupted glucose metabolism, compromised immunity, deficiencies in vitamins and nerve growth factors, as well as the Schwann cell hypothesis. Within the dorsal root ganglion (DRG), satellite glial cells (SGCs) envelop neuronal bodies, and it's observed that SGCs express the purinergic 2 (P2) Y12 receptor. Activation of SGCs emerges as a pivotal player in the progression of DNP. Curcumin, known for its anti-inflammatory and antioxidant properties, is harnessed for its therapeutic potential. Given curcumin's suboptimal metabolic stability and limited bioavailability in vivo, efforts have turned toward encapsulated curcumin nanoparticles to enhance its targeting precision and overall bioavailability. Researchers have delved into this avenue, discovering that nanoparticle-coated curcumin can effectively attenuate the elevation of P2Y12 receptor on SGCs within the DRG, subsequently mitigating mechanical and thermal hyperalgesia in diabetic rats (Parsamanesh et al., 2018). Similarly, the impact of nanocurcumin on sensorimotor polyneuropathy (DSPN) severity in type 2 diabetes mellitus (T2DM) patients has been investigated. The findings indicate that short-term supplementation with nanocurcumin can ameliorate and diminish DSPN severity in T2DM patients. Notably, serum fasting blood sugar (FBS) and HbA1c levels exhibited significant reductions, revealing an avenue to enhance DSPN through glycemic control in T2DM patients (Parsamanesh et al., 2018). Furthermore, nano-mir-146a-5p has shown promise in enhancing nerve conduction velocity and alleviating morphological damage and demyelination in the sciatic nerve of DPN rats. This nanoparticle-based treatment also curbed the expression of inflammatory cytokines, caspase-3, and cleaved caspase-3 in the sciatic nerve. In addition, nano-mir-146a-5p fostered the expression of myelin basic protein, implying a protective role in peripheral nerves within the DPN rat model. This protection potentially stems from the regulation of inflammatory responses and apoptosis (Parsamanesh et al., 2018).

e) **Impaired Wound Healing:** Diabetes can impair the body's ability to heal wounds properly. Elevated blood sugar levels can affect blood flow and damage the small blood vessels that supply oxygen and nutrients to the tissues. This can result in delayed wound healing, making individuals with diabetes more prone to infections, ulcers, and complications such as gangrene, which may require amputation in severe cases (Dubey et al., 2022).

f) **Other Complications:** Diabetes can also increase the risk of other complications, including:
   i. **Skin complications:** Diabetes can cause skin problems such as dry skin, itching, bacterial and fungal infections, and diabetic dermopathy (skin discoloration and patches).
   ii. **Oral health issues:** People with diabetes are more susceptible to gum diseases, oral infections, and tooth loss.
   iii. **Mental health disorders:** Diabetes is associated with an increased risk of mental health conditions like depression and anxiety.
   iv. **Pregnancy complications:** Uncontrolled diabetes during pregnancy can lead to complications for both the mother and the baby, including preeclampsia, premature birth, and increased risk of birth defects.
   v. **Increased susceptibility to infections:** High blood sugar levels weaken the immune system, making individuals with diabetes more prone to infections, including urinary tract infections, skin infections, and yeast infections.

Effective management of diabetes involves maintaining blood glucose levels within target ranges through a combination of healthy eating, regular physical activity, weight management, medication or insulin therapy as prescribed by healthcare professionals, and regular monitoring of blood sugar levels. Additionally, routine check-ups and screenings are essential to detect and manage potential complications at an early stage. By effectively managing diabetes and adopting a comprehensive approach to care, individuals with diabetes can reduce the risk of developing complications and lead a healthy, fulfilling life.

NEED FOR TARGETED THERAPIES IN DIABETIC COMPLICATIONS

The need for targeted therapies in diabetic complications arises from the limitations of conventional treatments and the complex pathophysiology of these complications. Targeted therapies offer the potential for more precise interventions, directly addressing the underlying mechanisms and specific affected sites in diabetic complications. This section discusses the rationale for targeted therapies and their potential benefits in the management of diabetic complications (Manimaran et al., 2021).

(a) **Limitations of Conventional Therapies:** Conventional therapies for diabetic complications, such as oral medications and injectable insulin, aim to control blood glucose levels and manage symptoms. However, they often have limitations in terms of their efficacy and safety profiles. For example, systemic administration of drugs may lead to off-target effects and adverse reactions in non-target tissues, reducing their therapeutic benefits. The blood-retinal and blood-brain barriers also pose challenges in delivering therapeutic agents to the eyes and the central nervous system, respectively (Manimaran et al., 2021).

(b) **Specificity and Efficacy:** Conventional therapies, such as oral medications or injectable insulin, primarily focus on controlling blood glucose levels. While important, these treatments may not effectively address the intricate molecular pathways and cellular abnormalities associated with diabetic complications. Targeted therapies, on the other hand, can be designed to selectively interact with specific molecules, receptors, or cells involved in the development and progression of complications. By precisely targeting these key factors, targeted therapies have the potential to enhance treatment efficacy and achieve more desirable outcomes (Mandal et al., 2023).

(c) **Minimization of Systemic Side Effects:** Systemic administration of drugs may result in off-target effects and adverse reactions in non-diseased tissues, leading to undesirable side effects. Targeted therapies aim to minimize such systemic effects by delivering therapeutic agents directly to the affected sites while sparing healthy tissues. This approach reduces the risk of toxicity and enhances the safety profile of the treatment, making it more favorable for long-term use (Manimaran et al., 2021).

(d) **Overcoming Physiological Barriers:** Certain diabetic complications, such as retinopathy and neuropathy, pose challenges in delivering therapeutic agents to the affected sites. The blood-retinal barrier and blood-nerve barrier limit the penetration of drugs into these areas, making it difficult to achieve therapeutic concentrations. Targeted therapies, particularly those utilizing nanomaterials or specialized delivery systems, can overcome these barriers. Nanoparticles or drug carriers can be engineered to traverse these barriers or be specifically designed to target the affected tissues, facilitating effective drug delivery to the desired sites (Manimaran et al., 2021).

(e) **Personalized Medicine:** Diabetic complications can vary among individuals due to genetic factors, underlying comorbidities, and lifestyle influences. Targeted therapies align with the concept of personalized medicine, allowing for tailored interventions based on individual patient characteristics. By considering patient-specific factors, such as genetic variations, biomarkers, or disease stage, targeted therapies can be customized to optimize treatment outcomes and improve patient care.

(f) **Targeted Therapies for Precise Intervention:** Targeted therapies offer the potential for precise intervention at the molecular and cellular levels, addressing the specific mechanisms underlying diabetic complications. By selectively delivering therapeutic agents to the affected sites, targeted therapies can enhance treatment efficacy while minimizing systemic side effects. This approach holds promise for improving patient outcomes and preventing the progression of diabetic complications.

(g) **Tailoring Treatment to Specific Complications:** Diabetic complications, such as cardiovascular disease, retinopathy, nephropathy, and neuropathy, have distinct pathophysiological processes. Targeted therapies can be designed to address the specific molecular pathways and cellular targets involved in each complication. For example, in diabetic retinopathy, targeting angiogenesis, inflammation, and oxidative stress pathways may help prevent or halt the progression of retinal damage. In diabetic nephropathy, interventions targeting renal fibrosis, inflammation, and oxidative stress can potentially slow down the decline in kidney function (Mandal et al., 2023).

(h) **Combination Therapies and Synergistic Effects:** Diabetic complications often involve complex pathophysiological processes, such as inflammation, oxidative stress, and aberrant angiogenesis. Targeted therapies can be developed to simultaneously target multiple pathways involved in these complications, offering the potential for synergistic effects and improved treatment outcomes. Combination therapies utilizing targeted approaches can address the multifactorial nature of diabetic complications, leading to enhanced therapeutic benefits (Manimaran et al., 2021).

(i) **Enhanced Site-Specific Drug Delivery:** Targeted nanotherapies offer advanced drug delivery systems that can overcome the limitations of conventional approaches. Nanomaterials, such as liposomes, polymeric nanoparticles, dendrimers, and carbon-based nanomaterials, can be engineered to encapsulate therapeutic agents and facilitate their targeted delivery to specific tissues and cells affected by diabetic complications. These nanocarriers can be surface-modified with ligands, antibodies, or receptors to improve tissue specificity and enhance cellular uptake, ensuring precise and efficient drug delivery.

Diabetic complications can vary among individuals due to genetic factors, underlying comorbidities, and lifestyle influences. Targeted therapies align with the concept of personalized medicine, allowing for tailored interventions based on individual patient characteristics. By considering patient-specific factors, such as genetic variations, biomarkers, or disease stage, targeted therapies can be customized to optimize treatment outcomes and improve patient care (Manimaran et al., 2021)

In conclusion, the development of targeted therapies is imperative for addressing the limitations of conventional treatments and improving the management of diabetic complications. By delivering therapeutic agents directly to the affected sites, targeted nanotherapies offer the potential for enhanced efficacy, reduced side effects, and personalized interventions. Further research and development in this field are crucial to harness the full potential of targeted therapies in mitigating the burden of diabetic complications (Manimaran et al., 2021).

NANOMATERIALS FOR TARGETED DRUG DELIVERY

Nanocarriers are specialized vehicles designed at the nanoscale to transport and deliver therapeutic agents, such as drugs or genes, to specific sites in the body. In the case of diabetes mellitus, nanocarriers play a crucial role in delivering antidiabetic drugs, insulin, or other therapeutic agents effectively. Here are the main types of nanocarriers used in drug delivery for diabetes:

Nanoparticles

Nanoparticles are solid colloidal particles with a size range typically between 1 and 100 nanometers. They can be made of various materials including polymers, lipids, metals, or inorganic compounds. Nanoparticles are versatile and can encapsulate both hydrophobic and hydrophilic drugs. They offer controlled release and protection of drugs against degradation, improving drug stability and bioavailability. Nanoparticles, which are tiny particles with dimensions typically in the nanometer range, have emerged as valuable tools in the field of diabetes mellitus research and treatment. Their unique properties and versatile applications make them promising for addressing various aspects of diabetes management. Here, we explore the role of nanoparticles in diabetes mellitus:

i. **Insulin Delivery:** Nanoparticles are being investigated as carriers for insulin delivery. These nanoscale carriers can encapsulate insulin molecules, protecting them from degradation in the body and allowing for controlled and sustained release. Nanoparticle-based insulin delivery systems offer the potential to replace or complement traditional insulin injections, improving patient compliance (Manimaran et al., 2021).
ii. **Oral Insulin Delivery:** A significant challenge in diabetes management is the oral delivery of insulin, as it is typically broken down by enzymes in the gastrointestinal tract. Nanoparticles can be designed to protect insulin during its journey through the digestive system, enabling its absorption in the intestines and mimicking the natural insulin release process (Mandal, et, al., 2023).

iii. **Glucose-Responsive Nanoparticles:** Smart nanoparticles are being engineered to respond to changes in blood glucose levels. These nanoparticles can release insulin or other therapeutic agents when glucose levels are elevated, providing an on-demand and closed-loop system for precise glycemic control.
iv. **Oral Drug Delivery:** Nanoparticles are used to enhance the oral delivery of various antidiabetic drugs. They can encapsulate hydrophobic drugs, improving their solubility and bioavailability. This approach can lead to better patient compliance and treatment outcomes.
v. **Targeted Therapy:** Functionalized nanoparticles can be designed to target specific cells or tissues involved in diabetes complications. For instance, nanoparticles can be directed to endothelial cells in blood vessels to address vascular complications commonly associated with diabetes. This targeted approach enhances drug delivery while minimizing side effects on healthy tissues.
vi. **Biomarker Detection:** Nanoparticles functionalized with specific receptors or enzymes are employed in biosensors for detecting diabetes-related biomarkers, including glucose and glycated hemoglobin (A1c). Their high surface area and customizable surface properties enhance the sensitivity and specificity of these biosensors.
vii. **Wound Healing:** Diabetic individuals often experience delayed wound healing. Nanoparticles loaded with growth factors, antimicrobial agents, or wound-healing agents can be applied topically to diabetic ulcers to promote faster and more efficient wound healing. The controlled release properties of nanoparticles create an optimal environment for tissue repair (Dubey et. al., 2022).
viii. **Imaging and Diagnostics:** Nanoparticles, especially those containing contrast agents, are used in diagnostic imaging techniques like magnetic resonance imaging (MRI) and computed tomography (CT) scans to visualize diabetes-related complications, such as organ damage and vascular changes. These nanoparticles enhance imaging contrast and enable early disease detection.
ix. **Biocompatibility and Safety:** Researchers are working on optimizing the biocompatibility and safety of nanoparticles for in vivo applications. Ensuring minimal toxicity is crucial for their use in diabetes management.
x. **Research Tools:** Nanoparticles serve as valuable tools in diabetes research, allowing scientists to create controlled environments for studying cellular and molecular processes relevant to the disease. They can be used in in vitro and in vivo experiments to gain insights into diabetes pathophysiology.

In summary, nanoparticles have emerged as versatile nanoscale structures with diverse applications in diabetes mellitus research and treatment. Their ability to encapsulate and deliver therapeutic agents, respond to glucose levels, enhance diagnostics, and promote targeted therapy makes them promising tools for improving diabetes management and advancing our understanding of the disease. Ongoing research in this field continues to explore new opportunities for nanoparticles in diabetes-related applications.

Liposomes

Liposomes are spherical vesicles with an aqueous core surrounded by a lipid bilayer. They are excellent carriers for both hydrophilic and lipophilic drugs due to their amphiphilic nature. Liposomes provide a biocompatible environment for drug encapsulation and can be surface-modified to achieve targeted drug delivery. They are advantageous for delivering insulin and other antidiabetic drugs. Liposomes, which are spherical vesicles composed of lipid bilayers, have gained prominence in the field of diabetes mellitus research and treatment. Their unique structure and properties make them valuable tools for addressing various aspects of diabetes management (Chalotra et al., 2023). Here, we explore the role of liposomes in diabetes mellitus:

i. **Insulin Delivery:** Liposomes have been investigated as carriers for insulin delivery. These lipid-based vesicles can encapsulate insulin molecules, protecting them from degradation in the body and allowing for controlled and sustained release. Liposome-based insulin delivery systems have the potential to replace or supplement traditional insulin injections, improving patient compliance.
ii. **Oral Insulin Delivery:** One of the challenges in diabetes management is the oral delivery of insulin, as it is typically broken down by enzymes in the gastrointestinal tract. Liposomes can be designed to protect insulin during its passage through the digestive system, enabling its absorption in the intestines and mimicking the natural insulin release process.
iii. **Glucose-Responsive Liposomes:** Researchers are developing glucose-responsive liposomes that can release insulin in response to elevated blood glucose levels. These "smart" liposomes offer the possibility of creating a closed-loop system for precise glycemic control.
iv. **Oral Drug Delivery:** Liposomes are used to improve the oral delivery of various antidiabetic drugs. They can encapsulate hydrophobic drugs, enhancing their solubility and bioavailability. This approach can lead to better patient compliance and treatment outcomes.
v. **Targeted Therapy:** Functionalized liposomes can be designed to target specific cells or tissues involved in diabetes complications. For instance, liposomes can be directed to endothelial cells in blood vessels to address vascular complications commonly associated with diabetes. This targeted approach enhances drug delivery while minimizing side effects on healthy tissues.
vi. **Biomarker Detection:** Liposomes functionalized with specific receptors or enzymes are employed in biosensors for detecting diabetes-related biomarkers, including glucose and glycated hemoglobin (A1c). Their high surface area and customizable surface properties enhance the sensitivity and specificity of these biosensors.
vii. **Wound Healing:** Diabetic individuals often experience delayed wound healing. Liposomes loaded with growth factors, antimicrobial agents, or wound-healing agents can be applied topically to diabetic ulcers to promote faster and more efficient wound healing. The controlled release properties of liposomes create an optimal environment for tissue repair.
viii. **Imaging and Diagnostics:** Liposomes, particularly those containing contrast agents, are used in diagnostic imaging techniques like magnetic resonance imaging (MRI) and computed tomography (CT) scans to visualize diabetes-related complications, such as organ damage and vascular changes. These liposomes enhance imaging contrast and enable early disease detection.
ix. **Biocompatibility and Safety:** Researchers are working on optimizing the biocompatibility and safety of liposomes for in vivo applications. Ensuring minimal toxicity is crucial for their use in diabetes management.
x. **Research Tools:** Liposomes serve as valuable tools in diabetes research, allowing scientists to create controlled environments for studying cellular and molecular processes relevant to the disease. They can be used in in vitro and in vivo experiments to gain insights into diabetes pathophysiology.

In summary, liposomes have emerged as versatile nanoscale structures with diverse applications in diabetes mellitus research and treatment. Their ability to encapsulate and deliver therapeutic agents, respond to glucose levels, enhance diagnostics, and promote targeted therapy makes them promising tools for improving diabetes management and advancing our understanding of the disease. Ongoing research in this field continues to explore new opportunities for liposomes in diabetes-related applications.

Polymeric Nanocarriers

These carriers are made of biocompatible polymers such as poly(lactic-co-glycolic acid) (PLGA), polyethylene glycol (PEG), and chitosan. Polymeric nanocarriers include nanoparticles and micelles that can encapsulate drugs and protect them from degradation. They offer controlled drug release and are suitable for both hydrophobic and hydrophilic drugs. Polymeric nanocarriers are nanoscale drug delivery systems composed of biocompatible polymers. They have emerged as promising tools in diabetes mellitus research and treatment due to their ability to encapsulate and release therapeutic agents, target specific cells or tissues, and improve drug bioavailability (Dehghani et al., 2023). Here, we explore the role of polymeric nanocarriers in diabetes mellitus:

i. **Insulin Delivery:** Polymeric nanocarriers are being investigated for the delivery of insulin, a crucial hormone in diabetes management. These nanocarriers can protect insulin from degradation, enable controlled release, and provide an alternative to traditional insulin injections. Some nanocarriers are designed to respond to glucose levels, releasing insulin when needed for precise glycemic control.
ii. **Oral Drug Delivery:** Many antidiabetic drugs are administered orally, but they may have low bioavailability. Polymeric nanocarriers can enhance the solubility and stability of these drugs, improving their absorption in the gastrointestinal tract and increasing overall therapeutic effectiveness. This is particularly valuable for patients who prefer oral medications over injections.
iii. **Targeted Therapy:** Functionalized polymeric nanocarriers can be designed to target specific cells or tissues involved in diabetes complications. For example, nanocarriers can be directed to endothelial cells in blood vessels to address vascular complications commonly associated with diabetes. This targeted approach enhances drug delivery while minimizing side effects on healthy tissues.
iv. **Glucose-Responsive Nanocarriers:** Smart polymeric nanocarriers are engineered to respond to changes in blood glucose levels. These nanocarriers release therapeutic agents, such as insulin, when glucose levels are elevated, providing an on-demand and closed-loop system for glycemic control.
v. **Biomarker Detection:** Polymeric nanocarriers functionalized with specific receptors or enzymes are employed in biosensors for detecting diabetes-related biomarkers, including glucose and glycated hemoglobin (A1c). Their high surface area and customizable surface properties enhance the sensitivity and specificity of these biosensors.
vi. **Wound Healing:** Diabetic individuals often experience delayed wound healing. Polymeric nanocarriers loaded with growth factors, antimicrobial agents, or wound-healing agents can be applied topically to diabetic ulcers to promote faster and more efficient wound healing. The controlled release properties of nanocarriers create an optimal environment for tissue repair.
vii. **Imaging and Diagnostics:** Polymeric nanocarriers, especially those loaded with imaging agents, are used in diagnostic imaging techniques like magnetic resonance imaging (MRI) and computed tomography (CT) scans to visualize diabetes-related complications, such as organ damage and vascular changes. These nanocarriers enhance contrast and enable early disease detection.

viii. **Biocompatibility and Safety:** Researchers are working on optimizing the biocompatibility and safety of polymeric nanocarriers for in vivo applications. This is essential to ensure their effectiveness and safety in diabetes management.

ix. **Research Tools:** Polymeric nanocarriers serve as valuable tools in diabetes research, allowing scientists to create controlled environments for studying cellular and molecular processes relevant to the disease. They can be used in in vitro and in vivo experiments to gain insights into diabetes pathophysiology.

x. **Personalized Medicine:** Polymeric nanocarriers offer the potential for personalized medicine in diabetes. Their tunable properties can be customized to individual patient needs, providing a more targeted and effective approach to treatment.

In summary, polymeric nanocarriers have a wide range of applications in diabetes mellitus research and treatment. Their ability to encapsulate and deliver therapeutic agents, respond to glucose levels, enhance diagnostics, and promote targeted therapy makes them promising tools for improving diabetes management and advancing our understanding of the disease. Ongoing research in this field continues to explore new opportunities for polymeric nanocarriers in diabetes-related applications.

Dendrimers

Dendrimers are highly branched, three-dimensional nanoparticles with a well-defined structure. They have a large number of functional groups on their surface, making them ideal for drug conjugation. Dendrimers can encapsulate drugs within their branches or conjugate drugs on their surface. They provide a precise drug release profile and can be tailored for targeted drug delivery. Dendrimers, highly branched and well-defined macromolecules with a symmetric, tree-like structure, have garnered attention for their potential applications in various fields, including diabetes mellitus research and treatment. Their unique characteristics make them versatile tools for addressing several aspects of diabetes management (Li et al., 2023). Here, we explore the role of dendrimers in diabetes mellitus:

i. **Drug Delivery:** Dendrimers are utilized as drug delivery vehicles in diabetes treatment. They can encapsulate and protect antidiabetic drugs, enhancing their solubility and stability. This controlled release system allows for prolonged drug activity and improved therapeutic outcomes.

ii. **Insulin Delivery:** Researchers are investigating dendrimers as carriers for insulin delivery. Their high surface area and ability to encapsulate insulin molecules make them promising candidates for developing non-invasive insulin delivery systems, such as nasal or pulmonary administration.

iii. **Glucose-Responsive Delivery:** Smart dendrimers are being engineered to respond to changes in blood glucose levels. These dendrimers can release insulin or other therapeutic agents when glucose levels are elevated, offering a potential closed-loop system for precise glycemic control.

iv. **Targeted Therapy:** Functionalized dendrimers can be designed to target specific cells or tissues associated with diabetes complications, such as endothelial cells in blood vessels. This targeted approach enhances the effectiveness of therapies while minimizing side effects on healthy tissues.

v. **Biomarker Detection:** Dendrimers functionalized with receptors or enzymes are employed in biosensors for detecting diabetes-related biomarkers, including glucose and glycated hemoglobin (A1c). Their high surface area and tailored functional groups enhance the sensitivity and specificity of these biosensors.

vi. **Wound Healing:** Dendrimers loaded with growth factors, antimicrobial agents, or wound-healing agents can be applied topically to diabetic ulcers and wounds to promote healing. Their controlled release properties create an optimal environment for tissue repair.
vii. **Imaging and Diagnostics:** Dendrimers, particularly those loaded with imaging contrast agents, are used in diagnostic imaging techniques like magnetic resonance imaging (MRI) and computed tomography (CT) scans to visualize diabetes-related complications, such as organ damage and vascular changes.
viii. **Biocompatibility and Safety:** Researchers are working on optimizing dendrimer composition and surface modifications to ensure biocompatibility and safety for in vivo applications. This is crucial for their use in diabetes management.
ix. **Research Tools:** Dendrimers serve as valuable tools in diabetes research, allowing scientists to create controlled environments for studying cellular and molecular processes relevant to the disease. They can be used in in vitro and in vivo experiments to gain insights into diabetes pathophysiology.
x. **Personalized Medicine:** Dendrimers offer the potential for personalized medicine in diabetes. Their tunable properties can be customized to individual patient needs, providing a more targeted and effective approach to treatment.

In summary, dendrimers present a range of applications in diabetes mellitus research and treatment. Their ability to encapsulate and deliver therapeutic agents, respond to glucose levels, enhance diagnostics, and promote targeted therapy makes them promising tools for improving diabetes management and advancing our understanding of the disease. Ongoing research in this field continues to explore new avenues for dendrimers in diabetes-related applications.

Micelles

Micelles are efficient carriers for hydrophobic drugs and offer improved drug solubility and stability. In an aqueous environment, they form a core-shell structure with a hydrophobic core and a hydrophilic shell. They can also be surface-modified for targeted drug delivery. Micelles, which are self-assembled nanostructures composed of amphiphilic molecules, have shown promise in various aspects of diabetes mellitus research and treatment. Their unique properties make them valuable tools for addressing challenges associated with this chronic condition (Attar et al., 2023). Here, we explore the role of micelles in diabetes mellitus:

i. **Drug Delivery:** Micelles are used as drug delivery carriers for antidiabetic drugs. Hydrophobic drugs, such as certain oral antidiabetic medications, can be encapsulated in the hydrophobic core of micelles, improving their solubility and bioavailability. This approach allows for controlled drug release and potentially reduces side effects.
ii. **Insulin Delivery:** Researchers are exploring micelles as carriers for insulin delivery. The hydrophobic core of micelles can protect insulin molecules from degradation in the body and allow for controlled release. This is particularly important for developing oral insulin delivery systems, which could replace or supplement traditional insulin injections.
iii. **Glucose-Responsive Micelles:** Smart micelles responsive to changes in blood glucose levels are under development. These micelles can release insulin or other therapeutic agents in response to elevated glucose concentrations, offering a closed-loop system for precise glycemic control.

iv. **Wound Healing:** Diabetic individuals often experience delayed wound healing. Micelles loaded with growth factors or antimicrobial agents can be applied topically to diabetic ulcers to promote wound healing. These micelles release their payload gradually, creating an optimal environment for tissue repair.
v. **Biomarker Detection:** Micelles functionalized with specific receptors or enzymes can be used in biosensors for detecting diabetes-related biomarkers, such as glucose and glycated hemoglobin (A1c). Their high surface area and unique properties enhance the sensitivity and accuracy of these biosensors.
vi. **Oral Delivery:** Micelles can improve the oral delivery of various antidiabetic drugs. By encapsulating these drugs, micelles protect them from degradation in the gastrointestinal tract and enhance their absorption, making them a viable option for improving patient compliance.
vii. **Targeted Therapy:** Functionalized micelles can be designed to target specific cells or tissues involved in diabetes-related complications, such as the endothelial cells of blood vessels. This targeted approach can enhance the efficacy of therapies while minimizing side effects on healthy tissues.
viii. **Biocompatibility and Safety:** Micelles can be engineered to be biocompatible and safe for in vivo applications. Researchers are working on optimizing the composition and surface properties of micelles to ensure minimal toxicity.
ix. **Research Tools:** Micelles serve as valuable tools for diabetes research, allowing scientists to create controlled environments for studying cellular and molecular processes relevant to the disease. They can be used in in vitro and in vivo experiments to gain insights into diabetes pathophysiology.
x. **Personalized Medicine:** Micelles offer the potential for personalized medicine in diabetes. Their tunable properties can be tailored to individual patient needs, providing a more targeted and effective approach to treatment.

In summary, micelles have emerged as versatile nanoscale structures with diverse applications in diabetes mellitus. Their ability to encapsulate and deliver therapeutic agents, respond to glucose levels, and enhance diagnostics makes them promising tools for improving diabetes management and advancing our understanding of the disease. Ongoing research in this field continues to explore new opportunities for micelles in diabetes research and treatment.

Nanogels

Nanogels are three-dimensional polymeric networks with a hydrophilic structure capable of absorbing water or biological fluids. They can encapsulate hydrophilic drugs and provide a controlled and sustained drug release. Nanogels are biocompatible and suitable for delivering insulin and other antidiabetic agents. Nanogels are a class of nanoscale materials with a three-dimensional network structure that can absorb and retain large amounts of water or biological fluids. They have gained significant attention in the field of diabetes mellitus due to their unique properties and versatile applications (Mandal et al., 2023). Here, we explore the role of nanogels in diabetes research and treatment:

i. **Insulin Delivery:** Nanogels are being investigated as carriers for insulin delivery. They can encapsulate insulin molecules, protecting them from degradation in the body and allowing for controlled and sustained release. This approach offers an alternative to traditional insulin injections, potentially improving patient compliance and overall glycemic control.

ii. **Oral Insulin:** One of the challenges in diabetes management is the oral delivery of insulin, as it is typically broken down by enzymes in the gastrointestinal tract. Nanogels can be designed to protect insulin during its journey through the digestive system, enabling its absorption in the intestines and mimicking the natural insulin release process.

iii. **Glucose-Responsive Nanogels:** Researchers are developing nanogels that can respond to changes in blood glucose levels. These "smart" nanogels release insulin in response to elevated glucose concentrations, providing a closed-loop system for precise glycemic control.

iv. **Topical Wound Healing:** Diabetic individuals often suffer from slow wound healing, which can lead to complications. Nanogels loaded with growth factors, antimicrobial agents, or other therapeutic agents can be applied topically to diabetic ulcers to promote faster and more efficient wound healing.

v. **Biomarker Detection**: Nanogels functionalized with specific receptors or enzymes can be used in biosensors for detecting diabetes-related biomarkers, such as glucose and A1c. Their high surface area and ability to retain a large volume of fluid enhance the sensitivity and accuracy of these biosensors.

vi. **Drug Delivery:** Besides insulin, nanogels can be used to deliver other antidiabetic drugs. They can encapsulate and release these drugs in a controlled manner, potentially reducing the frequency of drug administration and minimizing side effects.

vii. **Diagnostics and Imaging:** Nanogels can be employed as contrast agents in imaging techniques like magnetic resonance imaging (MRI) and computed tomography (CT) scans to visualize diabetes-related complications, such as vascular changes and organ damage.

viii. **Biocompatibility and Safety:** Nanogels can be designed to be biocompatible and safe for use in the human body. Researchers are working on optimizing the composition and surface properties of nanogels to ensure minimal toxicity.

ix. **Research Tools:** Nanogels are valuable tools for diabetes research, allowing scientists to create controlled environments for studying cellular and molecular processes relevant to the disease. They can be used in in vitro and in vivo experiments to gain insights into diabetes pathophysiology.

x. **Personalized Medicine:** Nanogels hold the potential for personalized medicine in diabetes. Their tunable properties can be tailored to individual patient needs, offering a more targeted and effective approach to treatment.

In summary, nanogels have emerged as versatile nanomaterials with various applications in diabetes mellitus. Their ability to encapsulate, protect, and release therapeutic agents, respond to glucose levels, and enhance diagnostics makes them promising tools for improving diabetes management and advancing our understanding of the disease. Ongoing research in this field continues to explore new opportunities for nanogels in diabetes research and treatment.

Inorganic Nanocarriers

Inorganic nanoparticles like gold, silver, silica, and magnetic nanoparticles are also employed as carriers in drug delivery. They offer unique properties for drug encapsulation and surface functionalization. Inorganic nanocarriers can be tailored for controlled drug release and imaging, enabling multifunctional applications in diabetes treatment. Inorganic nanocarriers play a significant role in the field of diabetes mellitus, offering innovative solutions for the diagnosis, treatment, and management of this chronic condition. These nanocarriers, often made from biocompatible and non-toxic materials, have unique properties that make them valuable tools in addressing various aspects of diabetes (Liu et al., 2023). Here, we explore the applications and contributions of inorganic nanocarriers in the context of diabetes mellitus:

i. **Drug Delivery:** Inorganic nanocarriers, such as nanoparticles made from materials like gold, silver, or silica, are employed to enhance drug delivery in diabetes treatment. They can encapsulate and protect therapeutic agents, such as insulin or oral antidiabetic drugs, ensuring controlled release and improved bioavailability. These carriers can be engineered to respond to specific triggers, such as glucose levels, enabling targeted drug release at the right time and place.
ii. **Insulin Delivery:** Nanocarriers are instrumental in developing innovative insulin delivery systems. For example, gold nanoparticles can be functionalized to carry insulin and respond to changes in glucose levels, offering a potential alternative to traditional insulin injections. This approach seeks to mimic the physiological release of insulin in response to blood sugar fluctuations.
iii. **Biomarker Detection:** Inorganic nanocarriers are utilized in the development of biosensors for detecting diabetes-related biomarkers, including glucose and glycated hemoglobin (A1c). Nanoparticles can be modified with receptors or enzymes that specifically bind to these biomarkers, enabling rapid and accurate detection. The small size and high surface area of nanocarriers enhance the sensitivity of such biosensors.
iv. **Imaging and Diagnostics:** Nanoparticles, particularly those containing contrast agents, are employed in diagnostic imaging techniques like magnetic resonance imaging (MRI) and computed tomography (CT) scans to visualize diabetes-related complications, such as diabetic retinopathy and nephropathy. These nanoparticles enhance the imaging contrast, allowing for earlier disease detection and monitoring.
v. **Wound Healing:** Inorganic nanocarriers can facilitate wound healing in diabetic patients, who often experience delayed wound repair. Nanoparticles loaded with growth factors or antimicrobial agents can be applied topically to chronic diabetic ulcers to promote healing and prevent infection.
vi. **Glucose-Responsive Materials:** Nanocarriers can be engineered to respond to changes in glucose levels, triggering the release of insulin or other therapeutic agents when needed. These "smart" nanomaterials hold promise for creating closed-loop systems that provide precise glucose control.
vii. **Reducing Side Effects:** Inorganic nanocarriers can minimize side effects associated with certain antidiabetic drugs by delivering them more selectively to target tissues. This can reduce the dosage required and limit adverse effects on other organs.
viii. **Research and Development:** Inorganic nanocarriers are invaluable tools in diabetes research, enabling scientists to investigate the cellular and molecular mechanisms underlying the condition. They are used in in vitro and in vivo studies to develop a deeper understanding of diabetes and test new treatment strategies.

In summary, inorganic nanocarriers represent a versatile and promising avenue for advancing the diagnosis and treatment of diabetes mellitus. Their unique properties, including tunable size, surface functionalization, and targeted drug delivery capabilities, make them valuable tools for improving the management of this prevalent chronic disease. Researchers continue to explore innovative applications of these nanocarriers to enhance the quality of life for individuals living with diabetes.

Utilizing these diverse nanocarriers provides a wide array of options for targeted drug delivery in diabetes management. Tailoring the properties of these nanocarriers to the specific needs of antidiabetic drugs and optimizing their characteristics for effective drug delivery holds great promise for enhancing the therapeutic outcomes in diabetes mellitus.

NANOMATERIALS AS CARRIERS

Nanomaterials Loaded With Natural Antidiabetic Extracts

In nature, there is an abundance of plants, marine organisms, and microorganisms, many of which contain substances with therapeutic potential (Elahi et al., 2018). Traditional remedies for diabetes have often utilized natural extracts from plants like *Allium sativum, Eugenia jambolana, Ficus glomerata, Momordica charantia, Murraya koenigii, Catharanthus roseus, Terminalia arjuna, and Brassica juncea*. When these natural antidiabetic compounds are combined with or incorporated into nanomaterials, they tend to exhibit excellent antidiabetic effects. This is likely due to increased biocompatibility and reduced toxicity compared to the use of these compounds alone. Currently, nanoparticles (NPs) employed for loading naturally occurring antidiabetic substances are primarily composed of inorganic elements such as gold (Au), platinum (Pt), silver (Ag), and zinc oxide (ZnO) (Liu et al., 2022). For example, gold nanoparticles (Au NPs) prepared from the potent antidiabetic herb Cassia auriculata yielded nano-sized Au particles with an average diameter ranging from 15 to 25 nanometers. These Au NPs remained stable across a wide pH range (from 3.4 to 10.2), indicating their high potential for antidiabetic treatment. In another study, Au NPs were employed in Wistar albino rats using an antidiabetic plant, *Gymnema sylvestre* R. Br. These Au NPs, with dimensions of approximately 50 nanometers and a negative charge of -17.5 mV, led to a significant reduction in blood glucose levels among the experimental group, consisting of diabetic rats treated with Au NPs at a dose of 0.5 milligrams per kilogram of body weight (Liu et al., 2022).

Additionally, platinum nanoparticles (Pt NPs) loaded with an extract from Whitania somnifera leaves (12 nanometers in size) produced a marked decrease in plasma glucose levels after administration to streptozotocin-induced diabetic rats at a dose of 1 milligram per kilogram. Silver nanoparticles (Ag NPs), ranging in size from 4 to 25 nanometers, were synthesized using an extract from Solanum nigrum, a medicinal plant historically used to treat diabetes. Administering these nanoparticles at a dosage of 10 milligrams per kilogram to alloxan-induced diabetic rats resulted in improvements in body weight, dyslipidemia, and a reduction in blood glucose levels. Similarly, compared to treatments with watercress leaf extract (150 milligrams per deciliter) and insulin (10 units per kilogram), diabetic Wistar rats induced with alloxan that received enriched zinc oxide nanoparticles (average pore diameter of 4.8 nanometers) loaded with watercress (*Nasturtium officinale*) leaf extract at a dosage of 8 milligrams per deciliter showed the most significant improvement in their diabetic condition. These findings suggest that inorganic nanoparticles loaded with extracts from naturally potent antidiabetic plants have the potential to serve as highly effective antidiabetic agents.

Nanomaterials Loaded With Recombinant Human Insulin

Apart from natural extracts, the U.S. Food and Drug Administration (FDA) has approved various synthetic antidiabetic medications, including sulfonylureas, biguanides (glucosidase/starch inhibitors), thiazolidinediones (insulin secretagogues), and, notably, recombinant human insulin, for regulating blood glucose levels in diabetic patients (Liu et al., 2022). These medications can be administered through two methods: subcutaneous injection and oral delivery. Small synthetic molecules can be taken orally or intravenously. However, oral insulin administration has limited effectiveness, making subcutaneous insulin injection the preferred method for managing patients requiring insulin (Dorokhov et al., 2016). It remains a challenge that subcutaneous insulin injections deliver insulin to the peripheral circulation rather than the portal circulation, while oral administration can alleviate the discomfort and trauma associated with injections while also closely mimicking insulin's natural physiological fate. Various nanosystems have been developed to enhance the oral bioavailability of insulin and other synthetic drugs, either by improving drug permeability or overcoming the first-pass effect.

Before orally administered insulin can become active, it must maintain its structure as it traverses the stomach, small intestine, and colon. However, the harsh conditions in the gastrointestinal (GI) tract and the acidic stomach environment pose significant challenges. Thus, an ideal nano-system for oral insulin delivery should prolong its presence in the intestines, enhance drug absorption by temporarily increasing mucosal epithelium permeability, and protect it from GI enzymes and the highly acidic stomach environment to ensure insulin remains active (Liu et al., 2022). According to Mukhopadhyay et al., effective oral insulin delivery systems must meet specific criteria, including:

- pH-sensitivity to protect the drug in the acidic stomach environment and release it in the intestines;
- targeted drug release near the absorption site to avoid intestinal proteases;
- selective and reversible opening of tight junctions, if possible;
- controlled release to achieve physiological insulin concentrations in the blood; and
- biocompatibility of the drug delivery vehicle.

In response to these challenges, various nanomaterials have been developed, incorporating features such as pH-sensitivity, targeted drug delivery to enhance cellular uptake, and even biofeedback mechanisms that release antidiabetic drugs in response to high glucose levels (glucose-responsiveness). These intelligent nanosystems offer a range of approaches to improve both oral bioavailability and subcutaneous injection of antidiabetic drugs.

Nanomaterials Loaded With Other Antidiabetic Drugs

The aforementioned studies have confirmed the potential for customizing insulin-loaded nanoparticles (NPs) to enhance insulin delivery. However, NPs can also enhance the bioavailability of various other antidiabetic drugs in vivo. For instance, stevioside, an FDA-approved sweetener with no toxicity concerns, possesses remarkable antidiabetic properties. Nevertheless, its practical use in humans is limited due to poor intestinal absorption and low bioavailability. Barwal et al. utilized biodegradable Pluronic-F-68 copolymer-based poly (lactic acid) NPs conjugated with stevioside through a nano-precipitation method to improve its intestinal absorption and bioavailability. These resulting spherical NPs (ranging from 110 to 130 nanometers) demonstrated enhanced delivery of stevioside (Barwal et al., 2013).

Similarly, metformin, a widely used antidiabetic medication, experiences limited absorption in the gastrointestinal tract, resulting in an oral bioavailability of 50-60%. Mirazi et al. developed metformin-conjugated nanotubes to reduce blood glucose levels, extend drug delivery duration, and enhance its efficacy in diabetic treatment compared to metformin alone (150 milligrams per kilogram, orally). Glibenclamide, another common treatment for Type II diabetes, faces challenges in its dissolution within a physiological medium, which restricts its absorption. A recent study revealed that zinc NPs loaded with glibenclamide (196 nanometers) induced a significant hypolipidemic effect in Caenorhabditis elegans worms, reducing approximately 15% of fat content. Notably, the NPs remained largely unaltered, suggesting that glibenclamide-loaded zinc NPs hold potential for diabetes treatment (Mirazi et al., 2015).

Moreover, glucagon-like peptide-1 (GLP-1), an incretin hormone used in Type II diabetes treatment, faces difficulties in oral administration due to the harsh conditions in the gastrointestinal tract and limited bioavailability. Martins et al. devised a nanosystem for GLP-1 delivery. They functionalized undecylenic acid-modified thermally hydrocarbonized porous silicon (UnPSi) nanoparticles (NPs) using the Fc fragment of immunoglobulin G and coated them with mucoadhesive chitosan for targeted applications. GLP-1 was loaded into these NPs, facilitating GLP-1 absorption across intestinal monolayers, demonstrating the FcRn transcytotic capacity, and making this nanosystem suitable for oral GLP-1 delivery (Zhu et al., 2021).

Furthermore, exendin-4, a GLP-1 mimetic for Type II diabetes treatment, faces challenges related to low patient compliance due to frequent injections. Ahn et al. discovered that the conjugation of low molecular weight chitosan (LMWC) with cysteinylated exendin-4 can maximize the availability of the active peptide. A pharmacokinetic study revealed that the bioavailability of the LMWC-exendin-4 conjugate (approximately 101 $\pm$ 41 nanometers) after oral administration (400 micrograms per kilogram) is 6.4% compared to subcutaneous administration. Additionally, the absorbed exendin-4 exhibited a significantly enhanced hypoglycemic effect, suggesting the potential of the LMWC-exendin-4 conjugate as an oral antidiabetic agent for Type II diabetes treatment.

Furthermore, Araújo et al. developed a multifunctional composite nanosystem using PLGA nanoparticles through the droplet microfluidics technique to enable dual delivery of GLP-1 and a dipeptidyl peptidase-4 inhibitor (iDPP4) in vivo. The PLGA nanoparticles in this system were functionalized with chitosan (CS) and a cell-penetrating peptide (CPP). Plasmatic insulin levels increased after 6 hours of oral administration of the system (equivalent to a GLP-1 content of 200 micrograms per kilogram of the rat's weight). Additionally, blood glucose levels were significantly lower compared to the control group (Araujo et al., 2016). Thus, NPs within delivery systems present a promising avenue for the development of novel oral formulations for antidiabetic agents.

CONCLUSION

The early detection, management, and treatment of diabetes and its associated complications pose an inevitable challenge for researchers and healthcare professionals. Fortunately, recent advancements in nanomedicine have opened up new possibilities for addressing the medical requirements related to diabetes. In this review, we offer an overview of the latest developments in nanomaterials for both detecting diabetic biomarkers and treating diabetes. Despite the numerous advantages associated with nanomaterial-assisted diabetic diagnosis and therapy, several challenges remain to be tackled.

Efficient, rapid, precise, and convenient detection of diabetic biomarkers stands as a pivotal area for future advancements in diabetes diagnosis. Researchers find this task relatively straightforward as the use of biosensors for diabetes diagnosis predominantly relies on in vitro or ex vivo detection methods. An intriguing approach is the noninvasive monitoring of acetone gas in human exhaled breath, which sets it apart from traditional blood-based biomarker detection (e.g., glucose and A1c). Consequently, there is ongoing work on developing acetone nanosensors with ultrafast response times and high accuracy. Future research should emphasize creating commercially available semiconductor oxide acetone sensors and streamlining the practical aspects of clinical testing.

In contrast to diabetic diagnosis, the use of nanomaterials for diabetes therapy invariably involves in vivo applications. While numerous studies demonstrate the antidiabetic properties of nanoparticles (NPs), several issues warrant investigation concerning their use in diabetes therapy. These include determining safe and effective NP dosages for patients, understanding the potential antidiabetic mechanisms of NPs, and assessing the epigenetic effects of NPs. Moreover, certain NPs, such as superparamagnetic NPs, may be recognized and engulfed by cells in the reticulocyte-endothelial system, including the liver, spleen, and lymph nodes. This accumulation in these cells can limit their therapeutic efficacy and may lead to toxicity, necessitating comprehensive scientific evaluation. Crucially, how can the phagocytosis of these endothelial systems be circumvented to enable NPs to precisely reach their intended targets? This is a common challenge in nanomedicine that requires resolution.

As previously mentioned, understanding the mechanisms underlying NP toxicity and their various roles in diabetes prevention and therapy is critical from both a foundational and practical perspective. To mitigate NP toxicity, it is imperative to optimize the raw materials and synthesis processes involved in their production. Reducing the use of toxic chemical reagents or opting for natural substances during synthesis can enhance biocompatibility. Furthermore, investigations into the in vivo regulation and control mechanisms of antidiabetic elements or oxides are essential for the application of NP-based therapies in diabetes. Maximizing the impact of nanoparticles will necessitate the development of innovative strategies for effectively targeting them to damaged tissues in diabetic patients. Ideally, an NP drug delivery system should possess the ability to locate, recognize, bind to, and deliver its payload to affected tissues while minimizing or avoiding harm to healthy tissues. Modifying NPs with specific targeting ligands is likely to be the simplest and most efficient strategy to achieve this goal.

In summary, nanoparticles exhibit significant promise in the realms of diabetes diagnosis and treatment. While there have been notable achievements in functional nanosystems for diabetes detection, treatment, and prevention, this field is still evolving and necessitates multidisciplinary collaboration encompassing chemistry, materials science, biology, medicine, electronics, and computer science. Ongoing efforts should focus on the discovery of new diabetic biomarkers, the development of advanced sensing mechanisms and point-of-care diagnostic devices, the design of highly effective nanocarriers for drug delivery, and the reduction of biotoxicity associated with current nanomaterials. We hope that the concepts outlined in this review, along with the existing challenges and emerging trends, will inspire researchers to create novel nanomaterials with unique functions and properties for improving diabetes diagnosis and therapy.

REFERENCES

Ahangarpour, A., Oroojan, A. A., Khorsandi, L., Kouchak, M., & Badavi, M. (2019). Antioxidant, anti-apoptotic, and protective effects of myricitrin and its solid lipid nanoparticle on streptozotocin-nicotinamide-induced diabetic nephropathy in type 2 diabetic male mice. *Iranian Journal of Basic Medical Sciences.*, *22*(12), 1424. PMID:32133060

Araujo, F., Shrestha, N., Gomes, M. J., Herranz-Blanco, B., Liu, D., Hirvonen, J. J., Granja, P. L., Santos, H. A., & Sarmento, B. (2016). In vivo dual-delivery of glucagon like peptide-1 (GLP-1) and dipeptidyl peptidase-4 (DPP4) inhibitor through composites prepared by microfluidics for diabetes therapy. *Nanoscale*, *8*(20), 10706–10713. doi:10.1039/C6NR00294C PMID:27150301

Attar, E. S., Chaudhari, V. H., Deokar, C. G., Dyawanapelly, S., & Devarajan, P. V. (2023). Nano Drug Delivery Strategies for an Oral Bioenhanced Quercetin Formulation. *European Journal of Drug Metabolism and Pharmacokinetics*, *48*(5), 1–20. doi:10.100713318-023-00843-7 PMID:37523008

Barwal, I., Sood, A., Sharma, M., Singh, B., & Yadav, S. C. (2013). Development of stevioside Pluronic-F-68 copolymer based PLA-nanoparticles as an antidiabetic nanomedicine. *Colloids and Surfaces. B, Biointerfaces*, *101*, 510–516. doi:10.1016/j.colsurfb.2012.07.005 PMID:23022553

Cao, X., Yao, F., Zhang, B., & Sun, X. (2023). Mitochondrial dysfunction in heart diseases: Potential therapeutic effects of Panax ginseng. *Frontiers in Pharmacology*, *14*, 1218803. doi:10.3389/fphar.2023.1218803 PMID:37547332

Chalotra, R., Gupta, T., Chib, S., Amanat, M., Kumar, P., & Singh, R. (2023). Treatment of diabetic complications: Do flavonoids holds the keys? *Critical Reviews in Food Science and Nutrition*, 1–22. doi:10.1080/10408398.2023.2232868 PMID:37435788

Dabla, P. K. (2010). Renal function in diabetic nephropathy. *World Journal of Diabetes*, *1*(2), 48. doi:10.4239/wjd.v1.i2.48 PMID:21537427

Dehghani, P., Rad, M. E., Zarepour, A., Sivakumar, P. M., & Zarrabi, A. (2023). An insight into the polymeric nanoparticles applications in diabetes diagnosis and treatment. *Mini-Reviews in Medicinal Chemistry*, *23*(2), 192–216. doi:10.2174/1389557521666211116123002 PMID:34784864

Dorokhov, Y. L., Sheshukova, E. V., Kosobokova, E. N., Shindyapina, A. V., Kosorukov, V. S., & Komarova, T. V. (2016). Functional role of carbohydrate residues in human immunoglobulin G and therapeutic monoclonal antibodies. *Biochemistry (Moscow)*, *81*(8), 835–857. doi:10.1134/S0006297916080058 PMID:27677552

Dubey, R., Prabhakar, P. K., & Gupta, J. (2022). Epigenetics: Key to improve delayed wound healing in type 2 diabetes. *Molecular and Cellular Biochemistry*, *477*(2), 371–383. doi:10.100711010-021-04285-0 PMID:34739665

Elahi, N., Kamali, M., & Baghersad, M. H. (2018). Recent biomedical applications of gold nanoparticles: A review. *Talanta*, *184*, 537–556. doi:10.1016/j.talanta.2018.02.088 PMID:29674080

Imig, J. D., & Ryan, M. J. (2013). Immune and inflammatory role in renal disease. *Comprehensive Physiology*, *3*(2), 957. doi:10.1002/cphy.c120028 PMID:23720336

Jia, G., Hill, M. A., & Sowers, J. R. (2018). Diabetic cardiomyopathy: An update of mechanisms contributing to this clinical entity. *Circulation Research*, *122*(4), 624–638. doi:10.1161/CIRCRESAHA.117.311586 PMID:29449364

Karthikeyan, A., Senthil, N., & Min, T. (2020). Nanocurcumin: A promising candidate for therapeutic applications. *Frontiers in Pharmacology*, *11*, 487. doi:10.3389/fphar.2020.00487 PMID:32425772

Li, S., Chen, L., & Fu, Y. (2023). Nanotechnology-based ocular drug delivery systems: Recent advances and future prospects. *Journal of Nanobiotechnology*, *21*(1), 1–39. doi:10.118612951-023-01992-2 PMID:37480102

Liu, M., Wei, X., Zheng, Z., Li, Y., Li, M., Lin, J., & Yang, L. (2023). Recent Advances in Nano-Drug Delivery Systems for the Treatment of Diabetic Wound Healing. *International Journal of Nanomedicine*, *18*, 1537–1560. doi:10.2147/IJN.S395438 PMID:37007988

Liu, Q., Wang, S., & Cai, L. (2014). Diabetic cardiomyopathy and its mechanisms: Role of oxidative stress and damage. *Journal of Diabetes Investigation*, *5*(6), 623–634. doi:10.1111/jdi.12250 PMID:25422760

Liu, Y., Zeng, S., Ji, W., Yao, H., Lin, L., Cui, H., Santos, H. A., & Pan, G. (2022). Emerging theranostic nanomaterials in diabetes and its complications. *Advancement of Science*, *9*(3), 2102466. doi:10.1002/advs.202102466 PMID:34825525

Mandal, D., Anand, K., & Prabhakar, P. K. (2023). Biomedical Applications of Nanofluids in Drug Delivery. In *Novel Technologies in Biosystems, Biomedical & Drug Delivery* (pp. 105–124). Springer Nature Singapore. doi:10.1007/978-981-99-5281-6_5

Manimaran, V., Sivakumar, P. M., Narayanan, J., Parthasarathi, S., & Prabhakar, P. K. (2021). Nanoemulsions: A Better Approach for Antidiabetic Drug Delivery. *Current Diabetes Reviews*, *17*(4), 486–495. doi:10.2174/1573399817666201209095205 PMID:33297917

Mirazi, N., Shoaei, J., Khazaei, A., & Hosseini, A. (2015). A comparative study on effect of metformin and metformin-conjugated nanotubes on blood glucose homeostasis in diabetic rats. *European Journal of Drug Metabolism and Pharmacokinetics*, *40*(3), 343–348. doi:10.100713318-014-0213-x PMID:24969688

Mrugacz, M., Bryl, A., & Zorena, K. (2021). Retinal vascular endothelial cell dysfunction and neuroretinal degeneration in diabetic patients. *Journal of Clinical Medicine*, *10*(3), 458. doi:10.3390/jcm10030458 PMID:33504108

Nankar, R., Prabhakar, P. K., & Doble, M. (2017). Hybrid drug combination: Combination of ferulic acid and metformin as anti-diabetic therapy. *Phytomedicine*, *37*, 10–13. doi:10.1016/j.phymed.2017.10.015 PMID:29126698

Parsamanesh, N., Moossavi, M., Bahrami, A., Butler, A. E., & Sahebkar, A. (2018). Therapeutic potential of curcumin in diabetic complications. *Pharmacological Research*, *136*, 181–193. doi:10.1016/j.phrs.2018.09.012 PMID:30219581

Prabhakar, P. K. (2016). Pathophysiology of secondary complications of diabetes mellitus. *Pathophysiology*, *9*(1), 32–36.

Prabhakar, P. K., & Sivakumar, P. M. (2019). Protein tyrosine phosphatase 1B inhibitors: A novel therapeutic strategy for the management of type 2 diabetes mellitus. *Current Pharmaceutical Design*, *25*(23), 2526–2539. doi:10.2174/1381612825666190716102901 PMID:31333090

Veith, A. P., Henderson, K., Spencer, A., Sligar, A. D., & Baker, A. B. (2019). Therapeutic strategies for enhancing angiogenesis in wound healing. *Advanced Drug Delivery Reviews*, *146*, 97–125. doi:10.1016/j.addr.2018.09.010 PMID:30267742

Xiong, J., Dong, X., Li, S., Jiang, F., Chen, J., Yu, S., Dong, B., & Su, Q. (2021). Effects of (Pro) renin receptor on diabetic cardiomyopathy pathological processes in rats via the PRR-AMPK-YAP pathway. *Frontiers in Physiology*, *12*, 657378. doi:10.3389/fphys.2021.657378 PMID:34122131

Zhu, Q., Chen, Z., Paul, P. K., Lu, Y., Wu, W., & Qi, J. (2021). Oral delivery of proteins and peptides: Challenges, status quo and future perspectives. *Acta Pharmaceutica Sinica. B*, *11*(8), 2416–2448. doi:10.1016/j.apsb.2021.04.001 PMID:34522593

Chapter 7
Nanomaterials in the Treatment of Infectious Diseases:
Treatment and Regulatory Aspect

Palwinder Kaur
Lovely Professional University, India

Manish Vyas
https://orcid.org/0000-0002-1426-2277
Lovely Professional University, India

Sandeep Sharma
Lovely Professional University, India

ABSTRACT

Infectious diseases are a major global burden according to the latest WHO reports. The problems of drug resistance, emergence, and reemergence cases are rising when treatment is given by conventional therapy. These therapeutic insufficiencies lead to treatment failure. Nanomaterials are a class of carrier systems that offer some desirable properties to combat the aforementioned problems related to the treatment of infectious diseases. They offer better targetability and better bioavailability than conventional systems. Thus, they are being explored to their full potential in the treatment of infectious diseases. The use of metallic nanoparticles, carbon dots, are a major area where research is being carried out to mark them as effective carriers. This book chapter gives an insight to various nanomaterials which are widely used and explored for the treatment of various diseases along with the safety and regulatory aspects of nanomaterials.

DOI: 10.4018/979-8-3693-0448-8.ch007

INTRODUCTION

Overview of Infectious Diseases

Infectious diseases are illnesses caused by pathogenic microorganisms such as bacteria, viruses, fungi, and parasites. These microorganisms can invade the body, multiply, and increases the incidence of morbidity. Infectious diseases can be transmitted from one person to another through direct or indirect contact, through the air, contaminated food or water, insect bites, or other means. Different types of microorganisms cause specific infectious diseases. For example, bacteria can cause diseases like tuberculosis (*Mycobacterium tuberculosis*), dental caries (*Streptococcus mutans*) and urinary tract infections (Poly microbial infection caused by *Escherichia coli, Klebsiella, Proteus, Enterococcus,* and *Staphylococcus).* Viruses are responsible for illnesses such as the common cold, influenza, and COVID-19. Fungi can cause conditions like athlete's foot and candidiasis, while parasites can lead to diseases like malaria and intestinal infections. Infectious diseases have a significant impact on global health. They can cause outbreaks and pandemics, leading to considerable morbidity, mortality, and economic consequences. The emergence and reemergence of infectious diseases present major challenges in disease management.

The peculiar problem with the management of infectious diseases lies in the fact that the microbes have short life span and grow rapidly in number (exponential growth) and does not have complex gene repair mechanism (unlike humans) so each new generation of microbes introduces the possibility of diverse genetic material. Thus the emergence of resistance is more in microbes. Resistant species in pathogens enable them to evade the host immune system and develop resistance to treatment therapy (Choi, 2021). Such adaptations can lead to the re-emergence of more virulent or drug-resistant forms. The irrational use of antibiotics has led to the development of antimicrobial resistance (AMR) in microbes. When microbes become resistant to multiple antibiotics, it becomes even more challenging to control the spread of these infections. At times, weaker immunity can render individuals more vulnerable to infections. This reduction in immunity may result in the resurgence of past infections as well as provide opportunities for new pathogens to invade and spread infection in the body(Nii-Trebi, 2017).

Significance of Nanomaterials in Treatment

Nanomaterials are materials that have nanoscale dimensions, typically ranging from 1 to 100 nanometers (nm). They possess unique properties and characteristics that differ from the same materials in bulk form, making them of significant interest in various fields. As the sizing scale shift to the nano size ranges many properties get altered e.g. mechanical, electrical, optical, thermal, and magnetic properties, etc. properties like quantum confinement and plasmonic effects come into the picture as size reduces to the nano range(Kambhampati, 2021).

Nanotechnology offers the ability to design targetted drug delivery systems that specifically target diseased cells or tissues, thus enhancing the effectiveness of treatments while minimizing side effects on healthy cells. For instance, in cancer treatment, the leaky nature of blood capillaries near tumor sites allows nanocarriers to accumulate locally. Nanocarriers can encapsulate drugs and be surface-modified with unique physicochemical properties, enabling them to selectively interact and bind with target agents. This targeted approach holds promise for more effective and less toxic therapies.(Wong, Sena-Torralba, Álvarez-Diduk, Muthoosamy, & Merkoçi, 2020). The smaller size of nanoscale drug delivery systems also provides advantages, such as overcoming biological barriers like the blood-brain barrier. These nanocarriers can more effectively penetrate tissues, cross cellular membranes, and accumulate at the intended site of action, resulting in elevated drug concentrations and improved treatment outcomes(Kumar et al., 2013).

Nanomaterials for Targeted Drug Delivery

Liposomes and Micelles

Liposomes are spherical vesicles composed of a lipid bilayer, and they can encapsulate drugs of contracsting solubility profiles within them. The lipid backbone can be made up of Phosphatidylcholine (PC), Phosphatidylethanolamine (PE), Phosphatidylserine (PS), or Phosphatidylinositol (PI). To further modify the properties of liposomes, cholesterol, edge activator or ethanol etc can be incorporated in the liposomal backbone. As they are biomimic nature and smaller in size, liposomes can efficiently penetrate cell membranes and can deliver their contents into the intracellular space.

Micelles, on the other hand, are spherical architectural moieties made up surfactants of double chain hydrophobic tail. They consisting of a hydrophobic core surrounded by a hydrophilic shell. This enable micelles to effectively solubilize and transport hydrophobic drugs to cells. Both liposomes and micelles are effective in delivering drugs to cells as they can mimic cellular bodies (Suhaimi et al., 2022) (Aderibigbe, 2017). Micelles can be used to deliver other nanocarriers like carbon dots, nanocrystals or quantum dots. As these nanocarriers are hydrophobic in nature, incorporation of them in micellar structure help in improved distribution of nanocarriers in biological fluids.

However, liposomes and micelles can be easily cleared from the body by the immune system. Another challenge is that they can be taken up by non-target cells, which can lead to side effects. To improve the targetability various ligands like small molecules, antibody fragments, peptides, etc, or surface coatings (stealth liposomes) can be done to avoid immune system clearance and improve the tissue, organ, or cellular targetability. For example, If the objective is to target a virus, opting for an antibody fragment that binds to the virus would be a suitable approach. On the other hand, if the goal is to target bacteria, a selected peptide that binds to a bacterial surface protein would be preferred. The use of ligands to target liposomes to specific cells or tissues can improve the effectiveness of drug delivery and reduce the risk of side effects. A recent example includes the attachment of tuftsin a tetrapeptide on liposomes. They help in targeting the liposomes to a specific site and are found effective against various infections like *tuberculosis, leishmaniasis, malaria, candidiasis* and *cryptococosis* (Khan, 2021).

Polymer Nanoparticles

Polymeric nanoparticles are made by polymerizing monomers together. The monomers can be natural or synthetic, and they can be organic or inorganic (Table 1). Polymeric nanoparticles have a number of advantages over other types of nanoparticles. They are biocompatible and biodegradable in nature. This makes them safe and effective to deliver drugs or other substances to the body. Polymeric nanoparticles are also very versatile. They can be loaded with a variety of functional groups to change their physicochemical behavious and thus they can be tailored to target site. This makes them a valuable tool for a variety of applications (Horvath & Basler, 2023).

Poly(lactic-co-glycolic acid) (PLGA) nanoparticles: PLGA is one of the most widely used biodegradable polymers in nanoparticle formulations. The are made up of lactic acid and glycolic acid copolymer.

Table 1. List of various polymeric nanomaterials based on their origin used in nanotherapeutics

	Natural Polymeric Nanoparticles	Synthetic Polymeric Nanoparticles
Organic Polymers	Chitosan Nanoparticles	PLGA Nanoparticles
	Alginate Nanoparticles	PEGylated Nanoparticles
	Gelatin Nanoparticles	Polyvinyl Alcohol (PVA) Nanoparticles
		Poly(caprolactone) (PCL) Nanoparticles
Inorganic Polymers		Silica Nanoparticles
		Titania Nanoparticles
		Zirconia Nanoparticles

It has been used to encapsulate various antimicrobial agents, such as antibiotics and antiviral drugs, for targeted and sustained release to combat bacterial and viral infections. For instance, a novel nanoparticle delivery system, known as ASP-PLGA-PEI, was developed by encapsulating the immunopotentiator Angelica sinensis polysaccharide (ASP) within Poly(lactic-co-glycolic acid) (PLGA) nanoparticles. To give the nanoparticles a positive charge, they were coated with a cationic polymer, polyethylenimine (PEI). The ASP-PLGA-PEI nanoparticles exhibited significant activation of macrophages, leading to increased expression of Major Histocompatibility Complex class II (MHCII), as well as enhanced production of Interleukins (IL-1β) and cytokines by the macrophages. Moreover, the presence of antigens on the surface of the ASP-PLGA-PEI nanoparticles facilitated antigen uptake by macrophages (Gu et al., 2019).

Chitosan nanoparticles: Chitosan, is a natural polysaccharide derived from chitin, is a natural polymer with excellent biocompatibility and biodegradability. Chitosan nanoparticles have been utilized for delivering antimicrobial peptides, nucleic acids (like siRNA or DNA vaccines), and other drugs for the treatment of various infectious diseases. Chitosan is Generally Recognized as Safe (GRAS) by the U.S. Food and Drug Administration (FDA). Chitosan nanoparticles (NPs) have found applications in drug delivery through various routes, including oral, ocular, pulmonary, nasal, mucosal, buccal, and vaginal administration(Boroumand et al., 2021).

Polymeric micelles: Amphiphilic polymers, such as poly(ethylene glycol)-poly(caprolactone) (PEG-PCL) and poly(ethylene glycol)-poly(lactic acid) (PEG-PLA), can self-assemble into micellar structures. These micelles can be loaded with antimicrobial agents and used to enhance drug delivery to infected sites. The micelles' can be made responsive to stimuli to deliver drug to the target. These stimuli can originate from the tumor microenvironment, such as changes in pH, hypoxia, or upregulated enzymes. Alternatively, external stimuli like light, ultrasound, and temperature can be applied to trigger micellar disassembly, leading to the release of the payload. Some varietyof polymers can be used to add varied functionalities to the micelles. A few hydrophilic and hydrophobic polymers are listed table 2.

Table 2. List of hydrophillic and hydrophobic polymers

Hydrophillic Polymers	Hydrophobic Polymers
Poly(ethylene glycol), poly(oxazolines), chitosan, dextran, and hyaluronic acids.	poly(lactide) (PLA), poly(caprolactone) (PCL), poly(lactide-co-glycolide) (PLGA), polyesters, poly(amino acids), lipids

(Ghosh & Biswas, 2021)

Dendrimers

Dendrimers offer promising potential in the treatment of infectious diseases due to their unique properties and versatility. They can be surface modified to allow controlled release kinetics. By actively targeting infected cells or pathogens, dendrimers enhance drug delivery efficiency, reduce systemic side effects, and increase the concentration of the drug at the infection site. Multivalent interactions provide an additional chance for functional groups to interact with a pathogen, its specific site, or protein. Moreover, they play a role in immunomodulation by engaging with the host's immune system as they increase the immunogenicity of vaccines. Dendrimers can be functionalized with imaging probes to serve as contrast agents in medical imaging techniques(Mhlwatika & Aderibigbe, 2018). Their unique properties, such as their large surface area and high payload capacity and multivalent interactions, enable efficient and accurate imaging of infectious target. This aids in the early detection and monitoring of infectious diseases. The design of dendrimers with multivalent interactions and unique modes of action can help overcome drug resistance mechanisms developed by pathogens. This ability to counteract resistance can improve the effectiveness of existing antimicrobial agents. Dendrimers are highly branched macromolecules with a well-defined structure, resembling a tree-like architecture. They have a core, branches, and terminal functional groups that can be modified for specific applications.

The core of a dendrimer can be made up of a variety of different materials, including metals, organic molecules, and inorganic compounds. The core is typically the first component of the dendrimer to be synthesized, and subsequent branches grow from it. There are several types of dendrimers, but one of the most common classes is the polyamidoamine (PAMAM) dendrimers, which have a well-defined core composed of amine groups and usually ethylenediamine. Other types of dendrimers may have different cores. For example, poly(propyleneimine) (PPI) dendrimers have a central core made of amines and methyl groups, while polyglycerol dendrimers have a core made of glycerol molecules.

Repeating units: The repeating units of a dendrimer are typically made up of monomers that are linked together by covalent bonds. The monomers can be the same or different, and they can be organic or inorganic. the choice of repeating units depends on the desired properties and functionalities of the dendrimer (Table 3). The sequential addition of repeating units allows for precise control over the size, shape, and surface chemistry of dendrimers, making them highly versatile and tunable for various applications in nanomedicine, drug delivery, imaging, and diagnostics.

Terminal functional groups: The terminal functional groups of a dendrimer are the groups that are attached to the outer shell. These groups can be used to attach other molecules, such as drugs, genes, or imaging agents. Usually hydroxyl, carboxyl, amine, polyethylene glycol group, azide, quaternary ammonium compound and sulfhydryl groups are attached.

Nanoemulsions and Nanocrystals

Nanoemulsions are a type of emulsion where small droplets of oil are dispersed in an aqueous medium with the aid of surfactants or emulsifiers. They have a core-shell structure, with the oil droplets encapsulated by surfactant molecules, stabilizing the emulsion (Juneja, Suthar, Pardhi, Ahmad, & Jain, 2022). Whereas, Nanocrystals are solid particles with a crystalline structure. They are typically formed by reducing the size of drug crystals to the nanoscale using techniques such as high-pressure homogenization or wet milling. Surface modifications can render the carrier system to offer better bioavailability, targetability, increase in solubility and improved stability. Nanoemulsions exhibit exceptional stability due

Table 3. Widely used dendrimers and their conjugated repeating units

Poly(amidoamine) (PAMAM) Dendrimers	Ethylenediamine	(Liu, Liang, Sun, Yang, & Cao, 2018)
	Methyl acrylate	
	Acetic anhydride	
	Diaminobutane	
	Ethylene diamine	
Poly(propyleneimine) (PPI) Dendrimers	Aziridine	(Fischer et al., 2010)
	Epichlorohydrin	
	Ethylenediamine	
	Diethylenetriamine	
	N-methyldiethylenetriamine	
Polyether Dendrimers	Ethylene oxide	(Cruz-Hernández, López-Méndez, & Guadarrama, 2022)
	Propylene oxide	
	Glycerol	
Poly(L-lysine) (PLL) Dendrimers	L-lysine	(Palmerston Mendes, Pan, & Torchilin, 2017)
	N,N'-Carbonyldiimidazole (CDI)	
	4-Methylmorpholine (NMM	
Carbosilane Dendrimers	Dihydrosilane	(Kim & Hong, 2009)
	Chloromethylsilane	
	Dendritic amines	

to the presence of surfactants or emulsifiers that prevent droplet coalescence. This stability allows them to remain dispersed for extended periods, even under various environmental conditions. Nanoemulsions can be engineered to be responsive to specific stimuli, such as changes in pH or temperature, enabling site-specific drug delivery. They can also be functionalized with ligands or antibodies to actively target infected tissues or cells, leading to enhanced drug accumulation at the site of infection.

Quantum Dots

Quantum dots (QDs) are semiconducting nanocrystals that have unique optical and electronic properties. Commonly used semiconductor materials for the core include cadmium selenide (CdSe), cadmium sulfide (CdS), indium phosphide (InP), lead selenide (PbSe), and others. QDs can be used to deliver drugs to specific cells or tissues (Matea et al., 2017). This can be done by loading QDs with antibiotics or other drugs and then targeting them to infected cells. The QDs cthe surface modifications can be done to promote directional targeting and thus release the drugs directly to the infected cells, killing the pathogens and preventing the spread of infection. QDs are a promising new technology for the diagnosis, treatment, and imaging of infectious diseases. However, more research is needed to fully understand the safety and efficacy of QDs for these applications (Ganesan & Nagaraaj, 2020).

Graphene Oxide

Graphene oxide, a derivative of graphene, has emerged as a promising material in the field of medical research, particularly in the treatment of infectious pathogens like *Klebsiella pneumoniae* and *P. aeruginosa* (Wu et al., 2017). Researchers have found that graphene oxide exhibits potent antimicrobial activity against a wide range of pathogens, including drug-resistant strains. Its unique properties, such as high surface area and strong oxidative potential, enable it to effectively disrupt bacterial cell membranes and inhibit their growth. A study demonstrated that graphene oxide-based nanocomposites can effectively kill *N. gonorrhoeae* bacteria (Khalil et al., 2020). The nanocomposites were able to penetrate the bacterial cells and disrupt their membrane integrity, leading to bacterial death. Furthermore, graphene oxide has shown promise as a drug delivery system for targeted treatment of infectious diseases. Its large surface area provides ample space for loading and delivering antimicrobial agents directly to infected sites, enhancing therapeutic efficacy while minimizing side effects on healthy tissues. Further studies are needed to determine optimal dosages, long-term safety profiles, and potential interactions with other medications. Nevertheless, the role of graphene oxide in combating infectious diseases like gonorrhea holds significant potential for future medical advancements.

Enhancing Drug Stability and Bioavailability

Drug encapsulation in nanomaterials offers significant advantages in enhancing drug stability and bioavailability. Nanomaterials, such as liposomes, nanoparticles, and nanocrystals, provide a protective environment for the encapsulated drug, leading to improved stability and controlled release. The nanomaterial acts as a barrier, preserving the drug's chemical integrity and therapeutic activity by shielding them from exposure to environmental factors, such as light, heat, and moisture, which can lead to drug degradation. Advantages like improving the solubility of poorly soluble drug with encapsulation in nanoemulsions or lipososmes offer improved bioavailability by improving drug distribution. Encapsulation of drug inside core of nanomaterials help in hiding the labile drug molecule from the environment, thus improving their bioavailability and stability (Colino, Lanao, & Gutierrez-Millan, 2021). Table 4 enlists various nanomaterials used for different infectious disesases to overcome problems like solubility, bioavailability, stability and release profile (Table 4).

Solubility Enhancement

The use of nanomaterials can significantly enhance the solubility of antibiotics, particularly for drugs with poor water solubility. By reducing the drug's particle size to the nanoscale, nanomaterials increase the surface area available for dissolution and improve drug dispersibility in aqueous solutions (Singh, Kruger, Maguire, Govender, & Parboosing, 2017). For example, Nanocrystals of clarithromycin were stabilized with a combination of poloxamer 407 with sodium lauryl sulfate (SLS) and cetyltrimethylammonium bromide giving positive and negative charge to nanocrystals respectively. It was observed that charge greatly affects the stability and dissolution profile of nanocrystals. The nanoscale particles enhance drug dissolution and allow for better drug absorption (Soisuwan, Teeranachaideekul, Wongrakpanich, Langguth, & Junyaprasert, 2019). Azithromycin is a widely used antibiotic, but its hydrophobic nature limits its solubility and bioavailability. Azithromycin-loaded nanoemulsions have been developed to improve drug solubility and enable transdermal permeation to answer skin infections. The emulsifica-

Table 4. Disease specific nanocarriers designed with specific area of improvement

Disease/Aim	Nanocarriers	Improvement	References
Tuberculosis	polymeric nanoparticles, solid lipid nanoparticles, liposomes	To improve plasma drug level and solubility	(Macêdo et al., 2022)
HIV/AIDS	Polymeric dendrimers, polyethylenimine-NPs, poly(lactic-co-glycolic acid)-NPs, chitosan nanoparticles, liposomal-based delivery systems and inorganic NPs, including gold and silver NPs	Enhanced solubility, sustained release, targeting abilities and facilitation of drug-dose reductions	(Asl et al., 2023)
Nanovaccines	Nanoparticles	in vivo instability, high toxicity and no multiple administrations.	(Gheibi Hayat & Darroudi, 2019)
Urinary tract infection	PAMAM dendrimers	Increase solubility and bioavailability	(Gürbüz, Ertürk, & Tülü, 2017)
COVID-19	Nanoparticles	Increase bioavailability, efficiency and decreased toxicity	(Rauf et al., 2022)

tion process increases the surface area of the drug, leading to enhanced dissolution, skin retention, and bioavailability. They also proved to provide prolonged effectiveness against bacterial skin infection (Abruzzo et al., 2022). Rifampicin is an essential antibiotic used to treat tuberculosis, but it has poor water solubility and variable oral bioavailability. Nanoparticles of rifampicin have been developed named mannose-anchored rifampicin-loaded solid lipid nanoparticles. They provided better solubility and better targetability to macrophages. This kills the intracellular pathogen thus offering improved drug delivery to infected tissues (Mistry, Bandyopadhyaya, & Mehra, 2022).

Controlled Release Systems

Controlled release systems of antibiotics using nanomaterials offer several advantages, including sustained drug release, reduced dosing frequency, and improved therapeutic outcomes. Nanomaterials can be engineered to release antibiotics in a controlled manner, ensuring a constant and targeted drug concentration at the infection site. Gentamicin is an aminoglycoside antibiotic used to treat severe bacterial infections. However, its short half-life requires frequent dosing, which can lead to toxicity. Gentamicin-loaded biodegradable polymer nanoparticles have been developed to provide controlled release of the antibiotic. The micronization of gentamicin-anionic surfactant yielded a particulated material by compressed antisolvent and sustained release of the drug over 70 days. These nanoparticles release the drug gradually over an extended period, reducing the need for frequent administration and minimizing systemic side effects. (Imbuluzqueta et al., 2013). Vancomycin is a glycopeptide antibiotic used to treat serious infections caused by methicillin-resistant Staphylococcus aureus (MRSA) and other bacteria. Frequent dosing is required to maintain effective therapeutic levels. Vancomycin-loaded niosomes have been designed to provide controlled release of the drug and giving 180 fold increase in activity as compared to untreated mice eye infection with MRSA strain. Liposomes can release the drug slowly, leading to sustained therapeutic levels and reducing the frequency of administration (Allam, El-Mokhtar, & Elsabahy, 2019). Tetracycline is a broad-spectrum antibiotic used to treat various infections, but its frequent dosing can lead to compliance issues.Tetracycline-loaded nanocrystals have been developed to achieve controlled release of the drug. Nanocrystals slowly release the drug, allowing for less frequent

Table 5. Role of different metallic nanoparticles in infectious disease management

Role of Metallic Nanoparticles in the Treatment of Infectious Diseases	Applications	Mechanisms of Action	References
Antimicrobial Activity	Wound dressings, Topical creams and ointments Implant coatings, Catheter coatings	Induce cell membrane disruption Generate reactive oxygen species (ROS), Interfere with microbial enzymes and DNA	(Kwiatkowska et al., 2022)
Drug Delivery	Oral, intravenous, or targeted drug delivery, Treatment of drug-resistant infections	Enhanced drug bioavailability, Targeted delivery to infected tissues, Overcoming drug resistance	(Allam et al., 2019)
Synergistic Effects with Antibiotics	Combination therapy with antibiotics, Treatment of multidrug-resistant infections	Enhanced antibiotic efficacy, Overcoming antibiotic resistance, Reduced antibiotic dosages	(Mishra et al., 2022)
Imaging and Diagnosis	Diagnostic imaging agents, Detecting pathogens and infections	Strong plasmonic properties for imaging, Specific targeting of pathogens, Improved sensitivity and specificity	(Boisselier & Astruc, 2009)
Biosensors	Rapid and sensitive pathogen detection, Point-of-care testing	Highly specific and sensitive detection, Real-time monitoring of infections	(Proniewicz, 2023)
Immunomodulation	Adjuvants for vaccines, Immune response modulation	Enhancing immune responses, Immunostimulatory effects	(Janic et al., 2021)

dosing and improved patient adherence. The use of Tetracycline-loaded mesoporous silica nanoparticles (MSNs) gel showed significantly lower colony forming units (CFU/ml) than tetracycline gel. When these were tested for periodontal infection, they found to release tetracycline from nanoparticles for a longer time compared to tetracycline gel. (Mirzaali, Dizaj, Shahi, Memar, & Parnia, 2023).

Antimicrobial Properties of Nanomaterials

Metallic Nanoparticles

Metallic nanoparticles, such as silver, copper, and gold nanoparticles, exhibit inherent antimicrobial properties and are even effective against drug-resistant strains. They can directly interact with microorganisms, including bacteria, viruses, and fungi, leading to cell membrane disruption, generation of reactive oxygen species (ROS), and inhibition of microbial growth. Metallic nanoparticles can be used in combination with traditional antibiotics to enhance their efficacy through synergistic action. This result in improved outcomes and may reduce chances of antibiotic resistance development. Some metallic nanoparticles possess strong plasmonic properties (They give different response to different light, due to special optical and electronic properties), making them useful as contrast agents in diagnostic imaging. They can be employed for detecting pathogens and infections in medical imaging and diagnostic techniques. Table 5 elaborates different roles of metallic nanoparticles in infectious disease management. They offer high specificity and sensitivity, making them valuable in point-of-care testing and surveillance of infectious diseases. Some metallic nanoparticles, such as silver and copper, are relatively abundant and cost-effective, which can contribute to their applicability in healthcare settings (Table 5).

Table 6. Applications of metal oxide nanoparticles in infectious disease management

Metal Oxide Nanoparticle	Applications in Infectious Diseases	References
Zinc Oxide (ZnO)	Antimicrobial coatings for medical devices and wound dressings, Antiviral agents, Antifungal treatments	(Pino, Bosco, Mollea, & Onida, 2023)
Copper Oxide (CuO)	Antimicrobial agents in wound dressings and Antiviral treatments, Methicillin resistant strains.	(Balcucho, Narváez, & Castro-Mayorga, 2020)
Titanium Dioxide (TiO_2)	Antimicrobial coatings for Photocatalytic disinfection, UV-protective coatings	(Alizadeh Sani et al., 2022)
Iron Oxide (Fe_2O_3, Fe_3O_4)	Magnetic resonance imaging (MRI) contrast agents, Drug delivery and targeting to infected tissues, Hyperthermia-based therapies	(Avasthi, Caro, Pozo-Torres, Leal, & García-Martín, 2020)
Cerium Oxide (CeO_2)	Antioxidant agents for reducing oxidative stress in infections	(Adebayo, Akinloye, & Adaramoye, 2020)

1.7.2 Metal Oxide Nanoparticles

Metal oxide nanoparticles are nanoscale particles composed of metal and oxygen atoms, forming various metal oxides. These nanoparticles have dimensions typically ranging from 1 to 100 nanometers (nm), making them smaller than 1000 times the diameter of a human hair. Metal oxide nanoparticles have unique physical, chemical, and biological properties due to their small size and high surface area-to-volume ratio. Oxides of various metals like zinc, titanium, copper, iron, magnesium and aluminium are explored for therapeutic management of the disease (Table 6). However, the potential risks associated with their use, such as toxicity and bioaccumulation, necessitate careful consideration and extensive research in their development and application.

SAFETY AND BIOCOMPATIBILITY CONSIDERATIONS

One of the main concerns regarding nanomaterials is their potential toxicity. Nanoparticles can exhibit different behavior from bulk materials due to their small size and large surface area, which can lead to interactions with biological molecules and tissues. For example, gold nanoparticles have shown size-specific toxicity in the human body. At a size of 1.4 nm, they were found to be toxic, but at a particle size of 12 nm, they did not exhibit any toxicity. Similarly, carbon nanotubes have been shown to induce mesothelioma, resembling the toxicity of asbestos, a naturally occurring carcinogenic mineral fiber. This toxicity is attributed to the specific shape of the nanoparticles. It is evident that factors such as shape, size, and surface charge significantly influence the toxicity profile of nanocarriers. To thoroughly understand the potential adverse effects, extensive toxicity studies are essential to assess how nanomaterials may impact cells, organs, and overall physiological processes. Proper evaluation of nanomaterials' safety is critical to ensure their safe application in various fields, including medicine, technology, and environmental applications.

Nanoparticles, owing to their elevated free surface energy, tend to interact with biological fluids, leading to the formation of a protein corona—a layer of proteins surrounding the nanoparticles. This interaction can cause alterations in the shape, size, surface charge, and zeta potential of the nanoparticles. Larger nanoparticles have a greater propensity to interact with biological proteins like albumin and fibrinogen, resulting in a strong binding that can lead to a permanent change in the protein structure. This binding can cause the proteins to unfold, rendering them incapable of fulfilling their biological functions effectively. Nanomaterials can interact with biological barriers, such as the blood-brain barrier, placental barrier, and mucosal barriers..Some nanomaterials like titanium dioxide, zinc oxide, polystyrene, and polycation particles interact with lysosomal membrane and release the proton, ions and hydrolytic enzymes. This causes cellular stress and damage to cellular organelles.

So It is essential to assess how nanomaterials may affect these barriers to ensure their safe application (Wolfram et al., 2015)(Patel & Shah, 2017). Biodegradability is essential for nanomaterials used in medical applications. Biodegradable nanoparticles can be broken down into harmless by-products and excreted from the body, minimizing long-term accumulation and potential adverse effects. Nanomaterials may trigger immune responses in the body, leading to adverse reactions. Biocompatible nanomaterials are designed to minimize immune recognition and reduce the risk of immune-related adverse effects. Change of physicochemical properties in vivo can alter the fate of nanoparticle in the body.

REGULATORY AND ETHICAL ASPECTS

Ensuring the safe application of nanomaterials in medicine requires a thorough understanding of their biocompatibility, potential toxic effects, and ethical considerations. Collaboration between scientists, clinicians, regulatory authorities, and ethicists is vital to harness the full potential of nanotechnology while minimizing risks and ensuring patient safety (Teunenbroek, Baker, & Dijkzeul, 2017).

Nanomedicines, including nanoparticles used for drug delivery, can be more complex than traditional small molecule drugs. They often involve intricate structures, surface modifications, and unique release mechanisms, making their characterization and evaluation more challenging. Defining critical quality attributes (CQA) for nanocarriers becomes crucial, as even minor changes in nanoparticle size, shape, or surface chemistry can impact their safety and performance.

Since the shape, size and surface mophology greatly influence the fate of nanomaterial in the body. Their safety profile need to be critically established to ensure efficient establishment of bioequivalency. Identification of appropriate assays for safety assessment is essential. Building nanoparticle safety libraries that link physicochemical characteristics to hazard potential can significantly enhance the understanding of nanoparticle safety and offer guidance during the initial stages of nanoparticle design. So, Adequate analytical techniques must be employed to ensure accurate characterization and comparability between the nanosimilars and the reference nanotherapeutic product. Standardization of methodologies becomes essential to ensure reproducibility and consistency(Wolfram et al., 2015).

CONCLUSION

Nanomaterials offer many advantages in the therapeutic management of infectious diseases. Due to special optical, electrical and magnetic properties, they are used to serve dual purpose of theranostics.

Polymeric nanoparticles, metallic nanoparticles and various subcategories of nanocrystals have been explored widely for therapeutic improvementof drug molecules. They have the capacity to cross various barriers like immunological clearance, renal clearance, enzymatic and mechanical degradation, vascular endothelium, the extracellular matrix, the cell membrane, the lysosome, and membrane pumps. This is due to nanosize range and special surface modifications provided with the aid of different ligands or functional groups. Nanomaterials can be harnessed to create controlled release systems for antibiotics. The controlled release of antibiotics using nanomaterials offers the potential for more effective and targeted treatment of infections, reducing the development of antibiotic resistance and improving patient outcomes. Allthough discovery of nanomaterials is more than four decade old, still some serious consideration about safety and toxicity of nanomaterials are unmet. More rigorous research and data libraries are needed to make them in comparison to conventional therapies. By adhering to rigorous safety assessments and employing standardized approaches, we can advance the responsible development and application of nanomaterials in medicine.

REFERENCES

Abruzzo, A., Parolin, C., Rossi, M., Vitali, B., Cappadone, C., & Bigucci, F. (2022). Development and Characterization of Azithromycin-Loaded Microemulsions: A Promising Tool for the Treatment of Bacterial Skin Infections. *Antibiotics (Basel, Switzerland)*, *11*(8), 1040. doi:10.3390/antibiotics11081040 PMID:36009909

Adebayo, O. A., Akinloye, O., & Adaramoye, O. A. (2020). Cerium Oxide Nanoparticles Attenuate Oxidative Stress and Inflammation in the Liver of Diethylnitrosamine-Treated Mice. *Biological Trace Element Research*, *193*(1), 214–225. doi:10.100712011-019-01696-5 PMID:30993490

Aderibigbe, B. A. (2017). Polymeric therapeutic delivery systems for the treatment of infectious diseases. *Therapeutic Delivery*, *8*(7), 557–576. doi:10.4155/tde-2017-0008 PMID:28633590

Alizadeh Sani, M., Maleki, M., Eghbaljoo-Gharehgheshlaghi, H., Khezerlou, A., Mohammadian, E., Liu, Q., & Jafari, S. M. (2022). Titanium dioxide nanoparticles as multifunctional surface-active materials for smart/active nanocomposite packaging films. *Advances in Colloid and Interface Science*, *300*, 102593. doi:10.1016/j.cis.2021.102593 PMID:34971916

Allam, A., El-Mokhtar, M. A., & Elsabahy, M. (2019). Vancomycin-loaded niosomes integrated within pH-sensitive in-situ forming gel for treatment of ocular infections while minimizing drug irritation. *The Journal of Pharmacy and Pharmacology*, *71*(8), 1209–1221. doi:10.1111/jphp.13106 PMID:31124593

Asl, F. D., Mousazadeh, M., Taji, S., Bahmani, A., Khashayar, P., Azimzadeh, M., & Mostafavi, E. (2023). Nano drug-delivery systems for management of AIDS: Liposomes, dendrimers, gold and silver nanoparticles. *Nanomedicine (London)*, *18*(3), 279–302. doi:10.2217/nnm-2022-0248 PMID:37125616

Avasthi, A., Caro, C., Pozo-Torres, E., Leal, M. P., & García-Martín, M. L. (2020). Magnetic Nanoparticles as MRI Contrast Agents. *Topics in Current Chemistry (Cham)*, *378*(3), 40. doi:10.100741061-020-00302-w PMID:32382832

Balcucho, J., Narváez, D. M., & Castro-Mayorga, J. L. (2020). Antimicrobial and Biocompatible Polycaprolactone and Copper Oxide Nanoparticle Wound Dressings against Methicillin-Resistant Staphylococcus aureus. *Nanomaterials (Basel, Switzerland)*, *10*(9), 1692. doi:10.3390/nano10091692 PMID:32872095

Boisselier, E., & Astruc, D. (2009). Gold nanoparticles in nanomedicine: Preparations, imaging, diagnostics, therapies and toxicity. *Chemical Society Reviews*, *38*(6), 1759–1782. doi:10.1039/b806051g PMID:19587967

Boroumand, H., Badie, F., Mazaheri, S., Seyedi, Z. S., Nahand, J. S., Nejati, M., Baghi, H. B., Abbasi-Kolli, M., Badehnoosh, B., Ghandali, M., Hamblin, M. R., & Mirzaei, H. (2021). Chitosan-Based Nanoparticles Against Viral Infections. *Frontiers in Cellular and Infection Microbiology*, *11*, 643953. doi:10.3389/fcimb.2021.643953 PMID:33816349

Choi, Y. K. (2021). Emerging and re-emerging fatal viral diseases. *Experimental & Molecular Medicine*, *53*(5), 711–712. doi:10.103812276-021-00608-9 PMID:33953321

Colino, C. I., Lanao, J. M., & Gutierrez-Millan, C. (2021). Recent advances in functionalized nanomaterials for the diagnosis and treatment of bacterial infections. *Materials Science and Engineering C*, *121*, 111843. doi:10.1016/j.msec.2020.111843 PMID:33579480

Cruz-Hernández, C., López-Méndez, L. J., & Guadarrama, P. (2022). Dendronization: A practical strategy to improve the performance of molecular systems used in biomedical applications. *European Journal of Medicinal Chemistry*, *229*, 113988. doi:10.1016/j.ejmech.2021.113988 PMID:34801269

Fischer, M., Appelhans, D., Schwarz, S., Klajnert, B., Bryszewska, M., Voit, B., & Rogers, M. (2010). Influence of surface functionality of poly(propylene imine) dendrimers on protease resistance and propagation of the scrapie prion protein. *Biomacromolecules*, *11*(5), 1314–1325. doi:10.1021/bm100101s PMID:20405854

Ganesan, M., & Nagaraaj, P. (2020). Quantum dots as nanosensors for detection of toxics: A literature review. *Analytical Methods*, *12*(35), 4254–4275. doi:10.1039/D0AY01293A PMID:32940270

Gheibi Hayat, S. M., & Darroudi, M. (2019). Nanovaccine: A novel approach in immunization. *Journal of Cellular Physiology*, *234*(8), 12530–12536. doi:10.1002/jcp.28120 PMID:30633361

Ghosh, B., & Biswas, S. (2021). Polymeric micelles in cancer therapy: State of the art. *Journal of Controlled Release*, *332*, 127–147. doi:10.1016/j.jconrel.2021.02.016 PMID:33609621

Gu, P., Wusiman, A., Wang, S., Zhang, Y., Liu, Z., Hu, Y., Liu, J., & Wang, D. (2019). Polyethylenimine-coated PLGA nanoparticles-encapsulated Angelica sinensis polysaccharide as an adjuvant to enhance immune responses. *Carbohydrate Polymers*, *223*, 115128. doi:10.1016/j.carbpol.2019.115128 PMID:31427012

Gürbüz, M. U., Ertürk, A. S., & Tülü, M. (2017). Synthesis of surface-modified TREN-cored PAMAM dendrimers and their effects on the solubility of sulfamethoxazole (SMZ) as an analog antibiotic drug. *Pharmaceutical Development and Technology*, *22*(5), 678–689. doi:10.1080/10837450.2016.1221425 PMID:27493125

Horvath, D., & Basler, M. (2023). PLGA Particles in Immunotherapy. *Pharmaceutics*, *15*(2), 615. doi:10.3390/pharmaceutics15020615 PMID:36839937

Imbuluzqueta, E., Gamazo, C., Lana, H., Campanero, M. Á., Salas, D., Gil, A. G., Elizondo, E., Ventosa, N., Veciana, J., & Blanco-Prieto, M. J. (2013). Hydrophobic gentamicin-loaded nanoparticles are effective against Brucella melitensis infection in mice. *Antimicrobial Agents and Chemotherapy*, *57*(7), 3326–3333. doi:10.1128/AAC.00378-13 PMID:23650167

Janic, B., Brown, S. L., Neff, R., Liu, F., Mao, G., Chen, Y., Jackson, L., Chetty, I. J., Movsas, B., & Wen, N. (2021). Therapeutic enhancement of radiation and immunomodulation by gold nanoparticles in triple negative breast cancer. *Cancer Biology & Therapy*, *22*(2), 124–135. doi:10.1080/15384047.2020.1861923 PMID:33459132

Juneja, M., Suthar, T., Pardhi, V. P., Ahmad, J., & Jain, K. (2022). Emerging trends and promises of nanoemulsions in therapeutics of infectious diseases. *Nanomedicine (London)*, *17*(11), 793–812. doi:10.2217/nnm-2022-0006 PMID:35587031

Kambhampati, P. (2021). Nanoparticles, Nanocrystals, and Quantum Dots: What are the Implications of Size in Colloidal Nanoscale Materials? *The Journal of Physical Chemistry Letters*, *12*(20), 4769–4779. doi:10.1021/acs.jpclett.1c00754 PMID:33984241

Khalil, W. F., El-Sayyad, G. S., El Rouby, W. M. A., Sadek, M. A., Farghali, A. A., & El-Batal, A. I. (2020). Graphene oxide-based nanocomposites (GO-chitosan and GO-EDTA) for outstanding antimicrobial potential against some Candida species and pathogenic bacteria. *International Journal of Biological Macromolecules*, *164*, 1370–1383. doi:10.1016/j.ijbiomac.2020.07.205 PMID:32735925

Khan, M. A. (2021). Targeted Drug Delivery Using Tuftsin-bearing Liposomes: Implications in the Treatment of Infectious Diseases and Tumors. *Current Drug Targets*, *22*(7), 770–778. doi:10.2174/1389450121999201125200756 PMID:33243117

Kim, C., & Hong, J. H. (2009). Carbosilane and carbosiloxane dendrimers. *Molecules (Basel, Switzerland)*, *14*(9), 3719–3730. doi:10.3390/molecules14093719 PMID:19783954

Kumar, A., Chen, F., Mozhi, A., Zhang, X., Zhao, Y., Xue, X., Hao, Y., Zhang, X., Wang, P. C., & Liang, X.-J. (2013). Innovative pharmaceutical development based on unique properties of nanoscale delivery formulation. *Nanoscale*, *5*(18), 8307–8325. doi:10.1039/c3nr01525d PMID:23860639

Kwiatkowska, A., Drabik, M., Lipko, A., Grzeczkowicz, A., Stachowiak, R., Marszalik, A., & Granicka, L. H. (2022). Composite Membrane Dressings System with Metallic Nanoparticles as an Antibacterial Factor in Wound Healing. *Membranes*, *12*(2), 215. doi:10.3390/membranes12020215 PMID:35207136

Liu, S., Liang, H., Sun, T., Yang, D., & Cao, M. (2018). A recoverable dendritic polyamidoamine immobilized TEMPO for efficient catalytic oxidation of cellulose. *Carbohydrate Polymers*, *202*, 563–570. doi:10.1016/j.carbpol.2018.09.016 PMID:30287037

Macêdo, D. C. D. S., Cavalcanti, I. D. L., Medeiros, S. M., Souza, J. B., Lira Nogueira, M. C. B., & Cavalcanti, I. M. F. (2022). Nanotechnology and tuberculosis: An old disease with new treatment strategies. *Tuberculosis (Edinburgh, Scotland)*, *135*, 102208. doi:10.1016/j.tube.2022.102208 PMID:35567896

Matea, C. T., Mocan, T., Tabaran, F., Pop, T., Mosteanu, O., Puia, C., Iancu, C., & Mocan, L. (2017). Quantum dots in imaging, drug delivery and sensor applications. *International Journal of Nanomedicine*, *12*, 5421–5431. doi:10.2147/IJN.S138624 PMID:28814860

Mhlwatika, Z., & Aderibigbe, B. A. (2018). Application of Dendrimers for the Treatment of Infectious Diseases. *Molecules (Basel, Switzerland)*, *23*(9), 2205. doi:10.3390/molecules23092205 PMID:30200314

Mirzaali, F., Dizaj, S. M., Shahi, S., Memar, M. Y., & Parnia, F. (2023). The Antibacterial Effect of Tetracycline-loaded Mesoporous Silica Nanoparticles in the Gingival Fluid at Implant-abutment Junction: A Randomized Clinical Trial Study. *Pharmaceutical Nanotechnology*, *11*(2), 208–216. doi:10.2174/2211738511666230106151403 PMID:36617708

Mishra, A., Pradhan, D., Halder, J., Biswasroy, P., Rai, V. K., Dubey, D., Kar, B., Ghosh, G., & Rath, G. (2022). Metal nanoparticles against multi-drug-resistance bacteria. *Journal of Inorganic Biochemistry*, *237*, 111938. doi:10.1016/j.jinorgbio.2022.111938 PMID:36122430

Mistry, N., Bandyopadhyaya, R., & Mehra, S. (2022). Enhancement of Antimycobacterial Activity of Rifampicin Using Mannose-Anchored Lipid Nanoparticles against Intramacrophage Mycobacteria. *ACS Applied Bio Materials*, *5*(12), 5779–5789. doi:10.1021/acsabm.2c00796 PMID:36441965

Nii-Trebi, N. I. (2017). Emerging and Neglected Infectious Diseases: Insights, Advances, and Challenges. *BioMed Research International*, *5245021*, 1–15. doi:10.1155/2017/5245021 PMID:28286767

Palmerston Mendes, L., Pan, J., & Torchilin, V. P. (2017). Dendrimers as Nanocarriers for Nucleic Acid and Drug Delivery in Cancer Therapy. *Molecules (Basel, Switzerland)*, *22*(9), 1401. doi:10.3390/molecules22091401 PMID:28832535

Patel, P., & Shah, J. (2017). Safety and Toxicological Considerations of Nanomedicines: The Future Directions. *Current Clinical Pharmacology*, *12*(2), 73–82. doi:10.2174/1574884712666170509161252 PMID:28486906

Pino, P., Bosco, F., Mollea, C., & Onida, B. (2023). Antimicrobial Nano-Zinc Oxide Biocomposites for Wound Healing Applications: A Review. *Pharmaceutics*, *15*(3), 970. doi:10.3390/pharmaceutics15030970 PMID:36986831

Proniewicz, E. (2023). Metallic nanoparticles as effective sensors of bio-molecules. *Spectrochimica Acta. Part A: Molecular and Biomolecular Spectroscopy*, *288*, 122207. doi:10.1016/j.saa.2022.122207 PMID:36502763

Rauf, A., Abu-Izneid, T., Khalil, A. A., Hafeez, N., Olatunde, A., Rahman, M., Semwal, P., Al-Awthan, Y. S., Bahattab, O. S., Khan, I. N., Khan, M. A., & Sharma, R. (2022). Nanoparticles in clinical trials of COVID-19: An update. *International Journal of Surgery*, *104*, 106818. doi:10.1016/j.ijsu.2022.106818 PMID:35953020

Singh, L., Kruger, H. G., Maguire, G. E. M., Govender, T., & Parboosing, R. (2017). The role of nanotechnology in the treatment of viral infections. *Therapeutic Advances in Infectious Disease*, *4*(4), 105–131. doi:10.1177/2049936117713593 PMID:28748089

Soisuwan, S., Teeranachaideekul, V., Wongrakpanich, A., Langguth, P., & Junyaprasert, V. B. (2019). Impact of uncharged and charged stabilizers on in vitro drug performances of clarithromycin nanocrystals. *European Journal of Pharmaceutics and Biopharmaceutics : Official Journal of Arbeitsgemeinschaft Fur Pharmazeutische Verfahrenstechnik e.V, 137*, 68–76. doi:10.1016/j.ejpb.2019.02.004

Suhaimi, N. A. A., Ahmad, S., Husna, S. M. N., Elena Sarmiento, M., Acosta, A., Norazmi, M. N., Ibrahim, J., Mohamud, R., & Kadir, R. (2022). Application of liposomes in the treatment of infectious diseases. *Life Sciences*, *305*, 120734. doi:10.1016/j.lfs.2022.120734 PMID:35760094

Van Teunenbroek, T., Baker, J., & Dijkzeul, A. (2017). Towards a more effective and efficient governance and regulation of nanomaterials. *Particle and Fibre Toxicology*, *14*(1), 54. doi:10.118612989-017-0235-z PMID:29258600

Wolfram, J., Zhu, M., Yang, Y., Shen, J., Gentile, E., Paolino, D., Fresta, M., Nie, G., Chen, C., Shen, H., Ferrari, M., & Zhao, Y. (2015). Safety of Nanoparticles in Medicine. *Current Drug Targets*, *16*(14), 1671–1681. doi:10.2174/1389450115666140804124808 PMID:26601723

Wong, X. Y., Sena-Torralba, A., Álvarez-Diduk, R., Muthoosamy, K., & Merkoçi, A. (2020). Nanomaterials for Nanotheranostics: Tuning Their Properties According to Disease Needs. *ACS Nano*, *14*(3), 2585–2627. doi:10.1021/acsnano.9b08133 PMID:32031781

Wu, X., Tan, S., Xing, Y., Pu, Q., Wu, M., & Zhao, J. X. (2017). Graphene oxide as an efficient antimicrobial nanomaterial for eradicating multi-drug resistant bacteria in vitro and in vivo. *Colloids and Surfaces. B, Biointerfaces*, *157*, 1–9. doi:10.1016/j.colsurfb.2017.05.024 PMID:28554055

Chapter 8
Nanomaterials in Cancer Therapy

Jayasree S. Kanathasan
https://orcid.org/0000-0001-7509-6746
Lincoln University College, Malaysia

Devi Nallappan
https://orcid.org/0000-0003-2673-5614
Lincoln University College, Malaysia

Sandeep Poddar
https://orcid.org/0000-0001-9771-877X
Lincoln University College, Malaysia

Andrew Ware
https://orcid.org/0000-0001-8596-2601
University of South Wales, Australia

ABSTRACT

Nanotechnology has been applied in healthcare to cure diseases, especially cancer. Cancer is one of the heterogenous diseases which lacks symptoms in the early stage thus has made it difficult to cure at a later stage. Despite early detection, effective treatment is regarded as one of the major solutions to cure cancer. Nanomaterials play a prominent role in enhancing or replacing conventional treatments with specific and less-toxic drug delivery or therapy. The requirement and properties of nanomaterials as well as their applications in cancer therapies are discussed in this chapter. Various types of nanoparticles are available on the bench side, but these nanoparticles may lack effectiveness to treat cancer using a single treatment mode. Hence, this chapter also explores the applications of various types of hybrid nanoparticles used in multiple therapies as they have shown more effective and safer outcomes for cancer patients. The combination of cancer therapies and their successes have been discussed in this chapter which is the cutting-edge applications of cancer treatment today.

DOI: 10.4018/979-8-3693-0448-8.ch008

INTRODUCTION

Cancer is one of the recalcitrant diseases which has a poor prognosis. It has a very low survival rate due to a lack of symptoms at the early stages (Murakami et al., 2019). Although variable leading treatment techniques are available, it is still cumbersome to treat cancer owing to the morphologies of the tumor microenvironment. Most of the tumors develop resistance towards cancer drugs due to their localization within the highly dense stroma. In addition, tumors become aggressive and metastasize to other organs at advanced stages not showing symptoms at the early stages. Despite being the most renowned treatment modalities, currently, available treatment options including chemotherapy and radiotherapy have been showing systemic adverse effects and side effects leading to healthy cells getting affected by exposure to the drugs or radiation. This creates a huge negative impact on the cancer patient's quality of life. The feeling of discomfort and complications arising from the therapy leads to a weakened immune system and makes their body not ready for the next therapy and resulting in the patients may give up on continuing these treatment options. Hence, a more sensitive and localized tumor treatment modality is expected to combat the currently existing challenges in treating a tumor. Despite the conventional tumor treatment modalities, a more specific and efficient treatment modality is desirable to gain access to the tumor microenvironment. Nanomedicine has been shown as an effective solution for localized treatment of the therapeutic agents in the tumor microenvironment owing to the excellent properties of the nanomaterials in cancer therapy (Govindan et al., 2023).

Applications of nanomaterials are diverse in treating chronic diseases, especially cancer. Its nanoscale size and excellent physicochemical properties enable it to be highly studied as a nanocarrier in drug delivery and targeted cancer therapy. Nanomaterial-based cancer medication faces leap progress from bench to bedside. Nanomaterials can be applied to target the tumour tissues via active and passive targeting. Passive targeting of nanomaterials involves their accumulation at the tumour tissues owing to their nanoscale and physicochemical properties (Bazak et al., 2015). This is because the distorted or abnormal vasculature system at the tumour region enables the accumulation of the nanosized nanomaterials at the tumour region. While active targeting of nanomaterials refers to specific targeting of the nanoparticle functionalised with biological components including antibody, peptide and protein component of nanoparticles to the compatible receptor of the overexpressed biomarker on the tumour region (Attia et al., 2019). There are some advantages offered by nanomaterials owing to their small size. One of them is their ability to escape the renal clearance system (Mundekkad & Cho, 2022). Escaping the kidney filtration system improves the half life of the nanoparticle in the blood circulation. In addition, the high surface-to-volume ratio makes it to be loaded with many biological compounds (Vinhas et al., 2017). Physicochemical properties such as pH, surface charge and hydrophilicity of the nanoparticles can be modified to make them as a more feasible carrier of therapeutic compounds.

There are various types of nanomaterial including organic, polymeric, semiconductor, magnetic and metals available in cancer nanomedicine, thanks to their respective abilities in aiding cancer treatment such as chemotherapy, radiotherapy, gene therapy, immunotherapy, photothermal and photodynamic therapy (Ali et al., 2022). Each type of nanomaterial can be used for varying purposes in cancer therapy. Organic nanomaterials such as liposomes have higher solubility and bioavailability in physiological environments which exhibit reduced toxicity towards living cells. Biodegradable nanomaterials such as carbon and silicon are widely studied nanomaterials, especially in brain tumours owing to several advantages posed by them such as their tuneable surface, non-toxic and longer half-life as they degrade at a slower rate compared to the organic nanomaterials which improved sustained release of drugs (Kashyap et al., 2023). Semiconductor and metal nanomaterials pose multifunctional properties as they can be occupied as theragnostic agents because of their fluorescence properties that enable live tracking of the therapeutic agent in living organisms.

Concerning improving the therapeutic effectiveness of cancer, it is important to note that the therapeutic agent can be combined with this nanoparticle system to specifically locate the target region for maximum delivery of the therapeutic agents at the tumour region. The expression of tumor biomarkers by the tumor cells creates an alarming situation in the physiological system. Hence, these biomarkers play a major role in aggravating tumor by contributing to the tumour growth (Edgington-Mitchell et al., 2017). A study by Yan et al. reported that functionalized porous silicon nanoparticle system which targets the biomarkers at the tumour region has reduced the metastatic rate of pancreatic ductal adenocarcinoma (Yan et al., 2018). Cancer cells' survival in human tissues and animal models has been linked to increased expression of apoptosis regulator of B-cell lymphoma-2 (BCL-2) and phosphoinositide 3-kinase (PI3K) signalling (Sun et al, 2020). Exosomes which are nanosized vesicles also serve an important role in cell regulation by controlling cell cycle and uncontrolled cell growth which leads to cancer. Hence, nanomaterials are regarded as one of the versatile tools used at the molecular level to target the tumor microenvironment. This chapter highlights the recent applications of various types of nanomaterials in cancer therapy.

In this chapter, the superior and exceptional properties of the nanomaterials which contribute to their immense roles in cancer therapy is reviewed. The various types of nanomaterials including organic, liposomal, polymeric, magnetic, semiconductor and metal-based nanomaterials available in cancer therapeutics will be explored. The applications of nanomaterials in the respective treatment modalities include (a) chemotherapy, (b) radiation therapy, (c) photothermal therapy, (d) photodynamic therapy, (e) gene therapy and (f) immunotherapy will be explored. Combination therapies which lead to enhanced tumour therapy are also explored. Moreover, the implications of Artificial Intelligence (AI) and artificial neural network-guided nanomedicine in the heightened efficacy of cancer therapy will be discussed in this chapter. This chapter which covers the current trends in applications as well as safety concerns of nanomaterials in cancer therapy is aimed to be a great source of basic and advanced knowledge for academia and industry professionals as well as policymakers who are interested to get themselves updated with the latest advances in nanomaterials in the field of biomedical sciences, especially cancer nanomedicine.

SUPERIOR QUALITIES OF NANOMATERIALS IN CANCER THERAPY

For the past several decades, nanomaterials hold significant hope to improve the diagnosis as well as treatment of cancer by resolving the challenges faced in the conventional delivery of drugs and therapeutics via chemotherapy and radiotherapy. One of the challenges faced by conventional cancer treatment is to overcome the cellular barrier and distribute the therapeutic compound at the target region via intracellular trafficking (Mitchell et al., 2021). The physical barriers faced in the delivery of nanoparticles include the blood-brain barrier, endothelial lining of blood vessels, tight epithelial cell layers and diffusion through the cytoplasm (Tharkar et al., 2019). Thus, some of the important requirements to be met by the nanomaterial in cancer treatment include specific targeting, improved biodistribution, longer bioavailability and better safety and efficacy.

Nanomaterials facilitate targeted drug delivery and effective anticancer therapy in cancer treatment. Compared to microparticles, nanoparticles are safer and biodegradable, making them a better option for cancer therapy (Cheng et al., 2021). Nanomaterials within the size range from tens to hundreds are known to be the most effective in light-to-heat therapy concerning their ability to evade the reticuloendothelial system (RES) (Hashimoto et al., 2012). The use of ultrasound in the production of nanoparticles improves the effectiveness of drug delivery with reduced side effects by improving the ability to overcome barriers in cancer therapy. Ultrasonic-sensitive polymeric nanoparticles have become an effective tool for cancer diagnosis and treatment. Tumor-induced angiogenesis produces immature vasculatures which block the lymphatic outflow as the tumour grows. Targeted cells can be accessed by nanoparticles due to reduced lymphatic drainage. The passive targeting of nanoparticles is heavily reliant on the increased permeability and retention effect characterised by distorted vasculature in the tumour microenvironment (Zhu et al., 2022).

Biocompatibility of the nanoparticles can be improved by conducting surface modifications using organic biomimetic biomolecules including protein, glycoproteins and peptides to the nanomaterials in cancer therapy (He et al., 2022). Paclitaxel has poor solubility despite being a strong inhibitor of microtubule growth, which causes capillary embolisms and quick drug aggregation. By encasing such drugs in micelles, their solubility can be raised to 0.0015–2 mg/ml (Majumder et al., 2020). Magnetic nanomaterials are often combined with a polymer matrix to improve the effective delivery of therapeutic drugs by improving the water solubility and bioavailability of the polymer coating to the polymer-magnetic hybrid nanostructures (Hu & Liu, 2015; Diaconu et al., 2019). Nanomaterials are used to deliver genes along with anticancer medications through gene therapy. The positive charges within the structure of cationic polymeric nanomaterials allow them to interact with anionic genetic material and attach to DNA to form polyplexes, which are smaller and more resistant to destruction than other polymers.

Particle size, surface charge, shape, and hydrophobicity are all important factors in how quickly nanoparticles reach their lymph node targets. It is also possible to use active transport to disperse nanoparticles more evenly by coating them with chemical ligands, such as mannose. The surface charge of the carrier has a substantial impact on immune response induction and cellular internalization (Foged et al., 2005). Moreover, both diagnosis and treatment can be carried out concurrently by using a theragnostic approach. Recently, novel theragnostic materials known as fluorescent polymeric nanoparticles have been discovered (Indoria et al., 2020). A fluorescent polymeric nanoparticle typically consists of fluorescent proteins, biocompatible biopolymers, inorganic quantum dots, and organic dyes. In fluorescence assays, drugs can be loaded by a π–π bond or hydrophobic interactions, increasing the anti-cancer efficiency of nanomedicine (Andreiuk et al., 2017; Kang et al., 2018). A peptide-protein docking simulation study has found that amongst the two types of similar peptides with varying orientations of linear and Y-shaped, the peptide in a linear orientation demonstrated enhanced binding efficiency towards a legumain, a tumour biomarker that was shown to be overexpressed in human and animal breast cancer cells (Kanathasan et al., 2020).

However, the nanoparticles pose a major challenge in heterogeneity in terms of the behaviour and functionality towards the patient's body (Blanco et al., 2015). Amongst the various types of nanomaterials discovered on the bench side, only a few of them are under consideration for bedside use in cancer treatment. This is due to the lack of understanding of the tumour microenvironment which may lead to alteration of the properties exhibited by the nanoparticles in the diseased tissue (Mitchell et al., 2021). One of the possible methods to improve the efficacy is by using combination therapies using nanomaterials owing to the limitations faced by single therapies. The combination of several therapies like chemotherapy, magnetic field and photothermal therapy effectively reduced metastasis in breast cancer (Govindan et al., 2023). Hyperthermia has been shown to treat various types of cancer, including brain

Figure 1. The types of nanomaterials used in various cancer therapies and the combination therapies that have been used in cancer treatment using nanoparticles

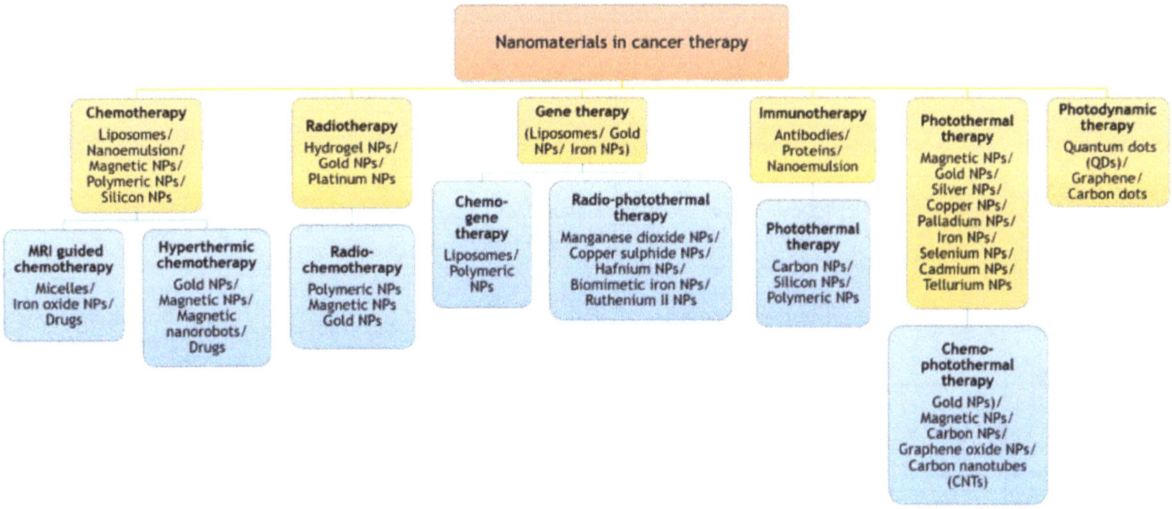

tumours and melanoma (Crezee et al., 2021). Hyperthermia is known to be effective when used in combination with other therapies including chemotherapy, radiation and magnetic field (Jha et al., 2016). Figure 1 shows the types of nanoparticles that have been used in cancer therapies and the combination therapies that have been occupied for better efficiency in cancer treatment.

VARIABLE TYPES OF NANOMATERIALS IN CANCER THERAPEUTICS

There are many nanomedicines have been approved by Food and Drug Administration (FDA), as there are about 13 of them were approved by the year 2015 (Malviya et al., 2021). Out of the nanomedicines in clinical trials, it is important to note that 53% of them are on cancer treatment (Shan et al., 2022). Among the different types of nanomedicines in clinical trials, 33% of them are lipid-based nanomaterials or liposomes, 15% of them are antibody-drug conjugates, 10% accounts for polymer nanoparticles and the remaining 10% is for polymer-drug or polymer-protein conjugations. Nanomaterial-based formulations have made their roles in the global pharmaceutical and healthcare as they have more than 100 of them approved by FDA and the European Medicines Agency (EMA). The transition of nanocarriers with approved drugs into clinical trials for the investigation of their efficiency shows the success of nanomaterials as a carrier. The nanomaterials which are approved by the FDA or EMA have been shown in Table 1.

Lipid-based nanomaterial research gains attention in cancer treatment. Phospholipid bilayer in the lipid-based nanomaterials enables to carry both hydrophilic and hydrophobic therapeutic compounds through the system. Lipid-based nanoparticles have many advantages including easy preparation, better bioavailability and biocompatibility and delivery of higher doses at the tumour region (Fonseca-Santos et al., 2015; Sercombe et al., 2015). The central cavity of liposome protects drugs from degradation thus reducing the multi-drug resistance which hinders the interaction of drugs to the tumour microenvironment (Samad et al., 2007, Zhang et al., 2008). Cancer drugs including paclitaxel, mitoxantrone, doxorubicin,

Table 1. List of FDA or EMA approved nanomaterials in cancer therapy

Type of nanomaterial	Product name	Therapeutic agent used	Company	Indication (s)	References
Liposome	Doxil®	Doxorubicin hydrochloride	Johnson and Johnson	Metastatic ovarian cancer, HIV-associated Kaposi's sarcoma	James (1995); Baren-holz (2012)
Liposome	DaunoXome®	Daunorubicin citrate	Galen Ltd	HIV-associated Kaposi's sarcoma	Gill P. S. et al., (1996)
PEGylated liposome	Caelyx®	Doxorubicin hydrochloride	Jansen Pharmaceutica NV	Metastatic breast cancer, ovarian cancer, Kaposi's sarcoma	Ranson et al., 2001
Liposome	Myocet®	Doxorubicin hydrochloride and an anthracycline cytotoxic agent	Teva Pharmaceutical Industries Ltd	Metastatic breast cancer	Brucker et al., (2016)
Liposome	Mepact®	Mifamurtide	Takeda France SAS	High grade non-metastatic osteosarcoma and myosarcoma	Frampton (2010)
Liposome	Marqibo®	Vincristine	Talon therapeutics	Philadelphia chromosome-negative acute lymphoblastic leukemia in adult patients	Silverman and Deithcher (2013)
Liposome	Lipodox®	Doxorubicin hydrochloride	Sun Pharmaceutical Industries Ltd (SPIL)	Kaposi's sarcoma, ovarian cancer, multiple myeloma	Chou et al. (2015)
Liposome	Onivyde®	Irinotecan	Merrimack Pharmaceuticals	Metastatic pancreatic cancer	Milano et al. (2022)
Liposome	Lipusu®	Paclitaxel	Luye Pgarna	Lung squamous cell carcinoma	Zhang et al. (2022)
Polymer-based nanomaterial	Oncaspar®	L-asparaginase	Enzon Pharamceuticals Inc	Acute lymphoblastic leukemia	Ettinger (1995)
Micelle	Genexol-PM®	Paclitaxel	Lupin Ltd	Breast cancer	Oerlemans et al. (2010)
Micelle	Apealea®	Paclitaxel	Oasmia Pharmaceutical AB	Ovarian cancer, peritonial cancer, fallopian tube cancer	Borga et al. (2019)
Hafnium oxide nanoparticles	Hensify®	Hafnium oxide	Nanobiotix	Locally advanced squamous cell carcinoma	Bonvalot et al. (2019)
Engineered fusion protein nanoparticle	Ontak®	Denileukin diftitox	Eisai Co., Ltd	Leukemia, T cell lymphoma	Duvic and Talpur (2008)
Albumin nanoparticle	Abraxane®	Paclitaxel	Eli Lilly	Metastatic breast cancer	Yuan et al. (2020)

irinotecan, daunorubicin and cytarabine are utilised in conjunction with liposome administration (Zeghoud et al., 2023). Lipid-based nanomaterials such as liposomes are most commonly approved by FDA include (Anselmo et al., 2019). Some of them include Doxil® and DaunoXome® to treat HIV-related Kaposi sarcoma (Cainelli & Vallone, 2009), Marqibo® to treat acute lymphoblastic leukemia and Onivyde® to treat metastatic pancreatic cancer. Advanced solid tumours were found to respond better to liposomes containing floxuridine and irinotecan.

Moreover, certain liposomes can release medications based on the pH level, as malignant parts are more acidic than healthy tissues. A pH-sensitive substance was used to make pH-sensitive cationic liposomes. For instance, the surface of the cationic liposome, which was preloaded with sorafenib and siRNA and coated with pH-sensitive carboxymethyl chitosan results in improved sorafenib release and cellular absorption at a pH of 6.5. (Yao et al., 2015). PEGylated liposome containing cobimetinib and NCL-240 was demonstrated to show a reduced cytotoxic profile and greater synergic effectiveness against colon carcinoma cells (Sriraman et al., 2015). Solid lipid nanoparticles are another type of lipid-based nanoparticles composed of solid components including emulsifiers, triglycerides, fatty acids, and PEGylated lipids (Ali et al., 2021). Lipid-based nanoparticles have been highly studied in cancer nanomedicine owing to a higher loading capacity of lipophilic drugs and can be delivered via a variety of routes including oral, inhalational, parenteral and ophthalmic (Selvamuthukumar & Velmurugan, 2012; Iqbal et al., 2012).

Lipid-based nanomaterials are most suitable for gene delivery owing to their components including ionizable positively charged lipids that aid endosomal escape and phospholipid bilayers and cholesterol which provides the stability of the nanostructures (Cheng et al., 2016). Liposome which carries multilayer siRNA molecules and doxorubicin has improved the efficacy of the drug, reducing the tumour bulk in breast cancer (Batist et al., 2009; Deng et al., 2013). However, a major challenge posed by lipid-based nanomaterials includes the entrapment by the reticuloendothelial system which require the surface modifications such as PEGylation and additions of inorganic or biomimetic nanostructures.

Polymeric nanoparticles are composed of colloidal organic macromolecules at submicron sizes between 10 and 1000 nm which possess a high surface-to-volume ratio. They serve as drug carriers by delivering chemical drugs to malignant sites. Polymeric nanomaterials consist of natural or synthetic materials which makes them a great option for drug delivery to malignant tumours thanks to their biocompatibility and simple preparation (Mitchell et al., 2021; Cheng et al., 2021). There are several types of polymeric nanoparticles including polymersome, dendrimer, polymer micelle and nanosphere. The unique properties of polymeric nanoparticles include biocompatibility, hydrophilicity, biodegradability, colloidal stability and flexibility owing to their chemical structures which create space for various types of surface modifications and conjugation of hydrophobic and hydrophilic compounds (Zhang et al., 2020). Among the FDA-approved polymeric nanomaterials include Oncaspar® which is used to treat acute lymphoblastic leukemia, Eligard® to treat prostate cancer and Abraxane® which was used in the treatment of lung cancer, metastatic breast cancer and metastatic pancreatic cancer.

One of the properties exhibited by polymeric nanoparticles like polymersomes includes better stability and retention of the drug compound (Rideau et al., 2018). While polymeric nanomaterials such as polymeric micelles and dendrimers are used to load various types of molecules owing to the presence of active functional groups on the exterior of the nanostructures (Liu et al., 2020). The charged form of polymers and polyelectrolytes such as Poly(ethylenimine) (PEI) and poly(amidoamine) (PAMAM) has gained attention for the development of pH-sensitive nanomaterials which results in improved bioavailability and mucosal transport (Cao et al., 2019; Tian et al., 2018). Despite their easily modified surface characteristics, the stability and toxicity issues of these polymeric nanomaterials are questionable in the physiological environment (Anselmo et al., 2019).

Dendrimers are unique nanoarchitectures with distinctive features including monodispersed unimicellar nature, a nanometric size range, and a spherical three-dimensional shape. Several dendrimers, including polypropylenimine, polyamidoamine (PAMAM), triethanolamine, 5-and aminolevulinic acid have been studied for cancer therapy by aligning ligands on their surfaces (Lo et al., 2013). The biocompatibility of dendrimers facilitates the administration of potent drugs such as doxorubicin. Dendrimers have been extensively studied for the delivery of contrast agents for magnetic resonance imaging because the surface coating of the gold nanoparticles with dendrimers lowered the toxicity of the gold nanoparticles without affecting their size. In addition, it serves as a ligand that binds to high-affinity targeting molecules in the tumour microenvironment (Kher & Kumar, 2022). Dendrimers have also been used for co-delivery of an essential component of the apoptotic pathway, the Tumor Necrosis Factor (TNF)-related apoptosis-inducing ligand (TRAIL) and doxorubicin in the treatment of colon cancer. The TRAIL and doxorubicin-loaded dendrimers demonstrated improved anticancer effects in comparison to modified carriers containing just the TRAIL or doxorubicin plasmids (Pishavar et al., 2019).

Protein molecules such as antibodies and peptides can be used to target the tumour through tumour immunotherapy. Monoclonal antibody (mAbs)-functionalized nanoparticles have been widely used in targeted cancer therapy owing to their specific targeting ability to the overexpressed receptors or biomarkers at the tumour microenvironment. Binding of the mAbs)-coated and cytotoxic drugs loaded nanoparticles to the specific antigens expressed in cancer cells enhance the therapeutic effectiveness of anticancer medications by achieving less toxicity and greater specificity (Zhu et al., 2022). Herceptin® or trastuzumab, an example of an antibody-drug conjugate which targets the human epidermal growth factor receptor-2 (HER2) which exhibited potential therapeutic effects have led researchers to consider it as potential nanomedicine for the treatment of HER2 receptor-positive cancer such as early-stage breast cancer (Fu et al., 2020; Liang et al., 2020).

Besides, nanoemulsions are also regarded as colloidal nanoparticles which are formed from oil, emulsifying agents and aqueous phase which can range in size from 10 to 1000 nm. Their lipophilic surface and negatively charge nature facilitate greater biocompatibility and bioavailability to be frequently employed as drug nanocarriers (Jaiswal et al., 2015). An earlier investigation revealed that paclitaxel and spirulina polysaccharides-based nanoemulsion enhanced the anticancer effects by controlling the TLR4/NF-B signalling pathways (Du et al., 2020). A nanoemulsion system containing bevacizumab and rapamycin showed prevention in tumour migration and angiogenesis as well as better cytotoxicity against advanced melanoma cancer cells (Dianzani et al., 2020). Moreover, interferon- γ loaded nanoemulsions have been applied in immunological therapy by reducing the viability of MCF-7 breast cancer cells and increasing the activity of phagocytes. Baicalein and paclitaxel incorporated nanoemulsion resulted in increased oxidative stress and lowered glutathione levels thereby improving the sensitivity of *in vivo* MCF-7/Tax cells to paclitaxel as compared to traditional paclitaxel (Sánchez-López et al., 2019; Meng et al., 2016). These findings suggest that nanoemulsions contribute to the efficient treatment of cancer (Ribeiro et al., 2020). However, these nanoparticles have some disadvantages including shorter circulation time in the bloodstream due to their organic ingredients which are easily biodegradable over a certain period.

Graphene has been extensively researched for application in cancer treatment due to its significant mechanical and electrical properties. Single-layer and multi-layer graphene, graphene oxide and reduced graphene oxide have all been characterised in terms of their compositions, structures, and properties (Chung et al., 2013). Graphene exhibits direct immunogenicity in contrast to other nanomaterials. The degree of immunostimulatory ability can be altered by adjusting its lateral size. Graphene can also activate macrophages and dendritic cells, demonstrating their potential for use in cancer therapy (Ma et al., 2015).

Silicon is one of the abundant semiconductor materials which exhibit a huge potential in nanomedicine. The properties stored by silicon include excellent biocompatibility, biodegradability, bioavailability, photostability and non-toxicity making it a leading nanomaterial in cancer theragnostic (Park et al., 2009). Various types of silicon nanomaterials are used in cancer therapy including porous silicon, silicon dioxide and silicon dots. Surface functionalised porous silicon exhibit great photostability and can have been used as a light-emitting nanostructure. The flexible surface area facilitates further modifications of the surface with antibodies, proteins and even peptides (Kanathasan et al., 2016). Porous silicon has shown reduced cytotoxicity in various types of cancers including brain tumours (Turan et al., 2019).

Metal nanoparticles exhibit photothermal and electronic properties which have been shown to kill cancer cells. Exposure to near-infra-red light towards the affected cancer cells has been shown to induce local toxic effects on the cancer cells (Wang et al., 2016). Gold nanoparticles are flexible nanomaterials that can be hybridized with other types of nanomaterials for improved cancer treatment. Gold nanoparticles are known to be an effective option for radiotherapy owing to their strong absorption of radiation owing to their high atomic number (Alamzadeh et al., 2020; Hainfeld et al., 2010; Piccolo et al., 2022). In line with this, gold nanoparticles emerged as a promising drug delivery system for the treatment of prostate and breast cancer owing to their ability to scatter and absorb light and convert optical energy into heat (Yang et al., 2019).

Magnetic nanomaterials are considered for targeted delivery owing to the magnetic properties that can be monitored using external magnetic field-based devices (Bonilla & Gonzalez, 2017). The superparamagnetic properties of nanomaterials improve cancer diagnosis and treatment. For instance, superparamagnetic iron oxide nanoparticles are capable of treating cancer because they have a strong ability to evade the immune system, thus providing great targeting specificity (Horst et al., 2017). There are various shapes of magnetic nanoparticles are designed according to the type of intervention. Magnetic nanoparticles in rod shape result in better magnetic torque and alternation magnetic field, which increases the intensity of the hyperthermic effect (Govindan et al., 2023). The qualities and characteristics of these nanomaterials have been identified and occupied aiming to improve cancer treatment.

APPLICATIONS OF NANOMATERIALS IN CANCER THERAPY: RECENT ADVANCES

Chemotherapy

Chemotherapy is one of the commonly used treatment modes to treat cancer by delivering anti-cancer drugs to the tumour region through traditional administration such as intravenous and oral administration. Traditionally used drugs for chemotherapy include doxorubicin and docetaxel (Govindan et al., 2023). Chemotherapeutic drugs can kill the cancer cells. Systemic delivery of chemotherapeutic drugs has a huge impact on the overall systemic functions. Generally, patients often refuse from taking chemotherapy as a treatment option for cancer treatment due to the adverse effects induced by the chemotherapeutic drugs on healthy cells including alopecia, nausea, severe body pain and reduced immune system (Gholami et al., 2020). The development of nanotechnology in medicine field has led to targeted therapy with the use of nanoparticles to deliver drugs to the tumour microenvironment owing to the nanoscale materials which offer effective drug delivery properties. Recent research on the use of nanomaterials for chemotherapy demonstrated tremendous progress to reduce the side effects of chemotherapy. Various types of nanoparticles have been used in chemotherapy including magnetic nanoparticles, polymer-magnetic nanoparticles and lipid-based nanoparticles. One of them is magnetic nanoparticles which have been used for chemotherapy (Govindan et al., 2023). Micelles have been used as a nanocarrier of ultra-small superparamagnetic iron oxide nanoparticles (USPION) and small interfering RNA (siRNA) for magnetic resonance imaging (MRI) guided chemotherapy and gene silencing (Lee et al., 2016).

Poly(lactic acid) (PLA)-poly(ethylene glycol)- (PEG)-Folic Acid (FA)-magnetic nanoparticles were used to deliver DOX drug for chemotherapeutic and hyperthermic purposes (Khaledian et al., 2020). Ferum oxide nanoparticles (Fe3O4 NPs) were used to load therapeutic compounds like folic acid (FA) and curcumin to treat cervical cancer (Ramezani et al., 2022). In another study by Dai et al. (2016), gold nanoparticles were found to improve the biocompatibility of the hydrophobic drug curcumin (Dai et al., 2016). One of the recent advances in chemotherapy is the use of multifunctional nanorobots which performs chemotherapeutic drug delivery, photothermal therapy and diagnosis using a magnetic contrast agent (Jin Z et al., 2019). These nanorobots have successfully delivered doxorubicin to cancer cells *in vitro* resulting significant reduction of cancer cells and reduced toxicity of chemotherapeutic drugs to the healthy cells (Kim et al., 2013). Magnetic nanorobots have been shown to deliver cisplatin to lung cancer cells in vitro (Ma et al., 2019). In another study, nanorobots have killed more than 63.7% of liver carcinoma cells (Hep3b cells) both *in vitro* and *in vivo* (Govindan et al., 2023). Recently studied exceedingly small magnetic iron oxide nanoparticles (ES-MIONs) at 3.6 nm have shown tremendous efficacy in liver cancer cell-targeted tumour imaging and chemotherapy (Shen et al., 2017).

Hybrid nanoparticles contribute to better therapeutic efficiency due to the masking effect of one type of nanomaterial with the complimenting property of another category of nanoparticle. For example, Bao et al. (2014) have developed a liposome-gold hybrid nanoparticle for sustained release of chemotherapeutic drug, paclitaxel through targeted drug delivery (Bao et al., 2014). Polymeric gold hybrid nanoparticles were used to heat-triggered release of chemotherapeutic drugs. The gold nanoparticles-polyrotaxane nanohybrid resulted in sustained release compared to free drugs (Adeli et al., 2011). Multiple chemotherapeutic drugs can be loaded into the nanomaterials for a more effective drug delivery system (Pushpalatha et al., 2017).

Resistance to drugs most commonly occurs in chemotherapy in which when the characteristics of the antineoplastic drug and the specific tumour combine to create inhibition of the drug in destroying the tumour cells. There are two types of drug resistance. Firstly, natural drug resistance results in the unresponsiveness of a tumor to a drug at the first exposure. While acquired resistance refers to the unresponsiveness of a tumor to a drug after the first round of successful treatment (Dey et al., 2022). Multidrug resistance refers is one of the biggest challenges posed by chemotherapy in treating cancer, with over 90% of failure rates. There are several factors which lead to the development of cancer chemoresistance including the complexity of cancer, inhibition of apoptosis, alteration of the metabolism of the drug, detoxification of the drug, drug inactivation before reaching the target site and drug efflux. There are several types of nanomaterials found to be used to overcome the multidrug resistance of these drugs, with most of them entering clinical trials. Organic nanomaterials like liposome were used to deliver the siRNAs that inhibit the overexpression of efflux-related protein pumps and enhances the delivery of the loaded drugs (Eloy et al., 2016). Polymeric nanoparticles result in enhanced drug accumulation in tumors, and increased cellular uptake (Saneja et al., 2019). Often, the tumour microenvironment becomes as a physical and biological barrier to the chemotherapeutic drugs. Combination therapies have been developed to overcome the multidrug resistance. Nanomaterials like liposomes, polymer-based, zinc oxide were loaded with drugs and have shown to reach the tumor site efficiently through downregulation and bypassing of protein pumps, synergistic autophagy and generation of reactive oxygen species, and controlled drug release (Dey et al., 2022)

Radiation Therapy

Radiotherapy is a cancer treatment mode which uses high-energy ionizing radiation to kill cancer cells. Radiotherapy is commonly used with chemotherapy to enhance the effective eradication of tumour cells (Sekar et al., 2023). However, radiation therapy also kills healthy cells and negatively affects the immune system. Tumour microenvironments are known to impose resistance towards radiation therapy. Hence, multimodal therapeutic platforms have been shown to improve the effectiveness of chemo-radiotherapy with the combination of hyperthermic effects. Hydrogels possess thermoresponsive properties which enable them to be used for radiotherapy (Alamzadeh et al., 2020). Cisplatin loaded Gold-alginate hybrid nanoparticles which were used for radiotherapy demonstrated apoptotic cell death results in tumour growth inhibition up to 95% and 51% of enhancement in anti-tumor activity in colon cancer cells *in vivo* as compared to standard chemotherapy (Mirrahimi et al., 2019). Nanomaterials that can illuminate upon radiation exposure has shown to enhance radiation therapy by activation of the nanoparticles at tumour regions which are located in deeper tissues (Mosleh-Shirazi et al., 2022). Gold nanoparticles are known as radiosensitizers that enhance radiotherapy (Fang et al., 2017). Platinum nanoparticles also have been shown to improve radiotherapy owing to their hyperthermic property with light irradiation by not exceeding the temperature of 46°C upon heating which is safer for healthy cells as well (Zhu et al., 2017).

The efficacy of radiotherapy is often enhanced by photothermal therapy (Shi et al., 2022). Lack of effectiveness of radiation therapy is often due to challenges in distinguishing normal cells and hypoxic cells (Baskar et al., 2012). The combination of photothermal therapy with radiotherapy improves the blood flow to the tumour microenvironment, reducing its resistance to the tumour region thereby improving the efficiency of radiotherapy (Mao et al., 2016). In a recent study, irradiation of near infra-red light to the manganese dioxide (MnO_2) and copper sulphide (CuS) coated upconversion nanoparticles improved the therapeutic efficacy of radiotherapy through the interaction of MnO_2 with overexpressed hydrogen peroxide (H_2O_2), causing oxygenation in the tumour region as well as inhibition of tumour growth (Ni et al., 2022). Folic acid-coated hafnium-based manganoprphyrin metal-organic nanoparticles (MnTCPP-Hf-FA) have improved radiotherapy with reduced relapse (Chen et al., 2019). Biomimetic iron-coated hafnium-porphyrin metal-organic frameworks (Hf-DBP-Fe) helps to destroy primary tumour as well as distant tumours (Ni et al., 2020). Another study used hafnium-bis(2,2'-bipyridine)(5,5'-di(4-benzoate)-2,2'-bipyridine)ruthenium(II) chloride (Hf-DBB-Ru) to irradiate mitochondria resulted in apoptosis of colon cancer cells (Ni et al., 2018).

Photothermal Therapy

Photothermal has been shown as one of the applicable treatment methods for various diseases, especially cancer. It uses a specific laser injected by a photothermal agent which transforms the light energy into heat that can be focused on the tumour region to kill the cancer cells when the temperature reaches above 48°C (Zhang M. et al., 2018; Ma & Xue, 2021). This therapy has shown great progress in creating local toxic effects on cancer cells than traditional cancer treatments like chemotherapy and radiotherapy. Many photothermal-based cancer treatment studies are currently being tested under clinical trials. Photothermal therapy is used to complement the existing chemotherapy by enhancing the drug release from the nanoparticles with increasing laser irradiation in various types of cancer, including brain tumours and melanoma (Crezee et al., 2021). Photothermal therapy is known to enhance the currently existing traditional therapies when used in combination with other therapies including chemotherapy, radiation and magnetic field (Jha et al., 2016). Magnetic nanoparticles are extensively used to treat cancer using photothermal therapy owing to their photothermic property. Nanoparticles like iron oxide nanoparticles are injected into the body and activated by a specific wavelength of light that induces heat generation to kill the cancer cells. A study which used human serum albumin (HAS) loaded redox-responsive magnetic nanovectors (RMNs) showed enhanced delivery of the proteins at the perinuclear region of cancer cells (Yang et al., 2017).

Photothermal therapy is often combined with chemotherapy to kill cancer cells using gold nanoparticles, thanks to the heat-emitting property of gold nanomaterials (Wang et al., 2016). Photothermal therapy can be used in combination with gene delivery to deliver DNA-embedded DOX in polyethylenimine (PEI) nanoparticles to make the chemotherapy more effective (Chen et al., 2021). In a photothermal therapeutic study, Xu et al. used glucose oxidase (Gox) modified N-doped carbon nanoparticles to improve chemotherapy (Xu et al., 2022). Gold nanorods are combined with DOX and reduced graphene oxide for effective photothermal effects (Song et al., 2015). Another study used nanoparticles which consist of DOX-loaded folic acid, gold nanoparticles, carbon quantum dots and multi-walled carbon nanotubes (FA-GdN@CQDs-MWCNTs) for multimodal theragnostic of fluorescent imaging, magnetic resonance imaging, chemotherapy and photothermal therapy has shown low toxicity and better compatibility than single treatment mode (Zhang et al.,2018). Hybrid nanoparticles of albumin and small gold nanorods (AuNRs-Alb-NPs) have reached up to 57°C and have shown better removal of brain tumour tissue (Seo et al.,2019).

Silver nanomaterials also have been used to treat cancer through photothermal effects by inducing cell death through the apoptosis process (Bian et al., 2018). Copper (Cu) and polyethylene glycol (PEG) coated gold nanorods have demonstrated improved photostability (Sun et al., 2014). Surface-modified palladium nanoparticles have shown better results in photothermal therapy. Arginylglycylaspartic acid (RGD) peptide-functionalized chitosan-modified palladium nanoparticles have been shown to improve tumour targeting via photothermal effect (Bharathiraja et al., 2018). Poly(lactic-co-glycolic acid) (PLGA) nanoparticles have the potential to be used as thermosensitive nanocarriers for multimodal therapy of chemotherapy and photothermal therapy. Copper, iron and selenium compound nanoparticles (CuFeSe2) which possess absorption up to the NIR range were found to be used for MRI or CT imaging-guided photothermal therapy (Jiang et al., 2017). The combination of CdTeS quantum dots and mesoporous SiO2 with Fe3O4 has demonstrated a great platform for fluorescence imaging, MRI and photothermal therapy (Yin et al., 2021).

Photodynamic Therapy

Photodynamic therapy involves an injection of nanoparticles inside the body which leads to chemical reactions including the generation of oxygen radicals upon irradiation of light that diminishes the tumour cells (Itoo et al., 2022; Revia & Zhang, 2016). This therapy has been used in treating certain types of cancer including head and neck cancer, bladder cancer and skin cancer (Zhang & Li, 2018). These techniques are more effective in treating cancer cells as this application creates a local effect which only kills the tumour cells while not diminishing the healthy cells (Govindan et al., 2023). Quantum dots, carbon dots, graphene and hybrid nanomaterials are mostly used in photodynamic therapy (Zhou et al., 2016). Carbon-based nanomaterials including carbon dots and graphene quantum dots exhibit stronger photostability and fluorescent properties which enable them to have been used in combination with magnetic nanomaterials for enhanced photodynamic therapy (Molaei & Salimi et al., 2022; Hassani et al., 2022).

Gene Therapy

Gene therapy has many benefits over conventional cancer treatments, including high specificity and potency, low off-target damage, and delivery of numerous genes that simultaneously target drug resistance, carcinogenesis, and recurrence. Gene therapy has made significant development over the past few decades and is now ready to replace other cancer treatments as the first choice. Nanoparticles have garnered a lot of interest among the numerous gene delivery technologies due to their desirable qualities, such as low toxicity profiles, well-controlled and high gene delivery efficiency, and multi-functionalities which enable multimodal therapies (Mirza & Karim, 2021; Wang et al., 2016).

Gold nanoparticles are increasingly being employed for gene therapy applications due to their high payload (caused by their huge surface area), low toxicity, improved absorption, quick endosomal escape, increased half-life, and effective and selective gene silencing. Successful use of gold nanoconjugates and oligonucleotides in gene therapy has also been reported (Mendes et al., 2017). Based on the previous findings, gold nanoparticles when functionalized with an antisense oligonucleotide against BCR-ABL mRNA, a fusion mRNA that upon translation results in a constitutively active tyrosine kinase that is essential for leukemogenesis, exhibited an increase in K562 cell death and effective silencing (Vinhas et al., 2017).

Besides, iron magnetic nanoparticles are used in a variety of cancer treatment and diagnosis procedures (Israel et al., 2020; Xie et al., 2019). Magnetic iron nanoparticles loaded with DNA in mitochondrial therapies exerted cell death by reacting with the mitochondrial translocation protein (Kim et al., 2016). Iron nanoparticles loaded with siRNA for silencing gene therapy can be developed due to their small size and variable functionalization. These nanoparticles have a net positive surface charge, which enhances the action of siRNA at the tumour region. In another study, Fe_3O_4-synthesized nanoparticles were employed in combination with magnetotherapy to enhance the gene-silencing effect of B-cell lymphoma-2 (BCL-2), an antiapoptotic protein on Ca9-22 oral cancer cells and (Jin et al., 2019).

In addition, liposomes have been widely applied in gene therapy owing to their ability to incorporate genetic materials and drugs inside (Sheoran et al., 2019). An effective liposomal nanoformulation was found to target TMPRSS2/ERG fusion mRNA and improved docetaxel treatment in prostate cancer (Shao et al., 2020). A previous study demonstrated that p53/C-rNC/L-FA liposome induced apoptosis in tumor cell lines and inhibited tumor growth in a breast cancer mouse model (Chen et al., 2019). PEG-coated polyplexes made of poly(2-aminoethyl methacrylate) (PAMA) enhanced transfection activity while reducing cytotoxicity in African green monkey kidney cells (COS-7) and human liver cancer (HepG2) cell lines (Santo et al., 2019). Besides, the investigation of biological vesicles for gene delivery has resulted in new and efficient therapeutic approaches for the treatment of cancer (Lee et al., 2012). The major drawbacks of gene delivery were fixed through the engineering of allogenic exosomes with miRNAs, mRNAs and proteins for targeted delivery, allowing the administration of the therapy to the target cells with a suppressed immune response (Gilligan & Dwyer, 2017).

Nanovectorization of genes for cancer therapy is essential for efficient gene transport with no side effects. The development of precision medicine focusing on targeted gene delivery via nanoparticles could help to treat cancer. However, the field of cancer gene therapy using nanotechnology is still in its infancy, with just a few numbers of phase I and phase II clinical trials planned, primarily using organic nanoparticles. Drug-liposome formulations containing doxorubicin are currently approved by the FDA for cancer therapy, such as Doxil (US), pegylated liposomes with doxorubicin Caelyx (EU) and non-pegylated liposome with doxorubicin (Myocet). This shows the extensive applications of liposomes in clinical trials (Mirza & Karim, 2019). Liposomal gold nanoparticles are also used for gene delivery (Deng et al., 2018). The main goals of liposomal nanomaterials in gene therapy include targeting the proto-oncogene cRAF with or without adjuvant chemotherapy, delivery of tumour suppressor genes (FUS1, NCT00059605, and TP53, NCT02354547), or delivery of mRNA vaccines for the treatment of ovarian cancer (NCT04163094) or melanoma (NCT02410733). The solid-lipid nanoformulation ALN-VSP02 used in phase I clinical trial NCT01158079 contained siRNAs that targeted the VEGF-A gene to suppress neo-angiogenesis and the kinesin spindle protein gene to cause cell cycle arrest. Following the treatment of the nanoformulation with 31 patients with advanced solid tumours, anti-tumor efficacy and tolerance to the medicines were reported to be consistent with the effect of anti-vascular endothelial growth factor (VEGF) (Cervantes et al., 2011).

Immunotherapy

The application of nanomaterials in cancer immunotherapy enhanced the efficacy and safety of therapeutic cancer vaccines (Bockamp et al., 2020). Nanomaterials can be coated with different ligands, including antibodies, aptamers, proteins, peptides and nucleic acids which are specific to the extracellular and sometimes intracellular receptor expressed in the tumour region. Owing to the flexible surface-to-volume ratio, these ligand-conjugated drug-loaded nanomaterials are readily used in targeted drug delivery which leads to the release of high-dose therapeutic compounds in the target area. The nanotechnology-based immunotherapy inhibits tumour growth through two distinct mechanisms, by triggering a powerful anti-tumor immune response during tumorigenesis and by enhancing tumour immune defence by modifying the immune suppression mechanism in the tumour microenvironment (Gao et al., 2021; Li et al., 2022). This ligand-engineered nanomaterial system benefits various cell-based therapeutic solutions in cancer immunotherapy (Golchin et al., 2018; Sebestyen et al., 2020). They promote the effective accumulation of adjuvants and antigens in draining lymph nodes, which delays their rapid dissemination into circulation (Goldberg, 2019; Gong et al., 2021). Recent investigation indicated that a nano vaccine system constructed using Poly(lactic-co-glycolic acid) (PLGA) nanoparticles with phospholipid membranes has efficiently concentrated in lymph nodes and elicited an antigen-specific adaptive T cell response, which inhibited the metastasis of B16-OVA melanoma cells, as evidenced by the significantly reduced number of metastatic nodules (Song et al., 2018).

The development of tumour immunity, characterized by the natural cascade of the immune system against tumour cells requires recognition of tumour antigens by antigen-presenting cells, to hint the immune cells to kill the tumour cells. Tumor antigens can be safely delivered to lymph nodes using nanoparticle delivery methods (Zhang et al., 2018). Moreover, tumors may promote the growth and dissemination of cancer cells by producing an immunosuppressive tumour microenvironment. The modification of this environment is frequently included as a key strategy in the immunotherapy treatment of cancer (Jeanbart & Swartz, 2015). The tumor microenvironment consists of tumor-associated macrophages and suppressor T-lymphocytes, which suppress anti-cancer immune responses by producing inflammatory cytokines like IL-12, IL-1b, TNF-, and IL-6. Moreover, the Transforming Growth Factor (TGF), a cytokine that is overexpressed in breast, liver, and lung cancer, may impair immune cell activation, maturation, and differentiation (Park et al., 2018). It is known that nanotechnology has been used in several immunotherapy and immunoprevention methods. It has a number of benefits, including enhanced lymph node access and improved antigen presentation, which further increases the anti-tumor immune response (Finn & Beatty, 2016). Overexpression of protein-based cellular components can be made of good use for targeted theragnostic to monitor the prognosis as well as treatment of various types of cancer. Legumain is one of the recently studied asparaginyl endopeptidases which is found to be overexpressed in various types of cancer, namely breast, oral, colon and skin cancers (Ke et al., 2022). Therefore, a specific type of asparagine-containing peptide has been conjugated onto porous silicon nanomaterials which have shown high binding specificity towards legumain was developed to target the legumain in a 4T1-solid tumour-induced mice model study (Kanathasan et al., 2022).

SAFETY, TOXICITY, AND REGULATORY SYSTEM OF NANOMATERIALS IN CANCER THERAPY

Applications of functional nanomaterials in cancer lead to the development of various types of nanomaterials in use as a nanocarrier of therapeutic drugs. Organic and polymeric nanomaterials are highly recommended and easily approved at the clinical trials due to their lower toxicity (Bhatia et al., 2022). However, they may impose issues on lower bioavailability and higher possibility in degradation. These limitations led to alternatives include inorganic nanoparticles. Inorganic nanomaterials include heavy metals like gold, silver and heavy metal-based semiconductors include Cadmium (Cd) and Selenium (Se) possess excellent intrinsic luminescence property, enabling their use as natural dye for live bioimaging (Zhong et al., 2012). However, they pose toxicity issue upon release of toxic ions that could intercalate between DNA causing DMA damages and have reduced renal clearance causing them to be deposited in the organs leading to organ dysfunction (Poon et al., 2020). With a concern to release of nontoxic by-products with the qualities of nanomaterials exhibited, semiconductor nanomaterials made from carbon and silicon were found to be a solution for previously based problem. These nanomaterials are more stable, totally non-toxic and exhibit various properties include excellent photostability and biocompatibility (Wang et al., 2014). Cytotoxicity tests are recommended to determine the toxicity level of the developed nanomaterial. One of the commonly used cytotoxicity tests to test a compound towards 2D cell culture is colorimetric assays such as MTT assay (Egbuna et al., 2021). While toxicity studies for animal work is conducted through histopathology study. The tumour regions and other organs like brain, heart, liver, kidney, spleen, stomach and lung will be examined for cell death due to toxicity of the compound.

Apart from the safety of the nanomaterials, the regulatory process for approval of the nanomedicine-based therapy for cancer treatment is a major concern to ensure the nanomedicine is safe to the consumed. There are several factors to be taken into consideration by regulatory bodies such as Food and Drug Administration (FDA) including the proper characterization and physicochemical stability of the nanomedicine, the pharmacokinetics of the nanomedicine, and the toxicity profiles of the developed nanomedicine before approval of the nanomedicine by the regulatory bodies. Due to its invisible size of the nanomedicine, the development of the nanoparticle system owing to its unique design requires specialized delivery system. (Thapa & Kim, 2023). Hence, more time and cost will be involved for testing of these nanomedicine for a safer use for humans. There are many nanomedicines that have been approved recently which gives a good hope for the nanomedicine to treat cancer.

ARTIFICIAL INTELLIGENCE FOR CANCER TREATMENT

Artificial intelligence (AI) has been one of the technologies which have been occupied in applications of almost all fields, not denying the medical field. AI is believed to contribute to finding solutions for currently existing challenges in tumor treatment modalities by using machine learning algorithms (Farina et al., 2022). Application of AI is expected to improve early tumour detection as well as localized therapy which could resolve the major challenges faced by oncologists. Image analysis of currently existing imaging modalities could help to predict the possibility of relapse occurring after surgery (Bi et al., 2019). AI has also improved in prediction of the risk of developing cancer among patients by analyzing patients' health records (Kumar et al., 2022). AI has been occupied in cancer treatment by targeted drug delivery, optimization of drug dose, real-time monitoring, and prediction of the effectiveness of the drug used. This paves for the development of tailored medicine and treatment modes based on the various types of adverse effects faced by the patient, with the use of AI-assisted software. In addition, AI-based deep learning algorithms known as CancerSEEK software are developed to detect liquid biopsies of eight types of cancer by tracing the circulating tumour DNA or cell-free DNA (cfDNA) for early detection of cancer which can have a huge impact on the prognosis of cancer (Cohen et al., 2018).

The combination of AI with nanoparticles leads to discoveries in cancer diagnosis as well as treatment. Recent advancements in AI in cancer nanotechnology result in AI-assisted nanoparticle synthesis and nanoparticle delivery systems (Osial et al.,2022). AI-based nanoparticle platform assists in tracking drug-loaded magnetic nanoparticles and monitoring of toxicity of the drug delivery, contributing to the reduced size of tumour growth in animal models (Horak et al., 2022; Tang et al., 2021). Currently, available AI-based nanosystems such as DeepCare, HyperView and ThermAI have led to precision medicine through enhanced optimization in photothermal and photodynamic therapies (Tran et al., 2021; Kourou et al., 2015). AI-based nanomaterial system has enabled the prediction of the response of a drug towards the patient which drives towards customized healthcare in cancer treatment which hopes for an overall positive impact in cancer treatment.

CHALLENGES AND FUTURE PERSPECTIVES

Nanoparticle drug delivery system plays an integral role to replace or improve traditional cancer treatment methods such as chemotherapy, radiotherapy and surgery which are non-specific and raises concerns over undesirable toxicity profiles. In line to achieve reduced adverse side effects, nanotechnology in cancer treatment also has achieved a higher concentration of drug delivery at the tumour region. Nanoparticles improve the delivery of drug-loaded nanoparticles to the cancer sites via nanotechnology-mediated chemotherapy and radiotherapy by exposing the tumour region to irradiation that facilitates the anti-cancer drugs to gain access and have closer interaction with the tumour cells. Various types of nanomaterials exhibit unique physicochemical properties to ensure the successful delivery of the therapeutic drug to the target region. For example, an organic nanoparticle system is the most preferred choice for drug delivery owing to its biocompatibility and non-toxicity nature. However, easily biodegradable organic nanoparticles like liposomal and polymeric nanoparticles may not have bioavailability and a half-life shorter than inorganic nanoparticles, making it not efficient. While the inorganic and metal nanomaterial systems which have great photostability and magnetic properties may face toxicity issues, limiting their potential from getting approved in clinical trials. Therefore, hybrid nanoparticles such as liposomal-coated magnetic nanoparticles must be explored in future clinical trials to reduce the bioavailability and toxicity issues. Some of the limitations posed by nanomaterials include smaller size that causes difficulty in handling, particles aggregation, limited drug loading and burst release (Thapa & Kim, 2023).

Moreover, not all nanoparticle-based cancer therapy is effective as a single treatment regime because nanoparticles still pose limitations in sustained delivery at the tumour microenvironment. Despite making good use of the individual nanoparticle drug delivery system using a single treatment mode, a combination of multiple therapies has significantly proven to reduce tumour growth and improve the survival rate of patients. Therefore, a nanoparticle system which can be activated through multiple cancer therapies may lead to an improved prognosis for the patients and have a greater possibility of getting accepted in clinical trials. For example, a drug-loaded nanoparticles system which consists of magnetic or metallic nanostructures can be used for multiple therapies including chemotherapy, radiotherapy and photothermal therapy as the irradiation from radiotherapy and hyperthermic effects shown by the heat energy of the nanoparticles would increase the efficiency at the similar dose of drugs compared to non-photothermal nanoparticle drug delivery system.

Artificial intelligence-based nanoparticle system is at the infancy level in cancer research. It offers attractive solutions for improved efficiency in drug delivery which can be tailored to every patient. This solution hits on the direct issue faced by the nanoparticle drug delivery system which has varying responses for various types of cancer owing to the heterogenous nature of cancer in every case. However, more investigations on the precision and reliability of the applications of AI-assisted algorithms in nanoparticle systems are required to ensure the successful use of AI in cancer treatment.

CONCLUSION

This chapter revolves around the cutting-edge applications of nanomaterials in cancer therapy. The desirable qualities expected in a leading nanoparticle system include the nanoscale size within 1000 nm, greater biocompatibility, hydrophilicity, bioavailability and non-toxicity. The various types of nanoparticles possess unique qualities such as the flexible surface modifiable ability and biocompatibility of the organic nanoparticles including liposomal, polymeric, silicon and carbon nanoparticles, the magnetic property of iron oxide and gold nanoparticles, absorption of light and radiation properties exhibited by metallic nanoparticles and carbon dots were explored. the applications of nanoparticle systems in treatment therapies including chemotherapy, radiotherapy, photothermal and photodynamic therapies, gene therapy and immunotherapy were discussed. Limitations posed by the application of a single treatment mode were found to be resolved by combination therapies as discussed in this chapter. These therapies including chemotherapy, radiotherapy, gene delivery and immunotherapy have shown better efficiency and reduced effect of multidrug resistance proving thier potential in combination therapies for cancer treatment. Lastly, the application of artificial intelligence-assisted algorithms has opened up a new avenue to precision medicine in cancer treatment with further evaluations required.

REFERENCES

Adeli, M., Sarabi, R. S., Yadollahi Farsi, R., Mahmoudi, M., & Kalantari, M. (2011). Polyrotaxane/Gold Nanoparticle Hybrid Nanomaterials as Anticancer Drug Delivery Systems. *Journal of Materials Chemistry*, *18686*(21), 18686. doi:10.1039/c1jm12412a

Alamzadeh, Z., Beik, J., Mirrahimi, M., Shakeri-Zadeh, A., Ebrahimi, F., Komeili, A., Ghalandari, B., Ghaznavi, H., Kamrava, S. K., & Moustakis, C. (2020). Gold Nanoparticles Promote a Multimodal Synergistic Cancer Therapy Strategy by Co-Delivery of ThermoChemo-Radio Therapy. *European Journal of Pharmaceutical Sciences*, *105235*(145), 105235. doi:10.1016/j.ejps.2020.105235

Ali, A. A., Abuwatfa, W. H., Al-Sayah, M. H., & Husseini, G. A. (2022). Gold-Nanoparticle Hybrid Nanostructures for Multimodal Cancer Therapy. *Nanomaterials (Basel, Switzerland)*, *3706*(12), 3706. doi:10.3390/nano12203706

Ali, E. S., Sharker, S. M., Islam, M. T., Khan, I. N., Shaw, S., Rahman, M. A., Uddin, S. J., Shill, M. C., Rehman, S., Das, N., Ahmad, S., Shilpi, J. A., Tripathi, S., Mishra, S. K., & Mubarak, M. S. (2021). Targeting cancer cells with nanotherapeutics and nanodiagnostics: Current status and future perspectives. *Seminars in Cancer Biology*, *69*, 52–68. doi:10.1016/j.semcancer.2020.01.011

Andreiuk, B., Reisch, A., Lindecker, M., Follain, G., Peyriéras, N., Goetz, J. G., & Klymchenko, A. S. (2017). Fluorescent polymer nanoparticles for cell barcoding in vitro and in vivo. *Small*, *13*(38), 1701582. doi:10.1002mll.201701582

Anselmo, A. C., & Mitragotri, S. (2019). Nanoparticles in the clinic: An update. *Bioengineering & Translational Medicine*, *4*(3), e10143. Advance online publication. doi:10.1002/btm2.10143

Attia, M. F., Anton, N., Wallyn, J., Omran, Z., & Vandamme, T. F. (2019). An overview of active and passive targeting strategies to improve the nanocarriers efficiency to tumour sites. *The Journal of Pharmacy and Pharmacology*, *71*(8), 1185–1198. doi:10.1111/jphp.13098

Bao, Q.-Y., Zhang, N., Geng, D.-D., Xue, J.-W., Merritt, M., Zhang, C., & Ding, Y. (2014). The Enhanced Longevity and Liver Targetability of Paclitaxel by Hybrid Liposomes Encapsulating Paclitaxel-Conjugated Gold Nanoparticles. *International Journal of Pharmaceutics*, *477*(1-2), 408–415. doi:10.1016/j.ijpharm.2014.10.040

Barenholz, Y. (2012). Doxil®—the first FDA-approved nano-drug: Lessons learned. *Journal of Controlled Release*, *160*(2), 117–134. doi:10.1016/j.jconrel.2012.03.020

Baskar, R., Lee, K. A., Yeo, R., & Yeoh, K. W. (2012). Cancer and Radiation Therapy: Current Advances and Future Directions. *International Journal of Medical Sciences*, *9*(3), 193–199. doi:10.7150/ijms.3635

Batist, G., Gelmon, K. A., Chi, K. N., Miller, W. H. Jr, Chia, S. K., Mayer, L. D., Swenson, C. E., Janoff, A. S., & Louie, A. C. (2009). Safety, pharmacokinetics, and efficacy of CPX-1 liposome injection in patients with advanced solid tumors. *Clinical Cancer Research*, *15*(2), 692–700. doi:10.1158/1078-0432.CCR-08-0515

Bazak, R., Houri, M., El Achy, S., Kamel, S., & Refaat, T. (2015). Cancer active targeting by nanoparticles: A comprehensive review of literature. *Journal of Cancer Research and Clinical Oncology*, *141*(5), 769–784. doi:10.100700432-014-1767-3

Bharathiraja, S., Bui, N. Q., Manivasagan, P., Moorthy, M. S., Mondal, S., Seo, H., Phuoc, N. T., Vy Phan, T. T., Kim, H., Lee, K. D., & Oh, J. (2018). Multimodal tumor-homing chitosan oligosaccharide-coated biocompatible palladium nanoparticles for photo-based imaging and therapy. *Scientific Reports*, *8*(1), 500. doi:10.103841598-017-18966-8

Bhatia, S. N., Chen, X., Dobrovolskaia, M. A., & Lammers, T. (2022). Cancer nanomedicine. *Nature Reviews. Cancer*, *22*(10), 550–556. doi:10.103841568-022-00496-9

Bi, W. L., Hosny, A., Schabath, M. B., Giger, M. L., Birkbak, N. J., Mehrtash, A., Allison, T., Arnaout, O., Abbosh, C., Dunn, I. F., Mak, R. H., Tamimi, R. M., Tempany, C. M., Swanton, C., Hoffmann, U., Schwartz, L. H., Gillies, R. J., Huang, R. Y., & Aerts, H. J. W. L. (2019). Artificial intelligence in cancer imaging: Clinical challenges and applications. *CA: a Cancer Journal for Clinicians*, *69*(2), 127–157. doi:10.3322/caac.21552

Bian, K., Zhang, X., Liu, K., Yin, T., Liu, H., Niu, K., Cao, W., & Gao, D. (2018). Peptide-Directed Hierarchical Mineralized Silver Nanocages for Anti-Tumor Photothermal Therapy. *ACS Sustainable Chemistry & Engineering*, *6*(6), 7574–7588. doi:10.1021/acssuschemeng.8b00415

Blanco, E., Shen, H., & Ferrari, M. (2015). Principles of nanoparticle design for overcoming biological barriers to drug delivery. *Nature Biotechnology*, *33*(9), 941–951. doi:10.1038/nbt.3330

Bockamp, E., Rosigkeit, S., Siegl, D., & Schuppan, D. (2020). Nano-enhanced cancer immunotherapy: Immunology encounters nanotechnology. *Cells*, *9*(9), 2102. doi:10.3390/cells9092102

Bonilla, A. M., & Gonzalez, P. H. (2017). Hybrid polymeric-magnetic nanoparticles in cancer treatments. *Current Pharmaceutical Design*, *23*(35), 5392–5402. doi:10.2174/1381612823666170519115601

Bonvalot, S., Rutkowski, P. L., Thariat, J., Carrère, S., Ducassou, A., Sunyach, M. P., Agoston, P., Hong, A., Mervoyer, A., Rastrelli, M., Moreno, V., Li, R. K., Tiangco, B., Herraez, A. C., Gronchi, A., Mangel, L., Sy-Ortin, T., Hohenberger, P., de Baère, T., & Le Jvmg Bovée, C. (2019). NBTXR3, a first-in-class radioenhancer hafnium oxide nanoparticle, plus radiotherapy versus radiotherapy alone in patients with locally advanced soft-tissue sarcoma (Act. In.Sarc): A multicentre, phase 2–3, randomised, controlled trial. *The Lancet. Oncology*, *20*(8), 1148–1159. doi:10.1016/S1470-2045(19)30326-2

Borgå, O., Lilienberg, E., Bjermo, H., Hansson, F., Heldring, N., & Dediu, R. (2019). Pharmacokinetics of total and unbound paclitaxel after administration of paclitaxel micellar or nab-paclitaxel: An open, randomized, cross-over, explorative study in breast cancer patients. *Advances in Therapy*, *36*(10), 2825–2837. doi:10.100712325-019-01058-6

Brucker, J., Mayer, C., Gebauer, G., Mallmann, P., Belau, A. K., Schneeweiss, A., Sohn, C., & Eichbaum, M. (2016). Non-pegylated liposomal doxorubicin for patients with recurrent ovarian cancer: A multicentric phase II trial. *Oncology Letters*, *12*(2), 1211–1215. doi:10.3892/ol.2016.4740

Cainelli, F., & Vallone, A. (2009). Safety and efficacy of pegylated liposomal doxorubicin in HIV-associated Kaposi's sarcoma. *Biologics*, 385–390. doi:10.2147/BTT.S3915

Cao, S. J., Xu, S., Wang, H. M., Ling, Y., Dong, J., Xia, R. D., & Sun, X. H. (2019). Nanoparticles: Oral delivery for protein and peptide drugs. *AAPS PharmSciTech*, *190*(20), 190. doi:10.120812249-019-1325-z

Cervantes, A., Alsina, M., Tabernero, J., Infante, J. R., LoRusso, P., Shapiro, G., Paz-Ares, L. G., Falzone, R., Hill, J., Cehelsky, J., White, A., Toudjarska, I., Bumcrot, D., Meyers, R., Hinkle, G., Svrzikapa, N., Sah, D. W., Vaishnaw, A., Gollob, J., & Burris, H. A. (2011). Phase I dose-escalation study of ALN-VSP02, a novel RNAi therapeutic for solid tumors with liver involvement. *Journal of Clinical Oncology*, *29*(15, suppl), 3025–3025. doi:10.1200/jco.2011.29.15_suppl.3025

Chen, C., Ma, Y. P., Du, S. Y., Wu, Y. Y., Shen, P. L., Yan, T., Li, X. Q., Song, Y. J., Zha, Z. B., & Han, X. (2021). Controlled CRISPR-Cas9 ribonucleoprotein delivery for sensitized photothermal therapy. *Small*, *2101155*(17), 2101155. doi:10.1002mll.202101155

Chen, Y., Zhong, H., Wang, J., Wan, X., Li, Y., Pan, W., Li, N., & Tang, B. (2019). Catalase-like metal-organic framework nanoparticles to enhance radiotherapy in hypoxic cancer and prevent cancer recurrence. *Chemical Science (Cambridge)*, *10*(22), 5773–5778. doi:10.1039/C9SC00747D

Cheng, X., & Lee, R. J. (2016). The role of helper lipids in lipid nanoparticles (LNPs) designed for oligonucleotide delivery. *Advanced Drug Delivery Reviews*, *99*, 129–137. doi:10.1016/j.addr.2016.01.022

Cheng, Z., Li, M., Dey, R., & Chen, Y. (2021). Nanomaterials for cancer therapy: Current progress and perspectives. *Journal of Hematology & Oncology*, *14*(1), 1–27. doi:10.118613045-021-01096-0

Chou, H., Lin, H., & Liu, J. M. (2015). A tale of the two PEGylated liposomal doxorubicins. *OncoTargets and Therapy*, *8*, 1719–1720. doi:10.2147/OTT.S79089

Chung, C., Kim, Y. K., Shin, D., Ryoo, S. R., Hong, B. H., & Min, D. H. (2013). Biomedical applications of graphene and graphene oxide. *Accounts of Chemical Research*, *46*(10), 2211–2224. doi:10.1021/ar300159f

Cohen, J. D., Li, L., Wang, Y., Thoburn, C., Afsari, B., Danilova, L., Douville, C., Javed, A. A., Wong, F., Mattox, A., Hruban, R. H., Wolfgang, C. L., Goggins, M. G., Dal Molin, M., Wang, T.-L., Roden, R., Klein, A. P., Ptak, J., Dobbyn, L, & Papadopoulos, N. (2018). Detection and localization of surgically resectable cancers with a multi-analyte blood test. *Science*, *359*(6378), 926–930. doi:10.1126cience.aar3247

Crezee, J., Franken, N. A., & Oei, A. L. (2021). Hyperthermia-based anti-cancer treatments. *Cancers (Basel)*, *1240*(13), 1240. doi:10.3390/cancers13061240

Dai, M., & Ja, F. (2016). Engineered Protein Polymer-Gold Nanoparticle Hybrid Materials for Small Molecule Delivery. *Journal of Nanomedicine & Nanotechnology*, *356*(7). doi:10.4172/2157-7439.1000356

Deng, W., Chen, W., Clement, S., Guller, A., Zhao, Z., Engel, A., & Goldys, E. M. (2018). Controlled Gene and Drug Release from a Liposomal Delivery Platform Triggered by X-Ray Radiation. *Nature Communications*, *2713*(9), 2713. doi:10.103841467-018-05118-3

Deng, Z. J., Morton, S. W., Ben-Akiva, E., Dreaden, E. C., Shopsowitz, K. E., & Hammond, P. T. (2013). Layer-by-layer nanoparticles for systemic codelivery of an anticancer drug and siRNA for potential triple-negative breast cancer treatment. *ACS Nano*, *7*(11), 9571–9584. doi:10.1021/nn4047925

Dey, N., Kamatchi, C., Vickram, A. S., Anbarasu, K., Thanigaivel, S., Palanivelu, J., Pugazhendhi, A., & Ponnusamy, V. K. (2022). Role of Nanomaterials in Deactivating Multiple Drug Resistance Efflux Pumps - A Review. *Environmental Research, 204*, 111968. doi:10.1016/j.envres.2021.111968

Diaconu, A., Chiriac, A.P., Neamtu, I., Nita, L.E. (2019). Magnetic Polymeric Nanocomposites. *Polymeric Nanomaterials in Nanotherapeutics*, 359–386. doi:10.1016/B978-0-12-813932-5.00010-8

Dianzani, C., Monge, C., Miglio, G., Serpe, L., Martina, K., Cangemi, L., Ferraris, C., Mioletti, S., Osella, S., Gigliotti, C. L., Boggio, E., Clemente, N., Dianzani, U., & Battaglia, L. (2020). Nanoemulsions as delivery systems for poly-chemotherapy aiming at melanoma treatment. *Cancers (Basel), 12*(5), 1198. doi:10.3390/cancers12051198

Du, M., Yang, Z., Lu, W., Wang, B., Wang, Q., Chen, Z., Chen, L., Han, S., Cai, T., & Cai, Y. (2020). Design and development of spirulina polysaccharide-loaded nanoemulsions with improved the antitumor effects of paclitaxel. *Journal of Microencapsulation, 37*(6), 403–412. doi:10.1080/02652048.2020.1767224

Duvic, M., & Talpur, R. (2008). Optimizing denileukin diftitox (Ontak) therapy. *Future Oncology (London, England), 4*(4), 457–469. doi:10.2217/14796694.4.4.457

Edgington-Mitchell, L. E., Barlow, N., Aurelio, L., Samha, A., Szabo, M., Graham, B., & Bunnett, N. (2017). Fluorescent diphenylphosphonate-based probes for detection of serine protease activity during inflammation. *Bioorganic & Medicinal Chemistry Letters, 27*(2), 254–260. doi:10.1016/j.bmcl.2016.11.064

Egbuna, C., Parmar, V. K., Jeevanandam, J., Ezzat, S. M., Patrick-Iwuanyanwu, K. C., Adetunji, C. O., Khan, J., Onyeike, E. N., Uche, C. Z., Akram, M., Ibrahim, M. S., El Mahdy, N. M., Awuchi, C. G., Saravanan, K., Tijjani, H., Odoh, U. E., Messaoudi, M., Ifemeje, J. C., Olisah, M. C., & Ibeabuchi, C. G. (2021). Toxicity of Nanoparticles in Biomedical Application: Nanotoxicology. *Journal of Toxicology, 9954443*, 1–21. doi:10.1155/2021/9954443

Eloy, J. O., Petrilli, R., Topan, J. F., Antonio, H. M. R., Barcellos, J. P. A., Chesca, D. L., Serafini, L. N., Tiezzi, D. G., Lee, R. J., & Marchetti, J. M. (2016). Co-loaded paclitaxel/rapamycin liposomes: Development, characterization and in vitro and in vivo evaluation for breast cancer therapy. *Colloids and Surfaces. B, Biointerfaces, 141*, 74–82. doi:10.1016/j.colsurfb.2016.01.032

Ettinger, A. R. (1995). Pegaspargase (Oncaspar). *Journal of Pediatric Oncology Nursing, 12*(1), 46–48. doi:10.1177/104345429501200110

Fang, X., Wang, Y., Ma, X., Li, Y., Zhang, Z., Xiao, Z., Liu, L., Gao, X., & Liu, J. (2017). Mitochondria-targeting Au nanoclusters enhance radiosensitivity of cancer cells. *Journal of Materials Chemistry. B, 5*(5), 4190–4197. doi:10.1039/C7TB00422B

Farina, E., Nabhen, J. J., Dacoregio, M. I., Batalini, F., & Moraes, F. Y. (2022). An overview of artificial intelligence in oncology. *Future Science OA, 8*(8), FSO787. doi:10.2144/fsoa-2021-0074

Finn, O. J., & Beatty, P. L. (2016). Cancer immunoprevention. *Current Opinion in Immunology, 39*, 52–58. doi:10.1016/j.coi.2016.01.002

Foged, C., Brodin, B., Frokjaer, S., & Sundblad, A. (2005). Particle size and surface charge affect particle uptake by human dendritic cells in an in vitro model. *International Journal of Pharmaceutics*, *298*(2), 315–322. doi:10.1016/j.ijpharm.2005.03.035

Fonseca-Santos, B., Gremião, M. P. D., & Chorilli, M. (2015). Nanotechnology-based drug delivery systems for the treatment of Alzheimer's disease. *International Journal of Nanomedicine*, *10*, 4981–5003. doi:10.2147/IJN.S87148

Frampton, J. E. (2010). Mifamurtide. *Paediatric Drugs*, *12*(3), 141–153. doi:10.2165/11204910-000000000-00000

Fu, Q., Wang, J., & Liu, H. (2020). Chemo-immune synergetic therapy of esophageal carcinoma: Trastuzumab modified, cisplatin and fluorouracil co-delivered lipid–polymer hybrid nanoparticles. *Drug Delivery*, *27*(1), 1535–1543. doi:10.1080/10717544.2020.1837294

Gao, S., Yang, X., Xu, J., Qiu, N., & Zhai, G. (2021). Nanotechnology for boosting cancer immunotherapy and remodeling tumor microenvironment: The horizons in cancer treatment. *ACS Nano*, *15*(8), 12567–12603. doi:10.1021/acsnano.1c02103

Gholami, A., Mousavi, S. M., Hashemi, S. A., Ghasemi, Y., Chiang, W.-H., & Parvin, N. (2020). Current trends in chemical modifications of magnetic nanoparticles for targeted drug delivery in cancer chemotherapy. *Drug Metabolism Reviews*, (52), 205–224. doi:10.1080/03602532.2020.1726943

Gill, P. S., Wernz, J., Scadden, D. T., Cohen, P., Mukwaya, G. M., von Roenn, J. H., Jacobs, M., Kempin, S., Silverberg, I., Gonzales, G., Rarick, M. U., Myers, A. M., Shepherd, F., Sawka, C., Pike, M. C., & Ross, M. E. (1996). Randomized phase III trial of liposomal daunorubicin versus doxorubicin, bleomycin, and vincristine in AIDS-related Kaposi's sarcoma. *Journal of Clinical Oncology*, *14*(8), 2353–2364. doi:10.1200/JCO.1996.14.8.2353

Gilligan, K. E., & Dwyer, R. M. (2017). Engineering exosomes for cancer therapy. *International Journal of Molecular Sciences*, *18*(6), 1122. doi:10.3390/ijms18061122

Golchin, A., Rekabgardan, M., Taheri, R. A., & Nourani, M. R. (2018). *Promotion of cell-based therapy: special focus on the cooperation of mesenchymal stem cell therapy and gene therapy for clinical trial studies. Cell Biology and Translational Medicine* (Vol. 4). Stem Cells and Cell Based Strategies in Regeneration. doi:10.1007/5584_2018_256

Goldberg, M. S. (2019). Improving cancer immunotherapy through nanotechnology. *Nature Reviews. Cancer*, *19*(10), 587–602. doi:10.103841568-019-0186-9

Gong, N., Sheppard, N. C., Billingsley, M. M., June, C. H., & Mitchell, M. J. (2021). Nanomaterials for T-cell cancer immunotherapy. *Nature Nanotechnology*, *16*(1), 25–36. doi:10.103841565-020-00822-y

Govindan, B., Sabri, M. A., Hai, A., Banat, F., & Haija, M. A. (2023). A Review of Advanced Multifunctional Magnetic Nanostructures for Cancer Diagnosis and Therapy Integrated into an Artificial Intelligence Approach. *Pharmaceutics*, *15*(3), 868. doi:10.3390/pharmaceutics15030868

Hainfeld, J. F., Dilmanian, F. A., Zhong, Z., Slatkin, D. N., Kalef-Ezra, J. A., & Smilowitz, H. M. (2010). Gold Nanoparticles Enhance the Radiation Therapy of a Murine Squamous Cell Carcinoma. *Physics in Medicine and Biology*, *55*(11), 3045–3059. doi:10.1088/0031-9155/55/11/004

Hashimoto, S., Werner, D., & Uwada, T. (2012). Studies on the interaction of pulsed lasers with plasmonic gold nanoparticles toward light manipulation, heat management, and nanofabrication. *Journal of Photochemistry and Photobiology C, Photochemistry Reviews*, *13*(1), 28–54. doi:10.1016/j.jphotochemrev.2012.01.001

Hassani, S., Gharehaghaji, N., & Divband, B. (2022). Chitosan-coated iron oxide/graphene quantum dots as a potential multifunctional nanohybrid for bimodal magnetic resonance/fluorescence imaging and 5-fluorouracil delivery. *Materials Today. Communications*, *103589*(31), 103589. doi:10.1016/j.mtcomm.2022.103589

He, P., Yang, G., Zhu, D., Kong, H., Corrales- Ureña, Y. R., Ciacchi, L. C., Wei, G. (2022). *Journal of Nanobiotechnology,* (20), 483. doi:10.1186/s12951-022-01691-4

Horak, P., Leichsenring, J., Goldschmid, H., Kreutzfeldt, S., Kazdal, D., Teleanu, V., Endris, V., Gieldon, L., Allgaeuer, M., Volckmar, A. L., Dikow, N., Renner, M., Kirchner, M., Penzel, R., Ploeger, C., Brandt, R., Seker-Cin, H., Budczies, J., & Heilig, C. E. (2022). Assigning evidence to actionability: An introduction to variant interpretation in precision cancer medicine. *Genes, Chromosomes & Cancer*, *61*(6), 303–313. doi:10.1002/gcc.22987

Horst, M. F., Coral, D. F., van Raap, M. B. F., Alvarez, M., & Lassalle, V. (2017). Hybrid nanomaterials based on gum Arabic and magnetite for hyperthermia treatments. *Materials Science and Engineering C*, *74*, 443–450. doi:10.1016/j.msec.2016.12.035

Hu, X., & Liu, S. (2015). Recent advances towards the fabrication and biomedical applications of responsive polymeric assemblies and nanoparticle hybrid superstructures. *Dalton Transactions (Cambridge, England)*, *44*(9), 3904–3922. doi:10.1039/C4DT03609C

Indoria, S., Singh, V., & Hsieh, M. F. (2020). Recent advances in theranostic polymeric nanoparticles for cancer treatment: A review. *International Journal of Pharmaceutics*, *119314*(582), 119314. doi:10.1016/j.ijpharm.2020.119314

Iqbal, M. A., Md, S., Sahni, J. K., Baboota, S., Dang, S., & Ali, J. (2012). Nanostructured lipid carriers system: Recent advances in drug delivery. *Journal of Drug Targeting*, *20*(10), 813–830. doi:10.3109/1061186X.2012.716845

Israel, L. L., Galstyan, A., Holler, E., & Ljubimova, J. Y. (2020). Magnetic iron oxide nanoparticles for imaging, targeting and treatment of primary and metastatic tumors of the brain. *Journal of Controlled Release*, *320*, 45–62. doi:10.1016/j.jconrel.2020.01.009

Itoo, A. M., Paul, M., Padaga, S. G., Ghosh, B., & Biswas, S. (2022). Nanotherapeutic Intervention in Photodynamic Therapy for Cancer. *ACS Omega*, *7*(7), 45882–45909. doi:10.1021/acsomega.2c05852

Jaiswal, M., Dudhe, R., & Sharma, P. K. (2015). Nanoemulsion: an advanced mode of drug delivery system. *3 Biotech, 5*, 123-127. doi:10.1007/s13205-014-0214-0

James, J. S. (1995). DOXIL approved for KS. *AIDS Treatment News*, (236), 6.

Jeanbart, L., & Swartz, M. A. (2015). Engineering opportunities in cancer immunotherapy. *Proceedings of the National Academy of Sciences of the United States of America*, *112*(47), 14467–14472. doi:10.1073/pnas.1508516112

Jha, S., Sharma, P. K., & Malviya, R. (2016). Hyperthermia: Role and risk factor for cancer treatment. *Achievements in the Life Sciences*, *10*(10), 161–167. doi:10.1016/j.als.2016.11.004

Jiang, X., Zhang, S., Ren, F., Chen, L., Zeng, J., Zhu, M., Cheng, Z., Gao, M., & Li, Z. (2017). Ultrasmall magnetic CuFeSe2 ternary nanocrystals for multimodal imaging guided photothermal therapy of cancer. *ACS Nano*, *11*(6), 5633–5645. doi:10.1021/acsnano.7b01032

Jin, L., Wang, Q., Chen, J., Wang, Z., Xin, H., & Zhang, D. (2019). Efficient delivery of therapeutic siRNA by Fe3O4 magnetic nanoparticles into oral cancer cells. *Pharmaceutics*, *11*(11), 615. doi:10.3390/pharmaceutics11110615

Jin, Z., Nguyen, K. T., Go, G., Kang, B., Min, H. K., Kim, S. J., Kim, Y., Li, H., Kim, C. S., Lee, S., Park, S., Kim, K. P., Huh, K. M., Song, J., Park, J. O., & Choi, E. (2019). Multifunctional Nanorobot System for Active Therapeutic Delivery and Synergistic Chemo-photothermal Therapy. *Nano Letters*, *19*(12), 8550–8564. doi:10.1021/acs.nanolett.9b03051

Kanathasan, J. S., Gunasagaram, D., Khan, S. U., Palanisamy, U. D., Radhakrishnan, A. K., Ahemad, N., & Swamy, V. (2020). Linear versus branched peptide with same amino acid sequence for legumain-targeting in macrophages: Targeting efficiency and bioimaging potential. *ChemistrySelect*, *5*(32), 9911–9919. doi:10.1002lct.202002161

Kanathasan, J. S., Palanisamy, U. D., Radhakrishnan, A. K., Chakravarthi, S., Thong, T. B., & Swamy, V. (2022). Protease-targeting peptide-functionalized porous silicon nanoparticles for cancer fluorescence imaging. *Nanomedicine (London)*, *17*(21), 1511–1528. doi:10.2217/nnm-2022-0017

Kanathasan, J. S., Swamy, V., Palanisamy, U. D., & Radhakrishnan, A. K. G. K. (2016). Legumain Targeting Peptide Conjugated Fluorescent Porous Silicon Nanoparticles for Breast Cancer Imaging. In P. Vincenzini (Ed.), *7th Forum on New Materials: Part F* (pp. 45-50). Trans Tech Publications. 10.4028/www.scientific.net/AST.102.45

Kang, E. B., Lee, J. E., Mazrad, Z. A. I., In, I., Jeong, J. H., & Park, S. Y. (2018). pH-Responsible fluorescent carbon nanoparticles for tumor selective theranostics via pH-turn on/off fluorescence and photothermal effect in vivo and in vitro. *Nanoscale*, *10*(5), 2512–2523. doi:10.1039/C7NR07900A

Kashyap, B. K., Singh, V. V., Solanki, M. K., Kumar, A., Ruokolainen, J., & Kesari, K. K. (2023). Smart Nanomaterials in Cancer Theranostics: Challenges and Opportunities. *ACS Omega*, *8*(16), 14290–14320. doi:10.1021/acsomega.2c07840

Ke, C. H., Sio, K. M., Wang, S. L., Kuo, Y., Huang, W. H., & Lin, C. S. (2022). The High Expression of Legumain in Canine Neoplasms: A Retrospective Analysis of 100 Cases. *Animals (Basel)*, *12*(4), 504. doi:10.3390/ani12040504

Khaledian, M., Nourbakhsh, M. S., Saber, R., Hashemzadeh, H., & Darvishi, M. H. (2020). Preparation and evaluation of doxorubicin-loaded pla–peg–fa copolymer containing superparamagnetic iron oxide nanoparticles (Spions) for cancer treatment: Combination therapy with hyperthermia and chemotherapy. *International Journal of Nanomedicine*, *6167*(15), 6167–6182. doi:10.2147/IJN.S261638

Kher, C., & Kumar, S. (2022). The application of nanotechnology and nanomaterials in cancer diagnosis and treatment: A review. *Cureus*, *14*(9), e29059. doi:10.7759/cureus.29059

Kim, K.-R., Kim, D.-R., Lee, T., Yhee, J. Y., Kim, B.-S., Kwon, I. C., & Ahn, D.-R. (2013). Drug delivery by a self-assembled DNA tetrahedron for overcoming drug resistance in breast cancer cells. *Chemical Communications (Cambridge)*, *49*(20), 2010–2012. doi:10.1039/c3cc38693g

Kim, Y. K., Zhang, M., Lu, J. J., Xu, F., Chen, B. A., Xing, L., & Jiang, H. L. (2016). PK11195-chitosan-graft-polyethylenimine-modified SPION as a mitochondria-targeting gene carrier. *Journal of Drug Targeting*, *24*(5), 457–467. doi:10.3109/1061186X.2015.1087527

Kourou, K., Exarchos, T. P., Exarchos, K. P., Karamouzis, M. V., & Fotiadis, D. I. (2015). Machine learning applications in cancer prognosis and prediction. *Computational and Structural Biotechnology Journal*, *13*, 8–17. doi:10.1016/j.csbj.2014.11.005

Kumar, Y., Koul, A., Singla, R., & Ijaz, M. F. (2023). Artificial intelligence in disease diagnosis: A systematic literature review, synthesizing framework and future research agenda. *Journal of Ambient Intelligence and Humanized Computing*, *14*(7), 8459–8486. doi:10.100712652-021-03612-z

Lee, S.-Y., Yang, C.-Y., Peng, C.-L., Wei, M.-F., Chen, K.-C., Yao, C.-J., & Shieh, M.-J. (2016). A theranostic micelleplex co-delivering SN-38 and VEGF siRNA for colorectal cancer therapy. *Biomaterials*, *86*, 92–105. doi:10.1016/j.biomaterials.2016.01.068

Lee, Y., El Andaloussi, S., & Wood, M. J. (2012). Exosomes and microvesicles: Extracellular vesicles for genetic information transfer and gene therapy. *Human Molecular Genetics*, *21*(R1), R125–R134. doi:10.1093/hmg/dds317

Li, Q., Liu, Y., Huang, Z., Guo, Y., & Li, Q. (2022). Triggering Immune System with Nanomaterials for Cancer Immunotherapy. *Frontiers in Bioengineering and Biotechnology*, *10*, 878524. doi:10.3389/fbioe.2022.878524

Liang, S., Sun, M., Lu, Y., Shi, S., Yang, Y., Lin, Y., Feng, C., Liu, J., & Dong, C. (2020). Cytokine-induced killer cells-assisted tumor-targeting delivery of Her-2 monoclonal antibody-conjugated gold nanostars with NIR photosensitizer for enhanced therapy of cancer. *Journal of Materials Chemistry. B*, *8*(36), 8368–8382. doi:10.1039/D0TB01391A

Liu, X., Li, C., Lv, J., Huang, F., An, Y., Shi, L., & Ma, R. (2020). Glucose and H_2O_2 dual-responsive polymeric micelles for the self-regulated release of insulin. *ACS Applied Bio Materials*, *3*(3), 1598–1606. doi:10.1021/acsabm.9b01185

Lo, S. T., Kumar, A., Hsieh, J. T., & Sun, X. (2013). Dendrimer nanoscaffolds for potential theranostics of prostate cancer with a focus on radiochemistry. *Molecular Pharmaceutics*, *10*(3), 793–812. doi:10.1021/mp3005325

Ma, H., & Xue, M. A. Q. (2021). Recent advances in the photothermal applications of two-dimensional nanomaterials: Photothermal therapy and beyond. *Journal of Materials Chemistry. A, Materials for Energy and Sustainability*, *9*(9), 17569–17591. doi:10.1039/D1TA04134G

Ma, J., Liu, R., Wang, X., Liu, Q., Chen, Y., Valle, R. P., Zuo, Y. Y., Xia, T., & Liu, S. (2015). Crucial role of lateral size for graphene oxide in activating macrophages and stimulating pro-inflammatory responses in cells and animals. *ACS Nano*, *9*(10), 10498–10515. doi:10.1021/acsnano.5b04751

Ma, W., Zhan, Y., Zhang, Y., Shao, X., Xie, X., Mao, C., Cui, W., Li, Q., Shi, J., Li, J., Fan, C., & Lin, Y. (2019). An intelligent DNA nanorobot with in vitro enhanced protein lysosomal degradation of HER2. *Nano Letters*, *19*(7), 4505–4517. doi:10.1021/acs.nanolett.9b01320

Majumder, N., Das, N. G., & Das, S. K. (2020). Polymeric micelles for anticancer drug delivery. *Therapeutic Delivery*, *11*(10), 613–635. doi:10.4155/tde-2020-0008

Malviya, R., Fuloria, S., Verma, S., Subramaniyan, V., Sathasivam, K. V., Kumarasamy, V., Hari Kumar, D., Vellasamy, S., Meenakshi, D. U., Yadav, S., Sharma, A., Fuloria, N. K. (2021). Commercial utilities and future perspective of nanomedicines. *PeerJ*, 9e12392. doi:10.7717/peerj.12392

Mao, F. X., Wen, L., Sun, C. X., Zhang, S. H., Wang, G. L., Zeng, J. F., Wang, Y., Ma, J., Gao, M., & Li, Z. (2016). Ultrasmall Biocompatible Bi_2Se_3 Nanodots for Multimodal Imaging-Guided Synergistic Radiophotothermal Therapy Against Cancer. *ACS Nano*, *10*(12), 11145–11155. doi:10.1021/acsnano.6b06067

Mendes, R., Fernandes, A. R., & Baptista, P. V. (2017). Gold nanoparticle approach to the selective delivery of gene silencing in cancer—The case for combined delivery? *Genes*, *8*(3), 94. doi:10.3390/genes8030094

Meng, L., Xia, X., Yang, Y., Ye, J., Dong, W., Ma, P., Jin, Y., & Liu, Y. (2016). Co-encapsulation of paclitaxel and baicalein in nanoemulsions to overcome multidrug resistance via oxidative stress augmentation and P-glycoprotein inhibition. *International Journal of Pharmaceutics*, *513*(1-2), 8–16. doi:10.1016/j.ijpharm.2016.09.001

Milano, G., Innocenti, F., & Minami, H. (2022). Liposomal irinotecan (Onivyde): Exemplifying the benefits of nanotherapeutic drugs. *Cancer Science*, *113*(7), 2224–2231. doi:10.1111/cas.15377

Mirrahimi, M., Khateri, M., Beik, J., Ghoreishi, F. S., Dezfuli, A. S., Ghaznavi, H., & Shakeri-Zadeh, A. (2019). Enhancement of Chemoradiation by Co-incorporation of Gold Nanoparticles and Cisplatin into Alginate Hydrogel. *Journal of Biomedical Materials Research. Part B, Applied Biomaterials*, *107*(8), 2658–2663. doi:10.1002/jbm.b.34356

Mirza, Z., & Karim, S. (2021, February). Nanoparticles-based drug delivery and gene therapy for breast cancer: Recent advancements and future challenges. *Seminars in cancer biology*, (69), 226-237. Academic Press. doi:10.1016/j.semcancer.2019.10.020

Mitchell, M. J., Billingsley, M. M., Haley, R. M., Wechsler, M. E., Peppas, N. A., & Langer, R. (2021). Engineering precision nanoparticles for drug delivery. *Nature Reviews. Drug Discovery*, *20*(2), 101–124. doi:10.103841573-020-0090-8

Molaei, M. J., & Salimi, E. (2022). Magneto-fluorescent superparamagnetic Fe_3O_4@ SiO_2@ alginate/carbon quantum dots nanohybrid for drug delivery. *Materials Chemistry and Physics*, *126361*(288), 126361. doi:10.1016/j.matchemphys.2022.126361

Mosleh-Shirazi, S., Abbasi, M., Moaddeli, M. R., Vaez, A., Shafiee, M., Kasaee, S. R., Amani, A. M., & Hatam, S. (2022). Nanotechnology Advances in the Detection and Treatment of Cancer: An Overview. In Nanotheranostics (Vol. 6, Issue 4, pp. 400–423). Ivyspring International Publisher. doi:10.7150/ntno.74613

Mundekkad, D., & Cho, W. C. (2022). Nanoparticles in Clinical Translation for Cancer Therapy. *International Journal of Molecular Sciences*, *23*(3), 1685. doi:10.3390/ijms23031685

Murakami, T., Hiroshima, Y., Matsuyama, R., Homma, Y., Hoffman, R. M., & Endo, I. (2019). Role of the tumor microenvironment in pancreatic cancer. *Annals of Gastroenterological Surgery*, *3*(2), 130–137. doi:10.1002/ags3.12225

Ni, K., Lan, G., Song, Y., Hao, Z., & Lin, W. (2020). Biomimetic nanoscale metal-organic framework harnesses hypoxia for effective cancer radiotherapy and immunotherapy. *Chemical Science (Cambridge)*, *11*(29), 7641–7653. doi:10.1039/D0SC01949F

Ni, K., Lan, G., Veroneau, S. S., Duan, X., Song, Y., & Lin, W. (2018). Nanoscale metal-organic frameworks for mitochondria-targeted radiotherapy-radiodynamic therapy. *Nature Communications*, *4321*(9), 4321. doi:10.103841467-018-06655-7

Oerlemans, C., Bult, W., Bos, M., Storm, G., Nijsen, J. F., & Hennink, W. E. (2010). Polymeric micelles in anticancer therapy: Targeting, imaging and triggered release. *Pharmaceutical Research*, *27*(12), 2569–2589. doi:10.100711095-010-0233-4

Osial, M., & Pregowska, A. (2022). The Application of Artificial Intelligence in Magnetic Hyperthermia Based Research. *Future Internet*, *356*(14), 356. doi:10.3390/fi14120356

Park, J. H., Gu, L., Von Maltzahn, G., Ruoslahti, E., Bhatia, S. N., & Sailor, M. J. (2009). Biodegradable luminescent porous silicon nanoparticles for in vivo applications. *Nature Materials*, *8*(4), 331–336. doi:10.1038/nmat2398

Park, W., Heo, Y. J., & Han, D. K. (2018). New opportunities for nanoparticles in cancer immunotherapy. *Biomaterials Research*, *22*(1), 1–10. doi:10.118640824-018-0133-y

Piccolo, O., Lincoln, J. D., Melong, N., Orr, B. C., Fernandez, N. R., Borsavage, J., Berman, J. N., Robar, J., & Ha, M. N. (2022). Radiation Dose Enhancement Using Gold Nanoparticles with a Diamond Linear Accelerator Target: A Multiple Cell Type Analysis. *Scientific Reports*, *1559*(12), 1559. doi:10.103841598-022-05339-z

Pishavar, E., Ramezani, M., & Hashemi, M. (2019). Co-delivery of doxorubicin and TRAIL plasmid by modified PAMAM dendrimer in colon cancer cells, in vitro and in vivo evaluation. *Drug Development and Industrial Pharmacy*, *45*(12), 1931–1939. doi:10.1080/03639045.2019.1680995

Poon, W., Kingston, B. R., Ouyang, B., Ngo, W., & Chan, W. C. W. (2020). A framework for designing delivery systems. *Nature Nanotechnology*, *15*(10), 819–829. doi:10.103841565-020-0759-5

Pushpalatha, R., Selvamuthukumar, S., & Kilimozhi, D. (2017). Nanocarrier mediated combination drug delivery for chemotherapy–A review. *Journal of Drug Delivery Science and Technology*, *39*, 362–371. doi:10.1016/j.jddst.2017.04.019

Ramezani Farani, M., Azarian, M., Heydari Sheikh Hossein, H., Abdolvahabi, Z., Mohammadi Abgarmi, Z., Moradi, A., Mousavi, S. M., Ashrafizadeh, M., Makvandi, P., Saeb, M. R., & Rabiee, N. (2022). Folic acid-adorned curcumin-loaded iron oxide nanoparticles for cervical cancer. *ACS Applied Bio Materials*, *5*(5), 1305–1318. doi:10.1021/acsabm.1c01311

Ranson, M. R., Cheeseman, S., White, S., & Margison, J. (2001). Caelyx (stealth liposomal doxorubicin) in the treatment of advanced breast cancer. *Critical Reviews in Oncology/Hematology*, *37*(2), 115–120. doi:10.1016/S1040-8428(00)00107-4

Revia, R. A., & Zhang, M. (2016). Magnetite nanoparticles for cancer diagnosis, treatment, and treatment monitoring: Recent advances. *Materials Today*, *19*(3), 157–168. doi:10.1016/j.mattod.2015.08.022

Ribeiro, E. B., de Marchi, P. G., Honorio-França, A. C., França, E. L., & Soler, M. A. (2020). Interferon-gamma carrying nanoemulsion with immunomodulatory and anti-tumor activities. *Journal of Biomedical Materials Research. Part A*, *108*(2), 234–245. doi:10.1002/jbm.a.36808

Rideau, E., Dimova, R., Schwille, P., Wurm, F. R., & Landfester, K. (2018). Liposomes and polymersomes: A comparative review towards cell mimicking. *Chemical Society Reviews*, *47*(23), 8572–8610. doi:10.1039/C8CS00162F

Samad, A., Sultana, Y., & Aqil, M. (2007). Liposomal drug delivery systems: An update review. *Current Drug Delivery*, *4*(4), 297–305. doi:10.2174/156720107782151269

Sánchez-López, E., Guerra, M., Dias-Ferreira, J., Lopez-Machado, A., Ettcheto, M., Cano, A., Espina, M., Camins, A., Garcia, M. L., & Souto, E. B. (2019). Current applications of nanoemulsions in cancer therapeutics. *Nanomaterials (Basel, Switzerland)*, *9*(6), 821. doi:10.3390/nano9060821

Saneja, A., Kumar, R., Mintoo, M. J., Dubey, R. D., Sangwan, P. L., Mondhe, D. M., Panda, A. K., & Gupta, P. N. (2019). Gemcitabine and betulinic acid co-encapsulated PLGA-PEG polymer nanoparticles for improved efficacy of cancer chemotherapy. *Materials Science and Engineering C*, *98*, 764–771. doi:10.1016/j.msec.2019.01.026

Santo, D., Mendonça, P. V., Lima, M. S., Cordeiro, R. A., Cabanas, L., Serra, A., Coelho, J. F. J., & Faneca, H. (2019). Poly (ethylene glycol)-block-poly (2-aminoethyl methacrylate hydrochloride)-Based Polyplexes as Serum-Tolerant Nanosystems for Enhanced Gene Delivery. *Molecular Pharmaceutics*, *16*(5), 2129–2141. doi:10.1021/acs.molpharmaceut.9b00101

Sebestyen, Z., Prinz, I., Déchanet-Merville, J., Silva-Santos, B., & Kuball, J. (2020). Translating gammadelta (γδ) T cells and their receptors into cancer cell therapies. *Nature Reviews. Drug Discovery*, *19*(3), 169–184. doi:10.103841573-019-0038-z

Sekar, R., Basavegowda, N., Thathapudi, J. J., Sekhar, M. R., Joshi, P., Somu, P., & Baek, K.-H. (2023). Recent Progress of Gold-Based Nanostructures towards Future Emblem of Photo-Triggered Cancer Theranostics: A Special Focus on Combinatorial Phototherapies. *Pharmaceutics*, *433*(15), 433. doi:10.3390/pharmaceutics15020433

Selvamuthukumar, S., & Velmurugan, R. (2012). Nanostructured lipid carriers: A potential drug carrier for cancer chemotherapy. *Lipids in Health and Disease*, *11*(1), 1–8. doi:10.1186/1476-511X-11-159

Seo, B., Lim, K., Kim, S. S., Oh, K. T., Lee, E. S., Choi, H. G., Shin, B. S., & Youn, Y. S. (2019). Small gold nanorods-loaded hybrid albumin nanoparticles with high photothermal efficacy for tumor ablation. *Colloids and Surfaces. B, Biointerfaces*, *1*(179), 340–351. doi:10.1016/j.colsurfb.2019.03.068

Sercombe, L., Veerati, T., Moheimani, F., Wu, S. Y., Sood, A. K., & Hua, S. (2015). Advances and challenges of liposome assisted drug delivery. *Frontiers in Pharmacology*, *286*(6). doi:10.3389/fphar.2015.00286

Shan, X., Gong, X., Li, J., Wen, J., Li, Y., & Zhang, Z. (2022). Current approaches of nanomedicines in the market and various stage of clinical translation. *Acta Pharmaceutica Sinica. B*, *12*(7), 3028–3048. doi:10.1016/j.apsb.2022.02.025

Shao, L., Kahraman, N., Yan, G., Wang, J., Ozpolat, B., & Ittmann, M. (2020). Targeting the TMPRSS2/ERG fusion mRNA using liposomal nanovectors enhances docetaxel treatment in prostate cancer. *The Prostate*, *80*(1), 65–73. doi:10.1002/pros.23918

Shen, Z., Chen, T., Ma, X., Ren, W., Zhou, Z., Zhu, G., Zhang, A., Liu, Y., Song, J., Li, Z., Ruan, H., Fan, W., Lin, L., Munasinghe, J., Chen, X., & Wu, A. (2017). Multifunctional Theranostic Nanoparticles Based on Exceedingly Small Magnetic Iron Oxide Nanoparticles for T_1-Weighted Magnetic Resonance Imaging and Chemotherapy. *ACS Nano*, *11*(11), 10992–11004. doi:10.1021/acsnano.7b04924

Sheoran, R., Khokra, S. L., Chawla, V., & Dureja, H. (2019). Recent patents, formulation techniques, classification and characterization of liposomes. *Recent Patents on Nanotechnology*, *13*(1), 17–27. doi:10.2174/1872210513666181127110413

Shi, X., Tian, Y., Liu, Y., Xiong, Z., Zhai, S., Chu, S., & Gao, F. (2022). Research Progress of Photothermal Nanomaterials in Multimodal Tumor Therapy. *Frontiers in Oncology*, *939365*(12), 939365. doi:10.3389/fonc.2022.939365

Shoaib, A., Azmi, L., Pal, S., Alqahtani, S. S., Rahamathulla, M., Hani, U., Alshehri, S., Ghoneim, M. M., & Shakeel, F. (2022). Integrating nanotechnology with naturally occurring phytochemicals in neuropathy induced by diabetes. *Journal of Molecular Liquids*, *350*, 118189. doi:10.1016/j.molliq.2021.118189

Silverman, J. A., & Deitcher, S. R. (2013). Marqibo® (vincristine sulfate liposome injection) improves the pharmacokinetics and pharmacodynamics of vincristine. *Cancer Chemotherapy and Pharmacology*, *71*(3), 555–564. doi:10.100700280-012-2042-4

Soliman, N. M., Shakeel, F., Haq, N., Alanazi, F. K., Alshehri, S., Bayomi, M., Alenazi, A. S. M., & Alsarra, I. A. (2022). Development and Optimization of Ciprofloxacin HCl-Loaded Chitosan Nanoparticles Using Box–Behnken Experimental Design. *Molecules (Basel, Switzerland)*, *27*(14), 4468. doi:10.3390/molecules27144468

Song, J., Yang, X., Jacobson, O., Lin, L., Huang, P., Niu, G., Ma, Q., & Chen, X. (2015). Sequential Drug Release and Enhanced Photothermal and Photoacoustic Effect of Hybrid Reduced Graphene Oxide-Loaded Ultrasmall Gold Nanorod Vesicles for Cancer Therapy. *ACS Nano*, *9*(9), 9199–9209. doi:10.1021/acsnano.5b03804

Song, N., Guo, H., Ren, J., Hao, S., & Wang, X. (2018). Synergistic anti-tumor effects of dasatinib and dendritic cell vaccine on metastatic breast cancer in a mouse model. *Oncology Letters*, *15*(5), 6831–6838. 10.3892%2Fol.2018.8188

Sriraman, S. K., Geraldo, V., Luther, E., Degterev, A., & Torchilin, V. (2015). Cytotoxicity of PEGylated liposomes co-loaded with novel pro-apoptotic drug NCL-240 and the MEK inhibitor cobimetinib against colon carcinoma in vitro. *Journal of Controlled Release*, *220*, 160–168. doi:10.1016/j.jconrel.2015.10.037

Sun, J., Russell, C. C., Scarlett, C. J., & McCluskey, A. (2020). Small molecule inhibitors in pancreatic cancer. *RSC Medicinal Chemistry*, *11*(2), 164–183. doi:10.1039/C9MD00447E

Sun, X., Huang, X., Yan, X., Wang, Y., Guo, J., Jacobson, O., Liu, D., Szajek, L. P., Zhu, W., Niu, G., Kiesewetter, D. O., Sun, S., & Chen, X. (2014). Chelator-Free 64CuIntegrated Gold Nanomaterials for Positron Emission Tomography Imaging Guided Photothermal Cancer Therapy. *ACS Nano*, *8*(8), 8438–8446. doi:10.1021/nn502950t

Tang, L., Li, J., Zhao, Q., Pan, T., Zhong, H., & Wang, W. (2021). Advanced and innovative nano-systems for anticancer targeted drug delivery. *Pharmaceutics*, *1151*(13), 1151. doi:10.3390/pharmaceutics13081151

Thapa, R. K., & Kim, J. O. (2023). Nanomedicine-based commercial formulations: Current developments and future prospects. *Journal of Pharmaceutical Investigation*, *53*(1), 19–33. doi:10.100740005-022-00607-6

Tharkar, P., Varanasi, R., Wong, W. S. F., Jin, C. T., & Chrzanowski, W. (2019). Nano-enhanced drug delivery and therapeutic ultrasound for cancer treatment and beyond. *Frontiers in Bioengineering and Biotechnology*, *7*, 324. doi:10.3389/fbioe.2019.00324

Tian, H., He, Z., Sun, C., Yang, C., Zhao, P., Liu, L., Leong, K. W., Mao, H. Q., Liu, Z., & Chen, Y. (2018). Uniform core-shell nanoparticles with thiolated hyaluronic acid coating to enhance oral delivery of insulin. *Advanced Healthcare Materials*, *7*(7), 1–12. doi:10.1002/adhm.201800285

Tran, K. A., Kondrashova, O., Bradley, A., Williams, E. D., Pearson, J. V., & Waddell, N. (2021). Deep learning in cancer diagnosis, prognosis and treatment selection. *Genome Medicine*, *152*(13), 152. doi:10.118613073-021-00968-x

Turan, O., Bielecki, P., Perera, V., Lorkowski, M., Covarrubias, G., Tong, K., Yun, A., Rahmy, A., Ouyang, T., Raghunathan, S., Gopalakrishnan, R., Griswold, M. A., Ghaghada, K. B., Peiris, P. M., & Karathanasis, E. (2019). Delivery of drugs into brain tumors using multicomponent silica nanoparticles. *Nanoscale*, *11*(24), 11910–11921. doi:10.1039/C9NR02876E

Vinhas, R., Mendes, R., Fernandes, A. R., & Baptista, P. V. (2017). Nanoparticles—Emerging potential for managing leukemia and lymphoma. *Frontiers in Bioengineering and Biotechnology*, *5*, 79. doi:10.3389/fbioe.2017.00079

Wang, H., Gu, W., Xiao, N., Ye, L., & Xu, Q. (2014). Chlorotoxin-conjugated graphene oxide for targeted delivery of an anticancer drug. *International Journal of Nanomedicine*, *9*(1), 1433–1442. doi:10.2147/IJN.S58783

Wang, L., Yuan, Y., Lin, S., Huang, J., Dai, J., Jiang, Q., Cheng, D., & Shuai, X. (2016). Photothermo-chemotherapy of cancer employing drug leakage-free gold nanoshells. *Biomaterials*, *78*, 40–49. doi:10.1016/j.biomaterials.2015.11.024

Xie, L., Jin, W., Chen, H., & Zhang, Q. (2019). Superparamagnetic iron oxide nanoparticles for cancer diagnosis and therapy. *Journal of Biomedical Nanotechnology*, *15*(2), 215–416. doi:10.1166/jbn.2019.2678

Xu, L., Wang, J., Wang, J., Lu, S.-Y., Yang, Q., Chen, C., Yang, H., Hong, F., Wu, C., Zhao, Q., Cao, Y., & Liu, H. (2022). Polypyrrole-iron phosphate-glucose oxidase-based nanocomposite with cascade catalytic capacity for tumor synergistic apoptosis-ferroptosis therapy. *Chemical Engineering Journal*, *131671*(427), 131671. doi:10.1016/j.cej.2021.131671

Yan, Q., Yuan, W., Sun, X., Zhang, M.-J., Cen, F., Zhou, S.-Y., Wu, W.-B., Xu, Y.-C., Tong, L.-H., & Ma, Z.-H. (2018). Asparaginyl endopeptidase enhances pancreatic ductal adenocarcinoma cell invasion in an exosome-dependent manner and correlates with poor prognosis. *International Journal of Oncology*, *52*(5), 1651–1660. doi:10.3892/ijo.2018.4318

Yang, H. Y., Jang, M. S., Li, Y., Lee, J. H., & Lee, D. S. (2017). Multifunctional and Redox-Responsive Self-Assembled Magnetic Nanovectors for Protein Delivery and Dual-Modal Imaging. *ACS Applied Materials & Interfaces*, *9*(22), 19184–19192. doi:10.1021/acsami.7b03747

Yang, W., Liang, H., Ma, S., Wang, D., & Huang, J. (2019). Gold nanoparticle based photothermal therapy: Development and application for effective cancer treatment. *Sustainable Materials and Technologies*, (22), e00109. doi:10.1016/j.susmat.2019.e00109

Yao, Y., Su, Z., Liang, Y., & Zhang, N. (2015). pH-Sensitive carboxymethyl chitosan-modified cationic liposomes for sorafenib and siRNA co-delivery. *International Journal of Nanomedicine*, 6185–6198. doi:10.2147/IJN.S90524

Yin, N., Wang, X., Yang, T., Ding, Y., Li, L., Zhao, S., Li, P., Xu, X., & Zhu, L. (2021). Multifunctional Fe_3O_4 cluster@ quantum dot-embedded mesoporous SiO_2 nanoplatform probe for cancer cell fluorescence-labelling detection and photothermal therapy. *Ceramics International*, *47*(6), 8271–8278. doi:10.1016/j.ceramint.2020.11.188

Zeghoud, S., Chandran, D., Amor, I. B., Hemmami, H., Mohankumar, P., & Emran, T. B. (2023). Nanotechnology and nanomaterials in the treatment and diagnosis of cancer: Correspondence. *Annals of Medicine and Surgery (London)*, *85*(5), 2258–2260. doi:10.1097/MS9.0000000000000677

Zhang, J., Pan, Y., Shi, Q., Zhang, G., Jiang, L., Dong, X., Gu, K., Wang, H., Zhang, X., Yang, N., Li, Y., Xiong, J., Yi, T., Peng, M., Song, Y., Fan, Y., Cui, J., Chen, G., Tan, W., & Zhou, C. (2022). Paclitaxel liposome for injection (Lipusu) plus cisplatin versus gemcitabine plus cisplatin in the frst-line treatment of locally advanced or metastatic lung squamous cell carcinoma: A multicenter, randomized, open-label, parallel controlled clinical study. *Cancer Communications (London, England)*, *42*(1), 3–16. doi:10.1002/cac2.12225

Zhang, L., Beatty, A., Lu, L., Abdalrahman, A., Makris, T. M., Wang, G., & Wang, Q. (2020). Microfluidic-assisted polymer-protein assembly to fabricate homogeneous functional nanoparticles. *Materials Science and Engineering C*, *110768*(111), 110768. doi:10.1016/j.msec.2020.110768

Zhang, L., Gu, F. X., Chan, J. M., Wang, A. Z., Langer, R. S., & Farokhzad, O. C. (2008). Nanoparticles in medicine: Therapeutic applications and developments. *Clinical Pharmacology and Therapeutics*, *83*(5), 761–769. doi:10.1038j.clpt.6100400

Zhang, L. X., Xie, X. X., Liu, D. Q., Xu, Z. P., & Liu, R. T. (2018). Efficient co-delivery of neo-epitopes using dispersion-stable layered double hydroxide nanoparticles for enhanced melanoma immunotherapy. *Biomaterials*, *174*, 54–66. doi:10.1016/j.biomaterials.2018.05.015

Zhang, M., Wang, W., Cui, Y., Zhou, N., & Shen, J. (2018). Magnetofluorescent Carbon Quantum Dot Decorated Multiwalled Carbon Nanotubes for Dual-Modal Targeted Imaging in Chemo-Photo-thermal Synergistic Therapy. *ACS Biomaterials Science & Engineering*, *4*(1), 151–162. doi:10.1021/acsbiomaterials.7b00531

Zhong, Y., Peng, F., Wei, X., Zhou, Y., Wang, J., Jiang, X., Su, Y., Su, S., Lee, T., & He, Y. (2012). Microwave-assisted synthesis of biofunctional and fluorescent silicon nanoparticles using proteins as hydrophilic ligands. *Angewandte Chemie International Edition*, *51*(34), 8485–8489. doi:10.1002/anie.201202085

Zhou, Z., Song, J., Nie, L., & Chen, X. (2016). Reactive oxygen species generating systems meeting challenges of photodynamic cancer therapy. *Chemical Society Reviews*, *45*(23), 6597–6626. doi:10.1039/C6CS00271D

Zhu, R., Zhang, F., Peng, Y., Xie, T., Wang, Y., & Lan, Y. (2022). Current progress in cancer treatment using nanomaterials. *Frontiers in Oncology*, *930125*(12), 930125. doi:10.3389/fonc.2022.930125

Zhu, Y. Y., Li, W., Zhao, X., Zhou, Z. J., Wang, Y. T., Cheng, Y. Y., Huang, Q., & Zhang, Q. (2017). Hyaluronic Acid-Encapsulated Platinum Nanoparticles for Targeted Photothermal Therapy of Breast Cancer. *Journal of Biomedical Nanotechnology*, *13*(11), 1457–1467. doi:10.1166/jbn.2017.2446

Chapter 9
Quantum Nanoscience in Targeted Drug Delivery:
Understanding the Mechanism of Bio-Nano Interactions in Targeting and Drug Delivery

Garima Shandilya
Bharati Vidhyapeeth, India

Kirtan Tarwadi
Bharati Vidhyapeeth, India

Sachin Chavan
Bharati Vidhyapeeth, India

ABSTRACT

Targeted drug delivery (TDD) is a concept to deliver drug elements directly to intended action site. TDD makes a system to specify drug moiety straight to specific location. TDD systems suggest synthesis, techniques and mechanisms associated with loading, transporting, and unloading of drug compounds at exact positions in body to get desired therapeutic results. To overcome the toxic behavior of conventional drug delivery methods, TDD was proposed. Nanotechnology is a science that deals with engineering, modifying, and dealing with structures at nanoscale range. Recent advances in nanomedicine have led to invention of TDD systems. To successfully understand science behind TDD, it is necessary to combine many fields together involving polymer science, pharmacology, chemistry, physics, and biology of nano structures, bio conjunction of nanoforms with desired sites, and many more. This review discusses quantum nanoscience behind the scenes enabling TDD. This may further inspire researchers to expand their vision of TDD systems and enhance the goal of nanotechnology in clinical translations.

DOI: 10.4018/979-8-3693-0448-8.ch009

1. INTRODUCTION AND EVOLUTION OF DRUG DELIVERY SYSTEMS

According to FDA, a *drug* is an active pharmaceutical ingredient (API) which is used in cure, treatment, diagnosis, mitigation and prevention of disease. A dosage form is the addition of drug (API) with non-drug components commonly called as additives or excipients (Langer, 1998). Drug delivery is an approach where the active ingredient of medication is delivered to patient in order to achieve some therapeutic approach in body by increasing the concentration of drug in some body parts (Benoit, 2020). Drug delivery system is highly integrated technique which requires integration of biologists, engineers, chemists and physicists to design proper dosage formation with suitable delivery mechanism (Mark SW, 2011).

1.1. Why We Need Drug Delivery Systems

Dosage form or ***unit doses*** are pharmaceutical formulations of drug product in specific mixture of API and inactive configuration. Direct clinical use of active drug substance "as it is" can be impractical and unfeasible as it is degraded by biological and chemical exposure to body's digestive system. Also, API's are sensitive to exposure to physical environmental factors such as pH, temperature, light, moisture etc. They have unpleasant organoleptic qualities such as taste, smell as well as potency and dosing handling issues which all leads to drug administration compliance (Langer, 1990). To overcome the difficulties of direct clinical use of API, role of excipients or additives come into play to provide organized structure, shaping formulation, enhancing bioavailability, masking bad taste, palatability and insuring safety during storage (Jain K, 2020) along with easing patient's acceptability of drug. In a way the non-drug components, excipients or additives act as delivery systems for active drug components (Ku M.S, 2008).

Through the years, there have been remarkable advances in the drug delivery approaches due to increase in molecular complexity of diseases/viruses, leading to change in cultivating therapeutic modalities.

1.2. Conventional Drug Delivery Systems vs. Targeted Drug Delivery Systems

Conventional drug delivery methods distribute drug substance throughout the body whether or not there is requirement of drug delivery to unaffected cells/tissues. This also led to requirement of more drug dosage to patient so that after distribution all over body requisite amount must be delivered to affected cells/tissues for treatment purpose. This was the particular reason for repeated dosages which also initiated other side effects of that drug by affecting healthy cells. To deal with the downside of conventional drug delivery approaches, such as uncontrolled drug release, unorganized distribution, side effects and frequent dose administration, targeted drug delivery mechanisms were thinked up (Felicity Thomas, 2022).

Thusly, targeted drug delivery approaches were considered which administered drug molecules in body through drug delivery systems to ensure transport of active therapeutic substance across biological membranes of diseased site only. The interface between patient's body and drug is managed by drug delivery systems. Thus, TDD also called "smart drug delivery" is a method to deliver medication in such a manner that increase dosage of medicine in only some parts of the body rather than distributing it throughout the body through systematic blood circulation.

1.3 Evolution of Drug Delivery Systems

Research on drug delivery systems (DDS) has been going since a long time and to mention them in a summary we can categorized them as generation of drug delivery systems. By taking considerations from previous generation DDS, new developments and research is still ongoing to adapt new generation delivery systems according to the need and impact required in that particular span of time. The development of drug delivery systems over the years (Deol P & Khuller GK, 1997) can be staircased as follows:

1. ***First Generation DDS***: Tablets, capsules, ointments, suspension, emulsions
2. ***Second Generation DDS***: Repeated dosage, prolong action tablets, coated tablets
3. ***Third Generation DDS***: Osmotically controlled system, swelling controlled system, controlled diffusion system
4. ***Fourth Generation DDS***: Targeted drug delivery systems, modulated drug delivery systems, self-regulated DDS
5. ***Fifth Generation DDS***: Gene therapy, nanotechnology based drug carriers

Evolution of TDD is a staircase of new approaches which were adapted along the way according to the requirements and available knowledge at that particular era (shown in Figure 1. Evolution of Targeted Drug Delivery). Today we are currently using the fourth generation of targeted drug delivery systems and enormous work and clinical trials are happening to approve fifth generation nano drug delivery tools.

The goal of TDD is to seek concentration of pharmaceutical agent to area of interest only for effective treatment while reducing the wastage of dosage to non- required regions. The TDD aims to have prolonged, localized, targeted and protected interactions with the affected organs or cells.

Figure 1. Evolution of targeted drug delivery

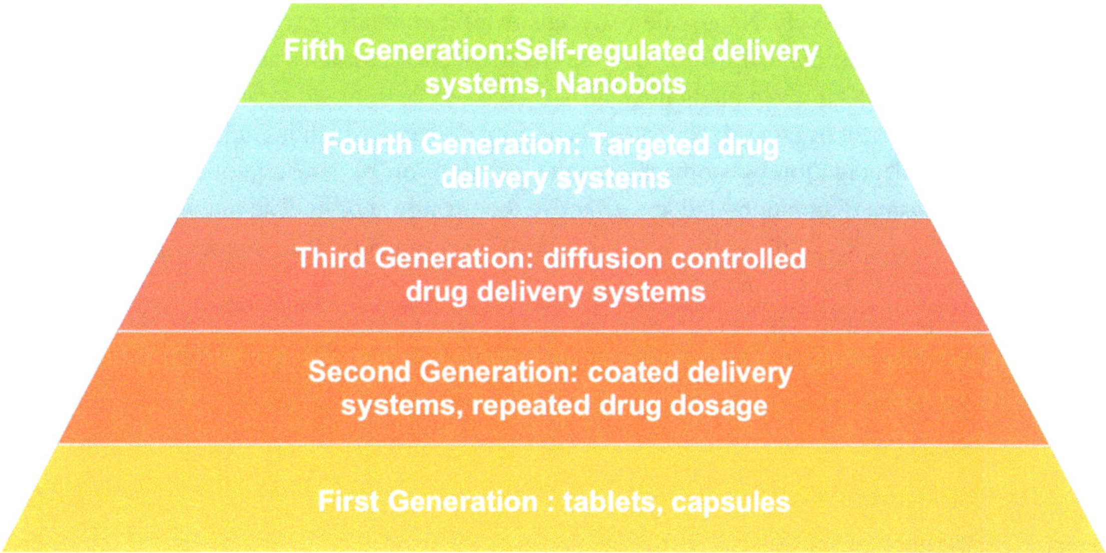

2. BASIC PRINCIPLES AND STRATEGIES OF TDD

Paul Ehrlich, the inventor of hypothetical abstraction of "***magic bullets***" suggested this name based on his vision considering two components: firstly, to recognize suitable target and binding drug entity to that location, secondly, releasing drug cargo and to ensure desired therapeutic action (Fahmy TM et al., 2005). Thus, "magic bullet" involves coordinated behavior of three components together: drug, moiety to target cells or tissues and delivery system to carry the drug (Benyettou F & Motte L.,2016).

(Zishan M. et al., 2017) mentions targeted drug delivery systems cite techniques, formulations, processes and technologies used in order to achieve transport of pharmaceutical molecules to specified location to obtain desired therapeutic effect. Targeted drug delivery (TDD) as the name suggests is designed to deliver the drug molecules to target or specific cells, tissues or organs in the body.

When a drug molecule selectively accumulates at targeted organs or tissues such that availability of drug molecules to diseased site is higher and its concentration is very low in non-targeted cells and tissues is termed as ***drug targeting***. (Valent et al., 2016) discusses prospects of attaining stress-free cure with drug targeting that focuses affinity towards causative bacteria, viruses or diseased cell with no affinity for host. As a consequence, a "magic bullet" exerts exclusive lethal action on parasite within organism at desired site of action. Over a century, this enthralling concept pressed researchers, scientists and scholars to investigate design and discovery of different drug delivery devices and carrier vehicles to implement stated hypothesis of Paul. (D. Peer et al.,2007), (V.P. Torchilin, 2000) has shown implementation of drug delivery using polymeric micelles, liposomes, carbon nanotubes, solid lipid nanoparticles (A. Grana et al.,2013), gold nanoparticles, quantum dots and other '***nanomaterials***' (Barz, 2015) to overcome drawbacks of traditional drug delivery systems. Nano medicine is the implementation of unique traits of nano systems in medicine. Being nanosized, these structures hold the capacity to easily pave their way in tissues and cells. Their ability to cross the blood brain barrier for carrying pharmaceutical compounds in the brain open new approaches to look for treatments related to nervous system. Due to these properties, we could use nanoscale materials in new and existing drugs by providing added traits of targeted, manageable and sustained delivery of the drug cargo along with fulfilling the actual demand of drug biology at site of action as well as appropriate linkage to the specific cells. Nanostructures being at nanoscale are easily amalgamated with the biologies of human body as they are designed by materials at atomic or molecular levels. Nanoscale materials exhibit enhanced properties at structural level, their chemical, physical, mechanical, biological and electrical characteristics are altered which could be utilized for amazing applications in medicine.

The challenges with use of large sized materials in drug delivery which includes in-vivo instability, poor bioavailability, degradation by stomach enzymes, absorption by intestine and liver, high doses, frequent dosages, plasma fluctuations and less effective therapeutic actions. The main principle of TDD is the reduction in frequency of dosages taken, to have uniform effect of drug, reduce drug side effects, balancing circulating fluctuations of drug in the body.

On the basis of permeability (intestinal absorption) and solubility (highest volume of water required to dissolve highest dose of drug), biopharmaceutical classification systems (Kewal, 2015) have categorized drugs in four types:

1. Type I: High solubility and high permeability
2. Type II: Low solubility and high permeability
3. Type III: High solubility and low permeability

4. Type IV: Low solubility and low permeability

3. NANOSCIENCE AND QUANTUM SCIENCE OF TARGETED DRUG DELIVERY

Nanoscience is the investigation, design, study and dealing with matter at molecular and atomic level usually below 100 nanometer. At bulk size, normal physics laws are taken into consideration but when we move to atomic and sub-atomic level, quantum physics that is principles, energy, frequency and vibrations of atoms come into play. Initial research studies were mainly focused on its chemical, physical, electrical, magnetic, biological applications, now attention has been towards exploring its pharmaceutical applications in the role of nano sized medicines or as drug delivery vehicles. (Mitchell, M. J et al., 2020) explains biologics of our body is also sized at atomic and sub-atomic level such as cells, cytoplasm, proteins and genetic materials so when integration of nanoscience with biology happens things can go pretty well with this interaction.

Quantum science might feel as a magical marvel materializing between atoms and molecules that might not be explained by classical physics. Importantly, research processes that biologists have used to study, measure and investigate living cells and organisms conclude that nanoscopic as well as short-lived quantum effects drives macroscopic physiological processes. Research results have shown that biological functions such as cell metabolism, electron transport, enzymatic activity, sensing magnetic fields, repair, reproduction and elimination are all influenced by quantum effects. We could utilize this concept to engineer future nano sized medicines and tools aiming drug targeting and delivery for obtaining précised and desired therapeutic outcomes (Clarice D. Aiello, 2023).

4. QUANTUM NANOSCIENCE AIDING PRECISION DRUG TARGETING

Quantum nanoscience is the basic research area at intersection of nanoscale that creates understanding about the quantum effects in nano world. It is the developing field with potential to revolutionize many aspects of our lives, including targeted drug delivery. It focuses on use of quantum mechanics in biology of body to explore and use coherent quantum effects in interaction mechanics of engineered nanostructures with human physiology for drug targeting (Arndt, M. et al., 2009).

4.1 Approaches for Targeted Drug Delivery

Drug delivery research over the years has offered multiple approaches to target drugs including local therapies, topical formulations, use of physical devices and now using nano drug delivery systems. To describe some of the approaches for targeted drug delivery (V.P. Torchilin, 2006) are as follows (shown in Figure 2. Describing targeted drug delivery systems with aspect to targeting approaches, drug considerations and physiology of nanocarriers):

4.1.1. Active Targeted Drug Delivery Mechanism

The covering material is decorated with ligand sites to have lock and key approach with its particular receptor only. Nano systems could also be triggered based on the site specific triggers for delivering the

Figure 2. Describing targeted drug delivery systems with aspect to targeting approaches, drug considerations and physiology of nanocarriers

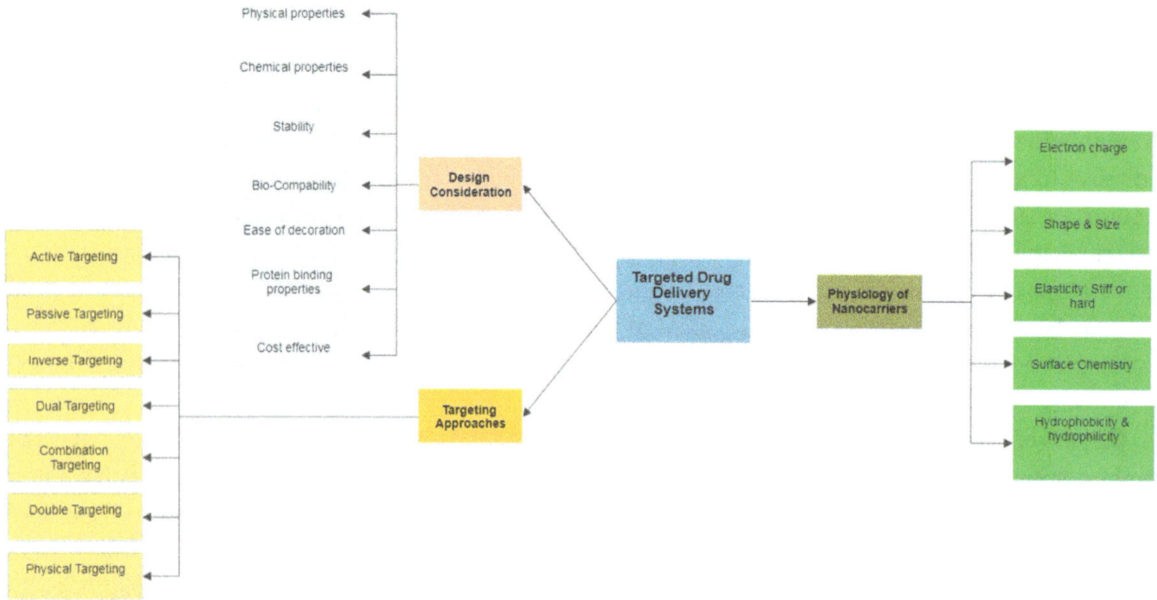

cargo to diseased cells or tissues. Active targeting ligands could be proteins, nucleic acids, or other molecules that bind to specific receptors on the surface of cells (Prasad, D & Harsh Chauhan, 2013). These carriers can be designed to have specific surface properties that allow them to bind to the target cells or tissues or organs. Once the carrier binds to cell, drug is released and can exert its therapeutic effect. However, there are still challenges that need to be addressed before this approach can be widely adopted.

- Developing ligands that are specific enough to target only the desired cells.
- Drafting drug carriers that are stable and can deliver drug to target cells with high efficiency.

There are a number of different ligands that can be used for active drug targeting, including:

- **Antibodies**: Antibodies are highly specific proteins that can bind to specific receptors on target cells.
- **Aptamers**: Aptamers are short, single-stranded DNA or RNA molecules that can bind to specific receptors on target cells.
- **Peptides**: Peptides are short chains of amino acids that can bind to specific receptors on target cells.
- **Carbohydrates**: Carbohydrates can bind to specific receptors on target cells.

4.1.2. Passive Targeted Drug Delivery Mechanism

It is achieved by encapsulating the drug in a shell which is formed of some nanoscale material. Engineering nanostructures that encapsulate the drug in nano moiety prove potential TDD vehicles as targeting strategy for drug delivery. Passive drug targeting is based on the enhanced permeability and retention (EPR) effect, a phenomenon that occurs in tumor tissues or diseased cells. The diseased tissues have leaky blood vessels that allow large drug molecules to enter tissues more easily than in healthy tissues. Additionally, two factors together are basis for passive drug targeting:

- Lymphatic drainage of tumor tissues creates an environment that prevents drug delivery molecules from being cleared from diseased tissue.
- Drug carriers that are large enough to be removed through bloodstream create possibility to accumulate in tumor cells even if they do not specifically target diseased cells/tissues.

Passive drug targeting is a promising approach for improving safety, efficiency and efficacy of drug delivery and could be used to deliver a variety of drugs to tumor tissues (Attia, M. F et al., 2019) including:

- ***Chemotherapy drugs***: used to kill cancer cells. Passive drug targeting can be used to deliver chemotherapy drugs to tumor tissues with reduced side effects.
- ***Radiotherapy drugs***: Passive drug targeting can be used to deliver radiotherapy drugs to tumor tissues with improved targeting strategies.
- ***Gene therapy drugs***: are used to deliver genes to cells to tumor cells with enhanced delivery mechanisms.

4.1.3. Inverse Targeted drug delivery mechanism

An inverse targeted drug delivery system is a type of drug delivery system that seeks to avoid passive uptake of colloidal carriers by the reticuloendothelial system (RES). The RES is a network of cells that are responsible for eliminating foreign particles from bloodstream. Colloidal carriers, such as liposomes and nanoparticles, are often taken up by the RES, which can limit their therapeutic efficacy. Achieving inverse targeted delivery by pre-injecting a large amount of blank colloidal carriers or macromolecules prevent RES from taking up the drug-loaded colloidal carriers. Due to this, drug-loaded carriers are able to circulate in the bloodstream for longer periods of time and reach their target tissues.

Inverse targeting has been shown to be effective in delivering drugs to a variety of tissues, including the brain, liver, and spleen. It has also been shown to be effective in delivering drugs to tumors or affected cells.

4.1.4. Dual targeting drug delivery mechanism

Dual targeted drug delivery is a promising new technology that has immense potential to improve efficacy and safety of drug therapy. Dual targeting uses two different targeting mechanisms to deliver drugs to specific cells or tissues. It is done by using two different ligands or by using a single ligand that can bind to two different receptors. Several advantages for dual TDD are:

- Improve specificity of drug delivery by targeting two different receptors thus reducing side effects by targeting the drug to desired cells or tissues and avoiding other cells that do not express target receptors.
- Enhancing efficiency of drug delivery by increasing binding affinity of drug to the target receptors. This can help to ensure that drug is delivered to target cells or tissues in a more efficient way.
- To deliver drugs to cells or tissues that is difficult to target with single targeted drug delivery. Dual targeted drug delivery can be used to deliver drugs even to the brain crossing blood-brain barrier.

4.1.5. Combination Targeting

Combination drug delivery systems (CDDS) are drug delivery systems that contain two or more drugs that are designed to work together to improve the efficacy or safety of the treatment. There are several different types of CDDSs, including:

- **Liposomes:** Liposomes are spherical vesicles that are made of phospholipids. They can be used to encapsulate drugs and deliver them to specific cells or tissues.
- **Dendrimers:** Dendrimers are highly branched polymers that can be used to carry drugs. They can be designed to target specific cells or tissues, and they can also be programmed to release drugs at a controlled rate.
- **Polymeric nanoparticles**: Polymeric nanoparticles are small particles that are made of polymers. They can be used to carry drugs and deliver them to specific cells or tissues.
- **Microspheres:** Microspheres are small beads that are made of polymers or other materials. They can be used to carry drugs and deliver them to specific cells or tissues.

4.1.6. Double Targeted Drug Delivery

In double targeting, temporal and spatial methodologies are combined, spatial placement to specific sites and temporal delivery occurs at a controlled rate. Double targeted drug delivery (DTDD) is a type of drug delivery system that combines two or more targeting mechanisms to deliver drugs to specific cells or tissues (Strategies of Drug Targeting, 2022). The two targeting mechanisms can be either spatial or temporal, or a combination of both.

- ***Spatial targeting*** involves delivering the drug to a specific location in body. This is done by using a carrier system that is designed to target specific cells or tissues. For example, liposomes can be targeted to cancer cells by using ligands that bind to specific receptors on the surface of the cells.
- ***Temporal targeting*** involves delivering drug at a specific time. This can be done by using a carrier system that is designed to release drug at a controlled rate. For example, polymeric nanoparticles can be loaded with a drug that is released over time.

4.1.7. Physical Targeting drug delivery mechanism

Physically facilitating drug-delivery (PFDD) systems emerge as manipulation of physical targeting tools where delivered drug could be handled or directed by applying various physical mechanisms in an in-vivo environment. Physical factors such as pH, temperature or electric charge factor have been explored for targeted drug delivery. In physical targeting drug carrier is distributed in systemic circulation in proper way that it will not accumulate at target site. However, drug carrier system will start to degrade at target site when drug is released (S. Ganta et al., 2008). Some of them are mentioned below:

- pH sensitive systems
- magnetic-sensitive systems
- ultrasound-sensitive systems
- temperature-sensitive systems

5. QUANTUM-NANO KINETICS BEHIND TARGETED DRUG SYSTEMS: GETTING INTO CELLS AND THEIR RELEASING MECHANISM

For drug delivery systems, bloodstream is the main transporting pathway from site of administration to intended targeted site of action. Drug release mechanism involves quantum interactions of drug delivery vehicles with the biological anatomy as well as physiological aspects of human body. On getting deep with the mechanisms happening in individual cells and their signaling with neighboring cells is a mesmerizing orchestra of cells performing complex sensations in seamless way. To list some of the release mechanism come to pass drugs into human body includes following processes (Wong PT & hoi SK, 2015):

1. Multivalent receptor-ligand interactions of nanosystems with target cells receptors
2. With the endocytosis nano- drug carrier enters in the cell
3. Ensuring drug release

The transfer of signals between molecular circuits allow binding to intracellular diseased targets, escaping undruggable cells and entry into cell via cell membranes. By some simple quantum molecular rules, cellular uptake happens in favorable chemical characteristics with help of sticky surface decorations of nanocarriers.

Nano-engineered carriers are the potential carriers of drug coupled with ligands to travel to their anticipated cellular targets. Due to size benefit of nanotechnology, drugs are able to pass the complex geometry of biological systems, paving way to contact targets, entering cells and releasing their cargo load for the therapeutic action. Mainly drug release mechanisms as shown in Figure 3. Quantum-nanoscience mechanisms in Targeted Drug Delivery systems manifests with following quantum processes in cells (Saltzman, M.W & Torchilin, V.P., 2021):

1. Linker cleavage process
2. Control carrier
3. Absorption
4. Distribution
5. Metabolism
6. Elimination
7. Toxicity

Figure 3. Quantum-nanoscience mechanisms in targeted drug delivery systems manifests with following quantum processes in cells
(Saltzman, M.W & Torchilin, V.P., 2021)

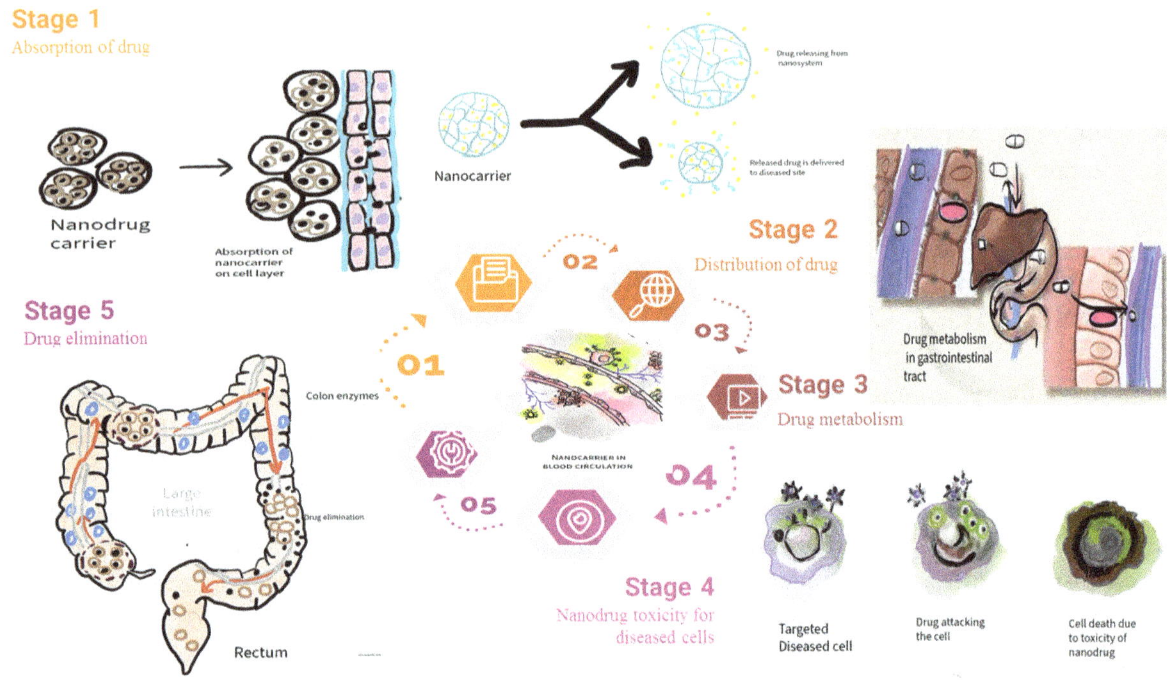

5.1. Linker Cleavage

In cells is a process of breaking bonds between two molecules that are linked together by a linker. This can be done by a variety of methods, including enzymatic cleavage, chemical cleavage and physical cleavage. In cells, linker cleavage is often used to release a payload from a carrier molecule.Linker cleavage can also be used to control release of molecule from cell. Some proteins are tagged with a linker to get cleaved by protease that is only active in certain tissues or under certain conditions. This allows protein to be released only when it is needed (Bargh JD et al., 2019). Methods that can be used for linker cleavage in cells are:

- **Enzymatic cleavage**: This is the most common method for linker cleavage in cells. Enzymes that can cleave linkers are often specific to certain tissues or conditions, which allows for the controlled release of molecules.
- **Chemical cleavage**: This method uses chemicals to break the bonds between two molecules. Chemical cleavage is often used to cleave linkers that are not susceptible to enzymatic cleavage.
- **Physical cleavage**: This method uses physical forces such as ultrasound or light to break the bonds between two molecules. Physical cleavage is often used to cleave linkers that are not susceptible to enzymatic or chemical cleavage.

5.2. Control of Carrier

The control of carrier in drug delivery systems and cells is a rapidly developing field. As our understanding of factors that affect carrier control improves, development of many effective and targeted drug delivery systems would increase (Zhao, Z et al., 2020). Some of the most important factors that can affect the control of carrier in drug delivery systems and cells include:

- Size and shape of the carrier
- Surface properties of the carrier
- Degradability of the carrier
- Environment in which the carrier is being delivered:.

5.3. Absorption of Drug in Cells

Once a drug enters a cell, it must be transported to the bloodstream in order to reach its target tissues. This process is called absorption. There are two main mechanisms of drug absorption: passive diffusion and carrier-mediated transport.

- ***Passive diffusion***: most common mechanism for drug absorption. It occurs when drug molecules move from an area of high concentration to low concentration. The rate of passive diffusion is determined by molecular weight, lipid solubility and the concentration gradient of drug.
- ***Carrier-mediated transport***: is a specialized mechanism of drug absorption. It occurs when drug molecules gets bind to carrier protein in cell membrane. The carrier protein then transports drug molecules across cell membrane. The rate of carrier-mediated transport is determined by drug's affinity for carrier protein and concentration of drug carrier protein into cell membrane.

The rate of distribution is determined by drug's solubility in blood, its affinity for plasma proteins and blood flow to tissues (Couvreur P., 2013). In this aspect, size of nanoparticles matters as they could interfere with their circulatory ability, persistence in blood to target pathological cells, coagulation may occur due to nanoparticle which may cause capillary occlusions (Su C. et al., 2019). When drug is taken, it is transported through the porous membranes into systematic circulation wherein they are absorbed by macrophages and lymphocytes and partially by phagocytized to enter circulatory systems through lymph vessels (Fu C et al.,2013, Zhao Y et al.,2012, Darville N et al., 2014, Wei X et al.,2013). After oral administration, nanoparticles gets absorbed into blood through chemical and enzymatic barriers in gastrointestinal tract by crossing barriers presented in intestinal epithelium via diffusion carrier medicated transcytosis or M cell absorption (Jin Y et al.,2012, Zhang Z et al.,2012).The factors that can affect drug absorption from cells to the body's circulating system are discussed as:

- **Drug's physicochemical properties**: The drug's molecular weight, lipid solubility, and ionization state all affect its absorption. Such as drugs that are highly lipid-soluble are more likely to be absorbed by passive diffusion.
- **Route of administration**: The route of administration can also affect the absorption of drugs. Drugs that are administered orally are absorbed through the gastrointestinal tract. Drugs that are administered subcutaneously or intramuscularly are absorbed through the tissues.

- **Patient's individual characteristics**: The patient's age, health status, and genetic makeup can all affect the absorption of drugs. For example, older adults may have a slower rate of absorption than younger adults. Patients with certain health conditions, such as liver or kidney disease may also have a slower rate of absorption.

5.4. Distribution of Drug in Cellular Mechanics

The distribution of drugs through cellular uptake is a complex process that is affected by a number of factors which includes drug's physicochemical properties, cell type along with presence of specific receptors or transporters on the cell surface. There are two main mechanisms of cellular uptake: passive diffusion and receptor-mediated endocytosis.

- ***Passive diffusion*** is most common mechanism of cellular uptake. It occurs when the drug molecules move from an area of high concentration to an area of low concentration across the cell membrane. The rate of passive diffusion is determined by the drug's molecular weight, lipid solubility, and concentration gradient.
- ***Receptor-mediated endocytosis*** is a more specialized mechanism of cellular uptake. It occurs when the drug molecules bind to specific receptors on and to cell surface. The receptor-drug complex is then internalized by the cell through endocytosis. The rate of receptor-mediated endocytosis is determined by drug's affinity for number of receptors on surface of cells.

Nanocarrier distribution is related to their biological distribution in regional lymph nodes, liver, spleen, kidney for retention and permeability in diseased cells showing EPR effect (Lee JH et al., 2015). Formation of protein-corona on nanoparticle in blood, EPR effect, targeted therapy as well as surface characteristics also affects distribution. To mention some factors that can affect drug distribution through cellular uptake are:

- **Drug's physicochemical properties**: The drug's molecular weight, lipid solubility, and ionization state all affect its uptake. Drugs that are highly lipid-soluble are more likely to be internalized by receptor-mediated endocytosis.
- **Cell type** can also affect uptake of drugs. For example, some cells have more receptors for certain drugs than other cells.
- **Presence of specific receptors or transporters**: The presence of specific receptors or transporters on the cell surface can also affect uptake of drugs. Cells that have receptors for a certain drug will take up that drug more readily than cells that do not have those specific receptors.

5.5. Metabolism of Drug in the Body

In the process of metabolism, nanocarriers lose their original forms as degradation of drug delivery system takes place due to chemical environment, drug payload is released as van-der-waals bonds of drug and excipients are loosen to lesions of unhealthy cells to reduce side effects. The "drug cargo" is released via dissolution of active pharmaceutical agent through enzymatic activity, pH dependent hydrolysis as well as presence of biological milieu in surrounding environment (Ren Q et al., 2019, Lee SY et al., 2019). Cells uptake the drug, process it, digest it at different levels and then push it further to the excretion zone.

Metabolism of nanosystems for drug delivery systems plays significant role in drug efficacy and sustained release mechanism. Thus more research is needed to understand pharmacodynamics of nanoparticles to improve their sustained release. Premature metabolism may also lead to drug leakage at non-intended sites and non-sustained release of drug may happen. An excessive slow mechanism may lead to long-term drug leakage which may result in accumulation in body by causing toxic side effects (Gao D et al.,2008).

5.6. Diseased Cell Death by Nanodrug Toxicity

Nanodrugs are a type of drug delivery systems that uses nanoparticles to carry drugs to specific cells or tissues. This can be used to target diseased cells and induce cell death which can be a useful treatment for cancer and other diseases.

There are a number of different ways that nanodrugs can induce cell death.

- One way is by triggering apoptosis; a programmed cell death process. ***Apoptosis*** is a tightly regulated process that involves activation of number of genes and proteins. By interfering with this process nanodrugs lead to death of the diseased cell.
- Another way that nanodrugs can induce cell death is by triggering ***necrosis***; a type of cell death that is not programmed. Necrosis is often causing damage to cell membrane which can lead to release harmful substances that intends to kill the cell. Nanodrugs can cause damage to the cell membrane which lead to necrosis.
- In addition to apoptosis and necrosis, nanodrugs can also induce other types of cell death, such as ***ferroptosis*** and ***pyroptosis.*** These are less well-understood than apoptosis and necrosis but they are also potential targets for nanodrug therapy.

Research on nanodrugs is still in its infancy and there is great potential for this technology to be used to treat numerous diseases (Liu, J et al., 2019). Nanodrugs have the potential to be more effective and less toxic than traditional drugs as well as they could also be used to target specific cells or tissues reducing side effects.

5.7. Elimination of Drug From Body

The elimination of drugs from body is a complex process that involves a number of organs and systems. The main organs involved in drug elimination are the liver, kidneys, lungs, and gastrointestinal tract. The liver is responsible for metabolizing drugs. This means that the liver breaks down drugs into smaller molecules that can be more easily eliminated from body. The kidneys are responsible for excreting drugs from the body in urine. The lungs are responsible for excreting drugs in the breath. The gastrointestinal tract is responsible for excreting drugs in feces. The elimination processes is carried by liver and kidney and are closely related to the efficacy, circulation duration, side effects of nanoparticles. After filtration process taking place in liver and kidneys, hepatocytes (Jiang X et al., 2019) help in removal of bile mostly through the renal or urine pathway. The physiochemical properties, surface charge and size negatively affect the excretion of nanoparticles from the body.Some factors that affect rate of drug elimination from body are:

- **Drug's physicochemical properties**: The drug's molecular weight, lipid solubility, and ionization state all affect its elimination. For example, drugs that are highly lipid-soluble are more likely to be eliminated by the liver.
- **Dose of the drug**: The dose of drug can also affect its elimination. Higher dose of a drug will be eliminated more slowly than a lower dose.
- **Patient's individual characteristics**: Patient's age, health status and genetic makeup can all affect the elimination of drugs. As older people may have a slower rate of elimination than younger adults. Patients with certain health conditions such as liver or kidney disease may also show a slower rate of elimination.

The elimination of drugs from body is an important process that determines duration and action of drug. By understanding factors that affect drug elimination, we could pave new ways in engineering more effective drug dosing regimens along with improving safety of drug therapies.

6. STRATEGIES ASSISTING ENGINEERING OF NANOSYSTEMS AS DRUG DELIVERY VEHICLES

Nanomedicine; a new developing field of nanoengineering with medicine where scientists and researchers engineer nanoparticles for their application in diagnosis as well as treatment of diseases (B.Y.S. Kim et al.,2005, B. Pelaz et al., 2017). Nanotechnology based drug delivery systems, diagnostics tools, imaging devices as well as nanotherapeutics are the future of healthcare. To bring these new concepts in real-time applications is a challenging process. To procure desired biological therapeutic action at desired site, it is critical to know the basic concepts behind how nanoparticles are responded by the biological systems and how their pathway to destination and curative aim is achieved. Engineered nanomaterials (ENM) possess incredible physiochemical properties that could be used in medicinal purposes such as imaging, drug delivery, diagnosis, clinical and therapeutic purposes (M. Björnmalm et al., 2017), D. Rosenblum et al.,2018). To achieve the goal of nanomedicine for efficient and effective delivery systems are required to fully control nanoparticle transport in body to specific cells. ENM has targeted drug delivery candidates allows precisely controlling delivery of active pharmaceutical ingredient to the desired lesion site of patient.

The major quest is to learn the fundamental concepts of nanoparticle interaction with biological system (C. von Roemeling et al.,2017). Factors contributing for designing the TDD systems as well as effective delivery of nanomedicines must be well understood to withstand the complex nano-bio interactions. (P.C. Ke et al., 2017)) explains some complexities of nano-bio interface which include:

i. Physiochemical properties of nanoparticles (shape, size, surface chemistry, composition, architecture, density, modulus)
ii. Interplay interactions between individual nanoparticle properties and biological parameters (biological composition, pH and other biochemical interactions in milieu)
iii. Kinetics and quantum physics of drug with biological factors

(C.D. Walkey et al., 2012), C.D. Walkey et al.,2012) demonstrates that when a nanomedicine is administered into body, it gets in contact with blood and serum proteins which starts cellular pathway responses by non-specifically getting absorbed onto nanoparticle surface forming protein-corona. This outer layer formation leads to change in nanoparticle physiochemical properties by giving them unintentional brand new decoration (M.P. Monopoli et al., 2012). Now this new layer determines fate of nanosystem interaction with the biological entities cells, tissues, organs, cellular and sub-cellular organelles. This nano-bio interaction influence pristine bio-identities of the nanocarrier systems elicitating numerous cellular and biological responses which ultimately determines the targeted efficiency and outcome of nanomedicine (Yaling Wang et al.,2019).

To describe the active ENM interactions are –

1. Adsorption
2. Dissolution
3. Surface reconstruction of nanocarrier in form of protein –corona in order to minimize free energy
4. Redox reactions with contact component of ENM

(C.C. Fleischer & C.K. Payne, 2014), S. Ritz et al., 2015), C.D. Walkey et al., 2014), C.D. Walkey et al., 2012), Q. Dai et al., 2018), S. Wilhelm et al., 2016)) states that upon biological interlinkage of nanoparticles with the mechanics of cells and tissues impose a challenge for designing, grooming and engineering nanocarriers as delivery systems. There is utmost need to address the fundamental concepts behind essential mechanisms of nanosystems interaction with the biologies of body. Previous studies (E. Blanco et al., 2015, B. Du et al., 2017, S. Barua & S. Mitragotri, 2014, B. Pelaz et al., 2015, S. Behzadi et al., 2017, J. Xu et al., 2018, K.M. Tsoi et al., 2016)) shows that we need to divide these studies majorly into three subsections:

- Interaction at organ-tissue level
- Interaction at cellular-subcellular level
- Role of physical, chemical and bio-molecular parameters for these quantum biomechanics

6.1. Why We Need Nano-Bio Interaction Understanding

Our goal is to deliver active therapeutic drug load to the specific location in body. For this, firstly nanosystems or nanocarriers must be able to distinguish between healthy cells and diseased cells. In order to manifest this goal we engineer nanoparticles either with bio-markers to locate its linker in biological swimming pool inside body or to decorate nanocrriers with analyte-ligand mechanism. This concept helps to recognize specific location, getting attached to complementary cell surface and delivering payloads to diseased sites (M.E. Davis et al., 2010, C. V. Pecot et al., 2011, K. Lee et al., 2017), M. Kodiha et al.,2015), M.R.K. Ali et al., 2017). These kinetics of targeted drug delivery focuses mainly on following interactions

- Cell uptake of nanoparticles
- Intracellular trafficking of nanoparticles into cells
- Mastering quantum dynamics and kinetics of nano-bio interactions

6.2. Determining Driving Forces Between Nano-Bio Interface

The "nano-bio" interactions hold the power of navigating nano drug delivery systems through biofluids of human body to targeted cells or non-targetd cells. Physiochemcial properties of the ENM, components surrounding them, quantum parameters at which nanocarriers make contact with the biological zones of body are involved in drug movement as well as its targeting mechanism. This chapter discusses these quantum nano-bio interfaces to achieve the desired outcome of nanomedicine as targeted drug delivery systems.

Starting with the nanomedicine drug administration, earlier studies have shown evidences indicating interactions with biological systems such as biofluids, biomolecules, proteins, DNA/RNA, lipids and cell membranes. The biophysiochemical interactions are mainly determined by the non-covalent interactions, van der-waals force, electrostatic interactions, hydrophobic interactions, hydrogen bonding, stereo-elective interaction, metal-ligand coordination, increasing complexity of nano-bio interactions (Yaling Wang et al., 2019). These forces are the key factors deciding the fate of bioindentity of nanocarriers in such dynamic physiology of body.

6.2.1. Nano-Protein Interface

Role of each driving forces such as electrostatic interaction, hydrophobic, hydrogen bonding, stereoselectivity is dependent on charge, sequence of distribution, size, and structure of protein. The physiochemical properties of nanoparticles including surface charge, molecular structure, hydrophobicity or hydrophilicity are also affected by the temperature, pH, and ionic strength of surrounding biofluid (Monopoli, M. P et al., 2012). The nano-protein interface can be sub- categorized as:

1. Hydrophobic Interaction
2. Electrostatic Interaction
3. Molecular Recognition
4. Metal-ligand Coordination

6.2.1.1. Hydrophobic Interaction: Serum protein binds to the surface of nanocarrier through $\pi-\pi$ stacking interactions between them (Ge, C et al., 2011). The π-cation or $\pi-\pi$-cation interactions also appear as driving forces to interact with serum albumin mostly through hydrophobic forces (Abraham, A. N et al., 2018) which are predominantly depended on the shape and size of the nanocarrier system.

6.2.1.2. Electrostatic Interaction: At nano-protein interface, (Wang, X et al., 2018) projects that amino acids are distributed along the linkage line where hydrogen bonding along with electrostatic forces forms strong salt bridges at the interface. Due to these amino acid sequences, targeting nanosystems have more affinity towards protein or polypeptide binding.

6.2.1.3. Molecular Recognition: For sustained release of drugs, molecular recognition, ligand-cognate receptors, antigens- antibodies, substances-enzymes are mostly used for specific target recognition. Different electrolyte environments caused by polyelectrolyte effect and hydrophobic interactions tends to change binding force between antigen-antibody interactions. The native steric conformation of proteins results in specific absorption of proteins on the surface of nanomedincine. (Gu, X et al., 2018) stereoselectivity, chirality and orientation of transferin determines recognition of receptors on cell membrane.

6.2.1.4. Metal-ligand Coordination: Electron charge of atoms of proteins and other biomolecules shows attraction towards presence of metal nanoparticles due to electrostatic pull. This force makes protein getting absorbed on the nanosystem by increasing their dissolution rate as well as physiochemical characterstics (Miclăuş, T et al., 2016, Nel, A. E et al., 2009).

6.2.2. Nano-Membrane Interface

A nano-membrane interface is the boundary between a nano-membrane and another material, such as a liquid, gas, or solid. The properties of nano-membrane interface can have a significant impact on performance of nano-membrane, such as its permeability, selectivity, and stability. The nano-membrane interface is typically characterized by its surface energy, roughness, and chemistry. The surface energy of nano-membrane, roughness and chemistry determines how well it will interact with other materials (Lou HY et al., 2018).

The nano-membrane interface can be modified in a number of ways to improve performance of nano-membrane. The roughness modified by etching or polishing, chemistry is modified by functionalizing it with specific molecules. As our understanding of nano-membrane interfaces improves, we will be able to design and fabricate nano-vehicles with even better performance, accurate traits and desired characteristics for various drug targeting channels.Nano-membranes enacts mainly two interactions:

6.2.2.1. Electrostatic Interaction: Internalization of nanosystems into cell is dependent on decoration of negatively charged proteins and self-assembled lipid bilayers on cell membranes. On other hand, electrostatic force, hydrophobic interactions, hydrogen bonding and charge on the outer coat of nano drug delivery system ensures connection with cell membranes to proceed with endocytosis once everything connects in order (Wang, J et al., 2018). (Peng, F et al., 2019) check successful interaction at cell junction, endothelial leakiness, repulsion-sedimentary interactions as well as electrostatic repulsions all play their roles specifically for entry of nanosystem into specific targeted cell.

6.2.2.2. Membrane Curvature: Biological membranes are structured in curved manner thus the initial curvature of cell membrane drives adsorption of nanoparticles and secure their behavior in cell. Other driving forces, local curvature, receptors, rafts, distribution, mobility, heterogeneity, stiffness as well as attractive or repulsive forces of cell membranes warrant fate of nanoparticles or nanosystems inside cell (Bahrami, A. H et al., 2018).

6.2.3. Nano-Biofluid Interface

A nano-biofluid interface is boundary between nanomaterial and biofluid, such as blood, lymph, or cerebrospinal fluid. The properties of nano-biofluid interface can have a significant impact on interaction between nanomaterial and biofluid, such as rate of transport of molecules across interface, adhesion of cells to nanosurface and activation of cells by nanomaterial contact.

Omnipresent biofluid is a combination of water, carbon dioxide, oxygen and ions to transport energy and substances as well as for carrying out vital life functions. Presence of water and oxygen in biofluid influence hydrogen bonding, electrostatic forces, hydrophobic interaction and stereoselectivity with nanosystems decide type of driving force for moving nano-drug carrier towards its final destination (Zhao W et al., 2017). Additionally, viscosity, flow velocity, stiffness, diffusivity greatly influence transportation as well as interaction of nanosytem with cell biology. The physiological properties of nanomedicine ascertain their biological providence in interaction with quantum mechanics of cells.

The protein-corona formation, time to be circulated in blood, interaction with liver linning and kidney internal surface, desired targets, cell functionalization, biocatalysis, interaction with DNA and removal through renal pathway (Wang, Y et al., 2016). Therefore, estimating underlying nano–bio interface mechanisms guide us to design and engineer prudent targeted drug delivery nanosystems in accordance with the fundamental traits of biological systems.

6.2.4. Sway of Chemical Redox Reactions on NANO–BIO Interface

Chemical redox reactions at the nano-bio interface can have a significant impact on the behavior of both the nanomaterial and biological system. These reactions can be used to control adhesion of cells to nanomaterial, activation of cells by the nanomaterial, and delivery of drugs to desired cells.When these nanoparticles are exposed to biofluid molecules on surface of the nanoparticles interacts with biofluid. If biofluid has a different charge than nanoparticles then they are attracted to biofluid adheration.

The dynamic identity of nano drug delivery systems as well as the biofludic pathway guides them inside cells. Cellular redox equilibrium, cell survival metabolism, intracellular signaling cascades, innate immunity regulation and chemical reactivity are all maintained by the reactive oxygen and nitrogen species (ROS and RNS). Intracellular ROS/RNS shows higher chemical reactivity with lipids, proteins and genetic materials eliciting series of downstream biological events (Catalano, F et al., 2015). It is also seen that accumulation of intracellular ROS/RNS leads to dysfunction of enzymes, insufficient antioxidants may lead to cascade of oxidative stress stimulating antioxidant defense, inflammatory response, cytotoxicity and cell death (Nel, A et al., 2006). Neutral molecular oxygen and water can readily cross membranes of cells in biological radical generation process but some changes occur when smart ENM try to invade cells. ENM are designed to be able to target unhealthy cells by two of the either processes: first, they will serve as pro-oxidants (producing ROS/RNS), blocking ROS/RNS or inducing cell death of diseases cell; secondly, it may act as antioxidant for hunting ROS/RNS or be an oxygen supplier to diminish hypoxic situations. (Chong, Y et al., 2017), Zhou, H et al., 2014) exclaims that nanodrug might also decrease the mitochondrial electron-transfer activity by acting as an antioxidant or pro-oxidant via four processes:

- Supplying molecular oxygen or reducing oxidative stress while interacting with radical ROS/RNS species
- Free molecules of oxygen, water reacting with ENM to produce ROS/RNS
- Reacting directly with the electronegative atoms of antioxidant biomolecules
- Detoxification of ROS/RNS by interaction with prosthetic group of oxidoreductase limiting enzyme activity

6.2.5. Electron Transfer Appliance of Redox Couplings at the NANO-BIO Interface

The efficacy and safety of nano delivery systems in humans is determined by the ROS/RNS generating capacity of engineered nano drug delivery systems. In order to discover the ROS/RNS generation capacity of nanomedicine, (Zhang, H et al., 2012), Burello, E. & Worth, A. P, 2011) redox potential, aqueous redox couples, energy levels of conduction and valence band were analyzed to predict thermodynamic nature of redox reactions with ENM in biospecial environment. The electron-transfer processes arising between nanosystems and bio species in the cell solubilize only if suitable orbital energies of electron donors and acceptors are just about at the same level (Xu, Y et al., 2000). Three prominent appliances involved in nano–bio interfacial electron-transfer processes can be mentioned as:

(i) ***direct electron injection***

Electrons can directly transfer to ENM making them sufficient to lessen ROS/RNS only when reactive species in biological medium has redox potential higher than energy levels of ENM.

(ii) surface sorbate (protein, photosensitizer)-mediated electron transfer

There are some ENM which are unable to react with or produce redox species then surface sorbate comes into play. Interaction of ENM with biological components of oxygen, water, thiol containing molecules induce change on the surface properties of nanosystems enabling dissolution of surface atoms, electron donation, oxygen reduction or other reduction reactions.

(iii) ***irradiation-induced electron transfer***

ENM with semiconducting properties possess energy levels in form of conduction band and valence band. When ENM has fulfilled valence band, direct transfer of redox cell species becomes unfavourable. However, when external stimulants such as UV light, X-ray provide sufficient energy, electrons in valence band are excited to conduction band leaving a hole in valence band (Yi, Z et al., 2010) to generate space for ROS activity. This paves a new way for photoinduced changes in the physiochemical properties of ENM. Thus, induced ROS activity could start a cascade of further reactions to deal with the drug in presence of bio environment (Wang, L et al., 2015).

7. EFFECTS OF THE PHYSICOCHEMICAL ATTRIBUTES OF ENGINEERED NANOMATERIALS AND SURROUNDING MICROENVIRONMENT ON REDOX PROCESSES

When energy levels of engineered nanocarriers are close to intracellular redox couples, active atoms in ENM perform redox reactions to make surface atoms or adsorbed biomolecules until chemical atom electrons and biomolecules gets equalized. The shape, size, facets and structural decorations of ENM make subsequent changes in energy states and redox reaction potential. The stability of ROS, surface redox potential, antioxidant or pro-oxidant behavior correlates to pH of solution, ROS generating capacity as well as electronic structure of drug carrying nano delivery systems (Hartmann, P et al., 2013, He, W et al., 2012).

8. SAFE ENGINEERING OF NANOCARRIERS BY ARIFICING NANO-BIO INTERATIONS

(Chen, H et al., 2018) says quantum-biological reactions and interactions taking place at nano-bio interfaces synergistically in physiological microenvironments influence pathway of nanocarriers in human system. A comprehensive understanding of pH, redox reaction mechanisms, quantum biomolecular properties enable key factors to rationally design nano TDD vehicles. Progress for development of smart nano-drug delivery vehicles is feasible once following oppositions of nano-bio interfaces is conquered. Surface properties such as electronic structure, active sites, orientation, distribution, surface grafting of individual nanocarriers. Qualitative and quantitative relationship between physiochemical properties of nanocarriers, their functions and toxicity synergy between nano-bio interactions requires advanced technologies as well as devices which are dynamic, high resolute, high speed and avails real-time monitoring of drug action. Accordingly, nano-quantitative structure – activity, relationship, high throughput selection, in-silico methods for drug activity predictions and better understanding of nanoinformatics will facilitate designing and engineering of nanovehicles to accelerate foundation for safe, effective and efficient nano-bio interaction. These obstacles will be resolved soon to delineate nano-bio interactions and to level-up in innovating nano-drug delivery vehicles.

9. CONCLUSION

The current knowledge and understanding of nano-bio interactions is very useful for engineering smart nano delivery systems but more research studies are essential to increase the depth of significant nano-bio interface for designing the future drug delivery vehicles. In this paper, different mechanisms of bio-nano interactions are inferred to prove quantum nanoscience has potential to revolutionize field of targeted drug delivery. However, there are still number of challenges that need to be addressed before quantum nanoscience can be widely used for targeted drug delivery. These challenges include requirement to develop more efficient methods for synthesizing quantum nanomaterials, entailing biocompatibility of quantum nanomaterials together with need to develop more accurate methods for targeting drugs to specific cells or tissues. Despite these challenges, quantum nanoscience holds a promise to revolutionize nanotechnology for targeted drug delivery. Thusly, further research, exploration, development and engineering with understanding of quantum nanoscience will have a major impact on treatment of diseases in the future.

REFERENCES

Abraham, A. N., Sharma, T. K., Bansal, V., & Shukla, R. (2018). Phytochemicals as Dynamic Surface Ligands to Control Nanoparticle-Protein Interactions. *ACS Omega*, *3*(2), 2220–2229. doi:10.1021/acsomega.7b01878 PMID:30023827

Aiello, C. D. (2023, May 15). Quantum physics proposes a new way to study biology – and the results could revolutionize our understanding of how life works. *The Conversation UK*. https://theconversation.com/quantum-physics-proposes-a-new-way-to-study-biology-and-the-results-could-revolutionize-our-understanding-of-how-life-works-204995

Albanese, A., Tang, P. S., & Chan, W. C. W. (2012). The Effect of Nanoparticle Size, Shape, and Surface Chemistry on Biological Systems. *Annual Review of Biomedical Engineering*, *14*(1), 1–16. doi:10.1146/annurev-bioeng-071811-150124 PMID:22524388

Ali, M. R. K., Wu, Y., Ghosh, D., Do, B. H., Chen, K., Dawson, M. R., Fang, N., Sulchek, T. A., & El-Sayed, M. A. (2017). Nuclear Membrane-Targeted Gold Nanoparticles Inhibit Cancer CellMigration and Invasion. *ACS Nano*, *11*(4), 3716–3726. doi:10.1021/acsnano.6b08345 PMID:28333438

Arndt, M., Juffmann, T., & Vedral, V. (2009). Quantum physics meets biology. *HFSP Journal*, *3*(6), 386–400. doi:10.2976/1.3244985 PMID:20234806

Attia, M. F., Anton, N., Wallyn, J., Omran, Z., & Vandamme, T. F. (2019). An overview of active and passive targeting strategies to improve the nanocarriers efficiency to tumour sites. *The Journal of Pharmacy and Pharmacology*, *71*(8), 1185–1198. doi:10.1111/jphp.13098 PMID:31049986

Bahrami, A. H., & Weikl, T. R. (2018). Curvature-Mediated Assembly of Janus Nanoparticles on Membrane Vesicles. *Nano Letters*, *18*(2), 1259–1263. doi:10.1021/acs.nanolett.7b04855 PMID:29281291

Bargh, J. D., Isidro-Llobet, A., Parker, J. S., & Spring, D. R. (2019, August 12). Cleavable linkers in antibody-drug conjugates. *Chemical Society Reviews*, *48*(16), 4361–4374. doi:10.1039/C8CS00676H PMID:31294429

Barua, S., & Mitragotri, S. (2014). Challenges associated with penetration of nanoparticles across cell and tissue barriers: A review of current status and future prospects. *Nano Today*, *9*(2), 223–243. doi:10.1016/j.nantod.2014.04.008 PMID:25132862

Barz, M. (2015). Complexity and simplification in the development of nanomedicines. *Nanomedicine (London)*, *10*(20), 3093–3097. doi:10.2217/nnm.15.146 PMID:26446374

Behzadi, S., Serpooshan, V., Tao, W., Hamaly, M. A., Alkawareek, M. Y., Dreaden, E. C., Brown, D., Alkilany, A. M., Farokhzad, O. C., & Mahmoudi, M. (2017). Cellular uptake of nanoparticles: Journey inside the cell. *Chemical Society Reviews*, *46*(14), 4218–4244. doi:10.1039/C6CS00636A PMID:28585944

Benoit, D. S., Overby, C. T., Sims, K. R., Jr., & Ackun-Farmmer, M. A. Biomaterials Science. Elsevier; Amsterdam, The Netherlands:2020. Drug delivery systems; pp. 1237–1266.

Benyettou F, Motte L. Nanomedicine: towards the "magic bullet" science. J Bioanal Biomed. 2016;8:2.11.

Björnmalm, M., Thurecht, K. J., Michael, M., Scott, A. M., & Caruso, F. (2017). Bridging Bio-Nano Science and Cancer Nanomedicine. *ACS Nano*, *11*(10), 9594–9613. doi:10.1021/acsnano.7b04855 PMID:28926225

Blanco, E., Shen, H., & Ferrari, M. (2015). Principles of nanoparticle design for overcoming biological barriers to drug delivery. *Nature Biotechnology*, *33*(9), 941–951. doi:10.1038/nbt.3330 PMID:26348965

Burello, E., & Worth, A. P. (2011). A Theoretical Framework for Predicting the Oxidative Stress Potential of Oxide Nanoparticles. *Nanotoxicology*, *5*(2), 228–235. doi:10.3109/17435390.2010.502980 PMID:21609138

Catalano, F., Accomasso, L., Alberto, G., Gallina, C., Raimondo, S., Geuna, S., Giachino, C., & Martra, G. (2015). Factors Ruling the Uptake of Silica Nanoparticles by Mesenchymal Stem Cells: Agglomeration Versus Dispersions, Absence Versus Presence of Serum Proteins. *Small*, *11*(24), 2919–2928. doi:10.1002mll.201400698 PMID:25689227

Chen, H., Gu, Z., An, H., Chen, C., Chen, J., Cui, R., Chen, S., Chen, W., Chen, X., Chen, X., Chen, Z., Ding, B., Dong, Q., Fan, Q., Fu, T., Hou, D., Jiang, Q., Ke, H., Jiang, X., ... Zhao, Y. (2018). Precise Nanomedicine for Intelligent Therapy of Cancer. *Science China. Chemistry*, *61*(12), 1503–1552. doi:10.100711426-018-9397-5

Chong, Y., Ge, C., Fang, G., Wu, R., Zhang, H., Chai, Z., Chen, C., & Yin, J. J. (2017). Light-Enhanced Antibacterial Activity of Graphene Oxide, Mainly via Accelerated Electron Transfer. *Environmental Science & Technology*, *51*(17), 10154–10161. doi:10.1021/acs.est.7b00663 PMID:28771330

Couvreur, P. (2013). Nanoparticles in drug delivery: Past, present and future. *Advanced Drug Delivery Reviews*, *65*(1), 21–23. doi:10.1016/j.addr.2012.04.010 PMID:22580334

Dai, Q., Wilhelm, S., Ding, D., Syed, A. M., Sindhwani, S., Zhang, Y., Chen, Y. Y., Macmillan, P., & Chan, W. C. W. (2018). Quantifying the Ligand-Coated Nanoparticle Delivery to Cancer Cells in Solid Tumours. *ACS Nano*, *12*(8), 8423–8435. doi:10.1021/acsnano.8b03900 PMID:30016073

Darville, N., van Heerden, M., Vynckier, A., De Meulder, M., Sterkens, P., Annaert, P., & Van den Mooter, G. (2014). Intramuscular Administration of Paliperidone Palmitate Extended-Release Injectable Microsuspension Induces a Subclinical Inflammatory Reaction Modulating the Pharmacokinetics in Rats. *Journal of Pharmaceutical Sciences*, *103*(7), 2072–2087. doi:10.1002/jps.24014 PMID:24845884

Davis, M. E., Zuckerman, J. E., Choi, C. H. J., Seligson, D., Tolcher, A., Alabi, C. A., Yen, Y., Heidel, J. D., & Ribas, A. (2010). Evidence of RNAi in humans from systemically administered siRNA via targeted nanoparticles. *Nature*, *464*(7291), 1067–1070. doi:10.1038/nature08956 PMID:20305636

Deol, P., & Khuller, G. K. (1997). Lung specific stealth liposomes: Stability, biodistribution and toxicity of liposomal antitubercular drugs in mice. *Biochimica et Biophysica Acta*, *1334*(2-3), 161–172. doi:10.1016/S0304-4165(96)00088-8 PMID:9101710

Du, B., Jiang, X., Das, A., Zhou, Q., Yu, M., Jin, R., & Zheng, J. (2017). Glomerular barrier behaves as an atomically precise bandpass filter in a sub-nanometre regime. *Nature Nanotechnology*, *12*(11), 1096–1102. doi:10.1038/nnano.2017.170 PMID:28892099

Fahmy, T.M., Fong, P.M., Goyal, A., & Saltzman, W.M. (2005). Targeted for drug delivery. Mater Today, 8, 18–26. doi: 71033-610. doi:10.1016/S1369-7021(05)

Fleischer, C. C., & Payne, C. K. (2014). Nanoparticle-cell interactions: Molecular structure of theprotein corona and cellular outcomes. *Accounts of Chemical Research*, *47*(8), 2651–2659. doi:10.1021/ar500190q PMID:25014679

Fu, C., Liu, T., Li, L., Liu, H., Chen, D., & Tang, F. (2013). The absorption, distribution, excretion and toxicity of mesoporous silica nanoparticles in mice following different exposure routes. *Biomaterials*, *34*(10), 2565–2575. doi:10.1016/j.biomaterials.2012.12.043 PMID:23332175

Ganta, S., Devalapally, H., Shahiwala, A., & Amiji, M. (2008). A review of stimuli-responsive nanocarriers for drug and genedelivery. *Journal of controlled release: official journal of the Controlled Release Society, 126*, 87-204.

Gao, D., Xu, H., Philbert, M. A., & Kopelman, R. (2008). Bioeliminable Nanohydrogels for Drug Delivery. *Nano Letters*, *8*(10), 3320–3324. doi:10.1021/nl8017274 PMID:18788823

Ge, C., Du, J., Zhao, L., Wang, L., Liu, Y., Li, D., Yang, Y., Zhou, R., Zhao, Y., Chai, Z., & Chen, C. (2011). Binding of Blood Proteins to Carbon Nanotubes Reduces Cytotoxicity. *Proceedings of the National Academy of Sciences of the United States of America*, *108*(41), 16968–16973. doi:10.1073/pnas.1105270108 PMID:21969544

Ghosh Tapash K. & Jasti Bhaskar R. (2009). *Oral controlled release Solid Dosage Forms; In theory and practice of contemporary Pharmaceutics*. CRC Press.

Grana, A., Limpach, A., & Chauhan, H. (2013). Formulation considerations and applications of solid lipid nanoparticles. *American Pharmaceutical Review*, 16.

Gu, X., Zhou, J., Zhou, L., Xie, S., Petti, L., Wang, S., & Wang, F. (2018). Specific Binding of Antigen-Antibody in Physiological Environments: Measurement, Force Characteristics and Analysis. *Optics and Lasers in Engineering*, *104*, 252–258. doi:10.1016/j.optlaseng.2017.09.016

Hartmann, P., Brezesinski, T., Sann, J., Lotnyk, A., Eufinger, J. P., Kienle, L., & Janek, J. (2013). Defect Chemistry of Oxide Nanomaterials with High Surface Area: Ordered Mesoporous Thin Films of the Oxygen Storage Catalyst CeO2-ZrO2. *ACS Nano*, *7*(4), 2999–3013. doi:10.1021/nn400255w PMID:23514447

He, W., Zhou, Y. T., Wamer, W. G., Boudreau, M. D., & Yin, J. J. (2012). Mechanisms of the pH Dependent Generation of Hydroxyl Radicals and Oxygen Induced by Ag Nanoparticles. *Biomaterials*, *33*(30), 7547–7555. doi:10.1016/j.biomaterials.2012.06.076 PMID:22809647

Jain, K. K. (2020). An overview of drug delivery systems. *Drug Delivery System*, *2059*, 1–54. PMID:31435914

Jiang, P. (2018). Dose Dependencies and Biocompatibility of Renal Clearable Gold Nanoparticles: From Mice to Non-human Primates. *Angewandte Chemie International Edition*, *57*(1), 266–271. doi:10.1002/anie.201710584 PMID:29160029

Jiang, X., Du, B., & Zheng, J. (2019). Glutathione-mediated biotransformation in the liver modulates nanoparticle transport. *Nature Nanotechnology*, *14*(9), 874–882. doi:10.103841565-019-0499-6 PMID:31308501

Jin, Y., Song, Y., Zhu, X., Zhou, D., Chen, C., Zhang, Z., & Huang, Y. (2012). Goblet cell-targeting nanoparticles for oral insulin delivery and the influence of mucus on insulin transport. *Biomaterials*, *33*(5), 1573–1582. doi:10.1016/j.biomaterials.2011.10.075 PMID:22093292

Ke, P. C., Lin, S., Parak, W. J., Davis, T. P., & Caruso, F. (2017). A Decade of the Protein Corona. *ACS Nano*, *11*(12), 11773–11776. doi:10.1021/acsnano.7b08008 PMID:29206030

Kewal, K. (2014). Drug Delivery System. Methods in Molecular Biology. Springer. , doi:10.1007/978-1-4939-0363-4_1

Kim, B. Y. S., Rutka, J. T., & Chan, W. C. W. (2010). Nanomedicine. *The New England Journal of Medicine*, *365*(25), 2434–2442. doi:10.1056/NEJMra0912273 PMID:21158659

Kodiha, M., Wang, Y. M., Hutter, E., Maysinger, D., & Stochaj, U. (2015). Off to the Organelles -Killing Cancer Cells with Targeted Gold Nanoparticles. *Theranostics*, *5*(4), 357–370. doi:10.7150/thno.10657 PMID:25699096

Ku, M. S. (2008). Use of the biopharmaceutical classification system in early drug development. *The AAPS Journal*, *10*(1), 208–212. doi:10.120812248-008-9020-0 PMID:18446521

Langer, R. (1990). New methods of drug delivery. *Science*, *249*(4976), 1527–1533. doi:10.1126cience.2218494 PMID:2218494

Langer, R. (1998). Drug delivery and targeting. *Nature*, *392*, 5–10. PMID:9579855

Lee JH, Sahu A, Jang C, Tae G. J Control Release 2015;209:219–28. undefined. doi:10.1016/j.jconrel.2015.04.035

Lee, K., Conboy, M., Park, H. M., Jiang, F., Kim, H. J., Dewitt, M. A., Mackley, V. A., Chang, K., Rao, A., Skinner, C., Shobha, T., Mehdipour, M., Liu, H., Huang, W. C., Lan, F., Bray, N. L., Li, S., Corn, J. E., Kataoka, K., & Murthy, N. (2017). Nanoparticle delivery of Cas9 ribonucleoprotein and donor DNA in vivo induces homology-directed DNA repair. *Nature Biomedical Engineering*, *1*(11), 889–901. doi:10.103841551-017-0137-2 PMID:29805845

Lee, S. Y., Hong, E., Jeong, J. Y., Cho, J., Seo, J., Ko, H., & Cho, H.-J. (2019). Esterase-sensitive cleavable histone deacetylase inhibitor-coupled hyaluronic acid nanoparticles for boosting anticancer activities against lung adenocarcinoma. *Biomaterials Science*, *7*(11), 4624–4635. doi:10.1039/C9BM00895K PMID:31451819

Liu, J., Miao, L., Sui, J., Hao, Y., & Huang, G. (2019). Nanoparticle cancer vaccines: Design considerations and recent advances. *Asian Journal of Pharmaceutical Sciences*, *15*(5), 576–590. doi:10.1016/j.ajps.2019.10.006 PMID:33193861

Lou, H. Y., Zhao, W., Zeng, Y., & Cui, B. (2018). The Role of Membrane Curvature in Nanoscale Topography-Induced Intracellular Signaling. *Accounts of Chemical Research*, *51*(5), 1046–1053. doi:10.1021/acs.accounts.7b00594 PMID:29648779

Mark, S. W. (2011). *Torchilin., Vladimir P., Drug delivery systems*. Access Science, McGraw-Hill Companies.

Miclăuş, T., Beer, C., Chevallier, J., Scavenius, C., Bochenkov, V. E., Enghild, J. J., & Sutherland, D. S. (2016). Dynamic Protein Coronas Revealed as a Modulator of Silver Nanoparticle Sulphidation In Vitro. *Nature Communications*, *7*(1), 11770. doi:10.1038/ncomms11770 PMID:27278102

Mitchell, M. J., Billingsley, M. M., Haley, R. M., Wechsler, M. E., Peppas, N. A., & Langer, R. (2020). Engineering precision nanoparticles for drug delivery. *Nature Reviews. Drug Discovery*. doi:10.103841573-020-0090-8 PMID:33277608

Monopoli, M. P., Åberg, C., Salvati, A., & Dawson, K. A. (2012). Biomolecular coronas provide the biological identity of nanosized materials. *Nature Nanotechnology*, *7*(12), 779–786. doi:10.1038/nnano.2012.207 PMID:23212421

Monopoli, M. P., Aberg, C., Salvati, A., & Dawson, K. A. (2012). Biomolecular Coronas Provide the Biological Identity of Nanosized Materials. *Nature Nanotechnology*, *7*(12), 779–786. doi:10.1038/nnano.2012.207 PMID:23212421

Nel, A., Xia, T., Mädler, L., & Li, N. (2006). Toxic Potential of Materials at the Nanolevel. *Science*, *311*(5761), 622–627. doi:10.1126cience.1114397 PMID:16456071

Nel, A. E., Madler, L., Velegol, D., Xia, T., Hoek, E. M., Somasundaran, P., Klaessig, F., Castranova, V., & Thompson, M. (2009). Understanding Biophysicochemical Interactions at the Nano-Bio Interface. *Nature Materials*, *8*(7), 543–557. doi:10.1038/nmat2442 PMID:19525947

Pecot, C. V., Calin, G. A., Coleman, R. L., Lopez-Berestein, G., & Sood, A. K. (2011). RNA interference in the clinic: Challenges and future directions. *Nature Reviews. Cancer*, *11*(1), 59–67. doi:10.1038/nrc2966 PMID:21160526

Peer, D., Karp, J. M., Hong, S., Farokhzad, O. C., Margalit, R., & Langer, R. (2007). Nanocarriers as an emerging platform forcancer therapy. *Nature Nanotechnology*, *2*(12), 751–760. doi:10.1038/nnano.2007.387 PMID:18654426

Pelaz, B., Alexiou, C., Alvarez-Puebla, R. A., Alves, F., Andrews, A. M., Ashraf, S., Balogh, L. P., Ballerini, L., Bestetti, A., Brendel, C., Bosi, S., Carril, M., Chan, W. C. W., Chen, C., Chen, X., Chen, X., Cheng, Z., Cui, D., Du, J., & Parak, W. J. (2017). Diverse Applications of Nanomedicine. *ACS Nano*, *11*(3), 2313–2381. doi:10.1021/acsnano.6b06040 PMID:28290206

Pelaz, B., Del Pino, P., Maffre, P., Hartmann, R., Gallego, M., Rivera-Fernández, S., De La Fuente, J. M., Nienhaus, G. U., & Parak, W. J. (2015). Surface Functionalization of Nanoparticles with Polyethylene Glycol: Effects on Protein Adsorption and Cellular Uptake. *ACS Nano*, *9*(7), 6996–7008. doi:10.1021/acsnano.5b01326 PMID:26079146

Peng, F., Setyawati, M. I., Tee, J. K., Ding, X., Wang, J., Nga, M. E., Ho, H. K., & Leong, D. T. (2019). Nanoparticles Promote In Vivo Breast Cancer Cell Intravasation and Extravasation by Inducing Endothelial Leakiness. *Nature Nanotechnology*, *14*(3), 279–286. doi:10.103841565-018-0356-z PMID:30692675

Prasad, D & Harsh Chauhan, (2013, October 25). *Key targeting approaches for Pharmaceutical Drug Delivery*. American Pharmaceutical Review. https://www.americanpharmaceuticalreview.com/Featured-Articles/148744-Key-Targeting-Approaches-for-Pharmaceutical-Drug-Delivery/

Ren, Q., Liang, Z., Jiang, X., Gong, P., Zhou, L., Sun, Z., Xiang, J., Xu, Z., Peng, X., Li, S., Li, W., Cai, L., & Tang, J. (2019). Enzyme and pH dual-responsive hyaluronic acid nanoparticles mediated combination of photodynamic therapy and chemotherapy. *International Journal of Biological Macromolecules*, *130*, 845–852. doi:10.1016/j.ijbiomac.2019.03.030 PMID:30844454

Ritz, S., Schöttler, S., Kotman, N., Baier, G., Musyanovych, A., Kuharev, J., Landfester, K., Schild, H., Jahn, O., Tenzer, S., & Mailänder, V. (2015). Protein Corona of Nanoparticles: Distinct Proteins Regulate the Cellular Uptake. *Biomacromolecules*, *16*(4), 1311–1321. doi:10.1021/acs.biomac.5b00108 PMID:25794196

Rosenblum, D., Joshi, N., Tao, W., Karp, J. M., & Peer, D. (2018). Progress and challenges towards targeted delivery of cancer therapeutics. *Nature Communications*, *9*(1), 1410. doi:10.103841467-018-03705-y PMID:29650952

Saltzman, M. W., & Torchilin, V. P. (2021, April). *Drug delivery system*. AccessScience. . https://www.accessscience.com/content/article/a757275 doi:10.1036/1097-8542.757275

Su, C., Liu, Y., Li, R., Wu, W., Fawcett, J.P., & Gu, J. (2019). Absorption, distribution, metabolism and excretion of the biomaterials used in Nanocarrier drug delivery systems. *Adv Drug Deliv. Rev*, *143*, 97-114. undefined. doi:10.1016/j.addr.2019.06.008

Thomas, F. (2022, May). An Evolving Approach to Drug Delivery, Published on: May 3, 2022, Pharmaceutical Technology. *Pharmaceutical Technology*, *46*(5), 26–27.

Torchilin, V. (2000). Drug targeting. *European journal of pharmaceutical sciences: official journal of the European Federation for Pharmaceutical Sciences*.

Torchilin, V. P. (2006). Multifunctional nanocarriers. *Advanced Drug Delivery Reviews*, *58*(14), 1532–1555. doi:10.1016/j.addr.2006.09.009 PMID:17092599

Tsoi, K. M., Macparland, S. A., Ma, X. Z., Spetzler, V. N., Echeverri, J., Ouyang, B., Fadel, S. M., Sykes, E. A., Goldaracena, N., Kaths, J. M., Conneely, J. B., Alman, B. A., Selzner, M., Ostrowski, M. A., Adeyi, O. A., Zilman, A., McGilvray, I. D., & Chan, W. C. W. (2016). Mechanism of hard-nanomaterial clearance by the liver. *Nature Materials*, *15*(11), 1212–1221. doi:10.1038/nmat4718 PMID:27525571

Valent, P., Groner, B., Schumacher, U., Superti-Furga, G., Busslinger, M., Kralovics, R., Zielinski, C., Penninger, J. M., Kerjaschki, D., Stingl, G., Smolen, J. S., Valenta, R., Lassmann, H., Kovar, H., Jäger, U., Kornek, G., Müller, M., & Sörgel, F. (2016). Paul Ehrlich (1854–1915) and his contributions to the foundation and birth of translational medicine. *Journal of Innate Immunity*, *8*(2), 111–120. doi:10.1159/000443526 PMID:26845587

von Roemeling, C., Jiang, W., Chan, C. K., Weissman, I. L., & Kim, B. Y. S. (2017). Breaking Down the Barriers to Precision Cancer Nanomedicine. *Trends in Biotechnology*, *35*(2), 159–171. doi:10.1016/j.tibtech.2016.07.006 PMID:27492049

Walkey, C. D., & Chan, W. C. W. (2012). Understanding and controlling the interaction of nanomaterials with proteins in a physiological environment. *Chemical Society Reviews*, *41*(7), 2780–2799. doi:10.1039/C1CS15233E PMID:22086677

Walkey, C. D., Olsen, J. B., Guo, H., Emili, A., & Chan, W. C. W. (2012). Nanoparticle size and surface chemistry determine serum protein adsorption and macrophage uptake. *Journal of the American Chemical Society*, *134*(4), 2139–2147. doi:10.1021/ja2084338 PMID:22191645

Walkey, C. D., Olsen, J. B., Song, F., Liu, R., Guo, H., Olsen, D. W. H., Cohen, Y., Emili, A., & Chan, W. C. W. (2014). Protein corona fingerprinting predicts the cellular interaction of gold and silver nanoparticles. *ACS Nano*, *8*(3), 2439–2455. doi:10.1021/nn406018q PMID:24517450

Wang, J., Zhang, L., Peng, F., Shi, X., & Leong, D. T. (2018). Targeting Endothelial Cell Junctions with Negatively Charged Gold Nanoparticles. *Chemistry of Materials*, *30*(11), 3759–3767. doi:10.1021/acs.chemmater.8b00840

Wang, L., Sun, Q., Wang, X., Wen, T., Yin, J. J., Wang, P., Bai, R., Zhang, X. Q., Zhang, L. H., Lu, A. H., & Chen, C. (2015). Using Hollow Carbon Nanospheres as a Light-Induced Free Radical Generator to Overcome Chemotherapy Resistance. *Journal of the American Chemical Society*, *137*(5), 1947–1955. doi:10.1021/ja511560b PMID:25597855

Wang, X., Wang, X., Wang, M., Zhang, D., Yang, Q., Liu, T., Lei, R., Zhu, S., Zhao, Y., & Chen, C. (2018). Probing Adsorption Behaviors of BSA onto Chiral Surfaces of Nanoparticles. *Small*, *14*(1703982), 1703982. doi:10.1002mll.201703982 PMID:29573549

Wang, Y., Cai, R., & Chen, C. (2019). The Nano–Bio Interactions of Nanomedicines: Understanding the Biochemical Driving Forces and Redox Reactions. *Accounts of Chemical Research*, *52*(6), 1507–1518. doi:10.1021/acs.accounts.9b00126 PMID:31149804

Wang, Y., Cai, R., & Chen, C. (2019). The Nano–Bio Interactions of Nanomedicines: Understanding the Biochemical Driving Forces and Redox Reactions. *Accounts of Chemical Research*, *52*(6), 1507–1518. doi:10.1021/acs.accounts.9b00126 PMID:31149804

Wang, Y., Qin, Z., Buehler, M. J., & Xu, Z. (2016). Intercalated Water Layers Promote Thermal Dissipation at Bio-Nano Interfaces. *Nature Communications*, *7*(1), 12854. doi:10.1038/ncomms12854 PMID:27659484

Wei, X., Han, Y., Quan, L., Liu, C., Liao, Y., & Eur, J. (2013). Oily nanosuspension for long-acting intramuscular delivery of curcumin didecanoate prodrug: Preparation, characterization and in vivo evaluation. *Pharmaceutical Sciences*, *49*(2), 286–293. doi:10.1016/j.ejps.2013.03.010 PMID:23542494

Wilhelm, S., Tavares, A. J., Dai, Q., Ohta, S., Audet, J., Dvorak, H. F., & Chan, W. C. W. (2016). Analysis of nanoparticle delivery to tumours. *Nature Reviews. Materials*, *1*(5), 16014. doi:10.1038/natrevmats.2016.14

Wong, P. T., & Choi, S. K. (2015, May 13). Mechanisms of drug release in nanotherapeutic delivery systems. *Chemical Reviews*, *115*(9), 3388–3432. doi:10.1021/cr5004634 PMID:25914945

Xu, Y., & Schoonen, M. A. A. (2000). The Absolute Energy Positions of Conduction and Valence Bands of Selected Semiconducting Minerals. *The American Mineralogist*, *85*(3-4), 543–556. doi:10.2138/am-2000-0416

Yi, Z., Ye, J., Kikugawa, N., Kako, T., Ouyang, S., Stuart-Williams, H., Yang, H., Cao, J., Luo, W., Li, Z., Liu, Y., & Withers, R. L. (2010). An Orthophosphate Semiconductor with Photooxidation Properties under Visible-Light Irradiation. *Nature Materials*, *9*(7), 559–564. doi:10.1038/nmat2780 PMID:20526323

Zhang, H., Ji, Z., Xia, T., Meng, H., Low-Kam, C., Liu, R., Pokhrel, S., Lin, S., Wang, X., Liao, Y.-P., Wang, M., Li, L., Rallo, R., Damoiseaux, R., Telesca, D., Mädler, L., Cohen, Y., Zink, J. I., & Nel, A. E. (2012). Nel, A. E. Use of Metal Oxide Nanoparticle Band Gap To Develop a Predictive Paradigm for Oxidative Stress and Acute Pulmonary Inflammation. *ACS Nano*, *6*(5), 4349–4368. doi:10.1021/nn3010087 PMID:22502734

Zhang, Z., Gao, F., Bu, H., Xiao, J., & Li, Y. (2012). Solid lipid nanoparticles loading candesartan cilexetil enhance oral bioavailability: In vitro characteristics and absorption mechanism in rats. *Nanomedicine (London)*, *8*(5), 740–744. doi:10.1016/j.nano.2011.08.016 PMID:21930110

Zhao, W., Hanson, L., Lou, H. Y., Akamatsu, M., Chowdary, P. D., Santoro, F., Marks, J. R., Grassart, A., Drubin, D. G., Cui, Y., & Cui, B. (2017). Nanoscale manipulation of membrane curvature for probing endocytosis in live cells. *Nature Nanotechnology*, *12*(8), 750–756. doi:10.1038/nnano.2017.98 PMID:28581510

Zhao, Y., Wang, C., Wang, L., Yang, Q., Tang, W., She, Z., & Deng, Y. (2012). A frustrating problem: Accelerated blood clearance of PEGylated solid lipid nanoparticles following subcutaneous injection in rats. *European Journal of Pharmaceutics and Biopharmaceutics*, *81*(3), 506–513. doi:10.1016/j.ejpb.2012.04.023 PMID:22580209

Zhao, Z., Ukidve, A., Kim, J., & Mitragotri, S. (2020). Targeting Strategies for Tissue-Specific Drug Delivery. *Cell*, *181*(1), 151–167. doi:10.1016/j.cell.2020.02.001 PMID:32243788

Zhou, H., Zhang, B., Zheng, J., Yu, M., Zhou, T., Zhao, K., Jia, Y., Gao, X., Chen, C., & Wei, T. (2014). The Inhibition of Migration and Invasion of Cancer Cells by Graphene via the Impairment of Mitochondrial Respiration. *Biomaterials*, *35*(5), 1597–1607. doi:10.1016/j.biomaterials.2013.11.020 PMID:24290441

Zishan, M., Zeeshan, A., & Faisal, S. (2017). Vesicular drug delivery system used for liver diseases. *World J Pharm Sci.*, *5*(4), 28–35.

Chapter 10
Nanomaterials in Imaging and Diagnostics

Swati Changdeo Jagdale
School of Health Sciences and Technology, Dr. Vishwanath Karad MIT World Peace University, Pune, India

Purva Uday Chandorkar
School of Health Sciences and Technology, Dr. Vishwanath Karad MIT World Peace University, Pune, India

Akash Anil Podutwar
School of Health Sciences and Technology, Dr. Vishwanath Karad MIT World Peace University, Pune, India

Satish A. Polshettiwar
School of Health Sciences and Technology, Dr. Vishwanath Karad MIT World Peace University, Pune, India

Aniruddha R. Chabukswar
School of Health Sciences and Technology, Dr. Vishwanath Karad MIT World Peace University, Pune, India

ABSTRACT

In the last two decades, application of nanomaterials as a tool for imaging and diagnosis has gained the attention of many researchers, as they have showed promising results in every aspect of disease management right from the diagnosis, delivering and real time tracking of the drug and monitoring the diseased condition to the in-vivo imaging. In-vivo imaging helps in early diagnosis of lethal diseases like, cancer, cardiovascular diseases, and renal failure, which can improve patient's lifestyle. Nanomaterials offer properties like enhanced diagnostic specificity, increased blood circulation time, and organ specific delivery just with the help of functionalization and conjugation with desired materials. Nanomaterials like dendrimer, silica nanoparticles, and some magnetic nanoparticles are used as contrast agents in imaging technology such as magnetic resonance imaging (MRI), computed tomography (CT) and radiopharmaceuticals. This chapter covers nanomaterials (NPs) as a biomedical tool for imaging and diagnosis of various diseases.

DOI: 10.4018/979-8-3693-0448-8.ch010

Figure 1. General considerations of nanomaterials used in imaging

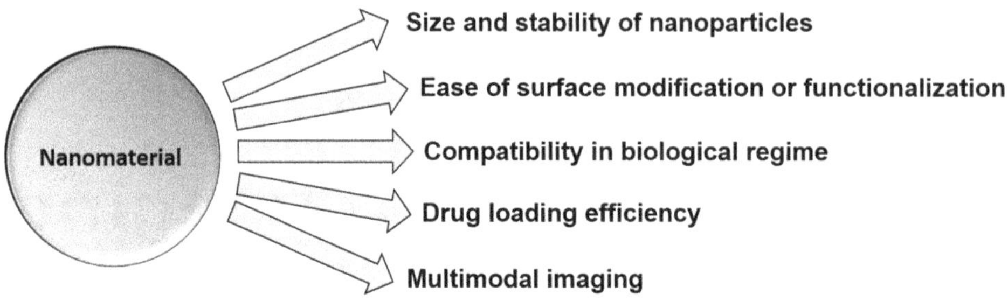

INTRODUCTION

Nanomaterials are the essential part of nanotechnology which have been extensively studied by the scientists for its use in the field of nanomedicine for imaging, diagnosis and treatment (Rani et al., 2019). Nanomaterials are defined as the substances whose at least one external dimension measures 100 nanometers or less (Turney, 2009). Nanomaterials offer properties like enhanced diagnostic specificity, increased blood circulation time and organ specific delivery (Patra et al., 2018).

Nanomaterials can be functionalized or conjugate with variety of agents that would increase their compatibility in a biological environment, can enhances targeting capability and better cellular uptake in desired cancerous cells. Physiochemical properties of nanomaterials like size and shape, texture of surface, atomic arrangement, composition of materials, charge of particles and system in which they are suspended are the most important consideration for better design and formulation of nanoparticles.

Bio-imaging or medical imaging is a method to visualize into the body non-surgically to gain predictive data about the affected region. From last 20 years, nanomaterials-based drugs have altered the way of bio-imaging (Subhra et al., 2021). Figure 1 depicts the general considerations of designing nanomaterials used for imaging.

Recent advance in bioimaging is multimodal imaging, it overcomes the limitations of existing bioimaging (visualizing one organ at a time). Multimodal imaging allows simultaneous production of signals for several imaging techniques at a time. Multimodal imaging is defined as combination of images from several modalities to form one combined image, it allows combinative structure and efficient information about the disease. To overcome the disadvantages associated with individual modality, multi-modal imaging systems such as Proton Emission Tomography-Computed Tomography (PET-CT), Computed Tomography-optical Proton Emission Tomography-Magnetic Resonance Imaging (CT-oPET-MRI) are currently in clinical usage (Subhra et al., 2021).

Every diagnostic method is designed to generate accurate results in early stage of disease. For this high quality, sensitive, specific imaging probe are required. Contrast agents, also known as imaging probes, are the substances that aids in visualization of X-rays or other imaging tools' interactions with the body for a definite period of time. They assist in enhancement of the diagnostic value of the imaging techniques. Prior to imaging, these agents are administered in the body which makes certain body tissues to be seen different than without introduction of the contrast media. It helps the doctors to diagnose the medical conditions by increasing the organ or tissue visibility (Richard Heller, 2022). The prerequisite properties for contrast agents are (Rani et al., 2019):

Figure 2. Types of nanomaterials

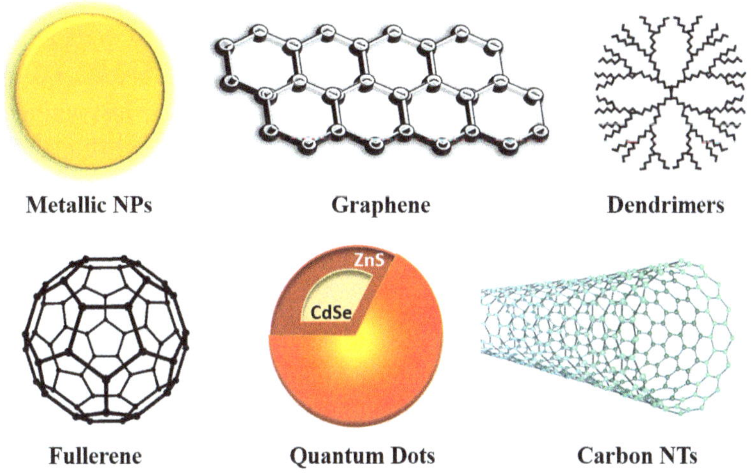

1. It must be stable in physiological environment in different pH, temperature and ionic strength.
2. It must keep colloidal solution stable with proper dispersion.
3. It must have high retention time in bloodstream to achieve high quality imaging.
4. Along with high retention it needs to be excrete from body via suitable route to minimize toxicological events.
5. It must have proper retention time within specific organ or location with proper contrast to ensure high quality imaging.
6. It must be biocompatible to minimize adverse reactions.

Figure 2 shows types of nanomaterials.

NANOPARTICLES

Nanoparticles (NPs) are the particles with size range of 10 to 100 nm. The anatomy of NPs is complex and they are composed of three layers:

a) The superficial layer, which can be easily conjugated with variety of molecules like different polymers, surfactants, metal ions and biological molecules like DNA, RNA or siRNA, etc.
b) Inner shell layer, it is different material from core in every aspect.
c) Innermost core, it is the important and central portion of any nanoparticle, considered as nanoparticle itself.

Nanoparticles are widely classified into several categories based upon their size, shape, morphology, and chemical properties (Khan et al., 2019).

Based upon chemical and physical characteristics, some distinguished classes of nanoparticles are as follows:

Gold Nanoparticles

Gold nanoparticles (AuNPs) are one of the most explored nanoparticles among all other nanoparticles serving tool for bioimaging and optical biosensing, as they are easy to fabricate, chemically stable, having extraordinary biocompatibility and with adaptable optical properties. Just with desired manufacturing the shape and size of AuNPs, several properties like Surface Enhanced Raman Scattering (SERS), Localized Surface Plasma Resonance (LSPR), ratio between light absorption and scattering coefficient and fluorescence (Si et al., 2021).

Applications of AuNPs are discussed in three aspects which are as follows (Wu et al., 2019):

a) Precise imaging of AuNPs within the biological system: This optical imaging includes Differential interference contrast (DIC) microscopy, Interferometric scattering (iSCAT) microscopy, photothermal imaging and Dark field (DF) microscopy. DIC microscopy makes use of double beam interferometry where in phase shift of the light beam occurs which produces a shadow-cast, false 3D image. It helps in direct visualization of subcellular organs like microtubules. Use of AuNPs as contrast media in DIC microscopy helps in imaging of cellular features and nanoparticles at the same time. iSCAT microscopy has advantage of greater spatial resolution and sensitivity. In this, the object is lightened and the reflected and scattered light is captured by the detector. Hancock, et.al, used AuNPs as imaging probes for the direct visualization of binding process of single tubulin dimers to develop microtubules (Mickolajczyk et al., 2019). Photothermal imaging uses a green heating laser beam, aimed on the object, which generates a heat wave absorbed by the AuNPs. A red beam is fragmented into two polarized light beams by a prism, one of them overlaps with the green laser. Both beams combine and the relative phase difference is detected by the detector. DF microscopy is a method, based on scattering, which yields a bright image on a dark background (Wu et al., 2019).

b) Monitoring of physiological processes and biological events: Monitoring of physiological processes and biological events can be carried out using Surface-enhanced Raman Spectroscopy (SERS) and Plasmon Enhanced Fluorescence (PEF) for ultra-sensitive detection. SERS provides extremely sensitive and extensive structural data of the objects. It help in detection of biomolecules which surround nanoparticles. Sensitivity of the SERS signals increase when distance between AuNPs and the Raman reporters decrease which makes it best to study bio-nano interactions. AuNPs possess plasmonic properties which allows studying samples with weak fluorescence emission. It is used for ultra-sensitive detection of the molecules (Wu et al., 2019).

c) Deep *in-vivo* tissue imaging: This imaging makes use of techniques such as Optical Coherence Tomography (OCT), Photoacoustic Imaging (PAI) and Two-photon or multi-photon imaging (TPI). OCT depends on interference of light where in a light beam is bifurcated into two, one of which traverse through the sample and other is utilized as a reference. A photon is conducted through or reflected from a tissue which contains spatial information about the tissue microstructure. The obtained interference is used to construct a 2D image which contains the data of internal microstructure of the tissue. It is particularly effective in bioimaging of eyes, breast and skin. PAI is based on the principle of ultrasound waves, produced using elastic expansion induced thermally which is caused due to photon pulses traversing through the tissues. TPI makes use of two near-infrared (NIR) or longer wavelengths to excite a fluorophores within the visible range. NIR light excitation helps in reducing background scattering in the tissue, thus enhances imaging depth (Wu et al., 2019).

Figure 3. Aspects of AuNPs considered for their application

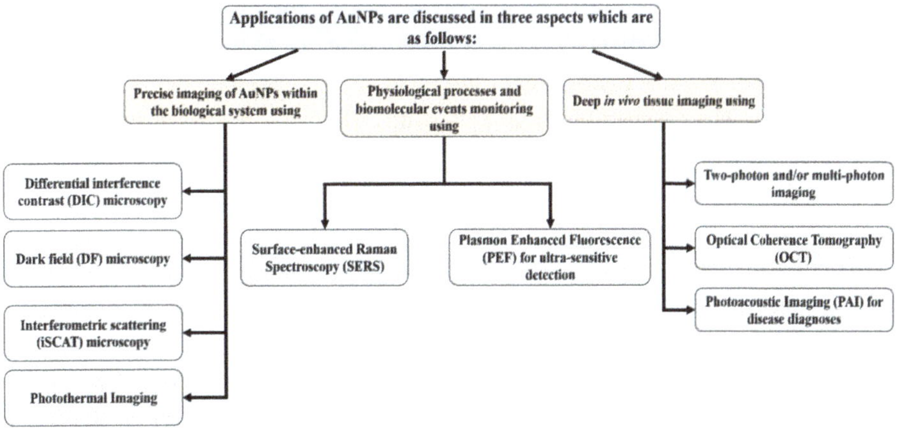

Silver Nanoparticles

Silver nanoparticles (AgNPs) possess superior chemical, physical, and biological properties, and they are differentiated due to shape, size, structure, composition, crystallinity of AgNPs in comparison with their bulk forms. Silver has several fascinating metallic properties with low cost compared to gold and abundant natural resource. Up till now the use of silver-based nanomaterials has been restricted due to their low stability, easy oxidation in oxygen containing fluid (Lee & Jun, 2019). Ruman T, et.al, ascertained use of Ag nanoparticles in laser ionization/desorption mass spectroscopy imaging helped in differentiating healthy renal tissue from cancerous renal cell proficiently (Arendowski et al., 2018).

Number of various techniques used for biomolecular imaging are listed in table no. 1 (Tan et al., 2021).

Magnetic Nanoparticles

Magnetic nanoparticles (MNPs) are newly discovered for research and MNPs are getting more attention these days due to their applications in the field of medical science. The applications of MNPs are in targeted drug delivery, catalysis and biological imaging as they have exceptional properties like high surface area, tunability of structure compositions and metal rich moieties (Mirza et al., 2019).

Table 1. Use of AgNPs in bioimaging

Sr. No.	Target	Used probe	Imaging technique
1	Leukemia	Glycine	Photo-luminescence
2	Immunoglobulin	IgG	SPR imaging
3	Renal cell carcinoma	Riboflavin	MS imaging
4	Neuroblastoma	Aptamer	Light Scattering Microscopy
5	Prion protein	Aptamer	Dynamic light scattering
6	Primary T-cells	Protein corona	X-ray microscopy
7	Glycoprotein	Aptamers	Forster resonance energy transfer

Iron oxide nanoparticles (IONPs) have been extensively explored in the field of nanomedicine because of their high biodegradability, biocompatibility and magnetic properties. IONPs are widely used in Magnetic Resonance Imaging (MRI) as negative contrast agents that elevates MRI contrast in darker images (i.e., T2-weighted). Several researchers found that IONPs can also be used in hyperthermia and nucleic drug delivery. For MRI assisted nucleic acid drug delivery, certain cationic IONPs are used (Y. Li et al., 2020). Mohapatra et al. formulated dual purpose magnetic micelles to achieve simultaneous delivery of contrast agent in MRI imaging and therapeutic agent in nucleic acid therapy. They have formulated magnetic micelles which are composed of mixture of polyethylene glycol and poly lactic acid having innermost core of super-para-magnetic iron oxide nanocrystal (Wang et al., 2012).

Manganese oxide nanoparticles (MONs) are testified as MRI T1 contrast agent which shows promising effect of overcoming obstacles of magnetic susceptibility and/or negative contrast enhancement, which is the common problem faced by the T2 contrast agents. One of the major advantages of MONs are they have high loading capacity with imaging as well as therapeutic agents. Several properties of MONs make them capable of using as theranostic agents for treatment of deadly diseases like cancers (Kim et al., 2011; Shin et al., 2009).

Silica Nanoparticles (SNPs)

Silica nanoparticles (SNPs) possess the superior position among other nanoparticles due to their easy synthesis, better surface chemistry, lesser toxicity and controllable properties like chemical, mechanical, physical and optoelectronic stability (Bharti et al., 2015).

SNPs can be easily used for molecular imaging techniques like:

a) Optical imaging for example, MRI, fluorescence and bioluminescence.
b) Radionuclide imaging for example, Computed Tomography (CT), Single Proton Emission Computed Tomography (SPECT), Proton Emission Tomography (PET), Ultrasound, Photoacoustic and Raman imaging.

In medical imaging, SNPs are also used as contrast agents to encapsulate other contrasting particles like gold, silver, organic dyes, iron oxide and quantum dots (Prabha et al., 2021).

Choi J, et.al, observed high specificity and high intensity due to immunofluorescent labeling of cancer cell surface using dye doped SNPs leading to immediate observation for rapid diagnosis (Choi et al., 2008).

Carbon Allotropic Nanomaterials

Carbon nanomaterials (CNs) are typically made from carbon and its allotropes such as graphene and fullerene. They possess distinctive characteristics like more flexibility, high optical transparency, greater specific surface area, better electrical conductivity and high carrier movement. Due to these properties, CNs are extensively used in the fields like bio-sensing, tissue engineering, bio-imaging and drug delivery. Commonly used CNs are graphene, carbon nanotubes, carbon or graphene quantum dots and fullerene (Speranza, 2021).

Quantum Dots

Quantum dots (QDs) are the fluorescent nanoparticles possessing high optical properties. Generally, they are the metallic NPs ranging from 2 to 20 nanometers in size. They emit fluorescence depending upon its size because of quantum confinement effect. As the size of QDs decreases, the energy required for activation increases which results in color change from red to blue. QDs can be bio-conjugated using biomolecules like DNA, RNA, siRNA, antibodies, proteins, etc. to target them at various cellular organelles for achieving localized effects (Pandey & Bodas, 2020).

The use of QDs in biomedicine can be divided in three general groups as; i) sensing and detection, ii) *in-vitro* labelling and imaging, and iii) *in-vivo* imaging. In sensing and detection, a visual display is utilized for both solution-based detection homogeneous assays and solid supports based heterogeneous assays. Secondly, QDs find a wide-spread use in fluorescent *in-vitro/in-vivo* labelling and imaging. In this, the bio-conjugated QDs, which are immobilized in the gels, paper strips, biochips, cells or membranes, are utilized for labeling of the targeted molecules. The particular interaction between the labelled molecule and the ligand is attained by molecular recognition; and the targeted location is brought to light by fluorescence (Robert H. Pierce, 2019).

Akerman et.al, used QDs coated with peptide for targeting them to the lung tumor vessels in live mice. They further analyzed the tissues of different organs to find presence of imaging probes. QDs were amassed in reticuloendothelial system related organs like spleen and liver. The polyethylene glycol (PEG) coating helped in avoiding excretion by this path which in turn extended its circulation half-life (Åkerman et al., 2002).

Fullerene

Fullerene-based nanomaterials finds great interest in the field of nanotechnology owing to its exceptional characteristics and non-rigid, flexible dimensional arrangement. Fullerene possess excellent optical, electrical and thermal characteristics which makes them favorable agent for tissue engineering, bio-sensing, drug delivery and bio-imaging (Gaur et al., 2021). Various types of fullerenes include buckyball cluster, nanotubes, mega tubes and nano-onions. Buckyball cluster is a hollow structure in which other atoms can be trapped within it. Nano-onions are the spherical structures, made of multiple carbon layers with buckyball center between the layers. Nanotubes are hollow tube like structures with single or multiple boundaries, having much smaller dimensions. Mega-tubes possess large diameter when compared with nanotubes (Bhakta & Barthunia, 2020).

The hexagonal and pentagonal cage forming structure of fullerene shows high resistance against metabolism of the body and are relatively non-toxic. Fullerenes find better application than metal chelates in diagnosis. Some metal atoms like scandium, yttrium, cerium, uranium, barium etc. when enclosed within the inner spheres of fullerene, forms endo-fullerenes, which are used as X-ray imaging agents, radiopharmaceuticals and MRI contrasting agents (Bakry R. et al., 2007).

Chen, et.al, constructed ploy (L-lactide) nanofibers packed with hydrophilic fullerene nanoparticles by electrospinnng blend technique. Human liver cancer cells were used for evaluating the *in-vitro* bioimaging characteristics of the fibers. The cell penetration of fullerene nanoparticles was confirmed using florescence imaging. Further, these nanocomposites were loaded with paclitaxel, an anticancer agent, and the drug release was observed by fluorescent imaging (Liu et al., 2013).

Graphene

Graphene and its derivatives like graphene oxide (GO), graphene quantum dots (GQDs), reduced graphene oxide (rGO), fluorographene, etc. are widely studied for its applications in the field of bioscience as diagnostic, drug delivery, photothermal therapy and bio-imaging agents, due to its excellent solubility, selectivity and biocompatibility. Bio-imaging has a major role in clinical practice as well as in research which permits the observational study of the physiological processes at the cell level in animals. With the help of particular contrasting substances or molecular probes, bio-imaging can help in detection and characterization of diseases in primary phase. It can offer a quick technique to observe the treatment response minutely (Banerjee, 2018; Lin et al., 2016).

According to a recent study Yang et al. developed a novel label free highly sensitive imaging technique for rapid visualization and layer analysis of graphene and GO, along with real time in-vivo imaging of GO with cell and ex-vivo in circulating blood by means of transient absorption. In that technique they used megahertz modulation which efficiently dodged the low frequency laser noise and a resonant circuit that amplified the heterodyne detected signal electronically. Using this imaging tool, they successfully achieved high speed imaging of GO in living cells, tissues, organs and animal with quantitative evaluation of concentration of dispersed Graphene Oxide functionalized by Poly Ethylene Glycol (GO-PEG). This opens up new possibilities for employing GO as a bioimaging agent via the transient absorption imaging approach (J. Li et al., 2015).

Carbon Nanotubes (CNTs)

CNTs are the cylindrical molecules, having hexagonal hybridized carbon atoms, believed to be the most unique discovery in the field of nanoscience. They possess exceptional thermal, mechanical, electrical and optical characteristics (H Sadegh et al., 2015). Hydrophobicity of CNTs make them insoluble in water and challenging to solubilize them in any other solvents, thus limiting its use in the industries. Many molecules with different chemical structures can be attached to CNTs leading to its use in the field of bioscience (Gerasimenko et al., 2015).

CNTs finds potential to be used as contrasting materials in MRI, photoacoustic (PA), nuclear imaging, optical detection, Raman scattering and fluorescent video imaging methods (Gong et al., 2013). Gambhir, et.al, used indocyanine green (ICG) molecules on PEGylated single-walled nanotubes (SWNTs) by π-π stacking for enhancing PA imaging using dyes. This helped in increasing the optical density of the imaging probe by 20 times. They further expanded their work by developing multiplexed PA probes with the incorporation of 5 NIR dyes. Among all, ICG-SWNTs showed separated and prominent absorbance which can be used for *in-vivo* PA imaging with better sensitivity (Zerda et al., 2010).

Dendrimers

Dendrimers belong to a group of highly branched man-made polymers which form spherical shaped macromolecules. They can be manufactured to a definite size in a reproducible way. They play an important role in the field of biomedical nanotechnology. They are formulated to be used in the area of bio-imaging as contrasting agents. Some external amine containing dendrimers can be modified and functionalized which permits the attachment of contrasting agents for the use in nuclear medicine, MRI, CT and optical imaging. They can be bio-conjugated using antibodies for targeting specific ligands (Barrett et al., 2009).

Iron oxide or gadolinium needs to be incorporated for creating MRI contrasting agents since dendrimers by themselves are not paramagnetic. These are called as magneto-dendrimers which are used for labelling as well as tracking the cells (Kiessling et al., 2006). Gadolinium dendrimers are advantageous over iron oxide dendrimers as they are a positive contrasting agent; whereas the iron oxide dendrimers generate Differential Enhancement (DE) with the help of reduction in signal. Very less research has been carried out on the use of dendrimers as CT contrasting agents due to high amount of iodine conjugated agents which can cause toxicity when multiple CT scans are required (Barrett et al., 2009).

For cancer research and theranostics application, fluorescent labelled dendrimers are promising labelling system as well as drug delivery system. During scientific study, over expression of folate receptor was found, so folic acid (FA) has been used for targeting purpose. Quintana et al. used the exceptional application of dendrimers which is multi-functionalization, and using it they manufacture Poly (amidoamine) - Generation 5 (PAMAM-G5) dendrimer with FA, fluorescein isothiocyanate (FITC) and methotrexate. Further in-vitro experiment with KB cells (human epithelial carcinoma cell) demonstrates their ability of uptake by bioimaging. The prepared conjugate was found to be 100 times more cytotoxic than drug alone (Quintana et al., 2002).

CONCLUSION

Nanomaterials, due to its controllable size, high surface area, easy surface modifications, enhanced specificity and better blood circulation time, offers extensive use in imaging and diagnosis in the field of nanomedicine. Various nanomaterials includes gold, silver, magnetic, silica nanoparticles, etc. and several carbon allotropic nanomaterials like, quantum dots, fullerene, graphene, carbon nanotubes and dendrimers. Nanomaterials can be functionalized or conjugate with variety of agents that would increase their compatibility in a biological environment, can enhances targeting capability and better cellular uptake in desired cancerous cells. Physiochemical properties of nanomaterials like size and shape, texture of surface, atomic arrangement, composition of materials, charge of particles and system in which they are suspended are the most important consideration for better design and formulation of nanoparticles. The major challenge of nanomaterials is their retention ability and the binding ability to the proteins. Thus this urges the scientists to do more research on the drawbacks so as to offer improved designs to help the mankind. Advancement in the development of nanoprobes would help in improved imaging and early diagnosis of the diseases.

REFERENCES

Åkerman, M. E., Chan, W. C. W., Laakkonen, P., Bhatia, S. N., & Ruoslahti, E. (2002). Nanocrystal targeting in vivo. *Proceedings of the National Academy of Sciences of the United States of America*, *99*(20), 12617–12621. doi:10.1073/pnas.152463399 PMID:12235356

Arendowski, A., Nizioł, J., Ossoliński, K., Ossolińska, A., Ossoliński, T., Dobrowolski, Z., & Ruman, T. (2018). Laser desorption/ionization MS imaging of cancer kidney tissue on silver nanoparticle-enhanced target. *Bioanalysis*, *10*(2), 83–94. doi:10.4155/bio-2017-0195 PMID:29239663

Bakry, R., Vallant, R. M., Najam-ul-Haq, M., Rainer, M., Szabo, Z., Huck, C. W., & Bonn, G. K. (2007). Medicinal applications of fullerenes. *International Journal of Nanomedicine*, *2*(4), 639–649. doi:10.2147/IJN.S2.4.639 PMID:18203430

Banerjee, A. N. (2018). Graphene and its derivatives as biomedical materials: Future prospects and challenges. *Interface Focus*, *8*(3), 20170056. Advance online publication. doi:10.1098/rsfs.2017.0056 PMID:29696088

Barrett, T., Ravizzini, G., Choyke, P., & Kobayashi, H. (2009). Dendrimers in medical nanotechnology. *IEEE Engineering in Medicine and Biology Magazine*, *28*(1), 12–22. doi:10.1109/MEMB.2008.931012 PMID:19150767

Bhakta, P., & Barthunia, B. (2020). Fullerene and its applications: A review. *Journal of Indian Academy of Oral Medicine and Radiology*, *32*(2), 159–163. doi:10.4103/jiaomr.jiaomr_191_19

Bharti, C., Gulati, N., Nagaich, U., & Pal, A. (2015). Mesoporous silica nanoparticles in target drug delivery system: A review. *International Journal of Pharmaceutical Investigation*, *5*(3), 124. doi:10.4103/2230-973X.160844 PMID:26258053

Choi, J., Burns, A. A., Williams, R. M., Zhou, Z., Flesken-Nikitin, A., Zipfel, W. R., Wiesner, U., & Nikitin, A. Y. (2008). Core-shell silica nanoparticles as fluorescent labels for nanomedicine. *Journal of Biomedical Optics*, *12*(06), 1. doi:10.1117/1.2823149 PMID:18163823

Gaur, M., Misra, C., Yadav, A. B., Swaroop, S., Maolmhuaidh, F., Bechelany, M., & Barhoum, A. (2021). Biomedical applications of carbon nanomaterials: Fullerenes, quantum dots, nanotubes, nanofibers, and graphene. *Materials (Basel)*, *14*(20), 5978. doi:10.3390/ma14205978 PMID:34683568

Gerasimenko, A. Y., Ichkitidze, L. P., Podgaetsky, V. M., & Selishchev, S. V. (2015). Biomedical Applications of Promising Nanomaterials with Carbon Nanotubes. *Biomedical Engineering*, *48*(6), 310–314. doi:10.100710527-015-9476-z

Gong, H., Peng, R., & Liu, Z. (2013). Carbon nanotubes for biomedical imaging: The recent advances. *Advanced Drug Delivery Reviews*, *65*(15), 1951–1963. doi:10.1016/j.addr.2013.10.002 PMID:24184130

Khan, I., Saeed, K., & Khan, I. (2019). Nanoparticles: Properties, applications and toxicities. *Arabian Journal of Chemistry*, *12*(7), 908–931. doi:10.1016/j.arabjc.2017.05.011

Kiessling, F., Morgenstern, B., & Zhang, C. (2006). Contrast Agents and Applications to Assess Tumor Angiogenesis In Vivo by Magnetic Resonance Imaging. *Current Medicinal Chemistry*, *14*(1), 77–91. doi:10.2174/092986707779313516 PMID:17266569

Kim, T., Momin, E., Choi, J., Yuan, K., Zaidi, H., Kim, J., Park, M., Lee, N., Mcmahon, M. T., Quinones-hinojosa, A., Bulte, J. W. M., Hyeon, T., & Gilad, A. A. (2011). *116 jacs 2011 T Kim Mesoporous Silica-Coated Hollow Manganese Oxide Nanoparticles.pdf*. 2955–2961.

La Zerda, A. D., Liu, Z., Bodapati, S., Teed, R., Vaithilingam, S., Khuri-Yakub, B. T., Chen, X., Dai, H., & Gambhir, S. S. (2010). Ultrahigh sensitivity carbon nanotube agents for photoacoustic molecular imaging in living mice. *Nano Letters*, *10*(6), 2168–2172. doi:10.1021/nl100890d PMID:20499887

Lee, S. H., & Jun, B. H. (2019). Silver nanoparticles: Synthesis and application for nanomedicine. *International Journal of Molecular Sciences*, *20*(4), 865. Advance online publication. doi:10.3390/ijms20040865 PMID:30781560

Li, J., Zhang, W., Chung, T. F., Slipchenko, M. N., Chen, Y. P., Cheng, J. X., & Yang, C. (2015). Highly sensitive transient absorption imaging of graphene and graphene oxide in living cells and circulating blood. *Scientific Reports*, *5*(June), 1–9. doi:10.1038rep12394 PMID:26202216

Li, Y., Wang, X., Zhang, Y., Nie, G., Nie, G., & Nie, G. (2020). Recent Advances in Nanomaterials with Inherent Optical and Magnetic Properties for Bioimaging and Imaging-Guided Nucleic Acid Therapy. *Bioconjugate Chemistry*, *31*(5), 1234–1246. doi:10.1021/acs.bioconjchem.0c00126 PMID:32302478

Lin, J., Chen, X., & Huang, P. (2016). Graphene-Based Nanomaterials for Bioimaging Graphical abstract HHS Public Access. *Advanced Drug Delivery Reviews*, *105*, 242–254. doi:10.1016/j.addr.2016.05.013 PMID:27233213

Liu, W., Wei, J., Chen, Y., Huo, P., & Wei, Y. (2013). Electrospinning of poly(L-lactide) nanofibers encapsulated with water-soluble fullerenes for bioimaging application. *ACS Applied Materials & Interfaces*, *5*(3), 680–685. doi:10.1021/am400037s PMID:23327807

Mickolajczyk, K. J., Geyer, E. A., Kim, T., Rice, L. M., & Hancock, W. O. (2019). Direct observation of individual tubulin dimers binding to growing microtubules. *Proceedings of the National Academy of Sciences of the United States of America*, *116*(15), 7314–7322. doi:10.1073/pnas.1815823116 PMID:30804205

Mirza, S., Ahmad, M. S., Shah, M. I. A., & Ateeq, M. (2019). Magnetic nanoparticles: Drug delivery and bioimaging applications. In *Metal Nanoparticles for Drug Delivery and Diagnostic Applications*. Elsevier Inc., doi:10.1016/B978-0-12-816960-5.00011-2

Pandey, S., & Bodas, D. (2020). High-quality quantum dots for multiplexed bioimaging: A critical review. *Advances in Colloid and Interface Science*, *278*, 102137. doi:10.1016/j.cis.2020.102137 PMID:32171116

Patra, J. K., Das, G., Fraceto, L. F., Campos, E. V. R., Rodriguez-Torres, M. D. P., Acosta-Torres, L. S., Diaz-Torres, L. A., Grillo, R., Swamy, M. K., Sharma, S., Habtemariam, S., & Shin, H. S. (2018). Nano based drug delivery systems: Recent developments and future prospects. *Journal of Nanobiotechnology*, *16*(1), 1–33. doi:10.118612951-018-0392-8 PMID:30231877

Prabha, S., Durgalakshmi, D., Rajendran, S., & Lichtfouse, E. (2021). Plant-derived silica nanoparticles and composites for biosensors, bioimaging, drug delivery and supercapacitors: A review. *Environmental Chemistry Letters*, *19*(2), 1667–1691. doi:10.100710311-020-01123-5 PMID:33199978

Quintana, A., Raczka, E., Piehler, L., Lee, I., Myc, A., Majoros, I., Patri, A. K., Thomas, T., Mulé, J., & Baker, J. R. Jr. (2002). Design and function of a dendrimer-based therapeutic nanodevice targeted to tumor cells through the folate receptor. *Pharmaceutical Research*, *19*(9), 1310–1316. doi:10.1023/A:1020398624602 PMID:12403067

Rani, R., Sethi, K., & Singh, G. (2019). Nanomaterials and Their Applications in Bioimaging. *Nanotechnology in the Life Sciences*, (October), 429–450. doi:10.1007/978-3-030-16379-2_15

Robert, H., & Pierce, X. G. (2019). Applications of Quantum Dots in Bioimaging and Bioassays. *Material Matters : Chemistry Driving Performance.*

H. Sadegh;R. Shahryari-ghoshekandi. (2015). Functionalization of carbon nanotubes and its application in nanomedicine: A review. *Nanomedicine Journal, 2*(4), 231–248. https://doi.org/. 2015.04.001 doi:10.7508/nmj

Shin, J., Anisur, R. M., Ko, M. K., Im, G. H., Lee, J. H., & Lee, I. S. (2009). Hollow manganese oxide nanoparticles as multifunctional agents for magnetic resonance imaging and drug delivery. *Angewandte Chemie International Edition*, *48*(2), 321–324. doi:10.1002/anie.200802323 PMID:19040234

Si, P., Razmi, N., Nur, O., Solanki, S., Pandey, C. M., Gupta, R. K., Malhotra, B. D., Willander, M., & De La Zerda, A. (2021). Gold nanomaterials for optical biosensing and bioimaging. *Nanoscale Advances*, *3*(10), 2679–2698. doi:10.1039/D0NA00961J PMID:36134176

Speranza, G. (2021). Carbon nanomaterials: Synthesis, functionalization and sen[1] Speranza, G., Carbon nanomaterials: Synthesis, functionalization and sensing applications, Nanomaterials 11 (2021).sing applications. *Nanomaterials (Basel, Switzerland)*, *11*(4). PMID:33918769

Subhra, T., Loganathan, S., Nanomaterials, M. E., & Applications, T. B. (2021). *Springer Series in Biomaterials Science and Engineering, 16*. Springer. https://www.springer.com/series/10955

Tan, P., Li, H. S., Wang, J., & Gopinath, S. C. B. (2021). Silver nanoparticle in biosensor and bioimaging: Clinical perspectives. *Biotechnology and Applied Biochemistry*, *68*(6), 1236–1242. doi:10.1002/bab.2045 PMID:33043496

Turney, D. J. (2009). *Nanomaterials*. EC. https://ec.europa.eu/health/scientific_committees/opinions_layman/nanomaterials/en/l-2/1.htm

Wang, C., Ravi, S., Martinez, G. V., Chinnasamy, V., Raulji, P., Howell, M., Davis, Y., Mallela, J., Seehra, M. S., & Mohapatra, S. (2012). Dual-purpose magnetic micelles for MRI and gene delivery. *Journal of Controlled Release*, *163*(1), 82–92. doi:10.1016/j.jconrel.2012.04.030 PMID:22561339

Wu, Y., Ali, M. R. K., Chen, K., Fang, N., & El-Sayed, M. A. (2019). Gold nanoparticles in biological optical imaging. *Nano Today*, *24*, 120–140. doi:10.1016/j.nantod.2018.12.006

Chapter 11
Nanotechnology and Its Application in Medical Sciences

Rahul Saxena
https://orcid.org/0000-0002-4517-8529
Sharda School of Allied Health Sciences, Sharda University, India

Suyash Saxena
Sharda School of Allied Health Sciences, Sharda University, India

Ajit pal Singh
Sharda School of Allied Health Sciences, Sharda University, India

Vandana Singh
Sharda School of Allied Health Sciences, Sharda University, India

ABSTRACT

Materials with 10-9m dimensions are considered nanomaterials, which exhibit beneficial aspects against health-related complications and thus have received much attention. Modern knowledge of the various functions of nanomaterials has advanced it to a new level of revolution. Several chemical, physical, and biological techniques can be used to create nanomaterials. A variety of methods are available for figuring out their physical characteristics and chemical makeup. Their unique physical and chemical properties, due to nanoscale size, enhance their utilization and applications in the field of medicine and biomedical sciences. However, glimpse of certain harmful paradigms offered by nanoparticles forces us to rethink the negative impacts against the human health. This chapter reviews an introductory overview covering the current concepts related to the properties and application of various sorts of nanomaterials used in the field of medical science, with special reference to their metabolic and physiological influence in many types of pathophysiological disorders.

DOI: 10.4018/979-8-3693-0448-8.ch011

INTRODUCTION

Since ancient times, people have been interested in their health and wellbeing, and many scientific endeavors have been made to lead prosperous and healthy lives. However, the mystery of immortality has not yet been solved, and it is now widely understood that physical and mental health will gradually deteriorate over time, followed by a cloud of health-related problems and ultimately death. Due to their distinctive qualities, such as their high surface to volume ratio, stable physical and chemical properties, good permeability, bioavailability, and biocompatibility, materials with sub-micrometer scales (1x10-9 nm) have drawn a lot of attention in a variety of fields, including those of agriculture, engineering, medicine, and biomedical sciences. The creation, synthesis, evaluation, and use of materials with dimensions on the nanoscale scale (1x 10^{-9} m) are all part of the multidisciplinary field of nanotechnology and such materials are known as nanoparticles or nanomaterials. The Greek word "nanos," which meaning "a dwarf," is the source of the prefix "nano". Nanotechnology has revolutionized a wide range of scientific disciplines during the last few decades, includes food production, engineering, health care, the pharmaceutical sector, and the biomedical sciences (Baig et al., 2021).

History of nanotechnology: Despite the fact that scientific research on nanotechnology is a relatively new development, its fundamental ideas developed over a longer period of time. Carbon nanotubes have been discovered in Keeladi, India, pottery between 600 and 300 BC, while it is unknown how they developed or whether the substance that contained them was used on purpose. Around 900 AD, Damascus steel has been found to contain cementite nanowires, albeit its origin and method of production are unknown. As early as the ninth century B.C., artisans in Mesopotamia utilized nanoparticles to give vessels a sparkling appearance. The speech "There's Plenty of Room at the Bottom," delivered by American physicist Richard Feynman in 1959 at a conference of the American Physical Society held at Caltech, is frequently cited as the source of inspiration for the discipline of nanotechnology. In a 1974 symposium, a Japanese scientist by the name of Norio Taniguchi from Tokyo University of Science was the first to introduce the phrase "nano-technology" to characterize semiconductor techniques with characteristic control on the order of a nanometer, such as thin film deposition and ion beam milling. According to his explanation, the basic components of nanotechnology are the processing, separation, consolidation, and deformation of materials by a single atom or molecule. Interestingly, the phrase was not used once more until 1981, when Eric Drexler published his first work on nanotechnology. At the time, he was not aware of Taniguchi's earlier use of the phrase. Pottery from the Middle Ages and the Renaissance frequently displays a distinctive gold or copper-colored metallic shimmer today. This lustre is brought on by a metallic coating that was placed to the clear surface of a ceramic glaze that has silver and copper nanoparticles evenly scattered throughout its glassy matrix (Bayda et al., 2019).

SYNTHESIS AND TYPES OF NANOPARTICLES

Nanomaterials have been prepared using a variety of approaches, including physical, chemical, biological, and hybrid ones. The kind, size, and intended quantity of the nanomaterial are typically taken into consideration when choosing a synthesis technique (Elias et al., 2017). Either a top-down or a bottom-up technique can be used to complete the synthesis. The top-down strategy uses physical (such as mechanical) or chemical means for the generation of nanoparticles, whereas the bottom-up approach mostly uses chemical and biological processes (Figure 1).

Figure 1. Synthesis of nanoparticles

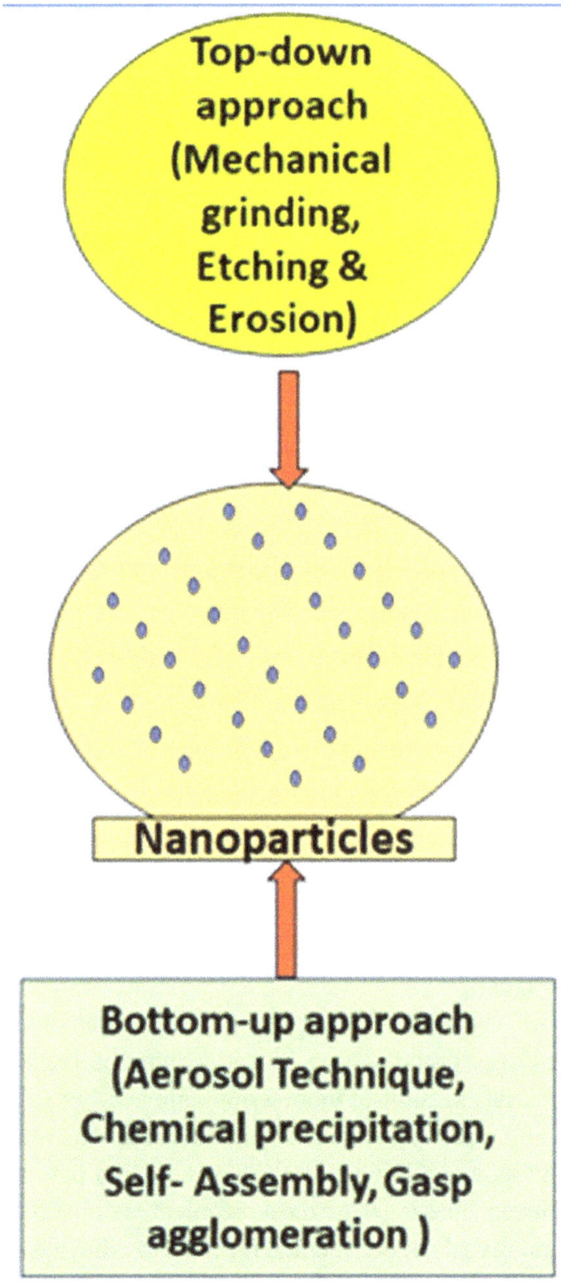

A core ingredient and surface additives that give nanomaterials their physicochemical features, such as charge, hydrophobicity, or other surface chemical properties, are the usual components of nanomaterials (Mansoori et al., 2005). Surface modifiers can be particular chemical compounds, peptides, or proteins. According to their chemical composition, nanomaterials can be divided into three groups: organic nanomaterials, which are predominantly comprised of organic macromolecule polymers such

Table 1. Classification of nanomaterials on the basis of core structure

Category	Types of Nanoparticles
Carbon nanomaterials	Carbon dots, Graphene and its derivatives, Nanodiamonds, Fullerene, Nanotubes, Chitosan nanoparticles.
Organic nanomaterials	Nanogels, Dendrimers, Nanolipidic EGCG particles, Hyperbranched polymers, Polymer nanocomposites, Poly (lactic-co-glycolic acid) nanoparticles.
Inorganic nanomaterials	Au nanoparticles, Ag nanoparticles, CuO nanoparticles, ZnO nanoparticles, TiO2 nanoparticles, Selenium nanoparticles, Silica nanoparticles.

as carobhydrates, lipids and proteins etc.; carbon nanomaterials, which are primarily made of carbon; and inorganic nanomaterials, which are predominantly comprised of inorganic components (Table 1; Zman et al., 2014).

Role of nanotechnology in medical science: Nanotechnology acceptance and advancement are anticipated to have a significant impact on human civilization and provide solutions to many of the problems that humans is now facing, notably in the field of medical sciences. In addition, wide range of medical applications of nanotechnology, in terms of diagnosis, treatment, and prevention, has shown its great potential. In the past several years, the field of medicine has made extensive use of various forms of nanomaterials including dendrimers, cubosomes, fullerenes, nanocrystals, liposomes, nanocapsules, solid lipid nanoparticles, and niosomes. Thus, the advancements in nanotechnology and other sectors make it possible to treat patients and enhance their health in a far more efficient and productive manner. Amazing contribution of nanotechnology in healthcare is evidenced by their application in various ways, as well represented in Figure 2.

a) **Dermatology:** Skin, the largest organ, is prone to a wide range of illnesses, conditions, and injuries, from relatively mild microbial infections to more serious ailments like skin cancer. Nanodermatology, one of the rapidly expanding subspecialties of nanomedicine, has transformed the detection and treatment of a number of skin conditions. More than a million new instances of skin cancer are recorded worldwide each year, making it the most prevalent malignant condition, especially among Caucasians. Based on quantum dots, one method for the early diagnosis of melanoma. Engineered fluorescent nanoparticles known as quantum dots (QDs) have special optical characteristics like high brightness, photobleach resistance, and variable wavelength. Despite the foreseeable future of nanodermatology, the potential hazardous consequences and associated safety worries could not be ignored. The most extensively studied QDs are cadmium/selenide (Cd/Se) QDs (Antonio et al., 2014). The quantum dots immunofluorescent label has been widely used as a promising method for biomedical imaging in cancer cells due to the high specificity and sensitivity. High-resolution photoacoustic tomography (PAT) and gold nanocages (AuNCs) were first combined by Kim et al. They claim that once AuNCs are bioconjugated with [Nle4,D-Phe7]-melanocyte-stimulating hor-

Figure 2. Role of nanoparticles in medical sciences

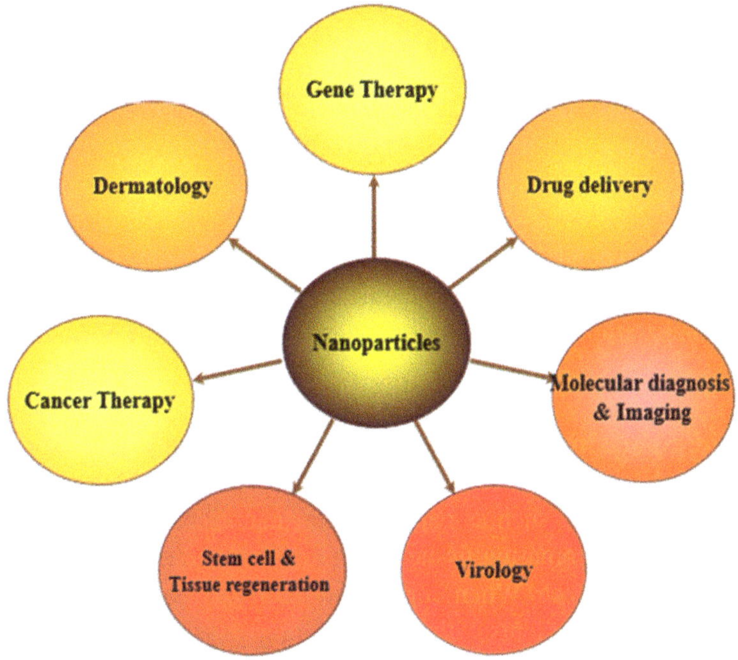

mone, they can act as a new contrast agent for in vivo molecular PAT of melanomas with exquisite sensitivity and great specificity (Chamcheu et al., 2018). Similar to this, in a mouse psoriasis-like dermatitis condition caused by imiquimod (IMQ), therapeutic efficacy of chitosan-based polymeric nanoparticle formulation of epigallocatechin-3-gallate (i.e. nanoEGCG) was seen.[8] Additionally, nanomaterials have had an impact on the cosmeceutical industry due to the distinct and improved qualities that the nanoscale particles have over the bulk materials.

b) **Wound healing and Tissue regeneration**: In last few decades, the possible uses of nanotechnology in the field of Wound healing and Tissue regeneration is expanding fast. After an injury, a series of biological processes begin in order to regenerate and repair the injured tissue; this process is known as wound healing. As a temporary physical barrier to defend against harmful microorganism invasion and to avoid wound dehydration while promoting healing, wound dressings have been developed. Nanomaterials have recently become a source for creating cutting-edge and very effective wound treatments. While some metal nanoparticles have the potential to be included into wound dressings due to their inherent antibacterial qualities, numerous polymeric nanofibres have demonstrated encouraging outcomes as scaffolds for skin regeneration (Chen et al., 2008).

The primary reason that nanoparticles are used in wound dressing materials is because they are naturally antibacterial. Metal nanoparticles with antibacterial qualities can aid in the healing of wounds. Examples include silver, gold, copper, copper oxide, iron oxide, zinc oxide, and titanium dioxide. The aforementioned metal nanoparticles' antibacterial activity is brought on by the production of reactive oxygen species (ROS), as well as interactions with biomolecules including DNA, proteins, or the suppression of enzymes. Both silver nanoparticles (AgNPs) and gold nanoparticles (AuNPs) have several antimicrobial effects. These nanoparticles have the ability to damage bacterial cell membranes, leak into the cytosol, and disrupt or destabilise enzymes, cytoplasmic proteins, and membrane proteins. This would ultimately result in bacterial cell death and metabolic dysfunction (Mihai et al., 2019).

Reactive oxygen species (ROS) mediated Oxidative stress can be produced by gold nanoparticles (AuNPs) and AgNPs. ROS can harm proteins and nucleic acids in bacterial cells and also prevent the electron transport chain from functioning properly, both of which can result in bacterial cell death. Moreover, nanocarriers that contain medications, biomolecules, and growth factors are providing new therapy modalities, particularly for chronic wounds. By preventing the degradation of drug and enhancing the drug's entry into the wound, the nanomaterials' small size and physicochemical characteristics make intracellular delivery of biomolecules or medications easier (Joshi et al., 2020). This allows for topical medication administration and increases the half-life, lowering the need for as many administrations and expenditures.

c) **Physiotherapy & Sports medicine:** Recently, there has been a lot of promise in the use of nanotechnology in physiotherapy, rehabilitation management, and sports medicine. The potential of various nanomaterials, such as nanoparticles, nanofibers, and nanocomposites, has been investigated in regards to promoting tissue repair and regeneration, reducing inflammation, and enhancing athletic performance. When opposed to traditional military uses, nanotechnology has a number of advantages for patients with muscular injuries, such as lighter, stronger accessories, and comfortable and secure workout equipment. Flexible and breathable sports wears also boosts confidence and improvement in performance of athletes. The healing of muscles that have been strained, injured, or worn out by physical activity, particularly in strenuous workouts connected to running, bodybuilding, wrestling, and powerlifting, can be aided by functional devices, accessories, and sportswear that offers therapeutic benefits.

Germanium and ceramic nanoparticles with far-infrared radiation properties, such as alumina, titanium dioxide, and silicon dioxide, can be combined with textile materials that meet the skin to create a variety of products that can be used for therapeutic purposes, such as knee bands, elbow bands, and back belts. Additionally, nanotechnology-based drug delivery systems have the potential to provide tailored medication administration to body regions, enhancing treatment effectiveness and reducing side effects. Nanotechnology has enormous potential for managing muscle injuries and enhancing general function (Singh et al., 2017). Even if there are obstacles to be overcome, it is expected that further research and development of nanotechnology-based interventions in physiotherapy and sports medicine will result in substantial improvements in the field that will help patients and athletes as well.

d) **Drug delivery:** The persistence of these molecules in the desired target site plays a key role in the potency and effectiveness of these bioactive compounds/drugs. These compounds may come into contact with various chemicals that could interact with them throughout the delivery process, which could affect the drug's efficacy or occasionally cause unanticipated reactions to be seen. Therefore, a medicine must overcome challenging physiological conditions during the distribution process and the right amount of active component must reach and enter the target site in order to have a true therapeutic impact. In this regard, drug delivery that is targeted and site-specific, especially for medications with low solubility and absorption, is possible thanks to nanotechnology. Biocompatibility, lack of adverse effects, stability, loss-free transport to the affected portion, and biodegradability are all qualities that a perfect medicine carrier should have. In reality, nanoparticles smaller than 100 nanometers in at least one dimension are used as nanocarriers. These nanoparticles may be constructed from a variety of biodegradable substances, including metals, lipids, and synthetic or natural polymers. To target a drug to a certain spot or to accomplish a controlled release of the medicine to a specific place, the nanoparticles used to transport medicine are created. There can be various mechanisms by which these nanoparticles can deliver the medicine which include Physical encapsulation, Chemical conjugation and Self-delivery method.

e) **Gene Therapy:** Through the introduction of genes, gene therapy involves altering the genetic makeup of the cell. By introducing therapeutic genes through either integrative or non-integrative vectors, gene therapy is utilized to treat a monogenic hereditary or acquired disease. Integrative vectors are secure modified viral carriers (such as lentiviruses, gamma retroviruses, foamy viruses, and adeno-associated viruses) that allow the delivery of a therapeutic transgene to the target cell's DNA. The therapeutic transgene is not persistently expressed in the target cell when using non-integrative vectors. Adenoviruses, herpesviruses, poxviruses, and vaccinia viruses are a few examples of viruses that can be utilised as nonviral or viral vectors for non-integrative vectors. Nonviral vectors are predominantly based on lipids or cationic polymers.

The use of nanoparticles to transfer nucleic acids and viral vectors (such as adenoviruses and retroviruses) has been reported by numerous groups in recent years, giving rise to novel techniques known as magnetofection and theranostics. Superparamagnetic nanoparticles are used in the viral and non-viral technique known as magnetofection to enhance gene transport in the presence of a magnetic field. Adding a magnetic field to a mixture of genetic material and nanoparticles accelerates the kinetics of transfection and raises the density of vectors at the cell surface. Prior to mixing the gene vectors with the magnetic particles, the gene vector is conventionally prepared as part of the magnetic vector complexing process. The majority of studies have found that additional substances are required to create the association between the nanoparticles and the gene delivery vector. Polymers can serve as a connection between the nanoparticles and the nucleic acid in the case of DNA (Herranz et al., 2011). Iron oxide nanoparticles (SPIOs) have been linked to DNA and coated with transfection agents like polyethyleneimine (PEI). Transfection efficiency improves 40-fold when the mix is conducted in a magnetic field, either permanent or pulsing (Kamau et al., 2006). This method offers novel, highly effective alternatives to integrative vectors while avoiding negative effects associated with their integration and requiring a small amount of DNA to reach high transfection levels.

f) **Antimicrobial activity:** The creation of new pharmaceutical products is very interested in the preparation of homogenous nanosized drug particles with specified specifications for size, shape, and physical and chemical properties. Due to their effective antibacterial capabilities, highly ionic metal oxide nanofluids like zinc oxide, magnesium oxide, calcium oxide, copper oxide, and titanium dioxide have gained a lot of attention. The benefit of using these inorganic oxide nanofluids as antibacterial agents is that they are stable under difficult process conditions and are typically regarded as essential mineral elements for people and animals at a lower concentration. Since ancient times, inorganic antimicrobials like silver and copper have been utilised to treat microbial diseases. According to early research, the antibacterial properties of silver, magnesium oxide, calcium oxide, and zinc oxide were robust against both Gram-positive and Gram-negative bacteria. In order to create a new generation of bactericidal materials, nanosized inorganic particles must be prepared, characterised, surface modified, and functionalized. As an antibacterial agent, ZnO nanofluid has recently piqued the interest of several researchers. According to several studies, ZnO nanosuspensions with relatively tiny particle sizes have demonstrated the strongest antibacterial activity against a variety of microorganisms, including important pathogens, among metal oxide nanoparticles including MgO, TiO2, and CuO (Zhang et al, 2007; Qi et al., 2020; Naser et al., 2021). ZnO nanoparticles have been shown to be highly effective antibacterial agents against both Gram-positive and Gram-negative bacteria (Sawai et al., 1998; Patil et al., 2019; Wu et al., 2010).

g) **Virology:** There are various methods available for the identification of different viruses such as culturing, electron microscopy, Radioimmuno assay (RIA), Enzyme Linked Immunosorbant assay (ELISA) etc. Despite the high sensitivity and high reproducibility of these conventional methods for pathogen identification, some drawbacks, such as the need for sophisticated, extremely expensive instruments, trained personnel, high costs, and extended run times, make the development of novel methods for pathogen detection necessary. As a result, utilising nanomaterials, current detecting techniques are developed that are rapid, quick and affordable. Due to their distinctive qualities, including as their magnetic, electrical, and catalytic capabilities, nanomaterials are used in these processes (Shinde et al., 2012). Diagnostic procedures typically utilise bioreceptors and transducers. An enzyme, protein, antibody, or biological system like a tissue, cell, or a whole organism can selectively connect with the pathogen. These biological molecules are known as bioreceptors. It is often immobilised on a suitable support medium, and a change in physicochemical properties is brought on by a particular interaction between the pathogen and the bioreceptor. The transducer notices and measures this change. Bioreceptors include things like dendrimers, liposomes, carbon nanotubes etc.

In order to develop treatment plans for infectious disorders brought on by viruses, extensive study is being done on the interactions between various nanomaterials and viruses. Gaikwad et al., for instance, assessed the antiviral efficacy of biogenic AgNPs against types 1 and 2 of the herpes simplex virus and type 3 of the human parainfluenza virus. This study showed that the size and zeta potential of the AgNPs affected how well they interacted with the tested viruses. Additionally, the activity was reliant on the source that was employed to create the AgNPs. The AgNPs made by Fusarium oxysporum and Curvularia species, which were smaller in size than the AgNPs made from other fungal sources, clearly exhibited antiviral action. It was hypothesised that smaller nanoparticles could adhere to viruses, preventing the interface between the virus and the host cell and weakening viral replication (Gaikwad et al., 2013).

Approaches utilising nanotechnology have the potential to significantly increase the potency of antiviral medications. Antiviral medications that have been encapsulated with nanoparticles typically have characteristics like regulated release kinetics, increased bioavailability, changed pharmacokinetics, and fewer side effects. Additionally, the physical characteristics of nanocarriers might enable the targeting of particular regions and contact with virus structures (Lembo et al., 2018). Acyclovir (ACV), an antiviral medication used to treat HSV infections, chicken pox, and shingles, has a brief half-life and only partial absorption. To extend the drug's plasma half-life after intravenous delivery, Kamel et al. created stealthy ACV nanoparticles using PLGA 85/15, a polylactic acid, polylactic-co-glycolic, and polylactic acid blend. This strategy boosted the drug's average residence time by 29 times (Kamel et al., 2009).

Figure 3. Nanomaterials mediated risk in human health

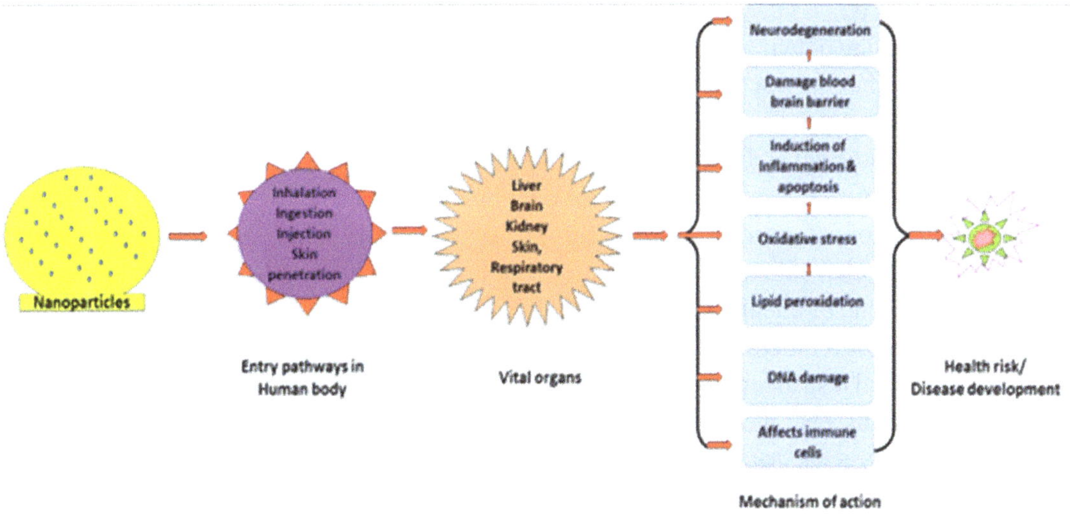

NANOMATERIAL MEDIATED HEALTH RISK

Despite that the advantages of nanotechnology predominate our thinking, the risks associated with the application of nanomaterials to human health cannot be ignored. Glimpse of certain harmful paradigms offered by nanoparticles forces us to rethink about the negative impacts against the positive ones. The application of nanotechnology in medicine and human health is thereby raising safety concerns. Due to their reduced size, nanoparticles can enter the body through a variety of methods, including ingestion, inhalation, injection, and skin penetration. Because of their incredibly small sizes, nanoparticles can passively diffuse through human membranes and readily pass through them. The brain, liver, kidneys, respiratory tract, and other organs and tissues can be accessed by nanoparticles after they enter the systemic circulation (Figure 3).

Exposure to silver nanoparticles and soluble silver compounds is known to have hazardous consequences on human health, including kidney and liver damage, blood cell alterations, irreversible skin and eye discoloration (argyria and argyrosis), irritation of the skin, eyes, digestive tract, and respiratory system. Nanoparticles' small size gives them the potential to pass across the blood-brain barrier, which could lead to central nervous system neurotoxicity, neuroinflammation, and neurodegeneration. Welding fumes, diesel exhaust particles, and other combustion-derived nanoparticles, as well as synthetic or created nanoparticles (such as carbon nanotubes, copper oxide, carbon black, etc.), have been implicated as potential important risk factors in the etiology of neurodegenerative illnesses. Moreover, reactive oxygen species (ROS) are mostly produced by nanoparticles (such as carbon nanotubes and ultrafine particles) when they are exposed to UV light or transition metals. Neurodegenerative diseases including Alzheimer disease and Parkinson disease have been linked to oxidative stress and ROS caused by nanoparticles.

When enough carbon nanotubes enter the lungs, they cause a hazardous reaction that develops in a time- and dose-dependent way. Technological breakthroughs and the beginning of the industrial revolution have led to an increase in the manufacturing of nanoparticles and their subsequent discharge into the environment that humans share. In addition, large sections of the atoms that make up nanoparticles are exposed to the outside of the particle due to their small size and would be free to engage in a variety of chemical processes (Gavas et al., 2021).

Therefore, identifying potential threats to the environment and human health is necessary for the successful use of nanotechnology in the future. To encourage nanotechnology for its financial benefits and potential medical uses, the government must provide safety regulations for the sector's manufacturing, worker exposure monitoring, ambient release of nanoparticles, and risk assessments.

Challenges and future prospective: It is conceivable that nanotechnology will keep developing and expanding in the field of nanomedicine. The scientific advancements made possible by nanotechnology involve mysterious mechanisms for strengthening and motivating accomplishments in the disciplines of tissue engineering and biomedicine. But before these inventions are introduced for use in healthcare, thorough investigation is required. In the near future, there are a number of other intriguing concepts for putting nanomechanical instruments to use in therapeutic settings. Additionally, it has been proposed that nanomachines might disperse medications throughout the patient's body. Such micro structures could carry medications to specific locations, enabling more accurate and adequate treatment. Interestingly, the key challenges in converting nanotechnology into treatments for medication delivery is the design and testing of novel techniques for managing the interaction of nanomaterials with the body. The major issues that need to be resolved include ways to direct these nanomaterials to locations in the body while preventing them from being absorbed by organs like the liver and spleen (Mushtaq et al., 2015).

Furthermore, future developments in nanomedicine will include items like miniature nanofluidic systems and devices that transport fluids more effectively to the point of delivery while minimizing turbulence and mixing (since fluids move with laminar flow through micro/nanochannels). To achieve the benefits that nanotechnology promises, we anticipate that major research will be carried out with increased financing, coordination efforts from numerous agencies, and the need for international cooperation.

Summary: Over the past few decades, numerous intriguing physical and chemical characteristics of nanoparticles have been discovered. An overview of current advances in nanoparticles in the field of medical sciences was provided in this chapter. A new line of defense against pathophysiological hazards can be developed using these novel features and behaviors in biological systems. The application of nanoparticles in drug delivery and prevention of disease development has enormous potential. The significant challenges in medical science, however, demand more focus in the future. For both medical research and therapeutic applications, the stability of the nanoparticles is a critical concern. There hasn't been much consensus among therapeutic interventions for many types of health concerns up until now. To explain the variance in the clinical setups, it is crucial to methodically define the precise biochemical characteristics of nanoparticles. Although numerous benefits have been associated with nanotechnology, several challenges remain to be addressed. These include worries about nanomaterial safety and the need for more thorough clinical research to assess the efficacy of interventions based on nanotechnology. Additionally, the expensive cost of nanotechnology-based therapies may prevent them from being widely used in performance enhancement and injury care. Moreover, in order to conduct therapeutic interventions and biomedical research in this area, healthcare professionals, clinicians and biomedical scientists must understand how nanoparticles and its related biomolecules interact with biological system.

REFERENCES

Antonio, J. R., Antônio, C. R., Cardeal, I. L., Ballavenuto, J. M., & Oliveira, J. R. (2014). Nanotechnology in dermatology. *Anais Brasileiros de Dermatologia*, *89*(1), 126–136. doi:10.1590/abd1806-4841.20142228 PMID:24626657

Baig, N., Kammakakam, I., & Falath, W. (2021). Nanomaterials: A review of synthesis methods, properties, recent progress, and challenges. *Materials Advances*, *2*(6), 1821–1871. doi:10.1039/D0MA00807A

Bayda, S., Adeel, M., Tuccinardi, T., Cordani, M., & Rizzolio, F. (2019). The History of Nanoscience and Nanotechnology: From Chemical-Physical Applications to Nanomedicine. *Molecules (Basel, Switzerland)*, *25*(1), 112. doi:10.3390/molecules25010112 PMID:31892180

Chamcheu, J. C., Siddiqui, I. A., Adhami, V. M., Esnault, S., Bharali, D. J., Babatunde, A. S., Adame, S., Massey, R. J., Wood, G. S., Longley, B. J., Mousa, S. A., & Mukhtar, H. (2018). Chitosan-based nanoformulated (-)-epigallocatechin-3-gallate (EGCG) modulates human keratinocyte-induced responses and alleviates imiquimod-induced murine psoriasiform dermatitis. *International Journal of Nanomedicine*, *13*, 4189–4206. doi:10.2147/IJN.S165966 PMID:30057446

Chen, X., & Schluesener, H. J. (2008). Nanosilver: A nanoproduct in medical application. *Toxicology Letters*, *176*(1), 1–12. doi:10.1016/j.toxlet.2007.10.004 PMID:18022772

Ealias, A. M., & Saravanakumar, M. P. (2017). A review on the classification, characterisation, synthesis of nanoparticles and their application. IOP Conf. Ser. *Materials Science and Engineering*, *263*, 032019.

Gaikwad, S., Ingle, A., Gade, A., Rai, M., Falanga, A., Incoronato, N., Russo, L., Galdiero, S., & Galdiero, M. (2013, November 6). Antiviral activity of mycosynthesized silver nanoparticles against herpes simplex virus and human parainfluenza virus type 3. *International Journal of Nanomedicine*, 4303–4314. PMID:24235828

Gavas, S., Quazi, S., & Karpiński, T. M. (2021). Nanoparticles for Cancer Therapy: Current Progress and Challenges. *Nanoscale Research Letters*, *16*(1), 173. doi:10.118611671-021-03628-6 PMID:34866166

Herranz, F., Almarza, E., Rodríguez, I., Salinas, B., Rosell, Y., Desco, M., Bulte, J. W., & Ruiz-Cabello, J. (2011, July). The application of nanoparticles in gene therapy and magnetic resonance imaging. *Microscopy Research and Technique*, *74*(7), 577–591. doi:10.1002/jemt.20992 PMID:21484943

Joshi, A. S., Singh, P., & Mijakovic, I. (2020). Interactions of gold and silver nanoparticles with bacterial biofilms: Molecular interactions behind inhibition and resistance. *International Journal of Molecular Sciences*, *21*(20), 7658–7664. doi:10.3390/ijms21207658 PMID:33081366

Kamau, S. W., Hassa, P. O., Steitz, B., Petri-fink, A., Hofmann, H., Hofmann-Amtenbrink, M., & Hottiger, M. O. (2006). Enhancement of the efficiency of non-viral gene delivery by application of pulsed magnetic field. *Nucleic Acids Research*, *34*(5), e40. doi:10.1093/nar/gkl035 PMID:16540591

Kamel, A. O., Awad, G. A., Geneidi, A. S., & Mortada, N. D. (2009, December). Preparation of intravenous stealthy acyclovir nanoparticles with increased mean residence time. *AAPS PharmSciTech*, *10*(4), 1427–1436. doi:10.120812249-009-9342-y PMID:19949904

Kim, C., Cho, E. C., Chen, J., Song, K. H., Au, L., Favazza, C., Zhang, Q., Cobley, C. M., Gao, F., Xia, Y., & Wang, L. V. (2010). In vivo molecular photoacoustic tomography of melanomas targeted by bioconjugated gold nanocages. *ACS Nano*, *4*(8), 4559–4564. doi:10.1021/nn100736c PMID:20731439

Lembo, D., Donalisio, M., Civra, A., Argenziano, M., & Cavalli, R. (2018, January 2). Nanomedicine formulations for the delivery of antiviral drugs: A promising solution for the treatment of viral infections. *Expert Opinion on Drug Delivery*, *15*(1), 93–114. doi:10.1080/17425247.2017.1360863 PMID:28749739

Mansoori, G. A., & Soelaiman, T. A. F. (2005). Nanotechnology—An introduction for the standards community. *Journal of ASTM International*, *2*(6), 1–22.

Mihai, M. M., Dima, M. B., Dima, B., & Holban, A. M. (2019). Nanomaterials for wound healing and infection control. *Materials (Basel)*, *12*(13), 2176. doi:10.3390/ma12132176 PMID:31284587

Mushtaq, G., Khan, J. A., Joseph, E., & Kamal, M. A. (2015). Nanoparticles, Neurotoxicity and Neurodegenerative Diseases. *Current Drug Metabolism*, *16*(8), 676–684. doi:10.2174/1389200216666150812122302 PMID:26264205

Naser, R., Abu-Huwaij, R., Al-khateeb, I., Abbas, M. M., & Atoom, A. M. (2021, May). Green synthesis of zinc oxide nanoparticles using the root hair extract of Phoenix dactylifera: Antimicrobial and anticancer activity. *Applied Nanoscience*, *11*(5), 1747–1757. doi:10.100713204-021-01837-0

Patil, P. P., Bohara, R. A., Meshram, J. V., Nanaware, S. G., & Pawar, S. H. (2019, February 1). Hybrid chitosan-ZnO nanoparticles coated with a sonochemical technique on silk fibroin-PVA composite film: A synergistic antibacterial activity. *International Journal of Biological Macromolecules*, *122*, 1305–1312. doi:10.1016/j.ijbiomac.2018.09.090 PMID:30227212

Qi, K., Xing, X., Zada, A., Li, M., Wang, Q., Liu, S. Y., Lin, H., & Wang, G. (2020, February 1). Transition metal doped ZnO nanoparticles with enhanced photocatalytic and antibacterial performances: Experimental and DFT studies. *Ceramics International*, *46*(2), 1494–1502. doi:10.1016/j.ceramint.2019.09.116

Sawai, J,, Yamamoto, O., Hotta, M., Kojima, H., & Sasamoto, T. (1998). Antibacterial characteristics of heated zinc oxide powders on Escherichia coli and Staphylococcus aureus; Kanetsu shori sareta sanka aen funmatsu no daichokin oyobi oshoku budoukyukin ni taisuru kokin tokusei. *Nippon Kagaku Kaishi (Journal of the Chemical Society of Japan, Chemistry and Industrial Chemistry).*

Shinde, S. B., Fernandes, C. B., & Patravale, V. B. (2012, April 30). Recent trends in in-vitro nanodiagnostics for detection of pathogens. *Journal of Controlled Release*, *159*(2), 164–180. doi:10.1016/j.jconrel.2011.11.033 PMID:22192572

Singh, M., & Singh, N. (2017). Nanotechnology in sports medicine: A perspective on latest developments. *International Journal of Nanomedicine*, *12*, 871–881.

Wu, B., Wang, Y., Lee, Y. H., Horst, A., Wang, Z., Chen, D. R., Sureshkumar, R., & Tang, Y. J. (2010, February 15). Comparative eco-toxicities of nano-ZnO particles under aquatic and aerosol exposure modes. *Environmental Science & Technology*, *44*(4), 1484–1489. doi:10.1021/es9030497 PMID:20102184

Zaman, M., Ahmad, E., Qadeer, A., Rabbani, G., & Khan, R. H. (2014). Nanoparticles in relation to peptide and protein aggregation. *International Journal of Nanomedicine*, *9*, 899–912. PMID:24611007

Zhang, L., Jiang, Y., Ding, Y., Povey, M., & York, D. (2007, June). Investigation into the antibacterial behaviour of suspensions of ZnO nanoparticles (ZnO nanofluids). *Journal of Nanoparticle Research*, *9*(3), 479–489. doi:10.100711051-006-9150-1

Chapter 12
The Significance of Nanomaterials in Medical Imaging and Diagnostics

Amit Pratap Singh Chouhan
Sharda School of Allied Health Sciences, Sharda University, India

Ankush Verma
Sharda School of Allied Health Sciences, Sharda University, India

Vandana Singh
Department of Microbiology, Sharda School of Allied Health Sciences, Sharda University, India

ABSTRACT

A new era in healthcare has been ushered in by the development of nanotechnology. Materials with exceptional properties at the nanoscale are being used to enhance the accuracy and efficacy of diagnostic methods. In particular, nanoparticles have become potent tools with a variety of applications in medical imaging. They can be employed as contrast agents in a number of imaging techniques, such as ultrasounds, computed tomography, and magnetic resonance imaging (MRI), to increase tissue visibility and help diagnose diseases. Increased sensitivity and specificity are two benefits of using nanomaterials in medical diagnostics. They allow for the creation of novel biosensors and diagnostic platforms that can identify biomarkers at lower concentrations, enabling the early identification and monitoring of illnesses. Precision healthcare benefits from the use of drug delivery systems based on nanomaterials because they enable customised therapy, lessen side effects, and enhance patient outcomes.

DOI: 10.4018/979-8-3693-0448-8.ch012

INTRODUCTION

Introduction to Nanomaterials

Healthcare imaging and diagnostics have undergone a significant transformation recently, partly due to the creative incorporation of nanomaterials. It's important to first comprehend the historical context and issues that conventional tactics encountered in order to fully appreciate the significance of these advancements. The sensitivity, specificity, and ability to accurately target particular illness indications were commonly limited by traditional medical imaging techniques. The search for novel solutions has also been fuelled by the desire to reduce patient exposition to ionising radiation while improving diagnostic accuracy in difficult circumstances like early detection of cancer or neurological disorders (Baig et al., 2021).

Nanomaterials have demonstrated to be a disruptive force in the healthcare sector in this situation. Their unique nanoscale characteristics which includes size, surface chemistry, and optical behaviour have led to new imaging and diagnostic possibilities. In order to change our perception of healthcare, this chapter tries to present a thorough explanation of how nanoparticles address these ongoing problems. It will describe the fundamentals, applications, benefits, and limitations of nanomaterials in many contexts, highlighting their revolutionary potential to improve the accuracy of therapeutic interventions as well

Figure 1. Showing the applications of the nanomaterials in medical imaging and diagnostics

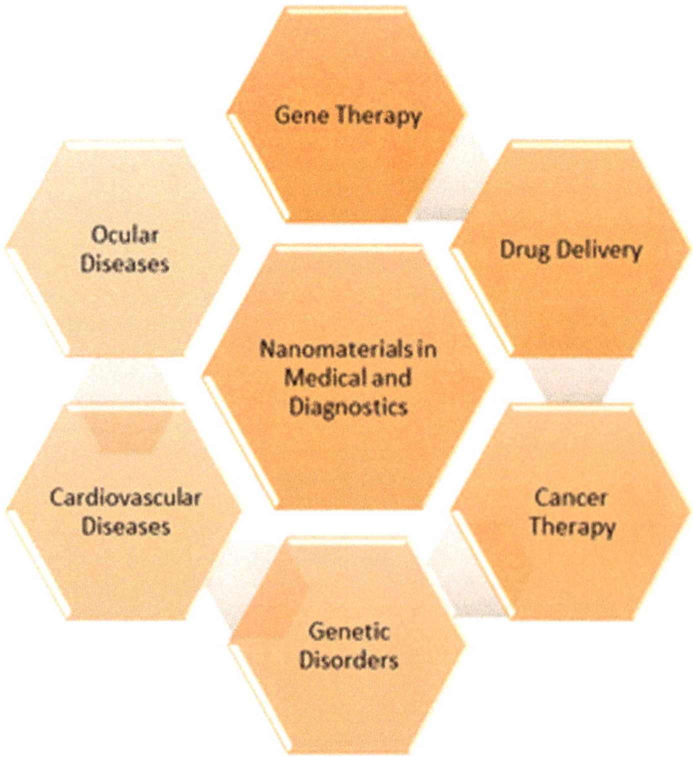

as the precision of medical diagnostics. Readers will gain a complete knowledge of the considerable influence that nanomaterials have had and will continue to have on the field of medical imaging and diagnostics from this investigation (Cheng et al., 2021).

Nanomaterials in Medical Imaging

The implementation of nanomaterials within medical imaging constitutes a significant achievement in the realm of healthcare (Pellico, Gawne, & de Rosales, 2021). Nanotechnology, which involves modifying materials at the nanoscale, has resulted in a new era of diagnostic imaging precision and creativity. Nanomaterials are establishing themselves as game-changing instruments in the creation of cutting-edge medical imaging systems due to their small size and outstanding characteristics (Ge, Zhang, Zeng, Gu, & Gao, 2020). Their unique capabilities, such as tunable optical properties, biocompatibility, and the potential to carry diagnostic chemicals, have opened up previously unexplored opportunities for increasing imaging modalities' accuracy, sensitivity, and specificity. This primer investigates the revolutionary role of nanomaterials in medical imaging, shedding light on their extraordinary potential for early illness identification, personalised treatment techniques, and improved patient care (Siddique & Chow, 2020) .As we learn more about the applications and consequences of these nanoscale treasures in medical diagnostics, it becomes clear that they are poised to revolutionise the way we visualise and comprehend the intricacies of the human body, eventually contributing to enhanced medical treatments (as shown in fig.1.1.) (Chow, 2022).

Nanomaterials in Diagnostics

In the discipline of diagnostics, nanoparticles have become a game-changing instrument with never-before-seen potential for early illness detection, accurate monitoring, and personalised medication. These materials, which usually range from nanoscale (1 to 100 nanometres) in size, possess special and favourable qualities that make them ideally suited for applications in diagnostics (Xie et al., 2021).

The enormous surface area-to-volume ratio of nanoparticles, which allows them to communicate with biological compounds and target analyses with exceptional sensitivity, constitutes one of their primary benefits in diagnostics (Mukhtar et al., 2020). For example, gold nanoparticles functionalized with certain antibodies or aptamers can attach to biological indicators in a sample, such as enzymes or nucleic acids, with high specificity. This interaction can be quickly and accurately diagnosed using a variety of methods, such as colour changes, fluorescence, or surface-enhanced Raman spectroscopy (Zeng et al., 2022).

Furthermore, the creation of multipurpose diagnostic platform is made possible by the variable size and surface chemistry of nanomaterials. Such platforms can act as both imaging agents and diagnostic payloads, such as contrast molecules or therapeutic medicines. For instance, superparamagnetic nanoparticles of iron oxide can be used in magnetic resonance imaging (MRI) for both therapy and diagnosis, allowing medical professionals to monitor the development of diseases and focus treatment on certain locations (Soufi & Iravani, 2020).

Point-of-care investigations have undergone a radical transformation thanks to nanomaterials. Complex diagnostic procedures may now be carried out outside of the confines of a standard laboratory setting thanks to the development of miniature gadgets that use nanoscale components like carbon nanotubes and quantum dots. In situations with limited resources, these portable and affordable devices can provide quick findings for a variety of ailments, from infectious pathogens to chronic conditions, improving access to healthcare (Ghaemi et al., 2021).

Nanomaterials also present the possibility of real-time monitoring of disease development and therapeutic response. Clinical decision-makers can use the information that functionalized nanoparticles can continually exchange with disease indicators in vivo to make informed judgements regarding treatment modifications (Gurav et al., 2019). In the setting of cancer therapy, where nanomaterial-based biological sensors can detect tumour growth and evaluate the efficacy of radiotherapy or targeted medicines, this capability is very essential (Arshad et al., 2021).

BASICS OF NANOMATERIALS

Nanomaterials are a fascinating domain at the convergence of technology and science, where matter is altered at the nanoscale, often at dimensions smaller than 100 nanometers. Because of their exceedingly small size, nanomaterials have distinct properties and behaviours that differ from the bulk materials they replace (Wu et al., 2020). Nanomaterials can be produced using a variety of materials, including metals, semiconductors, polymers, and carbon-based structures like nanotubes and graphene. They are excellent prospects for a wide range of potential uses in industries including computers and power storage to healthcare and environmental cleanup due to their distinctive features, which include a high surface area-to-volume ratio, quantum confinement effects, and improved reactivity (Saleh, 2020). Realising the potential of nanomaterials requires an understanding of their basics since doing so opens the door to concepts that have the potential to transform entire industries and enhance our quality of life (Pellico, Gawne, & de Rosales, 2021).

Types and Sizes of Nanomaterials

Nanomaterials are substances that have undergone nanoscale manufacturing or modification. They frequently have sizes between 1 and 100 nanometers. Materials have unique physical, chemical, and biological characteristics at this scale that distinguish them from their bulk counterparts. To appreciate the significance of nanomaterials in medical imaging and diagnosis, one must first understand their principles (Barabadi et al., 2019).

Size and Scale: Nanomaterials are unique in that they can interact with biological systems at both molecular and cellular levels due to their small size. Their small size-to-surface ratio makes them stand out.

Quantum Effects: The nanoscale reveals quantum interactions. As a result, nanomaterials may have changed electrical, optical, and magnetic characteristics, making them useful for a variety of applications, particularly imaging.

Surface Area: Nanomaterials' enormous surface area compared to volume allows for improved interactions between biological molecules, which makes them useful for tagging, focusing, and detecting specific cells or tissues.

Composition: Metals, as well semiconductors, polymers, and carbon-based materials such as nanomaterials and graphene can all be used to make nanostructures. The material used can have a considerable impact on its qualities and applications (Agathokleous et al., 2019).

Surface Chemistry: Surface alterations and functionalization's of nanoparticles can be tuned to establish particular interactions with biological entities, hence enhancing biocompatibility and targeting capabilities.

Biocompatibility: It is vital for medical usage of nanomaterials to ensure that they are biocompatible and non-toxic, particularly in diagnostic and therapeutic contexts.

Imaging Agents: Because of their propensity to absorb, scatter, or emit light or other signals when exposed to particular stimuli, such as electromagnetic energy or ultrasound, numerous nanomaterials can be used as imaging agents (Jandt & Watts, 2020).

Recognising the fundamental properties of nanomaterials is essential for realising their applications in medical imaging and diagnoses. In the following sections of this section, we will look at how these qualities are used to improve the methods of imaging, develop contrast agents, and enable targeted imaging for better disease diagnosis and monitoring (Saleh, 2020).

Types of Nanomaterials Used in Medical Imaging and Diagnostics

The varied range of nanomaterials used in contrast agents are each tailored to specific imaging techniques and therapeutic goals. the following are some of the most typical types of nanoparticles used as contrast agents:

1. Nanoparticles:

Nanoparticles, which typically range in size from one to one hundred nanometers, are adaptable and commonly employed in contrast media. Nanoparticles can be manufactured from a variety of materials, including metals, metal oxides, and polymers, allowing their properties to be customised (Siddique & Chow, 2020).

Gold Nanoparticles: Since gold nanoparticles have good X-ray attenuation qualities, they can be used as contrast agents for CT imaging. Their dimensions and form can be customised to meet the needs of individual applications.

Superparamagnetic Iron Oxide Nanoparticles (SPIONs): SPIONs are used to improve contrast in MRI by changing the relaxation periods of adjacent water protons. They are very useful for diagnosing liver abnormalities and visualising the vascular system (Soufi & Iravani, 2020).

2. Quantum Dots:

Quantum dots were tiny semiconductor nanoparticles with distinct optical characteristics. When activated by light, they produce fluorescence, and the wavelength of the emission is determined by their size. Quantum dots are gaining applications in the field of optical imaging and can allow for the simultaneous visualisation of many targets, a technique known as multiplexing.

3. Nanoliposomes and Nanovesicles:

Such lipid bilayer nanoscale vesicles are capable of holding contrast chemicals, allowing for controlled dispersion and targeted distribution. They're very handy for drug delivery and targeted imaging (Ge, Zhang, Zeng, Gu, & Gao, 2020).

4. Carbon-Based Nanomaterials:

Carbon-based nanomaterials, such as nanotubes made of carbon and graphene, have distinct features that can be utilised for medical imaging.

Carbon Nanotubes: The nanotubes of carbon have excellent X-ray attenuation qualities, making them useful contrast agents in CT imaging. Because of their small dimensions and high proportions, they are ideal for targeting specific cells or tissues.

Graphene and Graphene Oxide: Functionalized graphene and oxides of graphene can be employed in both magnetic resonance and computed tomography imaging. They have showed promise in imaging for cancer and pharmaceutical delivery applications, and their multifunctional roles have propelled them to the forefront of medical imaging.

5.Nanosensors:

Nanostructures or nanomaterials functionalized containing specific molecules can be used as sensors to detect a variety of analytes, including gases, ions, biological molecules, and pathogens.

Quantum Dots: Quantum dots constitute semiconductor nanoparticles with distinct optical characteristics that allow for real-time fluorescence detection. They're used for anything from environmental monitoring to disease detection.

Carbon Nanotubes: Carbon nanotubes are very sensitive materials capable of real-time detection of gases, biomolecules, and contaminants. They find application in gas sensors, biosensors, and monitoring the surroundings.

6. Nanoprobes:

Nanotechnology or nanostructures can be engineered to function as sensors for real-time imaging and tracking of biological techniques, cells, or tissues (Falahati et al., 1864).

Fluorescent Nanoparticles: When these nanoparticles connect to specific groups, they emit fluorescent indications, allowing for real-time monitoring of cellular processes and disease indicators.

Magnetic Nanoparticles: SPIONs (superparamagnetic iron oxide nanomaterials) are utilised in real-time MRI scans to monitor blood circulation, cellular behaviour, and medication delivery.

7. Nanoelectronics:

Nanomaterials can be used to produce tiny sensors and circuits for real-time electrical tracking by integrating them into electrical appliances.

Nanowires and Nanoscale Transistors: Nanowires and nanoscale semiconductors can be employed as sensors to detect biological substances, gases, or protons in real time. Applications like biological sensing and environment monitoring make use of them (Siafaka et al., 2021).

Role of Nanoparticles in Medical Imaging

With technical breakthroughs and the introduction of nanotechnology, medical imaging has seen a significant transformation over time, boosting our capacity to image and diagnose diseases. As useful tools for medical imaging, nanoparticles or nanoscale materials have evolved. They have become indispensable in a number of imaging modalities due to their distinctive characteristics, including as size, surface chemistry, and tunable optical properties. In this investigation, we delve into the various roles that nanoparticles play in medical imaging, highlighting their uses, advantages, and potential to revolutionise healthcare.

The ability to observe the human body non-intrusively has revolutionised medicine. Doctors can observe anatomical details, identify ailments, and monitor treatment outcomes thanks to medical imaging equipment. Technology like X-ray radiography, computed tomography (CT), magnetic resonance imaging (MRI), and ultrasound have historically been used in medical imaging. Despite their use in medical diagnosis, these techniques frequently have limitations in terms of their sensitivity, specificity, and ability to accurately target particular disease indicators (Lu & Hsiao, 2023).

A new era in medical imaging has been brought about by nanoparticles, which can be identified by their nanoscale size (typically 1 to 100 nanometers). These small materials have unique features that make them useful for a variety of imaging applications. Because of their adaptability and versatility, they have extended the possibilities for visualising diseases at the cellular and molecular levels. Let's look at the various roles that nanoparticles play in medical imaging.

Contrast Agents

Perhaps the most well-known uses of nanoparticles in medical imaging is as contrast agents. Contrast agents are substances that are injected into the body to make particular tissues or structures more visible in imaging investigations. Nanoparticles can be designed to be highly effective contrast agents for a variety of imaging modalities. Contrast media have long been used in medical imaging to help us visualise and diagnose illnesses. These agents were traditionally made of chemical compounds, but the advent of nanotechnology has heralded a new era of contrast media. Engineered at the nanoscale, nanomaterials have a plethora of unique features that make them essential in boosting contrast and precision in medical imaging. This investigation delves into the transforming role of nanomaterials in contrast media, clarifying their uses, benefits, and dramatic impact on diverse imaging modalities (Yue et al., 2023).

Medical imaging is a vital tool in modern healthcare, allowing clinicians and researchers to peek inside the human body without causing any harm. The use of contrast media is frequently required for the efficiency of imaging techniques such as X-ray, magnetic resonance imaging (MRI), computed tomography (CT), ultrasound, and optical imaging. When these chemicals are ingested, they improve the visibility of specific tissues, structures, or disorders in medical pictures.

Manufactured at the microscopic level nanomaterials have revolutionised the field of contrast materials by providing features previously unreachable with ordinary chemical substances. Their capacity to improve contrast, targeted particular cells or molecules, and serve a variety of functions (Alzoubi et al., 2023).

Applications of Nanomaterial-Based Contrast Media

Nanomaterial-based contrast agents have found use in a variety of medical imaging applications, providing various advantages:

1. Magnetic Resonance Imaging (MRI):

By changing the relaxation periods of protons, nanomaterials, particularly SPIONs and gadolinium-based nanoparticles, improve contrast in MRI. They improve visualisation of blood arteries, brain lesions, and soft tissues while lowering the amount of contrast agent required, potentially reducing adverse effects.

2. Computed Tomography (CT):

Nanomaterials, such as gold nanoparticles and iodine-based nanoparticles, improve X-ray attenuation, increasing the visibility of anatomical structures and abnormalities in CT images. Because of their high atomic number and adjustable characteristics, they are suitable for CT imaging.

3. Ultrasound Imaging:

In ultrasonic imaging, microbubbles, which are tiny gas-filled particles stabilised by lipid or protein shells, act as contrast agents. They improve the visualisation of blood flow and tissue perfusion by increasing the dispersion of ultrasound waves. These microbubbles have the potential to be functionalized for targeted imaging.

4. Optical Imaging:

In optical imaging, luminescent quantum dots and other fluorescent nanoparticles are useful. When activated, their capacity to emit specific wavelengths of light enables for the visualisation of specified cells or structures. This is especially helpful in fluorescence imaging and tracking particular target molecules.

5. Targeted Imaging:

Nanomaterials can be modified with ligands, antibodies, or peptides that attach to biomarkers or receptors precisely. This detailed imaging of disease-specific biomarkers or tracking particular cell populations improves diagnostic accuracy and reduces false positives.

6. Multimodal Imaging:

Nanomaterial-based contrast agents can be designed to serve different types of imaging at the same time, allowing for multifunctional imaging. This method combines the advantages of various imaging modalities to provide detailed information about a disease or condition (Jiang et al., 2023).

Through their superior targeting, increased contrast, and multifunctionality, nanomaterials have completely changed the way contrast media are used in medical imaging. Precision diagnostics and personalised medicine now have new avenues to explore thanks to these devices' adaptability across imaging modalities like MRI, CT, ultrasound, optical imaging, and targeted imaging. The promise of nanotechnology to revolutionise healthcare will be shown when nanomaterial-based contrast media become more and more important in enhancing illness identification, treatment monitoring, and patient outcomes. Clarity and accuracy are now at the forefront of diagnostics and patient care, thanks to the development of nanomaterials in the field of medical imaging (Hsu et al., 2023).

Targeted Imaging

Due to their ability for tailored imaging, nanoparticles have a special benefit in medical imaging. Nanoparticles can be made to preferentially attach to particular molecules or cells of interest by functionalizing their surface with particular ligands or antibodies. This focused strategy enables the monitoring of particular cell groups or the visualisation of disease-specific markers.

A cutting-edge technique in medical diagnosis called targeted imaging makes it possible to see particular biomarkers, cells, or tissues linked to diseases. This accuracy aids in early illness diagnosis and monitoring while also improving diagnostic precision. Targeted imaging has found use for nanomaterials that have been created at the nanoscale. They are incredibly successful at delivering contrast agents to specific places throughout the body because of their special qualities, which include size, surface functionalization, and multifunctionality. In this investigation, we examine the amazing function of nanomaterials in focused imaging, clarifying their uses, benefits, and promise to transform healthcare (Pourmadadi, Eshaghi, Ostovar, Mohammadi, Sharma, Paiva-Santos, Rahmani, Rahdar, & Pandey, 2023).

Medical imaging is essential to contemporary healthcare because it provides non-invasive ways to identify and visualise disorders. Traditional imaging methods frequently give a general picture of anatomical structures, while focused imaging is more precise. It enables medical experts to specifically observe and track particular biomarkers, cancer cells, or diseased tissues. This degree of precision not only supports early diagnosis but also enables individualised treatment plans. Targeted imaging has undergone a paradigm shift thanks to nanomaterials, which are typically 1 to 100 nanometers in size. Nanoparticles can be functionalized for selective targeting and improved contrast in a variety of imaging modalities thanks to their adaptability and versatility (Goel et al., 2023).

Applications of Nanomaterials in Targeted Imaging

Nanomaterials may have many uses in focused imaging across many different types of imaging and provide a number of benefits:

1. Cancer Imaging:

One important use for nanomaterials is targeted radiography in oncology. Functionalized nanomaterials can characterise and monitor malignant lesions by preferentially binding to cancer cells or particular tumour markers.

2. Inflammatory Imaging:

In diseases like atherosclerosis, rheumatoid arthritis, and inflammatory bowel disease, the progression of inflammation has been visualised using nanomaterials. For accurate illness assessment, targeted imaging of inflammatory markers is necessary.

3. Neurological Imaging:

Nanomaterials are able to be functionalized to target particular neuronal structures or indicators in neurological diseases. This makes it possible to see neurodegenerative conditions like Parkinson's and Alzheimer's.

4. Cardiovascular Imaging:

Nanomaterials can be created to specifically target cardiovascular disease plaque constituents or vascular endothelial indicators. This facilitates the evaluation of vascular diseases such as atherosclerosis.

5. Infectious Disease Imaging:

Using targeted medical imaging, infectious diseases can be found and tracked. In order to specifically bind to viruses or infected cells, nanomaterials can be functionalized, which helps with illness detection and therapy monitoring.

Personalised targeted imaging in healthcare has undergone a radical change because to nanomaterials, which now offer diagnostic and disease monitoring with an unprecedented level of precision. They have established themselves as potent instruments in personalised medicine due to their adaptability, specificity, and capacity to fulfil numerous roles at once. Targeted imaging with nanomaterials presents the possibility of early illness identification, individualised treatment plans, and improved patient outcomes, demonstrating the potential for nanotechnology to completely transform healthcare (Bedhiafi et al., 2023).

Multimodal Imaging

Modern medical diagnostics now rests on the foundation of multimodal imaging, which combines many imaging modalities. It enables medical personnel to compile thorough and complementary knowledge regarding physiologic functions, anatomical structures, and diagnoses and treatment plans more precisely. Nanoscale-engineered materials have become essential elements in multimodal imaging. They can function as versatile contrast agents that improve imaging across several modalities at once thanks to their special features. In the present research, we examine the crucial part that nanomaterials play in multimodal imaging, emphasising their uses, benefits, and potential to revolutionise healthcare. Multimodal imaging is made easier by the adaptability of nanoparticles, which may be used in several imaging modalities at once. This method combines the advantages of various imaging techniques to offer thorough details on a disease or condition. An effective diagnosis and characterization of a tumour, for instance, may be made possible by the use of a nanoparticle-based contrast agent in MRI, CT, and optical imaging.

By giving non-invasive techniques to see visualize the anatomy of the human body, medical imaging has transformed healthcare. Each imaging technique, nevertheless, has its limits and only offers a fragmentary picture of the physiological and pathological processes. By fusing the advantages of many imaging methods, multimodal imaging overcomes this difficulty and enables a more thorough picture of the patient's health (Sobhanan et al., 2023).

Applications of Nanomaterials in Multimodal Imaging

Numerous multimodal imaging techniques use nanomaterials to improve the precision and specificity of diagnosis:

1. Oncology:

The diagnosis and monitoring of cancer treatments benefit greatly from multidimensional imaging. Targeting specific cancer markers or cells with nanomaterials can yield information from MRI, CT, optical imaging, and other sources concurrently.

2. Cardiovascular Imaging:

Nanoparticles and scanning with ultrasound, MRI, and CT enable for a thorough evaluation of cardiovascular conditions such atherosclerosis and aneurysms.

3. Neurological Imaging:

Nanomaterials enable the visualization of neural structures and biomarkers through MRI, CT, and optical imaging, contributing to the understanding of neurological disorders like Alzheimer's and Parkinson's disease.

4. Inflammatory Disease Imaging:

Multimodal imaging with nanomaterials aids in the assessment of inflammatory conditions, such as rheumatoid arthritis, by combining techniques like MRI, CT, and optical imaging.

5. Infectious Disease Imaging:

Nanomaterial-based multimodal imaging can help detect and monitor infectious diseases, enabling the visualization of pathogens or infected tissues across various modalities (Sowmiya et al., 2023).

Considering their vital role in multimodal imaging, nanomaterials have brought about a new era of accuracy and thoroughness in medical imaging. Healthcare workers can better understand diseases by integrating the benefits of several imaging modalities, which can lead to earlier and more accurate diagnoses, customised treatment plans, and better patient outcomes. An example of how nanoscale innovation can have a significant and transformational effect on healthcare is the incorporation of nanotechnology into multimodal imaging (Vazquez-Prada et al., 2023).

Theranostics

A new era of revolution in healthcare is being brought about through theranostics, which seamlessly combines diagnostics and therapy. It helps medical practitioners to detect illnesses and customise patient care based on unique patient features. Nanoscale-engineered materials have become essential tools in theranostics. These adaptable materials work simultaneously as imaging enhancers, medicinal carriers, and diagnostic agents. In this investigation, we examine the revolutionary role of nanomaterials in theranostics, clarifying their uses, benefits, and promise to revolutionise personalised medicine.

Theranostics, a science that combines diagnoses and therapy, is another application for nanoparticles beyond just diagnostic imaging. Theranostic nanoparticles are made to carry therapeutic payloads (such medications or genes) and act as imaging agents at the same time. This dual feature enables both the tailored administration of treatments to illness sites and the real-time monitoring of therapy responses.

Diagnostics and therapy have historically been distinct areas of practise in healthcare, frequently needing numerous processes and interventions. By uniting diagnostic and therapeutic tasks into a single, coordinated strategy, theranostics aims to dismantle these barriers. This strategy helps medical professionals to make wise choices based on current patient data, leading to individualised and accurate treatments (Wang et al., 2023).

Applications of Nanomaterials in Theranostics

Nanomaterials are substances which are having many uses in theranostics and provide a number of benefits:

1. Cancer Therapy:

In cancer treatment, theranostics holds great promise. Through the use of imaging methods like MRI, CT, or fluorescence imaging, nanoparticles enable the delivery of tailored treatments like chemotherapy or photothermal treatment.

2. Cardiovascular Disease Management:

By visualising atherosclerotic plaques and transferring therapeutic drugs to specific vascular locations, nanomaterials can help in the diagnosis and treatment of cardiovascular disorders.

3. Neurological Disorders:

Utilising nanomaterials for theranostics, neural networks can be seen by MRI or optical imaging to target and cure neurological illnesses like Parkinson's or Alzheimer's.

4. Infectious Disease Management:

By transporting antimicrobial or antibacterial medications and enabling real-time imaging of microorganisms, nanomaterials are used for the detection and treatment of infectious disorders.

5. Rheumatology and Inflammatory Diseases:

Targeted therapy for diseases like rheumatoid arthritis are made possible by nanomaterials, which also provide imaging tools to track the development of the disease.

Theranostics has advanced thanks to nanomaterials, ushering in a new era of medical care. Their versatility, targeting skills, and imaging improvements enable individualised and precise therapies, ultimately leading to better patient outcomes. Theranostics based on nanomaterials holds the potential to revolutionise healthcare by offering individualised, real-time diagnostic and therapeutic treatments for a variety of illnesses and ailments as research progresses (Pei et al., 2023).

Real-Time Monitoring

In addition to other industries, real-time monitoring is essential in manufacturing, environmental monitoring, and healthcare. It makes it possible to continuously observe variables including body functions, environmental contaminants, chemical interactions, and industrial operations. Real-time monitoring systems provide timely, precise data that is crucial for decision-making, problem-solving, and process improvement. In healthcare, it is essential to be able to track physiological processes and treatment outcomes in real time. The ability to image nanoparticles offers a way to track changes in the body dynamically. For instance, using magnetic nanoparticles to track cell mobility or measure blood flow changes in response to treatment.

Modern healthcare and many other businesses depend heavily on real-time monitoring. It involves gathering and analysing data continuously or nearly continuously to monitor a variety of metrics, processes, or circumstances. Engineered at the nanoscale, nanomaterials have become essential instruments for real-time monitoring in a variety of applications. They can offer in-the-moment insights on biological, environmental, and industrial processes thanks to their special qualities, which include sensitivity, adaptability, and responsiveness. In this investigation, we examine the revolutionary role of nanomaterials in real-time monitoring, clarifying their uses, benefits, and potential to influence monitoring in the future (NajafiKhoshnoo et al., 2023).

Applications of Nanomaterials in Real-Time Monitoring

Real-time monitoring using nanomaterials is used in many different fields and has significant benefits:

1. Healthcare and Biomedical Monitoring:

For the real-time monitoring of health conditions, glucose levels, infections, and cellular activities, nanomaterial-based detectors and probes are used. For diseases evaluation, therapy monitoring, and personalised medicine, these kinds of applications are essential.

2. Environmental Monitoring:

Nanomaterial-based detectors are used to measure environmental changes in real time, identify pollutants and harmful gases, and monitor the quality of the air and water. These facts are essential for protecting the environment and promoting public health.

3. Industrial Process Control:

For real-time monitoring of chemical responses, environmental conditions, pressure, and other variables in manufacturing operations, nanomaterials are incorporated into sensors. This enhances safety, raises product quality, and streamlines procedures.

4. Energy Management:

Energy systems use nanomaterial-based detectors to track the effectiveness of fuel cells, batteries, and renewable energy sources in real time. This supports energy security and dependability.

5. Structural Health Monitoring:

For real-time quality monitoring in construction, bridge, and aerospace industries, nanomaterial-based detectors are used. This makes early defect diagnosis and maintenance planning possible.

Real-time surveillance, made possible by nanomaterials, is revolutionising how we track and react to changes in numerous processes and circumstances. Their sensitivity, adaptability, and reactivity enable real-time data capture in a variety of operations, including industrial processes, environmental monitoring, and healthcare. We may anticipate more advancements in real-time monitoring systems as nanomaterials research and development proceed, which will eventually enhance decision-making processes, enhance safety, and increase efficiency across a variety of applications (Shruti et al., 2023).

Small Animal Imaging

A key component of preclinical studies involves small animal imaging, which enables researchers to examine diseases, gauge how treatments work, and create new treatments. Small animal imaging has been transformed by nanomaterials, which can act as diverse contrast agents and delivery systems. They are useful instruments for improving the sensitivity and precision of imaging techniques because of their special qualities, including size, surface functionalization, and multimodality. In this investigation, we dive into the critical function of nanomaterials in small animal imaging, clarifying their uses, benefits, and potential to improve our comprehension of disease and the creation of new treatments.

Through the use of small animal examination. nanoparticles have revolutionised preclinical research. Nanoparticles are used to identify cells, monitor the development of disease, and evaluate the effectiveness of treatments in studies involving mice, rats, or other small animals. This skill facilitates the transition from laboratory research to clinical applications, which expedites the discovery of new treatments.

Diagnostic imaging of small animals is essential for bridging the gap between fundamental research and clinical applications. In living species, usually rodents like mice and rats, it enables researchers to analyse diseases, look into treatment options, and gauge the safety and efficacy of new remedies. Imaging of small animals can be performed using a variety of methods, such as MRI, positron emission tomography (PET), computed tomography using single-photon emission (SPECT), computed neuroimaging (CT), and optical imaging (Ding et al., 2023).

Applications of Nanomaterials in Small Animal Imaging

Numerous small animal imaging techniques have used nanomaterials because they have several benefits.:

1. Magnetic Resonance Imaging (MRI):

SPIONs including gadolinium-based nanomaterials in particular, which are nanomaterials, enhance MRI contrast and allow for better visualisation of structures of the body and functional data in tiny animals.

2. Computed Tomography (CT):

The use of Gold and iodine-based nanoparticles improve X-ray attenuation, increasing the visibility of anatomical features and anomalies in small animal CT examinations.

3. Optical Imaging:

For following the activities of cells, analysing tumour progression, and determining the distribution of drugs in small model organisms, fluorescence nanoparticles such as quantum dots are useful in optical imaging.

4. Multimodal Imaging:

Complete evaluations of disease and therapy responses in small animals are made possible by the ability of nanomaterial-based contrast materials to serve numerous imaging modalities concurrently.

5. Targeted Imaging:

In small model organisms, nanomaterials with functional properties can be created to target certain cells, tissues, or biomarkers, improving diagnostic precision and lowering false positives (Yan et al., 2023).

Advantages of Nanoparticles in Medical Imaging

Due to their distinctive features, which provide various advantages over conventional contrast agents and imaging methods, nanomaterials have attracted considerable interest and have been used in medical imaging. The following are the main benefits of using nanoparticles in medical imaging (Joseph et al., 2023):

1. **Enhanced Contrast:** In a variety of imaging modalities, including magnetic resonance imaging (MRI), computed tomography (CT), and ultrasound, nanomaterials can greatly improve contrast. They are effective contrast agents with high surface area and customizable qualities that enhance the visibility of anatomical structures and disease abnormalities.
2. **Targeted Imaging:** Targeting particular cells, tissues, or biomarkers in the body is possible with the use of nanoparticle engineering. Nanoparticles can selectively attach to disease-related areas thanks to functionalization using ligands, antibodies, or peptides, providing incredibly accurate and focused imaging. This is especially useful in cancer and the early diagnosis of particular disorders.
3. **Multimodal Imaging:** Nanomaterials can act simultaneously as flexible contrast agents for a variety of imaging modalities. Healthcare experts can acquire comprehensive information about a medical condition or illness in a single scan because to the ability of some nanoparticles to generate contrast for both MRI and retinal imaging, for instance.
4. **Long Circulation Time:** For the benefit of imaging and specific drug delivery, nanomaterials can be made to circulate for a long time in the circulatory system. With more time, images can be acquired more effectively, and there are more opportunities for nanoparticle aggregation at particular places of interest.
5. **Drug Delivery and Theranostics:** Theranostics is the hypothesis that nanoparticles can deliver therapeutic payloads while acting as imaging agents. Real-time tracking of medication distribution and therapeutic responses is made possible by this method, which results in personalised medicine and improved therapeutic outcomes.
6. **Reduced Dosages:** In comparison to conventional agents, nanoparticles frequently enable the use of lower contrast agent dosages. This can lessen patient risks and potential negative effects while maintaining or even enhancing imaging quality.
7. **Biocompatibility:** Many nanomaterials can be made biocompatible and non-toxic by engineering, which lowers the possibility of negative patient reactions. Particularly crucial is biocompatibility for ongoing or repeated imaging investigations.
8. **Improved Spatial Resolution:** The use of nanoparticles can improve imaging systems' spatial resolution, enabling the identification of tiny lesions, early-stage illnesses, or subtle alterations in cellular or tissue architecture.

9. **Real-Time Imaging:** Real-time imaging abilities offered by certain nanoparticles allow for the observation of dynamic bodily processes as blood flow, cellular interactions, and medication distribution.
10. **Disease Detection and Early Diagnosis:** Nanomaterials can help in early identification of diseases and diagnosis, increasing the likelihood of effective therapy. The accuracy of the diagnosis is increased by their capacity to target particular disease indicators or cells.
11. **Research and Development:** Development and research professionals can examine disease causes, test potential new drugs, and assess treatment outcomes using nanoparticles in both preclinical and clinical trials.
12. **Non-Invasiveness:** Nanoparticle-based medical imaging methods are often non-invasive, negating the requirement for biopsies or invasive operations. This lessens dangers, discomfort, and recuperation times for patients.

By providing improved contrast, accuracy, and adaptability, nanoparticles have completely changed medical imaging. Improved illness detection, treatment monitoring, and patient care are made possible by their capacity to target specific locations, transport therapeutic substances, and offer real-time data (Tang et al., 2023).

Challenges and Considerations

While nanoparticles provide many benefits for medical imaging, there are also unique problems and issues that must be taken into account for safe and efficient utilisation. The main issues and questions surrounding the use of nanoparticles in medical imaging are listed below:

1. **Biocompatibility and Safety:** It is crucial to make sure nanoparticles are safe and biocompatible. The long-term impacts of certain nanoparticles on human health need to be carefully examined since they may cause toxicity or elicit immunological responses. To evaluate the potential dangers associated with exposure to nanoparticles, thorough testing is necessary.
2. **Biodistribution and Clearance:** It is essential to comprehend how nanoparticles are distributed throughout the body and removed from the system. Nanoparticles may occasionally build up in specific organs or tissues, which could have unforeseen effects. Controlling the biodistribution of nanoparticles by appropriate design and modification (Nguyen et al., 2023).
3. **Size and Shape Effects:** The size and structure of nanoparticles can affect how they behave in biological structures. For instance, the circulation times, absorption rates, and interactions of nanoparticles of particular sizes or shapes may vary. The creation of nanomaterials for imaging purposes must take into account these variances.
4. **Regulatory Approval:** Before being used in the clinic, nanoparticle-based contrast materials and imaging methods must pass stringent testing and receive regulatory approval. The process of meeting regulatory standards and proving the safety and effectiveness of these agents can be difficult and time-consuming.
5. **Standardization:** In order to guarantee uniform and dependable outcomes in medical imaging, standardising the synthesis, characterisation, and functionalization of nanoparticles is imperative. Diagnostic accuracy may be harmed by inconsistent imaging data caused by variations in nanoparticle characteristics.

6. **Cost:** It can be expensive to produce nanoparticles, especially ones with unique characteristics or functionalizations. Especially in hospital contexts, the cost-effectiveness of nanoparticle-based imaging techniques needs to be carefully evaluated.
7. **Imaging Techniques:** Various imaging methods could call for particular nanoparticle characteristics or alterations. The shape and function of nanoparticles are influenced by the imaging modality chosen (such as MRI, CT, or optical imaging). For their imaging objectives, researchers must carefully choose the suitable nanoparticles.
8. **Long-Term Stability:** Over the years, nanoparticles' characteristics can alter, potentially impacting how well they image. It's essential to guarantee the long-term stability of nanoparticles, especially for applications that call for storage or prolonged use.
9. **Immune Response:** The body's immune system may identify and remove nanoparticles from the bloodstream, reducing their ability to circulate and be imaged. It is necessary to investigate methods for immune evasion or for immunological compatibility modification of nanoparticles.
10. **Ethical and Privacy Concerns:** The concerns about privacy and ethics pertaining to patient data, particularly when using nanoparticles for personalised therapy, grow more significant as medical imaging technology progress. It is crucial to protect patient data and guarantee informed consent.
11. **Clinical Translation:** It can be difficult to bridge the knowledge gap between research and clinical application of nanoparticle-based imaging procedures. To get these ideas to the bedside, issues with scalability, pricing, and regulatory barriers must be resolved.

It takes interdisciplinary cooperation between scientists, doctors, regulatory bodies, and industry collaborators to address these issues. Researchers can fully utilise nanoparticles to develop medical imaging and enhance patient care by carefully weighing the hazards and advantages of nanoparticle-based imaging and applying best practises (Kumar et al., 2023).

Nanomaterials in Diagnostic Applications

Numerous industries, including medicine and diagnostics, have been completely transformed by nanotechnology, the science and engineering of materials at the nanoscale. Nanomaterials, which are defined as substances with a minimum of one dimension that are in the nanometer range (often 1-100 nanometers), have special physical and chemical characteristics that make them ideal for use in diagnostic applications. Nanomaterials are essential to the field of diagnostics because they increase the sensitivity, specificity, and general effectiveness of diagnostic procedures. This article examines the various functions of nanoparticles in diagnostic usage, emphasising their influence on healthcare, improvements in detection methods, and the difficulties associated with their implementation.

In the world of diagnostic applications, nanoparticles have become potent instruments that are revolutionising how we identify and track diseases. They have paved the way for highly sensitive and specialised diagnostic platforms thanks to their special qualities, which include configurable size and surface features, high surface area-to-volume ratios, and the capacity to hold payloads. For example, by targeting particular biomarkers with nanoparticles, diseases including cancer, viral infections, and autoimmune illnesses can be detected early. Nanomaterials can also be used as adaptable contrast agents in a variety of imaging modalities, which increases the clarity of images of tissues and boosts their accuracy. As nanotechnology research advances, the use of nanomaterials into diagnostic equipment promises to revolutionise healthcare by providing quick and accurate illness diagnosis, individualised treatment plans, and enhanced patient outcomes (Kumawat et al., 2023).

Types of Nanomaterials in Diagnostics

A vast variety of materials, each with unique characteristics and uses, are included in the category of nanomaterials utilised in diagnostic applications. Nanoparticles, nanowires, nanotubes, quantum dot particles, and other nanostructures are some of the nanomaterials that are most frequently used. Let's examine each of these groups in more detail to see how they play a part in diagnostics:

Nanoparticles: Small particles known as nanoparticles typically have sizes between 1 and 100 nanometers. They can be created from a variety of substances, including lipids, polymers, metals (such as gold and silver), metal oxides, and metals. Due to their adaptability and ability to be functionalized with biomolecules, nanoparticles are excellent for a variety of diagnostic purposes.

Gold Nanoparticles: In antibodies like the enzyme-linked immunosorbent assay (ELISA) and lateral flow tests, gold nanoparticles that have been functionalized with antibodies, DNA probes, or aptamers are frequently utilised. They offer a colorimetric readout to make detection easier.

Magnetic Nanoparticles: In the field of magnetic resonance imaging (MRI) and magnetic resonant-based tests, magnetic nanoparticles are used. For sensitive and non-intrusive imaging, they are also utilised in magnetic particle imaging (MPI).

Carbon Nanotubes and Nanowires: One-dimensional nanoparticles with a high aspect ratio, such as carbon nanotubes and nanowires, are advantageous for biosensors because of their remarkable electrical conductivity. By monitoring changes in electrical conductance after binding to target molecules, they are used in field-effect transistor (FET)-based biosensors to identify biomolecules.

Quantum Dots (QDs): Semiconductor nanocrystals called quantum dots have special optical characteristics. They discharge fluorescent signals that are exceptionally bright and have tunable colours. For the simultaneous identification of numerous analytes, QDs are utilised in multiplexed assays. They are utilised in DNA microarrays, flow cytometry, and cellular imaging.

Nanostructures: The features of various nanostructures, such as nanowires, nanorods, and nanoshells, are created to be suitable for diagnostics. For instance, nanoshells have tunable optical characteristics that are useful for scanning and identification, while nanowires can be employed as high-surface-area substrates for improved biomolecule binding (Vega et al., 2023).

Applications of Nanomaterials in Diagnostics

Nanomaterials have found use in a variety of medical procedures and diagnostic methods. Here are some major areas where nanomaterials have contributed significantly.

Cancer Diagnostics:

With their revolutionary approaches to early diagnosis, accurate characterisation, and ongoing monitoring of malignant situations, nanomaterials have created astonishing new opportunities in the field of cancer diagnostics.

Early Detection: For the early identification of cancer-causing agents in blood or tissue samples, nanomaterials and nanosensors are used. Early cancer diagnosis is made possible by functionalized nanomaterials' ability to specifically attach to cancer-specific chemicals.

Imaging: Nanoparticles improve imaging processes like fluorescence imaging and magnetic resonance imaging (MRI), particularly ones with distinctive optical features like quantum dots. They can aid in the precise visualisation of tumours and metastases.

Infectious Disease Detection:

In the field of infectious illness detection, nanomaterials have a wide range of uses and provide creative approaches for quick, accurate, and focused diagnostic tools.

Point-of-Care Tests: The creation of quick screening methods for infectious illnesses, including bacterial and viral infections, depends heavily on nanomaterials. In order to identify specific diseases, nanoparticles are used as labels in lateral flow tests and paper-based diagnostics.

Sensitivity Enhancement: Nanoparticles provide effective target molecule capture and amplification, increasing the sensitivity of nucleic acid-based diagnostics (such as PCR).

Cardiovascular Disease Monitoring:

Innovative technology and pressing healthcare demands have come together in a fascinating way with the use of nanomaterials in cardiovascular disease monitoring. The capacity of nanomaterials to functionalize surfaces for tailored binding to certain cardiac biomarkers, for example, enables highly sensitive and early detection of cardiovascular disorders. These materials can also be used to create miniature, implantable sensors that can track vital signs like blood pressure, glucose levels, and cardiac biomarkers in real-time. Additionally, the resolution and accuracy of diagnostic instruments like magnetic resonance imaging (MRI) and ultrasound for cardiovascular evaluation are greatly improved by the use of nanomaterials in medical imaging procedures. Nanomaterial-based innovations have the ability to change illness as we navigate the rising worldwide burden of cardiovascular diseases.

Biomarker Detection: The identification of cardiovascular biomarkers in specimens of blood, such as troponin and brain natriuretic peptide (BNP), is improved by nanoparticles. This helps in heart condition monitoring as well as initial diagnosis.

Imaging Modalities: Contrast materials for imaging procedures like computed tomography (CT) angiography and MRI employ nanoparticles to help visualise blood arteries and evaluate the condition of the heart (Pourmadadi, Eshaghi, Ostovar, Mohammadi, Sharma, Paiva-Santos, Rahmani, Rahdar, & Pandey, 2023).

Neurological Disorders:

One of the most complex and difficult conditions of the central nervous system can be addressed through the use of nanomaterials in the field of neurological illnesses. With the help of nanotechnology, new avenues for medication delivery have become possible, enabling precise targeting of therapeutic medicines to certain brain regions. This is crucial when managing illnesses like Parkinson's and Alzheimer's, when traditional drug delivery methods typically fall short. Additionally, nanoparticles can serve as delivery mechanisms for medicines based on genes or RNA, opening up the possibility to potentially revolutionary treatments for genetic neurological diseases. Additionally, early and more accurate diagnosis of diseases including brain tumours and neurodegenerative disorders is now achievable because to the advancement of diagnostic imaging techniques using nanomaterials. The incorporation of nanomaterials will likely have a crucial role in advancing our comprehension of neurological disorders and in the development of more efficient treatments, which will improve the quality of life for millions of people affected by these disorders.

Biomarker Detection: Nanomaterial-based sensors can identify biomarkers for neurological disorders including Alzheimer's and Parkinson's, allowing for early diagnosis and monitoring of disease development.

Neuroimaging: Nanoparticles, particularly those with magnetic properties, are used in MRI contrast materials to enhance the visibility of neural networks and illnesses.

Diabetes Management:

In the field of managing diabetes, nanomaterials have carved out a considerable niche by providing cutting-edge ways to track and manage this long-term ailment. The creation of nanosensors with real-time glucose monitoring capabilities is one noteworthy application. These tiny sensors can be inserted beneath the skin to assess glucose levels continually, doing away with the need for uncomfortable fingerstick testing. Furthermore, insulin therapy has a promising future thanks to medication delivery technologies based on nanomaterials.

Glucose Monitoring: Graphene-based sensors, for example, have showed promise for ongoing tracking of glucose, which would enhance the treatment of diabetes.

Insulin Delivery: A regulated release of insulin can be achieved using nanoparticles, perhaps resulting in more effective diabetic treatments.

Drug Delivery and Therapeutics:

The use of nanoparticles in drug delivery and treatments has changed how modern medicine is practised. These novel pharmaceutical chemical carriers, which range from nanoparticles and liposomes to dendrimers and nanotubes, are made of nanoscale materials. Precision drug targeting, controlled release, and improved bioavailability are all made possible by their compact size and adaptable characteristics. Systems for delivering drugs using nanomaterials shield delicate substances from deterioration in the body, lessen side effects by reducing interactions that aren't intended to be there, and boost therapeutic effectiveness. Additionally, these carriers can cross biological barriers like the blood-brain barrier, making it easier to treat disorders that were previously intractable.

Targeted Drug Delivery: To target particular cells or tissues and lessen side effects while increasing medication efficacy, drug carriers made of nanoparticles, such as polymeric and liposomal nanoparticles, are utilised.

Theranostics: Real-time tracking of drug delivery and therapeutic response is made possible by the engineering of nanoparticles for both therapy and diagnostics.

Challenges and Considerations

Although there is enormous potential for using nanomaterials in diagnostic applications, there are a number of issues that need to be taken into account:

Biocompatibility: Nanomaterials must be environmentally friendly and biodegradable to prevent negative effects on biological systems.

Regulatory Approval: Safety evaluations must be carried out and regulatory authorisation for the use of nanoparticles in investigations may be necessary.

Scalability: The possibility for nanomaterial-based therapies to scale towards mass production and commercialization must be taken into consideration.

Cost: It is crucial to consider the cost-effectiveness of diagnostic procedures based on nanoparticles as well as their availability in a range of medical settings and patient populations.

Stability: In specific situations, such as shifts in temperature or pH, there might be stability issues with nanoparticles that need to be handled.

Ethical Concerns: Ethics surrounding the use of nanomaterials for therapeutic purposes and concerns regarding privacy demand careful consideration and regulation.

Nanomaterials, which offer improved sensitiveness, specificity and adaptability in recognising a variety of illnesses and conditions, have altered diagnostics. Nanomaterials are essential for enhancing healthcare results, from cancer detection to the identification of viral illnesses and medication administration. As research advances, it will be necessary to resolve problems with biocompatibility, oversight, and scalability in order to fully realise the promise of nanoparticles in medical diagnostics. Furthering the use of nanotechnology in diagnostics has the potential to fundamentally alter how we diagnose and treat diseases, leading to more effective and customised healthcare (Muthoosamy & Manickam, 2023).

CONCLUSION

In conclusion, the application of nanomaterials to perform medical imaging and diagnostics has ushered in a new era of accuracy and efficacy in medicine. These amazing materials have paved the path for earlier detection of illnesses, more accurate diagnostics, and tailored treatment strategies thanks to their unique capabilities and versatility. From magnetic nanoparticles that enhance MRI in contrast with quantum dots that enhance fluorescence imaging, nanoparticles have expanded our diagnostic toolset. As we realise the potential of these developments, it is critical to address the problems of biological compatibility, regulatory compliance, and adaptability to ensure that these advancements will be advantageous to a wide range of patients and subsequently promise an improved and more beneficial future for medical treatment and diagnostics.

REFERENCES

Agathokleous, E., Feng, Z., Iavicoli, I., & Calabrese, E. J. (2019). The two faces of nanomaterials: A quantification of hormesis in algae and plants. *Environment International*, *131*, 105044. doi:10.1016/j.envint.2019.105044 PMID:31362152

Alzoubi, F. Y., Abu Noqta, O., Al Zoubi, T., Al-Khateeb, H. M., Alqadi, M. K., Abuelsamen, A., & Makhadmeh, G. N. (2023). A Novel One-Pot Synthesis of PVP-Coated Iron Oxide Nanoparticles as Biocompatible Contrast Agents for Enhanced T2-Weighted MRI. *Journal of Composites Science*, *7*(3), 131. doi:10.3390/jcs7030131

Arshad, R., Barani, M., Rahdar, A., Sargazi, S., Cucchiarini, M., Pandey, S., & Kang, M. (2021). Multi-functionalized nanomaterials and nanoparticles for diagnosis and treatment of retinoblastoma. *Biosensors (Basel)*, *11*(4), 97. doi:10.3390/bios11040097 PMID:33810621

Baig, N., Kammakakam, I., & Falath, W. (2021). Nanomaterials: A review of synthesis methods, properties, recent progress, and challenges. *Materials Advances*, *2*(6), 1821–1871. doi:10.1039/D0MA00807A

Barabadi, H., Najafi, M., Samadian, H., Azarnezhad, A., Vahidi, H., Mahjoub, M. A., Koohiyan, M., & Ahmadi, A. (2019). A systematic review of the genotoxicity and antigenotoxicity of biologically synthesized metallic nanomaterials: Are green nanoparticles safe enough for clinical marketing? *Medicina*, *55*(8), 439. doi:10.3390/medicina55080439 PMID:31387257

Bedhiafi, T., Idoudi, S., Alhams, A. A., Fernandes, Q., Iqbal, H., Basineni, R., Uddin, S., Dermime, S., Merhi, M., & Billa, N. (2023). Applications of polydopaminic nanomaterials in mucosal drug delivery. *Journal of Controlled Release*, *353*, 842–849. doi:10.1016/j.jconrel.2022.12.037 PMID:36529384

Cheng, Z., Li, M., Dey, R., & Chen, Y. (2021). Nanomaterials for cancer therapy: Current progress and perspectives. *Journal of Hematology & Oncology*, *14*(1), 1–27. doi:10.118613045-021-01096-0 PMID:34059100

Chow, J. C. (2022). Application of Nanomaterials in Biomedical Imaging and Cancer Therapy. *Nanomaterials (Basel, Switzerland)*, *12*(5), 726. doi:10.3390/nano12050726 PMID:35269214

Ding, S., Chen, L., Liao, J., Huo, Q., Wang, Q., Tian, G., & Yin, W. (2023). Harnessing Hafnium-Based Nanomaterials for Cancer Diagnosis and Therapy. *Small*, *19*(32), 2300341. doi:10.1002mll.202300341 PMID:37029564

Falahati, M., Attar, F., Sharifi, M., Saboury, A. A., Salihi, A., Aziz, F. M., Kostova, I., Burda, C., Priecel, P., Lopez-Sanchez, J. A., Laurent, S., Hooshmand, N., & El-Sayed, M. A. (1864). 2020. Gold nanomaterials as key suppliers in biological and chemical sensing, catalysis, and medicine. *Biochimica et Biophysica Acta (BBA)-. Biochimica et Biophysica Acta. G, General Subjects*, *1864*(1), 129435. doi:10.1016/j.bbagen.2019.129435 PMID:31526869

Ge, J., Zhang, Q., Zeng, J., Gu, Z., & Gao, M. (2020). Radiolabeling nanomaterials for multimodality imaging: New insights into nuclear medicine and cancer diagnosis. *Biomaterials*, *228*, 119553. doi:10.1016/j.biomaterials.2019.119553 PMID:31689672

Ge, J., Zhang, Q., Zeng, J., Gu, Z., & Gao, M. (2020). Radiolabeling nanomaterials for multimodality imaging: New insights into nuclear medicine and cancer diagnosis. *Biomaterials*, *228*, 119553. doi:10.1016/j.biomaterials.2019.119553 PMID:31689672

Ghaemi, F., Amiri, A., Bajuri, M. Y., Yuhana, N. Y., & Ferrara, M. (2021). Role of different types of nanomaterials against diagnosis, prevention and therapy of COVID-19. *Sustainable Cities and Society*, *72*, 103046. doi:10.1016/j.scs.2021.103046 PMID:34055576

Goel, M., Mackeyev, Y., & Krishnan, S. (2023). Radiolabeled nanomaterial for cancer diagnostics and therapeutics: Principles and concepts. *Cancer Nanotechnology*, *14*(1), 1–36. doi:10.118612645-023-00165-y PMID:36865684

Gurav, D. D., Jia, Y. A., Ye, J., & Qian, K. (2019). Design of plasmonic nanomaterials for diagnostic spectrometry. *Nanoscale Advances*, *1*(2), 459–469. doi:10.1039/C8NA00319J PMID:36132258

Hsu, J. C., Tang, Z., Eremina, O. E., Sofias, A. M., Lammers, T., Lovell, J. F., Zavaleta, C., Cai, W., & Cormode, D. P. (2023). Nanomaterial-based contrast agents. *Nature Reviews. Methods Primers*, *3*(1), 30. doi:10.103843586-023-00211-4

Jandt, K. D., & Watts, D. C. (2020). Nanotechnology in dentistry: Present and future perspectives on dental nanomaterials. *Dental Materials*, *36*(11), 1365–1378. doi:10.1016/j.dental.2020.08.006 PMID:32981749

Jiang, Z., Zhang, M., Li, P., Wang, Y., & Fu, Q. (2023). Nanomaterial-based CT contrast agents and their applications in image-guided therapy. *Theranostics*, *13*(2), 483–509. doi:10.7150/thno.79625 PMID:36632234

Joseph, T. M., Kar Mahapatra, D., Esmaeili, A., Piszczyk, Ł., Hasanin, M. S., Kattali, M., Haponiuk, J., & Thomas, S. (2023). Nanoparticles: Taking a unique position in medicine. *Nanomaterials (Basel, Switzerland)*, *13*(3), 574. doi:10.3390/nano13030574 PMID:36770535

Kumar, A., Das, N., & Rayavarapu, R. G. (2023). Role of Tunable Gold Nanostructures in Cancer Nanotheranostics: Implications on Synthesis, Toxicity, Clinical Applications and Their Associated Opportunities and Challenges. *Journal of Nanotheranostics*, *4*(1), 1–34. doi:10.3390/jnt4010001

Kumawat, T. K., Kumawat, V., Sharma, V., Pandit, A., & Biyani, M. (2023). *Applications of Nanomaterials in Diagnostics and Treatment of Cancer. Sustainable Nanomaterials for Biomedical Engineering: Impacts*. Challenges, and Future Prospects.

Lu, C. H., & Hsiao, J. K. (2023). Diagnostic and therapeutic roles of iron oxide nanoparticles in biomedicine. *Tzu-Chi Medical Journal*, *35*(1), 11. doi:10.4103/tcmj.tcmj_65_22 PMID:36866343

Mukhtar, M., Bilal, M., Rahdar, A., Barani, M., Arshad, R., Behl, T., Brisc, C., Banica, F., & Bungau, S. (2020). Nanomaterials for diagnosis and treatment of brain cancer: Recent updates. *Chemosensors (Basel, Switzerland)*, *8*(4), 117. doi:10.3390/chemosensors8040117

Muthoosamy, K., & Manickam, S. (2023). Nanomaterials for disease diagnostics. *Mikrochimica Acta*, *190*(4), 143. doi:10.100700604-023-05724-z PMID:36933103

NajafiKhoshnoo, S., Kim, T., Tavares-Negrete, J. A., Pei, X., Das, P., Lee, S. W., Rajendran, J., & Esfandyarpour, R. (2023). A 3D Nanomaterials-Printed Wearable, Battery-Free, Biocompatible, Flexible, and Wireless pH Sensor System for Real-Time Health Monitoring. *Advanced Materials Technologies*, *8*(8), 2201655. doi:10.1002/admt.202201655

Nguyen, P. H. D., Jayasinghe, M. K., Le, A. H., Peng, B., & Le, M. T. (2023). Advances in drug delivery systems based on red blood cells and their membrane-derived nanoparticles. *ACS Nano*, *17*(6), 5187–5210. doi:10.1021/acsnano.2c11965 PMID:36896898

Pei, Z., Lei, H., & Cheng, L. (2023). Bioactive inorganic nanomaterials for cancer theranostics. *Chemical Society Reviews*, *52*(6), 2031–2081. doi:10.1039/D2CS00352J PMID:36633202

Pellico, J., Gawne, P. J., & de Rosales, R. T. (2021). Radiolabelling of nanomaterials for medical imaging and therapy. *Chemical Society Reviews*, *50*(5), 3355–3423. doi:10.1039/D0CS00384K PMID:33491714

Pellico, J., Gawne, P. J., & de Rosales, R. T. (2021). Radiolabelling of nanomaterials for medical imaging and therapy. *Chemical Society Reviews*, *50*(5), 3355–3423. doi:10.1039/D0CS00384K PMID:33491714

Pourmadadi, M., Eshaghi, M. M., Ostovar, S., Mohammadi, Z., Sharma, R. K., Paiva-Santos, A. C., Rahmani, E., Rahdar, A., & Pandey, S. (2023). Innovative nanomaterials for cancer diagnosis, imaging, and therapy: Drug deliveryapplications. *Journal of Drug Delivery Science and Technology*, *82*, 104357. doi:10.1016/j.jddst.2023.104357

Pourmadadi, M., Eshaghi, M. M., Ostovar, S., Mohammadi, Z., Sharma, R. K., Paiva-Santos, A. C., Rahmani, E., Rahdar, A., & Pandey, S. (2023). Innovative nanomaterials for cancer diagnosis, imaging, and therapy: Drug deliveryapplications. *Journal of Drug Delivery Science and Technology*, *82*, 104357. doi:10.1016/j.jddst.2023.104357

Saleh, T. A. (2020a). Nanomaterials: Classification, properties, and environmental toxicities. *Environmental Technology & Innovation*, *20*, 101067. doi:10.1016/j.eti.2020.101067

Saleh, T. A. (2020b). Trends in the sample preparation and analysis of nanomaterials as environmental contaminants. *Trends in Environmental Analytical Chemistry*, *28*, e00101. doi:10.1016/j.teac.2020.e00101

Shruti, A., Bage, N., & Kar, P. (2023). Nanomaterials based sensors for analysis of food safety. *Food Chemistry*, 137284. PMID:37703589

Siafaka, P. I., Okur, N. Ü., Karantas, I. D., Okur, M. E., & Gündoğdu, E. A. (2021). Current update on nanoplatforms as therapeutic and diagnostic tools: A review for the materials used as nanotheranostics and imaging modalities. *Asian Journal of Pharmaceutical Sciences*, *16*(1), 24–46. doi:10.1016/j.ajps.2020.03.003 PMID:33613728

Siddique, S., & Chow, J. C. (2020). Application of nanomaterials in biomedical imaging and cancer therapy. *Nanomaterials (Basel, Switzerland)*, *10*(9), 1700. doi:10.3390/nano10091700 PMID:32872399

Sobhanan, J., Anas, A., & Biju, V. (2023). Nanomaterials for Fluorescence and Multimodal Bioimaging. *Chemical Record (New York, N.Y.)*, *23*(3), e202200253. doi:10.1002/tcr.202200253 PMID:36789795

Soufi, G. J., & Iravani, S. (2020). Eco-friendly and sustainable synthesis of biocompatible nanomaterials for diagnostic imaging: Current challenges and future perspectives. *Green Chemistry*, *22*(9), 2662–2687. doi:10.1039/D0GC00734J

Sowmiya, P., Dhas, T. S., Inbakandan, D., Anandakumar, N., Nalini, S., Suganya, K. U., Remya, R. R., Karthick, V., & Kumar, C. V. (2023). Optically active organic and inorganic nanomaterials for biological imaging applications: A review. *Micron (Oxford, England)*, *172*, 103486. doi:10.1016/j.micron.2023.103486 PMID:37262930

Tang, X., Fu, J., & Qin, H. (2023). Microwave-induced thermoacoustic imaging with functional nanoparticles. *Journal of Innovative Optical Health Sciences*, *16*(02), 2230014. doi:10.1142/S1793545822300142

Vazquez-Prada, K. X., Moonshi, S. S., Wu, Y., Akther, F., Tse, B. W., Sokolowski, K. A., Peter, K., Wang, X., Xu, G., & Ta, H. T. (2023). A Spiky Silver-Iron Oxide Nanoparticle for Highly Efficient Targeted Photothermal Therapy and Multimodal Imaging of Thrombosis. *Small*, *19*(11), 2205744. doi:10.1002mll.202205744 PMID:36634995

Vega, D. M., Di Meglio, M., del Valle Alonso, S., Alvira, F., & Montanari, J. (2023). *Nanomaterials for Diagnosis, Treatment, and Prevention of Human Cutaneous Leishmaniasis: A Review*. OpenNano.

Wang, Q., Du, J., Ouyang, R., Liu, B., Miao, Y., & Li, Y. (2023). Recent advances in functional bismuth chalcogenide nanomaterials: Cancer theranostics, antibacterial and biosensing. *Coordination Chemistry Reviews*, *492*, 215281. doi:10.1016/j.ccr.2023.215281

Wu, Q., Miao, W. S., Zhang, Y. D., Gao, H. J., & Hui, D. (2020). Mechanical properties of nanomaterials: A review. *Nanotechnology Reviews*, *9*(1), 259–273. doi:10.1515/ntrev-2020-0021

Xie, S., Ai, L., Cui, C., Fu, T., Cheng, X., Qu, F., & Tan, W. (2021). Functional aptamer-embedded nanomaterials for diagnostics and therapeutics. *ACS Applied Materials & Interfaces*, *13*(8), 9542–9560. doi:10.1021/acsami.0c19562 PMID:33595277

Yan, T., Su, M., Wang, Z., & Zhang, J. (2023). Second Near-Infrared Plasmonic Nanomaterials for Photoacoustic Imaging and Photothermal Therapy. *Small*, *19*(30), 2300539. doi:10.1002mll.202300539 PMID:37060228

Yue, N. N., Xu, H. M., Xu, J., Zhu, M. Z., Zhang, Y., Tian, C. M., Nie, Y. Q., Yao, J., Liang, Y. J., Li, D. F., & Wang, L. S. (2023). Application of Nanoparticles in the Diagnosis of Gastrointestinal Diseases: A Complete Future Perspective. *International Journal of Nanomedicine*, *18*, 4143–4170. doi:10.2147/IJN.S413141 PMID:37525691

Zeng, Q., Qi, X., Shi, G., Zhang, M., & Haick, H. (2022). Wound dressing: From nanomaterials to diagnostic dressings and healing evaluations. *ACS Nano*, *16*(2), 1708–1733. doi:10.1021/acsnano.1c08411 PMID:35050565

Chapter 13
The Importance of Nanomedicine and Its Prospects for the Public Health and Research Fields in the Present and Future

Abhishek Kumar
https://orcid.org/0000-0001-6114-1657
Institute of Pharmacy, Shri Ramswaroop Memorial University, Barabanki, India

Deepti Dwivedi
Institute of Pharmacy, Ram Manohar Lohia Avadh University, India

Ankur Srivastava
Institute of Pharmacy, Ram Manohar Lohia Avadh University, India

Juti Rani Devi
NETES Institute of Pharmaceutical Sciences, India

Shubham Tripathi
Institute of Pharmaceutical Sciences and Research (IPSR) Unnao (U.P.), India

Somesh Shukla
School of Pharmacy, Lingaya's Vidyapeeth, India

Chandan Kumar Singh
School of Pharmacy, Mangalayatan University, India

ABSTRACT

Recognizing and promoting contributions relevant to public health is crucial as the range of nanotechnology uses in medicine expands. Nanomedical advances promise to have far-reaching effects across the medical spectrum, revealing exciting new approaches to enhance health and lengthen life that can be quantified on both an individual and a societal scale. In the United States, for instance, cardiovascular disease and cancer account for over half of all deaths each year, yet there is promising evidence that improvements in nanomedicine can help cut these numbers. Nanomedicine's public health uses, like quicker and more portable diagnostics and more potent immunizations, could radically alter the state of global health. Diverse innovators from engineering, biology, medicine, and public health should collaborate to maximize the impact of their research on human health.

DOI: 10.4018/979-8-3693-0448-8.ch013

INTRODUCTION

The field of study where nanotechnology is used in healthcare is known as nanomedicine. It is an emerging area with the potential to significantly impact health in the twenty-first century on both an individual and societal level. Public health's goal is to promote, safeguard, and maintain populations' or groups' health instead of clinical medicine's focus on the individual. For the maximum number of people to reap the advantages and avoid the risks associated with nanomedicine, it is essential to analyze and investigate its uses and effects from a public health perspective. (West & Halas, 2000). Nanotechnology applications are appealing because of the distinctive properties and phenomena that result from their small scale. The scale for nanotechnology that is most frequently used is 1–100 nm. This level of material engineering enables the development of cutting-edge medical treatments, such as creating nanoparticle-based medications with more precise cell targeting and fewer adverse effects for patients. Other improvements in medical equipment and instruments are being produced for less invasive surgical operations, which means fewer complications and less time spent recuperating after surgery. These developments will improve people's quality of life, increase longevity, and possibly even reduce healthcare expenses. Research is being performed worldwide to find uses for nanotechnology in cardiology, neurology, and other areas of medicine. (Etheridge et al., 2013). Examples include the application of carbon nanotubes to imaging modalities and using nanoparticles in drug delivery systems. Research driven by experts with a deep appreciation for the demands of public health is crucial for making headway in the field and creating medical technology with practical applications. Knowledge gaps regarding the fate and transport of artificial nanoparticles in biological systems necessitate ongoing investigation. The Food and Drug Administration has not established uniform guidelines for including engineered nanomaterials in consumables like food and cosmetics. (Hare et al., 2016; S, Elger, Hunziker, & Shaw, 2015) However, Concerns about this technique's safety have been raised because of the lack of data needed to forecast and minimize the health implications of exposure to generated nanoparticles. More study is needed to determine the effects of artificial nanoparticles on the environment, human health, and safety. However, dialogue with stakeholders about possible dangers and advantages is essential to promote nanotechnology properly. Regulatory bodies, public concern organizations, insurance companies, and others will present numerous obstacles to integrating nanomedicine into standard clinical practice for various reasons. To address these issues early on, collaboration amongst people with a stake in advancing nanomedicine should be encouraged. However, according to Mg, Krenn, Huebner, Wagner, and Resch ((Mg et al., 2015), the lack of data available to forecast and minimize the impacts of exposure to artificial nanoparticles has spurred increased worries regarding potential health and safety issues. The life cycle effects on the environment, health, and safety of produced nanomaterials need more research (Chan, 2017).

NANOMEDICINE IN PUBLIC HEALTH

The field of nanomedicine will have far-reaching effects on public health. Public health goals include disease prevention, increased longevity, and community-wide health and productivity. Hygiene in the public sphere, prevention of communicable diseases, and therapeutic measures, including screening and early diagnosis, are common examples of such population- or community-level interventions. Public health, in this sense, is concerned with improving the health of an entire community rather than just

Figure 1. Public health relations

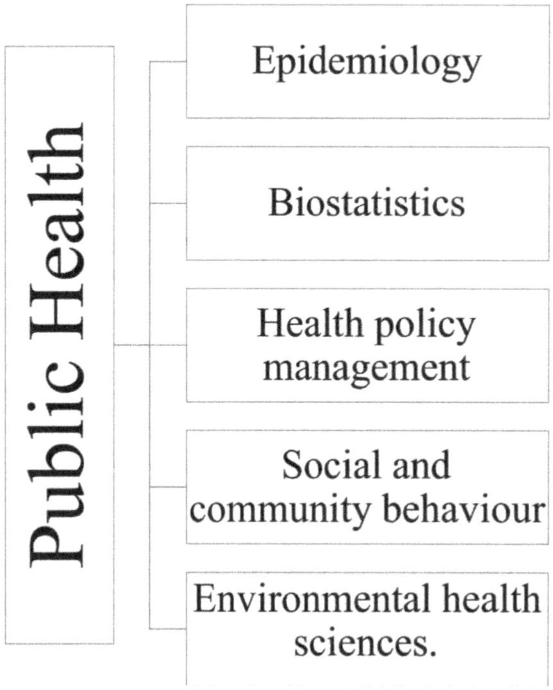

certain demographics within it. According to the Association of Schools of Public Health, there are five distinct areas within the larger field of public health.

The study of the causes and prevalence of the disease is known as epidemiology. It makes sense about biostatistics, which conducts quantitative analyses of the causes and distribution of disease. Legislation and guidelines are drafted with medical and public health community input. Social and communal behaviour research impacts health outcomes at all levels, from the individual to the organization, it shows in the above fig:1. (Mg et al., 2015; S et al., 2015). Environmental health is concerned with how people's health is impacted by their immediate surroundings, both physically and socially. A platform for analyzing, comprehending, and predicting the effects of nanomedicine on population health is provided for public health professionals by the knowledge base developed through these core disciplines. Public health technological advancements have shaped human history. For instance, vaccines have effectively eliminated or greatly reduced deadly infectious diseases worldwide. Side effects and health risks have influenced the creation and application of vaccines. As an illustration of how nanotechnology can be used to enhance current medical practice and significantly impact public health, consider hepatitis B immunization. Hepatitis B is a viral infection that affects over two billion people worldwide. A highly successful vaccination against this disease is already available. However, it requires three to four injections (Mg et al., 2015; S et al., 2015).

Particularly in third-world nations, noncompliance with the dosing schedule is a serious issue that can reduce or eliminate the vaccine's effectiveness. The vaccine can now be given in one dosage with the same efficiency because of advancements made by ongoing research and development (Hofmann-amtenbrink, Grainger, & Hofmann, 2015). One group is primarily looking into the efficiency of several PLGA microspheres for the single-dose administration of the hepatitis B vaccine. It is now possible to immunize a bigger population against an infectious illness that causes over 600,000 deaths yearly thanks to this sort of hepatitis B preventive therapy. Nanomedicine could have a major effect on public health on a global and local scale by revolutionizing the treatment of chronic diseases. With an estimated 1.48 million new cases in 2009, cancer was the second leading cause of death in the United States. Chemotherapy, surgery, and radiation therapy are examples of standard cancer treatment, but they can be detrimental to healthy and cancerous cells. When the NCI realized how much nanotechnology could help with cancer care, it formed the Alliance for Nanotechnology in Cancer that same year. This collaboration promotes the study and creation of more effective and unobtrusive nanotechnology-based cancer treatment and diagnosis options (Sandhiya, Dkhar, & Surendiran, 2009). Numerous medications and treatments that use nanotechnology are supported by the NCI throughout all stages of testing, including clinical trials. Abraxane® for breast cancer treatment and Doxia® for ovarian cancer treatment are two examples of nanotechnology-enabled cancer therapies approved by the FDA. Cancer, New treatments are being explored for Alzheimer's, cardiovascular, and other top US killers. Regenerative medicine uses carbon nanotubes, nano biers, nanopatterned extracellular matrices, and dendritic nano polymers. According to research, Nanomedicine can address major public health issues by treating several common ailments. (Boulaiz et al., 2011).

SCOPE OF NANOMEDICINE ANALYSIS

There is no universally accepted definition for "nanotechnology" or "nanomedicine," the terms continue to be the subject of heated discussion. Materials engineered to have unique medical effects due to their designs, such as those with at least one distinguishable dimension up to 300 nm, are the focus of nanomedicine. (Boulaiz et al., 2011; Chan, 2017), Because accomplishing the study's aims requires an operational definition. Two universal nanoscale phenomena in nanomedicine are changes in physiochemical characteristics and physiological relationships. The National Nanotechnology Initiative (NNI) employs 100 nm in the former situation, where quantum effects are frequently limited to structures of a few Nanometers to tens of Nanometers. The plasmon resonance in gold Nanoshells with a 150 nm diameter, which is being studied for cancer heat therapy, exhibits different physiochemical behaviour. Nanomedicine's benefits and limitations are linked to physiological interactions at the molecular-microscopic interface. Studies show that 150–200 nm diameter liposomes circulate in the bloodstream significantly longer than smaller liposomes (70 nm). Many 100-200 nm feature-size nanomedicine devices use the enhanced permeability and retention (EPR) phenomenon to target areas at the tissue level passively. However, it has been shown that particles as small as 400 nm can extravasate the blood-brain barrier and accumulate in tumors. (Lammers, 2018). Numerous factors influence the pathways for NP absorption and processing at the cellular level, but particle size plays a vital role. Although the best cellular absorption of colloidal gold has been demonstrated for diameters around 50 nm, macrophages can phagocytose polystyrene beads with a diameter of up to 200 nm. Since many nanomedicines use features with widths of 100 nm or less, this threshold rules out a wide range of potential uses. That has important implications for the field. In order to better capture the distinct physiological behaviour that is taking place at these sizes, we picked 300 nm. Additionally, while most of the discussion up to this point has focused on spherical NPs since they are the most frequently encountered, it is important to note that this behaviour is highly material- and geometry-specific. Our idea will still apply to many newly developed microscale systems that enhance vascular extravasation. Typically, five steps involve taking a medical application from the lab bench to the market. We concentrated on identifying applications currently or about to begin clinical testing in human subjects and goods that have already received FDA (or equivalent) approval in other countries to depict and analyze the nanomedicine landscape. This does not include earlier applications, such as laboratory experiments or preliminary tests on animals. Many revolutionary nanomedicine developments expected in the literature may take twenty years or more to reach the clinic. It is difficult to predict how things might be implemented and their effects. For instance, a 2006 survey predicted that by 2025 we would not have access to "nanomachines" that could perform theragnostic (combined therapy and diagnostics) on humans. Thus, the applications and products currently being tested on or utilized on humans are the subjects of our study. For the foreseeable future, these applications and products will most significantly impact industry, regulation, and society (Boulaiz et al., 2011; Bregoli et al., 2015).

THE DEVELOPMENT OF NANOMEDICINES IN PRECLINICAL AND CLINICAL RESEARCH FOR THE TREATMENT OF CANCER

Many anti-cancer nanomedicines in clinical trials are liposomes, polymeric conjugates, nanoparticles, micelles, and others. Antibody-drug conjugates are a therapeutic class distinct from particulate nanomedicine systems; This fig:2 shows the list of commercialized drugs (nanomedicines) that are clinically developed for anti-cancer properties. (Chan, 2017; Farokhzad & Langer, 2006; Lammers, 2018).

Figure 2. Clinically tested anti-cancer nanomedicines

Drug	Product Name	Indication	Clinical trial phase
Doxorubicin	Myocet™/ Teva UK	Breast cancer	Approved
	Doxil™/ Janssen	Ovarian cancer	Approved
	ThermoDox™/ Celsion	Primary hepatocellular carcinoma	Phase III
	2B3-101/ 2-BBB Medicines BV	Brain metastases Glioma	Phase II
Vincristine	Marqibo™/ Spectrum Pharmaceuticals	Acute lymphoblastic leukemia	Approved
Paclitaxel	LEP—ETU/ Insys	Breast cancer	Phase II
	EndoTAG-1/ MediGene	Breast cancer	Phase II
Camptothecin	CRLX101 (Cyclodextrin adamantane)/ Cerulean	Renal cancer Small cell lung cancer Ovarian cancer	Phase II
Asparaginase	Oncaspar™ (PEG)/ Baxalta	Acute lymphoblastic leukemia	Approved
Paclitaxel	Opaxio™ (Polyglycerol adipate)/ CTI Biopharma	Ovarian cancer Non-small cell lung cancer (women)	Phase III Phase II
Docetaxel + Prostate-Specific Membrane Antigen (PSMA)	BIND- 014 (Accurin™) / BIND Therapeutics	Cholangiocarcinoma Cervical cancer Bladder cancer Head and neck cancer Non-small cell lung cancer subtypes	Phase II

Only a few licensed anti-cancer nanomedicines (including BIND-014 from BIND Therapeutics and Merrimack Pharmaceuticals' MM-302) use ligand-mediated targeting to change nanomedicine behaviour rapidly. EPR-based medicines often modify pharmacokinetics and biodistribution to improve efficacy and tolerability. They can reduce the maximum free drug concentration (Coax) in the blood while increasing the total drug exposure (AUC) in the blood and the tumor. Several nanomedicines, such as CRLX101 (Cerulean) and AZD2811 nanoparticle (AstraZeneca), have enabled new inventive treatment procedures or conferred a greatly increased therapeutic index to an existing drug by reaching the right target and exposure. In order to reduce dose-limiting bone marrow toxicity, the Aurora-B kinase inhibitor used in the AZD2811 nanoparticle was ingeniously encapsulated in preclinical trials. (Bregoli et al., 2015; Pautler & Brenner, 2022; Webster & Webster, 2022). One of the main benefits of some nanomedicines is that they can be built without toxic dose-limiting excipients found in conventionally formulated drugs. This frequently improves tolerability and makes administering more medications to patients possible. For instance, because Abradant (Celgene) and the polymeric micelle formulation Genero-PM™ (Samyang Biopharmaceuticals) do not require the use of Reimport, which is required to produce Taxol, greater dosages of paclitaxel can be given to patients. Even though they are not frequently the main focus of nanomedicine research programs, these savings from solubilization can be substantial. By increasing the maximum tolerable dose of the active component while avoiding the tolerability difficulties brought on by solubilizing surfactants, this method might greatly affect the patients' experiences and the clinical results. (Duncan & Gaspar, 2011; Emerich & Thanos, 2003).

Nanomedicine systems may not become widely used due to their increasing cost until their effectiveness is improved from becoming a widespread treatment choice. Engaging physicians and other healthcare professionals are crucial for this new generation of therapies to show (what they see as) real clinical distinction. The discipline of nanomedicine has invested a lot of time and energy into understanding the benefits and drawbacks of various nanomedicine systems from a technological and biopharmaceutical perspective. The stability, pharmacokinetics/biodistribution, toxicity, and efficacy of cytotoxic and other types of payloads have all been enhanced by numerous innovative nanomedicines. There is a strong correlation between biodistribution and clearance of nanomedicine and its size, charge, shape, surface modification, and biocompatibility. Animal and human investigations have shown that patches of leaky vasculature can develop dramatically at concentrations of stealth nanomedicines with long half-lives. Nanomedicine systems with a size of less than 100 nm and low-molecular-weight macromolecules have more extravasation and vascular penetration than bigger systems. Suggesting a correlation between size and efficacy. This size dependence is analogous to the dependence on tumor size and nanomedicine, but it is too soon to generalize. (Park, 2019). Controlling the pace at which a drug is released from a nanomedicine is a key feature that can significantly improve therapeutic efficacy and patient safety. Using chemical conjugation linkers with different in vivo breakdown rates or changing diffusion via a polymer matrix makes it possible to time drug release to take advantage of the therapeutic window (such as hydrolysis).(Flühmann, Ntai, Brorchard, Simoens, & Mühlebach, 2018; Sahoo, Parveen, & Panda, 2007). The properties of the delivery system can be modified once the connection between disease biology and nanomedicine behaviour is more known. This article delves deeper into coordinating a delivery strategy, tumor, and medicine along a predetermined therapeutic trajectory (Sahoo, Parveen, & Panda, 2007).

PERCEIVED CHALLENGES IN THE FIELD OF NANOMEDICINE

It is crucial to understand why anti-cancer drugs fail so frequently in clinical trials if you want to increase your chances of success. The cause of failure for a few nanomedicines has been looked at. Phase III clinical trials were conducted to evaluate the paclitaxel polyglutamic acid conjugate OpaxioTM for treating incurable lung cancer. However, OpaxioTM treatment only positively affected female survival; It did not influence the survival of males. Since the clinical experiment, a link has been shown between estrogen levels and cathepsin B activity. (Sahoo et al., 2007), This is important because OpaxioTM depends on cathepsin B-mediated activation. As a result, women with estrogen levels above a set threshold were only allowed to participate in subsequent clinical investigations with OpaxioTM. OpaxioTM has created a sound plan to deal with the problem moving forward, focusing nanomedicine research and development on a single clinical focus, such as a delivery method, tumor, or drug, which is discussed in greater detail here. Furthermore, Complex biological variables likely contribute to inadequate clinical translation. In addition, persons with advanced metastatic cancer and co-morbidities who have received significant pre-treatment frequently participate in early-stage clinical studies. These features are difficult to predict from pre-clinical testing alone; interaction with clinicians is vital. It is believed that the success rate of nanomedicines is limited, similar to that of early antibody treatments. This article provides more detail on focusing nanomedicine development on a specific clinical line of sight by matching a delivery mechanism, tumor, and drug. (Lammers & Ferrari, 2020; Sahoo et al., 2007).

This circumstance ought to motivate us to improve the planning and execution of our projects. Focusing on how nanomedicine therapies are tested in clinical settings is crucial to benefit from the breakthroughs in nanomedicine engineering fully. The clinical results will be improved by investing in translational science, as it has been for other cancer treatments. Nanomedicines will become widely recognized as a reliable and practical medication development option after being proven to have better clinical performance. As was said above, traditional nanomedicine research initiatives have been designed to modify a delivery system's physical and chemical properties (loading, chemistry, size, charge, and surface modification) to manage it is in vivo behaviour. Understanding the characteristics of patient malignancies that pose particular difficulties for nanomedicines to work at their best has been mostly absent. Identifying the relationships between patient biology and nanomedicine behaviour has received less scientific attention. Even though the current emphasis on nanomedicine is focused on the enticing but frequently unproven premise of a positive correlation between EPR and efficacy, a greater emphasis on four critical areas will improve the clinical translation of nanomedicine initiatives.(Pautler & Brenner, 2022):

1. When the connection between the biology of the disease and the behaviour of nanomedicine has been better understood, it will be possible to alter the parameters of the delivery system based on the data. In this article, greater and more in-depth discussion is given on matching a delivery mechanism, tumor, and medicine to a particular clinical line of sight. (Sahoo, Parveen, & Panda, 2007).
2. Increasing the number of therapeutically relevant animal models used to fine-tune nanomedicine's properties and dosing regimens.(Flühmann, Ntai, Brorchard, Simoens, & Mühlebach, 2018; Flühmann et al., 2018).
3. Shift focus from studies motivated by formulations to those motivated by diseases.(Lammers & Ferrari, 2020).

4. Patients with the greatest possibility of benefiting from treatments based on nanomedicine are chosen in advance.(Lammers & Ferrari, 2020).

Patient-centred and disease-driven nanomedicine development is possible by applying the 5R principles and implementing these advancements in nanomedicine science(Duncan & Gaspar, 2011).

Figure 3. The effective implementation of nanomedicine in clinical practice

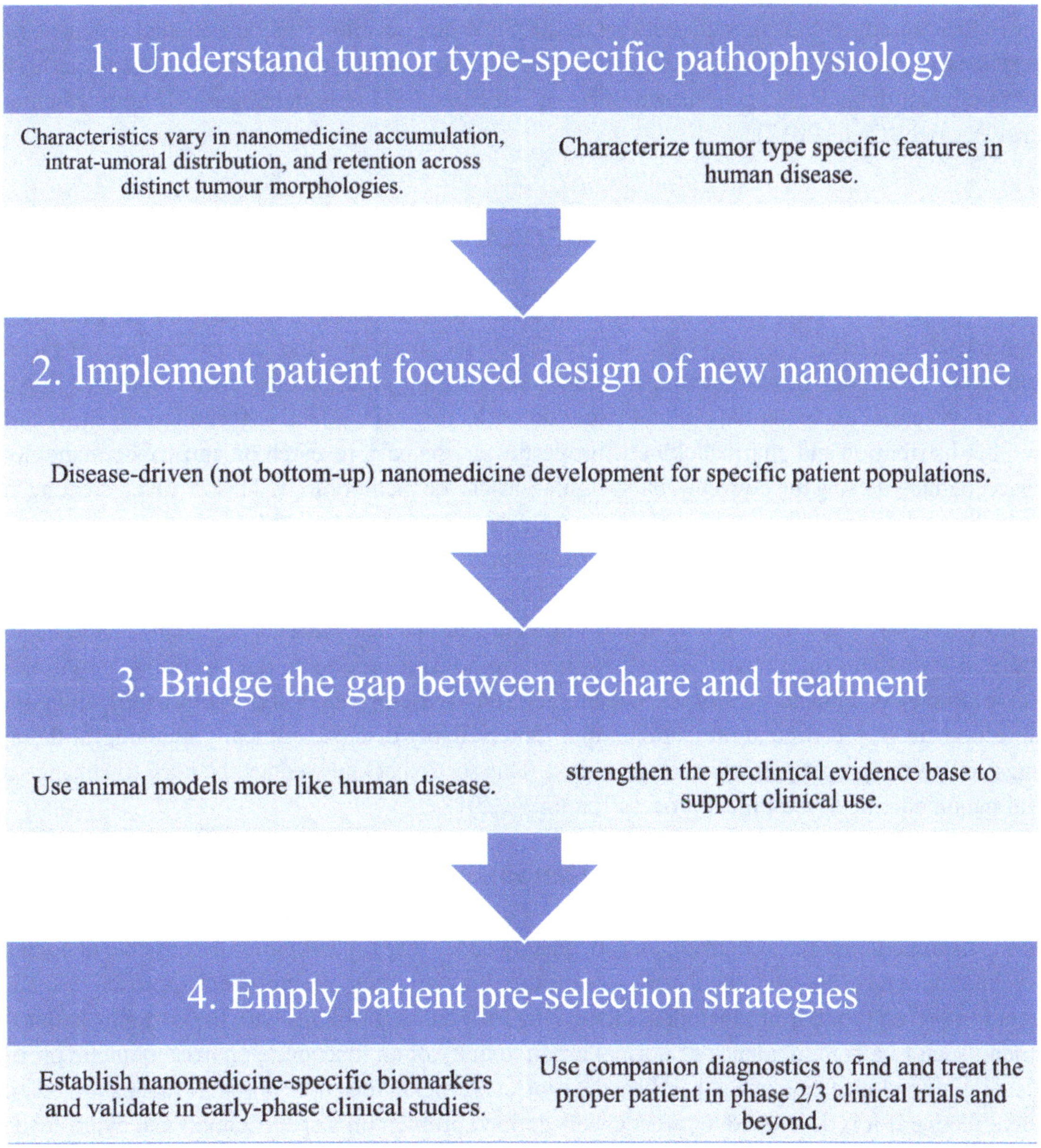

The selection of funding priorities is just as important as focusing on these four areas to speed up the clinical translation of nanomedicines. This will be determined by the specific difficulties encountered in creating each nanomedicine. Two prevalent situations in advancing nanomedicine are using novel delivery techniques with currently available medications and conventional delivery systems with novel payloads. Patients with the right characteristics can help speed up the process of creating a breakthrough nanomedicine with a clear delivery method. It is assumed here that the in vivo behavior and crucial delivery system quality parameters impacting in vivo performance are already understood, as are the factors determining the efficacy of the free medication (concentration vs. exposure time). Instead, while budgeting for evaluating a novel delivery method, it is important to learn how it performs in various cancer models to target your therapy better. (Jr, 2005). When developing a new medicine with a new delivery system, the most productive areas to concentrate on are patient-driven design and gathering solid pre-clinical data. The step is shown in fig:3(The Effective Implementation of Nanomedicine in Clinical Practice)(Chan, 2017).

INDUSTRIAL METHODS FOR NANOMEDICINE DEVELOPMENT

Successful proof-of-concept and optimization of novel nanomedicine technologies have been achieved through pre-clinical trials., but it is essential to recognize its limitations and retain objectivity regarding its significance for future development. Early preclinical testing should largely focus on identifying the therapeutic potential and potential clinical issues and selecting safe, effective formulations that exhibit desired biodistribution and pharmacokinetic properties. In the past, research on anti-cancer nanomedicine was conducted using the conventional formulation-driven methodology. This involved creating and evaluating novel nanomedicines through in vivo pharmacokinetics/biodistribution studies, anti-tumor experiments in xenograft models susceptible to the payload, and in vitro cytotoxicity assays. Unfortunately, this paradigm has not yielded the information necessary to address the major roadblocks inhibiting nanomedicines' safe and effective introduction into clinical practice. Instead, scientists should be able to determine whether or not to invest early in the development process before spending a substantial amount of money on clinical studies. (Koo et al., 2005). Disease-driven design is discussed, along with the development of pre-clinical project data that more reliably disclose clinically meaningful therapy findings so that the proper patients may be treated. This section acknowledges the need to enhance the present nanomedicine development process(Lammers, 2018).

Adopting a Systematic Strategy for Nanomedicine Initiatives

No single nanomedicine can effectively and adequately cure every type of tumor. Accessible nanomedicine technologies have allowed big pharma to shift to a disease-driven development approach instead of formulation-driven (bottom-up) methods. Identifying the precise problems with the current standard of treatment, such as a high incidence of normal organ toxicity or an inaccurate pharmacokinetic profile, and developing a clinical line of sight early in the project is crucial. It is more probable that nanomedicine will be effective if it is developed to target a well-defined problem in a specific malignancy; instead of first inventing a delivery mechanism and then attempting to match it with an existing clinical condition, this approach begins with the delivery mechanism. To enable the data-driven selection of nanomedicine systems best suited for certain disease types, it is necessary to consider the interaction between the pathophysiology of the illness, the patient, and the physicochemical features of various nanomedicines. This interaction must be taken into account. In addition, this necessitates that the clinic generates more specific data that can be used to improve development plans. Therefore, in order to generate clinically effective and transferrable nanomedicines, it is necessary to employ logical selection criteria. (Hare et al., 2016; Sandhiya et al., 2009). A disease-driven approach to drug development aims to maximize the effectiveness of a drug by coordinating its formulation, administration, and intended demographic of users. For instance, cancer medications have proven successful in treating humans. Different nanomedicine systems' physicochemical characteristics determine whether or not they are suitable for delivering particular medications and whether or not the "dose" of the delivery system causes undesirable side effects in patients. In addition, the characteristics of the target patient group's cancer will impact the system's capacity to achieve the drug release rate required to deliver the treatment to the tumor at therapeutic levels and exposures. The off-target accumulation of the carrier will determine whether or not the drug reaches an acceptable safety profile when administered in combination with standard-of-care regimens for the malignancy of interest. Although difficult, considering patient and illness specifics early in the design process may lead to more portable nanomedicines. (Bregoli et al., 2015; Farokhzad & Langer, 2006).

However, making individual nanomedicines for each patient is not feasible now. This methodically laid out plan aims to target a specific subset of patients in the creation of a nanomedicine. Drugs that target particular genetic reasons have been developed thanks to a patient-centred approach made possible by a comprehensive understanding of cancer genetics. An initial investment is required to understand the requirements outlined in Fig:4 (Disease-Driven et al. of Innovative Anticancer Nanomedicine: Delivery Method, Drug, and Patient Population) for research into patient-driven nanomedicine to advance. Despite its complexity, this knowledge can potentially enable targeted, expedited, and translational development

Figure 4. Disease-driven design and development of innovative anticancer nanomedicine: delivery method, drug, and patient population

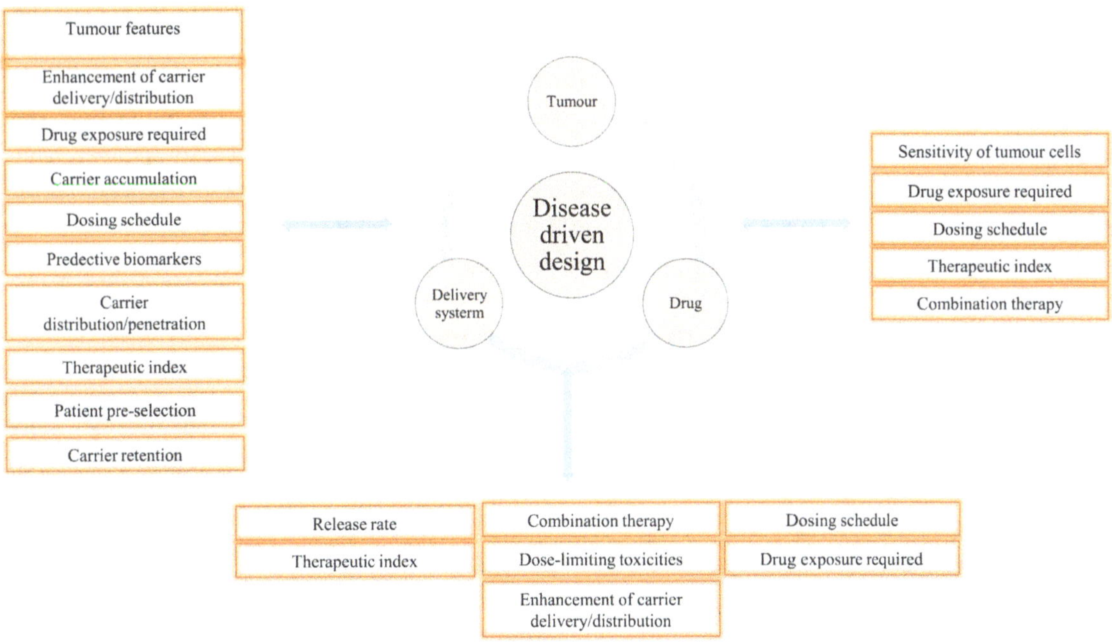

from a clinical standpoint. The genetic profile & inherent sensitivity of the target patient group are considered when a clinical line of sight has been established (Farokhzad & Langer, 2006).

The drug selection process entails several steps, including model selection, The optimization of the drug release rate (in order to reach the required high maximum concentration, the expanded area under the curve, enhanced therapeutic index, etc.), the optimization of the dosage schedule, and familiarity with combination therapy are all necessary. (Lammers, 2018). In vivo, research using realistic models is far more expensive. Thus, it is crucial to assess the value of the results thoughtfully. Evaluating models and nanomedicines that reflect the extremes of several factors can lead to a more in-depth understanding of the topic and the application of complementing in-silico modeling methodologies, which can lead to cost savings(Flühmann et al., 2018).

Utilizing Disease-Driven Design to Attain the Appropriate Effectiveness

Understanding how biology affects the behaviour of nanomedicine is the foundation of disease-driven design, which helps choose a carrier that can take advantage of the pathophysiology. Diverse tumors and diseases have diverse tumor microenvironments, which poses specific challenges for nanomedicine-based treatment. While some delivery systems can overcome these challenges, others may have issues. The disease-driven design considers the intended patient group early in the development process for optimal pathophysiology-based nanomedicine. (Hofmann-amtenbrink et al., 2015).

Some nanomedicines have physiological limitations that may be solved with therapies that change the cancer microenvironment in patients with strong stromal characteristics. (Farley, 2020). Nanomedicine has the potential to improve medical practice through combination techniques, including hyaluronidase, collagen lysis, control of collagen formation and cross-linking, and normalization of blood vessels are the goals of this treatment. Cancers of the kidney and other types of tumors that are highly vascularized frequently feature tumor cells that are positioned near blood vessels. However, the carrier's retention may be reduced or limited to the tumour's margins.

Nanomedicines have a drug release rate quick enough to make the payload accessible. Removing the delivery system from the tumor may be necessary before obtaining the desired exposure level. It is possible that cancers are not the ideal candidates for slow-release nanomedicines. Suppose the delivery mechanism is unlikely to be retained for an extended period. Increasing retention and avoiding this problem is also feasible by including a particular ligand in the carrier. Malignancies rich in macrophages can now be treated by employing the mononuclear phagocytic system and experimenting with immune-oncology therapies or combinations. These cases show why it may be beneficial to adapt a nanomedicine to the biological characteristics of a certain group of patients(Sahoo et al., 2007).

Utilizing Patient-Centred Design to Achieve Appropriate Safety

Evaluating the efficiency of nanomedicines is just as crucial as comprehending their off-target consequences. All tissues with characteristics, such as fenestrated vasculature that allow the accumulation of the delivery system, such as nanomedicines, will exhibit these traits. To boost effectiveness, it is equally important to define the characteristics governing the tissue localization of various delivery methods, particularly within the reticuloendothelial system. Nanomedicine can normalize blood vessel function, break down collagen, or control collagen synthesis and cross-linking as part of a combination strategy. Renal malignancies and other highly vascularized tumors frequently have cells placed close to the blood supply that supplies them. On the other hand, the carrier may be kept only at the tumour's periphery or, to a lesser extent, overall(Hare et al., 2016).

Suppose the delivery mechanism is removed from the tumor before the payload is accessible. In that case, a nanomedicine with a rapid enough drug release rate may be required to accomplish the desired level of targeted exposure. It is possible that slow-release nanomedicines are not the most effective treatment for certain forms of cancer. When extended retention of the delivery mechanism is improbable, on the other hand, this challenge may be avoided and retention enhanced by including a targeted ligand inside the carrier. For cancers rich in macrophages, it is now feasible to consider using the mononuclear phagocytic system and exploring therapies or combinations from the field of immunological oncology. These cases show why adjusting the biological makeup of nanomedicine for a certain patient population may be beneficial. (Kirtane, Siegel, & Panyam, 2014). Preclinical studies made advantage of the nanoparticle's-controlled drug release to lessen the harmful effects of the medication on bone marrow. (Hofmann-amtenbrink et al., 2015). Developing therapies based on nanomedicine will be greatly aided by expanding existing models to include a wider range of cancer types and normal tissues. By defining these characteristics across the nanomedicine toolkit, a drug's toxicity profile may be matched to an appropriate illness setting and delivery mechanism. Limiting a patient's cumulative dosage owing to doxorubicin-induced cardiotoxicity is one challenge that must be considered while designing a nanomedicine to treat it. A liposomal formulation of doxorubicin allows for greater cumulative dosages to be given to patients while reducing or eliminating their risk of cardiac toxicity. Nanomedicines that are generally well-tolerated, like DoxiaTM, may be especially effective in combination regimens, either by facilitating the administration of greater doses of the combination partners or by increasing tolerance to the individual components. (Boulaiz et al., 2011; Sandhiya et al., 2009). Due to changes in pharmacokinetics and biodistribution, the off-target toxicities of nanomedicines may be distinct from those of the parent medication(Etheridge et al., 2013).

Nanomedicine Project Advancement Requires Stronger Evidence

Typically, throughout the development of nanomedicine, the primary focus is on tumor accumulation based on the EPR effect. Although the accumulation of nanomedicines is low or highly variable in some cancer types, changing the drug's pharmacokinetics in peripheral plasma may still have therapeutic value. In order to evaluate the efficacy of nanomedicines, preclinical research must create data sets describing four Behavioral features. (Hare et al., 2016). Tumor accumulation, intratumorally distribution, tumor retention of the system, and the supplementary effect of the nanomedicine's peripheral pharmacokinetics are all examples of these features (or circulation). All of these characteristics are expected to play a role in the potential efficacy of each kind of cancer; however, the dominating characteristic may affect the most effective method of administration and the pace at which the drug is released. The following should be considered by informative and translatable data sets (Hare et al., 2016).

- Measure the time course of drug metabolism, drug release rates, and carrier retention inside tumors;(Hare et al., 2016).
- Determine the persistence of carriers within tumors, the rate of drug release, and the rate of drug metabolism over time (Hare et al., 2016).
- clarify the concentration of therapeutically active medication and drug metabolites within tumors. (Hare et al., 2016).

- Analyze the pharmacokinetics of the nanomedicine in plasma, off-target tissue, and tumors after repeated dosing. (Hare et al., 2016);
- assess therapy efficacy in cancers with decreased EPR content. (Delgado, Martin, Hare, Yates, & Barry, 2015).
- determine the therapeutic value of extravasation against simple buildup in the tumor's vasculature as opposed to changes in the pharmacokinetics of the medicine. (Hare et al., 2016).
- to what extent does extravasation occur, as opposed to straightforward accumulation or residence in the vascularity of the tumor., as well as changes to the drug's pharmacokinetics, provides a therapeutic advantage. (Etheridge et al., 2013).
- visualize the nanomedicine's ultimate clinical application (in conjunction with the standard of care) and evaluate its efficacy in this environment to arrive at an appropriate dose and dosing regimen.(Delgado et al., 2015).

To further comprehend how a payload eventually has a therapeutic impact, we must consider the payload's release, trafficking, and target engagement. In addition, it is necessary to invest in developing and enhancing essential analytical procedures since the capacity to distinguish between bioavailable and bound/encapsulated medicine concentrations in the body is crucial to the measurement of several of the metrics above. More strategic partnerships may be necessary to access these complex data sets. When used in the nanomedicine development process, buildup within the vasculature of the tumor as opposed to pharmacokinetic alteration of the drug(Hare et al., 2016).

More Clinically Relevant Models Improve Nanomedicine Translation

Therefore, for a number of the metrics above, it is vital to differentiate between the amounts of bioavailable medication and the quantity of drug bound or encapsulated in the body. You might need to form additional collaborations to access these intricate data sets. When put to use, the data packages that may be created while developing nanomedicine will be substantially more discriminatory and informative when selecting lead candidates and moving further toward the clinic. It is anticipated that keeping a steadfast eye on the end clinical usage of new nanomedicines and having a complete understanding of the therapeutic margin would greatly assist in translating these nanomedicines into clinical practice. (Gabizon & Martin, 1997). These models typically display diseases not representative of the complexity and variety of tumors seen in patients. The drug delivery field is predicated on the assumption that EPR-based effectiveness will hold for all human cancers. One major challenge to applying nanomedicine research is using unreliable models in pre-clinical testing. It is crucial to produce data sets in several models describing elements of the target clinical tumor population to depict the target patient tumor population accurately.

Multiple pre-clinical models are typically necessary to align medication and delivery system activity and determine whether the delivery system is suitable for a certain tumour's pathophysiology. Limitations that are recognized in advance might guide trial termination or patient selection. Early clinical trial success can be gleaned by calculating the therapeutic index of the nanomedicine in conjunction with the medications it will be used within clinical trials. In order to create nanomedicines and other anti-cancer therapies cost-effectively, early decision-making is essential. (Gabizon & Martin, 1997).

Therapeutically Relevant Models Are Advantageous

Cancer models employing patient-derived tumor explants (PDXs) or genetically altered mice closely mimic human tumours' appearance, complexity, and diversity (GEMMs). Although difficult to generate and maintain due to their sluggish growth rate and need for live passage, these models can evaluate the efficacy of nanomedicine in specific organs. Although they are not immediately predictive of the clinic, they enable the evaluation of nanomedicine performance and provide insight into potential dangers. Using these models, researchers have developed fresh perspectives on nanomedicines and GEMMs, in which the tumor develops in situ, which can provide additional information. With the availability of more therapeutically relevant and diverse models, it will be possible to provide evidence for the effectiveness of various nanomedicines across various tumor types by analyzing their accumulation, intra-tumoral distribution, and retention. (Kalra et al., 2014).

The mature vasculature of clinical tumors and PDX models is less permeable than the mature vasculature of xenografts, which develop over days and have features less influenced by the proliferation of cancer cells. (Song et al., 2014). For a more accurate understanding of potential outcomes across a wide range of human illness types, it is required to evaluate many models with diverse vascular distributions and tumor-to-tumor variance. (Kalra et al., 2014).

Therapeutically Relevant Models, Greater Variation, is Conceivable

Tumor architecture significantly affects the effectiveness of nanomedicine therapy in a cohort of tumors with similar inherent sensitivity. This highlights the need to develop patient pre-selection strategies through the development of biomarkers and imaging tools. (Delgado, Martin, Hare, Yates, & Barry, 2015). Xenografts produced from tumor cells retained more active SN-38 than tumor cell explants. The potential of liposomal irinotecan can be better understood, and more efficient development and population-specific strategies can be implemented if more models are explored. The work by Kalra et al. uses many models to provide light on the potential of liposomal irinotecan and to provide a database for targeted drug development and population-specific strategies. (Kirtane et al., 2014).

NANOMEDICINE AS A PHARMA PERSPECTIVE

Oncology projects confront obstacles such as inadequate pre-clinical testing, a disparity between animal models and human patients, and success determinants. To enhance translation and gain greater investments, project teams must describe tumor type, stage, dose, dosing regimen, and prospective medications that may be coupled with the novel agent. Answering these concerns is essential for translating oncology medicines and attracting further funding. To make a project appealing for pharmaceutical development, testing targeted hypotheses and making success determinations with low initial investment must be possible. The 5Rs are crucial to the success of any endeavour. (Cook, Brown, Alexander, March, & Morgan, 2014).

The Price of Victory and Defeat

About 6% of small molecule medicines make it from proof of concept in preclinical studies to market introduction. The industry has struggled to attract investment for nanomedicines and other therapeutic classes, including antibodies, peptides, and DNA/RNA-based therapeutics. Problems include complicated formulations, confusion over how quality attributes relate to drug effectiveness, and shifting perspectives among regulators., technical hurdles in manufacturing and scaling up, maturation of analytical methods, and high costs are obstacles for these medications. The cost-benefit ratio of nanotherapeutics should not be discounted due to the disproportionately high development expenses. Instead, producing active pharmaceutical compounds compatible with nanomedicine may be more sensible (Kalra et al., 2014).

Synthetic chemists can incorporate certain characteristics into the design of innovative tiny molecules in order to generate nanomedicine-compatible medications. However, moving a nanomedicine prototype into the clinic and beyond might be prohibitive for smaller biotech firms and academic laboratories. Due to increased technical sophistication, the risk associated with a novel medicine may be considered lower by large pharmaceutical corporations. (Cook et al., 2014). Therefore, nanomedicine therapies require stronger pre-clinical data sets than traditional pharmacological therapy (Cook et al., 2014).

Future Nanomedicine Development Requires Collaboration

Nanotherapeutics development involves biology and chemistry, nanotechnology, and medicine. Early in preclinical research, it is essential to build cooperation between giant pharma, smaller enterprises, and academia to generate translatable therapies. To develop data sets and insights relating the physicochemical features of nanomedicine systems to their biological consequences, Academia, industry, consortia, and cancer research hospitals must collaborate. The National Cancer Institute, NIST, and FDA developed Nanotechnology. In 2004, the Characterization Laboratory (NCL) was established. Their mission is to construct and standardize an analytical cascade for nanomaterial characterization, to enable the preclinical characterization of nanomaterial-based drug delivery devices, and to facilitate the clinical development and regulatory evaluation of nanomaterials for cancer clinical trials. EU-NCL, established in 2015, has the same goals as the Clothier Consortium. (Hare et al., 2016; Hofmann-amtenbrink et al., 2015).

FUTURE OPPORTUNITIES AND CONCLUDING REMARKS

Nanomedicines are increasingly being developed for cytotoxic applications, with future potential centred on the delivery of next-generation medications such as molecularly targeted agents, toxin-like agents, DNA/RNA-based therapies, and peptides. These medications confront obstacles, including off-target accumulation, transmembrane passage, synergistic drug ratios, and restricted therapeutic windows. To commercialize nucleic acid-based medications, pharmaceutical companies such as Alnylam and Calando, Avidity Nanomedicines, Merck, and Arrowhead Research Corporation are investing in more cost-effective distribution methods. Nanomedicines might become standard cancer treatments, including traditional and new pharmaceuticals, even if formulation-driven development has failed to benefit patients. Focused design and the 5Rs can make nanomedicines affordable. (Hare et al., 2016).

Without patient pre-selection methods, reaching the optimal cost-effectiveness for nanomedicine therapies remains problematic. The next wave of nanomedicines will be able to overcome the challenges encountered in present clinical trials due to a coordinated effort by the nanomedicine community to embrace new clinically focused methods of operation. Investing in the research underlying the fundamental ideas behind nanomedicine may play a significant role in creating successful treatments for patients using nanomedicine. (Hare et al., 2016).

CONCLUSION

The interdisciplinary discipline of nanotechnology is pushing the science of the nearly incomprehensibly tiny gadget ever closer and closer to the realm of possibility. The repercussions of these advancements will, at some time in the future, be so extensive that they will almost certainly impact the entirety of the scientific and technological communities. As a result, nanotechnology has the potential to provide the most significant technical advances in the annals of humanity. It is widely anticipated that nanotechnology will continue to develop and expand in various fields of life and science throughout the next few years. Furthermore, it is anticipated that the achievements of nanotechnology will be applied in the medical sciences, including diagnostics, drug delivery systems, and patient treatment.

The scope of nanomedicine's potential to advance health care is virtually unbounded. Incorporating public health professionals' knowledge and experience is necessary to achieve optimal results regarding individual and community health. This effect on the development of nanomedicine will assist in establishing how best to distribute resources, identify the largest areas of need for technical innovation and form policies to safeguard humans and the environment. Increasing the amount of cross-disciplinary training available to researchers, medical care providers, and public health experts employed by businesses, the government, and academic institutions is essential to improving nanomedicine. Regarding research and teaching in nanomedicine, adopting a strategy that emphasizes collaboration would expedite advancing the state of the science, resulting in a higher return on investment for the public's health. Research and development of innovative nanomedicine applications combined with the fundamentals of public health will revolutionize the state of human health across the globe.

REFERENCES

Chan, W. C. W. (2017). *Nanomedicine 2.0.* ACS. doi:10.1021/acs.accounts.6b00629

Delgado, J. A., Martin, S., Hare, J. I., Yates, J. W. T., & Barry, S. T. (2015). Tumour stromal morphology impacts nanomedicine cytotoxicity in patient-derived xenografts. *Nanomedicine; Nanotechnology, Biology, and Medicine*, *11*(5), 1247–1252. doi:10.1016/j.nano.2015.02.007 PMID:25752857

Duncan, R., & Gaspar, R. (2011). *Nanomedicine (s) under the Microscope*, 2101–2141. ACS. doi:10.1021/mp200394t

Etheridge, M. L., Campbell, S. A., Erdman, A. G., Haynes, C. L., Wolf, S. M., & Mccullough, J. (2013). The big picture on nanomedicine: The state of investigational and approved nanomedicine products. *Nanomedicine; Nanotechnology, Biology, and Medicine*, *9*(1), 1–14. doi:10.1016/j.nano.2012.05.013 PMID:22684017

Flühmann, B., Ntai, I., Brorchard, G., Simoens, S., & Mühlebach, S. (2018). SC. *European Journal of Pharmaceutical Sciences*. doi:10.1016/j.ejps.2018.11.019

Hare, J. I., Lammers, T., Ashford, M. B., Puri, S., Storm, G., & Barry, S. T. (2016). SC. *Advanced Drug Delivery Reviews*. doi:10.1016/j.addr.2016.04.025 PMID:27137110

Lammers, T. (2018). PT NU SC. *Journal of Controlled Release#*. doi:10.1016/j.jconrel.2018.11.031

Lammers, T., & Ferrari, M. (2020). Nano Today The success of nanomedicine. *Nano Today*, *31*, 100853. doi:10.1016/j.nantod.2020.100853 PMID:34707725

Pautler, M., & Brenner, S. (2022). *Nanomedicine: Promises and challenges for the future of public health*. Dove Press. doi:10.2147/IJN.S13816

Sahoo, S. K., Parveen, S., & Panda, J. J. (2007). The present and future of nanotechnology in human health care. *Nanomedicine, 3*, 20–31. doi:10.1016/j.nano.2006.11.008

Chapter 14
The Development of Nanomaterials for the Regulated and Sustained Delivery of Medications for Future Health and Research

Abhishek Kumar
https://orcid.org/0000-0001-6114-1657
Institute of Pharmacy, Shri Ramswaroop Memorial University, Barabanki, India

Deepti Dwivedi
Institute of Pharmacy, Ram Manohar Lohia Avadh University, India

Juti Rani Devi
NETES Institute of Pharmaceutical Sciences, India

Deepsikha Bharali
https://orcid.org/0000-0002-6619-4966
NETES Institute of Pharmaceutical Sciences, India

Babita Deka
NETES Institute of Pharmaceutical Sciences, India

Pooja Patowary
https://orcid.org/0000-0002-0476-2868
NETES Institute of Pharmaceutical Sciences, India

Bitu Gogoi
NETES Institute of Pharmaceutical Sciences, India

Shubham Tripathi
Institute of Pharmaceutical Sciences and Research (IPSR) Unnao (U.P.), India

ABSTRACT

Drug delivery research aims to deliver exact doses of anti-tumor drugs to tumors. Recent nanoparticle engineering trials have improved drug targeting, but results need to be better. Nanoparticles, like traditional medicine, target their target via blood circulation. The enhanced permeability and retention (EPR) effect helps most nanoparticles, PEGylated or not, reach their target. Nanoparticles with targeting moieties like antibodies or ligands do not deliver drugs to tumors, according to research. Targeted medicine delivery tumors created complicated biological, mechanical, chemical, and transport systems

DOI: 10.4018/979-8-3693-0448-8.ch014

with changing properties. However, most research has focused on making and modifying drug-carrying nanoparticle surfaces. Bioactive substances delivered utilizing stimuli-responsive controlled-release nanomedicine may reduce side effects and boost effectiveness.

INTRODUCTION

Targeted drug delivery involves the precise delivery of therapeutic agents to specific disease sites, thereby enhancing drug concentration at the target and minimizing systemic exposure (Koo, Rubinstein, & Onyuksel, 2005). This technique can potentially enhance therapeutic effectiveness while decreasing undesired side effects significantly. The advent of targeted medication delivery has radically altered the practice of medicine by providing a more targeted and effective method of administering medicinal substances. In contrast to conventional drug delivery systems, which disperse pharmaceuticals throughout the body, targeted drug delivery enables the selective distribution of therapies to unhealthy tissues or cells., sometimes resulting in systemic adverse effects and limited efficacy. (Koo et al., 2005; Singh & Lillard, 2009),(Koo et al., 2005; Singh & Lillard, 2009).

Differentiating between sick and healthy tissues is crucial to targeted medicine administration. Both passive and active targeting tactics can be used to accomplish this sort of discrimination. (Koo et al., 2005).

Targeted drug delivery technologies have advanced thanks to nanotechnology significantly. By engineering drug carriers at the nanoscale, researchers have achieved improved drug stability, prolonged circulation time, and enhanced targeting efficiency. As nanoscale technology becomes more widely available, it has the potential to radically alter how scientists approach illness detection, management, and prevention. (Li, Li, & Khashab, 2012). The National Institutes of Health coined "nanomedicines" to describe these cutting-edge medical technologies because of the potential clinical utility of molecular insights from genomics and proteomics. Infection, N nanoparticles can mimic or influence infection, tissue engineering, de novo synthesis, and other biological processes. Functionalized carbon nanotubes, nanomachines (built of swappable DNA components and DNA scaffold and s), Nano Dimension include things like nanofibers, self-assembling polymeric nanostructures, nanobeam branes, and similar dev.es. (Koo et al., 2005; Kreuter, 1994a). Preformed polymers have now been created and researched in addition to other polymerization techniques (Barratt, 2000; Kreuter, 1994a; Pitt et al., 1981).

Liposomes, polymeric nanoparticles, and inorganic nanoparticles are all examples of nanoparticles. They have been extensively studied as drug-delivery vehicles because of their malleability and adaptability. These nanocarriers can encapsulate or conjugate drugs, protect them from degradation, and facilitate their release at the target site (G. W. Liu, Guzman, Menon, & Langer, 2023; Li et al., 2012),(Zhang, Meng, Lu, Fei, & Dyson, 2009). Additionally, targeted drug delivery has shown promise in gene therapy, immunotherapy, and combination therapies, opening new avenues for personalized medicine and synergic treatment approaches Targeted delivery represents a paradigm shift in drug delivery strategies, offering the potential to enhance therapeutic efficacy and minimize side effects. By capitalizing on the unique characteristics of diseased tissues and leveraging nanotechnology, The utilized medication delivery systems allow targeted and controlled drug release. (Brayden, 2003).

For optimal treatment effects, sustained drug delivery's controlled and gradual release of medications over time has become an essential strategy in the pharmaceutical sciences. Sustained drug delivery systems provide a constant drug release profile, as opposed to the quick release and subsequent decrease seen with standard immediate-release formulations, this positively affects patient compliance, dose frequency, and therapeutic efficacy. (Jethara, Patel, & Patel, 2015). (Sampath, Bhowmik, & Srivastava, 2012).

Drug release rates can be modulated via diffusion or erosion in matrix systems, which entail incorporating medicines into a polymer matrix. Reservoir systems, conversely, consist of a drug reservoir encapsulated within a semipermeable membrane that regulates drug release through diffusion or osmotic pressure. Osmotic systems rely on osmotic gradients to release drugs from an osmotic core. Micro/nanoparticle-based delivery systems utilize carriers such as microspheres, nanoparticles, or liposomes to encapsulate and release drugs sustainably. Drug release rates can be modulated via diffusion or erosion in matrix systems, which entail incorporating medicines into a polymer matrix(Sampath, Bhowmik, & Srivastava, 2012).

Sustained drug delivery has wide-ranging applications in treating various diseases, including chronic conditions such as diabetes, cardiovascular diseases, neurological disorders, and cancer (Sampath, Bhowmik, & Srivastava, 2012). For instance, in diabetes management, sustained delivery systems provide a steady release of insulin or oral antidiabetic agents, mimicking the physiological insulin secretion pattern and enhancing glycaemic control. In cancer therapy, sustained drug delivery systems offer continuous and controlled release of chemotherapeutic agents, improving efficacy while minimizing systemic toxicity (Sampath et al., 2012).

Materials research, nanotechnology, and pharmaceutical formulation improvements have contributed considerably to creating long-lasting drug delivery systems. Researchers are continuously exploring innovative approaches to achieve precise control over drug release kinetics, enhance stability, improve biocompatibility, and enable personalized medicine through tailored drug delivery (Koo et al., 2005; Mukherjee, Ray, & Thakur, 2009; Zhang et al., 2009).

Sustained drug delivery systems, which allow for the slow and consistent release of medications over an extended period, are crucial to optimizing pharmacological therapy. There are many benefits to using these systems, including increased therapeutic efficiency, decreased side effects, and higher patient compliance. (Jethara et al., 2015; Sampath et al., 2012; Singh & Lillard, 2009). As research and development efforts continue in this field, sustained drug delivery holds tremendous potential for addressing current healthcare challenges and advancing personalized medicine by tailoring drug release profiles to individual patient needs(Jethara et al., 2015).

EXAMPLES OF NANOMATERIALS FOR NOVAL DRUG DELIVERY SYSTEM

This fig.1 briefly classifies its advantages and disadvantages, and below are some details given in specific drug delivery systems.

- **Liposomes**

Lipid bilayers are the building blocks of liposomes, which are spherical vesicles. Because of their biocompatibility and adaptability, they've been studied extensively for potential medication regulation. (Koo et al., 2005; Singh & Lillard, 2009).

- **Polymeric nanoparticles**

Polymeric nanoparticles refer to those crafted from either synthetic or natural polymers. They can be altered to encapsulate drugs for prolonged release. Polymeric nanoparticles' benefits include their ability to carry much medicine, be released slowly, and be directed where needed. Chitosan is just a few examples of well-known polymers...(Mukherjee et al., 2009)

- **Dendrimers:**

Dendrimers have the shape of trees and consist of multiple branches. Their size, surface functionality, and drug-loading capacity can all be precisely controlled during synthesis. Dendrimers can transport many medications and keep them stable. Their exterior can be tailored for precise drug administration and diagnostic imaging. (Koo et al., 2005).

- **Mesoporous Silica Nanoparticles (MSN)**

MSN has a very porous, structured structure that facilitates drug loading and release. Triggered and targeted drug delivery can be functionalized with targeting ligands. MSN also protect encapsulated pharmaceuticals from degradation and maintain their stability. (Slowing, Trewyn, & Lin, 2007).

- **Gold Nanoparticles**

Drugs may be efficiently loaded onto and released from MSN because of their organized porosity structure and high surface area. Drug delivery can be targeted and triggered by functionalizing them with targeting ligands or stimuli-responsive moieties. Encapsulated pharmaceuticals benefit from MSN because of the stability and protection they provide against degradation. (Li et al., 2012).

- **Carbon Nanotubes**

Due to their organized porosity, effective drug loading and release can occur in MSN. Targeting ligands or stimuli-responsive moieties can be attached to them to facilitate targeted and triggered medication delivery. In addition to protecting encapsulated pharmaceuticals from degradation, MSN ensures their stability(Li et al., 2012; Singh & Lillard, 2009; Slowing et al., 2007).

- **Metallic Nanoparticles**

Targeted drug delivery using iron oxide and silver nanoparticles has been investigated. Drugs and surface engineering can target specific cells and tissues. Magnetically directed medication delivery uses magnetic nanoparticles(Desai et al., 2021).

METHODS OF PREPARATION OF NANO FORMULATION

Several methods are used to prepare the Nano Formulation, which is given below in detail.

Figure 1. Advantages and disadvantages of NDDS and challenges of drug delivery with nanomaterial challenges

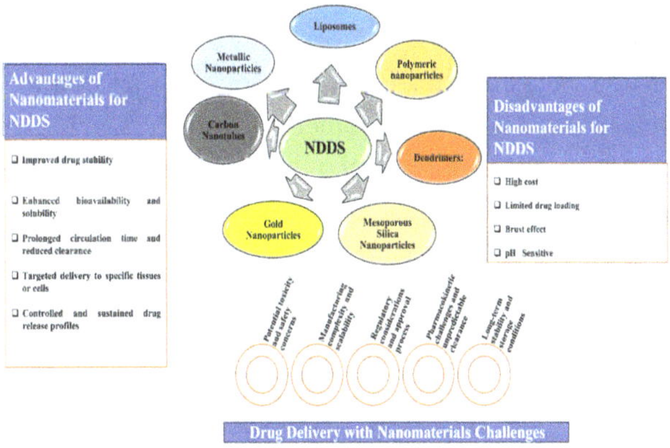

Figure 2. Methods of preparation of nano formulation

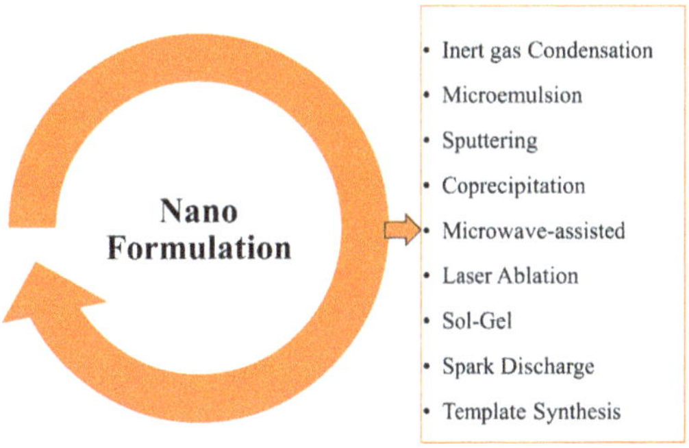

Coprecipitation

A coprecipitation occurs when nucleation, growth, coarsening, and agglomeration co-occur. Under very supersaturated circumstances, the products are often insoluble species. The production of small particles is known as the nucleation phase. Ostwald ripening and aggregation are examples of success that significantly affect the final products' size, shape, and features (Mascolo et al.,2013,D'Costa et al.,2012).

Inert Gas Condensation (IGC)

Nanoscale metal particles are most commonly made via inert gas condensation (IGC). High-pressure metal evaporation in a helium or argon container creates a vacuum. When metal atoms in the atmosphere collide with the gas, they lose energy and condense back into solid particles. In a Brownian motion, these particles clump together and crystallize into nanocrystals (Suryanarayana et al.,2007)

Metals and alloys with a nanocrystalline structure were first created using gas condensation. This process was initially designed to produce metallic and inorganic materials (Raffi et al.,2007,Safi et al.,2000).

Sputtering

Targets release their atoms when attacked with solid particles (Patamar et al.,2012). An electric field between two electrodes in a low-pressure gas produces glow discharge, the simplest method of generating ions for sputtering. Gas conducts electricity and degrades at a particular voltage. Plasma is an ion. Intense electric fields drive plasma ions toward something which is being aimed towards. Atoms and molecules are ejected into the plasma and deposited on the substrate when ions collide with a target. DC sputtering outlines this approach. Argon is frequently used as a sputtering gas because it prevents atomic reactions. Plasma ions become neutral atoms after hitting a target. (Grammatik Poulos et al., 2016)).

Microemulsion

When an electric field is established between two electrodes in a low-pressure gas, glow discharge produces ions for sputtering. If a threshold voltage is achieved, the gas degrades and conducts electricity. Plasma is ionized. A solid electric field throws plasma ions at the target. The plasma transports surface atoms (or molecules) from the target to the substrate when the ions smash against it. (Eslamian et al., 2009).

Microwave-Assisted

Biochemistry and nanotechnology both make extensive use of microwave-assisted synthesis. Chemical processes often have shorter reaction times, higher yields, and fewer byproducts than conventional convection heating methods. Reaction mixing in microwave reactors is easy to regulate, they can withstand high temperatures and pressures, and their results are consistent. When nanomaterial creation begins at room temperature, microwave-assisted approaches isolate the nucleation and growth stages well. Microwave-assisted heating can selectively activate nanomaterial precursors for scalability. Microwave synthesis selectively heats solvents or precursor compounds to make nanomaterials. (Chikan et al.,2016).

Laser Ablation

Laser ablation removes material from solid or liquid surfaces. Low laser flux causes sublimation or evaporation due to laser energy heating. Plasma forms at high laser flux. Continuous wave laser ablation is conceivable if the laser intensity is high enough, but pulsed laser ablation removes the material. This technique of nanoparticle synthesis is performed with the help of electrodes, as described in Fig:3. (Semaltianos et al.,2010).

Sol-Gel

Through "sol-gel manufacturing," tiny molecules can be formed into a solid. The sputtering gas is often argon because it prevents atomic reactions. Precipitation is a method for producing ceramic powders that are both exceedingly fine and homogeneous. Dental and biological applications for these nanoparticle-sized, single- and multi-component powders (Rane et al., 2018).

Figure 3. Laser ablation technique

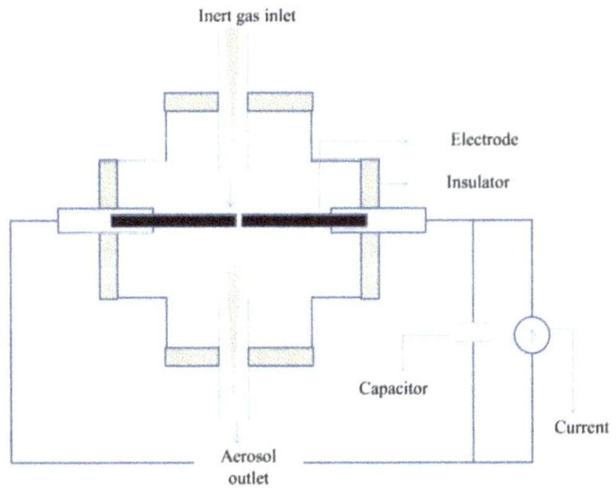

Spark Discharge

The "sol-gel" method joins molecular building components to form a solid. The sol (or solution) starts this chemical process to generate a gel-like biphasic system where the liquid and solid phases have unique morphologies (from discrete particles to continuous polymer networks). Precipitation of tiny, ceramic-like particles is possible. Dental and medical nanoparticle powders can be manufactured from a single component or several. Figure 4 shows the general setup for the spark discharge generator.(Efimov et al., 2016).

Template Synthesis

The development of an ecologically acceptable, straightforward approach to the production of nanoparticles is becoming increasingly relevant as the emphasis on green chemistry grows. Template synthesis, which uses porous materials' consistent void spaces to contain monodispersed inorganic nanoparticles, is a potential way to create them. The template has dual functionality. For starters, it allows the most precise recreation of the structure and serves as a framework for arranging a device's many functions, active components, and interfaces (Pantidos et al., 2014).

Figure 4. Spark discharge generator set up

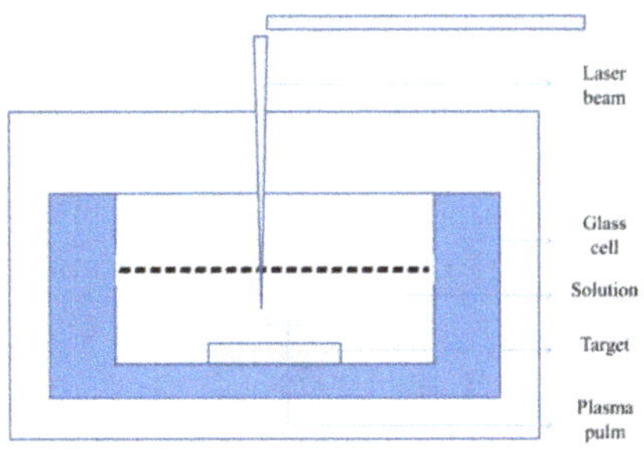

NANOPARTICLE MEDICATION DELIVERY: CRITICAL CHARACTERISTICS

Particle Size

In "sol-gel" technology, molecular building blocks are mixed to make a solid. A gel-like biphasic system forms a liquid phase and a solid phase with distinct morphology, with the sol (or solution) serving as the initiating phase (from discrete particles to continuous polymer networks). Tiny, uniform ceramic particles precipitate throughout the process. Dental and medical nanoparticle powders can be manufactured from one or more ingredients. Using Brownian motion and light scattering qualities, photon-correlation spectroscopy can determine a particle's diameter. However, this technique requires knowledge of the medium's viscosity(Singh et al., 2009). Scanning or transmission electron microscopy commonly validates photon-correlation spectroscopy results (SEM or TEM). Both the size and dispersion of nanoparticles are crucial. The distribution, fate of these factors control the distribution, toxicity, and specificity of various delivery modalities in vivo, and capacities factors influence nanoparticle stability, release, and capacity. (Dunne et al.,2000; Panyam et al., 2003).

Nanoparticle Surfaces

The MPS—liver, spleen, lungs, and bone marrow—receives most of the drug. This alters the drug's biodistribution profile. Nanoparticles are eliminated by phagocytes upon intravenous administration... (Muller et al., 1996). A drug's biodistribution profile is determined mainly by the liver, spleen, lungs, and bone marrow that comprise the MPS, or mononuclear phagocyte system...When administered intravenously, the human immune system can identify nanoparticles and clear them from the bloodstream using specialized cells called phagocytes. (Brigger et al.,2012).

Reducing opsonization and extending nanoparticles' circulation in vivo is critical for improving medicine-targeting success. Hydrophilic biodegradable copolymers such as PEG, PEO, poloxamer, poloxamine, and polysorbate 80 can coat or synthesize nanoparticles (Tween 80). According to the investigations, PEG on nanoparticles suppresses complement and serum opsonization (Grislain et al., 1983)

Zeta potential describes nanoparticle surface charge. Hydrophilic biodegradable copolymers. The investigations above on nanoparticles suppress complement and serum component opsonization (Couvreur et al.,2002). Their zeta potential describes nanoparticle surface charge.

Drug Loading

To minimize dose matrix material, nano-delivery devices need significant drug-loading capacities. Two techniques load drugs. The integration method requires incorporating the drug into the nanoparticle composition. Nanoparticles absorb drugs from a highly concentrated drug solution after production. Drug solubility in the excipient matrix material is affected by factors such as matrix composition, molecular weight, drug-polymer interactions, and the presence of end functional groups (ester or carboxyl) in either the drug or the matrix material (solid polymer or liquid dispersion agent. (Govender et al.,1999).

Since PEG has minimal effects on drug loading and interactions, it is frequently used in nanoparticle formulations. (Peracchia et al., 1997). In addition, the loading efficiency of nanoparticles containing macromolecules and medications. (Calvo et al., 1997).

Drug Release

Nanoparticle delivery systems must address drug release and polymer biodegradation. The drug's release rate depends on its solubility, ability to diffuse through the nanoparticle matrix, erosion or degradation rate, and erosion-diffusion combination. Particle matrix solubility, diffusion, and biodegradation control release. Due to their constant drug distribution, nanospheres release pharmaceuticals by matrix erosion or diffusion. Diffusion controls release if drug diffusion exceeds matrix degradation. Nanoparticles' enormous surface area gently binds or absorbs the medication, releasing it quickly (or "burst"). (Magenheim et al.,1993; Fresta et al.,1995).

Targeted Drug Delivery

You can either actively or passively target someone. An example of active targeting is converting a drug or carrier system to a ligand that recognizes a specific tissue or cell type. This was found by Lamprecht et al. (2001). Therapeutic agents can be incorporated into a macromolecule or nanoparticle and delivered to the target organ passively through a process known as passive targeting. Cancer cells can be passively targeted by drugs encapsulated in nanoparticles or macromolecules via the EPR effect. Nanoparticles may be transported throughout the body through a catheter. Nanoparticles can transport drugs through several biological barriers. (Fischer et al.,2002; Lockman et al., 2002).

The BBB poses a considerable barrier for many therapeutic agents, including those used to treat cancer, viruses, & other diseases. The use of nanoparticles to cross this barrier shows excellent promise. Since hyper-osmotic mannitol has been shown to open tight connections (Avgoustakis et al.,2002; Beletsi et al., 1999).

NANOTECHNOLOGY-BASED MEDICATION DELIVERY

Several nanotechnology-based medication delivery methods are now in use. Scientists consistently improve the medical field by developing new nano-based drug delivery systems. Below is a partial list of these: (P. Silva et al., 2013)

Liposomes

They are tiny vesicles composed of a lipid bilayer and an aqueous medium. Hydrophilic molecules are retained in the aqueous domain, whereas adsorbable lipophiles are introduced into the membrane. The alternative is to encapsulate both kinds of material. Phospholipids (natural or synthetic), sterols, and an antioxidant makeup comprise most vesicles (P. Silva et al., 2013). They are biodegradable, stabilizing therapeutic molecules, improving biodistribution, and enabling hydrophobic drugs. Liposomes can be broken down into four distinct types. (Patra et al., 2018).

Liposomes interact with cells primarily by adsorption, fusion, lipid exchange, leakage, endocytosis, and enzymatic breakdown. Liposomes can interact with cells in several ways, including through ligand/receptor or electrostatic interactions and by exchanging ions and fusing with the lipid components of cell membranes. An alternative is for the cells to ingest the liposomes through phagocytosis enclosed in liposomes released as they disintegrate. (Peng et al., 2023).

Figure 5. Drug diffusion through hydrogel membrane

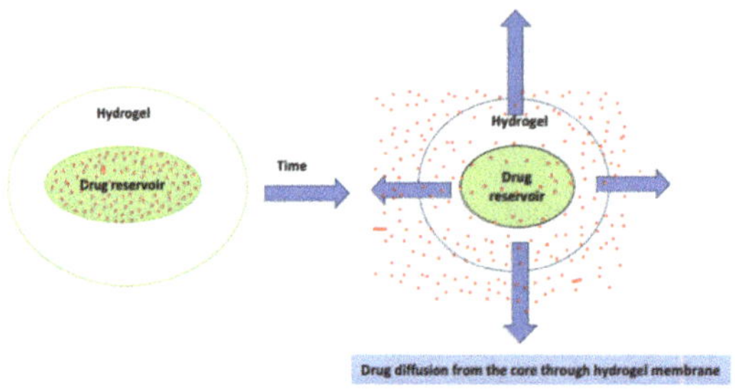

Liposomes are too large and lipophilic to pass BBB cells or cell membranes. Liposomes instead penetrate the BBB using transport mechanisms The improvement of brain tumor treatment based on this mechanism has been the subject of numerous cationic liposome-related investigations. Additionally, it is now well-accepted for cancer treatment. (Jamahiriya & de Lange, 2021).

Hydrogels

Hydrogels are polymeric materials with a three-dimensional mesh structure and can absorb water. Due to the ease with which the medication can be distributed throughout the matrix, these systems are frequently utilized for the controlled release of hydrophilic medicines. They also have physical biocompatible physical characteristics with biological tissues (Calixto et al., 2016). Hydrogels are either physical or chemical based on their production connections. Due to weak forces like ionic and H-bonding and molecular entanglements, physical hydrogels arise. This is because accessible chain endpoints and chain loops are reversible network defects. However, chemical hydrogels are often called permanent hydrogels when covalent connections are present. When covalent linkages are present, drug responsiveness, excellent drug loading efficiency, and the ability to create gel in situ are just a few of the excel over their chemical counterparts. (Vashist et al., 2014).

As shown in fig:5, the hydrogel releases the drugs from its reservoir by following the diffusion mechanism. Hydrogels' porous nature lets drugs gently release over time. A regulated release mechanism such as diffusion, swelling, chemicals, or environmental stimulation keeps the active therapeutic ingredient at a high local concentration for a long time(Narayanaswamy & Torchilin, 2019).

Micelles

Micelles with oppositely charged blocks can load hydrophilic charged macromolecules like peptides, proteins, and nucleic acids into the center of the micelle, forming a polygon complex (PIC) through electrostatic interactions and charge neutralization. The core-shell micellar structure formed by single polymer chains reduces the amount of water contact with the hydrophobic section. (Koo et al., 2005; Miyata et al., 2011).

Pluronic Micelles

Pluronic, an amphiphilic copolymer, is constructed from blocks of hydrophobic poly (propylene oxide) and hydrophilic poly (ethylene oxide). They develop nanoscale micellar structures above the critical micellar concentration (CMC). These systems contained hydrophobic chemicals that were either conjugated on the surface of nanoparticles or encapsulated within the micellar roomy core. The delivery systems based on Pluronic copolymers have several distinctive qualities and characteristics. First, contrary to acting as simplex vehicles like many drug delivery methods, poloxamers behave as pharmacologically active polymers that control the response of malignant cells. As polymerized pharmaceuticals, Pluronic are widely categorized. (Rahdar Abbas, 2018; Wang et al., 2018).

Dendrimers

Dendrimers were unintentionally found in 1978 by Vogtle and colleagues and are also known as arborio's, cascade molecules, or highly branched polymers. Dendrimers are chemically created polymeric molecules that resemble proteins in structure, size, and nanoscopic physicochemical properties. These polymers are nearly perfect spheres with sizes between 2 and 10 nm. Dendrimers are artificial. Therefore, they might be constructed from anything from peptides and lipids to polysaccharides and fatty acids. These new molecules are revolutionary because of their extracted regulated construction, which gives them properties such as a known molecular weight, biodegradability, and biocompatibility. (N. P., M. F. P., & C. M. Silva, 2012)(Lee & Yeo, 2015)

Nano Discs

Non-spherical nanocarriers like Nanodiscs (NDs) have recently received much interest. The Biologically derived strategies for lipids' poor water solubility in bloodstreams served as the basis for the concept of the ND constitution. The complex intercellular connections in the body are traversed by HDLs carrying signaling lipids, proteins, and microRNAs (Bariwal et al., 2022).

LNDs, or Lipid Nanodiscs

A lipid bilayer with a typical 10–20 nm diameter makes up LNDs. Amphiphilic biomacromolecules like apoA1 or membrane scaffold proteins surround and stabilize the lipid bilayer (Bariwal et al., 2022).

Lipid Nanoparticles Composed of Styrene and Maleic Acid (SMA) (SMALPs)

Replace LND amphiphilic membrane scaffold biomacromolecules with synthetic SMA or SMA-like copolymers (Bariwal et al., 2022).

PNDs, or Polymer Nanodiscs

Membrane scaffold polymers or biomacromolecules like MSPs are used in PNDs and LNDs; however, in PNDs, a synthetic membrane patch consisting of amphiphilic block copolymers takes the role of the lipid bilayer (Bariwal et al., 2022).

Hybrid Micelles or Hybrid Nanodiscs (HNDs)

Amphiphilic polymers do not stabilize these Nanodiscs. Short-chain phospholipids and long-chain keratome-forming lipids make up their composition (CFL)(Bariwal et al., 2022)

Qingxin Mu et al. safes' high-drug-loading biconcave carbon Nanodiscs can bypass physiological barriers and deliver therapeutically effective dosages of drugs to solid tumors, creating a biconcave carbon Nanodiscs (BCN) with an RBC-like geometric profile. Due to BCN surface carboxyl and hydroxyl groups interacting with charged functional groups of aromatic anticancer agent doxorubicin, drug release is pH-dependent (DOX) (Qingxin Mu et al., 2019)

Carbon Nanotubes (CNTs)

Carbon nanotubes (CNT) are ideal for field emission displays and strong fibers. In biology, modified CNT can operate as protein transporters or vaccine delivery systems (Bianco et al., 2005). Carbon nanostructures (CNSs) are incredibly versatile. Nanoparticles, nanotubes, Nanodiscs, Nanoshells, nanobuds, sp3-hybridized crystalline carbon flakes, and nanowires are some of the morphologies that can be synthesized. Carbon nanotubes (CNTs) are nanoscale nanostructures with distinctive graphene-based designs, substantial surface areas, and high mechanical stiffness. (Jha et al., 2020).

CNTs can be single-, multi-, or double-walled (DWCTs). CNTs have the strongest and stiffest tensile strength and elastic modulus due to their chemical bonding based on the sp2 orbital connection. Depending on chirality, tubes may be metallic or semiconducting. For in vivo stability, CNTs' sp2 carbon-carbon bonds boost mechanical strength. (Abdallah et al., 2020).Carbon nanotubes are small enough to enter cells and transport medications to their cytoplasm or nucleus. In addition to enhancing the drug's therapeutic profile and increasing its efficacy, drug delivery methods reduce its off-target effects.(Debnath & Srivastava, 2021).

Nanodiamonds

Nanodiamonds are widely regarded as the most biocompatible nanoparticles in the carbon family (ND). The last 20 years have seen a surge in interest, particularly in biomedicine and Theranostics applications. In particular, nanodiamond's spectroscopic qualities make them ideal for bio/medical imaging and labeling. The physical and chemical properties of nanodiamonds are unparalleled.(Perevedentseva et al., 2021)

NDs generated fewer reactive oxygen species (ROS) and affected the morphology of several cell types less than other Carbon Nanoparticles (CNPs). Because of its versatility and unique properties, ND has been studied for use in various drug delivery systems, in vivo imaging, and tissue engineering. (Jeong et al., 2016)

Quantum Dots

Quantum dots, a type of nanoscale semiconductor, are an essential substance that links nanotechnology with drug screening (QDs). They are ideal probe materials for (bio)sensing or immune-sensing platforms. Thanks to their unique physicochemical features, quantum dots (QDs) are used as luminous markers in drug delivery systems for monitoring drug metabolism. The biological applications are practically endless, including the development of fluorescence diagnostics for drug discovery and disease diagnosis.

(Badıllı et al., 2020) .The composition and size of a QD's metalloid crystalline core determines the type of fluorescence it will emit. Materials such as cadmium-selenium (CdSe), cadmium-tellurium (CdTe), indium-phosphate (InP), or indium-arsenate (InAs) make up the core. The material's optical, physical, and bioavailability qualities are further improved by a semiconductor shell stabilizing the core, most frequently zinc sulfide (ZnS). Biocompatible materials or polymer layers, such as POSSPCU and PEG, can be capped or coated to increase water solubility and desirable bioactivity (Polyhedral Oligomeric Silsesquioxane-Polycarbonate urethane)(Ghaderi et al., 2011; Iannazzo et al., 2017).

Nanowires

Platforms with magnetic sensitivity and release mechanisms, including sensitive systems, are utilized in tailored drug delivery technologies... NW is characterized architecturally by its one-dimensional shape, which includes lengths and nanometre-scale diameters (-10-200 nm). The considerable aspect ratio sets it apart from nanorods. Nanowires (NWs) stand out among other nanoparticles and nanocarriers due to their form, anisotropy, and colossal surface area. (Nana et al., 2019),(Pondman et al., 2015)

Nanorods

Gold nanorods have some intriguing applications, including drug delivery and photothermal therapy. Gold nanorods show promise due to their novel optical and photothermal capabilities, their adaptability (allowing for the modification of their surface and the conjugation of drugs/molecules to them), and their relative biocompatibility. Gold nanorods release pharmaceuticals by passive release from the nanoparticle surface and heat dissipation from absorbed light energy. For these reasons, gold nanoparticles have shown potential as laboratory drug delivery methods.(Alkilany et al., 2012), (Zong et al., 2021).

TARGETED AND SUSTAINED DELIVERY APPLICATIONS OF NANOMATERIALS

The various useful application of Targeted and sustained Delivery systems for Nanomedicine are dearer described.

Nanomaterials for Targeted and Sustained Delivery

Enhancing treatment outcomes across various diseases relies on the crucial aspect of targeted and sustained drug delivery. Nanomaterials possess distinctive advantages in this context, including their ability to carry leanings, adjustable properties, and capacity to target particular cells or tissues. The tables presented herein comprehensively summarize how nanomaterials are applied in targeted and sustained drug delivery(Patra et al., 2018).

Table 1 demonstrates the specificity and consistency of nanoparticle delivery. Benefits include high drug-loading capacity, tailored distribution to specific cells or tissues, and encapsulation of both hydrophilic and hydrophobic medicines(Zheng et al., 2021); Elsabahy & Wooley, 2012),(Craparo & Bondì, 2012); Cheng, Xie, & Sun, 2023).

Table 1. Nanomaterials for targeted and sustained delivery

Nanomaterial	Characteristics	Advantages	Applications	References
Liposomes	Biocompatible, versatile	Encapsulation of hydrophilic and hydrophobic drugs	Cancer therapy, gene delivery	(TORCHILIN, 2006)
Polymeric Biodegradable	Biodegradable tunable	controlled drug releaseSustained release	Chronic disease treatment tissue engineering	(Zheng et al., 2021)
Nanoparticles	High surface area, tunable properties	Targeted drug delivery, sustained release	Therapeutics, drug repurposing	(Elsabahy & Wooley, 2012)
Dendrimers	Precise structure, multifunctional	High drug-loading capacity, controlled release	Gene delivery, infectious disease treatment	(DUFES, UCHEGBU, & SCHATZLEIN, 2005)
Carbon-based	High surface area, tunable properties	Targeted delivery, sustained release	Neurological disorders, inflammatory diseases	(Gaur et al., 2021)

Table 2. Disease-specific applications of nanomaterials

Disease	Nanomaterial	Advantages	References
Cancer	Liposomes	Enhanced drug delivery to tumor tissues	(TORCHILIN, 2006)
Cardiovascular diseases	Polymeric Nanoparticles	Targeted drug delivery to atherosclerotic plaques	(Craparo & Bondì, 2012)
Inflammatory disorders	Nanoparticles	Sustained release of anti-inflammatory agents	(Cheng, Xie, & Sun, 2023)
Neurological disorders	Dendrimers	Blood-brain barrier penetration	(Pinheiro et al., 2021)
Gene therapy	Carbon-based	Efficient gene delivery	(Kościk, Jankowski, & Jagusiak, 2021)

Nanomaterials for Targeted and Sustained Drug Delivery in Cancer Therapy

Cancer therapy has greatly benefited from advancements in nanomaterial-based drug delivery systems. Nanomaterials offer unique properties that enable targeted and sustained release of therapeutic agents, improving drug efficacy while minimizing off-target effects. Cancer is a complex and heterogeneous disease that requires precise and efficient drug delivery strategies. Nanomaterials have emerged as promising tools in cancer therapy, offering controlled drug release, target specificity, and enhanced therapeutic outcomes (Wang et al., 2012; J. Liu et al., 2014).

Table 3 summarizes the various benefits of nanomaterials in cancer therapy. These advantages encompass targeted delivery of drugs, controlled release mechanisms, improved stability of drugs, and the ability to modify their surface to enhance drug effectiveness. Additionally, nanomaterials exhibit a multifunctional nature that enables combination therapies, allowing for simultaneous drug delivery and imaging (Maiti et al., 2019).

Table 3. Nanomaterials in cancer therapy

Nanomaterial	Characteristics	Advantages	Applications	References
Liposomes	Biocompatible versatile	Targeted drug delivery, Controlled release	Chemotherapy, gene therapy	(Wang et al., 2012)
Polymeric	Biodegradable tunable	Extended drug release, surface modification	Drug delivery, immunotherapy	(J. Liu et al., 2014)
Nanoparticles	High drug loading capacity	Sustained release, passive targeting	Photothermal therapy, immunotherapy	(Tong & Langer, 2015)
Dendrimers	Precise structure multifunctional	Controlled release, surface modification	Drug delivery, gene therapy, and siRNA delivery	(Sau et al., 2018)
Carbon-based	High surface area, tunable properties	Enhanced drug stability, imaging	Drug delivery, imaging, phototherapy	(Maiti, Tong, Mou, & Yang, 2019)

Nanomaterials for Targeted and Sustained Drug Delivery in Cardiovascular Diseases

Coronary artery disease, heart failure, and stroke are important health issues. Nanomaterial-based drug delivery systems allow precise medication targeting and controlled release, potentially improving cardiovascular therapy. Nanomaterials offer several advantages in cardiovascular disease treatment, as summarized in Table 4. These include targeted drug delivery to specific sites, controlled release for prolonged therapeutic effect, enhanced drug stability, and surface modification for improved compatibility and efficacy (Sahoo et al., 2003; Sahoo et al., 2003).

Nanomaterials present promising possibilities for precise and long-lasting drug delivery in cardiovascular disease. Table 4 outlines different nanomaterials' properties, benefits, and uses in treating CVD. (Chis et al., 2020).

Table 4. Nanomaterials in cardiovascular diseases

Nanomaterial	Advantages	Applications	References
Liposomes	Targeted drug delivery, controlled release	Gene therapy, antiplatelet therapy, Gene therapy for cardiovascular regeneration	(Sahoo & Labhasetwar, 2003)
Polymeric	Prolonged drug release, surface modification	Drug-eluting stents, tissue engineering scaffolds, Localized delivery of angiogenic factors	(Cicha, Singh, Garlichs, & Alexiou, 2016)
Nanoparticles	Enhanced drug stability, site-specific targeting	Imaging, anti-inflammatory therapy, and Imaging agents for early diagnosis of CVDs	(Libby & Ridker, 2004)
Dendrimers	Controlled releasesurface modification	Targeted drug delivery, Gene therapy for cardiac tissue regeneration	(Chis et al., 2020)
Carbon-based	Improved drug solubility imaging	Drug delivery diagnostics, Targeted drug delivery to atherosclerotic plaques	(Craparo & Bondì, 2012)

Table 5. Nanomaterials in infectious disease

Nanomaterial	Advantages	Applications	References
Liposomes	Targeted drug delivery, controlled release	Antiviral, antibacterial, and antifungal therapy	(Mura et al., 2013)
Polymeric	Extended drug release surface modification	Extended-release of antimicrobial agents	(Vasir & Labhasetwar, 2007)
Nanoparticles	Sustained release enhanced drug stability	Targeted delivery of antimicrobial agents	(Shete, Prabhu, & Patravale, 2014)
Dendrimers	Controlled releasesurface modification	Antiviral therapy against viral infections	(An, Deng, Wang, Xu, & Wang, 2023)
Carbon-based	Enhanced drug solubility, imaging	Diagnostic tools for infectious disease detection	(Cha, Shin, Annabi, Dokmeci, & Khademhosseini, 2013)

Nanomaterials for Infectious Disease Targeted and Long-Term Drug Delivery

Developing efficient medication delivery systems for treating infectious diseases is essential due to the global health concerns posed by these diseases. Nanomaterial-based drug delivery shows potential in delivering antimicrobial agents in a targeted and sustained manner, which leads to better therapeutic results and less medication resistance. Nanomaterials are examined regarding their features, benefits, problems, and recent progress in medicine delivery for infectious diseases (Mura, Nicolas, & Couvreur, 2013).

Nanomaterial-based medication delivery devices promise precision and continuity in infectious disease therapy. Table 5 concisely overviews nanomaterials' features, benefits, and applications in treating infectious diseases. (Shete et al., 2014; (Vasir et al., 2007).

Targeted and Long-Term Drug Delivery Using Nanomaterials for Neurological Disorders

Brain cancers and neurodegenerative diseases present formidable challenges because medications have difficulty penetrating the brain's protective barrier. Nanoparticles may deliver targeted and sustained CNS medications. Brain. This article highlights the utilization of nanomaterials in two crucial domains of CNS drug delivery:(Soni, Ruhela, & Medhi, 2016)

Blood-Brain Barrier Penetration

The blood-brain barrier (BBB) selectively blocks many therapeutic medications from reaching the brain. To overcome this obstacle and deliver medications to the brain and spinal cord, nanomaterials provide a novel potential (CNS) (Daneman & Prat, 2015). Approaches to enhance BBB penetration involve modifying the surface of nanomaterials with ligands that can interact with BBB transporters or receptors. By facilitating receptor-mediated transcytosis, these ligands enable nanomaterials to traverse. (Upadhyay, 2014).

Table 6. Nanomaterials in gene therapy

Nanomaterial	Advantages	Applications	References
Liposomes	Efficient gene encapsulation and delivery	Delivery of therapeutic genes for genetic diseases, Cancer gene therapy, and immunomodulation	(Verma & Weitzman, 2005)
Polymeric	Enhanced gene stability and release	Gene editing for precision medicine, RNA interference for targeted gene silencing	(Yin et al., 2014)
Nanoparticles	Cellular uptake and endosomal escape	Gene delivery for immunotherapy, Gene silencing, and modulation of cellular functions	(Peer & Lieberman, 2011)
Dendrimers	Controlled gene delivery and targeting	Gene editing for precise genome engineering	(Ouyang, Gao, Shen, & Shi, 2021)
Carbon-based	Efficient gene delivery and imaging	Molecular diagnostics for genetic diseases,	(Sun et al., 2014)

Targeted Brain Area Drug Administration

Nanomaterials can be designed to pass through the blood-brain barrier (BBB) and specifically target particular brain regions affected by neurological diseases (Pinheiro, Coutinho, Pinheiro, & Neves, 2021). This targeting is achieved by attaching ligands that recognize receptors or markers in the desired brain region. For instance, in the case of brain tumors, nanomaterials equipped with targeting ligands can accumulate selectively at the site of the tumor, enabling effective and localized delivery of drugs. (Dong, 2018). (Pinheiro et al., 2021).

Nanomaterials for Targeted and Sustained Drug Delivery in Gene Therapy

Gene therapy has great potential for genetic diseases and some malignancies. Therapeutic gene delivery remains difficult. Nanomaterial-based gene delivery technologies are promising. (Verma & Weitzman, 2005).

Nanomaterial-based drug delivery systems hold significant promise in facilitating targeted and long-term gene delivery for gene therapy. The provided tables 6 outlines the features, benefits, and applications of different nanomaterials in gene therapy. (Sun et al., 2014; Peer et al., 2011).

RECENT RESEARCH

Nanomaterials have several applications in the healthcare, pharmaceutical, and beauty industries. Natural polymers, especially polysaccharides, are the main focus of study in the aforementioned biological spheres. Biodegradability, safety, and physiological stability characterize polysaccharide-based natural polymers. They could enable drug delivery systems to deliver safe, effective doses over time. Nano-size carriers may increase bioavailability, pharmacokinetics, medication half-life, and administration frequency. This section in Table 7 summarises recent research in this field (Pomaded, M. et al., 2023):

Nanotechnology has successfully treated cancer by blocking the adverse effects of conventional therapeutic approaches, such as curcumin. Using chitosan could facilitate the selective destruction of tumor cells without harming normal ones. The capacity of the nano-scale vehicle to load curcumin is enhanced by the high specific area provided by magnetic iron oxide. Consequently, Curcumin was loaded with a 48.25% loading efficiency and an 87.50% entrapment efficiency into a double emulsion hydrogel made of Fe3O4/chitosan/agarose by Pourmadadi, M. et al., proving the nanocarrier is biocompatible. Furthermore, a high proportion of apoptosis demonstrated, via flow cytometry, that This curcumin-loaded double emulsion has a little toxic effect on cultured cells and has the potential to remove some of the hurdles now in the way of cancer treatment (Pourmadadi, M. et al. 2023, Pourmadadi M. et al., 2023).

Zhu, Y. et al. made dendritic, hollow, and mesoporous silica nanoparticles using simple methods. Nano-porous silica of varying pore shapes was tested for its efficacy as a stroma for Pueraria pharmaceuticals. Microwave scattering, Transmission electron microscopy, X-ray diffraction, and zeta potential were used to characterize MSN, DMSN, and HMSN. Those three mesoporous substances were then treated with Pueraria (PUE). MSN, DMSN, and HMSN loaded with PUE were tested for sustained release and drug delivery in PBS solutions of various pH values. MTT and hemolysis testing data assessed MSN, DMSN, and HMSN biocompatibility and stability (Zhu, Y. et al., 2023).

Mohammed, H. A. et al. (2015) discussed solid lipid nanoparticles (SLNs) and their possible future applications. Evidence suggests that reducing first-pass and intra-enterocyte metabolisms with SLNs as an oral medication delivery approach increases drug accumulation at the target region. Because of their improved physical stability, controlled drug release, enhanced drug accumulation in the targeted tissues and cells, increased drug bioactivity, extended blood circulation time, increased bioavailability, and improved delivery and retention in cancer cells, SLNs are a promising parenteral drug delivery system. They (Mohammed, H. A. et al., 2023, Jafernik, K. et al., 2023).

(Li, Z. et al., 2023).

Cervical carcinoma is a frequent gynecological malignancy. Cisplatin is a first-line cervical cancer treatment despite its disadvantages. Kousar et al. devised a green production method for hyaluronic acid-coated, thiolated chitosan nanocarriers for CD44-specific delivery and extended cisplatin release in cervical cancer cells. After ionic gelation synthesis, Zeta analysis revealed nanoparticles of 265.9 nm sizes, +22.3 mV zeta potentials, and PDIs of 0.226. SEM and TEM showed the nanoparticles' smooth, spherical form. They found that cisplatin may leak slowly over 72 hours. These data imply that a CD44-focused delivery method may reduce off-target toxicity, extend release, and increase cancer cell uptake (Kousar K. et al., 2023, Abbasi, M. et al., 2023).

Many females have breast cancer. Rajaei M. et al. created a potential drug loading and sustained release strategy using 5-fluorouracil (5-FU) to treat breast cancer. Glyoxal cross-linked a pH-sensitive, biocompatible CS/AG/GO hydrogel. (Rajaei M. et al., 2023).

Chemotherapy treats cancer. Doxorubicin kills cancer cells (DOX). Metal oxide nanoparticles can improve combination therapy for anti-cancer medications due to their unique features and minimal toxicity. Pourmadadi et al. created green synthetic pH-responsive nanocomposites with dioxane (DOX)-loaded polyvinylpyrrolidone (PVP), titanium dioxide (TiO2), and agarose (Ag)-modified macromolecules. The MTT experiment showed that the DOX-loaded PVP-Ag-TiO2 nanocomposite was much more dangerous than DOX. Flow cytometry demonstrated that PVP-Ag-DOX nanocarriers with TiO2 nanomaterials activated cell death more. These tests show that the nanocomposite loaded with DOX can replace conventional cancer therapy systems (Pourmadadi, M. et.al. 2023), (Spadari, C. et al. 2023).

Table 7. Recent research on nano formulation for different diseases

Sl No.	Formulation type	Materials used	Disease targeted	References
1.	Double emulsion hydrogel	Curcumin, Fe_3O_4/ chitosan/agarose	Cancer	(Pomaded, M. et.al. 2023)
2.	Mesoporous Silica Microspheres (mesoporous silica nanoparticles, dendritic mesoporous silica nanoparticles, hollow mesoporous silica nanoparticles)	Puerarin (PUE)	-	(Zhu, Y. et al., 2023)
3.	Solid lipid nanoparticles (SLNs)	Lipids, emulsifiers, stabilizers, co-surfactants, preservatives, cryoprotectants, and charge modifiers	Cancer, Alzheimer, Tuberculosis	(Mohammed, H. A., et al. 2023)
4.	Chitosan-based nanoparticles	Chitosan	-	(Jafernik, K. et.al. 2023)
5.	Hollow-structured nanomaterials (HSNMs)	protein/peptide, nucleic acid-based drugs	Antibiotics, Chemotherapeutic drugs, and imaging agents	(Li, Z. et al., 2023)
6.	Nanocarriers	Hyaluronic acid, thiolate chitosan	Cervical cancer	(Kousar, K. et.al. 2023)
7.	Folic acid decorated alginate nanoparticles loaded hydrogel	Diferourylmethane	Colorectal cancer	(Abbasi, M. et.al. 2023)
8	Hydrogel	chitosan/agarose/ graphene oxide, Glyoxal, 5-fluorouracil	Breast cancer	(Rajaei, M. et.al. 2023)
9	PVP-Ag-TiO_2 nanocomposite loaded with DOX	Polyvinylpyrrolidone (PVP), titanium dioxide (TiO2), agarose (Ag),	Cancer	(Pourmadadi, M. et.al. 2023)
10	Nanoparticles	Polysorbate 80 (P80),Miltefosine	Cryptococcal meningitis	(Spadari, C. C et.al. 2023)

CONCLUSION

In conclusion, the medical community has much to gain from exploring the potential of nanomaterials for targeted and long-term medication delivery. Thanks to advances in nanotechnology, scientists and researchers can now precisely control medication delivery processes and enhance treatment outcomes by engineering materials at the nanoscale.

There are several benefits to using nanoparticles for medicine delivery over more conventional methods. First, their diminutive stature promotes medication stability and solubility, leading to efficient transport to the desired location. Functionalizing nanomaterials with ligands and targeting moieties improves drug accumulation and marker interactions at particular sites. This specific strategy lessens the likelihood of unwanted side effects by reducing the dosage needed for therapeutic efficacy.

REFERENCES

Abbasi, M., Sohail, M., Minhas, M. U., Mahmood, A., Shah, S. A., Munir, A., & Kashif, M.-U.-R. (2023). Folic acid-decorated alginate nanoparticles loaded hydrogel for the oral delivery of diferourylmethane in colorectal cancer. *International Journal of Biological Macromolecules*, *233*, 123585. doi:10.1016/j.ijbiomac.2023.123585 PMID:36758757

Abdallah, B., Elhissi, A. M. A., Ahmed, W., & Najlah, M. (2020). Carbon nanotube drug delivery system for cancer treatment. In *Advances in Medical and Surgical Engineering* (pp. 313–332). Elsevier. doi:10.1016/B978-0-12-819712-7.00016-4

Ahmad, Z., Shah, A., Siddiq, M., & Kraatz, H.-B. (2014). Polymeric micelles as drug delivery vehicles. *RSC Advances*, *4*(33), 17028–17038. doi:10.1039/C3RA47370H

Alkilany, A. M., Thompson, L. B., Boulos, S. P., Sisco, P. N., & Murphy, C. J. (2012). Gold nanorods: Their potential for photothermal therapeutics and drug delivery is tempered by the complexity of their biological interactions. *Advanced Drug Delivery Reviews*, *64*(2), 190–199. doi:10.1016/j.addr.2011.03.005 PMID:21397647

An, H., Deng, X., Wang, F., Xu, P., & Wang, N. (2023). Dendrimers as Nanocarriers for the Delivery of Drugs Obtained from Natural Products. *Polymers*, *15*(10), 2292. doi:10.3390/polym15102292 PMID:37242865

Avgoustakis, K., Beletsi, A., Panagi, Z., Klepetsanis, P., Karydas, A. G., & Ithakissios, D. S. (2002). PLGA–mPEG nanoparticles of cisplatin: In vitro nanoparticle degradation, vitro drug release, and in vivo drug residence in blood properties. *Journal of Controlled Release*, *79*(1-3), 123–135. doi:10.1016/S0168-3659(01)00530-2 PMID:11853924

Badıllı, U., Mollarasouli, F., Bakirhan, N. K., Ozkan, Y., & Ozkan, S. A. (2020). Role of quantum dots in pharmaceutical and biomedical analysis, and its application in drug delivery. *Trends in Analytical Chemistry*, *131*, 116013. doi:10.1016/j.trac.2020.116013

Bariwal, J., Ma, H., Altenberg, G. A., & Liang, H. (2022). Nanodiscs: A versatile nanocarrier platform for cancer diagnosis and treatment. *Chemical Society Reviews*, *51*(5), 1702–1728. doi:10.1039/D1CS01074C PMID:35156110

Barratt, G. M. (2000). Therapeutic applications of colloidal drug carriers. *Pharmaceutical Science & Technology Today*, *3*(5), 163–171. doi:10.1016/S1461-5347(00)00255-8 PMID:10785658

Beletsi, A., Leontiadis, L., Klepetsanis, P., Ithakissios, D. S., & Avgoustakis, K. (1999). Effect of preparative variables on the properties of poly (dl-lactide-co-glycolide)–methoxy poly (ethylene glycol) copolymers related to their application in controlled drug delivery. *International Journal of Pharmaceutics*, *182*(2), 187–197. doi:10.1016/S0378-5173(99)00058-7 PMID:10341308

Bianco, A., Kostarelos, K., & Prato, M. (2005). Applications of carbon nanotubes in drug delivery. *Current Opinion in Chemical Biology*, *9*(6), 674–679. doi:10.1016/j.cbpa.2005.10.005 PMID:16233988

Boulaiz, H., Alvarez, P. J., Ramirez, A., Marchal, J. A., Prados, J., & Rodrí, F. (2011). *Nanomedicine : Application Areas and Development Prospects*, 3303–3321. MDPI. doi:10.3390/ijms12053303

Brayden, D. J. (2003). Controlled release technologies for drug delivery. *Drug Discovery Today*, *8*(21), 976–978. doi:10.1016/S1359-6446(03)02874-5 PMID:14643159

Brigger, I., Dubernet, C., & Couvreur, P. (2012). Nanoparticles in cancer therapy and diagnosis. *Advanced Drug Delivery Reviews*, *64*, 24–36. doi:10.1016/j.addr.2012.09.006 PMID:12204596

Calixto, G., Bernegossi, J., de Freitas, L., Fontana, C., & Chorilli, M. (2016). Nanotechnology-Based Drug Delivery Systems for Photodynamic Therapy of Cancer: A Review. *Molecules (Basel, Switzerland)*, *21*(3), 342. doi:10.3390/molecules21030342 PMID:26978341

Calvo, P., Remuñan-López, C., Vila-Jato, J. L., & Alonso, M. J. (1997). Chitosan and chitosan/ethylene oxide-propylene oxide block copolymer nanoparticles as novel carriers for proteins and vaccines. *Pharmaceutical Research*, *14*(10), 1431–1436. doi:10.1023/A:1012128907225 PMID:9358557

Cha, C., Shin, S. R., Annabi, N., Dokmeci, M. R., & Khademhosseini, A. (2013). Carbon-Based Nanomaterials: Multifunctional Materials for Biomedical Engineering. *ACS Nano*, *7*(4), 2891–2897. doi:10.1021/nn401196a PMID:23560817

Cheng, X., Xie, Q., & Sun, Y. (2023). Advances in nanomaterial-based targeted drug delivery systems. *Frontiers in Bioengineering and Biotechnology*, *11*, 1177151. doi:10.3389/fbioe.2023.1177151 PMID:37122851

Chikan, V., & McLaurin, E. J. (2016). Rapid nanoparticle synthesis by magnetic and microwave heating. *Nanomaterials (Basel, Switzerland)*, *6*(85), 85. doi:10.3390/nano6050085 PMID:28335212

Chis, A. A., Dobrea, C., Morgovan, C., Arseniu, A. M., Rus, L. L., Butuca, A., Juncan, A. M., Totan, M., Vonica-Tincu, A. L., Cormos, G., Muntean, A. C., Muresan, M. L., Gligor, F. G., & Frum, A. (2020). Applications and Limitations of Dendrimers in Biomedicine. *Molecules (Basel, Switzerland)*, *25*(17), 3982. doi:10.3390/molecules25173982 PMID:32882920

Cicha, I., Singh, R., Garlichs, C. D., & Alexiou, C. (2016). Nano-biomaterials for cardiovascular applications: Clinical perspective. *Journal of Controlled Release*, *229*, 23–36. doi:10.1016/j.jconrel.2016.03.015 PMID:26988601

Couvreur, P., Barratt, G., Fattal, E., & Vauthier, C. (2002). Nanocapsule technology: a review. *Critical Reviews™ in Therapeutic Drug Carrier Systems, 19*(2).

Craparo, E. F., & Bondì, M. L. (2012). Application of polymeric nanoparticles in immunotherapy. *Current Opinion in Allergy and Clinical Immunology*, *12*(6), 658–664. doi:10.1097/ACI.0b013e3283588c57 PMID:23095912

D'Costa, G., Pisal, D.S., Rane, D.S.(2012). *Report on Synthesis of nanoparticles and functionalization: Co-precipitation method.*

Daneman, R., & Prat, A. (2015). The Blood–Brain Barrier. *Cold Spring Harbor Perspectives in Biology*, *7*(1), a020412. doi:10.1101/cshperspect.a020412 PMID:25561720

Debnath, S. K., & Srivastava, R. (2021). Drug Delivery With Carbon-Based Nanomaterials as Versatile Nanocarriers: Progress and Prospects. *Frontiers in Nanotechnology*, *3*, 644564. doi:10.3389/fnano.2021.644564

Desai, N., Momin, M., Khan, T., Gharat, S., Ningthoujam, R. S., & Omri, A. (2021). Metallic nanoparticles as drug delivery system for the treatment of cancer. *Expert Opinion on Drug Delivery*, *18*(9), 1261–1290. doi:10.1080/17425247.2021.1912008 PMID:33793359

Dhull, A., Yu, C., Wilmoth, A. H., Chen, M., Sharma, A., & Yiu, S. (2023). Dendrimers in Corneal Drug Delivery: Recent Developments and Translational Opportunities. *Pharmaceutics*, *15*(6), 1591. doi:10.3390/pharmaceutics15061591 PMID:37376040

Dong, X. (2018). Current Strategies for Brain Drug Delivery. *Theranostics*, *8*(6), 1481–1493. doi:10.7150/thno.21254 PMID:29556336

Dufes, C., Uchegbu, I., & Schatzlein, A. (2005). Dendrimers in gene delivery. *Advanced Drug Delivery Reviews*, *57*(15), 2177–2202. doi:10.1016/j.addr.2005.09.017 PMID:16310284

Efimov, A. A., Lizunova, A. A., Volkov, I. A., Mylnikov, D. A., Arsenov, P. V., & Ivanov, V. V. (2016). A new approach to the high-yield synthesis of nanoparticles by spark discharge. *Journal of Physics: Conference Series*, *741*, 741. doi:10.1088/1742-6596/741/1/012035

Elsabahy, M., & Wooley, K. L. (2012). Design of polymeric nanoparticles for biomedical delivery applications. *Chemical Society Reviews*, *41*(7), 2545. doi:10.1039/c2cs15327k PMID:22334259

Erdlenbruch, B., Jendrossek, V., Eibl, H., & Lakomek, M. (2000). Transient and controllable opening of the blood-brain barrier to cytostatic and antibiotic agents by alkylglycerols in rats. *Experimental Brain Research*, *135*(3), 417–422. doi:10.1007002210000553 PMID:11146820

Eslamian, M., & Shekarriz, M. (2009). Recent advances in nanoparticle preparation by spray and microemulsion methods. *Recent Patents on Nanotechnology*, *3*(2), 99–115. doi:10.2174/187221009788490068 PMID:19519594

Fisher, R. S., & Ho, J. (2002). Potential new methods for antiepileptic drug delivery. *CNS Drugs*, *16*(9), 579–593. doi:10.2165/00023210-200216090-00001 PMID:12153331

Fresta, M., Puglisi, G., Giammona, G., Cavallaro, G., Micali, N., & Furneri, P. M. (1995). Pefloxacine mesylate-and ofloxacin-loaded polyethylcyanoacrylate nanoparticles: Characterization of the colloidal drug carrier formulation. *Journal of Pharmaceutical Sciences*, *84*(7), 895–902. doi:10.1002/jps.2600840721 PMID:7562444

Gaur, M., Misra, C., Yadav, A. B., Swaroop, S., Maolmhuaidh, F. Ó., Bechelany, M., & Barhoum, A. (2021). Biomedical Applications of Carbon Nanomaterials: Fullerenes, Quantum Dots, Nanotubes, Nanofibers, and Graphene. *Materials (Basel)*, *14*(20), 5978. doi:10.3390/ma14205978 PMID:34683568

Ghaderi, S., Ramesh, B., & Seifalian, A. M. (2011). Fluorescence nanoparticles "quantum dots" as drug delivery system and their toxicity: A review. *Journal of Drug Targeting*, *19*(7), 475–486. doi:10.3109/1061186X.2010.526227 PMID:20964619

Govender, T., Stolnik, S., Garnett, M. C., Illum, L., & Davis, S. S. (1999). PLGA nanoparticles prepared by nanoprecipitation: Drug loading and release studies of a water-soluble drug. *Journal of Controlled Release*, *57*(2), 171–185. doi:10.1016/S0168-3659(98)00116-3 PMID:9971898

Grammatikopoulos, P., Steinhauer, S., Vernieres, J., Singh, V., & Sowwan, M. (2016). Nanoparticle design by gas-phase synthesis. *Advances in Physics: X, 1*(1), 81–100. doi:10.1080/23746149.2016.1142829

Grislain, L., Couvreur, P., Lenaerts, V., Roland, M., Deprez-Decampeneere, D., & Speiser, P. (1983). Pharmacokinetics and distribution of a biodegradable drug carrier. *International Journal of Pharmaceutics, 15*(3), 335–345. doi:10.1016/0378-5173(83)90166-7

Gupta, V., Mohapatra, S., Mishra, H., Farooq, U., Kumar, K., Ansari, M. J., & lqbal, Z. (2022). Nanotechnology in cosmetics and cosmeceuticals—A review of latest advancements. *Gels (Basel, Switzerland), 8*(3), 173. doi:10.3390/gels8030173 PMID:35323286

Iannazzo, D., Pistone, A., Salamò, M., Galvagno, S., Romeo, R., Giofré, S. V., Branca, C., Visalli, G., & Di Pietro, A. (2017). Graphene quantum dots for cancer targeted drug delivery. *International Journal of Pharmaceutics, 518*(1–2), 185–192. doi:10.1016/j.ijpharm.2016.12.060 PMID:28057464

Jafernik, K., Ladniak, A., Blicharska, E., Czarnek, K., Ekiert, H., Wiącek, A. E., & Szopa, A. (2023). Chitosan-Based Nanoparticles as Effective Drug Delivery Systems—A review. *Molecules (Basel, Switzerland), 28*(4), 1963. doi:10.3390/molecules28041963 PMID:36838951

Jeong, S. H., Lim, D., Kim, K., Kang, E., Lim, S., Ricci, J., Sung, S., & Kwon, M. (2016). A comprehensive evaluation of carboxylated nanodiamond as a topical drug delivery system. *International Journal of Nanomedicine, 2381*, 2381. doi:10.2147/IJN.S104859

Jethara, S., Patel, M., & Patel, Al. (2014). Sustained Release Drug Delivery Systems: A Patent Overview. *Aperito Journal of Drug Designing and Pharmacology, 1*, 1–14.

Jha, R., Singh, A., Sharma, P. K., & Fuloria, N. K. (2020). Smart carbon nanotubes for drug delivery system: A comprehensive study. *Journal of Drug Delivery Science and Technology, 58*, 101811. doi:10.1016/j.jddst.2020.101811

Juhairiyah, F., & de Lange, E. C. M. (2021). Understanding Drug Delivery to the Brain Using Liposome-Based Strategies: Studies that Provide Mechanistic Insights Are Essential. *The AAPS Journal, 23*(6), 114. doi:10.120812248-021-00648-z PMID:34713363

Koo, O. M., Rubinstein, I., & Onyuksel, H. (2005). Role of nanotechnology in targeted drug delivery and imaging: A concise review. *Nanomedicine; Nanotechnology, Biology, and Medicine, 1*(3), 193–212. doi:10.1016/j.nano.2005.06.004 PMID:17292079

Kościk, I., Jankowski, D., & Jagusiak, A. (2021). Carbon Nanomaterials for Theranostic Use. *C, 8*(1), 3. doi:10.3390/c8010003

Kousar, K., Naseer, F., Abduh, M. S., Kakar, S., Gul, R., Anjum, S., & Ahmad, T. (2023). Green synthesis of hyaluronic acid coated, thiolated chitosan nanoparticles for CD44 targeted delivery and sustained release of Cisplatin in cervical carcinoma. *Frontiers in Pharmacology, 13*, 1073004. doi:10.3389/fphar.2022.1073004 PMID:36712656

Kreuter, J., Ramge, P., Petrov, V., Hamm, S., Gelperina, S. E., Engelhardt, B., Alyautdin, R., von Briesen, H., & Begley, D. J. (2003). Direct evidence that polysorbate-80-coated poly(butyl cyanoacrylate) nanoparticles deliver drugs to the CNS via specific mechanisms requiring prior binding of the drug to the nanoparticles. *Pharmaceutical Research*, *20*(3), 409–416. doi:10.1023/A:1022604120952 PMID:12669961

Kumar, K. P. S., Bhowmik, D., Srivastava, S., Paswan, S., & Dutta, A. S. (2012). Sustained Release Drug Delivery System Potential. *The Pharma Innovation*, *1*(2), 48–60.

Lamprecht, A. L. F., Ubrich, N., Yamamoto, H., Schäfer, U., Takeuchi, H., Maincent, P., & Lehr, C. M. (2001). Biodegradable nanoparticles for targeted drug delivery in the treatment of inflammatory bowel disease. *The Journal of Pharmacology and Experimental Therapeutics*, *299*(2), 775–781. PMID:11602694

Lee, J. H., & Yeo, Y. (2015). Controlled drug release from pharmaceutical nanocarriers. *Chemical Engineering Science*, *125*, 75–84. doi:10.1016/j.ces.2014.08.046 PMID:25684779

Li, S., Li, W., & Khashab, N. (2012). Stimuli-responsive nanomaterials for controlled release applications. *Nanotechnology Reviews*, *1*(6), 493–513. doi:10.1515/ntrev-2012-0033

Li, Z., Xu, K., Qin, L., Zhao, D., Yang, N., Wang, D., & Yang, Y. (2023). Hollow Nanomaterials in Advanced Drug Delivery Systems: From Single-to Multiple Shells. *Advanced Materials*, *35*(12), 2203890. doi:10.1002/adma.202203890 PMID:35998336

Libby, P., & Ridker, P. M. (2004). Inflammation and atherosclerosis: Role of C-Reactive protein in risk assessment. *The American Journal of Medicine*, *116*(6), 9–16. doi:10.1016/j.amjmed.2004.02.006 PMID:15050187

Liu, G. W., Guzman, E. B., Menon, N., & Langer, R. S. (2023). Lipid Nanoparticles for Nucleic Acid Delivery to Endothelial Cells. *Pharmaceutical Research*, *40*(1), 3–25. doi:10.100711095-023-03471-7 PMID:36735106

Liu, J., Huang, Y., Kumar, A., Tan, A., Jin, S., Mozhi, A., & Liang, X.-J. (2014). pH-Sensitive nanosystems for drug delivery in cancer therapy. *Biotechnology Advances*, *32*(4), 693–710. doi:10.1016/j.biotechadv.2013.11.009 PMID:24309541

Lockman, P. R., Mumper, R. J., Khan, M. A., & Allen, D. D. (2002). Nanoparticle technology for drug delivery across the blood-brain barrier. *Drug Development and Industrial Pharmacy*, *28*(1), 1–13. doi:10.1081/DDC-120001481 PMID:11858519

Magenheim, B., Levy, M. Y., & Benita, S. (1993). A new in vitro technique for evaluating drug release profile from colloidal carriers-ultrafiltration technique at low pressure. *International Journal of Pharmaceutics*, *94*(1-3), 115–123. doi:10.1016/0378-5173(93)90015-8

Maiti, D., Tong, X., Mou, X., & Yang, K. (2019). Carbon-Based Nanomaterials for Biomedical Applications: A Recent Study. *Frontiers in Pharmacology*, *9*, 1401. doi:10.3389/fphar.2018.01401 PMID:30914959

Mascolo, M. C., Pei, Y., & Ring, T. A. (2013). Room temperature co-precipitation synthesis of magnetite nanoparticles in a large pH window with different bases. *Materials (Basel)*, *6*(12), 5549–5567. doi:10.3390/ma6125549 PMID:28788408

Mihranyan, A., Ferraz, N., & Stromme, M. (2012). Current status and prospects of nanotechnology in cosmetics. *Progress in Materials Science*, *57*(5), 875–910. doi:10.1016/j.pmatsci.2011.10.001

Miyata, K., Christie, R. J., & Kataoka, K. (2011). Polymeric micelles for nano-scale drug delivery. *Reactive & Functional Polymers*, *71*(3), 227–234. doi:10.1016/j.reactfunctpolym.2010.10.009

Mohammed, H. A., Khan, R. A., Singh, V., Yusuf, M., Akhtar, N., Sulaiman, G. M., & Al-Subaiyel, A. M. (2023). Solid lipid nanoparticles for targeted natural and synthetic drugs delivery in high-incidence cancers, and other diseases: Roles of preparation methods, lipid composition, transitional stability, and release profiles in nanocarriers' development. *Nanotechnology Reviews*, *12*(1), 20220517 doi:10.1515/ntrev-2022-0517

Mukherjee, S., Ray, S., & Thakur, R. S. (2009). Solid lipid nanoparticles: A modern formulation approach in drug delivery system. *Indian Journal of Pharmaceutical Sciences*, *71*(4), 349–358. doi:10.4103/0250-474X.57282 PMID:20502539

Müller, R., Maaben, S., Weyhers, H., & Mehnert, W. (1996). Phagocytic uptake and cytotoxicity of solid lipid nanoparticles (SLN) sterically stabilized with poloxamine 908 and poloxamer 407. *Journal of Drug Targeting*, *4*(3), 161–170. doi:10.3109/10611869609015973 PMID:8959488

Mura, S., Nicolas, J., & Couvreur, P. (2013). Stimuli-responsive nanocarriers for drug delivery. *Nature Materials*, *12*(11), 991–1003. doi:10.1038/nmat3776 PMID:24150417

Nana, A. B. A., Marimuthu, T., Kondiah, P. P. D., Choonara, Y. E., Du Toit, L. C., & Pillay, V. (2019). Multifunctional Magnetic Nanowires: Design, Fabrication, and Future Prospects as Cancer Therapeutics. *Cancers (Basel)*, *11*(12), 1956. doi:10.3390/cancers11121956 PMID:31817598

Narayanaswamy, R., & Torchilin, V. P. (2019). Hydrogels and Their Applications in Targeted Drug Delivery. *Molecules (Basel, Switzerland)*, *24*(3), 603. doi:10.3390/molecules24030603 PMID:30744011

Ouyang, Z., Gao, Y., Shen, M., & Shi, X. (2021). Dendrimer-based nanohybrids in cancer photomedicine. *Materials Today. Bio*, *10*, 100111. doi:10.1016/j.mtbio.2021.100111 PMID:34027382

Pantidos, N., & Horsfall, L. E. (2014). Biological synthesis of metallic nanoparticles by bacteria, fungi, and plants. *Journal of Nanomedicine & Nanotechnology*, *5*(233). Advance online publication. doi:10.4172/2157-7439.1000233

Panyam, J., & Labhasetwar, V. (2003). Biodegradable nanoparticles for drug and gene delivery to cells and tissue. *Advanced Drug Delivery Reviews*, *55*(3), 329–347. doi:10.1016/S0169-409X(02)00228-4 PMID:12628320

Patra, J. K., Das, G., Fraceto, L. F., Campos, E. V. R., Rodriguez-Torres, M. del P., Acosta-Torres, L. S., Diaz-Torres, L. A., Grillo, R., Swamy, M. K., Sharma, S., Habtemariam, S., & Shin, H.-S. (2018). Nano based drug delivery systems: Recent developments and prospects. *Journal of Nanobiotechnology*, *16*(1), 71. doi:10.118612951-018-0392-8 PMID:30231877

Peer, D., & Lieberman, J. (2011). Special delivery: Targeted therapy with small RNAs. *Gene Therapy*, *18*(12), 1127–1133. doi:10.1038/gt.2011.56 PMID:21490679

Peng, T., Xu, W., Li, Q., Ding, Y., & Huang, Y. (2023). Pharmaceutical liposomal delivery—Specific considerations of innovation and challenges. *Biomaterials Science*, *11*(1), 62–75. doi:10.1039/D2BM01252A PMID:36373563

Peracchia, M. T., Gref, R., Minamitake, Y., Domb, A., Lotan, N., & Langer, R. (1997). PEG-coated nanospheres from amphiphilic diblock and multiblock copolymers: Investigation of their drug encapsulation and release characteristics. *Journal of Controlled Release*, *46*(3), 223–231. doi:10.1016/S0168-3659(96)01597-0

Perevedentseva, E., Lin, Y.-C., & Cheng, C.-L. (2021). A review of recent advances in nanodiamond-mediated drug delivery in cancer. *Expert Opinion on Drug Delivery*, *18*(3), 369–382. doi:10.1080/17425247.2021.1832988 PMID:33047984

Pinheiro, R. G. R., Coutinho, A. J., Pinheiro, M., & Neves, A. R. (2021). Nanoparticles for Targeted Brain Drug Delivery: What Do We Know? *International Journal of Molecular Sciences*, *22*(21), 11654. doi:10.3390/ijms222111654 PMID:34769082

Pitt, C. G., Gratzl, M. M., Kimmel, G. L., Surles, J., & Schindler, A. (1981). Aliphatic polyesters II. The degradation of poly (DL-lactide), poly (epsilon-caprolactone), and their copolymers in vivo. *Biomaterials*, *2*(4), 215–220. doi:10.1016/0142-9612(81)90060-0 PMID:7326315

Pondman, K. M., Bunt, N. D., Maijenburg, A. W., van Wezel, R. J. A., Kishore, U., Abelmann, L., ten Elshof, J. E., & ten Haken, B. (2015). Magnetic drug delivery with FePd nanowires. *Journal of Magnetism and Magnetic Materials*, *380*, 299–306. doi:10.1016/j.jmmm.2014.10.101

Pourmadadi, M., Ahmadi, M., & Yazdian, F. (2023). Synthesis of a novel pH-responsive Fe3O4/chitosan/agarose double nanoemulsion as a promising Nanocarrier with sustained release of curcumin to treat MCF-7 cell line. *International Journal of Biological Macromolecules*, *235*, 123786. doi:10.1016/j.ijbiomac.2023.123786 PMID:36828092

Pourmadadi, M., Yazdian, F., Koulivand, A., & Rahmani, E. (2023). Green synthesized polyvinylpyrrolidone/titanium dioxide hydrogel nanocomposite modified with agarose macromolecules for sustained and pH-responsive anticancer drug release. *International Journal of Biological Macromolecules*, *240*, 124345. doi:10.1016/j.ijbiomac.2023.124345 PMID:37054860

Raffi, M., Rumaiz, A. K., Hasan, M. M., & Shah, S. I. (2007). Studies of the growth parameters for silver nanoparticle synthesis by inert gas condensation. *Journal of Materials Research*, *22*(12), 3378–3384. doi:10.1557/JMR.2007.0420

Rahdar Abbas, K. S. A. F. (2018). Pluronic as nano-carrier platform for drug delivery systems. *Nanomed Res J*, *3*(4), 174–179.

Rajaei, M., Rashedi, H., Yazdian, F., Navaei-Nigjeh, M., Rahdar, A., & Díez-Pascual, A. M. (2023). Chitosan/agarose/graphene oxide nanohydrogel as drug delivery system of 5-fluorouracil in breast cancer therapy. *Journal of Drug Delivery Science and Technology*, *82*, 104307. doi:10.1016/j.jddst.2023.104307

Rane, A. V., Kanny, K., Abitha, V. K., & Thomas, S. (2018). Methods for synthesis of nanoparticles and fabrication of nanocomposites. In *Synthesis of inorganic nanomaterials* (pp. 121–139). Woodhead Publishing. doi:10.1016/B978-0-08-101975-7.00005-1

Redhead, H. M., Davis, S. S., & Illum, L. (2001). Drug delivery in poly (lactide-co-glycolide) nanoparticles surface modified with poloxamer 407 and poloxamine 908: In vitro characterisation and in vivo evaluation. *Journal of Controlled Release*, *70*(3), 353–363. doi:10.1016/S0168-3659(00)00367-9 PMID:11182205

Safi, I. (2000). Recent aspects concerning DC reactive magnetron sputtering of thin films: A review. *Surface and Coatings Technology*, *127*(2-3), 203–218. doi:10.1016/S0257-8972(00)00566-1

Sahoo, S. K., & Labhasetwar, V. (2003). Nanotech approaches to drug delivery and imaging. *Drug Discovery Today*, *8*(24), 1112–1120. doi:10.1016/S1359-6446(03)02903-9 PMID:14678737

Sau, S., Alsaab, H. O., Bhise, K., Alzhrani, R., Nabil, G., & Iyer, A. K. (2018). Multifunctional nanoparticles for cancer immunotherapy: A groundbreaking approach for reprogramming malfunctioned tumor environment. *Journal of Controlled Release*, *274*, 24–34. doi:10.1016/j.jconrel.2018.01.028 PMID:29391232

Semaltianos, N. G. (2010). Nanoparticles by laser ablation. *Critical Reviews in Solid State and Material Sciences*, *35*(2), 105–124. doi:10.1080/10408431003788233

Shete, H. K., Prabhu, R. H., & Patravale, V. B. (2014). Endosomal Escape: A Bottleneck in Intracellular Delivery. *Journal of Nanoscience and Nanotechnology*, *14*(1), 460–474. doi:10.1166/jnn.2014.9082 PMID:24730275

Silva, N. P., M. F. P., & C. M. (2012). Dendrimers as potential platforms in nanotechnology-based drug delivery systems. *IOSR Journal of Pharmacy*, *2*(5), 23–30. doi:10.9790/3013-25602330

Silva, P., Bonifácio, B., Ramos, M., Negri, K., Maria Bauab, T., & Chorilli, M. (2013). Nanotechnology-based drug delivery systems and herbal medicines: A review. *International Journal of Nanomedicine*, *1*, 1. doi:10.2147/IJN.S52634

Singh, R., & Lillard, J. W. Jr. (2009). Nanoparticle-based targeted drug delivery. *Experimental and Molecular Pathology*, *86*(3), 215–223. doi:10.1016/j.yexmp.2008.12.004 PMID:19186176

Slowing, I. I., Trewyn, B. G., & Lin, V. S. (2007). Mesoporous silica nanoparticles for intracellular delivery of membrane-impermeable proteins. *Journal of the American Chemical Society*, *129*(28), 8845–8849. doi:10.1021/ja0719780 PMID:17589996

Soni, S., Ruhela, R. K., & Medhi, B. (2016). Nanomedicine in Central Nervous System (CNS) Disorders: A Present and Future Prospective. *Advanced Pharmaceutical Bulletin*, *6*(3), 319–335. doi:10.15171/apb.2016.044 PMID:27766216

Spadari, C. C., Lanser, D. M., Araújo, M. V., De Jesus, D. F., Lopes, L. B., Gelli, A., & Ishida, K. (2023). Oral delivery of brain-targeted miltefosine-loaded alginate nanoparticles functionalized with polysorbate 80 to treat cryptococcal meningitis. *The Journal of Antimicrobial Chemotherapy*, *78*(4), 1092–1101. doi:10.1093/jac/dkad053 PMID:36881722

Sun, Q., Sun, X., Ma, X., Zhou, Z., Jin, E., Zhang, B., Shen, Y., Van Kirk, E. A., Murdoch, W. J., Lott, J. R., Lodge, T. P., Radosz, M., & Zhao, Y. (2014). Integration of Nanoassembly Functions for an Effective Delivery Cascade for Cancer Drugs. *Advanced Materials*, *26*(45), 7615–7621. doi:10.1002/adma.201401554 PMID:25328159

Suryanarayana, C., & Prabhu, B. (2007). Synthesis of nanostructured materials by inert-gas condensation methods. In *Nanostructured materials* (pp. 47–90). William Andrew Publishing. doi:10.1016/B978-081551534-0.50004-X

Tojo, C., de Dios, M., & Barroso, F. (2010). Surfactant effects on microemulsion-based nanoparticle synthesis. *Materials (Basel)*, *4*(1), 55–72. doi:10.3390/ma4010055 PMID:28879976

Tong, R., & Langer, R. (2015). Nanomedicines Targeting the Tumor Microenvironment. *Cancer Journal (Sudbury, Mass.)*, *21*(4), 314–321. doi:10.1097/PPO.0000000000000123 PMID:26222084

Torchilin, V. (2006). Multifunctional nanocarriers☆. *Advanced Drug Delivery Reviews*, *58*(14), 1532–1555. doi:10.1016/j.addr.2006.09.009 PMID:17092599

Upadhyay, R. K. (2014). Drug Delivery Systems, CNS Protection, and the Blood Brain Barrier. *BioMed Research International*, *2014*, 1–37. doi:10.1155/2014/869269 PMID:25136634

Vashist, A., Vashist, A., Gupta, Y. K., & Ahmad, S. (2014). Recent advances in hydrogel based drug delivery systems for the human body. *Journal of Materials Chemistry. B*, *2*(2), 147–166. doi:10.1039/C3TB21016B PMID:32261602

Vasir, J., & Labhasetwar, V. (2007). Biodegradable nanoparticles for cytosolic delivery of therapeutics☆. *Advanced Drug Delivery Reviews*, *59*(8), 718–728. doi:10.1016/j.addr.2007.06.003 PMID:17683826

Verma, I. M., & Weitzman, M. D. (2005). GENE THERAPY: Twenty-First Century Medicine. *Annual Review of Biochemistry*, *74*(1), 711–738. doi:10.1146/annurev.biochem.74.050304.091637 PMID:15952901

Wang, A. Z., Langer, R., & Farokhzad, O. C. (2012). Nanoparticle Delivery of Cancer Drugs. *Annual Review of Medicine*, *63*(1), 185–198. doi:10.1146/annurev-med-040210-162544 PMID:21888516

Wang, Z., Deng, X., Ding, J., Zhou, W., Zheng, X., & Tang, G. (2018). Mechanisms of drug release in pH-sensitive micelles for tumor-targeted drug delivery system: A review. *International Journal of Pharmaceutics*, *535*(1–2), 253–260. doi:10.1016/j.ijpharm.2017.11.003 PMID:29113804

Yin, H., Kanasty, R. L., Eltoukhy, A. A., Vegas, A. J., Dorkin, J. R., & Anderson, D. G. (2014). Non-viral vectors for gene-based therapy. *Nature Reviews. Genetics*, *15*(8), 541–555. doi:10.1038/nrg3763 PMID:25022906

Zhang, X., Meng, L., Lu, Q., Fei, Z., & Dyson, P. J. (2009). Targeted delivery and controlled release of doxorubicin to cancer cells using modified single-wall carbon nanotubes. *Biomaterials*, *30*(30), 6041–6047. doi:10.1016/j.biomaterials.2009.07.025 PMID:19643474

Zheng, Y., Hong, X., Wang, J., Feng, L., Fan, T., Guo, R., & Zhang, H. (2021). 2D Nanomaterials for Tissue Engineering and Regenerative Nanomedicines: Recent Advances and Future Challenges. *Advanced Healthcare Materials*, *10*(7), 2001743. doi:10.1002/adhm.202001743 PMID:33511775

Zhu, Y., Li, J., Li, W., Zhang, Y., Yang, X., Chen, N., Sun, Y., Zhao, Y., Fan, C., & Huang, Q. (2012). The Biocompatibility of Nanodiamonds and Their Application in Drug Delivery Systems. *Theranostics*, *2*(3), 302–312. doi:10.7150/thno.3627 PMID:22509196

Zhu, Y., Wang, B., Chen, J., He, J., & Qiu, X. (2023). Facile Synthesis of Three Types of Mesoporous Silica Microspheres as Drug Delivery Carriers and their Sustained-Release Properties. *Current Drug Delivery*, *20*(9), 1337–1350. doi:10.2174/1567201819666220616121602 PMID:35713141

Zong, Q., Dong, N., Yang, X., Ling, G., & Zhang, P. (2021). Development of gold nanorods for cancer treatment. *Journal of Inorganic Biochemistry*, *220*, 111458. doi:10.1016/j.jinorgbio.2021.111458 PMID:33857697

Chapter 15
Bacterial Exopolysaccharides-Based Nanomaterials for Targeting Biofilm-Associated Infections:
Bacterial Nanomaterials

Anand Ravichandran
Rajalakshmi Engineering College, India

D. Shobana
Rajalakshmi Engineering College, India

S. Visudha
Rajalakshmi Engineering College, India

Yazhini
Rajalakshmi Engineering College, India

S. Niveditha
Rajalakshmi Engineering College, India

P. Saravanan
https://orcid.org/0000-0002-1935-4381
Centre of Excellence in Biofilms, Department of Biotechnology, Rajalakshmi Engineering College, India

ABSTRACT

Bacteria that secrete exopolysaccharides (EPS) when colonised on living and non-living surfaces also protect from stressors in a variety of environments. EPS is considered a complex carbohydrate, which is part of their extracellular matrix. EPS play magnificent roles in microbial biofilm formation, providing structural integrity and protection for microbial communities. Chemically synthesised nanomaterials are not ideal for use as antimicrobial agents because they are harmful to environments and also ineffective. An alternative, sustainable approach is needed to control biofilm-related infections. Therefore, in this chapter, the authors discuss the techniques of optimisation and characterization of bacterial exopolysaccharide-mediated nanoparticles and nanomaterials for targeting oral biofilm-forming pathogens. It will be essential for the use of exopolysaccharide-mediated nanoparticles in biomedical applications to prevent biofilm-associated infections such as urinary catheter devices and biofilm-related chronic wounds.

DOI: 10.4018/979-8-3693-0448-8.ch015

1. INTRODUCTION

Bacteria that secrete exopolysaccharides (EPS) when colonized or attached to living and non-living surfaces also protect from stressors in a variety of environments. EPS is considered a complex carbohydrate that is part of their extracellular matrix and plays a magnificent role in microbial biofilm formation, providing structural integrity and thus allowing cell-cell contact and protection for microbial communities. The main functions of EPS are involved in the survival strategy of bacteria, allowing them to withstand harsh conditions and resist antimicrobial agents. Biofilm-related infections are broadly categorised into medical dwelling device-related infections and non-device-related infections. Studying biofilms is crucial for developing effective strategies to combat infections and maintain a disease-free environment. Bacterial EPS possess unique chemical compositions and structures, including variations in monosaccharide composition, glycosidic linkages, and branching arrangement of structure patterns. These structural characteristics can be tailored using recent advanced genetic engineering technology, resulting in EPS with specific properties suitable for nanomaterial applications. EPS has biocompatibility, biodegradability, self-assembly capabilities, and functional groups that allow for further modification. Bacterial EPS can be easily connected to fabricate nanoparticles and nanostructures with controlled sizes and shapes. For instance, EPS can serve as templates for the synthesis of metal or metal oxide nanoparticles, such as gold or iron oxide, by either reducing or complexing metal ions. EPS-based nanomaterials can also be produced through self-assembly or crosslinking methods, yielding nanogels, nanofibers, or nanoporous materials (Umut et al. 2020). EPS-based nanomaterials play a significant role in various biomedical applications (Sivakumar et al. 2014). EPS can be used as scaffolds or coatings in tissue engineering to promote cellular activity. Also, EPS's ability to easily react with the host, restrict the immune rejections, and mimic the extracellular matrix make them valuable in wound healing and tissue regeneration applications (Vaningelgem et al. 2004).

Researchers critically examined the aquatic biofilms, which primarily contained exopolysaccharides (EPS) with other small particles of silt, clay, oxidised products, etc.; the composition of these matrix components also differed from the nature of the environments in which the biofilm formed (Rodney M. 2016). The cellular components of the aquatic biofilm matrix consist of multispecies bacteria and water diatoms. These multispecies bacteria provide numerous functions, such as i) structural support, ii) sharing their nutrients, iii) evading the immune system, and iv) resisting different antibiotics to protect them from external shear forces. The biofilm matrix is usually made up of exopolysaccharides, proteins, lipids, nucleic acids (eDNA), metal ions, etc. (Jefferson 2004). Most of the substances present in the matrix are called extracellular polymeric substances, or exopolysaccharides (EPS). The EPS act as the molecular support to develop complex, three-dimensional structures that are resilient and attached to the biofilm's communities. The main advantages of the secreted EPS are its ability to survive in harsh environmental conditions, especially in terms of protection, which may have possible commercial applications in industrial processes. The main advantages of the secreted EPS are its ability to survive in harsh environmental conditions, especially in terms of protection, which may have possible commercial applications in industrial processes. Also, proteins, pili proteins, and extracellular DNA were majorly involved in causing the virulence for biofilm formation. These proteins and DNA were primarily involved in cell-cell signalling in the biofilm, which is part of communication between the species to co-habit mutually and strongly (Flemming et al., 2007; McDougald et al., 2012). In addition, the biofilm matrix possesses numerous virulence factors to protect it from harsh conditions (Govindarajan and Kandaswamy, 2022, 2023).

Figure 1. Matrix disruption by random enzymatic reactions and dispersion to start a new cycle

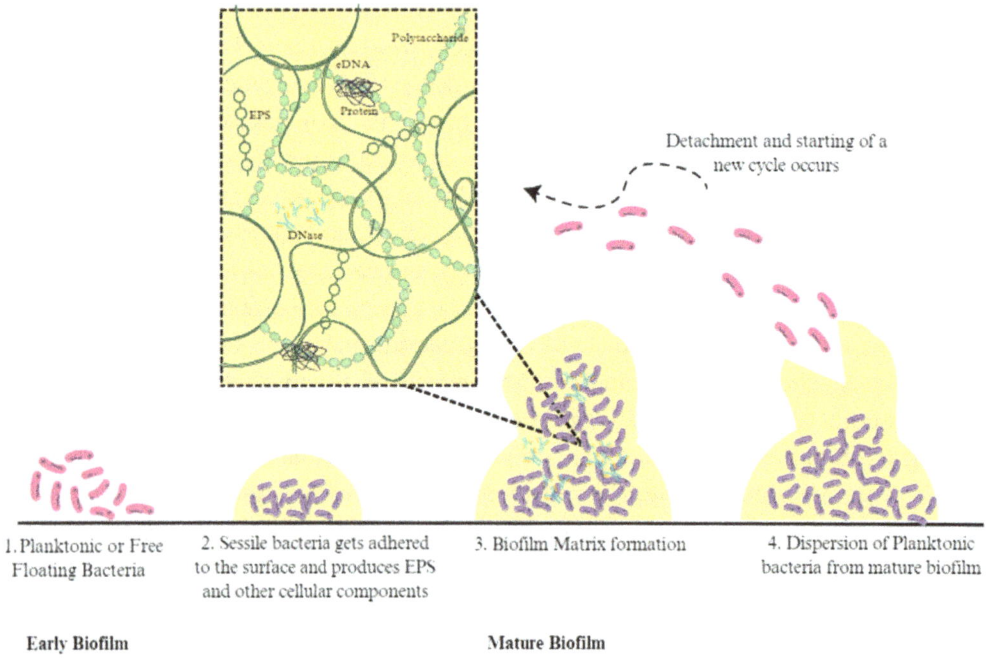

There are five steps involved in the formation of biofilms on surfaces: (1) It begins with the temporary colonisation of planktonic bacteria in wet, conditioned areas; (2) the establishment of cell aggregates leads to monolayer formation and the secretion of extracellular polysaccharides (slime). (3) formation of microcolonies and multilayer clustered cells (4) growth of three-dimensional mushroom-shaped biofilms and mature biofilms; (5) matrix disruption by random enzymatic reactions and dispersion to start a new cycle as shown in Figure 1.

The use of antibiotics to treat several biofilm related infections results become antibiotics resistance and ineffective treatment. There is an alternative sustainable approach is needed to eradicate the biofilm associated infection with low cost. EPS-based nanomaterials have shown great promise not only in biomedical applications but also in the fields of environmental remediation and nanobiotechnology. These nanomaterials possess unique properties, allowing them to encapsulate and protect therapeutic agents, leading to improved drug delivery systems with controlled release capabilities manner(Makabenta et al. 2021). Through genetic engineering and strain selection, researchers can tailor the composition and structure of EPS to create nanoparticles that enhance drug binding efficiency, increase bioavailability, and target specific cells or tissues, thereby reducing side effects and improving therapeutic outcomes (Li et al. 2017). Additionally, EPS-based nanomaterials exhibit excellent potential in water purification and pollutant removal, owing to their biodegradability and ability to bind to heavy metals and pollutants. These nanocomposites can selectively capture and sequester contaminants, contributing to effective environmental remediation and safer water sources (Verastegui et al. 2014). Furthermore, EPS modifications enable the production of nanomaterials with specific electronic and catalytic properties, suitable for applications in sensors, energy storage devices, and catalytic reactors, thereby advancing various technological fields. However, careful consideration of safety and biocompatibility is paramount for medical and environmental uses, necessitating rigorous testing and assessment to ensure they are safe integration into practical applications. In the field of nanobiotechnology it is essential to address scaling up production challenges and fully unlock the potential of EPS-based nanomaterials for a wide range of applications without compromising safety and efficiency.

In order to control the biofilm bacteria causing infections, it is essential to consume antibiotics that could eradicate the infections. There is a lot of attention focused on biofilm-associated infection-causing microorganisms increased resistance to antimicrobial agents and host immune evasion, leading to persistent infection. Due to the complexity of the biofilm community that resides in the human oral cavity, antimicrobial agents are not retained at the proper concentrations for long durations. Therefore, it is becoming very necessary to choose an alternative solution to the infections caused by biofilm. Nanotechnology is a fast-emerging and growing field in medicine and pharmaceuticals that uses metals to synthesise nanoparticles. The broad spectrum of metallic nanoparticles, their small size and shape, and their biocidal properties greatly influence their antimicrobial activity and also act as drug delivery vehicles for anti-biofilm therapeutics. This chapter aims to characterise nanoparticles and nanomaterials from novel bacterial exopolysaccharides through green synthesis to develop new therapeutic strategies or treatments for the control of biofilm-associated infections.

2. THE ROLE OF EXOPOLYSACCHARIDES IN BIOMEDICAL APPLICATIONS

Antibiofilm Agents:

EPS can act as carriers for drug targets due to their encapsulation characteristics and controlled release capabilities. The main role of EPS is to enhance their stability and provide sustainability and release at the specific target site. EPS or EPS-based nanoparticles can exhibit antimicrobial properties, which can mitigate bacterial infections. EPS can disrupt biofilm formation, inhibit bacterial adhesion, and enhance the efficacy of antimicrobial agents (Sutherland 1996; Chew et al. 2014).

Nanomaterials or Nanoparticles based exopolysaccharides can physically interact with the target EPS matrix of specific pathogen and compromise its stability and integrity. Loss of EPS stability leads to weakens the biofilm structure, when it interacts vulnerably by antimicrobial agents or the host's immune system. Intercellular channels and EPS of the biofilm matrix prevent bacterial dehydration and offer defence against external threats, such as antibiotics and other stresses (Karnwal et al. 2023). EPS of the biofilm matrix also facilitate horizontal gene transfer which results to increased antibiotic resistance (Netrusov et al. 2023). Some exopolysaccharide-based nanomaterials can obstruct the early adhesion of microbes to surfaces, preventing the biofilm development process in its tracks. These nanoparticles can facilitate the separation of existing biofilms from surfaces. The germs, which can be pathogenic bacteria, fungi, and maybe viruses are more easily removed and destroyed when the biofilm structure is compromised (Karnwal et al. 2023).

Antibiotics or antimicrobial peptides are only a few examples of antimicrobial agents that can be enclosed in EPS-based nanomaterials to increase the efficiency of the interact with biofilm matrix easily. Due to the distribution of antimicrobial agents and quickly respond to the biofilm location made possible by this encapsulation, treatment effectiveness is increased while the potential for side effects on nearby tissues is reduced(Zhang et al. 2010). Bacteria produce quorum sensing molecule involved in cell-cell communication when it reaches threshold limit of cell numbers during biofilm formation. It has been discovered that some exopolysaccharides interfere with this process. EPS-based nanomaterials

Figure 2. Exopolysaccharides in biomedical applications

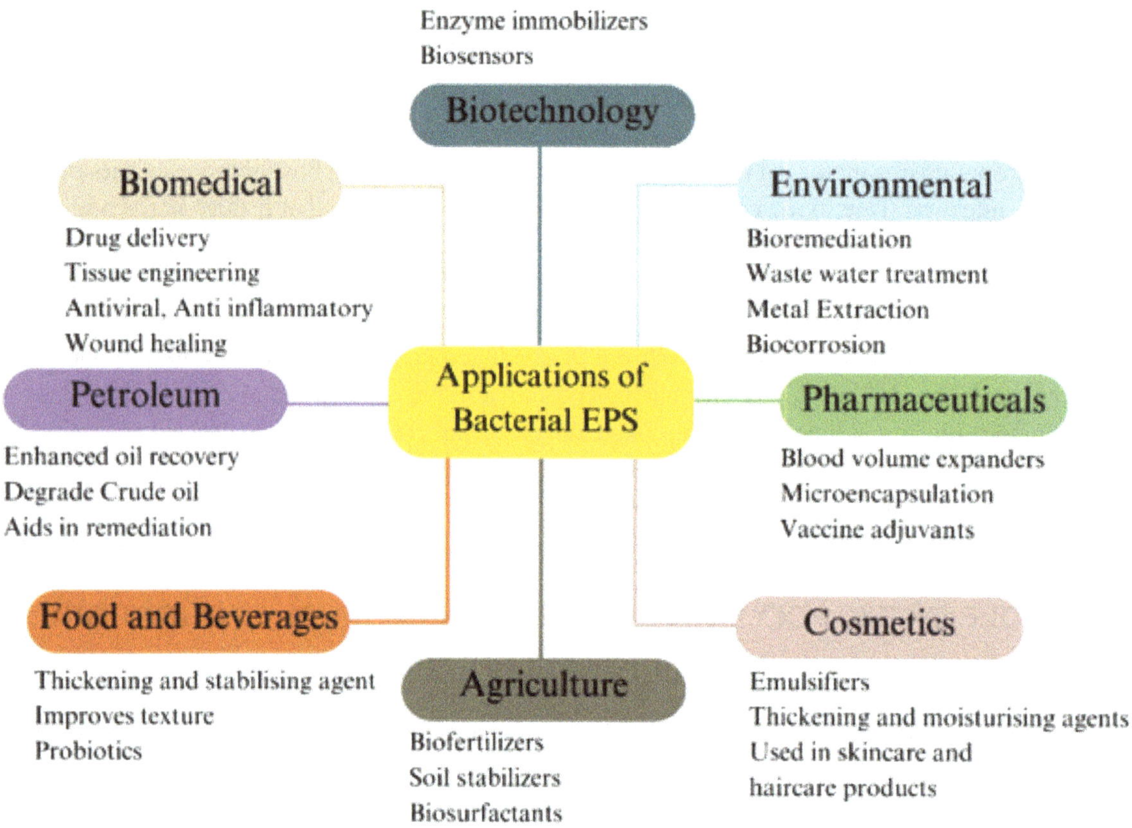

can obstruct the maturation and development of biofilms by interfering with quorum sensing (Abdalla et al. 2021). Exopolysaccharides are frequently found in nature and are biocompatible, making them appropriate for use in biomedical applications as shown Figure 2.

Biosensors:

EPS-based biosensors have been developed for the detection of pathogens, toxins, or other analytes. EPS can provide a stable and selective sensing platform due to their recognition properties, which can be used for diagnostic purposes. EPS have been investigated for dental applications, including remineralization of enamel, prevention of dental caries, and inhibition of biofilm formation on teeth surfaces. EPS-based materials can be incorporated into dental products for improved oral health (Rao et al. 2013).

Wound healing agents:

EPS can be incorporated into dressings and wound care products to modulate the immune response, promote tissue regeneration, and prevent infections. EPS-based dressings can create a favourable environment for wound healing. It is necessary to pay an attention is required to fully to know the properties, mechanisms of action, and safety profiles of bacterial EPS in biomedical applications. However, the unique characteristics of EPS make them promising candidates for various biomedical purposes, and ongoing studies are exploring their potential for improved therapeutic strategies. EPS nanomaterials can be employed to penetrate and disrupt the biofilm matrix, improve the targets of specific antibacterial agents to eradicate the bacteria causing the infection and enhanced the wound healing. EPS can modulate the immune response, making them potential candidates for immunotherapeutic applications. They can stimulate or suppress immune cells, regulate cytokine production, and enhance wound healing by promoting angiogenesis and tissue regeneration (Algburi et al. 2021).

Dwelling Medical device related infections:

Bacteria colonized in medical related surfaces causing severe infections resulting become very difficult to eradicated it. There are many numbers of microorganism strictly attached to cause in both medical instruments (devices) and non-instrument (devices) or tissue related infections for examples lungs, skin and oral enamel surfaces. In medical practice, catheters are also widely used. Urinary catheter-associated infections are the most frequent among them and are typically brought on by species of gram negative, positive organisms and inner cross kingdom *Candida* (Nicolle, 2014). Contrarily, the bacterial species that are often detected in central venous catheters are gram positive pathogens such as *S. epidermidis* and *S. aureus* (Donlan & Costerton, 2002). EPS nanomaterials can be utilized to prevent biofilm adhesion to the catheter surface or to disrupt the established biofilm, reducing the risk of catheter-associated infections. The unique properties of EPS nanomaterials, including their ability to penetrate biofilm matrices, interact with bacteria, and deliver therapeutic agents, make them attractive candidates for combating biofilm infections.

EPS-based nanomaterials can disrupt the EPS matrix that protects bacteria in biofilms by targeting and degrading it. The advantage of nanomaterials is their ability to permeate through the compartments of biofilms and quickly connect the components of bacteria in the interior parts of the matrix since the pore width of biofilms typically ranges between 50 and 100 nm (Sahli et al. 2022). Consequently, bacteria are successfully eliminated, and further infections are avoided. Recent developments in nanomaterial-based methods have made it possible for the EPS-based nanomaterials to control trained immunity, which is the body's immune system's ability to better protect against pathogens found in oral biofilms, such as dental plaque, and a type of innate immunological memory that offers improved defence against recurrent infections (van Leent et al. 2022). Some EPS constituents have immunomodulatory effects that can encourage immune cells to react with the site of infection, boosting the body's antibacterial defences.

Additionally, EPS-based nanomaterials can be utilised to improve the efficacy of target delivery of antibacterial agents to eradicate infections. For instance, to improve the biocompatibility and effectivity of coated nanoparticles of EPS. Important properties of EPS include excellent biocompatibility, low cytotoxicity, and a potent capacity to penetrate cancer cells. The EPS-coated magnetic nanoparticles (MNPs) have been employed for magnetic hyperthermia therapy, imaging of cancer cells, and quick delivery of specific targets. For industry application, it is important to optimize their efficacy, ethical, and clinical translation (Sivakumar et al. 2014).

METHODOLOGY

Synthesis of Nanoparticles Cum Nanomaterials

The EPS can undergo modification and processing techniques to obtain nanoscale forms, such as nanoparticles, nanofibers, or nanogels.

Nanoparticles: EPS can be processed into nanoparticles through techniques like nanoprecipitation, emulsion, or solvent evaporation. These nanoparticles can be tailored to improve quick delivery, enhance drug stability, or enhance the solubility of the drug, which can lead to better reachability of the drug in the body and increased bioavailability. They can also be functionalized with ligands or molecules that specifically target diseased cells, further reducing the overall drug dose as expected, potentially decreasing side effects, and improving therapeutic outcomes. EPS nanoparticles are versatile carriers that can encapsulate a wide range of molecules, opening up opportunities for various drug delivery systems and gene therapy applications. Bacillus-derived EPS is generally considered biocompatible, reducing the risk of adverse reactions when used as a drug delivery vehicle, which is a crucial factor in improving the delivery system safely.

Nanofibers: Electrospinning is commonly employed to fabricate EPS into nanofibers. The electro spun EPS nanofibers can serve as scaffolds for tissue engineering applications, wound healing, or drug delivery systems. They provide a good volume surface and can mimic the extracellular matrix, promoting cell adhesion, proliferation, and tissue regeneration.

Nanogels: EPS can be chemically crosslinked or self-assembled into nanogels. These nanogels have a three-dimensional network structure capable of encapsulating bioactive compounds, such as drugs or growth factors, for controlled release applications. The nanogels can provide sustained release profiles and protect the encapsulated agents from degradation.

The synthesis of EPS as nanomaterials offers opportunities to improve their unique properties and tailor them for specific applications. These nanomaterials can exhibit improved physicochemical properties, increased stability, enhanced bioactivity, and controlled release profiles (Unal et al. 2022)

In this chapter we concise the Exopolysaccharides from *Bacillus amyloliquefaciens* MCC 4424 and its role against oral biofilm causing bacterial pathogen. The exopolysaccharides from the *B.amyloliquefaciens* MCC 4424 were extracted using cold ethanol precipitation method. The EPS were dialysed and homogenized. Nano gels were synthesised using Gum acacia (10%), 1Mm Silver nitrate and Bacillus exopolysaccharides. These nano gels were characterised and studied against the biofilm causing bacteria. (Figure 3)

Figure 3. Nano gels were characterised and studied against the biofilm causing bacteria

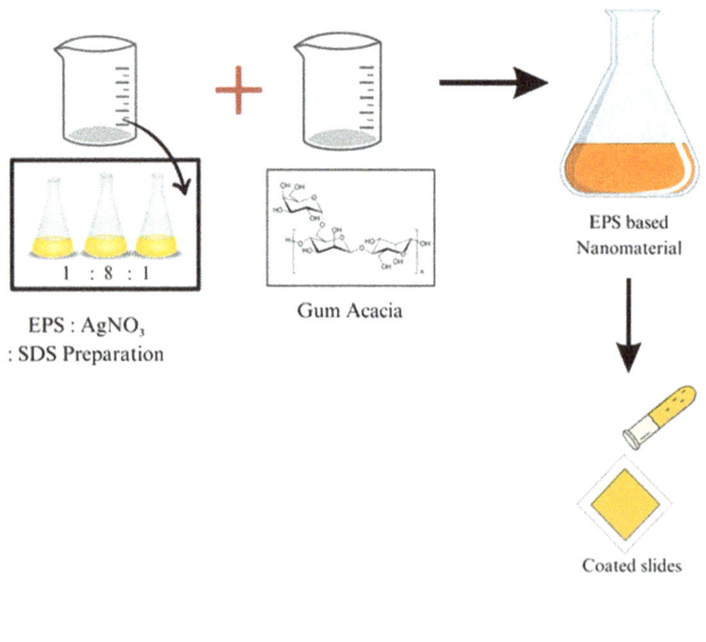

3. CHARACTERIZATION OF BACTERIAL EXOPOLYSACCHARIDES NANOMATERIALS

Spectroscopy Analysis by UV visible:

The biosynthesised EPS-mediated nanoparticles were exposed to sunlight and observed for the characteristic colour change to occur. Consecutively, the samples were stored in sterile falcon tubes. The spectrophotometer wavelength ranges from 200–800 nm, with the peaks corresponding to the capping capability of exopolysaccharides.

Fourier Transform Infra-Red (FTIR) spectrum analysis:

To identify functional groups and chemical bonds present in EPS nanomaterials, the IR-FTIR was used. The samples were prepared for FTIR spectrum within the range of 400-4000 cm^{-1}. With isopropyl alcohol as the standard being used, the resulting peaks observed were used to interpret the chemical alterations of Exopolysaccharides.

Field Emission Scanning Electron Microscopy (FESEM) analysis:

For the determination of the shape and size of the biosynthesized nanoparticles, FESEM analysis and scanning electron microscopy are widely used to examine the morphology and surface characteristics of biosynthesized EPS nanomaterials. These techniques provide high-resolution images, enabling visualisation of the nanomaterial structure, such as nanoparticles, nanofibers, or nanogels.

Confocal Laser Scanning microscopy (CLSM) analysis:

Confocal laser scanning microscopy (CLSM) can be used to visualize and characterize EPS nanomaterials labelled with fluorescent probes or dyes. This enables the investigation of their distribution, localization, and interactions within biofilms. (Rai et al. 2009). The visible biofilm aggregates were observed onto the slides, they were later stained with 33.4 μM Propidium iodide and 400 μM Syto-9-Green and further allowed to incubate for roughly about 3-4 hours for the stain to be absorbed into the matrices.

The other characterization of bacterial exopolysaccharide (EPS) nanomaterials is essential for understanding their properties and optimising their performance in treating biofilm-driven diseases. Nanoparticle tracking analysis (NTA) and dynamic light scattering (DLS) can be used to determine the particle size and size distribution of EPS nanoparticles. These techniques measure the Brownian motion of nanoparticles in solution, providing information about their hydrodynamic size. The zeta potential of EPS nanomaterials can be measured using techniques like electrophoretic mobility or laser Doppler velocimetry. Zeta potential provides insights into the surface charge and stability of the nanomaterials, which can influence their interactions with biological systems.

Antibiofilm activity of Bacterial EPS Nanomaterials:

In vitro models play a critical role in studying biofilm forming pathogens and evaluating the efficacy of exopolysaccharide (EPS) nanomaterials for targeting and combating these infections. They provide a controlled environment where researchers can simulate biofilm formation. These models often feature the development of biofilms on a variety of surfaces, including glass, plastic, or specialized assay plates for biofilms. Researchers can employ well-characterized laboratory strains or clinical isolates to study particular diseases. The growth of biofilms can be affected by a number of variables, including the growth media selected, temperature, pH, and shear pressures. In vitro, models aid in clarifying the methods through which EPS nanoparticles exert their antibiofilm activities in addition to evaluating results. This can involve direct antibacterial activity, breakdown of the biofilm matrix, suppression of adhesion factors, or interference with quorum sensing.

Static Biofilm Models:

Static biofilm models can construct controlled settings that resemble the surfaces on which biofilms grow. The capacity of nanoparticles to stop biofilm formation from the start by cultivating biofilms on surfaces like microtiter plates, coverslips, or silicone discs(Lebeaux et al. 2013) The role of synthesized nanoparticles to stop or disrupt the formation of biofilms by exposing them to biofilms produced in static models. This sheds light on the ability of EPS nanoparticles to fight biofilm-related illnesses and their antibacterial capabilities. The structural alterations in biofilms treated with nanoparticles using microscopy and other imaging methods. This aids in determining whether the biofilm's architecture has been altered by the nanomaterials, potentially making it more vulnerable to antibiotic remedies(Santos et al. 2019). The lowest effective concentration needed for antibiofilm action is established as a result. It helps to determine which applicants are most likely to benefit from additional research. When evaluating the potential of nanoparticles as antibiofilm agents, these models might be used as a starting point (Berger et al., 2018). Positive outcomes in static models may call for additional research with more complicated models or clinical trials.

Multi-well Plate Method:

A platform for the creation of biofilms is provided by multi-well plates with pegs or pins put into the wells. It studies how EPS nanoparticles affect the early stages of biofilm formation and establishment by letting biofilms grow on these pegs. Multi-well plate models provide more dynamic interactions between nanoparticles and biofilm formation. The structure of biofilms that have been exposed to nanoparticles using microscopy and imaging methods (Lee et al., 2014; Nair et al., 2017). This sheds light on the possibility that the nanoparticles alter the architecture of biofilms, potentially rendering them more susceptible to antimicrobial therapies (Filoche et al., 2004). This enables the determination of whether the nanomaterials improve the efficacy of therapies intended to disrupt or eradicate biofilms. Similar to static models, multi-well plate models let to test various EPS nanomaterial concentrations and assess how they affect biofilm formation and susceptibility. With the flexibility to run experiments in numerous wells at once, multi-well plate models have the advantage of improving the accuracy of data and facilitating statistical analysis. This strengthens the validity of the conclusions on the impact of EPS nanoparticles on biofilm structure and growth. This aids in determining the most efficient methods for battling illnesses brought on by biofilms.

Ex-vivo typodont model:

In this chapter, to elaborate the role of nanomaterials against oral biofilm infections, The *ex-vivo* typodont model, known as a typodont, was used to replicate the structure and characteristics of a human tooth within a controlled setting. The typodont itself is a plastic or synthetic model that mimics the shape, anatomy, and properties of human teeth. It often includes features such as enamel, dentin, pulp chamber, and roots, providing a lifelike representation. This model is commonly employed to examine and evaluate the impact of various dental materials and procedures on dental pulp (Meglioli et al. 2023). The ex-vivo typodont model holds a significant advantage in the realm of dental research by reducing the need for live animals, aligning with the 3R philosophy of reduction, refinement, and replacement. This model enables controlled experiments to examine dental materials and procedures on dental pulp, contributing to advancing dental science and refining oral care practices. Its controlled environment reduces variables and stress on animals, while its insights can guide subsequent stages of research. The typodont model exemplifies a responsible and ethical approach to scientific advancement, enhancing our understanding of dental health without compromising animal welfare.

In the realm of dental material assessment, antimicrobial activity assumes a critical role, as it aids in preventing bacterial growth and curbing the formation of biofilm, both of which can give rise to oral infections and other dental complications. A potential antimicrobial agent that has gathered attention is $AgNO_3$, which exhibits suitability for controlled release local delivery in the oral cavity, predominantly for treating periodontitis(Samiei et al. 2016).

In preparation for experimentation, the typodont teeth are subjected to a thorough sterilization process using sodium hypochlorite. This sterilization, conducted over a duration of 3-4 hours as per the reports suggested by(Sethi et al. 2018), ensures that the typodont model is devoid of any pre-existing bacterial presence. The experimental phase commences by immersing the typodont model, coated with nanomaterial, into the bacterial broth. This strategic immersion allows for direct contact between the bacterial components and the simulated dental surface represented by the typodont teeth. This setup aims to replicate the conditions under which oral pathogens might interact with dental structures.

Subsequent to immersion, the model enters an incubation period spanning three days. This duration allows ample time for bacteria to proliferate and establish biofilm, a common occurrence in dental environments. This biofilm formation mimics real-world scenarios and sets the stage for evaluating the nanomaterials' ability to hinder bacterial growth and biofilm development. A compelling approach for analysing and evaluating the samples is the utilization of scanning electron microscopy (SEM) imaging. SEM offers an incredibly detailed examination of the typodont teeth at a microscopic level. This imaging technique enables researchers to scrutinize the nanomaterials' impact on bacterial adhesion, morphology, and the overall structure of the biofilm.

Quantfication of antibiofilm activity:

The quantification of biofilm biomass was examined by using crystal violet stain (0.1%) for in-vitro biofilms such as static and multi-well models. The biofilm attached to the surfaces was quantified using a UV-VIS spectrophotometer. The biofilm biomass was quantified between the treated and control samples. In addition, the colony-forming unit assay will also be carried out to quantify the antibiofilm activity. The control and treated biofilms were scraped from the surfaces and plated on fresh media plates to enumerate the bacterial colonies, which helps us understand the viability of bacteria (Govindarajan et al., 2022). Similarly, the architecture of the disrupted mature biofilm was stained with propidium iodide and syto-9 green and visualized under estimated confocal laser scanning microscopy (CLSM). The confocal Image z stacks were obtained from triplicates of untreated control and treated biofilms and analysed (surface architecture and three-dimensional architecture). The images were analysed using COMSTAT2 software (Dr. Claus Sternberg, Technical University of Denmark). Biofilm parameters such as biofilm's maximum thickness (µm), roughness coefficient, and biovolume (m3) were analysed in terms of antibiofilm activity.

4. RESULTS AND DISCUSSION

In this chapter, preliminary results suggest that bacterial EPS exhibit antibacterial activity against oral biofilm-causing bacterial pathogens. In order to enhance the activity of EPS, we prepared nanomaterials from Bacillus EPS using silver nanoparticles (AgNPs). The concentration of silver nitrate, reaction time, temperature, and presence of Bacillus EPS can influence the size and shape of the synthesised AgNPs. Bacillus EPS acts as a good agent and quickly reacts, also providing electrons to reduce silver ions ($Ag+$) to silver atoms (Ag), leading to nanoparticle formation. Bacillus EPS also acts as a stabilising agent, preventing agglomeration or aggregation of the synthesised AgNPs (Gomaa 2016).

Figure 4. Morphology and stability of synthesized AgNPs

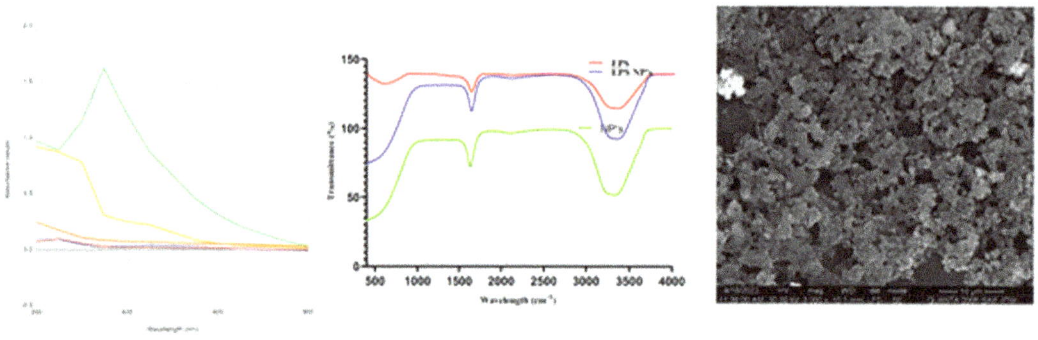

A B C

Characterization techniques such as spectrophotometers and microscopy can be employed to confirm the morphology (size, shape) and stability of the synthesised AgNPs, as shown in Figure 4. The characterization process helps assess the quality of the nanoparticles and ensures their suitability for further applications.

The synthesized AgNPs from Bacillus EPS exhibit antibiofilm efficacy against oral biofilm infection-causing pathogens. The AgNPs can disrupt biofilm formation, inhibit pathogen adherence, or directly target and disrupt existing biofilms, as shown in Figure 5. The small size and high surface volume ratio of AgNPs enhance their interaction with the biofilm structure, improving their efficacy against biofilm-associated pathogens (Rai et al. 2009; Kalishwaralal et al. 2010).

Overall, our data suggested that we successfully synthesised and characterised nanoparticles from Bacillus EPS and demonstrated their potential as antibiofilm agents against oral biofilm infections caused by bacterial pathogens. The synthesised AgNPs show promise for future applications in combating biofilm-related infections(Mohanty et al. 2012; Zhang et al. 2018; Vazquez-Rodriguez et al. 2020).

The use of bacterial exopolysaccharides (EPS) as nanomaterials possesses the diverse range of opportunities in variety of biological applications. Bacterial EPS, such as those derived from *B. amyloliquefaciens*, MCC 4424 have shown unique characteristics and functionalities that help in suitable for diverse applications. Synthesizing nanoparticles from Bacillus EPS offers an effective approach for use in potential biomedical applications. The process of synthesis involves utilizing the EPS act as good agent to quickly react and stabilizing agent, such as in the case of synthesizing silver nanoparticles (AgNPs) from silver nitrate. The resulting AgNPs exhibit antibiofilm activity against oral biofilm infection-causing pathogens, indicating their potential in combating biofilm-related infections. The successful synthesis and characterization of nanoparticles from Bacillus EPS is new avenue to check various applications. The synthesized nanoparticles can be engineered for targeted drug delivery, wound healing, tissue engineering, and antimicrobial applications. Their small size, stability, and ability to disrupt biofilm formation make them valuable tools in combating biofilm-associated infections.

Figure 5. AgNPs can disrupt biofilm formation, inhibit pathogen adherence, or directly target and disrupt existing biofilms

A) EPS-based Nanomaterial synthesized and coated on microscopic coverslips B) Antibacterial activity of Nanomaterial against biofilm-forming bacteria C) an ex vivo typodont model coated with nanomaterials; and D) an in vitro static biofilm model coated with EPS nanomaterials

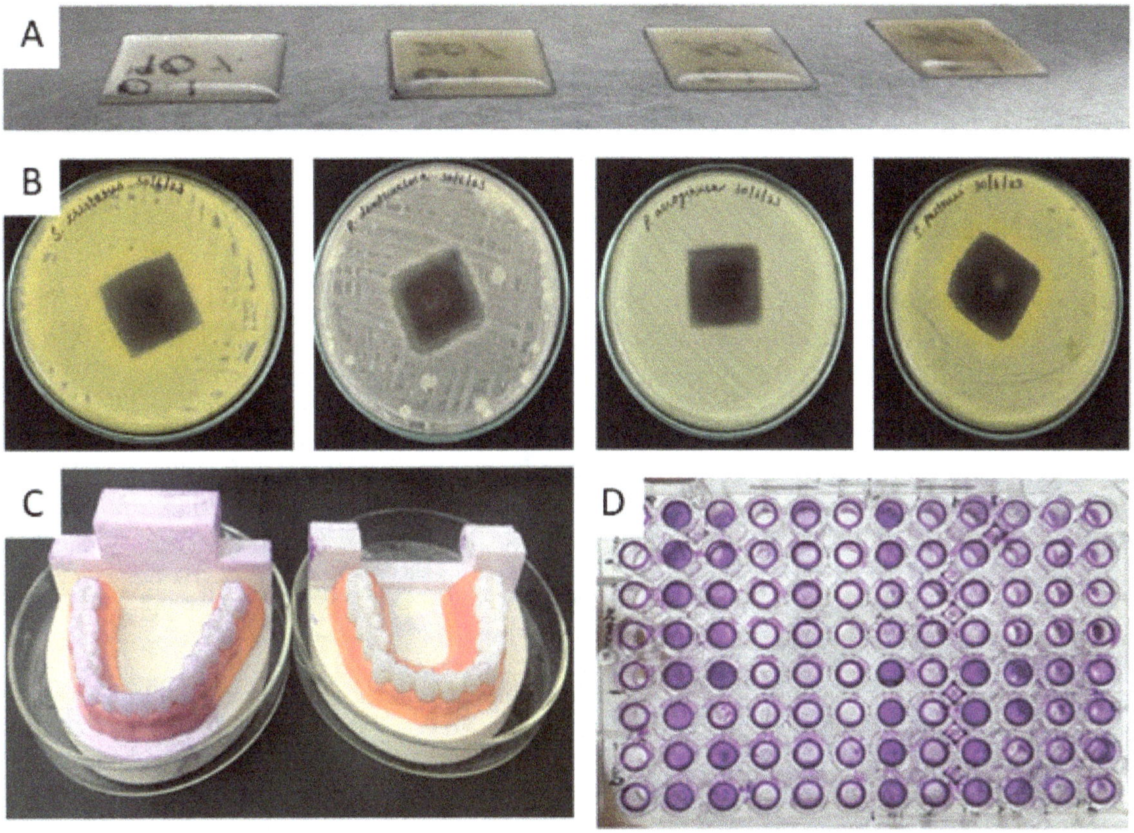

5. CONCLUSION

The use of bacterial exopolysaccharide (EPS)-mediated nanoparticles and nanomaterials in biomedical applications has shown promising results based on our preliminary studies. Our results indicated that EPS-mediated nanoparticles, particularly silver nanoparticles (AgNPs) synthesised from Bacillus EPS, exhibit substantial antibiofilm activity against pathogens responsible for oral biofilm infections. This finding suggests that their potential lies not only in addressing biofilm-related dental issues but also in other medical fields. The main benefit of using EPS-mediated nanoparticles is their biocompatibility, which is essential for biomedical applications.

For drug-targeted delivery systems, EPS-mediated nanoparticles make efficient use of specific ligands or conjugated molecules that quickly bind to target cells or tissues. This enables the nanoparticles to selectively deliver drugs to the specific target site, enhancing the therapeutic efficacy. In the context of wound healing and tissue engineering, EPS-based nanoparticles can be utilised to enhance the regenerative process. These nanoparticles can promote cellular activities thereby accelerating tissue repair and regeneration.

ACKNOWLEDGMENT

We would like to thank Department of Science and Technology & Science and Engineering Research Board for funding (ECR/2017/001335) and DST-FIST (File No.2021/1156). Also, we express our gratitude to Centre for Biotechnology, Anna University for collaborations.

REFERENCES

Abdalla, A. K., Ayyash, M. M., Olaimat, A. N., Osaili, T. M., Al-Nabulsi, A. A., Shah, N. P., & Holley, R. (2021). Exopolysaccharides as Antimicrobial Agents: Mechanism and Spectrum of Activity. *Frontiers in Microbiology*, *12*, 12. doi:10.3389/fmicb.2021.664395 PMID:34093478

Algburi, A., Al-Hasani, H. M., Ismael, T. K., Abdelhameed, A., Weeks, R., Ermakov, A. M., & Chikindas, M. L. (2021). Antimicrobial Activity of Bacillus subtilis KATMIRA1933 and Bacillus amyloliquefaciens B-1895 Against Staphylococcus aureus Biofilms Isolated from Wound Infection. *Probiotics and Antimicrobial Proteins*, *13*(1), 125–134. doi:10.100712602-020-09673-4 PMID:32556931

Berger, D., Rakhamimova, A., Pollack, A., & Loewy, Z. (2018). Oral Biofilms: Development, Control, and Analysis. *High-Throughput*, *7*, 1–8. doi:10.3390/ht7030024 PMID:30200379

Donlan, R. M., & Costerton, J. W. (2002). Biofilms: Survival mechanisms of clinically relevant microorganisms. *Clinical Microbiology Reviews*, *15*(2), 167–193. doi:10.1128/CMR.15.2.167-193.2002 PMID:11932229

dos Santos, D. M. S., Pires, J. G., & Braga, A. S. (2019). Comparison between static and semi-dynamic models for microcosm biofilm formation on dentin. *Journal of Applied Oral Science*, *27*, 1–6. doi:10.1590/1678-7757-2018-0163 PMID:30624468

Filoche, S. K., Zhu, M., & Wu, C. D. (2004). In situ biofilm formation by multi-species oral bacteria under flowing and anaerobic conditions. *Journal of Dental Research*, *83*(10), 802–806. doi:10.1177/154405910408301013 PMID:15381723

Flemming, H. C., Neu, T. R., & Wozniak, D. J. (2007). The EPS matrix: The "House of Biofilm Cells.". *Journal of Bacteriology*, *189*(22), 7945–7947. doi:10.1128/JB.00858-07 PMID:17675377

Govindarajan, D. K., & Kandaswamy, K. (2022). Virulence factors of uropathogens and their role in host pathogen interactions. *Cell Surface (Amsterdam, Netherlands)*, *8*, 100075. doi:10.1016/j.tcsw.2022.100075 PMID:35198842

Govindarajan, D. K., & Kandaswamy, K. (2023). Antimicrobial peptides: A small molecule for sustainable healthcare applications. *Medicine in Microecology*, *18*, 100090. doi:10.1016/j.medmic.2023.100090

Govindarajan, D. K., Meghanathan, Y., Sivaramakrishnan, M., Kothandan, R., Muthusamy, A., Seviour, T. W., & Kandaswamy, K. (2022). Enterococcus faecalis thrives in dual-species biofilm models under iron-rich conditions. *Archives of Microbiology*, *204*(12), 710. doi:10.100700203-022-03309-7 PMID:36383258

Kalishwaralal, K., BarathManiKanth, S., Pandian, S. R. K., Deepak, V., & Gurunathan, S. (2010). Silver nanoparticles impede the biofilm formation by Pseudomonas aeruginosa and Staphylococcus epidermidis. *Colloids and Surfaces. B, Biointerfaces*, *79*(2), 340–344. doi:10.1016/j.colsurfb.2010.04.014 PMID:20493674

Karnwal, A., Kumar, G., Pant, G., Hossain, K., Ahmad, A., & Alshammari, M. B. (2023). Perspectives on Usage of Functional Nanomaterials in Antimicrobial Therapy for Antibiotic-Resistant Bacterial Infections. *ACS Omega*, *8*(15), 13492–13508. doi:10.1021/acsomega.3c00110 PMID:37091369

Lebeaux, D., Chauhan, A., Rendueles, O., & Beloin, C. (2013). From in vitro to in vivo models of bacterial biofilm-related infections. *Pathogens (Basel, Switzerland)*, *2*(2), 288–356. doi:10.3390/pathogens2020288 PMID:25437038

Lee, K. W. K., Periasamy, S., Mukherjee, M., Xie, C., Kjelleberg, S., & Rice, S. A. (2014). Biofilm development and enhanced stress resistance of a model, mixed-species community biofilm. *The ISME Journal*, *8*(4), 894–907. doi:10.1038/ismej.2013.194 PMID:24152718

Li, C., Zhou, L., & Yang, H. (2017). *Self-assembled Exopolysaccharide Nanoparticles for Bioremediation and Green Synthesis of Noble Metal Nanoparticles.*

Makabenta, J. M. V., Nabawy, A., Li, C. H., Schmidt-Malan, S., Patel, R., & Rotello, V. M. (2021). Nanomaterial-based therapeutics for antibiotic-resistant bacterial infections. *Nature Reviews. Microbiology*, *19*(1), 23–36. doi:10.103841579-020-0420-1 PMID:32814862

McDougald, D., Rice, S. A., Barraud, N., Steinberg, P. D., & Kjelleberg, S. (2012). Should we stay or should we go: Mechanisms and ecological consequences for biofilm dispersal. *Nature Reviews. Microbiology*, *10*(1), 39–50. doi:10.1038/nrmicro2695 PMID:22120588

Meglioli, M., Mergoni, G., Artioli, F., Ghezzi, B., Manfredi, M., Macaluso, G. M., & Lumetti, S. (2023). A Novel Self-Assessment Method for Training Access Cavity on 3D Printed Endodontic Models. *Dentistry Journal*, *11*(6), 152. doi:10.3390/dj11060152 PMID:37366675

Mohanty, S., Mishra, S., Jena, P., Jacob, B., Sarkar, B., & Sonawane, A. (2012). An investigation on the antibacterial, cytotoxic, and antibiofilm efficacy of starch-stabilized silver nanoparticles. *Nanomedicine (London)*, *8*(6), 916–924. doi:10.1016/j.nano.2011.11.007 PMID:22115597

Nair, H. A. S., Periasamy, S., Yang, L., Kjelleberg, S., & Rice, S. A. (2017). Real Time, Spatial, and Temporal Mapping of the Distribution of c-di-GMP during Biofilm Development. *The Journal of Biological Chemistry*, *292*(2), 477–487. doi:10.1074/jbc.M116.746743 PMID:27899451

Netrusov, A. I., Liyaskina, E. V., Kurgaeva, I. V., Liyaskina, A. U., Yang, G., & Revin, V. V. (2023). Exopolysaccharides Producing Bacteria: A Review. *Microorganisms*, *11*(6), 1541. doi:10.3390/microorganisms11061541 PMID:37375041

Nicolle, L. E. (2014). Catheter associated urinary tract infections. *Antimicrobial Resistance and Infection Control, 3*(1), 1–8. doi:10.1186/2047-2994-3-23 PMID:25075308

Rai, M., Yadav, A., & Gade, A. (2009). Silver nanoparticles as a new generation of antimicrobials. *Biotechnology Advances, 27*(1), 76–83. doi:10.1016/j.biotechadv.2008.09.002 PMID:18854209

Rao,, B.P. (2013). Characterization of Exopolysaccharide from Bacillus amyloliquefaciens BPRGS for its Bioflocculant Activity. *International Journal of Scientific and Engineering Research, 4*, 1696–1704.

Samiei, M., Farjami, A., Dizaj, S. M., & Lotfipour, F. (2016). Nanoparticles for antimicrobial purposes in Endodontics: A systematic review of in vitro studies. *Materials Science and Engineering C, 58*, 1269–1278. doi:10.1016/j.msec.2015.08.070 PMID:26478430

Sethi, A. K., Samal, R., Lahiri, B., Das, A., Kumar, G., & Behera, S. (2018). Awareness, attitude and practice regarding disinfection and handling of extracted teeth among the students in a dental college in India. *Journal of International Society of Preventive & Community Dentistry, 8*(6), 488–494. doi:10.4103/jispcd.JISPCD_314_18 PMID:30596038

Unal, N., Bakirhan, N., Yucel, C., & Savluk, M. (2022). Antimicrobial effective nanoparticles: Mechanisms and recent achievements. Medicine Science |. *Medicine Science, 11*(2), 905. doi:10.5455/medscience.2021.12.401

Vazquez-Rodriguez, A., Vasto-Anzaldo, X. G., Leon-Buitimea, A., Zarate, X., & Morones-Ramirez, J. R. (2020). Antibacterial and Antibiofilm Activity of Biosynthesized Silver Nanoparticles Coated with Exopolysaccharides Obtained from Rhodotorula mucilaginosa. *IEEE Transactions on Nanobioscience, 19*(3), 498–503. doi:10.1109/TNB.2020.2985101 PMID:32248119

Verastegui, Y., Cheng, J., & Kolczynski, D. (2014). Multisubstrate Isotope Labeling and Metagenomic Analysis of Active. *mBio, 5*(4), e01157-14. Advance online publication. doi:10.1128/mBio.01157-14 PMID:25028422

Zhang, J., Yue, X., Zeng, Y., Hua, E., Wang, M., & Sun, Y. (2018). Bacillus amyloliquefaciens levan and its silver nanoparticles with antimicrobial properties. *Biotechnology, Biotechnological Equipment, 32*(6), 1583–1589. doi:10.1080/13102818.2018.1523690

Zhang, L., Pornpattananangkul, D., Hu, C.-M.J., & Huang, C.-M. (2010) *Development of Nanoparticles for Antimicrobial Drug Delivery*. Research Gate.

Chapter 16
Sustainable Use of Nanotechnology in Biomedical Sciences

Devi Nallappan
https://orcid.org/0000-0003-2673-5614
Lincoln University College, Malaysia

Jayasree S. Kanathasan
https://orcid.org/0000-0001-7509-6746
Lincoln University College, Malaysia

Sandeep Poddar
https://orcid.org/0000-0001-9771-877X
Lincoln University College, Malaysia

ABSTRACT

Researchers have directed their attention to the application of nanotechnology in the biomedical sciences owing to their promising effects. In light of this, the present chapter is a concerted effort to highlight the emerging application of nanotechnology in the field of biomedical sciences. The first part of the chapter describes the introduction to biomedical science, followed by an introduction to the development of nanotechnology, the types and characteristics of nanosized materials, and their potential therapeutic properties. Next, the present chapter describes the application of nanotechnology in biomedical sciences. It also highlights the current issues regarding the usage of nanotechnology in biomedical science, especially safety, regulation, and toxicity. This chapter aims to provide new insights into the extraordinary application of nanotechnology in the biomedical science field for researchers, policymakers, regulators, healthcare professionals, and others involved in the nano biomedical application field.

DOI: 10.4018/979-8-3693-0448-8.ch016

INTRODUCTION

Biomedical science is the field of study that emphasises the aspects of chemistry and biology that are relevant to the healthcare system. This is also referred to as biomedicine is the combination of medicine and biology fields that focuses on the health of humans and animals (Keating & Cambrosio, 2003). This is a very wide-ranging discipline, and there are a few general areas of speciality including biochemistry, bioengineering, physiological sciences, pharmacology, epidemiology and life sciences (Crinson & Crinson, 2021; Keating & Cambrosio, 2003). This field serves as a centralized platform to delve into fields including parasitology, cell and molecular biology and toxicology (Kumar, 2013).

Over the years, scientific discoveries in this field provide a valuable contribution to the medical field, especially clinical studies on cancer, diabetes, cardiovascular and infectious diseases (National Research Council, 2003; Duarte et al., 2018; Garcia-Gonzalez et al., 2020; Zhu et al., 2020). The prominent importance of this field is evident in the discovery of potent therapeutic drugs and underpinning the mechanism and delivery of drugs (Li et al., 2022). It is also important to note that biomedical science has been playing a pivotal role in the healthcare sector by facilitating effective diagnosis and imaging of diseases (Rhodes, 2011; Ng & Etehadtavakol, 2017).

Despite the effective diagnosis and treatment methods employed in the biomedical industry, it has been a great challenge for healthcare practitioners in providing better healthcare services with cost-effective diagnosis and treatment to patients. Thus, the biomedical industry rapidly shifts its direction toward developing potent therapeutic drugs and devices that satisfy the needs of both the healthcare industry and patients. In light of this, the application of nanotechnology and biomedicine has been a promising approach to revolutionising biomedical research including enzyme encapsulation, drug delivery, drug discovery, gene delivery, protein delivery, biosensor advancement and so forth (Machtakova et al., 2022;

Figure 1. Nanotechnology advances in the biomedical science field

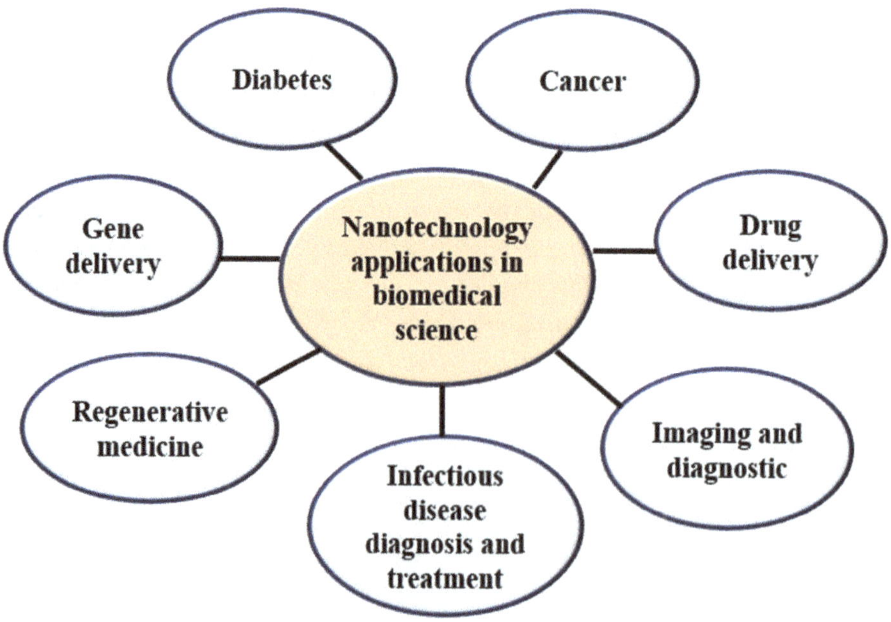

Deng et al., 2020; Wong et al., 2017; Yu et al., 2016; Mujawar et al., 2020). Today, nanoscale materials have successfully emerged as key players in advancing the healthcare sector and biomedicine with promising applications to curb ongoing healthcare crises as illustrated in Figure 1.

NANOTECHNOLOGY

Healthcare is one of the fields in which humankind finds challenges to treat diseases. One of the limitations in solving health-related problems is the lack of the ability to understand and monitor the biological and environmental systems of physiology at the molecular level (Zhang & James, 2023). Nanotechnology is a field comprised of techniques and tools developed at the nanoscale range using nanomaterials. Nanoparticles refer to materials synthesized at the nanoscale which range from 10 to 100 nm in size (Sakthi Devi et al., 2022). Nanomaterials are nanosized structures that exist in both organic, inorganic and combined forms that give space for flexibilities in various modifications and loading to perform their functions. Nanomaterials have been extensively used in biomedical applications such as therapy, imaging, biosensors, biomedical devices, intracellular trafficking and gene delivery (Diez-Pascual & Rahdar, 2022).

Organic nanoparticles are composed of natural or synthetic molecules or polymers. Examples of organic nanoparticles include polymer-based nanoparticles, lipid-based nanoparticles, molecular-based nanoparticles and protein-based nanoparticles. Polymeric nanoparticles are composed of single or multiple types of polymers including polymeric micelles, dendrimers, polyelectrolyte ionic complexes, nanocapsules and nanospheres. These polymeric nanoparticles exhibit a hydrophobicity nature which increases the bioavailability of the therapeutic compounds in physiological conditions. Lipid nanoparticles comprise nanovesicles, liposomes, quatsomes and micelles. Lipid nanoparticles are known for their unique combination of the ability to carry hydrophilic and hydrophobic drugs, allowing the drugs to reach the lipid-dense target sites in the body in the brain and skin (Marzi et al., 2022; Bueno et al., 2018).

Inorganic nanoparticles consist of semiconductor nanoparticles, non-metal nanoparticles and metal nanoparticles. Semiconductor-based nanoparticles include nanoporous silica, porous silicon, and carbonaceous nanomaterials. Semiconductor nanoparticles exist in quantum dots mostly due to their strong photoluminescence emission and photostability (Sun et al., 2006). Quantum dots are another type of nanostructure with sensitivity, selectivity and a wide range of optical properties that enable it to visualize brain structures while delivering the drugs. Metal nanoparticles are nanostructures formed by various metal structures. Metal nanoparticles like gold, silver, iron and heavy metals are some of the most commonly used metal nanoparticles for biomedical applications. Gold and silver nanoparticles possess biological properties including antibacterial, anti-inflammatory, antiviral, antiparasitic, antifungal, antiplatelet and anti-tumour activity (Marzi et al., 2022). Iron nanoparticles are also widely used in magnetic resonance imaging and thermal-based therapy. Metal nanoparticles which are used in nanotechnology include silver, copper, gold, platinum, osmium, palladium, rhodium, ruthenium, iridium and many more are renowned in biomedical applications owing to their resistance to corrosion and oxidation at higher temperatures (Sakthi Devi et al., 2022). Metal nanoparticles also exhibit photocatalytic and photothermal effects due to their reactiveness to varying wavelengths of energy (Ye et al., 2022). Additionally, silver nanoparticles are used as a component in dental implants, impregnated catheters, wound dressings, ventricular drainage catheters, treatment for orthopaedic infections as well as osteointegration (Sakthi Devi et al., 2022). Moreover, gold nanoparticles have been used in diagnosis, cancer treatment, and antibacterial and antiviral agents (Maleki et al., 2019). Gold has a strong history of medicinal usage in Chinese and Indian medicine, especially to treat arthritis. Gold nanoparticles exhibit some distinct features such as tuneable size, shape, optical and electrical characteristics and flexible surface functionalization properties (Giljohann et al., 2010). The urge for targeted diagnosis and treatment of healthcare issues demands a rising interest in nanotechnology in the biomedical field.

APPLICATION OF NANOTECHNOLOGY IN BIOMEDICAL SCIENCES

Drug Delivery

Treatment that utilized large-size material for drug delivery is accompanied by several issues including low solubility, poorly targeted delivery, and bioavailability as well as generalized side effects (Patra et al., 2018). Nanotechnology has been proven to bridge the gap between biological and physical sciences by using nanostructures and nanophases in various scientific fields, especially in nanomedicine and nano-based drug delivery systems, where such particles are of great importance (Mitchell et al., 2021). Nano-based drug delivery system offers benefits in the management and treatment of various chronic diseases including cancer (Cheng et al., 2021), diabetes (Samavati et al., 2022), cardiovascular diseases (Yang et al., 2022), asthma (da Silva et al., 2020) and acquired immunodeficiency syndrome (Asl et al., 2023). Recent studies indicated that nano architectures enhance the delivery of sparingly water-soluble therapeutic drugs and prevent oral drugs from degradation in the harsh gastrointestinal region. Nanodimentional materials facilitate the release of amalgamated drugs by staying in the blood circulatory system for a prolonged period, thus preventing plasma fluctuations with lowered adverse effects (Patra et al., 2018). Inorganic, organic, metallic, non-metallic and polymeric nanostructures, including micelles, liposomes and dendrimers attained attention in formulating target-specific drug delivery systems (Dristant et al., 2023). Inorganic nanoparticles such as magnetic and gold nanoparticles are generally incorporated in micelles and liposomes for efficient drug delivery (Yusuf et al., 2023). The Food and Drug Administration (FDA)-approved lipid-derived substances including micelles and liposomes are regarded as the very first generation of nanoparticle-based therapy (Patra et al., 2018). The polymer-drug conjugate showed a greater clinical potential in the treatment of ovarian, lung and breast cancers owing to the highly improved retention effect and permeability (Alven et al., 2020).

In light of emerging antibacterial resistance, the use of nanotechnology drug delivery in infection treatment is considered a promising strategy in clinical infection treatment by evading existing mechanisms involved in acquired drug resistance (Yeh et al., 2020). They become a promising "outside of the box" toolkit for controlling biofilm infection and resilient multidrug resistance planktonic bacteria (Makabenta et al., 2021). Besides, nanosized materials' physical properties and unique size enable them to target biofilms, hence curbing refractory infections. Nano architectures are novel to bacteria, thus able to circumvent the resistance mechanism against traditional antibiotics (Makabenta et al., 2021; Chakraborty et al., 2022). Carbon-based nanoparticles, polymeric nanoparticles, metal-based nanoparticles, liposomes, smart nanomaterials and nanocomposites are representative classes of nanomaterials for infection treatment applications (Fritea et al., 2021; Ren et al., 2022). The mechanisms employed by nanomaterials are including membrane disruption, production of reactive oxygen species, binding to intracellular components and delivery of therapeutics through membrane fusion (Makabenta et al., 2021). Nanomaterials-based antibacterial therapeutics including Silvasorb Silver® (Walia & Prasad, 2022),

Pulmaquin® (Cartlidge & Hill, 2017), Arikace® (Komalla & Haghi, 2020) and NanoAgCVC (Makvandi et al., 2023) exerted promising effect in clinical study.

In the same vein, the fabrication of nanomaterial has been widely applied for topical drug delivery. This is primarily focused on the local effect by reducing the need for systemic administration of drugs and minimizing the therapeutic dosage with potentially reduced side effects (Mustfa et al., 2021). Antiseptics, cutaneous anti-fungal treatments, keratolytic agents, local anaesthetics, sunscreens and anti-inflammatory agents for skin diseases are some examples of commercialized tropical dermatologic products (Mustfa et al., 2021; Goyal et al., 2016). In contrast, transdermal drug delivery is used for a systemic drug effect with the skin acting as the entry portal for the drugs including nicotine, fentanyl, clonidine and nitroglycerin into the body (Wong et al., 2023). In addition, electrospun nanofiber exhibits potency in the drug delivery system. The high surface area-to-volume ratio of fiber mats facilitates the efficient delivery of drugs owing to high porosity with interconnectivity, malleability, and sustained release with high patient compliance (Jiffrin et al., 2022). Recent scientific evidence highly suggests that nanomaterials offer a great deal of potential for use in drug delivery.

Gene Delivery

The use of cell and gene therapies has excellent chances for curing a variety of ailments that were previously thought to be incurable. This covers numerous malignancies, haematological issues, diabetes, inherited illnesses, including rare diseases, and other maladies (Hanna et al., 2017; Jensen et al., 2021). The demand for gene therapy is increasing in light of high-potential candidates for treatments. In gene therapy, exogenous nucleic acids, such as genes, oligonucleotides, gene segments, siRNAs or miRNAs are introduced into cells in order to alter the expression of a target gene, produce mRNA, or create an exogenous protein (Roma-Rodrigues et al., 2020). A safe, efficient, and controllable vector is important in gene therapy. The ideal vector is non-immunogenic, safe, and enables the expression of the gene product without inducing toxicity. It also accomplishes the level and duration of transgene expression required for the treatment (Mali et al., 2013).

The first platform for gene therapy that was suggested used viral vectors. Numerous clinical trials that resulted in the approval of some gene therapy drugs indicated that viruses were suitable vectors for delivering DNA and RNA to human cells (Zhao et al., 2022). However, the effectiveness of gene therapy involving viral vectors is limited due to several factors including immunogenicity and confined mass production of viral vectors, thus requiring the discovery and engineering of non-viral vectors, backed by nanomedicine (Tong et al., 2023). One of the most exciting developments in biomedical research is the use of nanoparticles as carriers for gene therapy owing to their simple and straightforward manufacturing, ability to be functionalized with various moieties, minimal immunogenicity, and low toxicity (Wang et al., 2022). The development of effective and compatible transfection systems to deliver Threose nucleic acid (TNA)s to cells and tissues, including RNA (microRNA, small interfering RNA (siRNA)) or DNA (plasmid DNA, antisense oligonucleotides) and short hairpin RNA into cells, is one of the areas of interest (Roma-Rodrigues et al., 2020). The use of functionalized nanoparticles can help overcome some of the drawbacks in the effectiveness of transfecting naked plasmid DNA or siRNAs (Pahle & Walther, 2016). However, there are several issues with this method that needs to be resolved, such as less effective transfection when compared to viral vectors or blood clearance before reaching the target site when administered systemically (Patil et al., 2019).

Natural polymers including dextran, chitosan, pullulan, gelatin and synthetic equivalents with advanced features like guanidinylated bio-reducible polymers have drawn interest in gene therapy owing to their simple manufacture and adaptive properties (Rai et al., 2019). In the same vein, lipid-based nanocarriers have been widely employed to encapsulate RNA into particles in recent years. Clinical trials are being conducted with drugs like ALN-PCS02 (which targets proprotein convertase subtilisin/Kexin type 9 (PCSK9) for the treatment of hypercholesterolemia) and ALN-TTRsc (which targets Transthyretin (TTR) for the treatment of transthyretin-mediated amyloidosis). In addition, ALN-TTR02 is a recently released clinical lipid-based nanocarrier for the prolonged alleviation of serum Transthyrétine protein (Hamimed et al., 2022). Recently, strong and adaptable inorganic nanomaterials have also become popular nanocarriers for effective gene delivery applications. In addition, inorganic nanomaterials can be readily functionalized with silane or thiol groups, which enhance interaction with biomolecules through chemical and thermal stability, as well as other desirable qualities for practical applications (Markman et al., 2013). Besides, protein-based nanoparticles are gaining interest as gene delivery vectors due to their biodegradability, biocompatibility, low toxicity, and amphiphilic nature. Several different proteins, including albumin, gelatin, ferritin, heat shock protein 16.5 and silk are employed for gene delivery (Lohcharoenkal et al., 2014; Faria et al., 2018; Riley & Vermerris, 2017). The scientific findings strongly suggest that nanocarriers have a lot of potential to be utilized in gene delivery.

Cancer

Chemotherapeutics have been used to treat cancer since 1930. However, these traditional treatments are accompanied by discomfort, unwanted side effects, and poor targeting. Nanomedicine has emerged as a promising alternative owing to its bioavailability, targeting, and low toxicity. Both active and passive strategies are used by nanoparticles to target cancer cells. Despite the currently available treatment choices for cancer such as surgical therapy, radiotherapy and chemotherapy, this cancer still has a poor prognosis due to factors including systemic toxicity, drug resistance and immunosuppression (Chen et al., 2022). Nanotechnology has been shown to resolve the limitations faced by the current treatment options whilst enhancing the efficacy of the therapies through targeted therapy. The excellent properties exhibited by nanomaterials including their structure, morphology, physicochemical properties and biological effects enable them to be used in cancer. Surface-modified liposomes with esterase-cleavable radionuclide anchors have been shown to enhance radiotherapy by reducing radionuclide retention in the spleen and liver but remain high radioactivity in the tumours (Llop et al., 2021). Nanoparticles have been a proposed solution for cancer treatment due to their ability to deliver a large dose of therapeutic compounds at the target site, avoiding nonspecific targets and unwanted damage occurring to the healthy cells.

In addition, the unique structure of the gastrointestinal tract poses challenges for treatment options like phototherapy for early stage and immunotherapy for gastrointestinal cancer with distant metastases to be really effective. The involuntary movement of the gastrointestinal tract results in low sensitivity and weak affinity of the therapeutic agents to the target site, causing a decrease in the survival rate at the advanced stage and recurrence of the disease (Deng et al., 2022). Studies have shown that silver nanoparticles are enabled to gain access inside the perinuclear space of cytoplasm and endo lysosomal regions of the cells through endocytosis (Asharani et al., 2009; Greulich et al., 2011). Hence, silver nanoparticle-conjugated therapeutic compounds could kill tumour cells by inducing oxidative stress, and damage to DNA leading to apoptosis of cancer cells. Silver nanoparticles could also disrupt the angiogenesis process in the cancer microenvironment (Yang et al., 2016).

Additionally, skin cancer is known as melanoma and nonmelanoma which include basal cell carcinoma and squamous cell carcinoma (Siegel et al., 2014). Despite various chemotherapeutic agents available to treat this cancer such as alkylating agents, antimetabolites, antimetabolites, terpenoids and plant alkaloids, the systemic effects of chemotherapy including toxicity against healthy cells like bone marrow, hair follicles and surrounding immune cells raise resistance towards chemotherapy, limiting the chances of treating the skin cancer. Paclitaxel-loaded N-isopropyl acrylamide/vinyl pyrrolidone heat-resistant nanopolymer micelles have been shown to kill the breast cancer cell line (MCF-7) and skin melanoma cell line (B16F10) with a sustained release of the therapeutic drug (Yadav et al., 2014).

Brain tumour has a rising prevalence and it leads to detrimental effects on the central nervous system, which is very vulnerable to the study due to the complications caused by the brain and central nervous system in daily routine. Owing to the semipermeable nature of the blood-brain barrier (BBB) which restricts almost 95% of the drugs and the concern to treat the brain tissue without side effects, most of the chemotherapeutic drugs are ruled out from treating brain tumours. The development of nanomedicine has been a great alternative to treat brain tumours of smaller size of nanomaterials such as quantum dots in nanometers which can cross the BBB and interact with the brain cells. Besides, antibody-targeted gold nanospheres have been shown to target epidermal growth factor receptors (EGFR) on carcinoma cells (Guo et al., 2017) as well as higher accumulation into the tumour tissue. While in cancer photodynamic therapy which uses photosensitizers to stimulate toxic reactive oxygen in the tumour microenvironment to kill malignant cells, gold nanoparticles are used to treat deep tumours (Ayala-Orozco et al., 2014; Vimaladevi et al., 2016).

On the other hand, nanotechnology is applied in cancer theranostics, the combination of diagnostics and therapy (Javed et al., 2019). The excellent feature of nanoparticles as bioimaging vectors makes them amenable to image-guided delivery the therapeutic agents to the target site. This combination allows the researchers for tracking the therapeutic compounds upon injection into the body. Antibody-conjugated silver nanoparticles have been used as a contrast agent in photoacoustic and ultrasonic imaging owing to their detection in one cm deep *ex vivo* pancreatic tissue with light energy radiated at 800 nm wavelength (Sakthi Devi et al., 2022). Numerous nanotherapeutics have been created since DoxilFDA ®'s approval, and a handful of them have been given the go-ahead for use in the treatment of cancer. Extracellular vesicles and thermal nanomaterials are currently being studied and used in practice, along with liposomes, solid lipid nanoparticles, polymeric nanoparticles and nanoemulsions.

Diabetes

Diabetes mellitus is a metabolic condition characterized by elevated blood glucose levels due to insulin deficiency and/or insulin resistance. Insulin is a peptide hormone secreted by β cells of the pancreatic islets of Langerhans that regulates normal blood glucose levels by mainly improving cellular glucose uptake (Dilworth et al., 2021; Rahman et al., 2021). Diabetes mellitus has several categories, including type 1, type 2, gestational diabetes and neonatal diabetes (Bukhari et al., 2022). Insulin replacement therapy has been widely prescribed for patients with type 1 diabetes which is believed to mimic the natural fluctuations in insulin levels (Janež et al., 2020). For patients with type 2 diabetes and prediabetes, regulation of meals and exercise are preferred for the initial treatment of type 2 diabetes (Syeda et al., 2023). In addition to lifestyle modification ways, patients with type 2 diabetes also receive oral first and/or second-line oral medications as well as injectable insulin via bolus route to improve insulin secretion and sensitivity in insulin-responsive organs (Padhi et al., 2020). There are various forms of insulin in the management of diabetes mellitus including short-acting insulin, rapid-acting insulin, intermediate-acting insulin and long-acting insulin. Nevertheless, insulin injections and glucose tests can be time-consuming and painful for diabetic patients (Liang et al., 2021; Jangam et al., 2013). Continuous glucose monitors and insulin pumps were improved to reduce the drawbacks of injection therapy and enhance patient compliance (Umpierrez & Klonoff, 2018; Ghazanfar et al., 2016). However, this is accompanied by difficulty in achieving euglycemia (basal level) as the insulin injection subcutaneous method is performed by measuring glucose levels in the interstitial fluid, which can consume more time. In addition, the major concern of this therapy would be the risk of exposure to patients' infections and inflammation due to implanted cannulas and sensors. In the same vein, this can also not be cost-effective for patients as frequent replacement and maintenance are required (Karakuş et al., 2021; Veiseh et al., 2015). Thus, warranting effective diagnosis and treatments in controlling diabetic complications by adopting safe and cost-effective therapies. Advances in nanotechnology have noteworthy applications in improving the care of diabetic patients. Over the span of years, nanotechnology has been employed in improving the non-invasive monitoring of blood glucose (Liu et al., 2022). Several different types of nanoparticles are currently being investigated for effective insulin delivery in diabetes treatment (Souto et al., 2019).

Polymeric nanoparticles are biodegradable polymers enveloped by nanoporous membranes and are widely applied as insulin transporter or carriers. They are found efficient compared to intravenous administration and traditional oral administration techniques. Insulin is released upon pH-induced changes in the polymer system (Xie et al., 2017). Copolymers including polyurethanes, polyacrylamide, polyanhydrides, polyacrylic acids and N, N-dimethylaminoethyl methacrylatem have been extensively explored for this application (Gupta, 2017). Polymeric nanoparticles can be incorporated with insulin, serving as a promising candidate for insulin therapy by transporting insulin (Mansoor et al., 2019). In addition, ceramic nanoparticles are reported to guard drug agents against denaturation caused by temperature and/or pH, thus serving as potential insulin carriers (Rashid et al., 2020). There are several inhaler systems applied to distribute inhaled products for dry powder formulations and solutions which are found effective over the gastrointestinal route as it requires a mild environment such as neutral pH and low enzyme concentration (Gupta, 2017; Qin et al., 2022). The encapsulation of insulin with nanoparticles in the dry powder formulation prevents insulin degradation as the dry powder preparation with insulin can be inhaled directly into the lungs and delivered to the bloodstream (Souto et al., 2019).

Additionally, dendrimers are used in the biomedical area as biocompatible nanocarriers to increase a pharmaceutical drug's effectiveness and decrease its toxicity (Sherje et al., 2018). The interaction between dendrimers and drugs improves solubility, thus enhancing the bioavailability and absorption of the drug molecule as well as improving its cytotoxicity (Chis et al., 2020). Recent studies unambiguously indicated amino-terminated poly(amido)amine (PAMAM) dendrimers have gained attention in diabetes studies owing to their protective effect as anti-carbonylation and anti-glycation agents, thus limiting the nonenzymatic modifications of biomacromolecules (Labieniec-Watala et al., 2013). On the other hand, liposomes are reported to play a significant role in diabetes management. Liposomes are mainly employed in improving the oral bioavailability of insulin (Wu et al., 2023). The physical characteristics of liposomes including size, drug release stability and zeta potential in formulation optimisation are warranted to improve the blood sugar alleviating effect (Guimarães et al., 2021).

Besides, oral insulin has emerged as an alternate option to invasive and painful subcutaneous injections, thus being a convenient therapeutic option in the management of diabetes (Wong et al., 2016). Nevertheless, insulin administration via the gastrointestinal route may promote insulin degradation in the stomach due to the presence of gastric enzymes. Insulin can be safeguarded from the harsh environment in the stomach by enveloping insulin in a matrix of calcium phosphate-polyethylene glycol with casein (Bajwa et al., 2018). Oral insulin administration can also be achieved using several polymeric nanoparticles including polyethylenimine, polymethacrylic acid, N-isopropylacrylamide, poly (-ε-caprolactone) and poly (isobutylcyanoacrylate) (Chordiya et al., 2021). Microspheres are proven to be a promising strategy for oral administration as they are capable of enhancing the permeation of insulin by inhibiting protease (Wong et al., 2018). In the management of type 2 diabetes, chitosan nanoparticles are regarded most promising method in inhalation delivery systems. Being a hydrophilic drug, insulin is not able to diffuse through the intestinal epithelium, thus requiring chitosan as a permeation enhancer for better adsorption (Pathomthongtaweechai & Muanprasat, 2021). The efficiency of insulin delivery can be improved by encapsulating insulin with the shell of carboxylated chitosan grafted poly(methylmethacrylated) nanoparticles (Sharma et al., 2015).

Recent investigations focus on insulin delivery by developing "smart" insulin patches which are potent in releasing insulin based on the body's needs (Wang et al., 2020; Veiseh & Langer, 2015). The commercialized nanoparticles used in the management of diabetes are GLP-1-based nanomaterials (chitosan nanoparticles), nano-DDP-4 inhibitors (polymeric, porous silicon and chitosan), metal nanoparticles (silver and zinc oxide) and nano-drug carriers (niosomes, chitosan, nanospheres and polymeric) (Ziebarth & Mainardes, 2023; Shrestha et al., 2016; Choudhury et al., 2020; Zolkepli et al., 2022).

Regenerative Medicine

The practice of regenerative medicine entails the discovery of techniques for replacing and repairing damaged or diseased cells, tissues, or organs in order to restore or establish normal tissue functions (Han et al., 2020). A potent technique for tissue regeneration involves mimicking the properties of tissues at the nanoscale, which can govern cellular adhesion, migration, and differentiation (Zhang et al., 2021). Additionally, nanomaterials differ from their bulk-level counterparts in terms of their special physical, chemical, optical, electrical, and magnetic capabilities (Baig et al., 2021). Nanomaterials are useful for *in vivo* cell tracking, stem cell treatment, scaffolds for tissue engineering and effective biomolecule delivery because of their small size and functional advantages (Peserico et al., 2022; Sun et al., 2020; Zheng et al., 2021; Fathi-Achachelouei et al., 2019). The use of nanoparticles for enhancing engineered tissues and removing barriers in tissue engineering and regenerative medicine has been made possible by their low toxicity, contrasting agent properties, tailorable characteristics, targeted/stimuli-response delivery potential, and precise control over behaviour (via external stimuli like magnetic fields) (Fathi-Achachelouei et al., 2019). In regenerative medicine, there are many different kinds of nanoparticles (polymeric, ceramic, and metallic) that can be applied for a variety of purposes, such as tissue targeting and imaging, the administration of bioactive agents, changing the mechanical properties of scaffolds, and having antibacterial and anticancer effects (Zheng et al., 2021; Serrano-Aroca et al., 2022; Bhutta et al., 2023). The advances in nanotechnology have changed traditional tissue engineering regenerative medicine techniques toward more complicated and effective solutions (Abdollahiyan et al., 2021). In addition to nanoparticles, the tissue engineering regenerative medicine field has exploited nanoscale technology's nanofibers and nanopatterned surfaces to control cell function (Rajendran et al., 2023). Nerve regeneration and nerve tissue engineering are two interesting tissue engineering regenerative medicine applications that could enhance the quality of life for patients with nerve damage (Li et al., 2021).

Stem cell therapy, commonly referred to as regenerative medicine, promotes the body's natural ability to repair damaged, incapacitated, or defective tissue using stem cells or their byproducts (Shan et al., 2023). A wide range of illnesses, including heart disease, cancer, neurological diseases and diabetes could be treated using stem cell therapy (Alnasser, 2022; Liu et al., 2021; Chen et al., 2020; Rahman et al., 2022). Notably, the fusion of two fields nanotechnology and stem cell sciences discloses new ways to explore the function of molecular machinery governing the differentiation of stem cells and elucidate more about stem cell-based treatment approaches for understanding human disease, prevention and theranostics (Alexander et al., 2019). The establishment of nanotechnology approaches in stem cell research was achieved by utilizing biodegradable, biocompatible, stability, solubility, specificity, multimodality and efficacy for undergoing attachment to cognate receptors (Samuel et al., 2023). Recent research has shown that various nanoparticles, including auto-assembled peptide, superparamagnetic iron oxide nanoparticles (ferucarbotran), magnetic nanoparticles, polyelectrolyte nanoparticles, cerium oxide nanoparticles, graphene oxide nanoparticles, gold nanoparticles, collagen nanofiber and carbon nanofiber have been developed for use in stem cell differentiation and regeneration therapy (Yao et al., 2020; Dong et al., 2021; Jian et al., 2018; Salvetti et al., 2020; Tashakori-Miyanroudi et al., 2023; Zhang et al., 2021).

Additionally, bone compositions made utilising tissue engineering techniques are now considered to be the best choice for the functional repair of segmental deossification (Xue et al., 2022). Titanium, nanohydroxyapatite, graphene oxide, calcium phosphate, carbon nanotubes, or a mix of them can all be utilised to make biomaterials and the scaffold that supports them for tissue engineering in orthopaedic surgery (Monte et al., 2023). Due to their combination of nanomaterials properties, good biocompatibility, and low toxicity, these composite scaffolds have a very broad range of potential applications in orthopaedic surgery and regenerative medicine (Zheng et al., 2021). The impact of various nanomaterials on stem cell research aimed at treating diseases of vital human organs, as well as their promising role in redefining the future of human medicine.

Imaging and Diagnostic

Probes that can sense the spatiotemporal changes in the cellular environments play a major role in the detection of any abnormality in the structure and function of cells, tissues and even the system (Zhang & James, 2023). These sensitive changes in the concentration of analytes have been detected at the molecular level using various imaging procedures including Magnetic Resonance Imaging (MRI), photoacoustic, Raman spectroscopy, and fluorescence or luminescence techniques. Recent advances in the diagnostic field led to the development of biosensors and molecular probes for molecular sensing and imaging. Hence, nanoprobes have been a promising solution for monitoring intracellular and extracellular microenvironment and spatiotemporal changes including temperature, polarity and membrane voltage.

One of the recently studied fluorescent probes offers a great deal of performance in the detection of pathogens (Wu et al., 2022). Fluorescence tools have been used as a bioimaging tool owing to their high sensitivity and specificity and ability to study the spatiotemporal conditions of the cells in real-time (Wu et al., 2017). Polyelectrolyte complex nanoparticles have been shown to improve stability in varying pH conditions (Porfiryeva et al., 2021). Dye-loaded quatsomes consists of ammonium surfactants and sterols which resulted in enhanced photostability with improved sensitivity in low dose (Ardizzone et al., 2018). Metal complexes such as iridium (III) (IrIII), rhenium (I) (RhI), ruthenium (II) (RuII), europium (III) (EuIII) and terbium (III) (TbIII) possess longer emission lifetimes that enable it to detect ions like aluminium ions, phosphates through biosensing and imaging (Zhang & James, 2023). Two-photon fluorescence imaging technique enables deep tissue imaging at near-infrared excitation owing to its longer wavelength. Fluorescent nanoparticles are combined with magnetic nanoparticles to form magneto fluorescent nanoparticles. With the magnetism controlled in the inner core, the external surface of the compounds can be attached with fluorescent quantum dots for image-guided diagnosis.

Light energy which can be transferred to other forms of energy plays an imminent role in photocatalysis, bioimaging and therapy. The light energy that arises from chemical reactions is known as chemiluminescence. Mechanoluminescence refers to the formation of non-thermal light energy from the stimulation of mechanical force to compounds. Some of the nanomaterials that act as force sensors include zinc sulfide doped nanoparticles, semiconducting polymer nanoparticles, naphthopyran derivatives, dioexetane derivatives and cyano-OPV derivatives (Wang et al., 2022). Integration of mechanoluminescence into ultrasound makes it possible for non-invasive deep imaging. Biophotonics is a multidisciplinary discipline which combines technologies which use light for biomedical applications including optical tomography, multiphoton microscopy, near-infrared microscopy and vibrational imaging. Integration of nanotechnology into biophotonics has emerged new ventures into understanding human physiology for improved diagnosis. At the nanoscale, nanophotonics offers tremendous benefits in better sensitivity and specificity. Fluorescent nanoparticles like quantum dots are used for molecular imaging of various types of disease including infectious diseases, cancer diagnosis, wound healing and metabolic diseases like diabetes mellitus.

Infectious Disease Diagnosis and Treatment

Infectious diseases have a big impact on morbidity and death all around the world. In the present time, the treatment of infectious health issues including tuberculosis, malaria and Human Immunodeficiency Virus (HIV) faces severe treatment problems due to their ongoing transmission and high death rates (Varo et al., 2020; Chakaya et al., 2021; Taiwo et al., 2023). The formulation of new and existing drugs in nano-sized carriers serves as a potential solution to a number of problems with treating these diseases, including low on-target bioavailability, sub-therapeutic drug accumulation in microbial sanctuaries and reservoirs and low patient adherence due to drug-related side effects and extensive therapeutic regimens (Kirtane et al., 2021). To enable targeted, sustained drug administration, medications can be encapsulated in nanocarriers like polymer nanoparticles, liposomes or synthetic drug nanocrystals (Jia et al., 2023). Vaccination has been the cheapest and most efficient way to prevent disease. Nanotechnology can be used to target particular cell types for vaccine administration as well as mimic the disease's actual target. Nanocarriers can be used to develop vaccines for infectious illnesses treatment (Cordeiro et al., 2021; Kirtane et al., 2021). There is no reliable vaccine that completely guards against contracting Tuberculosis. The only Tuberculosis vaccine licenced is Bacillus Calmette-Guerin (BCG), which was first introduced in 1921 but only provides mild protection (Li et al., 2021). Therefore, scientists are working to enhance the current BCG vaccine and create new vaccines to stop Tuberculosis. Chitosan, a biocompatible and biodegradable polycationic polymer, is also being investigated by researchers for its capacity as adjuvant therapy in tuberculosis (Pires et al., 2023). In addition, both RUTI and ID93+GLA-SE vaccination employ nanoparticle technology. This approach appears to be effective in enhancing the delivery, effectiveness, cost and storage conditions of the current tuberculosis vaccines (Saramago et al., 2021). The nano-formulated Tuberculosis medication in a single dose can lower the high frequency of administration (Kalombo et al., 2019).

A recent study demonstrated the use of nanoparticles as a physical barrier to stop the spread of disease. Heparin-polymersome combination inhibits malaria infection similarly to a medication and a vaccination

(Mondal et al., 2021). Additionally, the problems of vaccination instability and poor immunogenicity have been addressed using nanotechnology. The virus-like self-assembly and size of fullerenol nanoparticles make them great adjuvants. An HIV-1 vaccine was developed using the nanoadjuvant fullerenol as a plasmid DNA transporter and protector for this precious payload which improved immunological response (Mitchell et al., 2018).

A possible method to improve immune responses to vaccination and enhance the efficacy of medications for treatment is the use of customised nanoparticle vehicles designed to encapsulate therapeutic chemicals and deliver them to a target location. (Maus et al., 2021). In addition, there are now more than ten COVID-19 vaccine candidates based on nanotechnology in clinical trials, many of which are in Phase III and are already demonstrating promising outcomes (Al-Ahmady & Ali-Boucetta, 2020). Although there are such obvious distinctions, there are still no regulations specifically for nanomedicine approval, and any new nanomedicine product must still go through the entire clinical approval process (Mundekkad & Cho, 2022).

CURRENT ISSUES IN THE APPLICATION OF NANOTECHNOLOGY IN BIOMEDICAL SCIENCES

Safety and Toxicity

A completely new field of nanomedicine has emerged as a result of the development of drug and nutrient delivery systems, nanometer-scale contrasts as well as nanostructured materials for enhanced biocompatible interfaces (Patra et al., 2018). However, the expansion of nanoscale materials into the consumer environment, which is growing and is now mostly unregulated, has also sparked worries about the possible negative effects of uncontrolled exposure on human health (Thakur & Kathpalia, 2022). Numerous nanomedicines function by directly interacting with genetic material or by interacting with biomolecules necessary for normal cell division and genome function, all of which have the potential to be genotoxic and mutagenic (Md Anwar Nawaz et al., 2023). The inflammatory response of macrophages and neutrophils, which results in the formation of reactive nitrogen and oxygen species promotes oxidative stress-induced nanomedicine toxicity. Free radicals can seriously harm the body when they build up in the body (Manke et al., 2013; Missaoui et al., 2018). This harm may manifest in a number of ways, such as by inducing oxidative DNA damage that results in strand breaks, lipid peroxidation and protein denaturation that causes cancer, damage to mitochondrial membranes that results in cell death and necrosis and transcription of genes involved in fibrosis and cancer (Manke et al., 2013). There is a plethora of evidence that these particles accumulate in the liver after intravenous administration and go to other organs such as the cardiovascular, central nervous and renal systems (Missaoui et al., 2018). As a relatively established field, nanotoxicology is currently producing systematic knowledge for nanomaterials risk assessment as well as for the creation of safer-by-design nano-enabled goods, both of which are crucial milestones in the clinical translation of nanomedicines (Zielińska et al., 2020). Despite the relatively long history of nanomedicine, there were only about 50 FDA-approved nanomedicines on the market and 77 others in clinical studies, the majority of which were protein and liposome-based complexes (Sahu et al., 2021). Clinical translation of nanomedicine has been difficult due to low efficacy caused by incomplete knowledge of nanomaterial biocompatibility, nano-bio interactions, nanomaterial-specific toxicity, nanomaterial degradation and targeted delivery (Đorđević et al., 2022; Hua et al., 2018; Souri et al., 2022). Major advantages of nanomedicines over conventional medications include tumour targeting, release tunability, and good efficacy/toxicity ratios, which are crucial drivers driving the development of nanomedicine (Shan et al., 2022).

Additionally, it has been suggested that the field of nanotoxicology be changed to "nanosafety" since it is frequently seen from the viewpoint of nanomedicine as a subject that gives toxicity knowledge to direct the construction of safer nanomaterials (Zielińska et al., 2020). In addition, the host's physiological and pathological interactions with the microbiota have made the microbiota a crucial factor in defining the pharmacology and toxicity of nanomedicines (Zielińska et al., 2020; Utembe et al., 2022). At present, there is limited knowledge about how various nanomedicines interact with biological systems, making it difficult to fully comprehend and analyze their physical, chemical, and toxicological characteristics. However, not much will change in this area without consistent regulatory guidance (Nassiri Koopaei & Abdollahi, 2016; Soares et al., 2018).

Regulation

Nanomedicine regulation is crucial because, without it, manufacturers, medical practitioners, the public, and politicians lack legal certainty and clarity. The Nanotechnology Research and Development Act (NRDA), US Food and Drug Administration (FDA) and Environmental Protection Agency (EPA) have all made steps to address possible concerns posed by nanoparticles (Kumari et al., 2023). Local (or semi-local) community projects have been organised and supported which aim to identify the regulatory requirements for the clinical use of nanomedicines and nanomaterials (Ali et al., 2022). The potential environmental impact of nanomedicines during manufacture, usage and disposal is another aspect to take into account while analysing their potential effects. Since nanomedicines are anticipated to act similarly to traditional pharmaceuticals, which are commonly acknowledged to eventually be recovered in the environment, there is a possibility that they may have an adverse effect on the environment (Martínez et al., 2020). Based on estimated environmental consequences, there are inclusion and exclusion criteria used in the evaluation of medicinal items in the USA and the European Union (EU). In the EU, the permitted limit for surface water environmental concentrations is 0.01 ppb, and all marketing authorization applications must go through the pre-screening stage and an environmental risk assessment (Hansen & Baun, 2012). Therefore, no further steps are taken for the product in terms of environmental risk assessment if the estimated environmental concentration is below this and no additional environmental concerns are detected. If a new drug application is submitted in the USA, the FDA must do an environmental assessment unless an exemption applies. However, if the predicted environmental concentration is greater than 1 ppb, an exemption cannot be granted (Foulkes et al., 2020). The primary challenge for the regulation of nanomedicines is the utilisation of safety data from bulk materials by regulatory organisations like the FDA, which do not exhibit the same pharmacologic and pharmacokinetic activity as nanomedicines (Md Anwar Nawaz et al., 2023). Once the nanomedicine has been given marketing authorisation, the results of the safety and efficacy studies will not be a reliable indicator of what might actually happen when it is utilised in clinical settings. A non-nano version may meet regulatory criteria whereas a nanomedicine may not, which creates issues when rules are being established for the safety and efficacy of nanomedicines. More than 50 nanomedicines have been commercialised despite the lack of clear regulatory guidance and this number is continuously increasing (Foulkes et al., 2020; Farjadian et al., 2019). Globally, there is a lack of official control of the manufacture of nanomedicines and nanomaterials for medical uses. Some nanomedicines are classified as medical devices and others as medications due to inconsistencies among the various government agencies (Foulkes et al., 2020). Small compounds often lack global licensing because what is considered suitable in one jurisdiction may not be relevant in another. However, the nanomedicine community urgently needs uniformity across the government sector to enable development to proceed as planned. The manufacture of nanomaterials for use in healthcare applications is not formally regulated, which is regarded as a global problem (Foulkes et al., 2020; Fan et al., 2014).

THE FUTURE DIRECTION OF NANOTECHNOLOGY APPLICATION IN BIOMEDICAL SCIENCES

Nano(eco)toxicology studies provide information on the molecular processes through which nanomaterials interact with microbes that can be used to develop targeted nanomedicines with fewer adverse effects. For the development of targeted nanomedicines with fewer side effects, knowledge of the molecular mechanisms of nanomaterials interacting with microbes gathered from nano(eco)toxicology investigations will be helpful (Bondarenko et al., 2021). It is pertinent to explore the interlink between gut microbiota and metabolic disorders, especially the emerging roles of nanomaterials and modulating effects (Jalil et al., 2023; Lee et al., 2021). Future research in this area, which is pertinent to both nanomedicine and nanotechnology, should focus on analysing how nanomaterials, including potential nanomedicines, affect gut microbial metabolic pathways associated with human diseases by integrating targeted omics studies (Bondarenko et al., 2021; Domingues et al., 2022; Utembe et al., 2022).

Advanced omics technologies, such as epigenomics, culturomics, cellomics, genomics, functional genomics, lipidomics, glycomics, metagenomics, metabolomics, pharmacogenomics, proteomics, pharmacomicrobiomics, transcriptomics and toxicogenomics have greatly transformed medical research in recent years. Next-generation sequencing (NGS) is an emerging technology that holds great promise in generating and analyzing vast biomedical datasets. This breakthrough technology can help us explore fundamental nanotechnology questions such as how nanoscale chemical structures affect drug delivery *in vivo* and which biological pathways govern the delivery of nanoparticles *in vivo* (Paunovska et al., 2019). By integrating multi-omics technology and bionanotechnology, it becomes feasible to overcome challenges and discover innovative and effective biomedical applications for bionanomaterials (Virupannanavar et al., 2023). In the same vein, multi-omics analyses are potential techniques that assist in improving the drugs that nanomedicines are intended to deliver. One way is by enhancing the efficacy of RNA therapies through chemical modifications to the RNA (Abdelkader et al., 2023). Besides, cutting-edge mass spectrometry techniques at the nanoscale level offer a promising solution for more accurate and in-depth identification and quantification of proteins (Aydoğan et al., 2022). Both transcriptomics and proteomics analyses are promising techniques to identify disease-associated proteins or new drug transporters and cell surface antigens (Zou et al., 2022; Suhre et al., 2021). These advanced proteomics technologies can enable faster and more efficient investigation of critical biological inquiries, such as protein-binding signalling pathways and protein modifications, particularly in single-cell protein analysis (Ahmad & Budnik, 2023; Arias-Hidalgo et al., 2022). Advancements in nanotechnology have also made it possible to conduct high-throughput proteomics analysis by employing software tools like Data-driven Alignment of Retention Times for IDentification (DART-ID) and Data-driven Optimization of MS (DO-MS) (Arias-Hidalgo et al., 2022).

Additionally, there are upcoming challenges related to improving drug loading and release, as well as the need for further advancements in the diagnosis and treatment of metallic nanoparticles (Patra et al., 2018). In order to fully utilize the potential of nanomedicine, it is pertinent to carefully weigh the benefits against potential risks. Similar to all other medical devices or treatments, nanomedicine has to undergo strict control and comprehensive evaluation prior to its use for treating patients. This includes assessing its full potential, evaluating its toxicity and conducting multistage clinical studies (Đorđević et al., 2023). Nanotechnology is expected to be capable of detecting root causes without the need for medical expertise, external sensors or probabilistic diagnostic algorithms in the future. Furthermore, athletes can utilize nanotechnology to assess their muscles' circulation and decrease lactic acid production, enhancing their performance. By identifying their weaker muscles, they can adjust their training frequency and optimize their muscle potential (Haleem et al., 2023).

Apart from this, manufacturers, healthcare professionals, the general public and governments lack clarity as well as legal certainty in the absence of guidance (Subhan & Subhan, 2022; Zingg & Fischer, 2019; Schulte & Salamanca-Buentello, 2007). Although there have been some initiatives to establish National Characterization Laboratories among academic groups and government organisations, a more specific and strict direction is required from the major governing bodies, such as the FDA and The Medicines and Healthcare Products Regulatory Agency (MHRA). In order to advance these agendas and provide official direction to the research community, a global consortium for the regulation of nanomaterials should be established (Foulkes et al., 2020). Over the past two decades, billions of dollars have been invested in the creation of nanomedicine, but unless regulatory agencies provide clear leadership and direction, these efforts will fail to produce products that reach the market and future investment will be directed elsewhere (Foulkes et al., 2020; Roco, 2011; Kaur et al., 2014).

CONCLUSION

The development of nanomedicine research has tremendously benefited both the development of new pharmaceuticals and the reformulation of existing ones. Fast-moving developments in nanomedicine offer novel approaches that have the potential to revolutionise healthcare through improvements in efficacy, bioavailability, medication targeting and safety. Therefore, it is necessary to capitalise on current strength and facilitate the clinical development of nano products to address unmet clinical requirements outside of oncology. Additionally, it is essential to fill in the gaps that exist in the development of nanomedicine such as the mass production of Good Manufacturing Practices (GMP) standards, nanotoxicological aspect of new classes of nanomaterials and global regulatory approval clarification regarding both physicochemical characterization and biological activity.

REFERENCES

Abdelkader, Y., Perez-Davalos, L., LeDuc, R., Zahedi, R. P., & Labouta, H. I. (2023). Omics Approaches for the Assessment of Biological Responses to Nanoparticles. *Advanced Drug Delivery Reviews, 114992*, 114992. doi:10.1016/j.addr.2023.114992 PMID:37414362

Abdollahiyan, P., Oroojalian, F., Hejazi, M., de la Guardia, M., & Mokhtarzadeh, A. (2021). Nanotechnology, and scaffold implantation for the effective repair of injured organs: An overview on hard tissue engineering. *Journal of Controlled Release*, *333*, 391–417. doi:10.1016/j.jconrel.2021.04.003 PMID:33823222

Ahmad, R., & Budnik, B. (2023). A review of the current state of single-cell proteomics and future perspective. *Analytical and Bioanalytical Chemistry*, *415*(28), 1–11. doi:10.100700216-023-04759-8 PMID:37285026

Al-Ahmady, Z. S., & Ali-Boucetta, H. (2020). Nanomedicine & nanotoxicology future could be reshaped post-COVID-19 pandemic. *Frontiers in Nanotechnology*, *2*, 610465. doi:10.3389/fnano.2020.610465

Alexander, A., Saraf, S., Saraf, S., Agrawal, M., Patel, R. J., Agrawal, P., Khan, J., & Ajazuddin. (2019). Amalgamation of stem cells with nanotechnology: A unique therapeutic approach. *Current Stem Cell Research & Therapy*, *14*(2), 83–92. doi:10.2174/1574888X13666180703143219 PMID:29968543

Alnasser, S. M. (2022). Stem cell challenge in cancer progression, oncology and therapy. *Gene*, *146748*, 146748. doi:10.1016/j.gene.2022.146748 PMID:35868413

Alven, S., Nqoro, X., Buyana, B., & Aderibigbe, B. A. (2020). Polymer-drug conjugate, a potential therapeutic to combat breast and lung cancer. *Pharmaceutics*, *12*(5), 406. doi:10.3390/pharmaceutics12050406 PMID:32365495

Ardizzone, A., Kurhuzenkau, S., Illa-Tuset, S., Faraudo, J., Bondar, M., Hagan, D., & Ventosa, N. (2018). Nanostructuring Lipophilic Dyes in Water Using Stable Vesicles, Quatsomes, as Scaffolds and Their Use as Probes for Bioimaging. *Small*, *14*(16), e1703851. doi:10.1002mll.201703851 PMID:29573545

Arias-Hidalgo, C., Juanes-Velasco, P., Landeira-Viñuela, A., García-Vaquero, M. L., Montalvillo, E., Góngora, R., Hernández, A., & Fuentes, M. (2022). Single-Cell Proteomics: The Critical Role of Nanotechnology. *International Journal of Molecular Sciences*, *23*(12), 6707. doi:10.3390/ijms23126707 PMID:35743151

Asharani, P., Hande, M. P., & Valiyaveettil, S. (2009). Anti-proliferative activity of silver nanoparticles. *BMC Cell Biology*, *10*(1), 1–14. doi:10.1186/1471-2121-10-65 PMID:19761582

Asl, F. D., Mousazadeh, M., Taji, S., Bahmani, A., Khashayar, P., Azimzadeh, M., & Mostafavi, E. (2023). Nano drug-delivery systems for management of AIDS: Liposomes, dendrimers, gold and silver nanoparticles. *Nanomedicine (London)*, *18*(3), 279–302. doi:10.2217/nnm-2022-0248 PMID:37125616

Ayala-Orozco, C., Urban, C., Bishnoi, S., Urban, A., Charron, H., Mitchell, T., Shea, M., Nanda, S., Schiff, R., Halas, N., & Joshi, A. (2014). Sub-100nm gold nanomatryoshkas improve photo-thermal therapy efficacy in large and highly aggressive triple negative breast tumors. *Journal of Controlled Release*, *191*, 90–97. doi:10.1016/j.jconrel.2014.07.038 PMID:25051221

Aydoğan, C., Beltekin, B., Aslan, H., Yılmaz, F., Göktürk, I., Denizli, A., & El-Rassi, Z. (2022). Nanoscale separations: Recent achievements. *Journal of Chromatography Open*, *2*, 100066. doi:10.1016/j.jcoa.2022.100066

Baig, N., Kammakakam, I., & Falath, W. (2021). Nanomaterials: A review of synthesis methods, properties, recent progress, and challenges. *Materials Advances*, *2*(6), 1821–1871. doi:10.1039/D0MA00807A

Bajwa, K. S., Ali, M. A., Tahir, A., Abbas, H., Ahmad, H., Abid, L., Rana, M. B. U., & Rubab, W. (2018). Nanotechnology: A Triumphant Leap in Health Care and Medicine. *Life Science Journal*, *15*(7). doi:10.7537/marslsj150718.09

Bhutta, Z. A., Kulyar, M. F. E. A., Farooq, U., Ashar, A., Mahfooz, A., Kanwal, A., Akhtar, M., Asif, M., Nawaz, S., & Li, K. (2023). Applications of functionalized nanoparticles in tissue engineering. In *Antiviral and Antimicrobial Coatings Based on Functionalized Nanomaterials* (pp. 485–513). Elsevier. doi:10.1016/B978-0-323-91783-4.00006-1

Bondarenko, O., Mortimer, M., Kahru, A., Feliu, N., Javed, I., Kakinen, A., Lin, S., Xia, T., Song, Y., Davis, T. P., Lynch, I., Parak, W. J., Leong, D. T., Ke, P. C., Chen, C., & Zhao, Y. (2021). Nanotoxicology and nanomedicine: The Yin and Yang of nano-bio interactions for the new decade. *Nano Today*, *39*, 101184. doi:10.1016/j.nantod.2021.101184 PMID:36937379

Bueno, C. Z., Oliveira, C. A., & Rangel-Yagui, C. D. O. (2018). Polymeric and liposomal nanomaterials. In *Nanobiomaterials* (pp. 437–464). Woodhead Publishing. doi:10.1016/B978-0-08-100716-7.00017-9

Bukhari, I., Iqbal, F., & Thorne, R. F. (2022). Research advances in gestational, neonatal diabetes mellitus and metabolic disorders. *Frontiers in Endocrinology*, *13*, 969952. doi:10.3389/fendo.2022.969952 PMID:35966084

Cartlidge, M. K., & Hill, A. T. (2017). Inhaled or nebulised ciprofloxacin for the maintenance treatment of bronchiectasis. *Expert Opinion on Investigational Drugs*, *26*(9), 1091–1097. doi:10.1080/13543784.2017.1364728 PMID:28778139

Chakaya, J., Khan, M., Ntoumi, F., Aklillu, E., Fatima, R., Mwaba, P., Kapata, N., Mfinanga, S., Hasnain, S. E., Katoto, P. D. M. C., Bulabula, A. N. H., Sam-Agudu, N. A., Nachega, J. B., Tiberi, S., McHugh, T. D., Abubakar, I., & Zumla, A. (2021). Global Tuberculosis Report 2020–Reflections on the Global TB burden, treatment and prevention efforts. *International Journal of Infectious Diseases*, *113*, S7–S12. doi:10.1016/j.ijid.2021.02.107 PMID:33716195

Chakraborty, N., Jha, D., Roy, I., Kumar, P., Gaurav, S. S., Marimuthu, K., Ng, O. T., Lakshminarayanan, R., Verma, N. K., & Gautam, H. K. (2022). Nanobiotics against antimicrobial resistance: Harnessing the power of nanoscale materials and technologies. *Journal of Nanobiotechnology*, *20*(1), 375. doi:10.118612951-022-01573-9 PMID:35953826

Chen, S., Du, K., & Zou, C. (2020). Current progress in stem cell therapy for type 1 diabetes mellitus. *Stem Cell Research & Therapy*, *11*(1), 1–13. doi:10.118613287-020-01793-6 PMID:32641151

Chen, W., Liu, K., & Zhang, J. (2022). Functional nanomaterials: From structures to biomedical applications. *Molecules (Basel, Switzerland)*, *27*(21), 7492. doi:10.3390/molecules27217492 PMID:36364319

Cheng, Z., Li, M., Dey, R., & Chen, Y. (2021). Nanomaterials for cancer therapy: Current progress and perspectives. *Journal of Hematology & Oncology*, *14*(1), 1–27. doi:10.118613045-021-01096-0 PMID:34059100

Chis, A. A., Dobrea, C., Morgovan, C., Arseniu, A. M., Rus, L. L., Butuca, A., Juncan, A. M., Totan, M., Vonica-Tincu, A. L., Cormos, G., Muntean, A. C., Muresan, M. L., Gligor, F. G., & Frum, A. (2020). Applications and limitations of dendrimers in biomedicine. *Molecules (Basel, Switzerland)*, *25*(17), 3982. doi:10.3390/molecules25173982 PMID:32882920

Chordiya, K., Patwa, H., Walode, S. G., & Chatur, V. M. (2021). Role of Nanoparticles in the Management of Diabetes. *Int. Journal of Pharmaceutical Sciences and Medicine*, *6*(4), 83–91. doi:10.47760/ijpsm.2021.v06i04.007

Choudhury, H., Pandey, M., Lim, Y. Q., Low, C. Y., Lee, C. T., Marilyn, T. C. L., Loh, H. S., Lim, Y. P., Lee, C. F., Bhattamishra, S. K., Kesharwani, P., & Gorain, B. (2020). Silver nanoparticles: Advanced and promising technology in diabetic wound therapy. *Materials Science and Engineering C*, *112*, 110925. doi:10.1016/j.msec.2020.110925 PMID:32409075

Cordeiro, A. S., Patil-Sen, Y., Shivkumar, M., Patel, R., Khedr, A., & Elsawy, M. A. (2021). Nanovaccine delivery approaches and advanced delivery systems for the prevention of viral infections: From development to clinical application. *Pharmaceutics*, *13*(12), 2091. doi:10.3390/pharmaceutics13122091 PMID:34959372

Crinson, I., & Crinson, I. (2021). The Interdisciplinarity Field of Social Studies of Science and Technology (SSST). *The Biomedical Sciences in Society: An Interdisciplinary Analysis*, 1-16. doi:10.1007/978-981-15-9523-3_1

da Silva, A. L., Silva, L. A., Cruz, F. F., Rocco, P. R. M., & Morales, M. M. (2020). Application of novel nanotechnologies in asthma. *Annals of Translational Medicine*, *8*(5), 159. doi:10.21037/atm.2019.12.40 PMID:32309307

Deng, S., Gu, J., Jiang, Z., Cao, Y., Mao, F., Xue, Y., Wang, J., Dai, K., Qin, L., Wu, K., He, Q., & Cai, K. (2022). Application of nanotechnology in the early diagnosis and comprehensive treatment of gastrointestinal cancer. *Journal of Nanobiotechnology*, *20*(1), 415. doi:10.118612951-022-01613-4 PMID:36109734

Deng, Y., Zhang, X., Shen, H., He, Q., Wu, Z., Liao, W., & Yuan, M. (2020). Application of the nano-drug delivery system in treatment of cardiovascular diseases. *Frontiers in Bioengineering and Biotechnology*, *7*, 489. doi:10.3389/fbioe.2019.00489 PMID:32083068

Diez-Pascual, A. M., & Rahdar, A. (2022). Functional Nanomaterials in Biomedicine: Current Uses and Potential Applications. *ChemMedChem*, *17*(16), e202200142. doi:10.1002/cmdc.202200142 PMID:35729066

Dilworth, L., Facey, A., & Omoruyi, F. (2021). Diabetes mellitus and its metabolic complications: The role of adipose tissues. *International Journal of Molecular Sciences*, *22*(14), 7644. doi:10.3390/ijms22147644 PMID:34299261

Domingues, C., Santos, A., Alvarez-Lorenzo, C., Concheiro, A., Jarak, I., Veiga, F., Barbosa, I., Dourado, M., & Figueiras, A. (2022). Where is nano today and where is it headed? A review of nanomedicine and the dilemma of nanotoxicology. *ACS Nano*, *16*(7), 9994–10041. doi:10.1021/acsnano.2c00128 PMID:35729778

Dong, Y., Wu, X., Chen, X., Zhou, P., Xu, F., & Liang, W. (2021). Nanotechnology shaping stem cell therapy: Recent advances, application, challenges, and future outlook. *Biomedicine and Pharmacotherapy*, *137*, 111236. doi:10.1016/j.biopha.2021.111236 PMID:33486201

Đorđević, S., Gonzalez, M. M., Conejos-Sánchez, I., Carreira, B., Pozzi, S., Acúrcio, R. C., Satchi-Fainaro, R., Florindo, H. F., & Vicent, M. J. (2022). Current hurdles to the translation of nanomedicines from bench to the clinic. *Drug Delivery and Translational Research*, *12*(3), 1–26. doi:10.100713346-021-01024-2 PMID:34302274

Dristant, U., Mukherjee, K., Saha, S., & Maity, D. (2023). An Overview of Polymeric Nanoparticles-Based Drug Delivery System in Cancer Treatment. *Technology in Cancer Research & Treatment*, *22*, 15330338231152083. doi:10.1177/15330338231152083 PMID:36718541

Duarte, A. A., Mohsin, S., & Golubnitschaja, O. (2018). Diabetes care in figures: Current pitfalls and future scenario. *The EPMA Journal*, *9*(2), 125–131. doi:10.100713167-018-0133-y PMID:29896313

Fan, R. Z., Fei, D., D'Aurelio, R., & Ge, Y. (2014). The Impact of Nanopharmaceuticals on Healthcare and Regulation. *Nanomedicine: Principles and Perspectives*, 355-364. doi:10.1007/978-1-4614-2140-5_17

Faria, M., Björnmalm, M., Thurecht, K. J., Kent, S. J., Parton, R. G., Kavallaris, M., Johnston, A. P. R., Gooding, J. J., Corrie, S. R., Boyd, B. J., Thordarson, P., Whittaker, A. K., Stevens, M. M., Prestidge, C. A., Porter, C. J. H., Parak, W. J., Davis, T. P., Crampin, E. J., & Caruso, F. (2018). Minimum information reporting in bio–nano experimental literature. *Nature Nanotechnology*, *13*(9), 777–785. doi:10.103841565-018-0246-4 PMID:30190620

Farjadian, F., Ghasemi, A., Gohari, O., Roointan, A., Karimi, M., & Hamblin, M. R. (2019). Nanopharmaceuticals and nanomedicines currently on the market: Challenges and opportunities. *Nanomedicine (London)*, *14*(1), 93–126. doi:10.2217/nnm-2018-0120 PMID:30451076

Fathi-Achachelouei, M., Knopf-Marques, H., Ribeiro da Silva, C. E., Barthès, J., Bat, E., Tezcaner, A., & Vrana, N. E. (2019). Use of nanoparticles in tissue engineering and regenerative medicine. *Frontiers in Bioengineering and Biotechnology*, *7*, 113. doi:10.3389/fbioe.2019.00113 PMID:31179276

Foulkes, R., Man, E., Thind, J., Yeung, S., Joy, A., & Hoskins, C. (2020). The regulation of nanomaterials and nanomedicines for clinical application: Current and future perspectives. *Biomaterials Science*, *8*(17), 4653–4664. doi:10.1039/D0BM00558D PMID:32672255

Fritea, L., Banica, F., Costea, T. O., Moldovan, L., Dobjanschi, L., Muresan, M., & Cavalu, S. (2021). Metal nanoparticles and carbon-based nanomaterials for improved performances of electrochemical (Bio) sensors with biomedical applications. *Materials (Basel)*, *14*(21), 6319. doi:10.3390/ma14216319 PMID:34771844

Garcia-Gonzalez, I., Mühleder, S., Fernández-Chacón, M., & Benedito, R. (2020). Genetic tools to study cardiovascular biology. *Frontiers in Physiology*, *11*, 1084. doi:10.3389/fphys.2020.01084 PMID:33071802

Ghazanfar, H., Rizvi, S. W., Khurram, A., Orooj, F., & Qaiser, I. (2016). Impact of insulin pump on quality of life of diabetic patients. *Indian Journal of Endocrinology and Metabolism*, *20*(4), 506. doi:10.4103/2230-8210.183472 PMID:27366717

Giljohann, D. A., Seferos, D. S., Daniel, W. L., Massich, M. D., Patel, P. C., & Mirkin, C. A. (2010). Gold nanoparticles for biology and medicine. *Angewandte Chemie International Edition*, *49*(19), 3280–3294. doi:10.1002/anie.200904359 PMID:20401880

Goyal, R., Macri, L. K., Kaplan, H. M., & Kohn, J. (2016). Nanoparticles and nanofibers for topical drug delivery. *Journal of Controlled Release*, *240*, 77–92. doi:10.1016/j.jconrel.2015.10.049 PMID:26518723

Greulich, C., Diendorf, J., Simon, T., Eggeler, G., Epple, M., & Köller, M. (2011). Uptake and intracellular distribution of silver nanoparticles in human mesenchymal stem cells. *Acta Biomaterialia*, *7*(1), 347–354. doi:10.1016/j.actbio.2010.08.003 PMID:20709196

Guimarães, D., Cavaco-Paulo, A., & Nogueira, E. (2021). Design of liposomes as drug delivery system for therapeutic applications. *International Journal of Pharmaceutics*, *601*, 120571. doi:10.1016/j.ijpharm.2021.120571 PMID:33812967

Guo, J., Rahme, K., He, Y., Li, L. L., Holmes, J. D., & O'Driscoll, C. M. (2017). Gold nanoparticles enlighten the future of cancer theranostics. *International Journal of Nanomedicine*, *12*, 6131–6152. doi:10.2147/IJN.S140772 PMID:28883725

Gupta, R. (2017). Diabetes treatment by nanotechnology. *Journal of Biotechnology & Biomaterials*, *7*(3), 268. doi:10.4172/2155-952X.1000268

Haleem, A., Javaid, M., Singh, R. P., Rab, S., & Suman, R. (2023). Applications of Nanotechnology in Medical field. *Global Health Journal (Amsterdam, Netherlands)*, *7*(2), 70–77. Advance online publication. doi:10.1016/j.glohj.2023.02.008

Hamimed, S., Jabberi, M., & Chatti, A. (2022). Nanotechnology in drug and gene delivery. *Naunyn-Schmiedeberg's Archives of Pharmacology*, *395*(7), 769–787. doi:10.100700210-022-02245-z PMID:35505234

Han, F., Wang, J., Ding, L., Hu, Y., Li, W., Yuan, Z., Guo, Q., Zhu, C., Yu, L., Wang, H., Zhao, Z., Jia, L., Li, J., Yu, Y., Zhang, W., Chu, G., Chen, S., & Li, B. (2020). Tissue engineering and regenerative medicine: Achievements, future, and sustainability in Asia. *Frontiers in Bioengineering and Biotechnology*, *8*, 83. doi:10.3389/fbioe.2020.00083 PMID:32266221

Hanna, E., Rémuzat, C., Auquier, P., & Toumi, M. (2017). Gene therapies development: Slow progress and promising prospect. *Journal of Market Access & Health Policy*, *5*(1), 1265293. doi:10.1080/20016689.2017.1265293 PMID:28265348

Hansen, S. F., & Baun, A. (2012). European regulation affecting nanomaterials-review of limitations and future recommendations. *Dose-Response*, *10*(3), dose-response.1. doi:10.2203/dose-response.10-029.Hansen PMID:22942870

Hua, S., De Matos, M. B., Metselaar, J. M., & Storm, G. (2018). Current trends and challenges in the clinical translation of nanoparticulate nanomedicines: Pathways for translational development and commercialization. *Frontiers in Pharmacology*, *9*, 790. doi:10.3389/fphar.2018.00790 PMID:30065653

Jalil, A. T., Thabit, S. N., Hanan, Z. K., Alasheqi, M. Q., Al-Azzawi, A. K. J., Zabibah, R. S., & Fadhil, A. A. (2023). Modulating gut microbiota using nanotechnology to increase anticancer efficacy of the treatments. *Macromolecular Research*, *31*(8), 1–14. doi:10.100713233-023-00168-z

Janež, A., Guja, C., Mitrakou, A., Lalic, N., Tankova, T., Czupryniak, L., Tabak, A. G., Prazny, M. P., & Smircic-Duvnjak, L. (2020). Insulin therapy in adults with type 1 diabetes mellitus: A narrative review. *Diabetes Therapy : Research, Treatment and Education of Diabetes and Related Disorders*, *11*(2), 387–409. doi:10.100713300-019-00743-7 PMID:31902063

Jangam, S. R., Hayter, G., & Dunn, T. C. (2013). Impact of glucose measurement processing delays on clinical accuracy and relevance. *Journal of Diabetes Science and Technology*, *7*(3), 660–668. doi:10.1177/193229681300700311 PMID:23759399

Javed, R., Ahmad, M. A., & Ao, Q. (2019). Theranostic applications of nanobiotechnology in cancer. *Nanotheranostics: Applications and Limitations*, 277-295. doi:10.1007/978-3-030-29768-8_13

Jensen, T. L., Gøtzsche, C. R., & Woldbye, D. P. (2021). Current and future prospects for gene therapy for rare genetic diseases affecting the brain and spinal cord. *Frontiers in Molecular Neuroscience*, *14*, 695937. doi:10.3389/fnmol.2021.695937 PMID:34690692

Jia, Y., Jiang, Y., He, Y., Zhang, W., Zou, J., Magar, K. T., Boucetta, H., Teng, C., & He, W. (2023). Approved Nanomedicine against Diseases. *Pharmaceutics*, *15*(3), 774. doi:10.3390/pharmaceutics15030774 PMID:36986635

Jian, W. H., Wang, H. C., Kuan, C. H., Chen, M. H., Wu, H. C., Sun, J. S., & Wang, T. W. (2018). Glycosaminoglycan-based hybrid hydrogel encapsulated with polyelectrolyte complex nanoparticles for endogenous stem cell regulation in central nervous system regeneration. *Biomaterials*, *174*, 17–30. doi:10.1016/j.biomaterials.2018.05.009 PMID:29763775

Jiffrin, R., Razak, S. I. A., Jamaludin, M. I., Hamzah, A. S. A., Mazian, M. A., Jaya, M. A. T., Nasrullah, M. Z., Majrashi, M., Theyab, A., Aldarmahi, A. A., Aman, Z., Abdel-Daim, M. M., & Azad, A. K. (2022). Electrospun nanofiber composites for drug delivery: A review on current progresses. *Polymers*, *14*(18), 3725. doi:10.3390/polym14183725 PMID:36145871

Kalombo, L., Lemmer, Y., Semete-Makokotlela, B., Ramalapa, B., Nkuna, P., Booysen, L. L., Naidoo, S., Hayeshi, R., Verschoor, J. A., & Swai, H. S. (2019). Spray-dried, nanoencapsulated, multi-drug anti-tuberculosis therapy aimed at once weekly administration for the duration of treatment. *Nanomaterials (Basel, Switzerland)*, *9*(8), 1167. doi:10.3390/nano9081167 PMID:31443150

Karakuş, K. E., Sakarya, S., Yeşiltepe Mutlu, G., Berkkan, M., Muradoğlu, S., Can, E., Gökçe, T., Eviz, E., & Hatun, Ş. (2021). Benefits and drawbacks of Continuous Glucose Monitoring (CGM) use in young children with type 1 diabetes: A qualitative study from a country where the CGM is not reimbursed. *Journal of Patient Experience*, *8*, 23743735211056523. doi:10.1177/23743735211056523 PMID:34881352

Kaur, I. P., Kakkar, V., Deol, P. K., Yadav, M., Singh, M., & Sharma, I. (2014). Issues and concerns in nanotech product development and its commercialization. *Journal of Controlled Release*, *193*, 51–62. doi:10.1016/j.jconrel.2014.06.005 PMID:24933600

Keating, P., & Cambrosio, A. (2003). *Biomedical platforms: realigning the normal and the pathological in late-twentieth-century medicine*. Mit Press. doi:10.7551/mitpress/1622.001.0001

Kirtane, A. R., Verma, M., Karandikar, P., Furin, J., Langer, R., & Traverso, G. (2021). Nanotechnology approaches for global infectious diseases. *Nature Nanotechnology*, *16*(4), 369–384. doi:10.103841565-021-00866-8 PMID:33753915

Komalla, V., & Haghi, M. (2020). Liposomes in the treatment of chronic respiratory conditions. In *Targeting chronic inflammatory lung diseases using advanced drug delivery systems* (pp. 375–392). Academic Press. doi:10.1016/B978-0-12-820658-4.00018-2

Kumar, M. (2013). Molecular Biology Application in Biomedicine and Toxicology. *Annals of the Romanian Society for Cell Biology*, 15–26. doi:10.3389/fgeed.2023.1200987

Kumari, R., Suman, K., Karmakar, S., Lakra, S. G., Saurav, G. K., & Mahto, B. K. (2023). Regulation and safety measures for nanotechnology-based agri-products. *Frontiers in Genome Editing*, *5*, 1200987. doi:10.3389/fgeed.2023.1200987 PMID:37415849

Labieniec-Watala, M., Karolczak, K., Siewiera, K., & Watala, C. (2013). The Janus face of PAMAM dendrimers used to potentially cure nonenzymatic modifications of biomacromolecules in metabolic disorders—A critical review of the pros and cons. *Molecules (Basel, Switzerland)*, *18*(11), 13769–13811. doi:10.3390/molecules181113769 PMID:24213655

Lee, Y., Kamada, N., & Moon, J. J. (2021). Oral nanomedicine for modulating immunity, intestinal barrier functions, and gut microbiome. *Advanced Drug Delivery Reviews*, *179*, 114021. doi:10.1016/j.addr.2021.114021 PMID:34710529

Li, H., Wei, W., & Xu, H. (2022). Drug discovery is an eternal challenge for the biomedical sciences. *Acta Materia Medica*, *1*(1), 1–3. doi:10.15212/AMM-2022-1001

Li, Y., Ma, Z., Ren, Y., Lu, D., Li, T., Li, W., Wang, J., Ma, H. M., & Zhao, J. (2021). Tissue engineering strategies for peripheral nerve regeneration. *Frontiers in Neurology*, *12*, 768267. doi:10.3389/fneur.2021.768267 PMID:34867754

Liang, K., Xie, Q., Nie, J., & Deng, J. (2021). Study on the effect of education for insulin injection in diabetic patients with new simulation tools. *Medicine*, *100*(14), e25424. doi:10.1097/MD.0000000000025424 PMID:33832143

Liu, C., Han, D., Liang, P., Li, Y., & Cao, F. (2021). The current dilemma and breakthrough of stem cell therapy in ischemic heart disease. *Frontiers in Cell and Developmental Biology*, *9*, 636136. doi:10.3389/fcell.2021.636136 PMID:33968924

Liu, Y., Zeng, S., Ji, W., Yao, H., Lin, L., Cui, H., Santos, H. A., & Pan, G. (2022). Emerging theranostic nanomaterials in diabetes and its complications. *Advancement of Science*, *9*(3), 2102466. doi:10.1002/advs.202102466 PMID:34825525

Llop, J., & Lammers, T. (2021). Nanoparticles for Cancer Diagnosis, Radionuclide Therapy and Theranostics. *ACS Nano*, *15*(11), 16974–16981. doi:10.1021/acsnano.1c09139 PMID:34748314

Lohcharoenkal, W., Wang, L., Chen, Y. C., & Rojanasakul, Y. (2014). Protein nanoparticles as drug delivery carriers for cancer therapy. *BioMed Research International*, *2014*, 1–12. doi:10.1155/2014/180549 PMID:24772414

Machtakova, M., Thérien-Aubin, H., & Landfester, K. (2022). Polymer nano-systems for the encapsulation and delivery of active biomacromolecular therapeutic agents. *Chemical Society Reviews*, *51*(1), 128–152. doi:10.1039/D1CS00686J PMID:34762084

Makabenta, J. M. V., Nabawy, A., Li, C. H., Schmidt-Malan, S., Patel, R., & Rotello, V. M. (2021). Nanomaterial-based therapeutics for antibiotic-resistant bacterial infections. *Nature Reviews. Microbiology*, *19*(1), 23–36. doi:10.103841579-020-0420-1 PMID:32814862

Makvandi, P., Song, H., Yiu, C. K., Sartorius, R., Zare, E. N., Rabiee, N., Wu, W. X., Paiva-Santos, A. C., Wang, X. D., Yu, C. Z., & Tay, F. R. (2023). Bioengineered materials with selective antimicrobial toxicity in biomedicine. *Military Medical Research*, *10*(1), 8. doi:10.118640779-023-00443-1 PMID:36829246

Maleki, M., Pourhassan-Moghaddam, M., Karimi, A., Akbarzadeh, A., Zarghami, N., & Mohammadi, S. (2019). Synthesis, characterisation, and application of chamomile gold nanoparticles in molecular diagnostics: A new component for PCR kits. *Biointerface Research in Applied Chemistry*, *9*(6), 4635–4641. doi:10.33263/BRIAC96.635641

Mali, S. (2013). Delivery systems for gene therapy. *Indian Journal of Human Genetics*, *19*(1), 3. doi:10.4103/0971-6866.112870 PMID:23901186

Mansoor, S., Kondiah, P. P., Choonara, Y. E., & Pillay, V. (2019). Polymer-based nanoparticle strategies for insulin delivery. *Polymers*, *11*(9), 1380. doi:10.3390/polym11091380 PMID:31443473

Markman, J. L., Rekechenetskiy, A., Holler, E., & Ljubimova, J. Y. (2013). Nanomedicine therapeutic approaches to overcome cancer drug resistance. *Advanced Drug Delivery Reviews*, *65*(13-14), 1866–1879. doi:10.1016/j.addr.2013.09.019 PMID:24120656

Martínez, G., Merinero, M., Pérez-Aranda, M., Pérez-Soriano, E. M., Ortiz, T., Villamor, E., Begines, B., & Alcudia, A. (2020). Environmental impact of nanoparticles' application as an emerging technology: A review. *Materials (Basel)*, *14*(1), 166. doi:10.3390/ma14010166 PMID:33396469

Marzi, M., Osanloo, M., Vakil, M. K., Mansoori, Y., Ghasemian, A., Dehghan, A., & Zarenezhad, E. (2022). Applications of metallic nanoparticles in the skin cancer treatment. *BioMed Research International*, *2022*, 1–20. doi:10.1155/2022/2346941 PMID:36420097

Maus, A., Strait, L., & Zhu, D. (2021). Nanoparticles as delivery vehicles for antiviral therapeutic drugs. *Engineered Regeneration*, *2*, 31–46. doi:10.1016/j.engreg.2021.03.001

Md Anwar Nawaz, R., Darul Raiyaan, G. I., Sivakumar, K., & Arunachalam, K. D. (2023). Nanomedicine Regulation and Future Prospects. *Advances in Novel Formulations for Drug Delivery*, 67-80. doi:10.1002/9781394167708.ch4

Missaoui, W. N., Arnold, R. D., & Cummings, B. S. (2018). Toxicological status of nanoparticles: What we know and what we don't know. *Chemico-Biological Interactions*, *295*, 1–12. doi:10.1016/j.cbi.2018.07.015 PMID:30048623

Mitchell, M. J., Billingsley, M. M., Haley, R. M., Wechsler, M. E., Peppas, N. A., & Langer, R. (2021). Engineering precision nanoparticles for drug delivery. *Nature Reviews. Drug Discovery*, *20*(2), 101–124. doi:10.103841573-020-0090-8 PMID:33277608

Mitchell, S. L., & Carlson, E. E. (2018). Tiny things with enormous impact: Nanotechnology in the fight against infectious disease. *ACS Infectious Diseases*, *4*(10), 1432–1435. doi:10.1021/acsinfecdis.8b00138 PMID:30070819

Mondal, R. (2021). Nanotechnology in Microbiology. *Nanotechnology for Advances in Medical Microbiology*, 269-293. doi:10.1007/978-981-15-9916-3_11

Monte, J. P., Fontes, A., Santos, B. S., Pereira, G. A., & Pereira, G. (2023). Recent advances in hydroxyapatite/polymer/silver nanoparticles scaffolds with antimicrobial activity for bone regeneration. *Materials Letters*, *134027*, 134027. doi:10.1016/j.matlet.2023.134027

Mujawar, M. A., Gohel, H., Bhardwaj, S. K., Srinivasan, S., Hickman, N., & Kaushik, A. (2020). Nano-enabled biosensing systems for intelligent healthcare: Towards COVID-19 management. *Materials Today. Chemistry*, *17*, 100306. doi:10.1016/j.mtchem.2020.100306 PMID:32835155

Mundekkad, D., & Cho, W. C. (2022). Nanoparticles in clinical translation for cancer therapy. *International Journal of Molecular Sciences*, *23*(3), 1685. doi:10.3390/ijms23031685 PMID:35163607

Mustfa, S. A., Maurizi, E., McGrath, J., & Chiappini, C. (2021). Nanomedicine approaches to negotiate local biobarriers for topical drug delivery. *Advanced Therapeutics*, *4*(1), 2000160. doi:10.1002/adtp.202000160

Nassiri Koopaei, N., & Abdollahi, M. (2016). Opportunities and obstacles to the development of nanopharmaceuticals for human use. *Daru : Journal of Faculty of Pharmacy, Tehran University of Medical Sciences*, *24*, 1–6. 10.1186%2Fs40199-016-0163-8 PMID:27716350

National Research Council. (2003). *Large-scale biomedical science: exploring strategies for future research*. National Academies Press. doi:10.17226/10718

Ng, E. Y., & Etehadtavakol, M. (Eds.). (2017). *Application of infrared to biomedical sciences*. Springer., doi:10.1007/978-981-10-3147-2

Padhi, S., Nayak, A. K., & Behera, A. (2020). Type II diabetes mellitus: A review on recent drug based therapeutics. *Biomedicine and Pharmacotherapy*, *131*, 110708. doi:10.1016/j.biopha.2020.110708 PMID:32927252

Pahle, J., & Walther, W. (2016). Vectors and strategies for nonviral cancer gene therapy. *Expert Opinion on Biological Therapy*, *16*(4), 443–461. doi:10.1517/14712598.2016.1134480 PMID:26761200

Pathomthongtaweechai, N., & Muanprasat, C. (2021). Potential applications of chitosan-based nanomaterials to surpass the gastrointestinal physiological obstacles and enhance the intestinal drug absorption. *Pharmaceutics*, *13*(6), 887. doi:10.3390/pharmaceutics13060887 PMID:34203816

Patil, S., Gao, Y. G., Lin, X., Li, Y., Dang, K., Tian, Y., Zhnag, W. J., Jiang, S. F., Qadir, A., & Qian, A. R. (2019). The development of functional non-viral vectors for gene delivery. *International Journal of Molecular Sciences*, *20*(21), 5491. doi:10.3390/ijms20215491 PMID:31690044

Patra, J. K., Das, G., Fraceto, L. F., Campos, E. V. R., Rodriguez-Torres, M. D. P., Acosta-Torres, L. S., Torres, L. A., Grillo, R., Swamy, M. K., Sharma, S., Habtemariam, S., & Shin, H. S. (2018). Nano based drug delivery systems: Recent developments and future prospects. *Journal of Nanobiotechnology*, *16*(1), 1–33. doi:10.118612951-018-0392-8 PMID:30231877

Paunovska, K., Loughrey, D., Sago, C. D., Langer, R., & Dahlman, J. E. (2019). Using large datasets to understand nanotechnology. *Advanced Materials*, *31*(43), 1902798. doi:10.1002/adma.201902798 PMID:31429126

Peserico, A., Di Berardino, C., Russo, V., Capacchietti, G., Di Giacinto, O., Canciello, A., Rapini, C. C. S., & Barboni, B. (2022). Nanotechnology-Assisted Cell Tracking. *Nanomaterials (Basel, Switzerland)*, *12*(9), 1414. doi:10.3390/nano12091414 PMID:35564123

Pires, D., Mandal, M., Matos, A. I., Peres, C., Catalão, M. J., Azevedo-Pereira, J. M., Satchi-Fainaro, R., Florindo, H. F., & Anes, E. (2023). Development of Chitosan Particles Loaded with siRNA for Cystatin C to Control Intracellular Drug-Resistant Mycobacterium tuberculosis. *Antibiotics (Basel, Switzerland)*, *12*(4), 729. doi:10.3390/antibiotics12040729 PMID:37107091

Porfiryeva, N. N., Semina, I. I., Salakhov, I. A., Moustafine, R. I., & Khutoryanskiy, V. V. (2021). Mucoadhesive and mucus-penetrating interpolyelectrolyte complexes for nose-to-brain drug delivery. *Nanomedicine (London)*, *37*, 102432. doi:10.1016/j.nano.2021.102432 PMID:34186258

Qin, L., Cui, Z., Wu, Y., Wang, H., Zhang, X., Guan, J., & Mao, S. (2022). Challenges and strategies to enhance the systemic absorption of inhaled peptides and proteins. *Pharmaceutical Research*, 1–19. doi:10.100711095-022-03435-3 PMID:36385216

Rahman, M. M., Islam, M. R., Islam, M. T., Harun-Or-Rashid, M., Islam, M., Abdullah, S., Uddin, M. B., Das, S., Rahaman, M. S., Ahmed, M., Alhumaydhi, F. A., Emran, T. B., Mohamed, A. A. R., Faruque, M. R. I., Khandaker, M. U., & Mostafa-Hedeab, G. (2022). Stem cell transplantation therapy and neurological disorders: Current status and future perspectives. *Biology (Basel)*, *11*(1), 147. doi:10.3390/biology11010147 PMID:35053145

Rahman, M. S., Hossain, K. S., Das, S., Kundu, S., Adegoke, E. O., Rahman, M. A., Hannan, M. A., Uddin, M. J., & Pang, M. G. (2021). Role of insulin in health and disease: An update. *International Journal of Molecular Sciences*, *22*(12), 6403. doi:10.3390/ijms22126403 PMID:34203830

Rai, R., Alwani, S., & Badea, I. (2019). Polymeric nanoparticles in gene therapy: New avenues of design and optimization for delivery applications. *Polymers*, *11*(4), 745. doi:10.3390/polym11040745 PMID:31027272

Rajendran, A. K., Kim, H. D., Kim, J. W., Bae, J. W., & Hwang, N. S. (2023). Nanotechnology in tissue engineering and regenerative medicine. *Korean Journal of Chemical Engineering*, *40*(2), 286–301. doi:10.100711814-022-1363-1

Rashid, R., Naqash, A., Bader, G. N., & Sheikh, F. A. (2020). Nanotechnology and diabetes management: Recent advances and future perspectives. *Application of Nanotechnology in Biomedical Sciences*, 99-117. doi:10.1007/978-981-15-5622-7_6

Ren, R., Lim, C., Li, S., Wang, Y., Song, J., Lin, T. W., Muir, B. W., Hsu, H. Y., & Shen, H. H. (2022). Recent advances in the development of lipid-, metal-, carbon-, and polymer-based nanomaterials for antibacterial applications. *Nanomaterials (Basel, Switzerland)*, *12*(21), 3855. doi:10.3390/nano12213855 PMID:36364631

Rhodes, C. J. (2011). Electron Spin Resonance.: Part One: A Diagnostic Method in the Biomedical Sciences. *Science Progress*, *94*(1), 16–96. doi:10.3184/003685011X12982218769939 PMID:21548528

Riley, M. K. II, & Vermerris, W. (2017). Recent advances in nanomaterials for gene delivery—A review. *Nanomaterials (Basel, Switzerland)*, *7*(5), 94. doi:10.3390/nano7050094 PMID:28452950

Roco, M. C. (2011). The long view of nanotechnology development: The National Nanotechnology Initiative at 10 years. *Journal of Nanoparticle Research*, *13*(2), 427–445. doi:10.100711051-010-0192-z

Roma-Rodrigues, C., Rivas-García, L., Baptista, P. V., & Fernandes, A. R. (2020). Gene therapy in cancer treatment: Why go nano? *Pharmaceutics*, *12*(3), 233. doi:10.3390/pharmaceutics12030233 PMID:32151052

Sahu, T., Ratre, Y. K., Chauhan, S., Bhaskar, L. V. K. S., Nair, M. P., & Verma, H. K. (2021). Nanotechnology based drug delivery system: Current strategies and emerging therapeutic potential for medical science. *Journal of Drug Delivery Science and Technology*, *63*, 102487. doi:10.1016/j.jddst.2021.102487

Sakthi Devi, R., Girigoswami, A., Siddharth, M., & Girigoswami, K. (2022). Applications of gold and silver nanoparticles in theranostics. *Applied Biochemistry and Biotechnology*, *194*(9), 4187–4219. doi:10.100712010-022-03963-z PMID:35551613

Salvetti, A., Gambino, G., Rossi, L., De Pasquale, D., Pucci, C., Linsalata, S., Innocenti, A. D., Nitti, S., Prato, M., Ippolito, C., & Ciofani, G. (2020). Stem cell and tissue regeneration analysis in low-dose irradiated planarians treated with cerium oxide nanoparticles. *Materials Science and Engineering C*, *115*, 111113. doi:10.1016/j.msec.2020.111113 PMID:32600713

Samavati, S. S., Kashanian, S., Derakhshankhah, H., & Rabiei, M. (2022). Nanoparticle application in diabetes drug delivery. *Journal of Nanoparticle Research*, *24*(9), 178. doi:10.100711051-022-05547-8

Samuel, P., Sundarraj, S., & Sudarmani, D. N. P. (2023). *Nanotechnology-Based Stem Cell Therapy: Current Status and Perspectives*. IntechOpen. doi:10.5772/intechopen.109275

Saramago, S., Magalhães, J., & Pinheiro, M. (2021). Tuberculosis vaccines: An update of recent and ongoing clinical trials. *Applied Sciences (Basel, Switzerland)*, *11*(19), 9250. doi:10.3390/app11199250

Schulte, P. A., & Salamanca-Buentello, F. (2007). Ethical and scientific issues of nanotechnology in the workplace. *Environmental Health Perspectives*, *115*(1), 5–12. doi:10.1289/ehp.9456 PMID:17366812

Serrano-Aroca, Á., Cano-Vicent, A., Sabater i Serra, R., El-Tanani, M., Aljabali, A. A. A., Tambuwala, M. M., & Mishra, Y. K. (2022). Scaffolds in the microbial resistant era: Fabrication, materials, properties and tissue engineering applications. *Materials Today. Bio*, *100412*, 100412. Advance online publication. doi:10.1016/j.mtbio.2022.100412 PMID:36097597

Shan, S., Li, Q., Criswell, T., Atala, A., & Zhang, Y. (2023). Stem cell therapy combined with controlled release of growth factors for the treatment of sphincter dysfunction. *Cell & Bioscience*, *13*(1), 1–23. doi:10.118613578-023-01009-3 PMID:36927578

Shan, X., Gong, X., Li, J., Wen, J., Li, Y., & Zhang, Z. (2022). Current approaches of nanomedicines in the market and various stage of clinical translation. *Acta Pharmaceutica Sinica. B*, *12*(7), 3028–3048. doi:10.1016/j.apsb.2022.02.025 PMID:35865096

Sharma, G., Sharma, A. R., Nam, J. S., Doss, G. P. C., Lee, S. S., & Chakraborty, C. (2015). Nanoparticle based insulin delivery system: The next generation efficient therapy for Type 1 diabetes. *Journal of Nanobiotechnology*, *13*(1), 1–13. doi:10.118612951-015-0136-y PMID:26498972

Sherje, A. P., Jadhav, M., Dravyakar, B. R., & Kadam, D. (2018). Dendrimers: A versatile nanocarrier for drug delivery and targeting. *International Journal of Pharmaceutics*, *548*(1), 707–720. doi:10.1016/j.ijpharm.2018.07.030 PMID:30012508

Shrestha, N., Araujo, F., Shahbazi, M. A., Mäkilä, E., Gomes, M. J., Airavaara, M., Kauppinen, E. I., Raula, J., Salonen, J., Hirvonen, J., Sarmento, B., & Santos, H. A. (2016). Oral hypoglycaemic effect of GLP-1 and DPP4 inhibitor based nanocomposites in a diabetic animal model. *Journal of Controlled Release*, *232*, 113–119. doi:10.1016/j.jconrel.2016.04.024 PMID:27091697

Siegel, R., Ma, J., Zou, Z., & Jemal, A. (2014). Cancer statistics. *CA: a Cancer Journal for Clinicians*, *64*(1), 9–29. doi:10.3322/caac.21208 PMID:24399786

Soares, S., Sousa, J., Pais, A., & Vitorino, C. (2018). Nanomedicine: Principles, properties, and regulatory issues. *Frontiers in Chemistry*, *360*, 360. doi:10.3389/fchem.2018.00360 PMID:30177965

Souri, M., Soltani, M., Kashkooli, F. M., Shahvandi, M. K., Chiani, M., Shariati, F. S., Mehrabi, M. R., & Munn, L. L. (2022). Towards principled design of cancer nanomedicine to accelerate clinical translation. *Materials Today. Bio*, *13*, 100208. doi:10.1016/j.mtbio.2022.100208 PMID:35198957

Souto, E. B., Souto, S. B., Campos, J. R., Severino, P., Pashirova, T. N., Zakharova, L. Y., Silva, A. M., Durazzo, A., Lucarini, M., Izzo, A. A., & Santini, A. (2019). Nanoparticle delivery systems in the treatment of diabetes complications. *Molecules (Basel, Switzerland)*, *24*(23), 4209. doi:10.3390/molecules24234209 PMID:31756981

Subhan, M. A., & Subhan, T. (2022). Safety and global regulations for application of nanomaterials. In *Nanomaterials Recycling* (pp. 83–107). Elsevier. doi:10.1016/B978-0-323-90982-2.00005-6

Suhre, K., McCarthy, M. I., & Schwenk, J. M. (2021). Genetics meets proteomics: Perspectives for large population-based studies. *Nature Reviews. Genetics*, *22*(1), 19–37. doi:10.103841576-020-0268-2 PMID:32860016

Sun, Y., Lu, Y., Yin, L., & Liu, Z. (2020). The roles of nanoparticles in stem cell-based therapy for cardiovascular disease. *Frontiers in Bioengineering and Biotechnology*, *8*, 947. doi:10.3389/fbioe.2020.00947 PMID:32923434

Sun, Y. P., Zhou, B., Lin, Y., Wang, W., Fernando, K. A. S., Pathak, P., Meziani, M. J., Harruff, B. A., Wang, X., Wang, H., Luo, P. G., Yang, H., Kose, M. E., Chen, B., Veca, L. M., & Xie, S.-Y. (2006). Quantum-sized carbon dots for bright and colorful photoluminescence. *Journal of the American Chemical Society*, *128*(24), 7756–7757. doi:10.1021/ja062677d PMID:16771487

Syeda, U. A., Battillo, D., Visaria, A., & Malin, S. K. (2023). The importance of exercise for glycemic control in type 2 diabetes. *American Journal of Medicine Open*, *9*, 100031. doi:10.1016/j.ajmo.2023.100031

Taiwo, B. O., Romdhani, H., Lafeuille, M. H., Bhojwani, R., Milbers, K., & Donga, P. (2023). Treatment and comorbidity burden among people living with HIV: A review of systematic literature reviews. *Journal of Drug Assessment*, *12*(1), 1–11. doi:10.1080/21556660.2022.2149963 PMID:36582675

Tashakori-Miyanroudi, M., Janzadeh, A., Seifalian, A., Aboutaleb, N., Azizi, Y., & Ramezani, F. (2022). Will carbon nanotube/nanofiber bring new hope for the treatment of heart damage? A systematic review. *Nanomedicine (London)*, *17*(29), 2189–2205. doi:10.2217/nnm-2022-0113 PMID:36896892

Thakur, A., & Kathpalia, R. (2022). Engineered nanoparticles (ENPs): Unexplored potential and limitations. [IJBB]. *Indian Journal of Biochemistry & Biophysics*, *59*(12), 1163–1170. doi:10.56042/ijbb.v59i12.67304

Tong, L., Liu, D., Cao, Z., Zheng, N., Mao, C., Liu, S., He, L., & Liu, S. (2023). Research status and Prospect of non-viral vectors based on siRNA: A review. *International Journal of Molecular Sciences*, *24*(4), 3375. doi:10.3390/ijms24043375 PMID:36834783

Umpierrez, G. E., & Klonoff, D. C. (2018). Diabetes technology update: Use of insulin pumps and continuous glucose monitoring in the hospital. *Diabetes Care*, *41*(8), 1579–1589. doi:10.2337/dci18-0002 PMID:29936424

Utembe, W., Tlotleng, N., & Kamng'ona, A. W. (2022). A systematic review on the effects of nanomaterials on gut microbiota. *Current Research in Microbial Sciences*, *3*, 100118. doi:10.1016/j.crmicr.2022.100118 PMID:35909630

Varo, R., Chaccour, C., & Bassat, Q. (2020). Update on malaria. *Medicina Clínica (English Ed.)*, *155*(9), 395–402. doi:10.1016/j.medcle.2020.05.024 PMID:32620355

Veiseh, O., & Langer, R. (2015). A smart insulin patch. *Nature*, *524*(7563), 39–40. doi:10.1038/524039a PMID:26245577

Veiseh, O., Tang, B. C., Whitehead, K. A., Anderson, D. G., & Langer, R. (2015). Managing diabetes with nanomedicine: Challenges and opportunities. *Nature Reviews. Drug Discovery*, *14*(1), 45–57. doi:10.1038/nrd4477 PMID:25430866

Vimaladevi, M., Divya, K. C., & Girigoswami, A. (2016). Liposomal nanoformulations of rhodamine for targeted photodynamic inactivation of multidrug resistant gram negative bacteria in sewage treatment plant. *Journal of Photochemistry and Photobiology. B, Biology*, *162*, 146–152. doi:10.1016/j.jphotobiol.2016.06.034 PMID:27371913

Virupannavar, D., Shah, M. A., & Assad, R. (2023). Harnessing biomedical applications of bionanomaterials through omics approach. In *Synthesis of Bionanomaterials for Biomedical Applications* (pp. 379–394). Elsevier. doi:10.1016/B978-0-323-91195-5.00003-9

Walia, S. S., & Prasad, D. N. (2022). Silver sulfadiazine: Action on burn wound sepsis and infections. *Journal of Drug Delivery and Therapeutics*, *12*(4), 154–161. doi:10.22270/jddt.v12i4.5419

Wang, H., Qin, L., Zhang, X., Guan, J., & Mao, S. (2022). Mechanisms and challenges of nanocarriers as non-viral vectors of therapeutic genes for enhanced pulmonary delivery. *Journal of Controlled Release*, *352*, 970–993. doi:10.1016/j.jconrel.2022.10.061 PMID:36372386

Wang, W., Tasset, A., Pyatnitskiy, I., Mohamed, H. G., Taniguchi, R., Zhou, R., & Wang, H. (2022). Ultrasound triggered organic mechanoluminescence materials. *Advanced Drug Delivery Reviews*, *186*, 114343. doi:10.1016/j.addr.2022.114343 PMID:35580814

Wang, Y., Wang, H., Zhu, X. X., Guan, Y., & Zhang, Y. (2020). Smart microneedle patches for rapid, and painless transdermal insulin delivery. *Journal of Materials Chemistry. B*, *8*(40), 9335–9342. doi:10.1039/D0TB01822H PMID:32969458

Wong, C. Y., Al-Salami, H., & Dass, C. R. (2018). Microparticles, microcapsules and microspheres: A review of recent developments and prospects for oral delivery of insulin. *International Journal of Pharmaceutics*, *537*(1-2), 223–244. doi:10.1016/j.ijpharm.2017.12.036 PMID:29288095

Wong, C. Y., Martinez, J., & Dass, C. R. (2016). Oral delivery of insulin for treatment of diabetes: Status quo, challenges and opportunities. *The Journal of Pharmacy and Pharmacology*, *68*(9), 1093–1108. doi:10.1111/jphp.12607 PMID:27364922

Wong, J. K., Mohseni, R., Hamidieh, A. A., MacLaren, R. E., Habib, N., & Seifalian, A. M. (2017). Will nanotechnology bring new hope for gene delivery? *Trends in Biotechnology*, *35*(5), 434–451. doi:10.1016/j.tibtech.2016.12.009 PMID:28108036

Wong, W. F., Ang, K. P., Sethi, G., & Looi, C. Y. (2023). Recent Advancement of Medical Patch for Transdermal Drug Delivery. *Medicina*, *59*(4), 778. doi:10.3390/medicina59040778 PMID:37109736

Wu, D., Sedgwick, A. C., Gunnlaugsson, T., Akkaya, E. U., Yoon, J., & James, T. D. (2017). Fluorescent chemosensors: The past, present and future. *Chemical Society Reviews*, *46*(23), 7097–7472. doi:10.1039/C7CS00240H PMID:29019488

Wu, H., Nan, J., Yang, L., Park, H. J., & Li, J. (2023). Insulin-loaded liposomes packaged in alginate hydrogels promote the oral bioavailability of insulin. *Journal of Controlled Release*, *353*, 51–62. doi:10.1016/j.jconrel.2022.11.032 PMID:36410613

Wu, M., Zhang, Z., Yong, J., Schenk, P. M., Tian, D., Xu, Z. P., & Zhang, R. (2022). Determination and Imaging of Small Biomolecules and Ions Using Ruthenium (II) Complex-Based Chemosensors. *Topics in Current Chemistry (Cham)*, *380*(5), 29. doi:10.100741061-022-00392-8 PMID:35695976

Xie, J., Li, A., & Li, J. (2017). Advances in pH-sensitive polymers for smart insulin delivery. *Macromolecular Rapid Communications*, *38*(23), 1700413. doi:10.1002/marc.201700413 PMID:28976043

Xue, N., Ding, X., Huang, R., Jiang, R., Huang, H., Pan, X., Min, W., Chen, J., Duan, J. A., Liu, P., & Wang, Y. (2022). Bone tissue engineering in the treatment of bone defects. *Pharmaceuticals (Basel, Switzerland), 15*(7), 879. doi:10.3390/ph15070879 PMID:35890177

Yadav, D., Anwar, M. F., Garg, V., Kardam, H., Beg, M. N., Suri, S., Gaur, S., & Asif, M. (2014). Development of polymeric nanopaclitaxel and comparison with free paclitaxel for effects on cell proliferation of MCF-7 and B16F0 carcinoma cells. *Asian Pacific Journal of Cancer Prevention, 15*(5), 2335–2340. doi:10.7314/APJCP.2014.15.5.2335 PMID:24716980

Yang, F., Xue, J., Wang, G., & Diao, Q. (2022). Nanoparticle-based drug delivery systems for the treatment of cardiovascular diseases. *Frontiers in Pharmacology, 13*, 999404. doi:10.3389/fphar.2022.999404 PMID:36172197

Yang, T., Yao, Q., Cao, F., Liu, Q., Liu, B., & Wang, X. H. (2016). Silver nanoparticles inhibit the function of hypoxia-inducible factor-1 and target genes: Insight into the cytotoxicity and antiangiogenesis. *International Journal of Nanomedicine, 11*, 6679–6692. doi:10.2147/IJN.S109695 PMID:27994464

Yao, D., Liu, N. N., & Mo, B. W. (2020). Assessment of proliferation, migration and differentiation potentials of bone marrow mesenchymal stem cells labeling with silica-coated and amine-modified superparamagnetic iron oxide nanoparticles. *Cytotechnology, 72*(4), 513–525. doi:10.100710616-020-00397-5 PMID:32394163

Ye, L., Cao, Z., Liu, X., Cui, Z., Li, Z., Liang, Y., Zhu, S., & Wu, S. (2022). Noble metal-based nanomaterials as antibacterial agents. *Journal of Alloys and Compounds, 164091*, 164091. doi:10.1016/j.jallcom.2022.164091

Yeh, Y. C., Huang, T. H., Yang, S. C., Chen, C. C., & Fang, J. Y. (2020). Nano-based drug delivery or targeting to eradicate bacteria for infection mitigation: A review of recent advances. *Frontiers in Chemistry, 8*, 286. doi:10.3389/fchem.2020.00286 PMID:32391321

Yetisgin, A. A., Cetinel, S., Zuvin, M., Kosar, A., & Kutlu, O. (2020). Therapeutic nanoparticles and their targeted delivery applications. *Molecules (Basel, Switzerland), 25*(9), 2193. doi:10.3390/molecules25092193 PMID:32397080

Yu, M., Wu, J., Shi, J., & Farokhzad, O. C. (2016). Nanotechnology for protein delivery: Overview and perspectives. *Journal of Controlled Release, 240*, 24–37. doi:10.1016/j.jconrel.2015.10.012 PMID:26458789

Yusuf, A., Almotairy, A. R. Z., Henidi, H., Alshehri, O. Y., & Aldughaim, M. S. (2023). Nanoparticles as Drug Delivery Systems: A Review of the implication of nanoparticles' physicochemical properties on responses in biological systems. *Polymers, 15*(7), 1596. doi:10.3390/polym15071596 PMID:37050210

Zhang, R., & James, T. D. (2023). Responsive probes and molecular bioimaging. *Chemistry, an Asian Journal, 18*(5), e202300058. doi:10.1002/asia.202300058 PMID:36722771

Zhang, W., Yang, Y., & Cui, B. (2021). New perspectives on the roles of nanoscale surface topography in modulating intracellular signaling. *Current Opinion in Solid State and Materials Science, 25*(1), 100873. doi:10.1016/j.cossms.2020.100873 PMID:33364912

Zhang, Y., Wang, P., Wang, Y., Li, J., Qiao, D., Chen, R., Yang, W., & Yan, F. (2021). Gold nanoparticles promote the bone regeneration of periodontal ligament stem cell sheets through activation of autophagy. *International Journal of Nanomedicine*, *16*, 61–73. doi:10.2147/IJN.S282246 PMID:33442250

Zhao, Z., Anselmo, A. C., & Mitragotri, S. (2022). Viral vector-based gene therapies in the clinic. *Bioengineering & Translational Medicine*, *7*(1), e10258. doi:10.1002/btm2.10258 PMID:35079633

Zheng, X., Zhang, P., Fu, Z., Meng, S., Dai, L., & Yang, H. (2021). Applications of nanomaterials in tissue engineering. *RSC Advances*, *11*(31), 19041–19058. doi:10.1039/D1RA01849C PMID:35478636

Zhu, Y. G., Gillings, M., & Penuelas, J. (2020). Integrating biomedical, ecological, and sustainability sciences to manage emerging infectious diseases. *One Earth*, *3*(1), 23–26. doi:10.1016/j.oneear.2020.06.004 PMID:34173527

Ziebarth, J., & Mainardes, R. M. (2023). Preparation, characterization and in vitro evaluation of chitosan nanoparticles for the oral delivery of GLP-1 analog liraglutide. *Journal of Thermal Analysis and Calorimetry*, *148*(6), 2443–2455. doi:10.100710973-022-11909-0

Zielińska, A., Costa, B., Ferreira, M. V., Miguéis, D., Louros, J. M., Durazzo, A., Lucarini, M., Eder, P., Chaud, M. V., Morsink, M., Willemen, N., Severino, P., Santini, A., & Souto, E. B. (2020). Nanotoxicology and nanosafety: Safety-by-design and testing at a glance. *International Journal of Environmental Research and Public Health*, *17*(13), 4657. doi:10.3390/ijerph17134657 PMID:32605255

Zingg, R., & Fischer, M. (2019). The consolidation of nanomedicine. *Wiley Interdisciplinary Reviews. Nanomedicine and Nanobiotechnology*, *11*(6), e1569. doi:10.1002/wnan.1569 PMID:31240855

Zolkepli, H., Widodo, R. T., Mahmood, S., Salim, N., Awang, K., Ahmad, N., & Othman, R. (2022). A Review on the Delivery of Plant-Based Antidiabetic Agents Using Nanocarriers: Current Status and Their Role in Combatting Hyperglycaemia. *Polymers*, *14*(15), 2991. doi:10.3390/polym14152991 PMID:35893954

Zou, Z., Iwata, M., Yamanishi, Y., & Oki, S. (2022). Epigenetic landscape of drug responses revealed through large-scale ChIP-seq data analyses. *BMC Bioinformatics*, *23*(1), 51. doi:10.118612859-022-04571-8 PMID:35073843

Chapter 17
Emerging Applications of Nanomaterials With Less Toxicity and More Efficacy in Modern Biomedical Engineering

Ranjit Barua
https://orcid.org/0000-0003-2236-3876
Indian Institute of Engineering Science and Technology, Shibpur, India

Sudipto Datta
Indian Institute of Science, Bangalore, India

ABSTRACT

Understanding how nanomaterials (NMs) and biological systems interact at the interface is of great research interest. Nanoparticles (NPs) such as carbon nanotubes, graphene oxides, carbon dots, graphite nanopowders, and others are included in NMs. Through organic layers, medicinal compounds, proteins, DNA, and cellular matrices, these NPs exhibit a range of interactions with biological interfaces. The morphological surface of bio-nanoconjugates is influenced by a variety of biophysical and colloidal factors that control their biological responses, giving the NMs unique physical characteristics. Future-generation nano-tool design is essentially focused on the fundamental characteristics of NMs, such as shape, size, composition, functionality, etc., and substantial research has been done in this area. Understanding their characteristics encourages study in the biological and medical fields and enhances their relevance in the field of health management.

INTRODUCTION

After nearly two decades, a variety of NMs with varied shapes, sizes, and structures—such as nanowires, nanotubes, nanoclusters, nanocrystals, nano-coatings, nanocomposites, quantum dots, etc.—are currently being manufactured globally [Leary et al., 2006] [Barua et al., 2022]. Compared to their bulkier cousins,

DOI: 10.4018/979-8-3693-0448-8.ch017

they have improved their characteristics [Eldar boock et al., 2013] [Zhang et al., 2016]. They are used in a wide range of fields, including as robotics, biosensing, coating, electronics, optics, photonics, displays, magnetics, dot-circuits, cantilevers, QD-cellular automata, self-assembly, lithography, aerospace, and machining [Das et al., 2023] [Waidi et al., 2023]. Nanoscale synthesis has been motivated by research into bio-inspired naturally occurring materials. Building a nano-biological interface that bio-imitates the naturally occurring phenomenon is a key area for improving understanding [Datta et al., 2023]. In this regard, an interdisciplinary team of scientists organized the International Complex Adaptive Matter (ICAM) workshop on "Biologically inspired Nanomaterials" in November 2005 [Demirel et al., 2007]. The entire purpose was to facilitate the study of biological sciences using nanoscale materials. In this context, a variety of substances (such as polymers) that behave like antibodies are being produced widely [Yan]. Additionally, synthetic work harnessed by local power [Muthukrishnan et al., 2004] through emulating nano-architectures and tailored surfaces with cell-like capabilities [Pursel et al., 2005] are both being developed. This new frontier can result in systems that are environmentally friendly and crucial for reducing negative effects, where natural systems serve as models for the use of renewable resources. One of the nanotechnology fields with the fastest growing frontiers is the nano-bio interface. Understanding their physiochemical characterisation and biological medium is crucial because NMs differ from their counterparts in both biological and chemical characteristics [Barua et al., 2022]. Dynamic physiochemical interactions, kinetics, and thermodynamic exchanges are all present at this interface. As seen in Figure

Figure 1. Applications of diverse nanosystems in allied healthcare domains are presented schematically [Anjum et al., 2021]

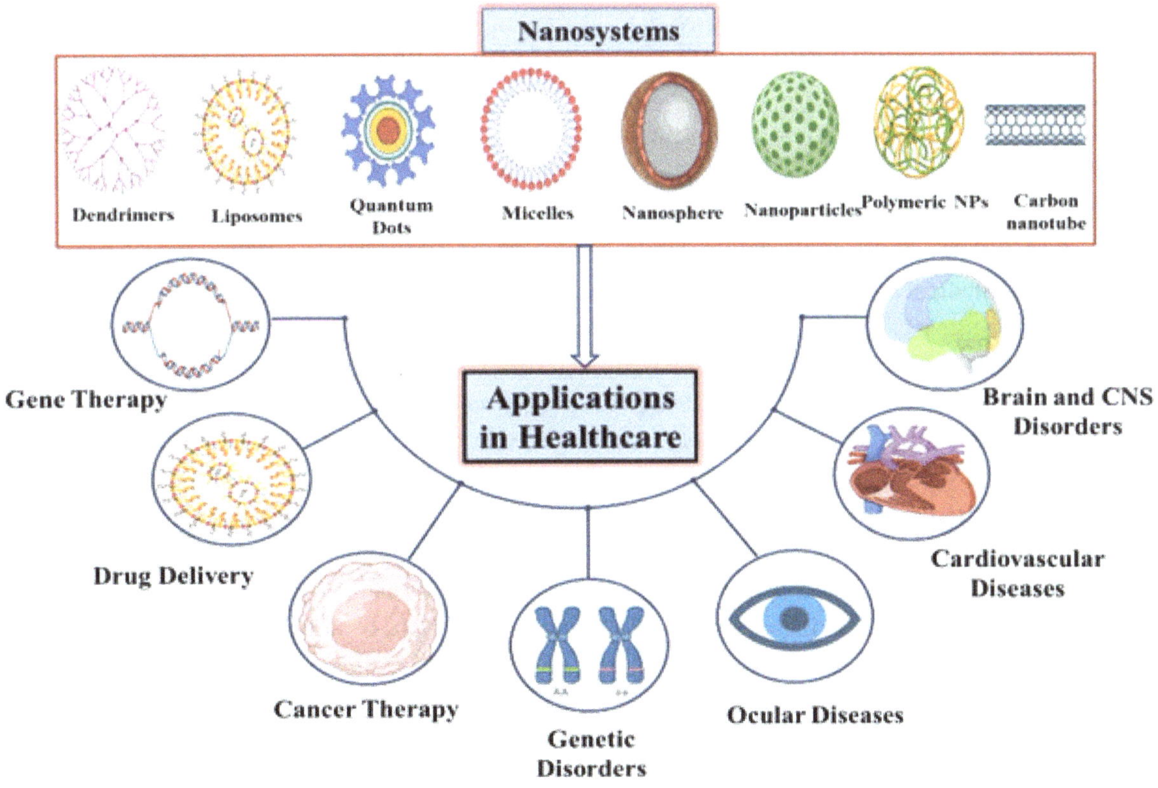

1, they have a range of biological applications, including medication delivery, bio-imaging, tissue engineering, bio-sensors, etc. This facilitates the creation of distinctive functionalities needed by biological systems. To control how forces interact with their molecular equivalents, both concepts must be understood equally. For diverse medicinal demands and electronic substitutes [You et al., 2005] [Barua et al., 2018] [Shim et al., 2002] [Reed et al., 2003], functionalized NPs are being produced. The primary goal of this paper is to give the reader a historical overview of NMs and an understanding of how they have been used in the interdisciplinary fields of biology, chemistry, electronics, and medicine. This chapter focuses on an in-depth and critical examination of the theoretical and experimental characteristics of nanoscale materials, which have served as the basis for many biological systems. Different self-assembled synthetic materials, bio-functionalized NMs, and their probing methods are used in the main analysis. In relation to diverse biological applications, the current review paper focuses on recently developing developments in the production and usage of nanomaterials. This page adds value to the literature by summarizing the most recent reports of nanomaterials, particularly in the field of health.

NANOMATERIALS' USE IN THE HEALTHCARE SECTOR

The World Health Organization (WHO) reports that 33.4 million persons had an HIV/AIDS diagnosis in 2008. According to estimates from 2011, there are about 5.5 million persons in the USA who have Alzheimer's disease, and their medical costs were USD 183 billion. By 2050, this figure will have increased to USD 1.1 trillion, or six times as much. According to another study, only 0.5% of cases of cancer are diagnosed and account for around 25% of fatalities. After cardiac illness, cancer is now the second biggest cause of death. All of this has a significant negative influence on human health, which causes society to collapse. Indeed, scientists, researchers, and medical professionals are looking for approximations of nanotechnological drugs to address the problem. Due to its potential to significantly increase illness detection, treatment, and prevention, the use of nanotechnology in medicine and pharmaceuticals has inspired a great deal of excitement. This shift from a fantastical world to a concrete one is an important advancement [Joseph et al., 2023]. In order to illustrate how silver nanoparticles can overcome biological barriers, Figure 2 has been provided. The study of the bio-compatibility and interaction between nanoscale biomaterials like cells, tissues, and organs as well as their application in a variety of medical and health sciences include the use of nanocarriers for drug, gene, and vaccine delivery, orthopedics, cardiovascular, and dental applications. Nanostructured biomaterials are made of polypeptides, proteins, nucleic acid, DNA-based self-assemblies, biopolymers, cells, and glycans. Due to the fact that nanoscale pharmaceuticals attach to specific receptors and activate those receptors, these NPs are crucial in the drug delivery process. In addition to this, the sector of pharmacology and medicine has seen NPs see significant growth. With the usage of these nanomedicines, new protocols are being adopted against traditional medical practices. Emulsions, polymers, vitamins, inorganic composites, liposomes, polymers, metal nanoparticles, etc. are some examples of innovative nanoformulations and nanocarriers for therapeutic treatments that aid in lowering the associated issues [Walia et al., 2019] [Ranjan et al., 2019]. For the delivery of micelles, nanoformulations, emulsions, solid lipid NPs, etc., the well-established lipid nanoparticulate technologies result in a wide variety of unique approaches. When compared to polymers, their attributes, such as eco-friendliness, biodegradability, tailorability of water-loving/hating features, biocompatibility, economical setup, ease of production, and dispersity limitations, play a significant impact. These qualities allow for improved status and make for one of the most popular platforms with simple scale-up choices. The development of inorganic nanoparticle-based systems has accelerated, particularly in the design of nanostructured materials with cohesive physical qualities to improve delivery in the context of both diagnosis and therapeutic modalities [Li et al., 2010]. With examples of AuNP-based alluring scaffolds for drug administration, their specialized qualities include functionalization alternatives, safer carrier capabilities, high surface area, and amphiphilicity. Glutathione (GSH), pH, light, temperature, and other internal and external stimuli-based systems are some examples of the triggers for the precondition for the spatio-temporal release of AuNPs [Hong et al., 2006]. A promising instrument, magnetic nanoparticles have a variety of special qualities that have broad uses. They include excellent solubility, low toxicity, and target-specific delivery with customized

Figure 2. (A) The role of nanoparticles in removing biological obstacles to the widespread use of nanomaterials in a variety of industries. (B) Microemulsions are used to synthesise silver nanoparticles with a tunable size and composition. The water-to-surfactant ratio is adjusted. Nanomaterials, Copyright and Permissions, 2023
[Joseph et al., 2023]

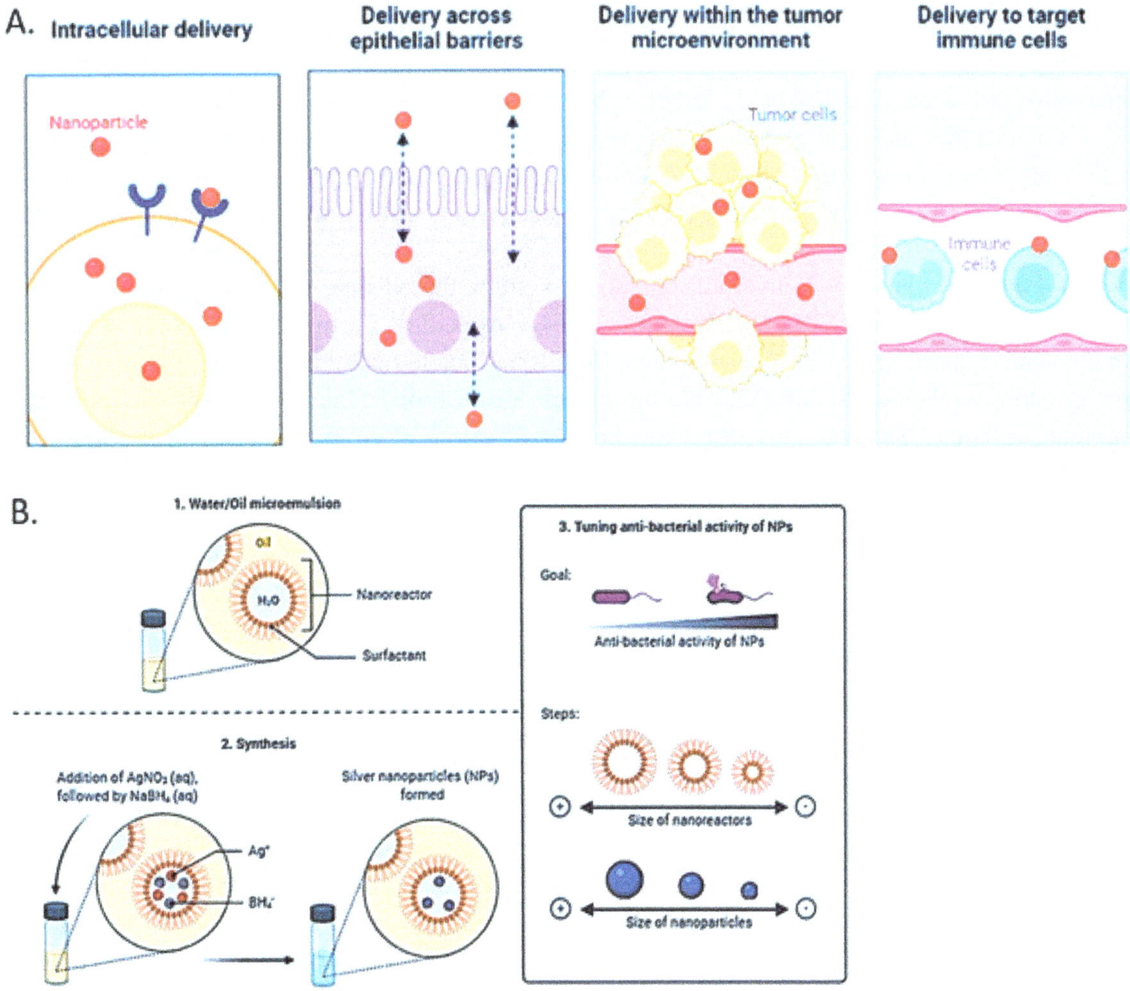

biocompatible versions for in vivo applications. They work well together due to their limited contact with solvent and effective magnetic core surface protection. One of the least expensive inorganic coatings is calcium carbonate [Popova et al., 2023]. For the investigation of labile nanomaterials and their advancement in the synthesis and uses in biomedicine, one review has been published [Chevallet et al., 2017].

Iron oxide nanoparticles, solid gold NPs, gold silica nanoshells, and carbon nanotubes have all demonstrated the ability to be used in targeted hyperthermic therapy [Cherukuri et al., 2010]. Iron oxide NPs have been used as both therapeutic and diagnostic nanoscale agents to treat deep tissue tumors [Samanta et al., 2008]. By labeling gold NPs with antibodies against particular tumor cells, more gold NPs could be produced. After the integration of NPs, the application of radio-frequency fields to cells resulted in the confinement of heat and the killing of tumor cells [Cherukuri et al., 2010]. Magnetic NPs offer a promising technique for the minimally invasive excision of tiny breast tumors by using magnetically produced heat [Jain., 2010]. This strategy is advantageous because it enables precise and targeted tuning of the degree of energy deposition, adequate temperature control at the target region, and also satisfies the growing demand for breast-conserving therapies [Hilger et al., 2005]. Anti-human epidermal growth factor receptor 2 antibodies can be used to deliver medications to tumors that overexpress human epidermal growth factor receptor 2, which can start an anticancer response [Jain., 2010]. The efficacy of thermal therapy has been demonstrated for CYT-6091, a pegylated colloidal GNP (gold nanoparticle) with tumor necrosis factor-attached to its surface, and it has received extensive adjuvant research [Pearce., 2011]. Superparamagnetic NPs also exhibit appealing features for the treatment of malignancies by inducing hyperthermia [Giustini et al., 2010]. When these NPs are exposed to an alternating magnetic field of sufficient frequency and strength, magnetic energy is converted into thermal energy. After that, the heat generated is transferred to the cells that revolve around the NPs. Apoptosis, which results in the death of tumor cells, can occur after the protein denatures and the limited temperature rises above 40 °C [Wust ey al., 2002].

In the event of a medicine delivery or diagnostic system, the NPs are artificially created and later connect to biological things and cells. When it comes to dyes, direct drug administration is common, with the primary particle being shielded by materials like silica to maintain its integrity until delivery. Particles carry out their duties after the outermost layers are adsorbed. One such use is the identification of proteins utilizing NPs, dyes, etc. comprehending the functions of proteins is crucial to comprehending the language, machinery, and structure of a cell. In immuno-histochemistry, AuNPs are utilized to detect protein-protein interactions. There have been advancements made in the screening of cancer therapies or cancer treatment choices. A laser is used to produce atomic oxygen, which is cytotoxic and used in photodynamic cancer therapy to kill cells. In contrast to healthy tissue, a significant amount of dye is required to produce atomic oxygen. The residual excess dye causes negative effects by migrating to the skin and eyes. The goal is to increase the effectiveness of photodynamic cancer therapy by laser-highlighting the target cells. The treatment utilizing a hydrophobic form of dye contained inside a porous nanoparticle is more efficient the higher the detection rate [Roy et al., 2003].

The best material with the perfect qualities is used to create human-made or cell-manipulated nanoparticles, which is what makes them so beautiful [Gertz et al., 2016]. Others employ magnets to use these particles and change the form of cells, while some carry and dispense materials to a specific location using capsules. Various ranges and metal thicknesses that are adaptable and mobile can be used to fine-tune the impact of the particles, their form, surface chemistry, and magnetic forces. In contrast to a one-size-fits-all approach to healthcare, it enables dealing with each case uniquely, as demonstrated by the use of liposomal targeted drug delivery (Figure 3). Commercial exploration will be a primary prior-

Figure 3. Nanoparticles' cellular absorption is influenced by physicochemical parameters, including surface charge, shape, size, and surface chemistry
[Foroozandeh et al., 2018]

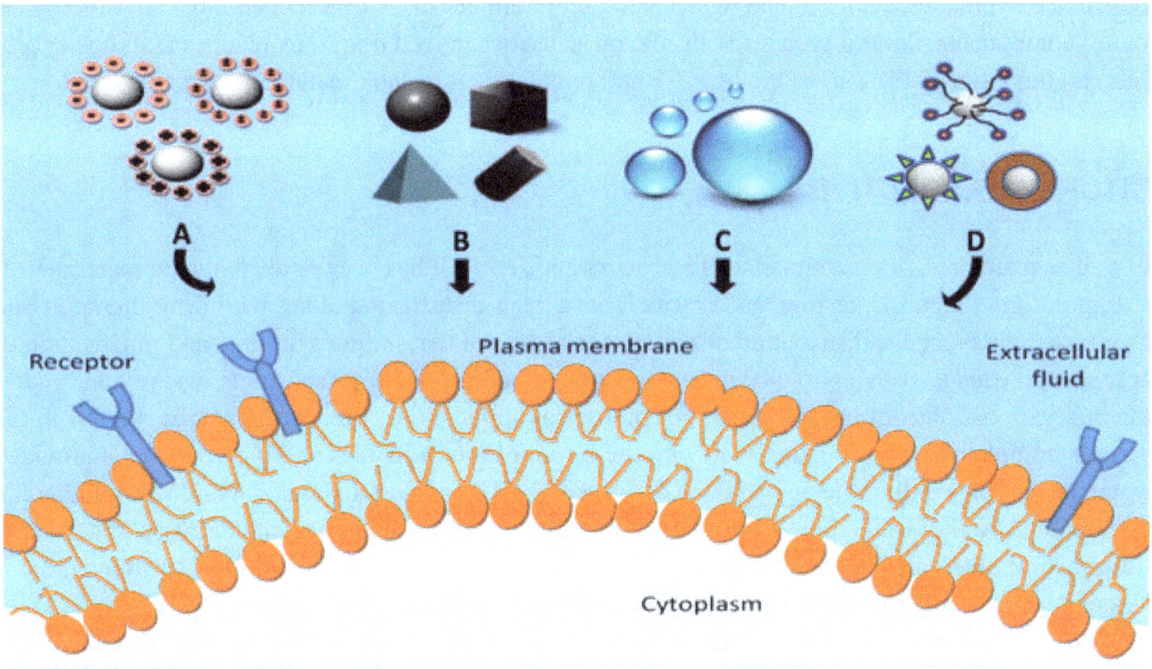

ity of the upcoming nanotechnology generation. It takes into account more than only biomaterials, drug delivery, and basic pharmaceuticals, which are the main areas of development. Band-Aids and dressings with colloidal silver nanoparticles and anti-microbial ingredients are some of the most recent inventions.

NANOMATERIALS AND BIOLOGICAL PHENOMENA ONE ANOTHER

It is common knowledge that living things are composed of cells, which are smaller units with an approximate 10 mm diameter. However, the organelles that make up cells are even smaller and are comparable in size to artificial nanoparticles (NPs). Therefore, these NPs can function as tiny probes that enable us to see cellular machinery unhindered. The precise control of particle size, their inner core (composition, size, and shape), stability, and functionalization of molecules leads to synthetic biology, a new subject that combines science, engineering, and technology [Rice et al., 2013]. Additionally, the NPs had anti-microbial characteristics. For instance, Rudramurthy et al., 2016 revealed that SWNTs are efficient antibiotics against drug-resistant and multi-resistant bacterial strains by demonstrating that they have antibacterial effects against Salmonella Enterica and E. coli. A new formulation of a curcumin lipid nano-emulsion with a size range of 47–55 nm was created by S. Anuchapreeda et al., 2012 and used for cancer chemotherapy [Anuchapreeda et al., 2012]. Delong et al. also described the specific characteristics of nucleic acid conjugates with protamine and AuNPs as nanorods in 2009 [DeLong et al., 2009]. Additionally, reports took into account the extraction of nucleic acids using various magnetic nanocomposites [Irkham, Bulgakova]. The second crucial strategy is based on biological and biomedical engineering signaling networks. Even the size of biogenic particles can be changed by changing the concentration of metal ions in the cellular environment. One of the most appropriate instances is the constructed synthetic circuit domain, which calls for a number of DNA-encoded molecular biological control components. Several proteins with enzyme activity can read this DNA blueprint, and other proteins can bind to metallic ions to produce NP and pass on their genetic material in the process.

FUTURE PERSPECTIVE

As well as many fatal disease situations like cancer and sepsis, it has been noted that nanomaterial uses in drug design, diagnosis, testing, and research have been investigated along with drug therapies and other possibilities for the distribution of nanomaterials. Even the routine synthesis and purification of these components is evolving to give us a more streamlined procedure. As a single resource for understanding various kinds of nanomaterials for biological applications, this paper may be helpful in the research community. A fascinating view into the future of biomechanics and biomedicine is provided by nanotechnology. All of the applications discussed in this study are operational and still undergoing development. Additionally, there is a ton of space for new developments in drug delivery systems and cell targeting, making them even more capable and efficient [Barua et al., 2020]. The foundation of the quickly developing field of nanotechnology, which has the potential to change medicines and diagnostics, is nanomaterials. The vast majority of commercially accessible nanoparticles are intended for simple pharmaceuticals. When replacing organic dyes, nanoparticles must have high multiplexing capacity and photo-stability. The use of magnetic nanoparticles to deliver drugs or heat tumor cells in order to kill or treat diseased cells is made possible by advances in the directing and remote control of nanoprobes. Making nonmaterials multipurpose and controlled by outside signals in order to turn them into nanodevices is a major development. There are still fresh developments to be made, particularly focused gadgets with multifunctional functions that can be helpful to medicine.

CONCLUSION

Currently, nanotechnology is being used in a broad variety of industries, including food, packaging, accessories, storage, transportation, and more. These applications offer several benefits for everyday use. These nano-based solutions can be used in everything from electronics to clothing to medical procedures and even surgery. Despite the technology' potential for good, there is also a great deal of room for evil. To prevent the misuse of scientific talents and research, it is imperative to establish a system of checks and balances. The foundation of ongoing discussions on the presence of nanotechnology in the world is a number of crucial issues, notwithstanding their growth and advancement. There are various drawbacks along with predicted threats and worrying difficulties. The standard of living has advanced at the same time as nano-pollution, which affects the air, soil, water, and food, has increased. The biotic components are substantially at risk.The dearth of employment prospects in traditional farming and the manufacturing and engineering sectors is a significant drawback. Although these sophisticated technologies and nanorobots have diminished the importance of labor, they nevertheless ensure quick and accurate results. For the first counter alert, cutting-edge and creative technologies for the detection and treatment of foreign diseases are being built. These are designed to improve the ability for a precise diagnosis and early treatment. They are based on the determination of changes in the vitals, changes in biomarker levels, hormonal imbalance, etc. Targeted delivery and healing acceleration are two changes made possible by technological advancements in nanostructure design. The pipelines to current medications, which subsequently increase their efficacy, are key functions of the new armamentarium of therapies in addition to the drug delivery mediated system. Numerous initiatives are being made to quickly review the status of physiologically active but unsatisfactory molecular systems that are supported by traditional sources. It's intriguing that these nano-objects' features are given to their potentially contaminating therapeutic properties. As a result, it's important to reduce the possibility of adversities being fine-tuned. Therefore, further in-depth research in these areas for a smarter, faster, eco-friendly, and sustainable system can overcome significant difficulties related to multiple platforms. Their properties are greatly impacted as the physical parameters vary. The most promising platforms include carbon nanotubes made of pure carbon (sp2 hybridized carbons), which have been employed as pencil graphite electrodes (PGE) and have the same chemical make-up as pencil graphite. Later, the material develops better mechanical and thermal properties due to the arrangement of the carbon in a layered tubular structure, making the system stiffer than steel.

ACKNOWLEDGMENT

The authors would like to thank IIEST-Shibpur, Centre for Healthcare Science and Technology lab, and thanks to Mrs. Nibedita Bardhan for language proof reading.

REFERENCES

Anjum, S., Ishaque, S., Fatima, H., Farooq, W., Hano, C., Abbasi, B. H., & Anjum, I. (2021). Emerging Applications of Nanotechnology in Healthcare Systems: Grand Challenges and Perspectives. *Pharmaceuticals (Basel, Switzerland)*, *14*(8), 707. doi:10.3390/ph14080707 PMID:34451803

Anuchapreeda, S., Fukumori, Y., Okonogi, S., & Ichikawa, H. (2012). Preparation of lipid nanoemulsions incorporating curcumin for cancer therapy. *Journal of Nanotechnology*, *2012*, 2012. doi:10.1155/2012/270383

Barua, R., Banerjee, D., & Bhowmik, S. (2022). Study of the Potential Impact of Microplastics and Additives on Human Health. In S. Joo (Ed.), *Assessing the Effects of Emerging Plastics on the Environment and Public Health* (pp. 128–147). IGI Global. doi:10.4018/978-1-7998-9723-1.ch007

Barua, R., Datta, S., Chowdhury, A. R., & Datta, P. (2018). Advances in MEMS and Micro-Scale technologies for application in controlled Drug-Dosing systems: MEMS-Based drug delivery systems. In *Design and Development of Affordable Healthcare Technologies* (pp. 165–179). IGI Global. doi:10.4018/978-1-5225-4969-7.ch007

Barua, R., Datta, S., & Das, J. (2020). Application of Nanotechnology in Global Issues. In M. Merviö (Ed.), *Global Issues and Innovative Solutions in Healthcare, Culture, and the Environment* (pp. 292–300). IGI Global. doi:10.4018/978-1-7998-3576-9.ch015

Barua, R., Roychowdhury, A., & Datta, P. (2022). Study of Different Additive Manufacturing Processes and Emergent Applications in Modern Healthcare. In R. Thanigaivelan, N. Rajan, & T. Argul (Eds.), *Advanced Manufacturing Techniques for Engineering and Engineered Materials* (pp. 239–259). IGI Global. doi:10.4018/978-1-7998-9574-9.ch014

Cherukuri, P., Glazer, E. S., & Curley, S. A. (2010). Targeted hyperthermia using metal nanoparticles. *Advanced Drug Delivery Reviews*, *62*(3), 339–345. doi:10.1016/j.addr.2009.11.006 PMID:19909777

Chevallet, M., Veronesi, G., Fuchs, A., Mintz, E., Michaud-Soret, I., & Deniaud, A. (2017). Impact of labile metal nanoparticles on cellular homeostasis. Current developments in imaging, synthesis and applications. *Biochimica et Biophysica Acta. G, General Subjects*, *1861*(6), 1566–1577. doi:10.1016/j.bbagen.2016.12.012 PMID:27993661

Das, S., Datta, S., Barman, A., & Barua, R. (2023). Smart Biodegradable and Bio-Based Polymeric Biomaterials for Biomedical Applications. In A. Kumar, P. Kumar, A. Srivastava, & V. Goyat (Eds.), *Modeling, Characterization, and Processing of Smart Materials* (pp. 56–82). IGI Global. doi:10.4018/978-1-6684-9224-6.ch003

Datta, S., & Barua, R. (2023). Fluorescent Nanomaterials and Its Application in Biomedical Engineering. In A. Rakha, A. Munawar, V. Khanna, & S. Bansal (Eds.), *Modeling and Simulation of Functional Nanomaterials for Forensic Investigation* (pp. 164–186). IGI Global. doi:10.4018/978-1-6684-8325-1.ch009

DeLong, R. K., Akhtar, U., Sallee, M., Parker, B., Barber, S., Zhang, J., Craig, M., Garrad, R., Hickey, A. J., & Engstrom, E. (2009). Characterization and performance of nucleic acid nanoparticles combined with protamine and gold. *Biomaterials*, *30*(32), 6451–6459. doi:10.1016/j.biomaterials.2009.07.067 PMID:19726081

Demirel, M., Parikh, A., Crespi, V., & Reed, S. (2007). *Biologically Inspired Nanomaterials: A Conference Report*. arXiv preprint arXiv:0708.0164.

Eldar-Boock, A., Polyak, D., Scomparin, A., & Satchi-Fainaro, R. (2013). Nano-sized polymers and liposomes designed to deliver combination therapy for cancer. *Current Opinion in Biotechnology*, *24*(4), 682–689. doi:10.1016/j.copbio.2013.04.014 PMID:23726153

Foroozandeh, P., & Aziz, A. A. (2018). Insight into cellular uptake and intracellular trafficking of nanoparticles. *Nanoscale Research Letters*, *13*(1), 1–12. doi:10.118611671-018-2728-6 PMID:30361809

Gertz, F., & Khitun, A. (2016). Biological cell manipulation by magnetic nanoparticles. *AIP Advances*, *6*(2), 025308. doi:10.1063/1.4942090

Giustini, A. J., Petryk, A. A., Cassim, S. M., Tate, J. A., Baker, I., & Hoopes, P. J. (2010). Magnetic Nanoparticle Hyperthermia In Cancer Treatment. *Nano LIFE, 1*(1n02), . https://doi.org/ doi:10.1142/S1793984410000067

Hilger, I., Hergt, R., & Kaiser, W. A. (2005). Use of magnetic nanoparticle heating in the treatment of breast cancer. *IEE Proceedings. Nanobiotechnology*, *152*(1), 33–39. doi:10.1049/ip-nbt:20055018 PMID:16441156

Hong, R., Han, G., Fernández, J. M., Kim, B. J., Forbes, N. S., & Rotello, V. M. (2006). Glutathione-mediated delivery and release using monolayer protected nanoparticle carriers. *Journal of the American Chemical Society*, *128*(4), 1078–1079. doi:10.1021/ja056726i PMID:16433515

Jain, K. K. (2010). Advances in the field of nanooncology. *BMC Medicine*, *8*(1), 83. doi:10.1186/1741-7015-8-83 PMID:21144040

Joseph, T. M., Kar Mahapatra, D., Esmaeili, A., Piszczyk, Ł., Hasanin, M. S., Kattali, M., Haponiuk, J., & Thomas, S. (2023). Nanoparticles: Taking a unique position in medicine. *Nanomaterials (Basel, Switzerland)*, *13*(3), 574. doi:10.3390/nano13030574 PMID:36770535

Leary, S. P., Liu, C. Y., & Apuzzo, M. L. (2006). Toward the emergence of nanoneurosurgery: part III—nanomedicine: targeted nanotherapy, nanosurgery, and progress toward the realization of nanoneurosurgery. *Neurosurgery*, *58*(6), 1009–1026. doi:10.1227/01.NEU.0000217016.79256.16 PMID:16723880

Li, S., Meng Lin, M., Toprak, M. S., Kim, D. K., & Muhammed, M. (2010). Nanocomposites of polymer and inorganic nanoparticles for optical and magnetic applications. *Nano Reviews*, *1*(1), 5214. doi:10.3402/nano.v1i0.5214 PMID:22110855

Muthukrishnan, G., Roberts, C. A., Chen, Y. C., Zahn, J. D., & Hancock, W. O. (2004). Patterning surface-bound microtubules through reversible DNA hybridization. *Nano Letters*, *4*(11), 2127–2132. doi:10.1021/nl048816b

Pearce, J. (2011). Mathematical models of laser-induced tissue thermal damage. *International journal of hyperthermia: The official journal of European Society for Hyperthermic Oncology. International Journal of Hyperthermia*, *27*(8), 741–750. doi:10.3109/02656736.2011.580822 PMID:22098359

Popova, V., Poletaeva, Y., Chubarov, A., & Dmitrienko, E. (2023). pH-Responsible Doxorubicin-Loaded Fe_3O_4@$CaCO_3$ Nanocomposites for Cancer Treatment. *Pharmaceutics*, *15*(3), 771. doi:10.3390/pharmaceutics15030771 PMID:36986632

Pursel, S., Horn, M. W., Demirel, M. C., & Lakhtakia, A. (2005). Growth of sculptured polymer submicronwire assemblies by vapor deposition. *Polymer*, *46*(23), 9544–9548. doi:10.1016/j.polymer.2005.07.092

Ranjan, S., Dasgupta, N., Singh, S., & Gandhi, M. (2019). Toxicity and regulations of food nanomaterials. *Environmental Chemistry Letters*, *17*(2), 929–944. doi:10.100710311-018-00851-z

Reed, S. M., Clegg, R. S., & Hutchison, J. E. (2003). *Tuning the electrical properties of monolayers by using internal peptide bonds.*

Rice, M. K., & Ruder, W. C. (2013). Creating biological nanomaterials using synthetic biology. *Science and Technology of Advanced Materials*. PMID:27877637

Roy, I., Ohulchanskyy, T. Y., Pudavar, H. E., Bergey, E. J., Oseroff, A. R., Morgan, J., Dougherty, T. J., & Prasad, P. N. (2003). Ceramic-based nanoparticles entrapping water-insoluble photosensitizing anticancer drugs: A novel drug-carrier system for photodynamic therapy. *Journal of the American Chemical Society*, *125*(26), 7860–7865. doi:10.1021/ja0343095 PMID:12823004

Rudramurthy, G. R., Swamy, M. K., Sinniah, U. R., & Ghasemzadeh, A. (2016). Nanoparticles: Alternatives against drug-resistant pathogenic microbes. *Molecules (Basel, Switzerland)*, *21*(7), 836. doi:10.3390/molecules21070836 PMID:27355939

Samanta, B., Yan, H., Fischer, N. O., Shi, J., Jerry, D. J., & Rotello, V. M. (2008). Protein-passivated Fe(3)O(4) nanoparticles: Low toxicity and rapid heating for thermal therapy. *Journal of Materials Chemistry*, *18*(11), 1204–1208. doi:10.1039/b718745a PMID:19122852

Shim, M., Shi Kam, N. W., Chen, R. J., Li, Y., & Dai, H. (2002). Functionalization of carbon nanotubes for biocompatibility and biomolecular recognition. *Nano Letters*, *2*(4), 285–288. doi:10.1021/nl015692j

Waidi, Y. O., Barua, R., & Datta, S. (2023). Metals, Polymers, Ceramics, Composites Biomaterials Used in Additive Manufacturing for Biomedical Applications. In A. Kumar, P. Kumar, A. Srivastava, & V. Goyat (Eds.), *Modeling, Characterization, and Processing of Smart Materials* (pp. 165–184). IGI Global. doi:10.4018/978-1-6684-9224-6.ch008

Walia, N., Dasgupta, N., Ranjan, S., Ramalingam, C., & Gandhi, M. (2019). Food-grade nanoencapsulation of vitamins. *Environmental Chemistry Letters*, *17*(2), 991–1002. doi:10.100710311-018-00855-9

Wust, P., Hildebrandt, B., Sreenivasa, G., Rau, B., Gellermann, J., Riess, H., Felix, R., & Schlag, P. M. (2002). Hyperthermia in combined treatment of cancer. *The Lancet. Oncology*, *3*(8), 487–497. doi:10.1016/S1470-2045(02)00818-5 PMID:12147435

You, C. C., De, M., & Rotello, V. M. (2005). Monolayer-protected nanoparticle–protein interactions. *Current Opinion in Chemical Biology*, *9*(6), 639–646. doi:10.1016/j.cbpa.2005.09.012 PMID:16226485

Zhang, W. (2016). Application of Fe 3 O 4 nanoparticles functionalized carbon nanotubes for electrochemical sensing of DNA hybridization. *Journal of Applied Electrochemistry*, *46*(5), 559–566. doi:10.100710800-016-0952-2

Chapter 18
Safety and Toxicity of Nanomaterials in Medicine

Vandana Singh
Department of Microbiology, Sharda School of Allied Health Sciences, Sharda University, India

Ankush Verma
Sharda School of Allied Health Sciences, Sharda University, India

Amit Pratap Singh Chouhan
Sharda School of Allied Health Sciences, Sharda University, India

Rahul Saxena
https://orcid.org/0000-0002-4517-8529
Sharda School of Allied Health Sciences, Sharda University, India

Sanjana Koranga
Sharda School of Allied Health Sciences, Sharda University, India

Takreem Husain
Sharda School of Allied Health Sciences, Sharda University, India

ABSTRACT

Nanomaterials' unique physicochemical features make them suitable for biological applications such medication delivery, imaging, and tissue engineering. However, there is growing concern regarding their safety and toxicity due to their small size and high surface area, which can result in unanticipated interactions with biological systems. Studies have demonstrated that cationic nanoparticles exhibit a propensity to interact with cellular membranes and elicit oxidative stress, while anionic nanoparticles have a tendency to accumulate within lysosomes and trigger inflammatory responses. Numerous methods have been developed to evaluate the safety and toxicity of nanomaterials, such as in-vitro, in-vivo assays, computational modeling, etc. Nanomaterials in medical sciences are subject to regulatory scaffolds that give guidelines/ policies for safety assessment and risk management, nonetheless more research is required to entirely comprehend the possible long-term effects or interactions of nanoparticles with other environmental elements.

DOI: 10.4018/979-8-3693-0448-8.ch018

INTRODUCTION

Nanomaterials comprise a diverse array of substances, such as nanotubes, nanoparticles, nanofibers, and nanocomposites, and exhibiting unique physico-chemical characteristics. These materials possess the capability to be custom-made in order to meet the requirements of different medical applications (Baig et al., 2021). Nanomaterials, as per the International Organization for Standardization (ISO), are described as materials that possess large dimensions within the nanoscale assortment or exhibit an internal or surface structure at the nanoscale. Nanomaterials, which typically have diameters ranging from 1 to 100 (nm) nanometers, have distinct physicochemical properties that set them apart from their bulk counterparts. These properties have attracted considerable attention in the medical sciences, owing to their capacity to potentially transform diagnostics, therapeutics, and medical device technologies. The significant surface area-to-volume ratio, adjustable surface chemistry, and molecular-level interaction capabilities of nanomaterials facilitate precise alteration of their interactions with biological systems (Cheng et al., 2021). Hence, they have been utilized in various capacities such as nanomedicines, drug delivery vehicles, imaging agents, scaffolds for tissue engineering, and biosensors. For example, quantum dots, which are semiconductor particles at the nanoscale, have demonstrated potential in the field of fluorescent labeling for cellular and molecular imaging diagnosis. The ability to adjust their emission possessions depending on their size enables the simultaneous detection of multiple specific biomolecules. Similarly, the utilization of iron oxide nanoparticles has been implemented in magnetic resonance imaging (MRI) for the purpose of augmenting contrast, thereby facilitating improved observation of anatomical morphologies and pathological alterations. These are few examples that highlight the significant impact that nanomaterials can have on enhancing medical diagnosis and treatment procedures (Saleh, 2020).

The astonishing potential of nanomaterials in the medicine is accompanied by the need for a thorough comprehension of their safety profiles due to their complex interactions with biological systems. This chapter emphasized on the crucial element of nanomaterial safety and toxicity in the context of medical applications. Furthermore, the various factors that contribute to nanotoxicity, including the mechanisms of exposure and absorption, methods for assessing toxicity in controlled laboratory settings and living organisms, considerations related to the immune system, existing regulatory frameworks, and approaches for minimizing the harmful effects of nanomaterials are also discussed (Wang et al., 2021).

CLASSIFICATION OF NANOMATERIALS EMPLOYED IN THE FIELD OF MEDICINE

The field of nanotechnology has facilitated a wide range of nanomaterials, and each of them possessing a distinct characteristic that render them well-suited for a variety of medical uses. These nanomaterials can be broadly classified into nanoparticles, nanotubes and nanofibers, nanocomposites, and nanoporous materials etc. These all types play a significant role in the progress of diagnostics, drug delivery, tissue engineering, and other related fields (Joudeh & Linke, 2022).

Nanoparticles

Metallic Nanoparticles: Metallic nanoparticles, such as gold, silver, and iron oxide nanoparticles etc., have garnered scientific interest owing to their unique optical, magnetic, and catalytic characteristics.

For instance, gold nanoparticles demonstrate a phenomenon known as surface plasmon resonance, in which its electrons undergo collective oscillation when exposed to particular wavelengths of light. The resonance can be adjusted by doing modification in the dimensions and morphology of the nanoparticle. Gold nanoparticles have been explored well in the field of bioimaging, wherein they exhibit the ability to improve contrast in various imaging techniques such as dark-field microscopy etc. Additionally, these nanoparticles have been employed in photothermal therapy, a method that involves converting absorbed light into heat (Jamkhande et al., 2019). This heat can be selectively targeted towards cancer cells, leading to their destruction. Similarly, Silver nanoparticles exhibit antimicrobial characteristics as a result of their capacity to liberate silver ions, which disrupt the integrity of bacterial cell membranes and impede their proliferation. The incorporation of nanoparticles into wound dressings, coatings for medical devices, and antimicrobial agents for diverse infections is observed. Another example is, Iron oxide nanoparticles exhibit magnetic properties, rendering them suitable for utilization as contrast agents in magnetic resonance imaging (MRI). Enhanced imaging contrast is achieved through the manipulation of the local magnetic field, which aids in the visualization of anatomical structures and pathological alterations (Gao et al., 2020).

Polymeric Nanoparticles: Polymeric nanoparticles are fabricated using biocompatible polymers, which endows them with exceptional adaptability in the field of drug delivery and targeting. For example, Poly (lactic-co-glycolic acid) nanoparticles are widely employed in pharmaceutical applications owing to their ability to regulate drug release and their biodegradable nature. The nanoparticles possess the ability to encapsulate a diverse array of therapeutic agents, thereby safeguarding them against degradation and facilitating controlled release over an extended duration (Zielińska et al., 2020).

Lipid-Based Nanoparticles: Lipid-Based Nanoparticles: Lipid-based nanoparticles refer to a class of nanoparticles that are composed primarily of lipids, which are organic molecules. Lipid-based nanoparticles emulate the composition and organization of cellular membranes and have emerged as crucial agents for the transportation of hydrophobic pharmaceuticals and genetic material. For example, Liposomes are lipid bilayer structures that exhibit a spherical shape. They have the ability to encapsulate hydrophilic drugs in their inner aqueous core and hydrophobic drugs within their lipid membrane. These advancements provide enhanced solubility, stability, and targeted delivery of pharmaceutical compounds. Similarly, Lipid nanoparticles (LNPs) have gained significant attention in the field of mRNA-based therapeutics approaches, such as in various COVID-19 vaccines. Lipid nanoparticles (LNPs) serve as a safeguard for delicate RNA molecules, enhancing its cellular absorption and rendering them as a highly promising framework for gene therapy and vaccination (Thi et al., 2021).

Nanotubes and Nanofibers

Carbon Nanotubes: Carbon nanotubes are cylindrical structures constituted of carbon atoms arranged in a hexagonal lattice. The extraordinary mechanical strength and electrical conductivity of carbon nanotubes (CNTs), which can be an attributed to their distinctive carbon lattice structure. Single-Walled Carbon Nanotubes (SWCNTs) and Multi-Walled Carbon Nanotubes (MWCNTs) are two forms of carbon nanotubes generally used in medical sciences. These structures exhibit high aspect ratios and are being explored for applications in drug delivery, biosensing, tissue engineering etc. Single-walled carbon nanotubes (SWCNTs) and multi-walled carbon nanotubes (MWCNTs) also have the capability to undergo functionalization by incorporating targeting ligands, this enables them to effectively carry the different drugs and facilitate the delivery of these drugs to specific sites within the body (Norizan et al., 2020).

Nanofibers: Nanofibers are enormously thin fibers, which allow resemblance to the extracellular matrix, exhibit significant promise in the field of medical science such as, tissue engineering and wound healing applications. For example, Electrospinning is a fabrication system that yields nanofibers characterized by a significantly enhanced surface area-to-volume ratio, which has been observed to positively influence cell adhesion and facilitate the process of tissue regeneration. The nanofibers also possess the capability to work with bioactive molecules and growth factors, thereby resulting in amplified therapeutic effects (Yadav et al., 2020).

Nanocomposites: These are materials that consist of a combination of nanoparticles and a matrix material. Nanocomposites are formed by integrating nanoparticles with matrix materials in order to leverage the advantageous characteristics exhibited by both constituents. For example, Polymer-metal nanocomposites are fabricated by integrating metallic nanoparticles into polymer matrices, resulting in materials that exhibit improved electrical conductivity and mechanical strength. The utilization of these nanocomposites is observed in biosensors, wearable medical devices, and tissue engineering scaffolds. Similarly, Ceramic-polymer nanocomposites are a class of materials where ceramic nanoparticles are incorporated into polymer matrices, resulting in enhanced mechanical properties and bioactivity. These composite materials are utilized in the field of bone tissue engineering and dental applications to improve the biocompatibility and mechanical strength of implants (Omanović-Mikličanin et al., 2020).

Nano-porous materials: This refers to substances that acquire a highly porous structure at the nanoscale. Nano-porous materials display a network of interconnected pores at the nano-level, which endows them with substantial surface areas and the capacity for precise regulation of drug delivery. For example, Mesoporous silica nanoparticles exhibit diverse pore structures that aid to the encapsulation of pharmaceutical drugs and therapeutic molecules. Moreover, Mesoporous silica nanoparticles are also employed as carriers for the purpose of controlled drug delivery and targeted therapy, and their surface chemical-harmony can be customized to suit specific applications in medical sciences. Another example is, Nano-porous hydrogels which possess a tridimensional lattice configuration that exhibits the ability to absorb and desorb water molecules. These Hydrogel nanomaterials have applications in wound dressings, drug delivery systems, and tissue engineering etc., owing to their inherent capacity to sustain a moist milieu and promote cellular interactions (Lou et al., 2023).

ROUTES OF EXPOSURE AND ABSORPTION

Determining the possible influence of nanoparticles on human health requires an understanding of the different pathways by which they can enter the body (Figure 1). Nanomaterials have the capability to engage with the human body via various routes, such as inhalation, contact with the skin, ingestion, injection, and absorption through the skin (Al Osman et al., 2019).

Inhalation: Nanomaterials, specifically in the form of aerosolized particles or nanoparticles, have the potential to be respired and subsequently distributed across various regions of the respiratory system. The magnitude of sedimentation is contingent upon the dimensions, morphology, and pulmonary airflow of the particles. Ultrafine nanoparticles, owing to their diminutive dimensions, possess the capability to infiltrate the pulmonary system at a profound level, thereby potentially accessing the alveoli. This pathway is of specific interest in occupational environments where workers may encounter airborne nanomaterials while engaged in production or handling activities (Praphawatvet et al., 2020).

Epidermal Exposure: Nanomaterials have the potential to interact with the skin either by direct application or by being exposed to products that contain nanoparticles. The integumentary system functions as a protective barrier, impeding the passage of substances. However, specific nanoparticles possess the capability to traverse the outer layers of the skin and access underlying tissues. These circumstances can elicit apprehension regarding the potential toxicological effects and long-term accumulation of nanoparticles. The utilization of nanomaterials in sunscreens and cosmetics has instigated investigations aimed at evaluating their potential for skin permeation and toxicity (Yuan et al., 2021).

Ingestion: The process of consuming or taking in substances through the mouth, typically for the purpose of nourishment or absorption into the body. Nanomaterials have the ability to infiltrate the human body via the process of ingestion, which can occur either deliberately (such as through the consumption of oral medications) or inadvertently (for instance, by consuming contaminated food or water). Nanoparticles have the potential to engage with the digestive system, wherein their absorption and potential toxicity can be influenced by factors such as particle size and surface chemistry. Gaining knowledge about the destiny of nanoparticles within the gastrointestinal tract holds significance in evaluating their systemic dispersion and potential impact on human health (Parenti et al., 2020).

Injection: The process of introducing a substance into a system or organism through a controlled and precise method, typically involving the use of a needle or cannulas. Injection is a method wherein nanomaterials are introduced directly into the body through intravenous, intramuscular, subcutaneous, or alternative pathways. Nanoparticles utilized in drug delivery systems, medical imaging, or targeted therapies are frequently introduced via intravenous injection. This pathway offers a regulated administration technique, circumventing obstacles such as the gastrointestinal system and enabling accurate localization. Nevertheless, the design of injected nanoparticles must be meticulously crafted in order to mitigate immune responses, prevent excessive accumulation, and minimize unintended distribution (Bagherzadeh et al., 2020).

Transdermal Uptake: Transdermal uptake pertains to the process of nanoparticles being absorbed through the skin in order to achieve systemic delivery. Nanoparticles specifically engineered for transdermal administration have the capability to permeate the epidermis, the outermost layer of the skin, and access the systemic circulation. This pathway provides a non-intrusive alternative for pharmaceutical delivery and is frequently employed for transdermal patches and topical therapies.

Every pathway of exposure and absorption poses distinct challenges and considerations. The properties of nanomaterials, such as their dimensions, surface characteristics, and chemical makeup, exert a substantial influence on their behavior within biological systems. In order to guarantee the secure utilization of nanomaterials in medical contexts, it is imperative to conduct thorough investigations that evaluate their potential interactions with various biological systems and identify any potential negative consequences that may arise from exposure via these pathways (Takeuchi et al., 2021).

FACTORS AFFECTING THE TOXICITY OF NANOMATERIALS

The toxicity of nanomaterials is intricately influenced by a multitude of factors that dictate their interactions with biological systems. Comprehending these variables is essential for forecasting and alleviating potential detrimental impacts of nanomaterials in medical contexts. For responsible and safe development, these things must be taken into account when designing and testing nanomaterials. Nanomaterials can behave in very different ways depending on the situation, including the application, the way they are

Figure 1. Pathways by which nanoparticles can enter biological systems

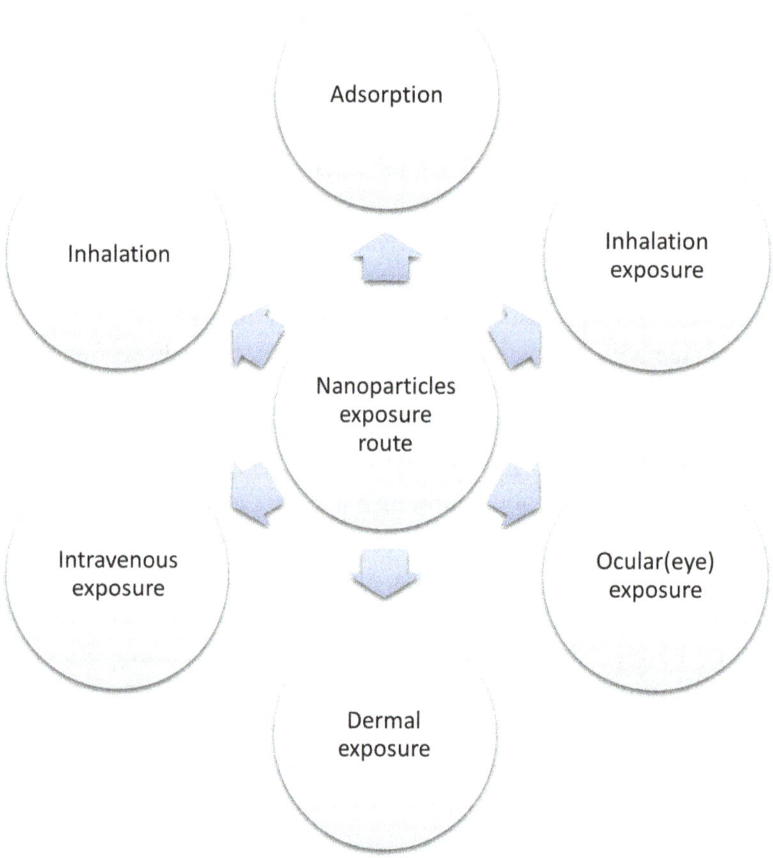

exposed, and the living things around them (Figure 2). To find potential hazards and make nanomaterials work best for medical uses while lowering risks, they need to be accord through a lot of evaluations and thoroughly characterized (Dugershaw et al., 2020).

Dimensions, Geometry, and Surface Area: The dimensions and morphology of nanomaterials have a substantial influence on their performance within biological systems. Nanoparticles of reduced size exhibit an augmented surface-to-volume ratio, resulting in heightened reactivity and the possibility of engaging with biomolecules. For example, nanoparticles of smaller size may exhibit enhanced cellular penetration capabilities, thereby influencing the mechanisms by which they are internalized by cells. Various geometric configurations (spheres, rods, tubes) can exhibit distinct interactions with cellular structures and biological tissues, which may consequently result in divergent profiles of toxicity (Qian et al., 2021).

Surface Chemistry and the Process of Functionalization: The surface chemistry of nanomaterials, encompassing the existence of functional groups or coatings, has the potential to impact their interactions with proteins, cells, and tissues. Surface modifications are frequently employed to augment biocompatibility, selectively target particular cell types, or regulate the release of drugs. Nevertheless, inadequate surface functionalization may result in heightened toxicity or unintended interactions (Zhang et al., 2020).

Agglomeration and Dispersion Phenomenon: Nanoparticles exhibit a propensity for agglomeration or aggregation as a result of the influence of van der Waals forces or electrostatic interactions. Agglomerated nanoparticles exhibit distinct characteristics compared to isolated nanoparticles, which can influence their cellular absorption, distribution within the body, and potential for toxicity. Optimal dispersion is of utmost importance in order to uphold uniformity and predictability within biological systems (Kishore et al., 2023).

Biodistribution and Bioaccumulation: Nanomaterials, upon administration, have the ability to disperse throughout different organs and tissues within the body. The biodistribution of particles is contingent upon various factors, including but not limited to particle size, surface properties, and the chosen route of administration. Certain nanomaterials have the potential to accumulate within specific organs, which could result in the manifestation of long-term effects. Gaining insights into the mechanisms by which nanomaterials are eliminated from the human body and determining their potential for accumulation is crucial in assessing their safety (Habumugisha et al., 2023).

Mechanisms of Cellular Internalization: Nanoparticles have the capability to infiltrate cellular structures via diverse mechanisms, including endocytosis or direct membrane permeation. The process of internalization can influence the subsequent intracellular destiny and potential harmful effects.

Figure 2. Factors affecting the toxicity of nanomaterials

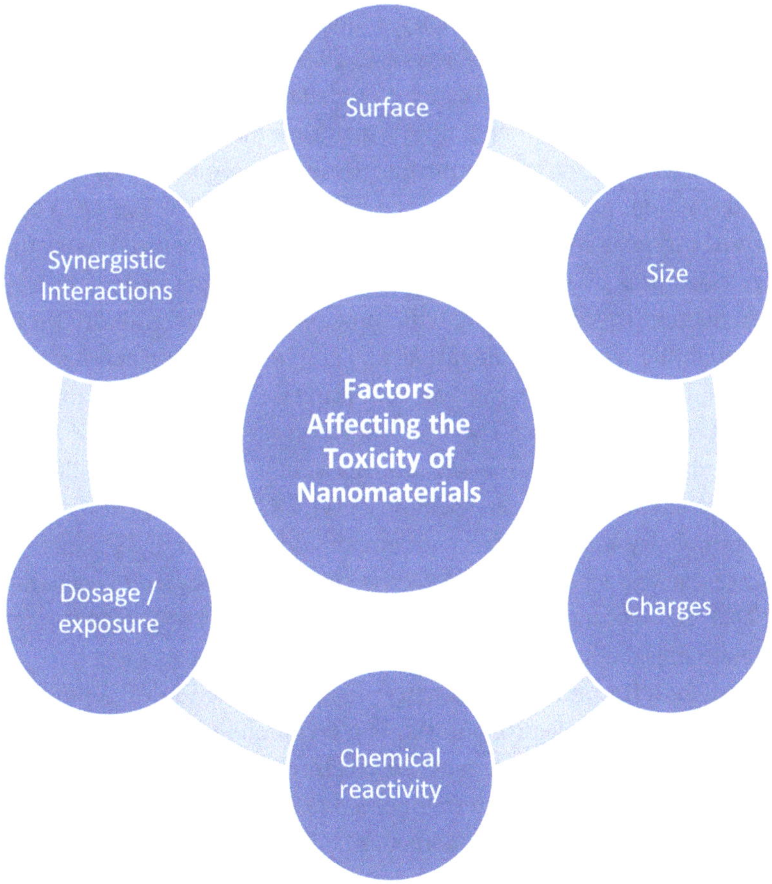

Nanoparticles that are internalized by cells through the process of endocytosis may come into contact with endosomal compartments, thereby potentially affecting their degradation and interaction with cellular constituents.

Synergistic Interactions: Toxicity of nanomaterials may also result from the synergistic interaction of various factors. As an illustration, the interplay between nanoparticles and various substances, such as pharmaceuticals or contaminants in the environment, can result in synergistic phenomena that intensify the level of toxicity. Investigating these intricate interconnections is crucial for comprehending real-life situations (Yang et al., 2020).

IN VITRO TOXICITY ASSESSMENT

Examining the possible negative effects of nanomaterials on cells isolated from a living organism is known as in vitro toxicity assessment. The aforementioned in vitro toxicity assessment methods play a crucial role as primary screening tools in the evaluation of nanomaterial safety. These experimental setups offer regulated environments to study the interactions between nanomaterials and cells, as well as their capacity to elicit cytotoxicity, genotoxicity, oxidative stress, or inflammation. Nevertheless, it is crucial to acknowledge that in vitro models may not entirely mimic the intricacy of in vivo systems, and their findings should be interpreted alongside other information, such as in vivo studies and physicochemical characterization, to formulate comprehensive conclusions regarding the safety of nanomaterials. Several important techniques for assessing in vitro toxicity include:

Assessment of Cellular Viability: The MTT assay (3-(4,5-dimethylthiazol-2-yl)-2,5-diphenyltetrazolium bromide assay), is commonly employed assay is predicated upon the metabolic activity exhibited by cells. Living cells contain functional mitochondria, which have the ability to convert MTT into formazan crystals, resulting in the manifestation of a purple hue. Researchers quantify the absorbance of the aforementioned pigmented solution in order to assess the viability of cells. A decline in absorbance indicates diminished cellular viability as a result of toxicity induced by nanomaterials. Another test named The Alamar Blue Assay, which utilizes Alamar Blue, a redox indicator that undergoes a color change (from blue to pink) upon reduction by cellular metabolic processes. The magnitude of chromatic alteration is directly correlated with the quantity of metabolically active and viable cellular entities. Through the quantification of chromatic alterations, researches are able to assess the cytotoxic impact of nanomaterials.

Quantification of Oxidative Stress: The Dichlorofluorescein Assay (DCF Assay) can be utilized for quantification of oxidative stress. DCF assay, utilizes a fluorescent probe called dichlorofluorescein (DCFH). In the presence of reactive oxygen species (ROS), DCFH undergoes a conversion process and transforms into a significantly more fluorescent compound known as DCF. Nanomaterials that elicit cellular oxidative stress can trigger augmented reactive oxygen species (ROS) generation, consequently leading to elevated DCF fluorescence levels. The assay quantifies the observed fluorescence augmentation as a metric for assessing the level of oxidative stress.

Evaluation of Genotoxicity and Mutagenicity: for the evaluation of genotoxicity the comet assay, also known as single cell gel electrophoresis, is a technique used to identify and quantify DNA damage at the cellular level. During the process of electrophoresis, cells that are enclosed within an agarose gel experience a phenomenon where fragmented DNA moves away from the nucleus, resulting in the formation of a structure resembling a "comet tail." The manifestation of genotoxicity caused by nanomaterials is discerned through the measurement of tail length and intensity. Increased tail length or greater intensity is indicative of a higher degree of DNA damage. Similarly, the Micronucleus Assay is a another scientific method used to evaluate genotoxicity. It involves the examination of micronuclei, which are smaller nuclei that form outside the main nucleus within a cell. When nanomaterials elicit DNA damage during cellular mitosis, segments of chromosomes have the potential to be excluded from the nuclei of daughter cells, resulting in the formation of micronuclei. The detection of micronuclei serves as a reliable indicator of the presence of genotoxicity.

Inflammatory Response Evaluation: to measure the inflammatory response, the Cytokine Release Assays is one of the most know methods. Nanomaterials have the ability to stimulate immune cells, specifically macrophages, resulting in the secretion of pro-inflammatory cytokines, including interleukins (such as IL-1β and IL-6) and tumor necrosis factor (TNF-α). Enzyme-linked immunosorbent assays (ELISAs) or bead-based assays are utilized for the quantitative measurement of these cytokines. Increased levels of cytokines are indicative of an immune response triggered by exposure to nanomaterials. Similarly, the Nitric Oxide (NO) Assay is utilized to measure the presence and activity of nitric oxide (NO), a crucial component involved in the process of inflammation. When cellular entities are subjected to nanomaterials, the inducible nitric oxide synthase (iNOS) enzyme has the capability to generate nitric oxide (NO) as a component of the immune system's reaction. Scientists quantitatively assess the levels of nitric oxide (NO), commonly employing the Griess assay, as a means to evaluate the inflammatory capacity of nanomaterials. Increased production of nitric oxide (NO) is indicative of an activated immune response and the possibility of inflammation (Jia et al., 2019).

IN VIVO TOXICITY STUDIES

In vivo investigations provide a comprehensive viewpoint on the toxicity of nanomaterials by taking into account intricate interactions within biological systems. Nevertheless, they also encounter ethical considerations and may not precisely reproduce human reactions. Researchers frequently combine controlled testing with real-world biological complexity by integrating in vitro and in vivo data to improve the trustworthiness of findings. In vivo toxicity studies encompass the evaluation of the impacts of nanomaterials on living organisms, commonly employing animal models. These studies offer a more holistic comprehension of the potential hazards and impacts of exposure to nanomaterials. Important components to in vivo toxicity studies involve:

Animal Models for the Evaluation of Nanotoxicity: The careful selection of suitable animal models is of utmost importance in order to accurately replicate human responses and extrapolate research findings. Frequently employed animal models encompass Mus musculus (mice), Rattus norvegicus (rats), and non-human primates. The selection of a model is contingent upon various factors, including the intended application of the nanomaterial, the potential pathways through which it may be encountered, and its resemblance to the physiological characteristics of humans.

Acute and Chronic Toxicity Studies: Acute toxicity studies investigate the immediate consequences of nanomaterial exposure, typically encompassing singular or brief exposures. Chronic toxicity studies estimate the potential long-term impacts that may occur over the period of time. These analyses aid in forming the highest tolerable dosage and detecting any potential cumulative or delayed toxicological impacts.

Immunological Responses: Nanomaterials also have the capability to engross with the immune system, resulting in the initiation of immunological responses or reactions. Evaluating these responses is critical for comprehending the likelihood of allergies, hypersensitivity reactions or immune-mediated adverse effects. Methods include quantification of cytokine concentrations, evaluating immune cell subsets, and scrutinizing antibody synthesis.

Evaluation of Toxicity Specific to Organs: Nanomaterials also exhibit an organ-specific effects. The evaluation of organ-specific toxicity entails the analysis of nanomaterial accumulation, distribution, and potential harm within specific organs. Histopathological-microscopic analysis of tissue samples to identify any structural abnormalities is one of the method to evaluate specific organ toxicity (Sani et al., 2021).

IMMUNOLOGICAL FACTORS TO BE TAKEN INTO ACCOUNT

The association of immunological responses is crucial in the assessment of the safety and effectiveness of nanomaterials employed in medical sciences. Acquisition insight into the mechanisms by which nanomaterials engross with the immune system is imperative in the pursuit of creating nanomedical interventions that are both safe and effective.

Immune Response to Nanomaterials: Nanomaterials have the potential to provoke various immune responses, which can extent from mild inflammation to more intricate reactions. The immune system has function to identifies foreign entities by discerning their distinct characteristics, such as sizes, morphology, surface composition, electrical charge etc. These properties exert an influence on the processing of nanomaterials by immune cells and perform their specific function.

Hypersensitivity Reactions: Hypersensitivity reactions manifest as an inflated response of the immune system to a specific stimulus or allergen, resulting in detrimental consequences. Susceptible individuals may experience hypersensitivity as a consequence of exposure to nanomaterials. For example, specific alterations to any instrument surface or the application of coatings may elicit allergic reactions or worsen pre-existing medical conditions of the patients.

Immunomodulatory Effects: Nanomaterials also possess the ability to regulate immune responses, manifesting either as augmentation or inhibition of immune action. Certain nanomaterials can be purposely engineered to boost immune responses, particularly for purposes such as tumor immunotherapy. Conversely, alternate nanomaterials may require deliberate alterations to mitigate immune activation, thereby averting any potential adverse reactions. Moreover, Nanomaterials have the capability to exert an influence on diverse populaces of immune cells, encircling macrophages, dendritic cells, T cells, and B cells. These interactions have the potential to stimulus the production of cytokines, the demonstration of antigens, and the triggering of immune cells.

Approaches to Mitigate Immunological Considerations

- Surface Modification: The alteration of surface characteristics of nanomaterials has the potential to control their interactions with immune cells. Through the manipulation of surface chemistry or the introduction of specific ligands, nanoparticles have the ability to decrease immune activation or improve targeting capabilities.
- Immunomodulatory Agents: Certain nanomaterials possess the capability to be persistently designed for the transportation of immunomodulatory agents, thereby permitting precise adjustment

of immune responses. For example, nanoparticles could be engineered with the tenacity of conveying anti-inflammatory medications to mitigate hyperactive immune responses.

- Preclinical Immunotoxicity Testing: The preclinical evaluations are very important for the assessment of the immune-toxic properties of nanoparticles or nanomaterials. This involves conducting in vitro trials to investigate interactions between immune cells, as well as in vivo analyses exploiting animal models to measure immune responses and potential negative outcomes.

Immunological Considerations Tailored to the Individual: The accomplishment of nanomedicine is depending upon its capability to accommodate individual variations in immune responses. The implementation of personalized medicine strategies may entail the customization of nanomaterial characteristics to align with individual patient profiles, thereby mitigating the potential for immune-related complications (Xu et al., 2022).

BLOOD-BRAIN BARRIER PENETRATION

The blood-brain barrier (BBB) is a specialized barrier that exhibits high selectivity, effectively segregating the central nervous system (CNS) from the circulatory system. It effectively impedes the ingress of numerous substances, encompassing specific pharmaceuticals and nanoparticles, into the cerebral region. Careful consideration is necessary when assessing the advantages of therapies that target the central nervous system (CNS) against the potential risks associated with their ability to penetrate the blood-brain barrier (BBB). Nanomaterials require cautious design and assessment and must take into account their intended uses, therapeutic payloads, and possible central nervous system impacts. The main goal is to develop effective strategies for utilizing nanomaterials to their maximum potential with simultaneously preserving neurological safety. Because of the potential risks and therapeutic benefits, it is imperative to consider how nanomaterials may pierce the blood-brain barrier (BBB) in medical settings.

Potential Hazards of Nanomaterials in the Central Nervous System: Although the blood-brain barrier (BBB) serves an essential role in protecting the brain, it can impede the passage of medication and the application of nanomaterial-based therapies. The potential concerns posed by nanomaterials to the central nervous system (CNS) include the following:

- Neurotoxicity: Nanomaterials or nanoparticles that penetrate the blood-brain barrier (BBB) have the potential to elicit neurotoxic consequences through their interfaces with nerves, neurons, glial cells, or by interfering with pathways of neural signaling.
- Accumulation: The gradual accrual of nanomaterials within the brain has the potential to persuade negative consequences/ toxicity or modify cerebral functionality.
- Inflammation: The potential passage of nanoparticles through the blood-brain barrier (BBB) could potentially elicit immune responses or aggravate inflammation within the brain segments, thereby impacting neural well-beingness of individual.

Techniques for Reducing Brain Exposure: Various methodologies are implemented to mitigate cerebral exposure to nanomaterials while preserving their therapeutic advantages:

- Surface Modification: Through the deliberate manipulation of nanomaterial surfaces, scientists have the ability to control their interactions with cells in the blood-brain barrier (BBB) and subsequently decrease their ability to penetrate the brain. Surface coatings have the potential to augment selectivity towards particular tissues or restrict interactions with brain endothelial cells.
- Optimization of Size and Charge: The permeability of the blood-brain barrier is influenced by the size and charge of nanomaterials. Nanoparticles of reduced size may exhibit enhanced permeability across the blood-brain barrier (BBB), whereas the surface charge of these particles can influence their interactions with BBB endothelial cells.
- Targeted Delivery: The process of developing nanomaterials equipped with ligands that possess the ability to selectively recognize receptors on the endothelial cells of the blood-brain barrier (BBB) can significantly improve the efficiency of delivering substances to the brain, while simultaneously reducing the occurrence of unintended effects on non-targeted areas.
- Intranasal Administration: Intranasal administration circumvents the blood-brain barrier (BBB) by directly entering the brain through the olfactory and trigeminal pathways. The investigation of this pathway is currently underway to facilitate the transportation of therapeutic nanoparticles to the central nervous system (CNS).
- Focused ultrasound is can induce temporary disruption of the blood-brain barrier (BBB), thereby easing the transient passage of nanoparticles. This procedure provides a non-intrusive method for augmenting the carriage of therapeutic substances to the brain.
- Carrier systems refer to the process of encapsulating drugs within nanomaterials, which are specifically engineered to efficiently traverse the blood-brain barrier (BBB). This approach has the potential to enhance the ability of drugs to penetrate the brain. Lipid-based nanoparticles and specific polymers serve as exemplars of carrier systems employed for central nervous system (CNS) drug delivery (Guo et al., 2021).

THE REGULATORY FRAMEWORK AND SAFETY GUIDELINES

The establishment of a regulatory framework and implementation of safety guidelines are crucial in the field of medical nanotechnology to guarantee the safety of patients and facilitate the successful integration of nanomaterial-based innovations into clinical settings. Following these norms and criteria guarantees that before being licensed for clinical use, nanomaterials employed in medical applications undergo thorough evaluations for quality, safety, and efficacy. It contributes to the preservation of patient trust and confidence in medical innovations facilitated by nanotechnology. These established protocols facilitate the comprehensive assessment and adherence to precise safety criteria for nanomaterial-based products prior to their authorization for utilization.

The Food and Drug Administration (FDA) and other international regulatory agencies: The United States Food and Drug Administration (FDA) and other regulatory agencies around the world have a vital role in evaluating the safety and effectiveness of medical nanomaterials. The regulation of nanomedicines and medical devices is overseen by the FDA's Center for Drug Evaluation and Research (CDER) and Center for Devices and Radiological Health (CDRH), respectively. These regulatory bodies offer protocols for conducting preclinical and clinical investigations, assessing the potential harmful effects of nanomaterials, and validating the safety and effectiveness of products based on nanotechnology. Globally, various regulatory bodies, including the European Medicines Agency (EMA), Health Canada, and Japan Pharmaceuticals and Medical Devices Agency (PMDA), have established distinct regulatory frameworks to assess medical products based on nanomaterials.

Risk Assessment and Safety Evaluation: A Comprehensive Analysis of Potential Hazards and the Examination of Measures to Ensure Safety and Mitigate Risks. The evaluation of nanomaterial safety encompasses a thorough examination of potential hazards and advantages. The essential elements comprise:

- Physicochemical Characterization: Thorough characterization of nanomaterials is imperative for comprehending their properties, encompassing dimensions, morphology, interfacial chemistry, and robustness. This data facilitates the anticipation of potential interactions with biological systems.
- Toxicity testing: Thorough in vitro and in vivo studies are performed to evaluate the effects of nanomaterials on cellular, tissue, organ, and immune system function. These scientific investigations aid in the identification of potential negative impacts and provide guidance for the development of safe designs.
- Biodistribution and Pharmacokinetics: The investigation of biodistribution and pharmacokinetics involves the examination of the distribution, metabolism, and excretion of nanomaterials within the human body. This analysis yields valuable information regarding the possible accumulation of these materials in particular organs and tissues.
- Clinical trials: these are systematically designed studies that aim to assess the safety and effectiveness of products containing nanomaterials in human subjects. These trials adhere to regulatory protocols and evaluate variables such as dosage, patient demographics, and therapeutic efficacy.

Biocompatibility Criteria for Medical Nanomaterials: Biocompatibility standards are implemented to ensure that nanomaterials utilized in medical applications do not elicit unfavorable biological reactions. Several widely utilized standards are commonly employed:

- ISO 10993 is a collection of standards established by the International Organization for Standardization (ISO) that offers a framework for assessing the biocompatibility of medical devices, encompassing those that utilize nanomaterials.
- The ASTM F1903 standard primarily concerns the characterization of the biological reaction to nanoparticles and nanomaterials in an artificial environment, specifically in vitro.
- The United States Pharmacopeia (USP) General Chapter <1088> outlines the protocols and criteria for evaluating the potential impact of nanomaterials on human health (Foulkes et al., 2020).

STRATEGIES FOR MITIGATING THE TOXICITY OF NANOMATERIALS

The assessment of nanomaterial toxicity is a crucial component in ensuring their safe utilization in medical contexts. Various processes are implemented to improve potential toxic consequences and to supplement the safety features of nanomaterials in medical sciences, some are listed below:

Surface Alteration of nanomaterial for Alleviated Toxicity: Surface modification encompasses the process of altering the external stratum or surface of nanomaterials with the objective of enhancing their biocompatibility and extenuating interactions with cells and tissues. Through the changes of surface chemistry, alteration in charges, or the implementation of biocompatible coatings, of nanomaterial, make them able to effectively reduce the potential toxicity associated with them. This particular approach has the potential to efficiently mitigate unsought interactions and decrease the probability of adverse immune reactions. For example, the implementation of polyethylene glycol (PEG) coatings has the potential to augment the "stealth" features of nanoparticles, thereby extenuating their detection by the immune system and fading their toxicity/clearance.

Encapsulation and Controlled Release: Encapsulation means to the process of enclosing therapeutic drugs/agents within nanomaterials, which serves the purpose of safeguarding the drugs/agents during transportation and permitting their controlled release at the anticipated site. This methodology has the potential to mitigate direct interaction amid the nanomaterial and biological components, thereby fading potential toxicity. Controlled release systems also assure the gradual release of therapeutic agents, thereby optimizing their therapeutic efficiency while minimizing any potential off-target effects. For example, liposomes and polymeric nanoparticles are frequently used as carriers for drug encapsulation, thereby augmenting the safety and efficacy of the drugs.

Rational Design: Rational design encompasses the deliberate customization of nanomaterial features in order to achieve precise therapeutic goals while simultaneously mitigating toxicity. This approach taken into account are variables such as dimensions, morphology, surface characteristics, and degradability. Through the optimization of these parameters, make them able to improve the interactions between specific cells and tissues, and also minimizes the potential risks or toxicity. For example, the strategic development of nanomaterials that mimic the structural characteristics of naturally existing substances can enhance their ability to interact with biological systems and minimize immune response/reactions.

Multifunctional Nanomaterials: Multifunctional nanomaterials have been engineered to perform multiple tasks, such as enabling precise therapeutic interventions, imaging capabilities, and diagnostic functionalities and many more. These materials can be controlled through engineering methods to possess distinct possessions that effectively reduces the toxicity. For example, a specifically engineered nanoparticle premeditated for cancer therapy has the capability to concurrently transport a therapeutic drug as well as imaging agent (used in radiological investigations). This enables accurate administration of the drugs while offering the ability to monitor the efficiency of the treatment in real-time.

Computational Modeling and Predictive Approaches: Contemporary advances in computational modeling and simulation methodologies have facilitated the ability of researchers to make accurate predictions concerning the behavior and interactions of nanomaterials with or within biological systems. Computational methods can be exploited to identify potential toxicity hazards and provides guidance for the development of safer nanomaterials prior to conducting trial assessments in medical sciences. This methodology optimizes the efficiency by conserving time and resources, while also facilitating the identification and prioritization of the most viable entrants for subsequent advancement (Buchman et al., 2019).

APPLICATIONS OF NANOMATERIAL IN MEDICAL SCIENCES

Several examples demonstrate the potential advantages and difficulties of using nanoparticles in a range of medical specialties.

Contrast Agents for Imaging in Medicine: In medical imaging, nanoparticles such as quantum dots and superparamagnetic iron oxide nanoparticles (SPIONs) have been used as contrast agents. By offering a clear contrast in soft tissues and facilitating accurate viewing of anatomical structures or clinical lesions, SPIONs improve magnetic resonance imaging (MRI). Contrarily, quantum dots have extremely luminous qualities that make imaging possible that is more sensitive and detailed, especially when using fluorescence-based imaging methods.

Drug Delivery System: Two well-known types of nanomaterials utilized in drug delivery systems are polymeric nanoparticles and liposomal formulations. Therapeutic compounds are encapsulated in liposomes, which shield them from deterioration and allow for regulated release at the intended location. These nanocarriers increase the therapeutic index, decrease adverse effects, and increase medication absorption. For example, liposomal doxorubicin formulations have demonstrated less cardiotoxicity and increased efficacy in the treatment of cancer.

Implantable Medical Devices: Nanomaterials are being used more and more to enhance the functionality and biocompatibility of implantable medical devices. For example, orthopedic implants with nanostructured coatings encourage cell adhesion and integration with the surrounding bone tissue, improving the stability and durability of the implant. Furthermore, drug-eluting stents use nanoscale drug carriers to deliver anti-inflammatory or anti-proliferative medications directly to the target region, preventing restenosis.

Materials in Regenerative Health Care: Nanomaterials that act as scaffolds for tissue engineering are beneficial to regenerative medicine. Biodegradable nanoscale scaffolds offer an environment conducive to tissue regeneration and cell proliferation. These scaffolds direct cell behavior and facilitate tissue repair by imitating the extracellular matrix. For example, scaffolds built on nanofibers have shown great promise in the regeneration of injured nerve tissue in spinal cord injuries (Yaqoob et al., 2020).

Targeted Cancer Therapy: Nanomaterials are essential to targeted cancer treatments. By binding to cancer cells specifically, functionalized nanoparticles can deliver drugs precisely and lessen systemic toxicity. Scientists have created nanoparticles that release therapeutic payloads only when cancer cells are present in response to particular cues from the tumor microenvironment. This focused strategy minimizes harm to healthy tissues while increasing the effectiveness of treatment.

Customized Health Care and Diagnostics: The creation of state-of-the-art diagnostic instruments depends heavily on nanomaterials. For example, biosensors that utilise gold nanoparticles are capable of quickly and accurately identifying biomarkers linked to a wide range of illnesses. By guiding treatment decisions based on unique patient profiles, these nanosensors can be customized for personalized medicine methods and allow for early illness diagnosis.

Wound Healing Scaffolds: Nanofibrous scaffolds have been found to enhance wound healing by facilitating efficient tissue regeneration. The nanoscale materials exhibit properties similar to the extracellular matrix, promoting cellular adhesion and aiding in the process of tissue regeneration. Growth factors or antimicrobial agents can be incorporated into them to augment the process of wound healing.

Nanomaterials in Ophthalmology: Nanomaterials are utilized in ocular drug delivery systems to facilitate the transportation of drugs to the eye. The utilization of nanoparticles has the capacity to augment the bioavailability of drugs when administered to the ocular region, thereby presenting promising therapeutic options for ailments such as glaucoma or age-related macular degeneration.

Nanomaterials in Dentistry: Nanostructured dental materials are widely employed in the field of dentistry, specifically in the development of dental composites, coatings, and biomaterials. These materials are composed of nanomaterials, which are substances with dimensions on the nanometer scale. The incorporation of nano-scale fillers enhances the mechanical characteristics of dental materials while simultaneously preserving their aesthetic attributes. These materials exhibit properties that contribute to the extended lifespan and improved functionality of dental restorations.

Nanomaterials in Dermatology: Nanoparticles, specifically zinc oxide and titanium dioxide, are incorporated into sunscreens to offer efficient ultraviolet (UV) shielding. The nanoscale dimensions of these particles enable the creation of transparent formulations that provide comprehensive sun protection, eliminating the conventional issue of visible white residue.

Nanomaterials in Cardiovascular Medicine: Targeted drug delivery for cardiovascular diseases involves the utilization of nanocarriers to specifically transport drugs to vascular sites that are impacted by atherosclerosis or thrombosis. These carriers have the capability to efficiently deliver anticoagulants or anti-inflammatory drugs to the specific target site, thereby minimizing any potential adverse effects on the entire system.

Nanomaterials in Neurology: The scientific community is currently exploring the potential of nanomaterials in circumventing the blood-brain barrier and facilitating the transportation of therapeutic agents to the brain. This holds significant potential for the therapeutic management of neurological disorders, including but not limited to Alzheimer's disease and brain tumors.

Nanomaterials in Gastroenterology: Nanomaterials have the ability to safeguard drugs from degradation within the acidic milieu of the stomach and subsequently release them in the intestine, thereby enhancing the efficacy of drug administration via the oral route. This is crucial for conditions necessitating precise interventions in the gastrointestinal tract.

Nanomaterials in Orthopedics: Nanocomposite materials, such as nanohydroxyapatite, are employed to augment the mechanical properties and biocompatibility of bone implants. They facilitate osseointegration and mitigate the likelihood of complications associated with implants.

Nanomaterials in Urology: Nanoparticles have the potential to be modified in order to specifically target cancerous cells within the urinary system. This targeted approach enables the localized administration of therapeutic drugs, thereby reducing the risk of harm to surrounding healthy tissues. This application is particularly relevant in the context of intravesical chemotherapy, a treatment method employed for bladder cancer.

These varied applications show the range of uses for nanomaterials in medicine, providing specialized solutions to solve particular issues in a range of medical specializations. The field of nanomedicine holds great promise for the development of new treatments, diagnostics, and medical devices with improved effectiveness and fewer adverse effects (Palit & Hussain, 2020).

FUTURE DIRECTIONS AND CHALLENGES

The domain of nanomaterials in medical applications is undergoing rapid advancement, yet it also encounters various significant future avenues and obstacles that necessitate attention to guarantee their secure and efficient assimilation into healthcare.

The Emergence of Nanomaterials and Their Potential Hazards: With the emergence and implementation of novel nanomaterials, it is imperative to conduct a comprehensive evaluation of their potential hazards. The distinctive characteristics of novel nanomaterials have the potential to elicit unforeseen interactions with biological systems. To ensure their safety, it is imperative to conduct thorough assessments of their physicochemical properties, toxicity profiles, and potential implications for human health prior to their extensive utilization.

Long-Term Safety Evaluation: The evaluation of nanomaterials' long-term safety poses a significant challenge owing to their relatively recent integration into medical applications. Gaining knowledge about the long-term behavior of nanomaterials within the human body, including their potential to accumulate and cause chronic toxicity, is crucial for ensuring the safety of patients. Complete safety precises require the accomplishment of long-term analyses that observe the behavior, distribution, and potential adverse or toxic effects of nanomaterials.

Nanotoxicology: The field of nanotoxicology, investigates the toxicity of nanomaterials, necessitates the utilization of a multidisciplinary approach. In order to execute an in-depth assessment of the efficacy of nanomaterials, it is essential to integrate knowledge from materials science, toxicology, chemistry, biology, and medicine. The integration of multidisciplinary knowledge facilitates the optimization of experimental design, the comprehension of complex data, and the establishment of informed decisions about the development and use of nanomaterials in the field of medicine.

Standardization and Regulatory Harmonization: The establishment of standardized protocols for the characterization of nanomaterials, assessment of their toxicity, and evaluation of their safety is of utmost importance. These established criteria can facilitate the maintenance of uniformity in the process of gathering and analyzing data, thereby enabling significant comparisons between different research studies and augmenting the effectiveness of regulatory decision-making. The harmonization of regulatory guidelines on an international scale has the potential to enhance the secure transition of nanomaterials from the realm of research to their application in clinical practice (Schuemann et al., 2020).

Ethical and Societal Considerations: With the increasing integration of nanomaterials into medical practice, there arises a need to address ethical and societal implications. Ensuring equitable access to nanotechnology-based medical interventions, mitigating potential disparities, and effectively communicating potential benefits and risks to patients and the public are crucial areas that require attention.

Quantification of Environmental Impact: While the primary emphasis is frequently placed on human health, it is imperative to not disregard the ecological ramifications of nanomaterials employed in medical applications. The appropriate disposal, potential environmental release, and comprehension of their impacts on ecosystems are crucial factors to be taken into account for the sustainable advancement of nanotechnology (Ma et al., 2021).

CONCLUSION

The investigation of nanomaterials in medical contexts has unveiled novel horizons in the field of healthcare, offering potential groundbreaking resolutions for diagnostics, therapeutics, and regenerative medicine. During the course of this discourse, a number of pivotal aspects have surfaced, underscoring the inherent possibilities and obligations linked to the field of nanotechnology in the realm of medicine. Nanomaterials possess distinct advantages attributable to their dimensions, surface characteristics, and customized functionalities, facilitating the implementation of targeted pharmaceutical administration, accurate medical imaging, and tissue regeneration. The incorporation of these technologies into medical devices and therapies presents significant potential for enhancing patient outcomes and overall quality of life. Nevertheless, the immense capacity for transformation must be counterbalanced by a meticulous dedication to the evaluation of safety. The discourse has elucidated diverse variables impacting the toxicity of nanomaterials, encompassing dimensions and surface chemistry, as well as biodistribution and immune reactions. Regulatory entities, such as the Food and Drug Administration (FDA) and international counterparts, have a pivotal role in formulating guidelines and standards to guarantee the secure progression of nanomaterial advancements from laboratory settings to clinical applications. Ongoing safety evaluation is of utmost importance as the field progresses. The continuous assessment of potential risks and the resolution of unforeseen challenges are imperative due to the presence of novel nanomaterials, emerging applications, and evolving manufacturing techniques. The integration of research, clinical practice, regulatory oversight, and interdisciplinary expertise is essential for achieving a holistic comprehension of the interactions between nanomaterials and biological systems. With the progression of nanomedicine, a comprehensive viewpoint encompassing the advantages and potential hazards will steer the responsible advancement of this field. Through the integration of diverse fields of expertise, the implementation of standardized protocols, and the prioritization of patient safety, nanomaterials have the potential to bring about a transformative impact on the field of medicine, all while upholding the utmost standards of ethical conduct and scientific rigor. The pursuit of secure and efficient nanomedicine signifies a fundamental transformation in the field of healthcare, wherein the intersection of groundbreaking advancements and the welfare of patients occurs.

REFERENCES

Al Osman, M., Yang, F., & Massey, I. Y. (2019). Exposure routes and health effects of heavy metals on children. *Biometals*, *32*(4), 563–573. doi:10.100710534-019-00193-5 PMID:30941546

Bagherzadeh, S. A., Jalali, E., Sarafraz, M. M., Ali Akbari, O., Karimipour, A., Goodarzi, M., & Bach, Q. V. (2020). Effects of magnetic field on micro cross jet injection of dispersed nanoparticles in a microchannel. *International Journal of Numerical Methods for Heat & Fluid Flow*, *30*(5), 2683–2704. doi:10.1108/HFF-02-2019-0150

Baig, N., Kammakakam, I., & Falath, W. (2021). Nanomaterials: A review of synthesis methods, properties, recent progress, and challenges. *Materials Advances*, *2*(6), 1821–1871. doi:10.1039/D0MA00807A

Buchman, J. T., Hudson-Smith, N. V., Landy, K. M., & Haynes, C. L. (2019). Understanding nanoparticle toxicity mechanisms to inform redesign strategies to reduce environmental impact. *Accounts of Chemical Research*, *52*(6), 1632–1642. doi:10.1021/acs.accounts.9b00053 PMID:31181913

Cheng, Z., Li, M., Dey, R., & Chen, Y. (2021). Nanomaterials for cancer therapy: Current progress and perspectives. *Journal of Hematology & Oncology*, *14*(1), 1–27. doi:10.118613045-021-01096-0 PMID:34059100

Dugershaw, B. B., Aengenheister, L., Hansen, S. S. K., Hougaard, K. S., & Buerki-Thurnherr, T. (2020). Recent insights on indirect mechanisms in developmental toxicity of nanomaterials. *Particle and Fibre Toxicology*, *17*(1), 1–22. doi:10.118612989-020-00359-x PMID:32653006

Foulkes, R., Man, E., Thind, J., Yeung, S., Joy, A., & Hoskins, C. (2020). The regulation of nanomaterials and nanomedicines for clinical application: Current and future perspectives. *Biomaterials Science*, *8*(17), 4653–4664. doi:10.1039/D0BM00558D PMID:32672255

Gao, C., Lyu, F., & Yin, Y. (2020). Encapsulated metal nanoparticles for catalysis. *Chemical Reviews*, *121*(2), 834–881. doi:10.1021/acs.chemrev.0c00237 PMID:32585087

Guo, Z., Zhang, P., Chakraborty, S., Chetwynd, A. J., Abdolahpur Monikh, F., Stark, C., Ali-Boucetta, H., Wilson, S., Lynch, I., & Valsami-Jones, E. (2021). Biotransformation modulates the penetration of metallic nanomaterials across an artificial blood–brain barrier model. *Proceedings of the National Academy of Sciences of the United States of America*, *118*(28), e2105245118. doi:10.1073/pnas.2105245118 PMID:34260400

Habumugisha, T., Zhang, Z., Fang, C., Yan, C., & Zhang, X. (2023). Uptake, bioaccumulation, biodistribution and depuration of polystyrene nanoplastics in zebrafish (Danio rerio). *The Science of the Total Environment*, *893*, 164840. doi:10.1016/j.scitotenv.2023.164840 PMID:37321508

Jamkhande, P. G., Ghule, N. W., Bamer, A. H., & Kalaskar, M. G. (2019). Metal nanoparticles synthesis: An overview on methods of preparation, advantages and disadvantages, and applications. *Journal of Drug Delivery Science and Technology*, *53*, 101174. doi:10.1016/j.jddst.2019.101174

Jia, H. R., Zhu, Y. X., Duan, Q. Y., Chen, Z., & Wu, F. G. (2019). Nanomaterials meet zebrafish: Toxicity evaluation and drug delivery applications. *Journal of Controlled Release*, *311*, 301–318. doi:10.1016/j.jconrel.2019.08.022 PMID:31446084

Joudeh, N., & Linke, D. (2022). Nanoparticle classification, physicochemical properties, characterization, and applications: A comprehensive review for biologists. *Journal of Nanobiotechnology*, *20*(1), 262. doi:10.118612951-022-01477-8 PMID:35672712

Kishore, K., Pandey, A., Wagri, N. K., Saxena, A., Patel, J., & Al-Fakih, A. (2023). *Technological challenges in nanoparticle-modified geopolymer concrete: A comprehensive review on nanomaterial dispersion, characterization techniques and its mechanical properties*. Case Studies in Construction Materials.

Lou, F., Dong, S., Zhu, K., Chen, X., & Ma, Y. (2023). Thermal Insulation Performance of Aerogel Nano-Porous Materials: Characterization and Test Methods. *Gels (Basel, Switzerland)*, *9*(3), 220. doi:10.3390/gels9030220 PMID:36975669

Ma, W., Zhan, Y., Zhang, Y., Mao, C., Xie, X., & Lin, Y. (2021). The biological applications of DNA nanomaterials: Current challenges and future directions. *Signal Transduction and Targeted Therapy*, *6*(1), 351. doi:10.103841392-021-00727-9 PMID:34620843

Norizan, M. N., Moklis, M. H., Demon, S. Z. N., Halim, N. A., Samsuri, A., Mohamad, I. S., Knight, V. F., & Abdullah, N. (2020). Carbon nanotubes: Functionalisation and their application in chemical sensors. *RSC Advances*, *10*(71), 43704–43732. doi:10.1039/D0RA09438B PMID:35519676

Omanović-Mikličanin, E., Badnjević, A., Kazlagić, A., & Hajlovac, M. (2020). Nanocomposites: A brief review. *Health and Technology*, *10*(1), 51–59. doi:10.100712553-019-00380-x

Palit, S., & Hussain, C. M. (2020). Functionalization of nanomaterials for industrial applications: recent and future perspectives. In *Handbook of functionalized nanomaterials for industrial applications* (pp. 3–14). Elsevier. doi:10.1016/B978-0-12-816787-8.00001-6

Parenti, C. C., Binelli, A., Caccia, S., Della Torre, C., Magni, S., Pirovano, G., & Casartelli, M. (2020). Ingestion and effects of polystyrene nanoparticles in the silkworm Bombyx mori. *Chemosphere*, *257*, 127203. doi:10.1016/j.chemosphere.2020.127203 PMID:32480083

Praphawatvet, T., Peters, J. I., & Williams, R. O. III. (2020). Inhaled nanoparticles–An updated review. *International Journal of Pharmaceutics, 587*, 119671. doi:10.1016/j.ijpharm.2020.119671 PMID:32702456

Qian, W., Xu, S., Zhang, X., Li, C., Yang, W., Bowen, C. R., & Yang, Y. (2021). Differences and similarities of photocatalysis and electrocatalysis in two-dimensional nanomaterials: Strategies, traps, applications and challenges. *Nano-Micro Letters, 13*(1), 1–38. doi:10.100740820-021-00681-9 PMID:34264418

Saleh, T. A. (2020). Nanomaterials: Classification, properties, and environmental toxicities. *Environmental Technology & Innovation, 20*, 101067. doi:10.1016/j.eti.2020.101067

Sani, A., Cao, C., & Cui, D. (2021). Toxicity of gold nanoparticles (AuNPs): A review. *Biochemistry and Biophysics Reports, 26*, 100991. doi:10.1016/j.bbrep.2021.100991 PMID:33912692

Schuemann, J., Bagley, A. F., Berbeco, R., Bromma, K., Butterworth, K. T., Byrne, H. L., Chithrani, B. D., Cho, S. H., Cook, J. R., Favaudon, V., Gholami, Y. H., Gargioni, E., Hainfeld, J. F., Hespeels, F., Heuskin, A.-C., Ibeh, U. M., Kuncic, Z., Kunjachan, S., Lacombe, S., & Krishnan, S. (2020). Roadmap for metal nanoparticles in radiation therapy: Current status, translational challenges, and future directions. *Physics in Medicine and Biology, 65*(21), 21RM02. doi:10.1088/1361-6560/ab9159 PMID:32380492

Takeuchi, I., Suzuki, T., & Makino, K. (2021). Iontophoretic transdermal delivery using chitosan-coated PLGA nanoparticles for transcutaneous immunization. *Colloids and Surfaces. A, Physicochemical and Engineering Aspects, 608*, 125607. doi:10.1016/j.colsurfa.2020.125607

Thi, T. T. H., Suys, E. J., Lee, J. S., Nguyen, D. H., Park, K. D., & Truong, N. P. (2021). Lipid-based nanoparticles in the clinic and clinical trials: From cancer nanomedicine to COVID-19 vaccines. *Vaccines, 9*(4), 359. doi:10.3390/vaccines9040359 PMID:33918072

Wang, X., Zhong, X., Li, J., Liu, Z., & Cheng, L. (2021). Inorganic nanomaterials with rapid clearance for biomedical applications. *Chemical Society Reviews, 50*(15), 8669–8742. doi:10.1039/D0CS00461H PMID:34156040

Xu, L., Wang, X., Wang, W., Sun, M., Choi, W. J., Kim, J. Y., Hao, C., Li, S., Qu, A., Lu, M., Wu, X., Colombari, F. M., Gomes, W. R., Blanco, A. L., de Moura, A. F., Guo, X., Kuang, H., Kotov, N. A., & Xu, C. (2022). Enantiomer-dependent immunological response to chiral nanoparticles. *Nature, 601*(7893), 366–373. doi:10.103841586-021-04243-2 PMID:35046606

Yadav, D., Amini, F., & Ehrmann, A. (2020). Recent advances in carbon nanofibers and their applications–a review. *European Polymer Journal, 138*, 109963. doi:10.1016/j.eurpolymj.2020.109963

Yang, J., Dai, D., Lou, X., Ma, L., Wang, B., & Yang, Y. W. (2020). Supramolecular nanomaterials based on hollow mesoporous drug carriers and macrocycle-capped CuS nanogates for synergistic chemo-photothermal therapy. *Theranostics, 10*(2), 615–629. doi:10.7150/thno.40066 PMID:31903141

Yaqoob, A. A., Ahmad, H., Parveen, T., Ahmad, A., Oves, M., Ismail, I. M., Qari, H. A., Umar, K., & Mohamad Ibrahim, M. N. (2020). Recent advances in metal decorated nanomaterials and their various biological applications: A review. *Frontiers in Chemistry, 8*, 341. doi:10.3389/fchem.2020.00341 PMID:32509720

Yuan, J., Zhang, Y., Zhang, Y., Mo, Y., & Zhang, Q. (2021). Effects of metal nanoparticles on tight junction-associated proteins via HIF-1α/miR-29b/MMPs pathway in human epidermal keratinocytes. *Particle and Fibre Toxicology*, *18*(1), 1–22. doi:10.118612989-021-00405-2 PMID:33407654

Zhang, J., Mou, L., & Jiang, X. (2020). Surface chemistry of gold nanoparticles for health-related applications. *Chemical Science (Cambridge)*, *11*(4), 923–936. doi:10.1039/C9SC06497D PMID:34084347

Zielińska, A., Carreiró, F., Oliveira, A. M., Neves, A., Pires, B., Venkatesh, D. N., Durazzo, A., Lucarini, M., Eder, P., Silva, A. M., Santini, A., & Souto, E. B. (2020). Polymeric nanoparticles: Production, characterization, toxicology and ecotoxicology. *Molecules (Basel, Switzerland)*, *25*(16), 3731. doi:10.3390/molecules25163731 PMID:32824172

Chapter 19
Thermo-Acoustic Investigations on Benzoate-Based Mixtures Using Ultrasonic Technique: A Review

Ashpinder Kaur Gill
Lovely Professional University, India

Nabaparna Chakraborty
https://orcid.org/0000-0003-3891-0408
Lovely Professional University, India

Kailash Chandra Juglan
https://orcid.org/0000-0002-8753-4843
Lovely Professional University, India

ABSTRACT

This chapter focuses on the viscometric, volumetric, and spectroscopic techniques to investigate the thermo-acoustic parameters and nature of molecular interactions. This in-depth analysis of the literature focuses on the properties and uses of benzoate-based combinations in aqueous solutions. Studies examining the density and volumetric properties, excess parameters, molecular interactions, and thermal properties of benzoate-based compounds like sodium benzoate, ethyl benzoate, and methyl benzoate are the main subject of interest. The current review presents research and studies on acoustic and thermodynamic investigations as well as molecular interactions of the mixtures. This review aims not only to consolidate the existing knowledge but also to inspire future investigations that contribute to the development of novel materials used in many applications of ultrasonic sound in the disciplines of medical, pharmacology, agricultural practices, etc.

DOI: 10.4018/979-8-3693-0448-8.ch019

INTRODUCTION

The ultrasonic method is one of the greatest methods for figuring out bulk characteristics, and intermolecular forces in mixtures of many liquid components. In both pure liquids and liquid components, ultrasonic measures are frequently employed to examine molecular interactions. Researchers have been undertaking more study in recent years as a result of the many applications of ultrasonic sound in the disciplines of medical, pharmacology, agricultural practises, material science, and biological research. To gain insight into the nature of intermolecular interactions, researchers are examining the acoustical and thermodynamic characteristics of liquid mixtures. Due to their wide range of thermodynamic properties and many commercial uses, benzoate-based mixtures have gained a lot of interest in scientific research. They inhibit the growth of bacteria, fungus, yeasts, and mould, helping to the shelf life of various products. This in-depth review attempts to offer a thorough examination of the substantial research on the thermo-acoustic parameters and uses of mixtures based on benzoates (Palani et al., 2009). Understanding the structural changes in relation to liquids requires measurements of thermodynamic and their excess properties, such excess acoustic impedance, isentropic compressibility, excess intermolecular free length, adiabatic compressibility, Lennard-Jones potential and Relative association which shed light on the benzoate based mixtures (Duraivathi et al., 2022). They can be utilized in various experimental techniques for different purposes like gas chromatography, electrochemistry, spectroscopy (NMR, FTIR, and IR), synthesis and reactions, and biological and biochemical studies. Benzoate- based mixtures hold significant importance in research due to their diverse applications and properties, as they can be used as substrates or inhibitors in enzymatic to study enzyme activity or inhibition mechanisms. Significant progress was made in recent years with the application of ultrasonic techniques to address thermodynamic, volumetric, physicochemical and acoustical properties of liquid blends. This approach is providing a substantial amount of insight into the diversity of interactions in liquid mixtures at both subatomic and molecular levels. Due to its nondestructive nature, this technique is usually preferred for the purpose of preserving the integrity, structure and configuration of samples. Ultrasonic velocity and density are key features that determine the overall molecular configuration. In order to examine the unique characteristics of liquid mixtures with more than one fragment, these ultrasonic properties are required in order to prevent any distortion. In order to examine the various molecular interactions of different components within these mixtures, acoustic and thermodynamic characteristics of liquids are essential tools. These properties are used to investigate the complex behavior and relationships of molecules in a mixture, which leads to comprehensive understanding of their interactions (Chakraborty et al.; 2018; Devunuri et al.; 2016; Thakur et al.; 2019). They are often used as components or solvents in the formulation of ionic liquids or deep eutectic solvent, electrolytes, or components in the energy storage and conversion systems. These interactions are crucial for determining the behavior and properties of substances at the molecular level. The research and studies on acoustic and thermodynamic investigations and molecular interactions of the Benzoate based mixtures are presented in the current review.

A REVIEW ON THE ACOUSTIC AND THERMODYNAMIC INVESTIGATIONS OF THE BENZOATE BASED MIXTURES

Thermo Acoustic Phenomena of Benzoate Based Mixtures

The term "benzoate-based mixtures" describes solutions or compositions that contain benzoic acid or its derivatives and have been employed in a variety of scientific and industrial applications. Benzoate-based mixtures have the potential to produce sound waves through the thermo acoustic effect in the context of thermo acoustic phenomena in ultrasonic techniques. Due to temperature gradients in a medium, thermo acoustic phenomena include the transformation of heat into acoustic waves. These phenomena can be used in ultrasonic techniques to produce and control high-frequency sound waves. The velocities of sound of mixtures of Benzyl Benzoate ($C_{14}H_{12}O_2$) + Gernyl Acetate ($C_{12}H_{20}O_2$) can be measured at 2 MHz frequency using ultrasonic methods. To analyze the interactions occurring amongst the liquid mixtures, various acoustical and thermodynamical properties from Redlich-Kister Polynomial equation, including velocity, molar volume and acoustic impedance. In addition, the antibacterial activity of both individual chemicals and liquid combinations and the importance of benzoate-based mixes in ultrasonic techniques lies in their capacity to effectively transform thermal energy into acoustic energy, enabling the generation of ultrasonic waves for a variety of applications such as non-destructive testing, medical imaging, and industrial operations (Chinnarao et al., 2023). In areas requiring exact control of ultrasonic signals, these combinations provide a controlled and controllable way of producing sound waves. In benzoate-based mixtures, a variety of thermo acoustic properties can be investigated effectively and without causing any damage using ultrasonic techniques. These techniques provide information on molecular interactions, density, compressibility, sound speed, and viscosity, all of which are vital for comprehending the behaviour of materials (Chakraborty et al., 2020). The study of thermo acoustic properties such as partial molar compressibility, isentropic compressibility, acoustic impedance, molecular interactions, sound speed, density, relaxation time, and viscosity of benzoate-based mixtures is greatly aided by ultrasonic techniques. These methods measure the sound wave propagation across the medium by using ultrasonic waves, which offers important information about the interactions and molecular behaviour of the mixture. Researchers can learn details about the mixture's thermodynamic characteristics, molecular composition, and intermolecular forces by examining changes in sound velocity and attenuation (Kaur et al.; 2023; Chakraborty et al.; 2022). Ultrasonic measurements support improvements in energy conversion, medical imaging, and industrial applications by tracking temperature changes, evaluating the effectiveness of thermo acoustic devices, and characterising the acoustic properties of materials.

Molecular Interactions and Thermo-Acoustic Investigations

Ultrasonic methods are used to investigate the properties of benzoate-based mixtures through thermodynamic and acoustic experiments. The molecular interactions, phase behaviour, and structural alterations of these mixtures can all be studied using ultrasonic techniques. Researchers can learn a lot about the mixtures by combining their thermodynamic and acoustic investigations. The measured values of sound speed, viscosities, and densities values of Para methoxy benzoic (benzoate) acid + amides with the help of interferometer, specific gravity bottle, and viscometer methods had been used to determine a number of thermoacoustic characteristics, including surface tension, acoustic impedance, partial molar volumes and associated excess parameters. The least squares method had been used to fit these extra parameters to the R-K equations. Additionally, to illustrate the partial molar volumes' effects on the chemical interactions between methoxy molecules and amides, FT-IR spectroscopy of the pure solvents and their mixtures had also been investigated (Nagarjuna et al., 2023). The density, ultrasonic velocity, and viscosity of aspartic acid ($C_4H_7NO_4$) and sodium benzoate ($C_7H_5NaO_2$) and acetic acid ammonium salt at constant temperature were measured in order to investigate the intermolecular interactions. From the experimental results, various acoustic and thermodynamic properties were then calculated, including impedance, surface tension, isothermal and isentropic compressibilities. They also observed that ASP occurs as zwitterions (- COO^-,-NH_3^+) with a totally deprotonated side chain carboxyl group when there are substantial anions present, such as carboxylates. Higher ASP and SB/AA concentrations cause more interactions between particles when they are near together (Dhal et al., 2023). The specific conductance of glutamic acid in H_2O and aqueous medium such as, Sodium Benzoate ($C_7H_5NaO_2$) and Potassium Sorbate ($C_6H_7O_2K$) had been obtained to better understand the types of intermolecular interactions between the carboxylate ions at different compositions and temperatures. Numerous acoustical and thermodynamic metrics, including internal pressure, relative association, and acoustic impedance were assessed with the experimental data. They noticed that strong ion-solvent interactions predominate in mixtures in all of these physicochemical and thermodynamic data that in the presence of sorbate/ benzoate (Dhal et al., 2022). The molecular arrangement and strength of the interactions within the mixtures can be determined by measuring ultrasonic velocity and attenuation. These acoustic characteristics may alter in response to intermolecular interactions, phase transitions, or molecular behaviour. Ultrasonic velocity of binary mixture of pure methyl benzoate($C_8H_8O_2$) + alcohols (1- propanol/1-butanol/ethanol) using DSA 5000 M at different temperatures and refractive index were obtained at 303.2K temperature using an abbe refractometer. Additionally, they looked at the impact of alkyl chain length on the interactions of ($C_8H_8O_2$) +alcohols at the molecular level. Determining excess properties like excess molar volume, excess adiabatic compressibility, and excess acoustic impedance may also be a part of the study. Researchers can acquire a thorough grasp of the characteristics, behaviour, and molecular interactions of benzoate-based mixtures by combining thermodynamic and acoustic techniques in the investigation of benzoate-based mixtures utilising ultrasonic methods. The Laplace equation was used to determine the isentropic compressibilities of the liquid mixes. The resulting excess values of the combinations were successfully matched to the R-K equation (Chen et al., 2020). Applications in many disciplines, such as chemistry, pharmacology, and materials science, can benefit from this understanding. By analyzing the ultrasonic velocity and attenuation, you can obtain information about various parameters like density, viscosity, adiabatic compressibility. The excess thermodynamical parameters from sound speed, and density were investigated with the help of specific gravity bottle, and interferometer method for binary liquid systems containing ethyl benzoate (Benzoic acid ethyl ester) at various temperatures and at atmospheric pressure. These additional parameters were adjusted to the R-K equation. Deviations in Excess adiabatic compressibility were shown to be negative over the mole fraction of $C_9H_{10}O_2$ indicated the existence of molecular interactions through dipole-dipole interactions. Changes in density can reflect changes in concentration and composition. Viscosity affects the velocity of sound waves (Nagarjuna et al., 2013). An increase in viscosity might indicate molecular interactions or structural changes in the mixture. Changes in compressibility reveal molecular interactions and changes in intermolecular forces within the mixture. Adiabatic Compressibility provides insights into changes in the free volume and compressibility of the mixture's components. Ultrasonic velocity changes with temperature, allowing you to calculate the thermal expansion coefficient. Deviations in ultrasonic velocity and attenuation from ideal behavior indicate interactions like hydrogen bonding, dipole-dipole interactions, and van der

Waals forces. Dielectric properties and conformation of Hydrogen-bonded propan-1-ol (1 PN) mixtures with benzoates (MB/EB) were obtained using LF impedance analyzer, plunger technique, and abbe's refractometer method. The thermodynamic parameters, relaxation time, excess inverse relaxation time, and Kirkwood's effective correlation factor were all calculated using the experimental data, along with the corrected Kirkwood correlation factor. Results showed that FT-IR spectra were used to confirm that a hydrogen bond exists between the propan1-ol's OH group and the CH groups of methyl and ethyl benzoates (Mohan et al., 2011).

APPLICATIONS OF BENZOATE BASED MIXTURES

Thermoacoustic measurements can offer valuable information about the physical and chemical properties of the liquid mixtures and liquids (Bhakri et al., 2023). Benzoate-based mixtures find a wide range of applications in various industries due to their versatile properties. One major application is in the food industry, where they are used as preservatives to inhibit the growth of bacteria, yeast, and mold in food products. These mixtures are particularly effective in acidic environments, making them suitable for items like fruit juices, soft drinks, and condiments (Bruna et al., 2018). In the pharmaceutical sector, benzoate-based compounds can be found in topical medications and ointments due to their antimicrobial properties. In the field of cosmetics, these mixtures are utilized as preservatives to extend the shelf life of personal care products such as lotions, creams, and shampoos (Kodsangma et al., 2020). They help maintain the product's quality and prevent microbial contamination. Additionally, Sodium benzoate have applications in industrial settings as well, where they serve as corrosion inhibitors for various metals, helping to protect machinery and equipment from degradation over time (Naveen et al., 2017)

Medical Applications

Benzoate-based mixtures have several medical applications due to their properties as preservatives, antimicrobial agents, and treatment enhancers. In certain medical conditions, benzoate-based mixtures are used in combination with other medications to enhance their effectiveness (Khoshnoud et al., 2018). For instance, in combination with salicylic acid, they can improve the efficacy of treatment for skin disorders like psoriasis. These mixtures are also used in medical imaging, typically involves technologies like X-rays, MRI, CT scans, ultrasound, and PET scans, which utilize contrast agents or techniques to visualize internal structures and diagnose conditions (Jakhmola et al., 2012).

Pharmaceuticals

Benzoate-based mixtures have several applications in the pharmaceutical industry. One common use is as a solubilizing agent in formulations. Sodium benzoate, for instance, can be used to enhance the solubility of poorly water-soluble drugs, improving their bioavailability. It can also act as a preservative in oral liquid medications, helping to extend their shelf life by inhibiting the growth of microorganisms (Agrawal et al., 2016;Sá et al., 2017). Additionally, benzoate derivatives like benzyl benzoate have applications in topical formulations, often as a vehicle or penetration enhancer in creams and lotions. They can aid in delivering active ingredients through the skin barrier for targeted therapeutic effects (Sharma et al., 2016).

Material Science

Benzoate-based mixtures have various applications in material science due to their unique properties. They can be used as plasticizers, additives in polymer formulations, and corrosion inhibitors. Additionally, they can act as stabilizers for polymers and resins, enhancing their durability and performance (Ambrogi et al., 2017). Benzoate compounds are also utilized in the production of liquid crystal displays (LCDs), where they aid in achieving precise alignment of liquid crystal molecules (Ziobro et al., 2012). Their low toxicity and compatibility with other materials make them versatile choices for improving the properties of various materials.

Biological Research

Benzoate-based mixtures have various applications in biological research. Sodium benzoate, for instance, is often used as a preservative in cell culture media to inhibit bacterial and fungal growth (Rojo et al., 2015). It's also utilized to study the effects of mitochondrial dysfunction, as it interferes with oxidative phosphorylation. Additionally, benzoate derivatives are essential intermediates in the metabolism of aromatic compounds by microorganisms. These compounds can be studied to understand microbial degradation pathways and environmental bioremediation (Elshahed et al., 2001).

CHALLENGES

Thermoacoustic investigations of benzoate-based compounds using ultrasonics have several limitations. These include: The composition and structure of benzoate compounds can vary widely, leading to differences in thermal and acoustic properties. This complexity can make it challenging to generalize findings across different compounds. Thermoacoustic properties can be temperature-dependent, affecting the accuracy and repeatability of measurements. Temperature fluctuations during experiments can introduce variability in results. Ultrasonic techniques are limited by their frequency range. If the chosen frequency does not match the natural frequencies of the material, certain phenomena may not be adequately detected or analyzed. Thermoacoustic techniques often assume homogeneous materials, but benzoate compounds could exhibit heterogeneity that affects the propagation of ultrasound waves and the resulting thermoacoustic signals. Ultrasonic waves are influenced by the surface characteristics of materials. For benzoate-based compounds with varying surface properties, the accuracy of measurements can be compromised. The effectiveness of ultrasound transmission through benzoate compounds depends on the quality of the coupling medium used between the transducer and the sample. If not properly matched, signal loss or distortion can occur. Thermoacoustic signals may be weak, especially for low-concentration samples, limiting the sensitivity of measurements and making it harder to detect small changes in properties. Background noise and interference can obscure the desired signals, particularly when working with low-amplitude thermoacoustic responses. Ensuring accurate and consistent measurements requires proper calibration and standardization of equipment, which can be challenging due to the unique characteristics of benzoate compounds (Petanovska-Ilievska et al., 2017). Thermoacoustic experiments often generate data that need post-processing, which might not provide real-time insights during experiments. In some cases, sample preparation for thermoacoustic investigations might involve invasive procedures that could alter the properties of benzoate compounds. The interpretation of thermoacoustic data can be complex and may involve the consideration of multiple parameters, leading to potential uncertainty in drawing conclusions.

FUTURE DIRECTIONS

There is great promise in studying benzoate-based compounds employing ultrasonic techniques for thermoacoustic research. Exploring the connection between molecular structure and thermoacoustic characteristics may be a future focus. This work may help create unique materials with specialised thermal and acoustic capabilities. Additionally, studying how various environmental factors and outside stimuli affect these substances may help in the development of sensors or other devices that can keep track of changes in temperature, pressure, or chemical composition. Material scientists, chemists, and engineers working together could develop this discipline and find innovative applications. In the future, these studies might focus on improving experimental designs to increase sensitivity and accuracy, applying cutting-edge signal processing algorithms to glean precise data from measurements, and investigating a wider variety of benzoate-based compounds to unearth novel properties and applications. By supplying useful information for creating and manufacturing novel materials with specialised thermal and mechanical properties, this research has the potential to have an impact on industries including materials science, pharmaceuticals, and energy storage.

CONCLUSION

Molecular Interactions play a crucial role in various biological, chemical and physical processes. Investigating the thermo-acoustic parameters and nature of molecular interactions in mixtures containing benzoates can provide valuable insights into their behavior, properties of molecules and materials and their potential applications. Benzoates are a class of compounds derived from benzoic acid, and they are extensively in many different industries, including those that produce food, medicine, animal feed, and cosmetics. Benzoate, specifically sodium benzoate, has several applications in medical sciences. One notable use is as a preservative in pharmaceutical formulations to increase shelf life and prevent microbial growth. Additionally, benzoate compounds, such as sodium phenyl acetate and sodium benzoate, are used to treat patients with urea cycle disorders, a group of genetic disorders affecting the body's ability to remove ammonia from the bloodstream. These compounds help convert ammonia into less harmful substances, reducing its toxicity. It's essential to follow medical guidelines and dosages when using benzoate in any medical context. They can also be used as corrosion inhibitors in oil-based systems, rust preventatives in metalworking fluids, and antifreeze agents in automotive cooling systems. When benzoates are used in mixtures with other components, such as solvents or other chemicals, excess thermodynamic parameters can be employed to describe the non-ideal behavior of these mixtures. Benzoates exhibit synergistic effects antimicrobial properties and inhibit the growth of microorganisms; they are very effective against bacteria, molds, and yeast.

ACKNOWLEDGEMENT

I want to acknowledge and extend my sincere gratitude to Dr. Nabaparna Chakraborty and my supervisor, Dr. Kailash Chandra Juglan, who made this effort possible. They provided me with guidance and suggestions throughout the entire writing process of this review paper, which I was able to accomplish.

REFERENCES

Agrawal, S., & Kasturi, M. (2016). Hydrotropic solubilisation technique to challenge the solubility of poorly water soluble drug valsartan. *World Journal of Pharmaceutical Research*, *5*(8), 833–845. doi:10.20959/wjpr20168-6722

Ambrogi, V., Carfagna, C., Cerruti, P., & Marturano, V. (2017). Additives in Polymers. In Modification of Polymer Properties (pp. 87–108). Elsevier. doi:10.1016/B978-0-323-44353-1.00004-X

Bhakri, K., Chakraborty, N., Juglan, K. C., Kumar, H., & Sharma, R. (2023). Thermodynamic behaviour and physicochemical characteristics of EG, DEG, TEG in aqueous gluconolactone solutions. *Journal of Thermal Analysis and Calorimetry*, *148*(14), 7185–7205. doi:10.100710973-023-12223-z

Bruna, G. O. L., Thais, A. C. C., & Lígia, A. C. C. (2018). Food additives and their health effects: A review on preservative sodium benzoate. *African Journal of Biotechnology*, *17*(10), 306–310. doi:10.5897/AJB2017.16321

Chakraborty, N., Kaur, K., Juglan, K. C., & Kumar, H. (2020). Volumetric and ultrasonic studies on interactions of glycols in aqueous solutions of xylitol at different temperatures. *Journal of Chemical & Engineering Data*, *65*(4), 1435–1446. doi:10.1021/acs.jced.9b00869

Chakraborty, N., Kumar, H., Kaur, K., & Juglan, K. C. (2018). Acoustic and thermodynamic study of D-Panthenol in aqueous solutions of glycol at different temperatures. *The Journal of Chemical Thermodynamics*, *126*, 137–146. doi:10.1016/j.jct.2018.07.006

Chakraborty, N., Lamba, M., Juglan, K. C., & Kumar, H. (2022). Temperature dependent thermodynamic studies of glycols in aqueous solutions of vitamin B3. In Journal of Physics: Conference Series, 2267(1), 012134). doi:10.1088/1742-6596/2267/1/012134

Chen, T., Feng, X., Yin, Y., & Xu, Y. (2020). Investigation of the Effect of Alkyl Chain Length on Molecular Interactions Between Methyl Benzoate with Alcohols: A Study of Physicochemical Properties. *Journal of Solution Chemistry*, *49*(11), 1402–1418. doi:10.100710953-020-01029-4

Chinnarao, D., Padmarao, C. V., Beena, C., Srilatha, M., Ramanjaneyulu, M. V. V., Choppara, P., Murali, N., & Rao, B. V. (2023). Acoustic, excess thermodynamical, molecular interaction and anti-microbial activity studies on binary liquid mixtures of geranyl acetate and benzyl benzoate in the temperature range of 303.15K–318.15K. *Journal of the Indian Chemical Society*, *100*(5), 100969. doi:10.1016/j.jics.2023.100969

Devunuri, N., Kancherla, S., Chennuri, B. K., & Gardas, R. L. (2016). Apparent molar volume and isentropic compressibilities of antidepressant drugs (Citalopram HBr and Escitalopram oxalate) with water. *Journal of Molecular Liquids*, *216*, 347–353. doi:10.1016/j.molliq.2016.01.058

Dhal, K., Das, P., Singh, S., & Talukdar, M. (2023). Analysis of ultraacoustic behavior of l-aspartic acid in aqueous sodium benzoate and ammonium acetate media. *Journal of Molecular Liquids*, *376*, 121413. doi:10.1016/j.molliq.2023.121413

Dhal, K., Singh, S., & Talukdar, M. (2022). Ultraacoustic and conductometric studies on the interactions of l-glutamic acid with potassium sorbate and sodium benzoate in aqueous media. *Journal of Molecular Liquids*, *368*, 120761. doi:10.1016/j.molliq.2022.120761

Duraivathi, C., Priya, J. J., Poongodi, J., & Jeyakumar, H. J. (2022). Ultrasonic study of molecular interactions in organic liquid with CCl4 at different temperature. *Materials Today: Proceedings*, *49*, 1968–1972. doi:10.1016/j.matpr.2021.08.140

Elshahed, M. S., Bhupathiraju, V. K., Wofford, N. Q., Nanny, M. A., & McInerney, M. J. (2001). Metabolism of Benzoate, Cyclohex-1-ene Carboxylate, and Cyclohexane Carboxylate by "Syntrophus aciditrophicus" Strain SB in Syntrophic Association with H_2-Using Microorganisms. *Applied and Environmental Microbiology*, *67*(4), 1728–1738. doi:10.1128/AEM.67.4.1728-1738.2001 PMID:11282627

Jakhmola, A., Anton, N., & Vandamme, T. F. (2012). Inorganic Nanoparticles Based Contrast Agents for X-ray Computed Tomography. *Advanced Healthcare Materials*, *1*(4), 413–431. doi:10.1002/adhm.201200032 PMID:23184772

Kaur, H., Thakur, R. C., & Kumar, H. (2020). Effect of proteinogenic amino acids lserine/l-threonine on volumetric and acoustic behavior of aqueous 1-butyl-3-propyl imidazolium bromide at T=(288.15, 298.15, 308.15, 318.15) K. *The Journal of Chemical Thermodynamics*, *150*, 106211. doi:10.1016/j.jct.2020.106211

Khoshnoud, M. J., Siavashpour, A., Bakhshizadeh, M., & Rashedinia, M. (2018). Effects of sodium benzoate, a commonly used food preservative, on learning, memory, and oxidative stress in brain of mice. *Journal of Biochemical and Molecular Toxicology*, *32*(2), e22022. doi:10.1002/jbt.22022 PMID:29243862

Kodsangma, A., Homsaard, N., Nadon, S., Rachtanapun, P., Leksawasdi, N., Phimolsiripol, Y., Insomphun, C., Seesuriyachan, P., Chaiyaso, T., Jantrawut, P., Inmutto, N., Ougizawa, T., & Jantanasakulwong, K. (2020). Effect of sodium benzoate and chlorhexidine gluconate on a bio-thermoplastic elastomer made from thermoplastic starch-chitosan blended with epoxidized natural rubber. *Carbohydrate Polymers*, *242*, 116421. doi:10.1016/j.carbpol.2020.116421 PMID:32564859

Mohan, T. M., Sastry, S. S., & Murthy, V. R. K. (2011). Thermodynamic, Dielectric and Conformational Studies on Hydrogen Bonded Binary Mixtures of Propan-1-ol with Methyl Benzoate and Ethyl Benzoate. *Journal of Solution Chemistry*, *40*(1), 131–146. doi:10.100710953-010-9634-6

Nagarjun, B., Sarma, A. V., Rao, G. V. R., & Rambabu, C. (2013). Thermodynamic and Acoustic Study on Molecular Interactions in Certain Binary Liquid Systems Involving Ethyl Benzoate. *Journal of Thermodynamics*, *2013*, 1–9. doi:10.1155/2013/285796

Nagarjuna, A., Raju, K., Kotilingaiah, N., & Praveen, B. (2023). Comparltive study of Binary liquid mixtures containing P-methoxy Benzoate Acid and Amides. *European Chemical Bulletin*, *12*, 3395–3407. doi:10.31838/ecb/2023.12.si6.3022023.06/06/2023

Naveen, E., Ramnath, B. V., Elanchezhian, C., & Nazirudeen, S. S. M. (2017). Influence of organic corrosion inhibitors on pickling corrosion behaviour of sinter-forged C45 steel and 2% Cu alloyed C45 steel. *Journal of Alloys and Compounds*, *695*, 3299–3309. doi:10.1016/j.jallcom.2016.11.133

Palani, R., & Geetha, A. (2009). Acoustical and excess thermodynamic studies of molecular interaction in aqueous mixed solvent systems at 303, 308 and 313 K. *Physics and Chemistry of Liquids*, *47*(5), 542–552. doi:10.1080/00319100802562862

Petanovska-Ilievska, B., Velkoska-Markovska, L., & Jankulovska, M. S. (2017). Development of reverse-phase high-performance liquid chromatography method for simultaneous determination of sodium benzoate and potassium sorbate in beverages. *Acta Chromatographica*, *29*(3), 345–358. doi:10.1556/1326.2017.29.3.05

Rojo, M. C., Arroyo López, F. N., Lerena, M. C., Mercado, L., Torres, A., & Combina, M. (2015). Evaluation of different chemical preservatives to control Zygosaccharomyces rouxii growth in high sugar culture media. *Food Control*, *50*, 349–355. doi:10.1016/j.foodcont.2014.09.014

Sá, A. G. A., de Meneses, A. C., de Araújo, P. H. H., & de Oliveira, D. (2017). A review on enzymatic synthesis of aromatic esters used as flavor ingredients for food, cosmetics and pharmaceuticals industries. *Trends in Food Science & Technology*, *69*, 95–105. doi:10.1016/j.tifs.2017.09.004

Sharma, G., Dhankar, G., Thakur, K., Raza, K., & Katare, O. P. (2016). Benzyl Benzoate-Loaded Microemulsion for Topical Applications: Enhanced Dermatokinetic Profile and Better Delivery Promises. *AAPS PharmSciTech*, *17*(5), 1221–1231. doi:10.120812249-015-0464-0 PMID:26669889

Thakur, A., Juglan, K. C., Kumar, H., & Kaur, K. (2019). Investigation on molecular interaction of glycols in methanol solutions of methylparaben (methyl 4–hydroxybenzoate) at different temperatures through thermo-acoustical analysis. *Journal of Molecular Liquids*, *288*, 111014. doi:10.1016/j.molliq.2019.111014

Ziobro, D., Dąbrowski, R., Tykarska, M., Drzewiński, W., Filipowicz, M., Rejmer, W., Kuśmierek, K., Morawiak, P., & Piecek, W. (2012). Synthesis and properties of new ferroelectric and antiferroelectric liquid crystals with a biphenylyl benzoate rigid core. *Liquid Crystals*, *39*(8), 1011–1032. doi:10.1080/02678292.2012.691560

Chapter 20
Thermo-Acoustic Investigations on Phosphate-Based Mixtures in Aqueous Solutions:
A Review

Sunita Devi
Lovely Professional University, India

Kailash Chandra Juglan
https://orcid.org/0000-0002-8753-4843
Lovely Professional University, India

Nabaparna Chakraborty
https://orcid.org/0000-0003-3891-0408
Central Instrumentation Facility, Lovely Professional University, Phagwara, India

ABSTRACT

Phosphate-based mixtures are widely used in various industries, and understanding their thermodynamic properties is crucial for optimizing their applications in medicine, pharmaceuticals, leather manufacturing, textiles, etc. This comprehensive review explores the literature on the thermodynamic characteristics and applications of phosphate-based mixtures in aqueous solutions. The focus is on studies investigating density and volumetric properties, phase equilibrium, molecular interactions, and thermal properties of phosphate compounds such as Disodium dihydrogen pyrophosphate and DiPotassium hydrogen phosphate. The chapter provides a comprehensive summary of the extensive research conducted on the thermodynamics of mixtures, specifically in aqueous solutions. The focus of these investigations has been on exploring the thermodynamic properties of various compounds containing phosphates. The findings presented in this review contribute to the existing knowledge base and provide a foundation for further research and optimization of phosphate-based mixtures in aqueous solutions.

DOI: 10.4018/979-8-3693-0448-8.ch020

INTRODUCTION

Investigations into the thermodynamic and ultrasonic characteristics of binary mixtures play a crucial role in enhancing our essential perceptive of how unlike molecules interact with each other. These studies are highly significant in unraveling the nature and behavior of these interactions between unlike molecules (Palaiologou et al., 2016). These mixtures have diverse uses in sectors such as medicine, pharmaceuticals, leather manufacturing, textiles, cleaning products, mineral fertilizers, and solvent solutions. In recent years, there has been notable progress in comprehending the thermodynamic, volumetric, physicochemical, and acoustical attributes of liquid blends through the application of ultrasonic methodologies. This approach offers a substantial volume of insights concerning the diverse interactions at both subatomic and molecular levels within the liquid mixture. This technique is commonly favored due to its non-destructive nature, which ensures the integrity, structure, and configurations of the sample remain intact. Among the crucial features shaping the entire molecular configuration, ultrasonic velocity and density play pivotal roles. These ultrasonic properties are indispensable for investigating the unique traits of liquid mixtures comprising multiple fragments, all while avoiding any form of distortion. Acoustic and thermodynamic properties of liquid mixtures serve as essential tools for examining distinct molecular interactions among different components within these mixtures. These properties are employed to investigate the intricate behaviors and relationships among the molecules in the mixture, leading to a comprehensive understanding of their interactions (Chakraborty et al., 2018; Devunuri et al., 2016; Thakur et al., 2019). This comprehensive review aims to provide a detailed inspection of the extensive literature on the thermodynamic characteristics. The determination of thermal expansion coefficients and molar volumes has played an essential role in understanding the performance of these mixtures. Moreover, investigations into phase equilibria, including ternary systems and the effects of temperature on solution behavior, have contributed to a deeper understanding of phosphate-based mixtures. The use of experimental techniques such as isothermal solution saturation and X-ray diffraction has provided valuable insights into the phase diagrams and density-composition relationships of these systems. Widespread research has been conducted to investigate the thermal behavior and heat storage capabilities of materials based on phosphates, highlighting their promising potential for various energy storage applications. Additionally, the influence of phosphate concentration on molecular interactions, viscosity, and acoustic parameters has been examined. These insights shed light on the solute-solvent and solute-solute interactions within phosphate mixtures. Researchers have conducted numerous investigations to explore the behavior and characteristics of different compounds, ranging from ionic liquids .These studies have contributed valuable insights into the thermodynamic, electrochemical properties, and molecular interactions of these systems. Measurements using ultrasonic technology reveal a lot about different polymer solution properties (Upmanyu et al., 2014)

THERMODYNAMIC INVESTIGATIONS: CHALLENGES IN UNDERSTANDING PHOSPHATE-BASED MIXTURES

Understanding the thermodynamic properties of phosphate-based mixtures presents several challenges. These challenges involve the complex nature of molecular interactions and the varying compositions of mixtures. Investigating these challenges is crucial for optimizing applications in diverse industries. The recent studies mentioned have delved into diverse aspects of phosphate-based mixtures, shedding light on their intriguing properties and potential applications. The physicochemical characteristics of methanolic mixtures containing deep ethylene glycols, revealing insights into proton conduction mechanisms and charge transport within these mixtures (Álvarez et al., 2023). This study not only examined ion conductivity and thermal characteristics but also introduced innovative categories of ionic liquids for potential use in energy storage devices (Bhowmick et al., 2022). The volumetric properties of diSodium di pyrohydrogenphosphate solutions, affirming the accuracy of their measurements (Alimov et al., 2021). These studies collectively contribute to a deeper understanding of the intricate behaviors of phosphate-based mixtures and their potential applications in various fields. The ultrasonic behaviour of (K_2HPO_4) and (Na_2HPO_4) in an aqueous solution that included ($C_6H_{11}NO_3$) at different temperatures. The team is using Anton Paar automated vibrating tube densimeter DSA 5000M and an automatic micro viscometer (AMVn), which are both manufactured by ANTON PAAR. Data on properties such as observed molar volume, as well as coefficients related to pair wise and triplet interactions, were collected by the researchers. The findings indicated that solute-solvent interaction played a dominant role compared to solute-solute interaction (Xu et al., 2020). In order to obtain broad information on the density and dynamic viscosity of liquid at a wide range of concentrations, researchers targeted binary systems that consisted of ionic liquids and ethanol. In normal atmospheric pressure conditions, the temperature between 293.15 and 338.15 K was measured. The study also demonstrated that the thermal behaviour of three solid ionic liquids, as well as their aqueous solutions, are influenced by temperature and composition. This investigation contributes valuable insights into the thermodynamic behavior and physicochemical characteristics of Dimethyl phosphate-based ionic liquids, providing essential data for their potential application in absorption refrigeration technology. Conducted a study to investigate the structural properties of glasses made of a combination of $NaPO_3$-MoO_3. The researchers have applied different methods of analysis. These methods allowed them to analyze and understand the characteristics and arrangement of the glassy materials at the molecular level. The investigation aimed to understand the properties and arrangement of the glassy materials through the analysis of their structural features. The findings provided valuable insights into the composition and organization of the $NaPO_3$-MoO_3 glasses using a range of spectroscopic and analytical methods the findings indicated the formation of a highly stable glass structure with a significantly increased glass transition temperature. Moreover, the glass demonstrated resistance to recrystallization under elevated heating conditions during thermal analysis. Thermodynamic investigations of phosphate-based mixtures are essential for revealing their behavior under different conditions. These investigations help explain the effects of temperature and composition on phase behavior, molecular interactions, and more .These studies collectively enhance our comprehension of phosphate-based mixtures. Their exploration of thermodynamic behaviors, molecular interactions, and structural properties is essential for diverse applications (Skonieczny et al., 2023; Sadeghi et al., 2008).

Molecular Interactions and Acoustic Parameters

The use of ultrasonic analysis has become essential for exploring the molecular arrangement and properties of substances due to its non-invasive nature. Acoustic investigation of liquid blends is employed to derive the thermodynamic features of compacted liquids (Chakraborty et al., 2021).To understand interactions between the solute and the cosolvents, measurements of volume and compressibility have been performed. The results revealed that the mixtures exhibited prevailing ion-hydrophilic and hydrophobic-hydrophilic interactions. Various characteristics, including apparent molar volume, partial molar volume, and apparent molar isentropic compression, were obtained to assess the properties of the solutions. The findings showed a progressive increase in the interactions between solute molecules as the amino acids changed from glycine to L-alanine to L-valine. This research provides valuable insights into the molecular associations in amino acid solutions containing DiSodium hydrogen phosphate, shedding light on the thermodynamic properties and interaction patterns in these mixtures Understanding molecular interactions within phosphate mixtures is crucial for optimizing their applications. Studies reveal the prevalence of ion-hydrophilic and hydrophobic-hydrophilic interactions, shedding light on the complex dynamics of solute-solvent interactions. In order to evaluate the balance between phases in Salty solutions containing Trisodium Phosphate at temperatures exceeding 100C, Scientists have carried out a study. The research aimed to evaluate the balance of components and their interactions within the system. The focus was on understanding the thermodynamic equilibrium state, where the various phases coexist at a given temperature and composition. The investigation provided valuable insights into the stability and distribution of substances within the solution, shedding light on the equilibrium phenomena occurring in the trisodium phosphate system. The scientists measured and determined several different parameters including Gibbs energies, enthalpies, heat capacities, activity coefficients, and heat of dilution (Kumar et al., 2014; Weber et al., 1999). Various thermodynamic and acoustic parameters are essential tools that significantly contribute to understanding the forces between molecules (Chakraborty et al., 2020).

Significance

Thermo-acoustic investigations of diverse mixtures in aqueous solutions play a pivotal role in offering invaluable insights into the complex interactions and behaviors inherent to these combinations. Such studies delve deep into the intricate interplay between temperature and composition, unraveling their effects on the physical and chemical attributes of aqueous solutions. Lately, there has been growing interest in studying acoustic properties in solutions containing polymers and liquids (Juglan et al., 2020). Studying how sound behaves in these mixtures helps scientists learn a lot about how the molecules are arranged, how different substances interact, and how things like changing from one phase to another happen. This knowledge is really important in areas like making better batteries, medicines, and solutions to environmental problems. Knowing how mixtures work is like having a strong base to build upon, which then helps make new materials, improve how things are made, and push forward in fields like energy, health, and taking care of the environment.

APPLICATIONS OF PHOSPHATE-BASED MIXTURES

Ultrasonic studies are widely used to analyze the physical and chemical characteristics of liquids and liquid mixtures (Kaur et al.,2017). Phosphate-based mixtures find applications in various industries, including medicine, pharmaceuticals, textiles, and more. The versatility of these mixtures makes them valuable in different contexts, from energy storage to biological research. Data on properties such as observed molar volume, observed molar isentropic compression, partial molar volume, partial molar volume of transfer, and partial molar expansivity, as well as coefficients related to pair wise and triplet interactions, were collected by the researchers. The findings indicated that solute-solvent interaction played a dominant role compared to solute-solute interaction (Kumar et al., 2016). Recent research studies have explored various aspects of phosphate-based materials, offering valuable insights into their structural characteristics and behavior under different conditions. A spectroscopic, UV-visible, and FT-

IR investigation of sodium nitrate and di sodium hydrogen orthophosphate. Their research showed how Biofield treatment affected the compounds' structural characteristics, which was especially clear from alterations in FT-IR results. Notably, UV analysis revealed a distinct influence of Biofield treatment on electron migration, with observable variations in connected and disconnected electrons within the substance, when compared to control samples (Trivedi et al., 2015). Scientists looked at how different things mix together in a liquid at a certain temperature, specifically with a mixture of three things: sodium dihydrogen phosphate, sodium sulfate, and water. The researchers employed a consistent temperature method for saturating the solution and employed X-ray diffraction (XRD) methods. The results of the investigation enabled the construction of a phase diagram and a chart illustrating the correlation between densities and composition in the system (Chen et al., 2014). The findings provided valuable insights into the composition and organization of the $NaPO_3$-MoO_3 glasses using a range of spectroscopic and analytical methods the findings indicated the formation of a highly stable glass structure with a significantly increased glass transition temperature. Moreover, the glass demonstrated resistance to recrystallization under elevated heating conditions during thermal analysis (Huang et al., 2013). Overall, these studies collectively contribute to the growing body of knowledge concerning phosphate-based materials. They shed light on the intricate structural characteristics and behaviors of these materials, offering insights that have implications for various applications in fields ranging from materials science to thermal analysis.

Medical Applications

Phosphate-based mixtures have significant medical applications. For instance, phosphates play a vital role in treating urinary tract infections by acidifying urine. A research examined heat capacities of sodium and tetra methyl ammonium salts in aqueous phosphate solutions at 250°C using specific equipment. The study explored the impact of interactions between phosphate ions and the sodium and tetramethylammonium cations. Moreover, they contribute to bone health and calcium regulation, particularly in individuals with phosphorus-deficient diets. Phosphate-containing mixtures have medical applications, helping regulate body functions, develop medications, and support medical research due to their distinct properties in interacting with biological systems (Bianchi et al., 1995). Thermodynamic, volumetric, physicochemical, and acoustical aspects of liquid mixtures utilized in many industries can be examined non-destructively using the ultrasonic approach. Liquids' acoustic and thermodynamic characteristics make it possible to examine numerous molecular interactions between distinct constituents. One of the best techniques for determining bulk properties and intermolecular forces in mixes of several liquid components is the ultrasonic technique. Ultrasonic measurements are commonly used in both pure liquids and liquid components to look at molecular interactions (Nain et al., 2014). Ultrasonic parameters, also referred to as ultrasonic parameters, include ultrasonic velocity and absorption. These characteristics can be measured using a variety of techniques (Kumar et al., 2016). Other important factors, including as bulk modulus, compressibility, and more, are required to understand how molecules interact in the liquid (Banipal et al., 2007). Basic variables like density, viscosity, and ultrasonic velocity affect these characteristics. Chemicals, automobiles, textiles, medicine, and other industries all use it (Kumar et al., 2014). This method has a wide range of applications in various fields and can teach us a lot about how liquids behave (Romero et al., 2004).

Energy Storage

The thermal characteristics and heat storage capabilities of phosphate-based materials make them promising candidates for energy storage applications. Conducted a study on the synthesis of (MEPCMs) using disodium hydrogen phosphate heptahydrate. The results revealed that microencapsulated phase change materials (MEPCMs) utilizing disodium hydrogen phosphate heptahydrate exhibit significant potential for thermal storage applications, particularly in the context of solar space heating These mixtures offer potential solutions for efficient heat storage, with implications for renewable energy systems (Santagneli et al.,2007). The study of the molecular interactions of polymers with solvents has been greatly accelerated by the widespread use of polymeric materials in technology (Dhiman et al., 2019).

Environmental Solutions

Phosphate-based mixtures are utilized in environmental applications, such as phosphate removal from water sources. The modification of dolomite using ultrasound to enhance its physicochemical properties for effective phosphate removal. The modified dolomite exhibited increased surface area, improving its adsorption capabilities. Over 90% of phosphates have been removed in the optimal operating conditions. Experimental and mathematical model analyses supported the physisorption and chemisorption mechanisms. Thermodynamic investigations indicated a spontaneous and endothermic process Studies demonstrate how modified materials, such as dolomite, exhibit enhanced adsorption capabilities for effective phosphate removal (Ivone et al., 2023).

Industrial Uses

The industrial sector benefits from the application of phosphate-based mixtures. These mixtures have roles in cleaning agents, mineral fertilizers, food production, and textiles. The researchers investigated the dissolution characteristics of Sodium orthophosphates (Na_3PO_4) and potassium orthophosphate (K_3PO_4) in ethylene glycol. The aim was to explore the potential applications of these compounds in various industries, including cleaning agents, mineral fertilizers, food production, animal feed additives, and textiles. The research highlighted the advantageous effects of utilizing ethylene glycol in these fields. The results demonstrated that the solubility of Sodium and potassium orthophosphates in ethylene glycol ($C_2H_6O_2$) exhibits a temperature-dependent increase, suggesting an elevation in solubility with rising temperatures Investigations into dissolution characteristics and solubility in solvents like ethylene glycol highlight their potential industrial benefits (Kurzin et al.,2012). The chemical industry uses the molecular interaction research in liquid mixtures to create a variety of transport and processing equipment (Upmanyu et al., 2021).

FUTURE DIRECTIONS AND OPTIMIZATIONS

Future pathways for phosphate-based mixtures include enhanced drug delivery, sustainable energy storage, and improved water treatment methods, driving innovation. While significant insights have been gained, there is still room for further research to fully exploit the potential of phosphate-based mixtures. The behaviour of liquid-liquid equilibria at different temperatures in a quaternary Biphasic system composed of both ionic liquids and dipotassium hydrogen phosphate. The researchers observed that the region where the two liquid phases coexist expanded as the temperature decreased, while the slope of the tie-lines, which represent the composition of each phase, slightly decreased as the temperature increased. The empirical observations of liquid-liquid equilibrium were effectively fitted using the NRTL thermodynamic model, demonstrating a satisfactory concurrence with the experimental findings. To reproduce the experimental binodal data, the researchers used the Merchuk equation, which required three fitting parameters. These parameters were further expressed as a linear function of temperature, with $(T - T_0)$ K as the variable. This approach allowed for a satisfactory reproduction of the experimental data. The researchers observed temperature-dependent changes in the biphasic region and tie-line slopes. They successfully correlated the experimental data using thermodynamic models and accurately reproduced the binodal data using the Merchuk equation with temperature-dependent parameters. The utilization of Disodium hydrogen phosphate in saline purgative, animal nutrition and the food sector has been observed. The procedures were determined through linear interpolation of published information, taking into account the respective range to which each solution belongs (Malekghasemi et al., 2016; Khaled et al.,2011).The Researchers Investigated the isopiestic molalities, which refer to the concentrations of solutes in solution, of elevated-temperature aqueous solutions containing different phosphate salts such as sodium dihydrogen phosphate (NaH_2PO_4), potassium phosphate (K_3PO_4), sodium phosphate (Na_3PO_4), and potassium dihydrogen phosphate (KH_2PO_4). The study involved the determination of osmotic pressures to acquire significant information. Future studies could focus on refining the understanding of interactions, exploring new applications, and optimizing mixture compositions for specific purposes (Holmes et al., 2000).

CONCLUSION

Extensive research has been conducted on the thermal characteristics and capacity for storing heat of materials based on phosphates, demonstrating their promising prospects in applications related to energy storage. Phosphate, the phosphorus salt, finds applications in medicine, fertilizers, and biological research. It helps treat urinary tract infections by acidifying urine and plays a vital role in bone strength and calcium control for those with phosphorus-deficient diets. The review article also explores the impact of phosphate concentration on molecular interactions, viscosity, and acoustic parameters, providing insights into the interactions between solute and solvent interactions within phosphate mixtures. This study yields crucial insights into thermodynamic and acoustic characteristics of these systems and underlining their wide applications in various industries. Additional research is required to enhance their utilization across various sectors and fully exploit their thermodynamic properties.

ACKNOWLEDGEMENT

I am immensely grateful to Dr. Kailash Chandra Juglan for his profound impact on my research work and personal development. His vast knowledge, expertise, and unwavering support have played a pivotal role throughout my Ph.D. journey. I am grateful to Dr. Nabaparna Chakraborty for her invaluable guidance and the research environment she has fostered. I am thankful to all who have contributed to my academic and personal growth.

REFERENCES

Alimov, U., Zhao, K., Hu, J., Guo, Y., Meng, L., Pan, X., & Deng, T. (2021). Volumetric properties of disodium dihydrogen pyrophosphate aqueous solution from 283.15 to 363.15 K at 101.325 kPa. *Food Chemistry*, *352*, 129410. doi:10.1016/j.foodchem.2021.129410 PMID:33677210

Álvarez, M. S., Deive, F. J., Longo, M. A., Rodriguez, A., Segade, L., & Cabeza, O. (2023). Physicochemical characterization of methanolic mixtures of cholinium dihydrogen phosphate-based DES. *Journal of Molecular Liquids*, *383*, 122024. doi:10.1016/j.molliq.2023.122024

Banipal, T. S., Kaur, D., Banipal, P. K., & Singh, G. (2007). Thermodynamic and transport properties of l-serine and l-threonine in aqueous sodium acetate and magnesium acetate solutions at T= 298.15 K. *The Journal of Chemical Thermodynamics*, *39*(3), 371–384. doi:10.1016/j.jct.2006.08.003

Bhowmick, S., Filippov, A., Khan, I. A., & Shah, F. U. (2022). Physical and electrochemical properties of new structurally flexible imidazolium phosphate ionic liquids. *Physical Chemistry Chemical Physics*, *24*(38), 23289–23300. doi:10.1039/D2CP03022E PMID:36156000

Bianchi, H., & Tremaine, P. R. (1995). Thermodynamics of aqueous phosphate solutions: Apparent molar heat capacities and volumes of the sodium and tetramethylammonium salts at 25°C. *Journal of Solution Chemistry*, *24*(5), 439–463. doi:10.1007/BF01004477

Chakraborty, N., Juglan, K. C., & Kumar, H. (2018). Acoustic and thermodynamic study of D-Panthenol in aqueous solutions of glycol at different temperatures. *The Journal of Chemical Thermodynamics*, *126*, 137–146. doi:10.1016/j.jct.2018.07.006

Chakraborty, N., Juglan, K. C., & Kumar, H. (2020). Study of thermodynamic and acoustic properties of niacin in aqueous hexylene glycol and propylene glycol at different temperatures. *ACS Omega*, *5*(50), 32357–32365. doi:10.1021/acsomega.0c04292 PMID:33376872

Chakraborty, N., Juglan, K. C., & Kumar, H. (2021). Volumetric and ultrasonic studies of molecular interactions of glycols in aqueous Niacin (vitamin B3) at different temperatures. *Journal of Molecular Liquids*, *332*, 115869. doi:10.1016/j.molliq.2021.115869

Chen, X. Z., Tang, J.-H., Cui, Y.-N., Liu, M., & Mao, D. (2014). Phase equilibrium for ternary system NaH2PO4 + Na2SO4 + H2O in aqueous solution at 298.15 K. *Journal of Chemical & Engineering Data*, *59*(2), 481–484. doi:10.1021/je400932e

Devunuri, N., Kancherla, S., Chennuri, B. K., & Gardas, R. L. (2016). Apparent molar volume and isentropic compressibilities of antidepressant drugs (Citalopram HBr and Escitalopram oxalate) with water. *Journal of Molecular Liquids*, *216*, 347–353. doi:10.1016/j.molliq.2016.01.058

Dhiman, M., Singh, K., Kaushal, J., Upmanyu, A., & Singh, D. P. (2019). Ultrasonic study of molecular interactions in polymeric solution of polypropylene glycol-400 and ethanol at 303 K. *Acta Acustica united with Acustica*, *105*(5), 743–752. doi:10.3813/AAA.919354

Holmes, H. F., Simonson, J. M., & Mesmer, R. E. (2000). Aqueous solutions of the mono-and di-hydrogenphosphate salts of sodium and potassium at elevated temperatures. Isopiestic results. *The Journal of Chemical Thermodynamics*, *32*(1), 77–96. doi:10.1006/jcht.1999.0571

Huang, J., Wang, T., Zhu, P., & Xiao, J. (2013). Preparation, characterization, and thermal properties of the microencapsulation of a hydrated salt as phase change energy storage materials. *Thermochimica Acta*, *557*, 1–6. doi:10.1016/j.tca.2013.01.019

Ivone Vanessa Jurado-Davila, I. A. H. S. (2023). Phosphate removal using dolomite modified with ultrasound: Mathematical and experimental analysis. *Journal of Environmental Science and Health. Part A, Toxic/Hazardous Substances & Environmental Engineering*, *58*(5), 469–482. doi:10.1080/10934529.2023.2196928 PMID:37005870

Juglan, K. C., & Kumar, H. (2020). Volumetric and ultrasonic investigation of polyethylene glycols (PEG-200 and PEG-600) in aqueous solutions of sodium methylparaben at various temperatures. *The Journal of Chemical Thermodynamics*, *140*, 105916. doi:10.1016/j.jct.2019.105916

Kaur, K., Juglan, K. C., & Kumar, H. (2017, July). Thermo-acoustical molecular interaction study in binary mixtures of glycerol and ethylene glycol. *AIP Conference Proceedings*, *1860*(1), 020026. doi:10.1063/1.4990325

Khaled, H. G. B., Khattech, I., & Jemal, M. (2011). Standard enthalpy of formation of disodium hydrogen phosphate hexahydrate and sodium diphosphate. *The Journal of Chemical Thermodynamics*, *43*(4), 521–526. doi:10.1016/j.jct.2010.11.008

Kumar, H., & Behal, I. (2016). Volumetric and ultrasonic investigation of molecular interactions of l-serine and l-threonine in aqueous nicotinamide solutions at T= (288.15–318.15) K. *Journal of Molecular Liquids*, *219*, 756–764. doi:10.1016/j.molliq.2016.04.019

Kumar, H., Singla, M., & Jindal, R. (2014). Investigations on solute–solvent interactions of amino acids in aqueous solutions of sodium dihydrogen phosphate at different temperatures. *Monatshefte für Chemie*, *145*(7), 1063–1082. doi:10.100700706-014-1183-z

Kumar, H., Singla, M., & Mittal, H. (2016). Volumetric, acoustic and viscometric behaviour of dipotassium hydrogen phosphate and disodium hydrogen phosphate in aqueous solution of N-acetyl glycine at different temperatures. *The Journal of Chemical Thermodynamics*, *94*, 204–220. doi:10.1016/j.jct.2015.10.017

Kurzin, A. V., Evdokimov, A. N., Golikova, V. S., & Fedorov, V. A. (2012). Solubility of potassium and sodium orthophosphates in ethylene glycol. *Russian Journal of Applied Chemistry*, *85*(5), 841–842. doi:10.1134/S1070427212050278

Malekghasemi, S., Mokhtarani, B., Hamzehzadeh, S., Sharifi, A., & Mirzaei, M. (2016). Liquid–liquid equilibria of aqueous biphasic systems of ionic liquids and dipotassium hydrogen phosphate at different temperatures: Experimental study and thermodynamic modeling. *Journal of Molecular Liquids*, *219*, 95–103. doi:10.1016/j.molliq.2016.03.026

Nain, A. K., Pal, R., & Neetu. (2014). Physicochemical study of solute–solute and solute–solvent interactions of l-phenylalanine in (water+ arabinose/glucose/sucrose) solutions at different temperatures. *The Journal of Chemical Thermodynamics*, *68*, 169–182. doi:10.1016/j.jct.2013.09.008

Palaiologou, M. M., Arianas, G. K., & Tsierkezos, N. G. (2006). Thermodynamic investigation of dimethyl sulfoxide binary mixtures at 293.15 and 313.15 K. *Journal of Solution Chemistry*, *35*(11), 1551–1565. doi:10.100710953-006-9082-5

Romero, C. M., & Negrete, F. (2004). Effect of temperature on partial molar volumes and viscosities of aqueous solutions of α-dl-Amino butyric acid, dl-Norvaline and dl-Norleucine. *Physics and Chemistry of Liquids*, *42*(3), 261–267. doi:10.1080/00319100410001659596

Sadeghi, R., Hosseini, R., & Jamehbozorg, B. (2008). Effect of sodium phosphate salts on the thermodynamic properties of aqueous solutions of poly (ethylene oxide) 6000 at different temperatures. *The Journal of Chemical Thermodynamics*, *40*(9), 1364–1377. doi:10.1016/j.jct.2008.05.007

Santagneli, S. H., de Araujo, C. C., Strojek, W., Eckert, H., Poirier, G., Ribeiro, S. J. L., & Messaddeq, Y. (2007). Structural studies of NaPO3– MoO3 glasses by solid-state nuclear magnetic resonance and Raman spectroscopy. *The Journal of Physical Chemistry B*, *111*(34), 10109–10117. doi:10.1021/jp072883n PMID:17683136

Skonieczny, M., Królikowska, M., & Królikowski, M. (2023). Investigation of thermodynamic properties of dimethyl phosphate-based ILs for use as working fluids in absorption refrigeration technology. *Molecules (Basel, Switzerland)*, *28*(4), 1940. doi:10.3390/molecules28041940 PMID:36838928

Thakur, A., Juglan, K. C., Kumar, H., & Kaur, K. (2019). Investigation on molecular interaction of glycols in methanol solutions of methylparaben (methyl 4–hydroxybenzoate) at different temperatures through thermo-acoustical analysis. *Journal of Molecular Liquids*, *288*, 111014. doi:10.1016/j.molliq.2019.111014

Trivedi, M., & Dahryn Trivedi, A. B. (2015). Spectroscopic characterization of disodium hydrogen orthophosphate and sodium nitrate after biofield treatment. *Journal of Chromatography & Separation Techniques*, *5*(6). doi:10.4172/2157-7064.1000282

Upmanyu, A., Dhiman, M., Singh, D. P., & Kumar, H. (2021). Thermo-viscous investigations of molecular interactions for the binary mixtures of polyethylene glycol-400 and polyethylene glycol-600 with dimethyl sulfoxide and water at different temperatures. *Journal of Molecular Liquids*, *334*, 115939. doi:10.1016/j.molliq.2021.115939

Upmanyu, A., & Singh, D. P. (2014). Ultrasonic studies of molecular interactions in polymer solution of the Polyisobutylene (PIB) and Benzene. *Acta Acustica united with Acustica*, *100*(3), 434–439. doi:10.3813/AAA.918723

Weber, C. F., Beahm, E. C., & Watson, J. S. (1999). Modeling thermodynamics and phase equilibria for aqueous solutions of trisodium phosphate. *Journal of Solution Chemistry*, *28*(11), 1207–1238. doi:10.1023/A:1021784515522

Xu, Q., Akkurt, N., Zou, Z., Liu, Y., Feng, J., Yu, C., Ding, Y., Xiong, Y., Zhou, J., Zang, Y., & Ding, Y. (2020). Synthesis and characterization of disodium hydrogen phosphate dodecahydrate-lauric-palmitic acid used for indoor energy storage floor units. *Journal of Thermal Science*, *29*(2), 477–485. doi:10.100711630-020-1273-7

Chapter 21
Thermodynamic Investigations of Vitamin B7 With Glycol Ethers as the Function of Temperature

Swati Bhathley
Lovely Professional University, India

Nabaparna Chakraborty
https://orcid.org/0000-0003-3891-0408
Lovely Professional University, India

Kailash Chandra Juglan
https://orcid.org/0000-0002-8753-4843
Lovely Professional University, India

Ambrish Singh
Nagaland University, India

ABSTRACT

Utilizing the ultrasonic speed of sound and density of ternary mixture of butoxyethanol (BE), phenoxyethanol(PE) in aqueous solution of biotin (Vitamin B7) at concentrations (0.0012, 0.0017, 0.0022) mol·⟦kg⟧^(-1)and varying temperature from (288.15 to 303.15 K) for constant frequency (3 MHz), various thermoacoustic parameters, such as acoustic impedance (Z), adiabatic compressibility (β), Wada's constant (W), Rao's constant (R), intermolecular free length (LF), and Vander Waal's constant (b) have been determined. The experimental work was carried out by using Anton Paar DSA 5000 M at constant pressure 0.1 MPa. The calculated values obtained from experimental values provided the understanding of intermolecular interaction between solute and solvent in liquid mixture. Variation in these parameters describes the understanding of behavior and interaction between the components in solution. Decrease in ultrasonic velocity depicts the weak interaction between molecules.

DOI: 10.4018/979-8-3693-0448-8.ch021

INTRODUCTION

Ultrasonic testing is a Non-destructive testing technique that utilizes high-frequency sound waves to detect and characterize internal flaws, defects, or properties of materials. It involves the generation of ultrasonic waves and their interaction with the material being examined. There are certain areas in which Ultrasonic waves have applications such as, medical diagnosis, imaging, cleaning, and the detection of submarines, etc. (Chakrabory et al., 2021). This nondestructive method reveals important details about the arrangement of molecules, their microscopic structures in the medium, hydrogen bonds, dipole interactions, complex formations, dispersive forces, molecular interactions with their strength and nature, structural arrangements of molecules with their shape, etc (Chakraborty et al., 2022). Along with this, Ultrasonic technique is very accurate and reliable for investigation of liquid mixture, electrolytic and polymeric solution, which are utilize to determine the thermodynamic properties of compressed liquids used in pharmaceutical, chemical, leather, textile and cosmetic and nuclear industries (Chakraborty et al., 2020; Kaur et al., 2021; Kumar et al., 2021) .

Volumetric and acoustic study of a liquid mixture is helpful in examining the physical characteristics and behavior of a liquid mixture. Butoxyethanol (having molecular formula $BuOC_2H_4OH$) can dissolve a wide range of materials, including oils, resins, waxes, paints, varnishes, and dyes. It can be used in a variety of formulations and industrial processes because of its high solubility in water and other polar solvents. It is a colorless liquid and has a ether-like smell used in many household and industrial products as a generally nonvolatile, affordable solvent due to its capabilities as a surfactant. A glycol ether known as 2-butoxyethanol is often used as a solvent in paints, paint thinners, glass cleaners, lacquers, herbicides (Arokiaraj et al., 2022), personal care products, and other items for use on the body as well as a chemical intermediary (Trüeb et al., 2016; Woiski et al., 2020) . Phenoxyethanol is an organic compound with formula $C_6H_5OC_2H_4OH$. Due to its commercial significance, phenoxyethanol (PE), aromatic glycol ether that is naturally formed in green tea, is also made in a laboratory by combining phenol with ethylene oxide. Being biocompatible and biodgradable it has been recognised as a secure organic solvent that is also environmentally friendly. Because of its pure chemical form, pleasant smell, and colorless appearance, it is frequently used in the production of cosmetic items such moisturizers, hand sanitizers, soaps, sunscreen creams, mascara, and perfumes etc. Phenoxyethanol can be used as a preservative for heavy flushing and residual cosmetics, however it has weaker antibacterial activity than other cosmetic chemical preservatives on normal skin (Akgunduz et al., 2020; Zhu et al., 2023; Li et al., 2022).

Biotin is a water-soluble vitamin that aids in metabolising food to produce energy. It is primarily present in a variety of foods, including milk, eggs, bananas, cheese, mushrooms, cauliflower, sweet potatoes, and almonds. It is utilized as a supplement for strengthening hair and nails. Deficiency of biotin is rather uncommon but it can cause skin rashes, cell growth, brittle nails and hair loss (Chakraborty et al., 2022). The risk of deficiency can, however, be increased by a number of circumstances or elements, including prolonged use of antibiotics, heavy alcohol use, specific hereditary abnormalities, and ailments that impair nutrient absorption (Zhang et al., 2020; Lamba et al., 2022) .The present study deals with the interrogation of physicochemical behavior of butoxyethanol and phenoxyethanol in aqueous solution of biotin with the help of density and velocity data taken at different temperature values. Various ultrasonic parameters have been calculated by utilizing the values of density and speed of sound such as acoustic impedance (Z), adiabatic compressibility (β), Wada's constant (W), Rao's constant (R), intermolecular free length, and Vander Waal constant.

MATERIALS AND METHODS

In the current study, the chemicals used are Butoxyethanol, Phenoxyethanol and biotin with molar masses of 118.18, 138.17 and 244.31 g•mol^{-1} respectively obtained from Loba Chemie Pvt. Ltd. Each chemical have mass fraction purity greater than 0.99. The chemicals were vacuum dried for 2 days to absorb the moisture.

With the aid of an Anton Paar DSA 5000M densimeter, the speed of sound of a liquid mixture containing (Biotin + Butoxy ethanol + Phenoxy ethanol) at a frequency of 3 MHZ is obtained. Constant pressure of 0.1 MPa is applied inside the instrument at various temperatures controlled by the built-in Peltier thermometer, and the experimental speed of sound and density are measured separately. With the help of a borosilicate glass Anton Paar oscillating U tube, it concurrently calculates the sound density and speed in distinct cells. An ultrasonic transducer is placed into the specimen in a measuring cell, resulting the speed of sound is calculated from the period of sound that is received at the receiver while taking into account the distance between the transmitter and receiver.

RESULTS AND DISCUSSION

The ternary mixture of butoxyethanol, phenoxyethanol and biotin with molar masses of 118.18, 138.17 and 244.31 g•mol^{-1} respectively is used to examine the intermolecular interaction between the solution. The ultrasonic velocity and density have measured from experiment at temperature values 293.15 K, 298.15, 303.15 K, 308.15 K. Acoustic parameters such as acoustic impedence (Z), adiabatic compressibility (β), Wada's constant (W), Rao's constant (R), intermolecular free length ($Lf_)$, and Van Der Waal constant (b) are calculated to understand the nature of solvent. With increase in concentration of Biotin, the speed of sound is found to be increase. The presence of more molecules with higher concentrations is indicated by an increase in density. Ion-solvent and solvent-solvent interactions are quantified by density. The observed behavior exhibits reductions with increasing mole fraction(Dixit et al., 2014; Kaur et al., 2016).

As the concentration of biotin increases, the values of acoustic impedance also increases linearly. With increase in molality and temperature, acoustic impedance is found to be increase while the value of adiabatic compressibility is found to be decrease which shows the strong interaction between the liquid mixture. The resistance provided to the propagation of an ultrasonic wave in a material is determined by its acoustic impedance (Z) (Duraivathi et al., 2022). Figure 1 depicts the variation in acoustic impedance with molality and Figure 2 depicting the fluctuations in adiabatic compressibility with molality following opposite trend to Z which demonstrate complex creation caused by the production of hydrogen bonds. When no heat is flowing in or out, the volume change caused by a change in pressure is indicated by adiabatic compressibility (Kumari et al., 2014; Dange et al., 2021). The reduced adiabatic compressibility results in closer packing of the molecules, causes a decrease in free length. Decrease in β indicates strengthening in bonds (Singh et al., 2010). The absence of specialised interactions like complex creation, as evidenced by the linear fluctuation in acoustic impedance.Strong molecular interaction is because of increase in viscosity, when biotin concentration increases, value of viscosity also increases indicating greater solute and solvent molecule (Lamba et al., 2022; Kaur et al., 2015). The values of Z and β are listed in [Table1] The expression for acoustic impedence and adiabatic compressibility is given by

Table 1. Values of acoustic impedance and adiabatic compressibility of ternary mixture of Butoxyethanol, Phenoxyethanol and Biotin at different temperature values

m_A/mol•kg^{-1}	Z×10^6/(kg•m^{-1}•s)				β×10^{-10}m2/N)			
	T=288.15K	T=293.15K	T=298.15K	T=303.15K	T=288.15K	T=293.15K	T=298.15K	T=303.15K
BE + 0.00 mol•kg^{-1}Biotin								
0.00000	1465.505	1479.988	1491.532	1502.286	4.653	4.557	4.482	4.412
0.10016	1466.772	1481.176	1492.879	1503.383	4.646	4.551	4.475	4.406
0.20147	1468.138	1482.471	1494.382	1504.594	4.638	4.544	4.466	4.400
0.29196	1469.289	1483.625	1495.953	1505.710	4.631	4.538	4.458	4.394
0.39510	1470.837	1485.001	1497.643	1506.974	4.622	4.530	4.448	4.387
0.49928	1472.225	1486.325	1499.408	1508.359	4.614	4.522	4.439	4.380
BE + 0.0012 mol•kg^{-1}Biotin								
0.00000	1468.678	1483.401	1494.619	1505.088	4.634	4.538	4.465	4.397
0.09999	1469.834	1484.399	1495.948	1506.061	4.628	4.533	4.458	4.393
0.20010	1471.134	1485.654	1497.371	1507.122	4.620	4.526	4.450	4.387
0.30120	1472.465	1486.930	1499.020	1508.322	4.613	4.519	4.441	4.381
0.39990	1473.760	1488.270	1500.678	1509.522	4.605	4.511	4.432	4.375
0.50008	1475.241	1489.553	1502.252	1510.805	4.597	4.504	4.423	4.368
BE+0.0017 mol•kg^{-1}Biotin								
0.00000	1469.968	1484.932	1495.790	1506.209	4.627	4.529	4.459	4.392
0.10062	1471.075	1485.974	1497.038	1507.134	4.620	4.524	4.452	4.387
0.19988	1472.302	1487.195	1498.445	1508.200	4.613	4.517	4.445	4.382
0.30009	1473.681	1488.392	1500.094	1509.464	4.606	4.511	4.435	4.375
0.40431	1475.000	1489.779	1501.892	1510.765	4.598	4.503	4.426	4.368
0.49999	1476.521	1490.989	1503.364	1512.024	4.589	4.496	4.417	4.361
BE+0.0022 mol•kg^{-1}Biotin								
0.00000	1471.143	1486.259	1497.120	1507.564	4.620	4.522	4.451	4.385
0.10000	1472.223	1487.211	1498.394	1508.402	4.614	4.517	4.445	4.381
0.19990	1473.450	1488.418	1499.797	1509.546	4.607	4.510	4.437	4.375
0.30010	1474.833	1489.594	1501.398	1510.778	4.599	4.504	4.428	4.368
0.40009	1476.083	1490.935	1503.110	1512.101	4.592	4.496	4.419	4.361
0.50121	1477.632	1492.203	1504.601	1513.466	4.583	4.489	4.411	4.354
PE+0.00 mol•kg^{-1}Biotin								
0.00000	1465.505	1479.988	1491.532	1502.286	4.653	4.557	4.482	4.412
0.09102	1467.895	1482.209	1493.762	1504.629	4.640	4.546	4.470	4.400
0.20047	1470.584	1485.041	1496.499	1507.521	4.625	4.531	4.456	4.385
0.29106	1473.059	1487.502	1498.760	1509.843	4.611	4.517	4.445	4.373
0.39951	1476.091	1490.233	1501.538	1512.592	4.594	4.503	4.430	4.359
0.49928	1478.502	1492.643	1504.121	1515.220	4.581	4.490	4.416	4.346
PE+0.0012 mol•kg^{-1}Biotin								
0.00000	1468.678	1483.401	1494.619	1505.088	4.634	4.538	4.465	4.397
0.09979	1471.054	1485.706	1496.808	1507.511	4.621	4.526	4.454	4.385
0.19999	1473.535	1488.328	1499.301	1510.147	4.608	4.512	4.441	4.372

continued on following page

Table 1. Continued

m_A/mol•kg^{-1}	$Z\times10^6$/(kg•m^{-1}•s)				$\beta\times10^{-10}$(m2/N)			
	T=288.15K	T=293.15K	T=298.15K	T=303.15K	T=288.15K	T=293.15K	T=298.15K	T=303.15K
0.30042	1476.150	1490.893	1501.837	1512.653	4.593	4.498	4.428	4.359
0.40008	1478.772	1493.533	1504.344	1515.171	4.579	4.484	4.415	4.346
0.50021	1481.232	1496.044	1506.774	1517.704	4.565	4.471	4.402	4.334
PE+0.0017 mol•kg^{-1}Biotin								
0.00000	1469.968	1484.932	1495.790	1506.209	4.627	4.529	4.459	4.392
0.09989	1472.353	1487.202	1497.836	1508.576	4.614	4.518	4.449	4.380
0.20020	1474.858	1489.828	1500.270	1511.160	4.600	4.503	4.436	4.367
0.30031	1477.407	1492.344	1502.795	1513.614	4.586	4.490	4.423	4.354
0.39993	1480.009	1494.893	1505.294	1516.153	4.571	4.477	4.410	4.341
0.50011	1482.382	1497.483	1507.688	1518.737	4.559	4.463	4.397	4.328
PE+0.0022 mol•kg^{-1}Biotin								
0.00000	1471.143	1486.259	1497.120	1507.564	4.620	4.522	4.451	4.385
0.09997	1473.455	1488.644	1499.216	1509.969	4.607	4.509	4.441	4.373
0.20012	1475.863	1491.126	1501.659	1512.552	4.594	4.496	4.428	4.360
0.30703	1478.666	1493.905	1504.427	1515.219	4.579	4.481	4.414	4.346
0.39979	1481.076	1496.201	1506.746	1517.664	4.565	4.469	4.402	4.334
0.50002	1483.375	1498.852	1509.208	1520.156	4.553	4.455	4.389	4.321

Acoustic impedance $Z = \rho \times c$ (1)

Adiabatic compressibity $\beta = 1/[\rho[c^2]]$ (2)

Where 'ρ' is the density and 'c' is the speed of sound

The constants such as Wada's constant and Rao's constant have computed and values of these constants are given in [Table.2]. Values are calculated using formulas

$$W = (\beta)^{-\frac{1}{7}}\left(\frac{M}{\rho}\right) \quad (3)$$

and

$$R = (c)^{\frac{1}{3}}\left(\frac{M}{\rho}\right) (4).$$

Variation in values of Wada's constant (W) presented in Figure 3 and Rao's constant (R) increases as the concentration increases as shown in Figure 4 which suggests the strong solute- solvent interaction between the molecules because of ion-dipole interaction and hydrogen bonding and the number of com-

Table 2. Values of Wada's constant (W) and Rao's constant (R) of Butoxyethanol and phenoxyethanol in solution of Biotin at different values of temperature

m_A/mol•kg^{-1}	W/(m^3/mol)(Pa)$^{1/7}$				R(m^3/mol)(m/s)$^{1/3}$			
	T=288.15K	T=293.15K	T=298.15K	T=303.15K	T=288.15K	T=293.15K	T=298.15K	T=303.15K
BE + 0.00 mol•kg^{-1}Biotin								
0.00000	94.947	95.328	95.667	96.017	1343.698	1349.999	1355.608	1361.390
0.10016	94.947	95.327	95.669	96.014	1343.709	1349.983	1355.640	1361.333
0.20147	94.951	95.330	95.676	96.014	1343.777	1350.029	1355.749	1361.343
0.29196	94.955	95.334	95.688	96.017	1343.845	1350.094	1355.941	1361.391
0.39510	94.966	95.342	95.701	96.023	1344.027	1350.223	1356.169	1361.485
0.49928	94.977	95.352	95.720	96.034	1344.208	1350.388	1356.474	1361.662
BE + 0.0012 mol•kg^{-1}Biotin								
0.00000	94.972	95.351	95.682	96.013	1344.111	1350.371	1355.848	1361.317
0.09999	94.972	95.348	95.686	96.010	1344.115	1350.322	1355.909	1361.266
0.20010	94.977	95.351	95.693	96.010	1344.193	1350.380	1356.029	1361.279
0.30120	94.983	95.356	95.706	96.015	1344.306	1350.467	1356.247	1361.360
0.39990	94.991	95.365	95.721	96.022	1344.438	1350.606	1356.493	1361.464
0.50008	95.004	95.374	95.736	96.031	1344.645	1350.759	1356.742	1361.614
BE + 0.0017 mol•kg^{-1}Biotin								
0.00000	94.981	95.362	95.683	96.011	1344.261	1350.565	1355.859	1361.288
0.10062	94.981	95.361	95.686	96.009	1344.272	1350.550	1355.922	1361.257
0.19988	94.986	95.365	95.695	96.011	1344.344	1350.613	1356.057	1361.290
0.30009	94.994	95.370	95.708	96.017	1344.474	1350.688	1356.275	1361.397
0.40431	95.000	95.378	95.724	96.024	1344.584	1350.820	1356.538	1361.506
0.49999	95.013	95.386	95.736	96.033	1344.803	1350.955	1356.747	1361.653
BE + 0.0022 mol•kg^{-1}Biotin								
0.00000	94.992	95.374	95.696	96.017	1344.441	1350.750	1356.076	1361.396
0.10000	94.992	95.372	95.701	96.014	1344.453	1350.720	1356.163	1361.347
0.19990	94.997	95.376	95.709	96.018	1344.526	1350.785	1356.303	1361.407
0.30010	95.005	95.380	95.722	96.024	1344.664	1350.855	1356.516	1361.506
0.40009	95.012	95.388	95.738	96.032	1344.777	1350.992	1356.773	1361.644
0.50121	95.025	95.396	95.750	96.043	1344.994	1351.123	1356.977	1361.815
PE + 0.00 mol•kg^{-1}Biotin								
0.00000	110.999	111.445	111.841	112.250	1570.869	1578.236	1584.792	1591.552
0.09102	110.996	111.437	111.833	112.243	1570.822	1578.110	1584.830	1591.432
0.20047	110.993	111.436	111.828	112.240	1570.769	1578.087	1584.958	1591.381
0.29106	110.998	111.440	111.827	112.239	1570.861	1578.161	1585.182	1591.371
0.39951	111.010	111.445	111.832	112.242	1571.056	1578.234	1585.448	1591.417
0.49928	111.017	111.452	111.841	112.252	1571.175	1578.351	1585.805	1591.576
PE + 0.0012 mol•kg^{-1}Biotin								
0.00000	111.028	111.471	111.858	112.245	1571.352	1578.670	1585.073	1591.467
0.09979	111.023	111.463	111.848	112.239	1571.264	1578.541	1584.896	1591.363
0.19999	111.022	111.464	111.846	112.239	1571.249	1578.558	1584.863	1591.373
0.30042	111.026	111.466	111.847	112.240	1571.320	1578.594	1584.885	1591.380

continued on following page

Table 2. Continued

m_A/mol•kg^{-1}	W/(m^3/mol)(Pa)$^{1/7}$				R(m^3/mol)(m/s)$^{1/3}$			
	T=288.15K	T=293.15K	T=298.15K	T=303.15K	T=288.15K	T=293.15K	T=298.15K	T=303.15K
0.40008	111.033	111.473	111.851	112.244	1571.441	1578.707	1584.951	1591.446
0.50021	111.040	111.481	111.857	112.251	1571.552	1578.831	1585.044	1591.567
PE + 0.0017 mol•kg^{-1}Biotin								
0.00000	111.038	111.485	111.859	112.243	1571.527	1578.897	1585.086	1591.433
0.09989	111.034	111.477	111.848	112.238	1571.457	1578.777	1584.906	1591.347
0.20020	111.034	111.480	111.847	112.239	1571.460	1578.819	1584.894	1591.370
0.30031	111.038	111.482	111.851	112.240	1571.516	1578.850	1584.956	1591.391
0.39993	111.046	111.488	111.857	112.246	1571.645	1578.947	1585.045	1591.477
0.50011	111.050	111.496	111.861	112.253	1571.720	1579.086	1585.120	1591.599
PE + 0.0022 mol•kg^{-1}Biotin								
0.00000	111.051	111.498	111.874	112.251	1571.738	1579.114	1585.340	1591.559
0.09997	111.046	111.493	111.864	112.245	1571.647	1579.043	1585.164	1591.476
0.20012	111.044	111.493	111.863	112.246	1571.626	1579.039	1585.142	1591.487
0.30703	111.050	111.498	111.867	112.247	1571.724	1579.117	1585.215	1591.507
0.39979	111.058	111.502	111.871	112.254	1571.844	1579.185	1585.283	1591.609
0.50002	111.061	111.513	111.876	112.259	1571.899	1579.358	1585.371	1591.704

Table 3. Values of intermolecular free length and Vander Waal's constant of Butoxyethanol and phenoxy-ethanol in Biotin solution at varying temperature values from 288.15 to 303.15 K

m_A/mol•kg^{-1}	Lf×10^{-10}m				b (m^3/mol)			
	T=288.15K	T=293.15K	T=298.15K	T=303.15K	T=288.15K	T=293.15K	T=293.15K	T=303.15K
BE + 0.00 mol•kg^{-1}Biotin								
0.00000	4.356	4.351	4.354	4.360	78.665	78.748	78.839	78.948
0.10016	4.352	4.348	4.351	4.357	78.649	78.731	78.823	78.932
0.20147	4.349	4.344	4.347	4.354	78.634	78.716	78.808	78.916
0.29196	4.346	4.341	4.343	4.351	78.621	78.704	78.796	78.904
0.39510	4.341	4.338	4.338	4.348	78.609	78.692	78.784	78.892
0.49928	4.338	4.334	4.333	4.344	78.599	78.682	78.774	78.882
BE + 0.0012 mol•kg^{-1}Biotin								
0.00000	4.347	4.342	4.346	4.352	78.641	78.719	78.809	78.909
0.09999	4.344	4.339	4.343	4.350	78.626	78.704	78.795	78.894
0.20010	4.340	4.336	4.339	4.347	78.612	78.690	78.781	78.881
0.30120	4.337	4.332	4.335	4.344	78.600	78.677	78.769	78.869
0.39990	4.333	4.329	4.330	4.341	78.588	78.666	78.759	78.858
0.50008	4.329	4.325	4.326	4.338	78.578	78.656	78.749	78.848
BE + 0.0017 mol•kg^{-1}Biotin								
0.00000	4.343	4.337	4.343	4.350	78.631	78.708	78.794	78.893
0.10062	4.341	4.335	4.340	4.347	78.617	78.693	78.781	78.880

continued on following page

Table 3. Continued

m_A/mol•kg^{-1}	Lf×10^{-10}m				b (m^3/mol)			
	T=288.15K	T=293.15K	T=298.15K	T=303.15K	T=288.15K	T=293.15K	T=293.15K	T=303.15K
0.19988	4.337	4.332	4.336	4.345	78.604	78.680	78.769	78.868
0.30009	4.334	4.328	4.332	4.341	78.591	78.668	78.757	78.856
0.40431	4.330	4.325	4.327	4.338	78.579	78.655	78.745	78.844
0.49999	4.326	4.322	4.323	4.335	78.568	78.646	78.735	78.834
BE + 0.0022 mol•kg^{-1}Biotin								
0.00000	4.340	4.334	4.340	4.346	78.623	78.698	78.787	78.880
0.10000	4.337	4.331	4.336	4.344	78.609	78.685	78.774	78.867
0.19990	4.334	4.328	4.332	4.341	78.596	78.672	78.762	78.855
0.30010	4.330	4.325	4.328	4.338	78.584	78.659	78.750	78.844
0.40009	4.327	4.322	4.324	4.334	78.573	78.648	78.739	78.833
0.50121	4.323	4.318	4.320	4.331	78.562	78.637	78.729	78.823
PE + 0.00 mol•kg^{-1}Biotin								
0.00000	4.356	4.351	4.354	4.360	91.964	92.061	92.168	92.296
0.09102	4.350	4.345	4.349	4.354	91.925	92.021	92.149	92.255
0.20047	4.343	4.338	4.342	4.346	91.881	91.977	92.132	92.209
0.29106	4.336	4.332	4.336	4.341	91.847	91.943	92.117	92.174
0.39951	4.328	4.325	4.329	4.334	91.809	91.904	92.103	92.134
0.49928	4.322	4.318	4.322	4.327	91.778	91.873	92.092	92.102
PE + 0.0012 mol•kg^{-1}Biotin								
0.00000	4.347	4.342	4.346	4.352	91.936	92.028	92.133	92.250
0.09999	4.341	4.336	4.341	4.346	91.896	91.987	92.092	92.208
0.20010	4.335	4.329	4.334	4.340	91.857	91.948	92.053	92.169
0.30120	4.328	4.323	4.328	4.334	91.820	91.910	92.015	92.132
0.39990	4.321	4.316	4.322	4.327	91.785	91.875	91.980	92.097
0.50008	4.314	4.309	4.315	4.321	91.752	91.842	91.948	92.064
PE + 0.0017 mol•kg^{-1}Biotin								
0.00000	4.343	4.337	4.343	4.350	91.924	92.014	92.116	92.231
0.09979	4.337	4.332	4.338	4.344	91.884	91.974	92.077	92.192
0.19999	4.331	4.325	4.332	4.337	91.846	91.936	92.039	92.154
0.30042	4.324	4.319	4.326	4.331	91.809	91.899	92.004	92.118
0.40008	4.318	4.312	4.319	4.325	91.775	91.865	91.970	92.084
0.50021	4.311	4.305	4.313	4.318	91.742	91.832	91.937	92.050
PE + 0.0022 mol•kg^{-1}Biotin								
0.00000	4.340	4.334	4.340	4.346	91.915	92.003	92.107	92.216
0.09989	4.334	4.328	4.334	4.340	91.876	91.964	92.067	92.176
0.20020	4.328	4.322	4.328	4.334	91.838	91.926	92.029	92.138
0.30031	4.321	4.314	4.321	4.327	91.799	91.887	91.991	92.099
0.39993	4.315	4.309	4.315	4.321	91.768	91.855	91.959	92.067
0.50011	4.309	4.302	4.309	4.314	91.735	91.823	91.926	92.034

ponents are increases that are closely packed together (Chakraborty et al., 2022; Dudhe). As the variation in values of W and R is linear, it shows that there is absence of complex formation in mixture (Bhakri et al., 2023). The concentration and temperature have an impact on Wada's constant. The molecules draw closer together as the temperature rises and the distance between solute and solvent molecules decrease as temperature and concentration rise, indicating that the molecules are moving closer to one another and indicating a significant solute-solvent interaction in the solution (Patnaik et al., 2021).

The intermolecular free length increases as the temperature rises but falls as the concentration rises which is because of compression of liquids. This implies the presence of strong interaction between solute and solvent within the mixture (Chakraborty et al., 2022). Free length must decrease as concentration increases since the ultrasonic velocity rises as concentration does, and vice versa. Dipole-dipole interactions, hydrogen bonding association, and complex formation between the constituent molecules cause a reduction in free length (Dhiman et al., 2019). The intermolecular free length is calculated by using

$$L_f = K_T \times \beta 1^{/2} \quad (5)$$

and values are given in Table 3. The value of Vander Waal's constant (b) varies with concentration of biotin. As the concentration increases in solution, value of Vander Waal constant decreases which leads to weaker binding forces and absence of complex formation. This shows the weak interaction between molecules of liquid mixture (Lamba et al., 2022; Chakraborty et al., 2020). Figure 5 depicting the variation in Vander Waal's constant correspond to molality at varying temperature. The value of b is calculated using formula

$$b = \left(\frac{M}{\rho}\right)[1-\left(\frac{RT}{Mc^2}\right)\sqrt{1+\left(\frac{Mc^2}{3RT}\right)}-1] \quad (6)$$

which are given in Table 3.

CONCLUSION

Various thermo- acoustic parameters have been calculated through experimental data for liquid solution containing Butoxyethanol (BE), phenoxyethanol (PE) in Biotin (Vitamin B7) at varying temperature from 288.15 to 303.15 K over Biotin concentration (0.012, 0.0017, 0.0022) $mol{\bullet}kg^{-1}$ are analyzed. Presence of molecular interaction between the solute and solvent is indicated through the variation in calculated parameters. It is observed that the ultrasonic velocity and density increases with increase in concentration of Biotin. Acoustic impedance and adiabatic compressibility shows the opposite behavior but adiabatic compressibility and intermolecular free length behaves in same and follows the same pattern. The acoustic impedance, Wada's constant, Rao's constant shows linearly increasing trend with rise in temperature and concentration which indicates, there is no formation of complexity. Whereas adiabatic compressibility and intermolecular free length follows linearly decreasing order as temperature and concentration increases which depicts the attractive behavior of molecules towards each other and there is strong molecular interaction in components of solution. Decrease in free length is because of dipole-dipole interactions, hydrogen bonding association. Linear variation of Wada's constant and Rao's constant indicate that there is no complex formation Vander Waal's constant decreases with increase in concentration shows the weak interaction. It is concluded that the components show strong molecular interaction in liquid solution and with decrease in ultrasonic velocity intermolecular interaction is weak.

ACKNOWLEDGMENT

The author (Swati Bhathley) is grateful to the Head, Department of Physics, Lovely proffessional, Phagwara, Punjab, India for providing the facilities for research.

REFERENCES

Akgunduz, M. C., Cavusoglu, K., & Yalsin, E. (2020). The Potential Risk Assessment of Phenoxyethanol with a Versatile Model System. *Journal of Experimental Orthopaedics*, *10*(1). PMID:31988350

Arokiaraj, R. G., Ravikumar, S., Raju, R., Losetty, V., Bhanuprakash, P., & Pandiyan, V. (2022). Investigation of solute-solvent interactions between 2-butoxyethanol and substituted ketones by volumetric, acoustic and FTIR studies at T=(303.15–318.15) K. *Chemical Thermodynamics and Thermal Analysis*, *6*, 100049. doi:10.1016/j.ctta.2022.100049

Bhakri, K., Chakraborty, N., Juglan, K. C., & Kumar, H. (2023). Investigation of Volumetric and Acoustical Properties of Polyethylene Glycols in Niacin Solutions. *Journal of Physics: Conference Series*, *12*(3).

Chakraborty, N., Bhakri, K., Juglan, K. C., & Kumar, H. (2022). Physicochemical studies of polyethylene glycols in aqueous biotin solutions at different temperatures and constant pressure. *Journal of Physics: Conference Series*, *2267*(1), 012124. doi:10.1088/1742-6596/2267/1/012124

Chakraborty, N., Juglan, K. C., & Kumar, H. (2020). Study of thermodynamic and acoustic properties of niacin in aqueous hexylene glycol and propylene glycol at different temperatures. *ACS Omega*, *5*(50), 32357–32365. doi:10.1021/acsomega.0c04292 PMID:33376872

Chakraborty, N., Juglan, K. C., Kumar, H., & Singla, M. (2022). Measurement of the Density and Ultrasonic Speed of the Sound of Poly (ethylene glycols)(600 and 6000) in Aqueous Vitamin B5 Solutions at Different Temperatures. *Journal of Chemical & Engineering Data*, *67*(9), 2292–2306. doi:10.1021/acs.jced.2c00260

Chakraborty, N., Juglan, K. C., Kumar, H., & Singla, M. (2022). Study of thermodynamic parameters of ternary solutions of polyethylene glycols in aqueous biotin solutions at multiple temperatures. *The Journal of Chemical Thermodynamics*, *174*, 106876. doi:10.1016/j.jct.2022.106876

Chakraborty, N., Lamba, M., Juglan, K. C., & Kumar, H. (2022). Temperature–dependent thermodynamic studies of glycols in aqueous solutions of vitamin B3. *Journal of Physics: Conference Series*, *2267*(1), 012134. doi:10.1088/1742-6596/2267/1/012134

Chakraborty, N., Rani, M., & Juglan, K. C. (2020). Ultrasonic Investigation of Dichloromethane with Ethanolamine at Various Temperatures. *Plant Archives*, *20*, 2825–2829.

Chakrabory, N., Juglan, K. C., & Kumar, H. (2021). Volumetric and ultrasonic studies of molecular interactions of glycols in aqueous Niacin (vitamin B3) at different temperatures. *Journal of Molecular Liquids*, *332*, 115869. doi:10.1016/j.molliq.2021.115869

Dange, S. P., Chimankar, O. P., & Borkar, P. D. (2021). Physico-chemical analysis on binary liquid mixture of Nicotinic acid at different temperatures. *Indian Journal of Pure and Applied Physics*, *59*(2), 132–137. doi:10.56042/ijpap.v59i2.33311

Dhiman, M., Singh, K., Kaushal, J., Upmanyu, A., & Singh, D. P. (2019). Ultrasonic study of molecular interactions in polymeric solution of polypropylene glycol-400 and ethanol at 303 K. *Acta Acustica united with Acustica*, *105*(5), 743–752. doi:10.3813/AAA.919354

Dixit, A., & Juglan, K. C., Sharma. (2014). Acoustic parameter investigation of ternary mixture of n-butanol, water and acetic acid by using ultrasonic technique. *Journal of Chemical and Pharmaceutical Research*, *6*(10), 93–104.

Duraivathi, C., Priya, J. J., Poongodi, J., & Jeyakumar, H. J. (2022). Ultrasonic study of molecular interactions in organic liquid with CCl4 at different temperature. *Materials Today: Proceedings*, *49*, 1968–1972. doi:10.1016/j.matpr.2021.08.140

Kaur, H., Chakraborty, N., Juglan, K. C., & Kumar, H. (2021). Volumetric and Acoustic Behavior of PEG-200 and PEG-600 in Aqueous D-Mannitol solutions at Different Temperatures. *Journal of Solution Chemistry*, *50*(8), 1079–1102. doi:10.100710953-021-01105-3

Kaur, K., & Juglan, K. C. (2015). Studies of molecular interaction in the binary mixture of chloroform and methanol by using ultrasonic technique. *Der Pharma Chem*, *7*(2), 160–167.

Kaur, K., & Juglan, K. C. (2016). Ultrasonic velocity, density and viscosity studies of the binary mixtures of ethyl acetate with hexane. *Journal of Chemical and Pharmaceutical Research*, *87*, 49–53.

Kumar, M., Khan, M. A., Yadav, C. P., Pandey, D. K., & Singh, D. (2021). Ultrasonic characterization of binary mixture of 2, 3-dichloroaniline and polyethylene glycols. *The Journal of Chemical Thermodynamics*, *161*, 106557. doi:10.1016/j.jct.2021.106557

Kumari, S., Juglan, K. C., & Sharma, A. (2014). Acoustic parameter investigation of tyrosine derivative in dimethyl sulpho oxide by ultrasonic technique. *Journal of Chemical and Pharmaceutical Research*, *6*(11), 782–794.

Lamba M., Chakraborty, N., Juglan, K. C., & Kumar, H. (2022). Thermodynamic-Acoustic Studies of Mixture Vitamin B7 Glycols at Different Temperatures. *Lett. Appl. NanoBioScience, 12*(4).

Li, Y., Xu, R., & Zuo, Y. (2022). Effects and Detection Methods of Potential Toxic Chemicals in Cosmetics: Metals, Phenoxyethanol and Aloe Vera. *Highlights in Science. Engineering and Technology*, *6*, 9–17.

Patnaik, P., Chakraborty, N., Kaur, P., Juglan, K. C., & Kumar, H. (2021). Thermodynamic and Acoustic Investigation of D-Panthenol in Homologous Series of Polyethylene Glycol at Different Temperatures. *Advances in fundamental and smart material: Select proceedings of ICFMMP*.

Singh, P. K., & Bhatt, S. C. (2010). Investigation of acoustical parameters of polyvinyl acetate. *Applied physics research, 2*(1)

Trüeb, R. M. (2016). Serum Biotin Levels in Women Complaining of Hair Loss. *International Journal of Trichology*, *8*(2), 73–77. doi:10.4103/0974-7753.188040 PMID:27601860

Woıski, C., Dobslaw, D., & Engesser, K. H. (2020). Isolation and characterization of 2-butoxyethanol degrading bacterial strains. *Biodegradation*, *31*(3), 153–169. doi:10.100710532-020-09900-3 PMID:32356147

Zhang, Y., Wang, R., Dong, Y., Huang, G., Ji, B., & Wang, Q. (2020). Assessment of biotin interference in thyroid function tests. *Medicine*, *99*(9), e19232. doi:10.1097/MD.0000000000019232 PMID:32118725

Zhu, Y., Tang, R., Yu, Y., Yu, Z., Wang, K., Wang, Y., & Han, D. (2023). Efficient co-production of xylooligosaccharides and glucose from vinegar residue by biphasic phenoxyethanol-maleic acid pretreatment. *Fermentation (Basel, Switzerland)*, *9*(1), 61. doi:10.3390/fermentation9010061

Chapter 22
A Review on the Acoustic and Thermodynamic Properties of Sugar Alcohols

Harsimaran Kaur
Lovely Professional University, India

Kailash Chandra Juglan
https://orcid.org/0000-0002-8753-4843
Lovely Professional University, India

Nabaparna Chakraborty
https://orcid.org/0000-0003-3891-0408
Lovely Professional University, India

ABSTRACT

In order to examine the non-ideal behaviour of a liquid, it is crucial to conduct investigations. To determine excess properties, a range of measurable properties can be utilized in experimental calculations. Major characteristics to consider in binary and ternary mixtures include density and apparent molar volume. From a thermodynamic standpoint, several combination characteristics, various thermodynamic features, such as partial molar volumes, at infinite dilution, hold great significance. The purpose of this review is to provide a summary of recent research on the acoustics and thermodynamics of sugar alcohols in various mixtures and temperatures. Sugar alcohols are widely used in the nutrition and pharmacological industries, and many medical applications. They function as low-calorie sweeteners, providing a sweet flavour without rapidly raising blood sugar levels. Specific sugar alcohols, like xylitol, support dental health. Furthermore, acoustics can be employed as a tool for particle sizing, as well as for revealing information about the microstructure of the dispersed system.

INTRODUCTION

DOI: 10.4018/979-8-3693-0448-8.ch022

Recently, there has been a significant surge in research on the volumetric, acoustical, physicochemical, and thermodynamic properties of fluid blends using ultrasonic techniques (Devunuri, et al. 2016). The non-destructive nature of this approach sets it apart from other methods, as it allows for analysis of the molecular interactions within the liquid system without altering the sample's shape or structure, making it a preferred option. The parameters of ultrasonic speed and density obtained using sound play a critical role in comprehending the atomic structure and combinations within the liquid mixture (Chakraborty, 2020). Studying ultrasonic properties is crucial for understanding the unique traits of multi-segment fluid blends in a non-intrusive manner. Liquid mixtures' acoustic and thermodynamic properties are used to explore the molecular interactions between their components. The correlation amid thermodynamic properties and the types of molecular interlinkage is an area of research that is both fascinating and worthy of investigation (Kumar, et al. 2016).

Sugar alcohols, which are also referred to as polyols, glycitols, and alditols, are substances that are derived from sugars and contain one hydroxyl group attached to each carbon atom (Park, et al 2016; Teo, 2006). Specific sugar alcohols, like xylitol, improve dental health by lowering the incidence of cavities in addition to their intrinsic hygroscopic qualities, which help bakeries keep moisture and textural quality. Although they have fewer calories than conventional sugars, it is important to take their caloric impact into account given that some people may experience gastrointestinal discomfort after excessive consumption. These compounds have numerous applications in various industries, especially in food production, where they serve as both thickeners and sweeteners, frequently used to replace sucrose (Naseem, et al. 2016; Warmińska, 2012). Some of the most commonly used sugar alcohols include inositol, maltitol, lactitol, erythritol, D-mannitol, glycerol, and xylitol, each with a broad range of uses. Inositol, for instance, is a carbocyclic sugar alcohol that is naturally produced in mankind from glucose, and it is roughly half as sweet as sucrose. It is abundant in the brain and commonly utilized in the manufacturing of explosives and cutting agents. Additionally, inositol has been found to be beneficial in treating PCOS (polycystic ovary syndrome) (Parthasarathy, et al. 2006). The food industry and personal care product manufacturers commonly use glycerol, which is a straightforward polyol compound. Unlike other sugar alcohols, xylitol occurs naturally in pumpkins, plums, strawberries, and cauliflower, and it is achiral. It is commonly used for preventing ear aches, diabetes, weight management, and dental care (Egas, et al. 2021). Low-calorie food products frequently use lactitol as a substitute bulk sweetener. Additionally, lactitol, erythritol, maltitol, sorbitol, D-mannitol, and xylitol are approved food additives and recognized for not causing an increase in blood glucose levels (Thirumaran, et al. 2009; Majka, J., et al 2017).

Sugar alcohols have a crucial significance in the food and pharmaceutical sectors owing to their artificial sweetening properties in dairy products and their capacity to substantially influence blood sugar levels. An expedient way of assessing the solvation conduct of polyol is by evaluating its volumetric and acoustic characteristics. This research is important for comprehending the underlying mechanisms of sweet taste chemoreception and for gaining significant insights into the stabilization of proteins and the interactions between solutes and solvents.

A COMPREHENSIVE REVIEW

Acoustic And Thermodynamic Investigation and Studies of Different Liquid Mixture With Sugar Alcohol

Chakraborty et. al. (2020) utilized velocity and density values to analyse several acoustical and volumetric variables for binary and ternary mixtures of glycols with xylitol at diverse concentrations and temperatures. Through their calculations, they determined, $V_{\phi 0}$, $K\phi_{,s,}$ pair and triplet coefficients and many more parameters. These findings indicated strong interactions among the solute (glycols) and the solvent (xylitol). The volumetric data gathered provided crucial insights into how the intermolecular interactions were affected by temperature, position, and chain length of the hydroxyl group of xylitol.

In a separate study, Kaur et al. (2021) and their colleagues conducted an experimental analysis to determine velocity and density values for binary as well as ternary blends of polyethylene glycol (PEG 200/ 600) with D-Mannitol. The researchers then used the obtained experimental data to calculate various parameters ($V\phi$, $V\phi 0$, $K\phi,s$, and $K0\phi,s$). The study demonstrated the potential applications of PEG's and D-mannitol in different industries like cosmetics, leather, food, and pharmaceuticals. Their findings showed that density values decreased as the temperature increased and increased with an increase in D-mannitol concentration . The researchers also observed strong interactions of solute-solvent based on the positive values of $V\phi$. Additionally, the study revealed that molecular interactions increased with the molar mass of PEG's (PEG 200 - PEG 600). Kaur et. al (2017). conducted an inquiry into the attributes of Sorbitol in both water and glycols, namely EG, DEG, and TEG. To obtain information about the sound speed and density, they utilized the Anton Paar Density Sound Analyzer 5000M. Their research also uncovered a variety of other thermodynamic and acoustical factors. The outcomes suggested solid solute-solvent relationships and various contacts existing within the liquid mix, such as dipole-dipole, hydrophilic-2, hydrophobic-2, and ion hydrophilic interactions. In another study, Bergua et. al (2018). focused on the features of sugar alcohol (Inositol) with natural deep eutectic solvent solutions (aqueous). They used velocity and density measurements to calculate several parameters, including the standard partial molar volume, compressibility, for the diluted mixtures. The examination of their findings was conducted by evaluating the temperature and concentration, revealing the prevalence of hydrophilic-2 and ionic-hydrophilic interactions.

Shi et. al. (2020) directed a study on the behaviour of maltitol in watered glycylglycine mixtures, using various techniques such as sound speed and density evaluation at diverse temperatures and pressures. Jones-Dole equation used to establish a correlation between solution viscosities and the viscosity B coefficient. By employing these methods, the researchers gained a better understanding of maltitol's solvation behaviour.

In a separate study, Shahaidy et. al (2022). investigated the potential applications of sugar alcohol in the pharmaceutical and food industries. They examined meso-erythritol's sound speed and density in water as well as watered- DMSO blends at five different temperatures (ranging from 20-300C) under ambient pressure. The evaluation of the physical properties of polyol through volumetric and acoustic analyses was utilized to characterize its solvation behaviour. The study of sweet taste chemoreception mechanisms is greatly aided by an understanding of the role played by certain proteins in this process. Moreover, investigating the stabilization of proteins and the interactions between solutes and solvents can yield valuable information in this area. These factors are critical to comprehending the mechanisms underlying the perception of sweetness, and to advancing our knowledge of the chemical processes involved in this phenomenon. The researchers observed various mixing effects resulting from the interlinkage among meso-erythritol in water as well as in watered DMSO solutions, Offering perspectives on the water-binding properties and solvent interactions of polyols. The collected data could be valuable in developing new applications for sugar alcohol in various industries.

Banipal et. al. (2015) conducted a study to examine viscosity and density evaluations on triplex mixtures composed of polyhydroxy solute, Ammonium bromide and water. The investigation was conducted under normal atmospheric conditions while examining a broad temperature spectrum of 15-450C. In order to evaluate the transfer characteristics of polyhydroxy compounds, the scientists employed information gathered from $V\phi 0_{at}$ infinite. Afterwards, the interaction factors were derived. The study found that the densities of all solutes studied increased linearly with the molalities of co-solute.

In another study, Longinotti, and Corti (2004) conducted an investigation on the esterification process involving borate ion and either sucrose or trehalose, with the aim of studying the reaction. The researchers measured the pH variations formed by adding the consistent sugar to sodium borate solutions to determine the reaction. The equilibrium information was used to speciation of the ternary system consisting of sugar, borate, and water was determined, and the electrical conductivity of the system was analysed by isolating the individual ionic species and examining their contributions. After analysing the results, it can be concluded that Walden's rule applies to the borate-trehalose and borate-sucrose ions in the studied viscosity range. However, the performance of the smaller borate ion is still uncertain.

Bama et al. (2010) conducted research to examine the thermal diffusivity and conductivity of watery solutions of D-mannitol at room temperature using ultrasonic and photoacoustic techniques. According to their findings, there was a minor concentration dependence. The velocities increased progressively up to 65°C for most concentrations and then started to decrease. The sound speed in DM for the diverse concentrations investigated in the present study displayed a temperature dependence that resembled that of velocities in water.

Jengathe et. al (2015) conducted a research study to determine the sound speed and density of DPH in solutions with varying compositions. Specifically, they investigated the behaviour of DPH in watered solutions and in sodium chloride as well as myo-inositol (MI) at diverse temperatures (T = 15, 25, and 350^{C}). During the study, the team of researchers measured the sound speed and density of the DPH solutions using various techniques. They analysed the data obtained from these measurements to determine the behaviour of DPH in the different solution compositions and temperatures. The results of the study showed that the sound speed and density of DPH in watered solution and in the aqueous solutions of sodium chloride and myo-inositol (MI) varied significantly with changes in temperature. The findings of the study provide valuable insights into the behaviour of DPH in solution and could have important implications in various industries, including pharmaceuticals and chemical engineering. The data acquired from the experiment were employed to assess diverse thermodynamic characteristics, and the authors elucidated the outcomes concerning the interplay between the molecules of the solute and the solvent .

Jiang et al (2013) also conducted a study on the viscosities and densities of binary (three polyols + water) and ternary solutions (three polyols + L-ascorbic acid + water) at atmospheric pressure and temperatures ranging from $20^{0}C$ to $50^{0}C$. The authors used the densities to calculate the ($V_{\phi,}$ $V\phi_{0,}$ $K\phi,_{s,}$ and $K0\phi,^{s}$). Furthermore, different equation was utilized to correlate the viscosities and densities of polyols in aqueous solutions containing L-ascorbic acid, respectively. The authors employed the viscosity B-coefficients in determining the free energy of activation for each mole of solvent and solute. These discoveries enhance our comprehension of the interactions present in ternary solutions of polyol, water and L-ascorbic acid.

Bernal et al. (2019) conducted a study in which they measured the densities and sound speeds of aqueous solutions of some polyols (Erythritol, Xylitol, Sorbitol, and Maltitol) at different temperatures using a DSA 5000M. The study aimed to characterize the hydration of sugar alcohols and investigate its relationship with sweet taste chemoreception. The researchers analysed the results to compute various parameters such as the (Vϕ, $_{V\phi}$0, $_{K\phi}$'s, $_{and}$ K0ϕ,s) $^{s}{}_{peci}$fic volumes and compressions, and hydration numbers, including their temperature dependence. In a separate study, Chawla et. al (2021) examined the co-relation between EG, DEG, TEG with d-mannitol at diverse four temperatures using volumetric and acoustic processes. The authors considered utilised values of sound speed and density of glycols at different three concentrations in d-mannitol watery mixtures at T=(20, 25, 30 and 35)0C. The^{y} determined the values of Vϕ, Vϕ0, $_{K}\phi$,$s_{,}$ ^{a}nd $_{K0\phi,}$s which $_{reve}$aled the relations among d-mannitol and glycols. The study found that the solute-solvent interlinkage increases from EG to DEG to TEG, indicating a strong solute-solvent interlinkage that increases with an increase in molar concentration as well as with a rise in molar mass of glycols. The calculated properties also suggest a strong solute-solvent interlinkage.

CONCLUSION

Studying solutions that contain both polyols and other chemicals such as saccharides and many more in mixed aqueous media is a subject that generates a great deal of interest in both fundamental research and practical applications. These applications span several industries, including food science, pharmacy, chemical engineering, crystallization, and desalination. To gain valuable insights into the behaviour of these solutions, their volumetric properties can be analysed using both acoustic and thermodynamic methods. It is worth noting that various factors, such as temperature and pressure, can distress the thermodynamic and volumetric properties of these mixtures. Numerous properties can be determined through this analysis, including thermal expansion coefficients, isothermal coefficients of pressure excess molar enthalpy, Vϕ, Vϕ0, $K_{\phi,}$s, $_{an}{}^{d}$ K$0_{\phi,s,}$ at inf$_{nite}$ dilution. All of these properties have significant thermodynamic implications.

REFERENCES

Banipal, P. K., Arti, S., & Banipal, T. S. (2015). Influence of NH4Br on solvation behavior of polyhydroxy solutes in aqueous solutions at different temperatures and atmospheric pressure. Journal *of Chemical & Engineering Data, 60(4),* 1023–1047. doi:10.1021/je500886a

Bergua, F., Nuez, M., Muñoz-Embid, J., Lafuente, C., & Artal, M. (2018). Volumetric and acoustic behaviour of myo-inositol in aqueous Natural Deep Eutectic Solvent solutions. Journa*l of Molecular Liquids, 258,* 106–113. doi:10.1016/j.molliq.2018.02.128

Bernal, P., Brown, S., Mera, M., & Bouchibti, Y. (2019). Partial molar volumes and isentropic compressions of sugar alcohols in aqueous solutions from 15° C to 40°C at atmospheric pressure. Foo*d Chemistry, 280,* 164–174. doi:10.1016/j.foodchem.2018.11.120 PMID:30642483

Chakraborty, N., Juglan, K. C., & Kumar, H. (2020). Study of thermodynamic and acoustic properties of niacin in aqueous hexylene glycol and propylene glycol at different temperatures. *ACS Omega*, *5*(50), 32357–32365. doi:10.1021/acsomega.0c04292 PMID:33376872

Chakraborty, N., Kaur, K., Juglan, K. C., & Kumar, H. (2020). Volumetric and ultrasonic studies on interactions of glycols in aqueous solutions of xylitol at different ttemperatures. *Journal of Chemical & Engineering Data*, *65*(4), 1435–1446. doi:10.1021/acs.jced.9b00869

Chawla, D., Chakraborty, N., Juglan, K. C., & Kumar, H. (2021). Temperature-dependent physico-chemical studies of some glycols in aqueous d-mannitol solution. *Chemical Papers*, *75*(4), 1497–1506. doi:10.100711696-020-01403-y

Devunuri, N., Kancherla, S., Chennuri, B. K., & Gardas, R. L. (2016). Apparent molar volume and isentropic compressibilities of antidepressant drugs (Citalopram HBr and Escitalopram oxalate) with water. *Journal of Molecular Liquids*, *216*, 347–353. doi:10.1016/j.molliq.2016.01.058

Egas, A. P., Talavera-Prieto, N. M., Ferreira, A. G., Santos, J. B., Santos, M. J., Almeida, Z. L., & Fonseca, I. M. (2021). Speed of sound and derived thermodynamic properties of glycerol. *The Journal of Chemical Thermodynamics*, *156*, 106367. doi:10.1016/j.jct.2020.106367

Jengathe, S. P., Dhondge, S. S., Paliwal, L. J., Tangde, V. M., & Mondal, S. (2015). Effect of sodium chloride and myo-inositol on diphenhydramine hydrochloride drug in aqueous solution at different temperatures: Volumetric and acoustic approach. *The Journal of Chemical Thermodynamics*, *87*, 78–87. doi:10.1016/j.jct.2015.03.020

Jiang, X., Zhu, C., & Ma, Y. (2013). Densities and viscosities of erythritol, xylitol, and mannitol in l-ascorbic acid aqueous solutions at T=(293.15 to 323.15) K. *Journal of Chemical & Engineering Data*, *58*(11), 2970–2978. doi:10.1021/je400395u

Kaur, H., Chakraborty, N., Juglan, K. C., & Kumar, H. (2021). Volumetric and acoustic behavior of PEG-200 and PEG-600 in aqueous D-mannitol solutions at different temperatures. *Journal of Solution Chemistry*, *50*(8), 1079–1102. doi:10.100710953-021-01105-3

Kaur, K., Juglan, K. C., & Kumar, H. (2017). Investigation on temperature-dependent volumetric and acoustical properties of homologous series of glycols in aqueous sorbitol solutions. *Journal of Chemical & Engineering Data*, *62*(11), 3769–3782. doi:10.1021/acs.jced.7b00501

Krishna Bama, G., Anitha, R., & Ramachandran, K. (2010). On the thermal properties of aqueous solution of D-mannitol. *Nondestructive Testing and Evaluation*, *25*(1), 67–75. doi:10.1080/10589750902994407

Kumar, H., Kaur, K., Arti, S., & Singla, M. (2016). Study of thermodynamic properties of sodium dodecyl sulphate in aqueous solutions of alkoxyalkanols at different temperatures. *Journal of Molecular Liquids*, *221*, 526–534. doi:10.1016/j.molliq.2016.06.027

Longinotti, M. P., & Corti, H. R. (2004). Electrical conductivity and complexation of sodium borate in trehalose and sucrose aqueous solutions. *Journal of Solution Chemistry*, *33*(8), 1029–1040. doi:10.1023/B:JOSL.0000048053.92048.7b

Majka, J., Babiński, L., & Olek, W. (2017). Sorption isotherms of waterlogged subfossil Scots pine wood impregnated with a lactitol and trehalose mixture. *Holzforschung*, *71*(10), 813–819. doi:10.1515/hf-2017-0006

Naseem, B., Khan, M., & Jamal, M. A. (2016). Acoustical studies of pharmaceutical excipients in binary solvent mixtures. *Journal of Molecular Liquids, 220*, 581–591. doi:10.1016/j.molliq.2016.04.091

Park, Y. C., Oh, E. J., Jo, J. H., Jin, Y. S., & Seo, J. H. (2016). Recent advances in biological production of sugar alcohols. *Current Opinion in Biotechnology, 37*, 105–113. doi:10.1016/j.copbio.2015.11.006 PMID:26723007

Parthasarathy, L. K., Ratnam, L., Seelan, S., Tobias, C., Casanova, M. F., & Parthasarathy, R. N. (2006). Mammalian inositol 3-phosphate synthase: Its role in the biosynthesis of brain inositol and its clinical use as a psychoactive agent. Biology of Inositols and Phosphoinositides. *Sub-Cellular Biochemistry, 39*, 293–314. doi:10.1007/0-387-27600-9_12 PMID:17121280

Shahazidy, U., Jamal, M. A., Muneer, M., Naseem, B., & Qureshi, A. K. (2022). Elucidation of molecular interactions between sugar alcohol and dimethyl sulfoxide in aqueous system: Volumetric and acoustic study. *Journal of Molecular Liquids, 350*, 118543. doi:10.1016/j.molliq.2022.118543

Shi, Y., Zhu, C., Fu, T., Gao, X., & Ma, Y. (2020). Volumetric and Viscometric Properties of Maltitol in Glycylglycine Aqueous Solutions at T= 293.15–333.15 K. *Journal of Chemical & Engineering Data, 66*(1), 360–367. doi:10.1021/acs.jced.0c00731

Teo, G., Suzuki, Y., Uratsu, S. L., Lampinen, B., Ormonde, N., Hu, W. K., DeJong, T. M., & Dandekar, A. M. (2006). Silencing leaf sorbitol synthesis alters long-distance partitioning and apple fruit quality. *Proceedings of the National Academy of Sciences of the United States of America, 103*(49), 18842–18847. doi:10.1073/pnas.0605873103 PMID:17132742

Thirumaran, S., Suguna, M., & Selvi, S. R. (2009). Acoustic and Thermodynamic Studies of Ternary Liquid Mixtures at Different Temperatures. *Research Journal of Chemistry and Environment, 13*(3), 81–89.

Warmińska, D. (2012). Volumetric and acoustic properties of D-mannitol in aqueous sodium or magnesium chloride solutions over the temperature range of 293.15–313.15 K. *Carbohydrate Research, 349*, 44–51. doi:10.1016/j.carres.2011.12.004 PMID:22221791

Compilation of References

Abbasi, M., Sohail, M., Minhas, M. U., Mahmood, A., Shah, S. A., Munir, A., & Kashif, M.-U.-R. (2023). Folic acid-decorated alginate nanoparticles loaded hydrogel for the oral delivery of diferourylmethane in colorectal cancer. *International Journal of Biological Macromolecules, 233*, 123585. doi:10.1016/j.ijbiomac.2023.123585 PMID:36758757

Abd El- Salam, A. M., Tahoun, A., & Hanafy, N. A. N. (2023). Evaluation of liposomal hydrocolloidal NPs loaded by tea tree oil as antifungal agent in vitro and in vivo investigations: Preclinical studies. *Food Hydrocolloids for Health, 3*, 100136. doi:10.1016/j.fhfh.2023.100136

Abdalla, A. K., Ayyash, M. M., Olaimat, A. N., Osaili, T. M., Al-Nabulsi, A. A., Shah, N. P., & Holley, R. (2021). Exopolysaccharides as Antimicrobial Agents: Mechanism and Spectrum of Activity. *Frontiers in Microbiology, 12*, 12. doi:10.3389/fmicb.2021.664395 PMID:34093478

Abdallah, B., Elhissi, A. M. A., Ahmed, W., & Najlah, M. (2020). Carbon nanotube drug delivery system for cancer treatment. In *Advances in Medical and Surgical Engineering* (pp. 313–332). Elsevier. doi:10.1016/B978-0-12-819712-7.00016-4

Abdelkader, Y., Perez-Davalos, L., LeDuc, R., Zahedi, R. P., & Labouta, H. I. (2023). Omics Approaches for the Assessment of Biological Responses to Nanoparticles. *Advanced Drug Delivery Reviews, 114992*, 114992. doi:10.1016/j.addr.2023.114992 PMID:37414362

Abdollahiyan, P., Oroojalian, F., Hejazi, M., de la Guardia, M., & Mokhtarzadeh, A. (2021). Nanotechnology, and scaffold implantation for the effective repair of injured organs: An overview on hard tissue engineering. *Journal of Controlled Release, 333*, 391–417. doi:10.1016/j.jconrel.2021.04.003 PMID:33823222

Abed, A., Derakhshan, M., Karimi, M., Shirazinia, M., Mahjoubin-Tehran, M., Homayonfal, M., Hamblin, M. R., Mirzaei, S. A., Soleimanpour, H., Dehghani, S., Dehkordi, F. F., & Mirzaei, H. (2022). Platinum Nanoparticles in Biomedicine: Preparation, Anti-Cancer Activity, and Drug Delivery Vehicles. *Frontiers in Pharmacology, 13*, 797804. doi:10.3389/fphar.2022.797804 PMID:35281900

Abraham, A. N., Sharma, T. K., Bansal, V., & Shukla, R. (2018). Phytochemicals as Dynamic Surface Ligands to Control Nanoparticle-Protein Interactions. *ACS Omega, 3*(2), 2220–2229. doi:10.1021/acsomega.7b01878 PMID:30023827

Abruzzo, A., Parolin, C., Rossi, M., Vitali, B., Cappadone, C., & Bigucci, F. (2022). Development and Characterization of Azithromycin-Loaded Microemulsions: A Promising Tool for the Treatment of Bacterial Skin Infections. *Antibiotics (Basel, Switzerland), 11*(8), 1040. doi:10.3390/antibiotics11081040 PMID:36009909

Acunzo, A., Scardapane, E., De Luca, M., Marra, D., Velotta, R., & Minopoli, A. (2022). Plasmonic Nanomaterials for Colorimetric Biosensing: A Review. *Chemosensors (Basel, Switzerland), 10*(4), 136. doi:10.3390/chemosensors10040136

Adebayo, O. A., Akinloye, O., & Adaramoye, O. A. (2020). Cerium Oxide Nanoparticles Attenuate Oxidative Stress and Inflammation in the Liver of Diethylnitrosamine-Treated Mice. *Biological Trace Element Research*, *193*(1), 214–225. doi:10.100712011-019-01696-5 PMID:30993490

Adedoja, O. S., Sadiku, E. R., & Hamam, Y. (2023). An Overview of the Emerging Technologies and Composite Materials for Supercapacitors in Energy Storage Applications. *Polymers*, *15*(10), 2272. doi:10.3390/polym15102272 PMID:37242851

Adeli, M., Sarabi, R. S., Yadollahi Farsi, R., Mahmoudi, M., & Kalantari, M. (2011). Polyrotaxane/Gold Nanoparticle Hybrid Nanomaterials as Anticancer Drug Delivery Systems. *Journal of Materials Chemistry*, *18686*(21), 18686. doi:10.1039/c1jm12412a

Aderibigbe, B. A. (2017). Polymeric therapeutic delivery systems for the treatment of infectious diseases. *Therapeutic Delivery*, *8*(7), 557–576. doi:10.4155/tde-2017-0008 PMID:28633590

Adeyemi, J., Adekoya, O. K. O., Oluwasegun, S. T., Olugbenga, D. E., & Neerish, R. (2018). Band Structure, Morphology, Functionality, and Size- Dependent Properties of Metal Nanoparticles. In S. M. Singh & D. Bristow Alan (Eds.), *Noble and Precious Metals*. IntechOpen.

Agathokleous, E., Feng, Z., Iavicoli, I., & Calabrese, E. J. (2019). The two faces of nanomaterials: A quantification of hormesis in algae and plants. *Environment International*, *131*, 105044. doi:10.1016/j.envint.2019.105044 PMID:31362152

Agrawal, N., Saha, C., Kumar, C., Singh, R., Zhang, B., Jha, R., & Kumar, S. (2020). Detection of L-Cysteine Using Silver Nanoparticles and Graphene Oxide Immobilized Tapered SMS Optical Fiber Structure. *IEEE Sensors Journal*, *20*(19), 11372–11379. doi:10.1109/JSEN.2020.2997690

Agrawal, N., Saha, C., Kumar, C., Singh, R., Zhang, B., & Kumar, S. (2020). Development of Uric Acid Sensor Using Copper Oxide and Silver Nanoparticles Immobilized SMSMS Fiber Structure-Based Probe. *IEEE Transactions on Instrumentation and Measurement*, *69*(11), 9097–9104. doi:10.1109/TIM.2020.2998876

Agrawal, N., Saxena, R., Singh, L., Saha, C., & Kumar, S. (2022). Recent advancements in plasmonic optical biosensors: A review. *ISSS Journal of Micro and Smart Systems*, *11*(1), 31–42. doi:10.100741683-021-00079-0

Agrawal, N., Zhang, B., Saha, C., Kumar, C., Kaushik, B. K., & Kumar, S. (2020). Development of Dopamine Sensor Using Silver Nanoparticles and PEG-Functionalized Tapered Optical Fiber Structure. *IEEE Transactions on Biomedical Engineering*, *67*(6), 1542–1547. doi:10.1109/TBME.2019.2939560 PMID:31494542

Agrawal, N., Zhang, B., Saha, C., Kumar, C., Pu, X., & Kumar, S. (2020). Ultra-Sensitive Cholesterol Sensor Using Gold and Zinc-Oxide Nanoparticles Immobilized Core Mismatch MPM/SPS Probe. *Journal of Lightwave Technology*, *38*(8), 2523–2529. doi:10.1109/JLT.2020.2974818

Agrawal, S., & Kasturi, M. (2016). Hydrotropic solubilisation technique to challenge the solubility of poorly water soluble drug valsartan. *World Journal of Pharmaceutical Research*, *5*(8), 833–845. doi:10.20959/wjpr20168-6722

Agrawal, Y. O., Patil, K. D., More, K. R., Mohd Siddique, M. U., Alkahtani, S., Aljarba, N. H., & Hasnain, M. S. (2022). Amelioration of bioavailability through formulating and optimizing Azilsartan Entrapped nanostructured lipid carriers and its pharmacokinetic assessment. *Journal of Drug Delivery Science and Technology*, *77*, 103894. doi:10.1016/j.jddst.2022.103894

Aguilera-Garrido, A., Graván, P., Navarro-Marchal, S. A., Medina-O'Donnell, M., Parra, A., Gálvez-Ruiz, M. J., Marchal, J. A., & Galisteo-González, F. (2023). Maslinic acid solid lipid nanoparticles as hydrophobic anticancer drug carriers: Formulation, in vitro activity and in vivo biodistribution. *Biomedicine and Pharmacotherapy*, *163*, 114828. doi:10.1016/j.biopha.2023.114828 PMID:37163783

Ahangarpour, A., Oroojan, A. A., Khorsandi, L., Kouchak, M., & Badavi, M. (2019). Antioxidant, anti-apoptotic, and protective effects of myricitrin and its solid lipid nanoparticle on streptozotocin-nicotinamide-induced diabetic nephropathy in type 2 diabetic male mice. *Iranian Journal of Basic Medical Sciences.*, *22*(12), 1424. PMID:32133060

Ahmad, R., & Budnik, B. (2023). A review of the current state of single-cell proteomics and future perspective. *Analytical and Bioanalytical Chemistry*, *415*(28), 1–11. doi:10.100700216-023-04759-8 PMID:37285026

Ahmad, Z., Shah, A., Siddiq, M., & Kraatz, H.-B. (2014). Polymeric micelles as drug delivery vehicles. *RSC Advances*, *4*(33), 17028–17038. doi:10.1039/C3RA47370H

Aiello, C. D. (2023, May 15). Quantum physics proposes a new way to study biology – and the results could revolutionize our understanding of how life works. *The Conversation UK*. https://theconversation.com/quantum-physics-proposes-a-new-way-to-study-biology-and-the-results-could-revolutionize-our-understanding-of-how-life-works-204995

Akagi, T., Kaneko, T., Kida, T., & Akashi, M. (2005). Preparation and characterization of biodegradable nanoparticles based on poly (γ-glutamic acid) with L-phenylalanine as a protein carrier. *Journal of Controlled Release*, *108*(2-3), 226–236. doi:10.1016/j.jconrel.2005.08.003 PMID:16125267

Åkerman, M. E., Chan, W. C. W., Laakkonen, P., Bhatia, S. N., & Ruoslahti, E. (2002). Nanocrystal targeting in vivo. *Proceedings of the National Academy of Sciences of the United States of America*, *99*(20), 12617–12621. doi:10.1073/pnas.152463399 PMID:12235356

Akgunduz, M. C., Cavusoglu, K., & Yalsin, E. (2020). The Potential Risk Assessment of Phenoxyethanol with a Versatile Model System. *Journal of Experimental Orthopaedics*, *10*(1). PMID:31988350

Akouibaa, A., Masrour, R., Jabar, A., Benhamou, M., Ouarch, M., & Derouiche, A. (2022). Study of the Optical and Thermoplasmonics Properties of Gold Nanoparticle Embedded in Al(2)O(3) Matrix. *Plasmonics*, *17*(3), 1157–1169. doi:10.100711468-022-01607-w PMID:35228839

Al Osman, M., Yang, F., & Massey, I. Y. (2019). Exposure routes and health effects of heavy metals on children. *Biometals*, *32*(4), 563–573. doi:10.100710534-019-00193-5 PMID:30941546

Al-Ahmady, Z. S., & Ali-Boucetta, H. (2020). Nanomedicine & nanotoxicology future could be reshaped post-COVID-19 pandemic. *Frontiers in Nanotechnology*, *2*, 610465. doi:10.3389/fnano.2020.610465

Alamzadeh, Z., Beik, J., Mirrahimi, M., Shakeri-Zadeh, A., Ebrahimi, F., Komeili, A., Ghalandari, B., Ghaznavi, H., Kamrava, S. K., & Moustakis, C. (2020). Gold Nanoparticles Promote a Multimodal Synergistic Cancer Therapy Strategy by Co-Delivery of ThermoChemo-Radio Therapy. *European Journal of Pharmaceutical Sciences*, *105235*(145), 105235. doi:10.1016/j.ejps.2020.105235

Alaniz, L., Cabrera, P. V., Blanco, G., Ernst, G., Rimoldi, G., Alvarez, E., & Hajos, S. E. (2002). Interaction of CD44 with different forms of hyaluronic acid. Its role in adhesion and migration of tumor cells. *Cell Communication & Adhesion*, *9*(3), 117–130. doi:10.1080/15419060214522 PMID:12521133

Al-Awsi, G. R. L., Alameri, A. A., Al-Dhalimy, A. M. B., Gabr, G. A., & Kianfar, E. (2024). Application of nano-antibiotics in the diagnosis and treatment of infectious diseases. *Brazilian Journal of Biology*, *84*, e114828. doi:10.1590/1519-6984.264946 PMID:36722677

Albanese, A., Tang, P. S., & Chan, W. C. W. (2012). The Effect of Nanoparticle Size, Shape, and Surface Chemistry on Biological Systems. *Annual Review of Biomedical Engineering*, *14*(1), 1–16. doi:10.1146/annurev-bioeng-071811-150124 PMID:22524388

Aldosari, F. M. M. (2022). Characterization of Labeled Gold Nanoparticles for Surface-Enhanced Raman Scattering. *Molecules (Basel, Switzerland)*, *27*(3), 892. doi:10.3390/molecules27030892 PMID:35164155

Alexander, A., Saraf, S., Saraf, S., Agrawal, M., Patel, R. J., Agrawal, P., Khan, J., & Ajazuddin. (2019). Amalgamation of stem cells with nanotechnology: A unique therapeutic approach. *Current Stem Cell Research & Therapy*, *14*(2), 83–92. doi:10.2174/1574888X13666180703143219 PMID:29968543

Algburi, A., Al-Hasani, H. M., Ismael, T. K., Abdelhameed, A., Weeks, R., Ermakov, A. M., & Chikindas, M. L. (2021). Antimicrobial Activity of Bacillus subtilis KATMIRA1933 and Bacillus amyloliquefaciens B-1895 Against Staphylococcus aureus Biofilms Isolated from Wound Infection. *Probiotics and Antimicrobial Proteins*, *13*(1), 125–134. doi:10.100712602-020-09673-4 PMID:32556931

Ali Abuderman, A., Syed, R., & Alyousef, A., A., S. Alqahtani, M., Shamsul Ola, M., & Malik, A. (2019). Green synthesized silver Nanoparticles of Myrtus communis L (AgMC) extract inhibits cancer hallmarks via targeting aldose reductase (AR) and associated signaling network. *Processes (Basel, Switzerland)*, *7*(11), 860. doi:10.3390/pr7110860

Ali, A. A., Abuwatfa, W. H., Al-Sayah, M. H., & Husseini, G. A. (2022). Gold-Nanoparticle Hybrid Nanostructures for Multimodal Cancer Therapy. *Nanomaterials (Basel, Switzerland)*, *3706*(12), 3706. doi:10.3390/nano12203706

Ali, E. S., Sharker, S. M., Islam, M. T., Khan, I. N., Shaw, S., Rahman, M. A., Uddin, S. J., Shill, M. C., Rehman, S., Das, N., Ahmad, S., Shilpi, J. A., Tripathi, S., Mishra, S. K., & Mubarak, M. S. (2021). Targeting cancer cells with nanotherapeutics and nanodiagnostics: Current status and future perspectives. *Seminars in Cancer Biology*, *69*, 52–68. doi:10.1016/j.semcancer.2020.01.011

Ali, M. R. K., Wu, Y., Ghosh, D., Do, B. H., Chen, K., Dawson, M. R., Fang, N., Sulchek, T. A., & El-Sayed, M. A. (2017). Nuclear Membrane-Targeted Gold Nanoparticles Inhibit Cancer CellMigration and Invasion. *ACS Nano*, *11*(4), 3716–3726. doi:10.1021/acsnano.6b08345 PMID:28333438

Alimov, U., Zhao, K., Hu, J., Guo, Y., Meng, L., Pan, X., & Deng, T. (2021). Volumetric properties of disodium dihydrogen pyrophosphate aqueous solution from 283.15 to 363.15 K at 101.325 kPa. *Food Chemistry*, *352*, 129410. doi:10.1016/j.foodchem.2021.129410 PMID:33677210

Alizadeh Sani, M., Maleki, M., Eghbaljoo-Gharehgheshlaghi, H., Khezerlou, A., Mohammadian, E., Liu, Q., & Jafari, S. M. (2022). Titanium dioxide nanoparticles as multifunctional surface-active materials for smart/active nanocomposite packaging films. *Advances in Colloid and Interface Science*, *300*, 102593. doi:10.1016/j.cis.2021.102593 PMID:34971916

Aljohani, A. A., Alanazi, M. A., Munahhi, L. A., Hamroon, J. D., Mortagi, Y., Qushawy, M., & Soliman, G. M. (2023). Binary ethosomes for the enhanced topical delivery and antifungal efficacy of ketoconazole. *OpenNano*, *11*, 100145. doi:10.1016/j.onano.2023.100145

Alkilany, A. M., Thompson, L. B., Boulos, S. P., Sisco, P. N., & Murphy, C. J. (2012). Gold nanorods: Their potential for photothermal therapeutics and drug delivery is tempered by the complexity of their biological interactions. *Advanced Drug Delivery Reviews*, *64*(2), 190–199. doi:10.1016/j.addr.2011.03.005 PMID:21397647

Allam, A., El-Mokhtar, M. A., & Elsabahy, M. (2019). Vancomycin-loaded niosomes integrated within pH-sensitive in-situ forming gel for treatment of ocular infections while minimizing drug irritation. *The Journal of Pharmacy and Pharmacology*, *71*(8), 1209–1221. doi:10.1111/jphp.13106 PMID:31124593

Allémann, E., Gurny, R., & Doelker, E. (1992). Preparation of aqueous polymeric nanodispersions by a reversible salting-out process: Influence of process parameters on particle size. *International Journal of Pharmaceutics*, *87*(1-3), 247–253. doi:10.1016/0378-5173(92)90249-2

Allen, R. P., Bolandparvaz, A., Ma, J. A., Manickam, V. A., & Lewis, J. S. (2018). Latent, Immunosuppressive Nature of Poly (lactic-co-glycolic acid) Microparticles. *ACS Biomaterials Science & Engineering*, *4*(3), 900–918. doi:10.1021/acsbiomaterials.7b00831 PMID:30555893

Allouche, J. (2013). Synthesis of organic and bioorganic nanoparticles: an overview of the preparation methods. *Nanomaterials: a danger or a promise?* 27-74.

Almawash, S. (2023). Solid lipid nanoparticles, an effective carrier for classical antifungal drugs. *Saudi Pharmaceutical Journal*, *31*(7), 1167–1180. doi:10.1016/j.jsps.2023.05.011 PMID:37273269

Alnasser, S. M. (2022). Stem cell challenge in cancer progression, oncology and therapy. *Gene*, *146748*, 146748. doi:10.1016/j.gene.2022.146748 PMID:35868413

Al-Sheddi, E. S., Farshori, N. N., Al-Oqail, M. M., Al-Massarani, S. M., Saquib, Q., Wahab, R., Musarrat, J., Al-Khedhairy, A. A., & Siddiqui, M. A. (2018). Anticancer Potential of Green Synthesized Silver Nanoparticles Using Extract of Nepeta deflersiana against Human Cervical Cancer Cells (HeLA). *Bioinorganic Chemistry and Applications*, *9390784*, 1–12. doi:10.1155/2018/9390784 PMID:30515193

Alvares, D., Wieczorek, L., Raguse, B., Ladouceur, F., & Lovell, N. H. (2013). Development of nanoparticle film-based multi-axial tactile sensors for biomedical applications. *Sensors and Actuators. A, Physical*, *196*, 38–47. doi:10.1016/j.sna.2013.03.021

Álvarez, M. S., Deive, F. J., Longo, M. A., Rodriguez, A., Segade, L., & Cabeza, O. (2023). Physico-chemical characterization of methanolic mixtures of cholinium dihydrogen phosphate-based DES. *Journal of Molecular Liquids*, *383*, 122024. doi:10.1016/j.molliq.2023.122024

Alven, S., Nqoro, X., Buyana, B., & Aderibigbe, B. A. (2020). Polymer-drug conjugate, a potential therapeutic to combat breast and lung cancer. *Pharmaceutics*, *12*(5), 406. doi:10.3390/pharmaceutics12050406 PMID:32365495

Alzoubi, F. Y., Abu Noqta, O., Al Zoubi, T., Al-Khateeb, H. M., Alqadi, M. K., Abuelsamen, A., & Makhadmeh, G. N. (2023). A Novel One-Pot Synthesis of PVP-Coated Iron Oxide Nanoparticles as Biocompatible Contrast Agents for Enhanced T2-Weighted MRI. *Journal of Composites Science*, *7*(3), 131. doi:10.3390/jcs7030131

Åmand, H. L., Rydberg, H. A., Fornander, L. H., Lincoln, P., Nordén, B., & Esbjörner, E. K. (2012). Cell surface binding and uptake of arginine- and lysine-rich penetratin peptides in absence and presence of proteoglycans. *Biochimica et Biophysica Acta. Biomembranes*, *1818*(11), 2669–2678. doi:10.1016/j.bbamem.2012.06.006 PMID:22705501

Ambrogi, V., Carfagna, C., Cerruti, P., & Marturano, V. (2017). Additives in Polymers. In Modification of Polymer Properties (pp. 87–108). Elsevier. doi:10.1016/B978-0-323-44353-1.00004-X

Andreani, T., Kiill, C. P., de Souza, A. L. R., Fangueiro, J. F., Doktorovová, S., Garcia, M. L., Gramião, M. P. D., Silva, A. M., & Souto, E. B. (2015). Effect of cryoprotectants on the reconstitution of silica nanoparticles produced by sol–gel technology. *Journal of Thermal Analysis and Calorimetry*, *120*(1), 1001–1007. doi:10.100710973-014-4275-4

Andreiuk, B., Reisch, A., Lindecker, M., Follain, G., Peyriéras, N., Goetz, J. G., & Klymchenko, A. S. (2017). Fluorescent polymer nanoparticles for cell barcoding in vitro and in vivo. *Small*, *13*(38), 1701582. doi:10.1002mll.201701582

An, H., Deng, X., Wang, F., Xu, P., & Wang, N. (2023). Dendrimers as Nanocarriers for the Delivery of Drugs Obtained from Natural Products. *Polymers*, *15*(10), 2292. doi:10.3390/polym15102292 PMID:37242865

Anjum, S., Ishaque, S., Fatima, H., Farooq, W., Hano, C., Abbasi, B. H., & Anjum, I. (2021). Emerging Applications of Nanotechnology in Healthcare Systems: Grand Challenges and Perspectives. *Pharmaceuticals (Basel, Switzerland)*, *14*(8), 707. doi:10.3390/ph14080707 PMID:34451803

Anselmo, A. C., & Mitragotri, S. (2019). Nanoparticles in the clinic: An update. *Bioengineering & Translational Medicine*, *4*(3), e10143. Advance online publication. doi:10.1002/btm2.10143

Antonio, J. R., Antônio, C. R., Cardeal, I. L., Ballavenuto, J. M., & Oliveira, J. R. (2014). Nanotechnology in dermatology. *Anais Brasileiros de Dermatologia*, *89*(1), 126–136. doi:10.1590/abd1806-4841.20142228 PMID:24626657

Anuchapreeda, S., Fukumori, Y., Okonogi, S., & Ichikawa, H. (2012). Preparation of lipid nanoemulsions incorporating curcumin for cancer therapy. *Journal of Nanotechnology*, *2012*, 2012. doi:10.1155/2012/270383

Araujo, F., Shrestha, N., Gomes, M. J., Herranz-Blanco, B., Liu, D., Hirvonen, J. J., Granja, P. L., Santos, H. A., & Sarmento, B. (2016). In vivo dual-delivery of glucagon like peptide-1 (GLP-1) and dipeptidyl peptidase-4 (DPP4) inhibitor through composites prepared by microfluidics for diabetes therapy. *Nanoscale*, *8*(20), 10706–10713. doi:10.1039/C6NR00294C PMID:27150301

Ardizzone, A., Kurhuzenkau, S., Illa-Tuset, S., Faraudo, J., Bondar, M., Hagan, D., & Ventosa, N. (2018). Nanostructuring Lipophilic Dyes in Water Using Stable Vesicles, Quatsomes, as Scaffolds and Their Use as Probes for Bioimaging. *Small*, *14*(16), e1703851. doi:10.1002mll.201703851 PMID:29573545

Arendowski, A., Nizioł, J., Ossoliński, K., Ossolińska, A., Ossoliński, T., Dobrowolski, Z., & Ruman, T. (2018). Laser desorption/ionization MS imaging of cancer kidney tissue on silver nanoparticle-enhanced target. *Bioanalysis*, *10*(2), 83–94. doi:10.4155/bio-2017-0195 PMID:29239663

Arias-Hidalgo, C., Juanes-Velasco, P., Landeira-Viñuela, A., García-Vaquero, M. L., Montalvillo, E., Góngora, R., Hernández, A., & Fuentes, M. (2022). Single-Cell Proteomics: The Critical Role of Nanotechnology. *International Journal of Molecular Sciences*, *23*(12), 6707. doi:10.3390/ijms23126707 PMID:35743151

Arikan, K., Burhan, H., Bayat, R., & Sen, F. (2022). Glucose nano biosensor with non-enzymatic excellent sensitivity prepared with nickel–cobalt nanocomposites on f-MWCNT. *Chemosphere*, *291*, 132720. doi:10.1016/j.chemosphere.2021.132720 PMID:34743867

Arndt, M., Juffmann, T., & Vedral, V. (2009). Quantum physics meets biology. *HFSP Journal*, *3*(6), 386–400. doi:10.2976/1.3244985 PMID:20234806

Arokiaraj, R. G., Ravikumar, S., Raju, R., Losetty, V., Bhanuprakash, P., & Pandiyan, V. (2022). Investigation of solute-solvent interactions between 2-butoxyethanol and substituted ketones by volumetric, acoustic and FTIR studies at T=(303.15–318.15) K. *Chemical Thermodynamics and Thermal Analysis*, *6*, 100049. doi:10.1016/j.ctta.2022.100049

Arshad, R., Barani, M., Rahdar, A., Sargazi, S., Cucchiarini, M., Pandey, S., & Kang, M. (2021). Multi-functionalized nanomaterials and nanoparticles for diagnosis and treatment of retinoblastoma. *Biosensors (Basel)*, *11*(4), 97. doi:10.3390/bios11040097 PMID:33810621

Asad, S., Jacobsen, A.-C., & Teleki, A. (2022). Inorganic nanoparticles for oral drug delivery: Opportunities, barriers, and future perspectives. *Current Opinion in Chemical Engineering*, *38*, 100869. doi:10.1016/j.coche.2022.100869

Asharani, P., Hande, M. P., & Valiyaveettil, S. (2009). Anti-proliferative activity of silver nanoparticles. *BMC Cell Biology*, *10*(1), 1–14. doi:10.1186/1471-2121-10-65 PMID:19761582

Asl, F. D., Mousazadeh, M., Taji, S., Bahmani, A., Khashayar, P., Azimzadeh, M., & Mostafavi, E. (2023). Nano drug-delivery systems for management of AIDS: Liposomes, dendrimers, gold and silver nanoparticles. *Nanomedicine (London)*, *18*(3), 279–302. doi:10.2217/nnm-2022-0248 PMID:37125616

Attama, A. A., Agbo, C. P., Onokala, O. B., Kenechukwu, F. C., Ugwueze, M. E., Mbah, C. C., Umeryor, C. E., Uronnachi, E. M., & Nnamani, P. O. (2023). Applications of nanoemulsions as drug delivery vehicle for phytoconstituents. In S. Thomas, A. O. Oyedeji, O. S. Oluwafemi, & R. Jaquilin Pj (Eds.), *Nanotechnology in Herbal Medicine* (pp. 119–194). Woodhead Publishing. doi:10.1016/B978-0-323-99527-6.00017-3

Attar, E. S., Chaudhari, V. H., Deokar, C. G., Dyawanapelly, S., & Devarajan, P. V. (2023). Nano Drug Delivery Strategies for an Oral Bioenhanced Quercetin Formulation. *European Journal of Drug Metabolism and Pharmacokinetics*, *48*(5), 1–20. doi:10.100713318-023-00843-7 PMID:37523008

Attia, M. F., Anton, N., Wallyn, J., Omran, Z., & Vandamme, T. F. (2019). An overview of active and passive targeting strategies to improve the nanocarriers efficiency to tumour sites. *The Journal of Pharmacy and Pharmacology*, *71*(8), 1185–1198. doi:10.1111/jphp.13098

Attia, M. S., Yahya, A., Monaem, N. A., & Sabry, S. A. (2023). Mesoporous silica nanoparticles: Their potential as drug delivery carriers and nanoscavengers in Alzheimer's and Parkinson's diseases. *Saudi Pharmaceutical Journal*, *31*(3), 417–432. doi:10.1016/j.jsps.2023.01.009 PMID:37026045

Avasthi, A., Caro, C., Pozo-Torres, E., Leal, M. P., & García-Martín, M. L. (2020). Magnetic Nanoparticles as MRI Contrast Agents. *Topics in Current Chemistry (Cham)*, *378*(3), 40. doi:10.100741061-020-00302-w PMID:32382832

Avgoustakis, K., Beletsi, A., Panagi, Z., Klepetsanis, P., Karydas, A. G., & Ithakissios, D. S. (2002). PLGA–mPEG nanoparticles of cisplatin: In vitro nanoparticle degradation, vitro drug release, and in vivo drug residence in blood properties. *Journal of Controlled Release*, *79*(1-3), 123–135. doi:10.1016/S0168-3659(01)00530-2 PMID:11853924

Ayala-Orozco, C., Urban, C., Bishnoi, S., Urban, A., Charron, H., Mitchell, T., Shea, M., Nanda, S., Schiff, R., Halas, N., & Joshi, A. (2014). Sub-100nm gold nanomatryoshkas improve photo-thermal therapy efficacy in large and highly aggressive triple negative breast tumors. *Journal of Controlled Release*, *191*, 90–97. doi:10.1016/j.jconrel.2014.07.038 PMID:25051221

Aydoğan, C., Beltekin, B., Aslan, H., Yılmaz, F., Göktürk, I., Denizli, A., & El-Rassi, Z. (2022). Nanoscale separations: Recent achievements. *Journal of Chromatography Open*, *2*, 100066. doi:10.1016/j.jcoa.2022.100066

Badıllı, U., Mollarasouli, F., Bakirhan, N. K., Ozkan, Y., & Ozkan, S. A. (2020). Role of quantum dots in pharmaceutical and biomedical analysis, and its application in drug delivery. *Trends in Analytical Chemistry*, *131*, 116013. doi:10.1016/j.trac.2020.116013

Baetke, S. C., Lammers, T., & Kiessling, F. (2015). Applications of nanoparticles for diagnosis and therapy of cancer. *The British Journal of Radiology*, *88*(1054), 20150207. doi:10.1259/bjr.20150207 PMID:25969868

Bagherzadeh, S. A., Jalali, E., Sarafraz, M. M., Ali Akbari, O., Karimipour, A., Goodarzi, M., & Bach, Q. V. (2020). Effects of magnetic field on micro cross jet injection of dispersed nanoparticles in a microchannel. *International Journal of Numerical Methods for Heat & Fluid Flow*, *30*(5), 2683–2704. doi:10.1108/HFF-02-2019-0150

Bahrami, A. H., & Weikl, T. R. (2018). Curvature-Mediated Assembly of Janus Nanoparticles on Membrane Vesicles. *Nano Letters*, *18*(2), 1259–1263. doi:10.1021/acs.nanolett.7b04855 PMID:29281291

Bahrami, B., Hojjat-Farsangi, M., Mohammadi, H., Anvari, E., Ghalamfarsa, G., Yousefi, M., & Jadidi-Niaragh, F. (2017). Nanoparticles and targeted drug delivery in cancer therapy. *Immunology Letters*, *190*, 64–83. doi:10.1016/j.imlet.2017.07.015 PMID:28760499

Baig, N., Kammakakam, I., & Falath, W. (2021). Nanomaterials: A review of synthesis methods, properties, recent progress, and challenges. *Materials Advances*, *2*(6), 1821–1871. doi:10.1039/D0MA00807A

Bajwa, K. S., Ali, M. A., Tahir, A., Abbas, H., Ahmad, H., Abid, L., Rana, M. B. U., & Rubab, W. (2018). Nanotechnology: A Triumphant Leap in Health Care and Medicine. *Life Science Journal*, *15*(7). doi:10.7537/marslsj150718.09

Bakr, E. A., Gaber, M., Saad, D. R., & Salahuddin, N. (2023). Comparative study between two different morphological structures based on polylactic acid, nanocellulose and magnetite for co-delivery of flurouracil and curcumin. *International Journal of Biological Macromolecules*, *230*, 123315. doi:10.1016/j.ijbiomac.2023.123315 PMID:36708892

Bakry, R., Vallant, R. M., Najam-ul-Haq, M., Rainer, M., Szabo, Z., Huck, C. W., & Bonn, G. K. (2007). Medicinal applications of fullerenes. *International Journal of Nanomedicine*, *2*(4), 639–649. doi:10.2147/IJN.S2.4.639 PMID:18203430

Balcucho, J., Narváez, D. M., & Castro-Mayorga, J. L. (2020). Antimicrobial and Biocompatible Polycaprolactone and Copper Oxide Nanoparticle Wound Dressings against Methicillin-Resistant Staphylococcus aureus. *Nanomaterials (Basel, Switzerland)*, *10*(9), 1692. doi:10.3390/nano10091692 PMID:32872095

Banerjee, A. N. (2018). Graphene and its derivatives as biomedical materials: Future prospects and challenges. *Interface Focus*, *8*(3), 20170056. Advance online publication. doi:10.1098/rsfs.2017.0056 PMID:29696088

Banik, B. L., Fattahi, P., & Brown, J. L. (2016). Polymeric nanoparticles: The future of nanomedicine. *Wiley Interdisciplinary Reviews. Nanomedicine and Nanobiotechnology*, *8*(2), 271–299. doi:10.1002/wnan.1364 PMID:26314803

Banipal, P. K., Arti, S., & Banipal, T. S. (2015). Influence of NH4Br on solvation behavior of polyhydroxy solutes in aqueous solutions at different temperatures and atmospheric pressure. *Journal of Chemical & Engineering Data*, *60*(4), 1023–1047. doi:10.1021/je500886a

Banipal, T. S., Kaur, D., Banipal, P. K., & Singh, G. (2007). Thermodynamic and transport properties of l-serine and l-threonine in aqueous sodium acetate and magnesium acetate solutions at T= 298.15 K. *The Journal of Chemical Thermodynamics*, *39*(3), 371–384. doi:10.1016/j.jct.2006.08.003

Bao, Q.-Y., Zhang, N., Geng, D.-D., Xue, J.-W., Merritt, M., Zhang, C., & Ding, Y. (2014). The Enhanced Longevity and Liver Targetability of Paclitaxel by Hybrid Liposomes Encapsulating Paclitaxel-Conjugated Gold Nanoparticles. *International Journal of Pharmaceutics*, *477*(1-2), 408–415. doi:10.1016/j.ijpharm.2014.10.040

Barabadi, H., Najafi, M., Samadian, H., Azarnezhad, A., Vahidi, H., Mahjoub, M. A., Koohiyan, M., & Ahmadi, A. (2019). A systematic review of the genotoxicity and antigenotoxicity of biologically synthesized metallic nanomaterials: Are green nanoparticles safe enough for clinical marketing? *Medicina*, *55*(8), 439. doi:10.3390/medicina55080439 PMID:31387257

Barcińska, E., Wierzbicka, J., Zauszkiewicz-Pawlak, A., Jacewicz, D., Dabrowska, A., & Inkielewicz-Stepniak, I. (2018). Role of oxidative and nitro-oxidative damage in silver nanoparticles cytotoxic effect against human pancreatic ductal adenocarcinoma cells. *Oxidative Medicine and Cellular Longevity*, *2018*, 1–15. doi:10.1155/2018/8251961 PMID:30186549

Barenholz, Y. (2012). Doxil®—the first FDA-approved nano-drug: Lessons learned. *Journal of Controlled Release*, *160*(2), 117–134. doi:10.1016/j.jconrel.2012.03.020

Bargh, J. D., Isidro-Llobet, A., Parker, J. S., & Spring, D. R. (2019, August 12). Cleavable linkers in antibody-drug conjugates. *Chemical Society Reviews*, *48*(16), 4361–4374. doi:10.1039/C8CS00676H PMID:31294429

Bariwal, J., Ma, H., Altenberg, G. A., & Liang, H. (2022). Nanodiscs: A versatile nanocarrier platform for cancer diagnosis and treatment. *Chemical Society Reviews*, *51*(5), 1702–1728. doi:10.1039/D1CS01074C PMID:35156110

Barratt, G. M. (2000). Therapeutic applications of colloidal drug carriers. *Pharmaceutical Science & Technology Today*, *3*(5), 163–171. doi:10.1016/S1461-5347(00)00255-8 PMID:10785658

Barrett, T., Ravizzini, G., Choyke, P., & Kobayashi, H. (2009). Dendrimers in medical nanotechnology. *IEEE Engineering in Medicine and Biology Magazine*, *28*(1), 12–22. doi:10.1109/MEMB.2008.931012 PMID:19150767

Barua, R., Banerjee, D., & Bhowmik, S. (2022). Study of the Potential Impact of Microplastics and Additives on Human Health. In S. Joo (Ed.), *Assessing the Effects of Emerging Plastics on the Environment and Public Health* (pp. 128–147). IGI Global. doi:10.4018/978-1-7998-9723-1.ch007

Barua, R., Datta, S., Chowdhury, A. R., & Datta, P. (2018). Advances in MEMS and Micro-Scale technologies for application in controlled Drug-Dosing systems: MEMS-Based drug delivery systems. In *Design and Development of Affordable Healthcare Technologies* (pp. 165–179). IGI Global. doi:10.4018/978-1-5225-4969-7.ch007

Barua, R., Datta, S., & Das, J. (2020). Application of Nanotechnology in Global Issues. In M. Merviö (Ed.), *Global Issues and Innovative Solutions in Healthcare, Culture, and the Environment* (pp. 292–300). IGI Global. doi:10.4018/978-1-7998-3576-9.ch015

Barua, R., Roychowdhury, A., & Datta, P. (2022). Study of Different Additive Manufacturing Processes and Emergent Applications in Modern Healthcare. In R. Thanigaivelan, N. Rajan, & T. Argul (Eds.), *Advanced Manufacturing Techniques for Engineering and Engineered Materials* (pp. 239–259). IGI Global. doi:10.4018/978-1-7998-9574-9.ch014

Barua, S., & Mitragotri, S. (2014). Challenges associated with penetration of nanoparticles across cell and tissue barriers: A review of current status and future prospects. *Nano Today*, *9*(2), 223–243. doi:10.1016/j.nantod.2014.04.008 PMID:25132862

Barwal, I., Sood, A., Sharma, M., Singh, B., & Yadav, S. C. (2013). Development of stevioside Pluronic-F-68 copolymer based PLA-nanoparticles as an antidiabetic nanomedicine. *Colloids and Surfaces. B, Biointerfaces*, *101*, 510–516. doi:10.1016/j.colsurfb.2012.07.005 PMID:23022553

Barz, M. (2015). Complexity and simplification in the development of nanomedicines. *Nanomedicine (London)*, *10*(20), 3093–3097. doi:10.2217/nnm.15.146 PMID:26446374

Bashkeran, T., Kamaruddin, A. H., Ngo, T. X., Suda, K., Umakoshi, H., Watanabe, N., & Nadzir, M. M. (2023). Niosomes in cancer treatment: A focus on curcumin encapsulation. *Heliyon*, *18710*(8), e18710. Advance online publication. doi:10.1016/j.heliyon.2023.e18710 PMID:37593605

Baskar, R., Lee, K. A., Yeo, R., & Yeoh, K. W. (2012). Cancer and Radiation Therapy: Current Advances and Future Directions. *International Journal of Medical Sciences*, *9*(3), 193–199. doi:10.7150/ijms.3635

Batist, G., Gelmon, K. A., Chi, K. N., Miller, W. H. Jr, Chia, S. K., Mayer, L. D., Swenson, C. E., Janoff, A. S., & Louie, A. C. (2009). Safety, pharmacokinetics, and efficacy of CPX-1 liposome injection in patients with advanced solid tumors. *Clinical Cancer Research*, *15*(2), 692–700. doi:10.1158/1078-0432.CCR-08-0515

Bayda, S., Adeel, M., Tuccinardi, T., Cordani, M., & Rizzolio, F. (2019). The History of Nanoscience and Nanotechnology: From Chemical-Physical Applications to Nanomedicine. *Molecules (Basel, Switzerland)*, *25*(1), 112. doi:10.3390/molecules25010112 PMID:31892180

Bazak, R., Houri, M., El Achy, S., Kamel, S., & Refaat, T. (2015). Cancer active targeting by nanoparticles: A comprehensive review of literature. *Journal of Cancer Research and Clinical Oncology*, *141*(5), 769–784. doi:10.100700432-014-1767-3

Bedhiafi, T., Idoudi, S., Alhams, A. A., Fernandes, Q., Iqbal, H., Basineni, R., Uddin, S., Dermime, S., Merhi, M., & Billa, N. (2023). Applications of polydopaminic nanomaterials in mucosal drug delivery. *Journal of Controlled Release*, *353*, 842–849. doi:10.1016/j.jconrel.2022.12.037 PMID:36529384

Begines, B., Ortiz, T., Pérez-Aranda, M., Martínez, G., Merinero, M., Argüelles-Arias, F., & Alcudia, A. (2020). Polymeric nanoparticles for drug delivery: Recent developments and future prospects. *Nanomaterials (Basel, Switzerland)*, *10*(7), 1403. doi:10.3390/nano10071403 PMID:32707641

Beheshtizadeh, N., Salimi, A., Golmohammadi, M., Ansari, J. M., & Azami, M. (2023). In-silico engineering of RNA nanoplatforms to promote the diabetic wound healing. *BMC Chemistry*, *17*(1), 52. doi:10.118613065-023-00969-4 PMID:37291669

Behzadi, S., Serpooshan, V., Tao, W., Hamaly, M. A., Alkawareek, M. Y., Dreaden, E. C., Brown, D., Alkilany, A. M., Farokhzad, O. C., & Mahmoudi, M. (2017). Cellular uptake of nanoparticles: Journey inside the cell. *Chemical Society Reviews*, *46*(14), 4218–4244. doi:10.1039/C6CS00636A PMID:28585944

Beletsi, A., Leontiadis, L., Klepetsanis, P., Ithakissios, D. S., & Avgoustakis, K. (1999). Effect of preparative variables on the properties of poly (dl-lactide-co-glycolide)–methoxy poly (ethylene glycol) copolymers related to their application in controlled drug delivery. *International Journal of Pharmaceutics*, *182*(2), 187–197. doi:10.1016/S0378-5173(99)00058-7 PMID:10341308

Bennet, D., & Kim, S. (2014). *Polymer nanoparticles for smart drug delivery* (*Vol. 8*).

Bennet, D., & Kim, S. (2013). A transdermal delivery system to enhance quercetin nanoparticle permeability. *Journal of Biomaterials Science. Polymer Edition*, *24*(2), 185–209. doi:10.1163/156856212X630258 PMID:23565597

Benoit, D. S., Overby, C. T., Sims, K. R., Jr., & Ackun-Farmmer, M. A. Biomaterials Science. Elsevier; Amsterdam, The Netherlands:2020. Drug delivery systems; pp. 1237–1266.

Benyettou F, Motte L. Nanomedicine: towards the "magic bullet" science. J Bioanal Biomed. 2016;8:2.11.

Berger, D., Rakhamimova, A., Pollack, A., & Loewy, Z. (2018). Oral Biofilms: Development, Control, and Analysis. *High-Throughput*, *7*, 1–8. doi:10.3390/ht7030024 PMID:30200379

Bergua, F., Nuez, M., Muñoz-Embid, J., Lafuente, C., & Artal, M. (2018). Volumetric and acoustic behaviour of myo-inositol in aqueous Natural Deep Eutectic Solvent solutions. *Journal of Molecular Liquids*, *258*, 106–113. doi:10.1016/j.molliq.2018.02.128

Bernabeu, S., Ratnam, K. C., Boutal, H., Gonzalez, C., Vogel, A., Devilliers, K., Plaisance, M., Oueslati, S., Malhotra-Kumar, S., Dortet, L., Fortineau, N., Simon, S., Volland, H., & Naas, T. (2020). A Lateral Flow Immunoassay for the Rapid Identification of CTX-M-Producing Enterobacterales from Culture Plates and Positive Blood Cultures. *Diagnostics (Basel)*, *10*(10), 764. doi:10.3390/diagnostics10100764 PMID:32998433

Bernal, P., Brown, S., Mera, M., & Bouchibti, Y. (2019). Partial molar volumes and isentropic compressions of sugar alcohols in aqueous solutions from 15° C to 40°C at atmospheric pressure. *Food Chemistry*, *280*, 164–174. doi:10.1016/j.foodchem.2018.11.120 PMID:30642483

Bernard, M.-C., Bazin, E., Petiot, N., Lemdani, K., Commandeur, S., Verdelet, C., Margot, S., Perkov, V., Ripoll, M., Garinot, M., Ruiz, S., Boudet, F., Rokbi, B., & Haensler, J. (2023). The impact of nucleoside base modification in mRNA vaccine is influenced by the chemistry of its lipid nanoparticle delivery system. *Molecular Therapy. Nucleic Acids*, *32*, 794–806. doi:10.1016/j.omtn.2023.05.004 PMID:37346973

Betancor, L., & Luckarift, H. R. (2008). Bioinspired enzyme encapsulation for biocatalysis. *Trends in Biotechnology*, *26*(10), 566–572. doi:10.1016/j.tibtech.2008.06.009 PMID:18757108

Beyene, H. D., Werkneh, A. A., Bezabh, H. K., & Ambaye, T. G. (2017). Synthesis paradigm and applications of silver nanoparticles (AgNPs), a review. *Sustainable materials and technologies*, *13*, 18-23.

Bhakri, K., Chakraborty, N., Juglan, K. C., & Kumar, H. (2023). Investigation of Volumetric and Acoustical Properties of Polyethylene Glycols in Niacin Solutions. *Journal of Physics: Conference Series*, *12*(3).

Bhakri, K., Chakraborty, N., Juglan, K. C., Kumar, H., & Sharma, R. (2023). Thermodynamic behaviour and physicochemical characteristics of EG, DEG, TEG in aqueous gluconolactone solutions. *Journal of Thermal Analysis and Calorimetry*, *148*(14), 7185–7205. doi:10.100710973-023-12223-z

Bhakta, P., & Barthunia, B. (2020). Fullerene and its applications: A review. *Journal of Indian Academy of Oral Medicine and Radiology*, *32*(2), 159–163. doi:10.4103/jiaomr.jiaomr_191_19

Bhandari, G., Dhasmana, A., Chaudhary, P., Gupta, S., Gangola, S., Gupta, A., Rustagi, S., Shende, S. S., Rajput, V. D., Minkina, T., Malik, S., & Slama, P. (2023). A Perspective Review on Green Nanotechnology in Agro-Ecosystems: Opportunities for Sustainable Agricultural Practices & Environmental Remediation. *Agriculture*, *13*(3), 668. doi:10.3390/agriculture13030668

Bharathala, S., & Sharma, P. (2019). Biomedical applications of nanoparticles. In *Nanotechnology in Modern Animal Biotechnology: Concepts and Applications*. Elsevier. doi:10.1016/B978-0-12-818823-1.00008-9

Bharathiraja, S., Bui, N. Q., Manivasagan, P., Moorthy, M. S., Mondal, S., Seo, H., Phuoc, N. T., Vy Phan, T. T., Kim, H., Lee, K. D., & Oh, J. (2018). Multimodal tumor-homing chitosan oligosaccharide-coated biocompatible palladium nanoparticles for photo-based imaging and therapy. *Scientific Reports*, *8*(1), 500. doi:10.103841598-017-18966-8

Bharti, C., Gulati, N., Nagaich, U., & Pal, A. (2015). Mesoporous silica nanoparticles in target drug delivery system: A review. *International Journal of Pharmaceutical Investigation*, *5*(3), 124. doi:10.4103/2230-973X.160844 PMID:26258053

Bhatia, S. N., Chen, X., Dobrovolskaia, M. A., & Lammers, T. (2022). Cancer nanomedicine. *Nature Reviews. Cancer*, *22*(10), 550–556. doi:10.103841568-022-00496-9

Bhattacharya, R., & Mukherjee, P. (2008). Biological properties of "naked" metal nanoparticles. *Advanced Drug Delivery Reviews*, *60*(11), 1289–1306. doi:10.1016/j.addr.2008.03.013 PMID:18501989

Bhowmick, S., Filippov, A., Khan, I. A., & Shah, F. U. (2022). Physical and electrochemical properties of new structurally flexible imidazolium phosphate ionic liquids. *Physical Chemistry Chemical Physics*, *24*(38), 23289–23300. doi:10.1039/D2CP03022E PMID:36156000

Bhutta, Z. A., Kulyar, M. F. E. A., Farooq, U., Ashar, A., Mahfooz, A., Kanwal, A., Akhtar, M., Asif, M., Nawaz, S., & Li, K. (2023). Applications of functionalized nanoparticles in tissue engineering. In *Antiviral and Antimicrobial Coatings Based on Functionalized Nanomaterials* (pp. 485–513). Elsevier. doi:10.1016/B978-0-323-91783-4.00006-1

Bianchi, H., & Tremaine, P. R. (1995). Thermodynamics of aqueous phosphate solutions: Apparent molar heat capacities and volumes of the sodium and tetramethylammonium salts at 25°C. *Journal of Solution Chemistry*, *24*(5), 439–463. doi:10.1007/BF01004477

Bianco, A., Kostarelos, K., & Prato, M. (2005). Applications of carbon nanotubes in drug delivery. *Current Opinion in Chemical Biology*, *9*(6), 674–679. doi:10.1016/j.cbpa.2005.10.005 PMID:16233988

Bian, K., Zhang, X., Liu, K., Yin, T., Liu, H., Niu, K., Cao, W., & Gao, D. (2018). Peptide-Directed Hierarchical Mineralized Silver Nanocages for Anti-Tumor Photothermal Therapy. *ACS Sustainable Chemistry & Engineering*, *6*(6), 7574–7588. doi:10.1021/acssuschemeng.8b00415

Bi, W. L., Hosny, A., Schabath, M. B., Giger, M. L., Birkbak, N. J., Mehrtash, A., Allison, T., Arnaout, O., Abbosh, C., Dunn, I. F., Mak, R. H., Tamimi, R. M., Tempany, C. M., Swanton, C., Hoffmann, U., Schwartz, L. H., Gillies, R. J., Huang, R. Y., & Aerts, H. J. W. L. (2019). Artificial intelligence in cancer imaging: Clinical challenges and applications. *CA: a Cancer Journal for Clinicians*, *69*(2), 127–157. doi:10.3322/caac.21552

Björnmalm, M., Thurecht, K. J., Michael, M., Scott, A. M., & Caruso, F. (2017). Bridging Bio-Nano Science and Cancer Nanomedicine. *ACS Nano*, *11*(10), 9594–9613. doi:10.1021/acsnano.7b04855 PMID:28926225

Blanco, E., Shen, H., & Ferrari, M. (2015). Principles of nanoparticle design for overcoming biological barriers to drug delivery. *Nature Biotechnology*, *33*(9), 941–951. doi:10.1038/nbt.3330

Bockamp, E., Rosigkeit, S., Siegl, D., & Schuppan, D. (2020). Nano-enhanced cancer immunotherapy: Immunology encounters nanotechnology. *Cells*, *9*(9), 2102. doi:10.3390/cells9092102

Bohrey, S., Chourasiya, V., & Pandey, A. (2016). Polymeric nanoparticles containing diazepam: Preparation, optimization, characterization, in-vitro drug release and release kinetic study. *Nano Convergence*, *3*(1), 1–7. doi:10.118640580-016-0061-2 PMID:28191413

Bohunicky, B., & Mousa, S. A. (2010). Biosensors: The new wave in cancer diagnosis. *Nanotechnology, Science and Applications*, *4*, 1–10. doi:10.2147/NSA.S13465 PMID:24198482

Boisselier, E., & Astruc, D. (2009). Gold nanoparticles in nanomedicine: Preparations, imaging, diagnostics, therapies and toxicity. *Chemical Society Reviews*, *38*(6), 1759–1782. doi:10.1039/b806051g PMID:19587967

Bolhassani, A., Javanzad, S., Saleh, T., Hashemi, M., Aghasadeghi, M. R., & Sadat, S. M. (2014). Polymeric nanoparticles: Potent vectors for vaccine delivery targeting cancer and infectious diseases. *Human Vaccines & Immunotherapeutics*, *10*(2), 321–332. doi:10.4161/hv.26796 PMID:24128651

Bondarenko, O., Mortimer, M., Kahru, A., Feliu, N., Javed, I., Kakinen, A., Lin, S., Xia, T., Song, Y., Davis, T. P., Lynch, I., Parak, W. J., Leong, D. T., Ke, P. C., Chen, C., & Zhao, Y. (2021). Nanotoxicology and nanomedicine: The Yin and Yang of nano-bio interactions for the new decade. *Nano Today*, *39*, 101184. doi:10.1016/j.nantod.2021.101184 PMID:36937379

Bonilla, A. M., & Gonzalez, P. H. (2017). Hybrid polymeric-magnetic nanoparticles in cancer treatments. *Current Pharmaceutical Design*, *23*(35), 5392–5402. doi:10.2174/1381612823666170519115601

Bonvalot, S., Rutkowski, P. L., Thariat, J., Carrère, S., Ducassou, A., Sunyach, M. P., Agoston, P., Hong, A., Mervoyer, A., Rastrelli, M., Moreno, V., Li, R. K., Tiangco, B., Herraez, A. C., Gronchi, A., Mangel, L., Sy-Ortin, T., Hohenberger, P., de Baère, T., & Le Jvmg Bovée, C. (2019). NBTXR3, a first-in-class radioenhancer hafnium oxide nanoparticle, plus radiotherapy versus radiotherapy alone in patients with locally advanced soft-tissue sarcoma (Act.In.Sarc): A multicentre, phase 2–3, randomised, controlled trial. *The Lancet. Oncology*, *20*(8), 1148–1159. doi:10.1016/S1470-2045(19)30326-2

Borgå, O., Lilienberg, E., Bjermo, H., Hansson, F., Heldring, N., & Dediu, R. (2019). Pharmacokinetics of total and unbound paclitaxel after administration of paclitaxel micellar or nab-paclitaxel: An open, randomized, cross-over, explorative study in breast cancer patients. *Advances in Therapy*, *36*(10), 2825–2837. doi:10.100712325-019-01058-6

Borhaninia, M., Zahiri, M., Abnous, K., Taghdisi, S. M., Ramezani, M., & Alibolandi, M. (2023). Self-targeted hyaluronic acid-b-poly (β-amino ester) pH-switchable polymersome for guided doxorubicin delivery to metastatic breast cancer. *International Journal of Biological Macromolecules*, *248*, 125882. doi:10.1016/j.ijbiomac.2023.125882 PMID:37473882

Boroumand, H., Badie, F., Mazaheri, S., Seyedi, Z. S., Nahand, J. S., Nejati, M., Baghi, H. B., Abbasi-Kolli, M., Badehnoosh, B., Ghandali, M., Hamblin, M. R., & Mirzaei, H. (2021). Chitosan-Based Nanoparticles Against Viral Infections. *Frontiers in Cellular and Infection Microbiology*, *11*, 643953. doi:10.3389/fcimb.2021.643953 PMID:33816349

Botcha, S., & Prattipati, S. D. (2020). Callus extract mediated green synthesis of silver nanoparticles, their characterization and cytotoxicity evaluation against MDA-MB-231 and PC-3 cells. *BioNanoScience*, *10*(1), 11–22. doi:10.100712668-019-00683-3

Boulaiz, H., Alvarez, P. J., Ramirez, A., Marchal, J. A., Prados, J., & Rodrí, F. (2011). *Nanomedicine : Application Areas and Development Prospects*, 3303–3321. MDPI. doi:10.3390/ijms12053303

Bozkaya, O., Ekici, H., Gün Gök, Z., Arat, E., Ekici, S., Yiğitoğlu, M., & Vargel, İ. (2023). Investigation of the in vitro antibacterial, cytotoxic and in vivo analgesic effects of silver nanoparticles coated with Centella asiatica plant extract. *Ankara Üniversitesi Veteriner Fakültesi Dergisi*, *70*(1), 87–96. doi:10.33988/auvfd.1014802

Brayden, D. J. (2003). Controlled release technologies for drug delivery. *Drug Discovery Today*, *8*(21), 976–978. doi:10.1016/S1359-6446(03)02874-5 PMID:14643159

Brigger, I., Dubernet, C., & Couvreur, P. (2012). Nanoparticles in cancer therapy and diagnosis. *Advanced Drug Delivery Reviews*, *64*, 24–36. doi:10.1016/j.addr.2012.09.006 PMID:12204596

Brindhadevi, K., Garalleh, H. A. L., Alalawi, A., Al-Sarayreh, E., & Pugazhendhi, A. (2023). Carbon nanomaterials: Types, synthesis strategies and their application as drug delivery system for cancer therapy. *Biochemical Engineering Journal*, *192*, 108828. doi:10.1016/j.bej.2023.108828

Brucker, J., Mayer, C., Gebauer, G., Mallmann, P., Belau, A. K., Schneeweiss, A., Sohn, C., & Eichbaum, M. (2016). Non-pegylated liposomal doxorubicin for patients with recurrent ovarian cancer: A multicentric phase II trial. *Oncology Letters*, *12*(2), 1211–1215. doi:10.3892/ol.2016.4740

Bruna, G. O. L., Thais, A. C. C., & Lígia, A. C. C. (2018). Food additives and their health effects: A review on preservative sodium benzoate. *African Journal of Biotechnology*, *17*(10), 306–310. doi:10.5897/AJB2017.16321

Bruna, T., Maldonado-Bravo, F., Jara, P., & Caro, N. (2021). Silver Nanoparticles and Their Antibacterial Applications. *International Journal of Molecular Sciences*, *22*(13), 7202. doi:10.3390/ijms22137202 PMID:34281254

Buchman, J. T., Hudson-Smith, N. V., Landy, K. M., & Haynes, C. L. (2019). Understanding nanoparticle toxicity mechanisms to inform redesign strategies to reduce environmental impact. *Accounts of Chemical Research*, *52*(6), 1632–1642. doi:10.1021/acs.accounts.9b00053 PMID:31181913

Bueno, C. Z., Oliveira, C. A., & Rangel-Yagui, C. D. O. (2018). Polymeric and liposomal nanomaterials. In *Nanobiomaterials* (pp. 437–464). Woodhead Publishing. doi:10.1016/B978-0-08-100716-7.00017-9

Bukhari, I., Iqbal, F., & Thorne, R. F. (2022). Research advances in gestational, neonatal diabetes mellitus and metabolic disorders. *Frontiers in Endocrinology*, *13*, 969952. doi:10.3389/fendo.2022.969952 PMID:35966084

Burello, E., & Worth, A. P. (2011). A Theoretical Framework for Predicting the Oxidative Stress Potential of Oxide Nanoparticles. *Nanotoxicology*, *5*(2), 228–235. doi:10.3109/17435390.2010.502980 PMID:21609138

Buttacavoli, M., Albanese, N. N., Di Cara, G., Alduina, R., Faleri, C., Gallo, M., Pizzolanti, G., Gallo, G., Feo, S., Baldi, F., & Cancemi, P. (2018). Anticancer activity of biogenerated silver nanoparticles: An integrated proteomic investigation. *Oncotarget*, *9*(11), 9685–9705. doi:10.18632/oncotarget.23859 PMID:29515763

Büyükbayraktar, H. K., Pelit Arayıcı, P., Ihlamur, M., Gökkaya, D., Karahan, M., Abamor, E. Ş., & Topuzoğulları, M. (2023). Effect of polycation coating on the long-term pulsatile release of antigenic ESAT-61–20 peptide from PLGA nanoparticles. *Colloids and Surfaces. B, Biointerfaces*, *228*, 113421. doi:10.1016/j.colsurfb.2023.113421 PMID:37356137

Caballero Gómez, N., Manetsberger, J., Benomar, N., & Abriouel, H. (2023). Novel combination of nanoparticles and metallo-β-lactamase inhibitor/antimicrobial-based formulation to combat antibiotic resistant Enterococcus sp. and Pseudomonas sp. strains. *International Journal of Biological Macromolecules*, *248*, 125982. doi:10.1016/j.ijbiomac.2023.125982 PMID:37499723

Cainelli, F., & Vallone, A. (2009). Safety and efficacy of pegylated liposomal doxorubicin in HIV-associated Kaposi's sarcoma. *Biologics*, 385–390. doi:10.2147/BTT.S3915

Cai, Y., Qi, J., Lu, Y., He, H., & Wu, W. (2022). The in vivo fate of polymeric micelles. *Advanced Drug Delivery Reviews*, *188*, 114463. doi:10.1016/j.addr.2022.114463 PMID:35905947

Calixto, G., Bernegossi, J., de Freitas, L., Fontana, C., & Chorilli, M. (2016). Nanotechnology-Based Drug Delivery Systems for Photodynamic Therapy of Cancer: A Review. *Molecules (Basel, Switzerland)*, *21*(3), 342. doi:10.3390/molecules21030342 PMID:26978341

Calvo, P., Remuñan-López, C., Vila-Jato, J. L., & Alonso, M. J. (1997). Chitosan and chitosan/ethylene oxide-propylene oxide block copolymer nanoparticles as novel carriers for proteins and vaccines. *Pharmaceutical Research*, *14*(10), 1431–1436. doi:10.1023/A:1012128907225 PMID:9358557

Calzoni, E., Cesaretti, A., Polchi, A., Di Michele, A., Tancini, B., & Emiliani, C. (2019). Biocompatible polymer nanoparticles for drug delivery applications in cancer and neurodegenerative disorder therapies. *Journal of Functional Biomaterials*, *10*(1), 4. doi:10.3390/jfb10010004 PMID:30626094

Cao, M., Su, J., Fan, S., Qiu, H., Su, D., & Li, L. (2021). Wearable piezoresistive pressure sensors based on 3D graphene. *Chemical Engineering Journal*, *406*, 126777. doi:10.1016/j.cej.2020.126777

Cao, S. J., Xu, S., Wang, H. M., Ling, Y., Dong, J., Xia, R. D., & Sun, X. H. (2019). Nanoparticles: Oral delivery for protein and peptide drugs. *AAPS PharmSciTech*, *190*(20), 190. doi:10.120812249-019-1325-z

Cao, X., Lai, S., & James Lee, L. (2001). Design of a self-regulated drug delivery device. *Biomedical Microdevices*, *3*(2), 109–118. doi:10.1023/A:1011494008729

Cao, X., Yao, F., Zhang, B., & Sun, X. (2023). Mitochondrial dysfunction in heart diseases: Potential therapeutic effects of Panax ginseng. *Frontiers in Pharmacology*, *14*, 1218803. doi:10.3389/fphar.2023.1218803 PMID:37547332

Caraway, C. A., Gaitsch, H., Wicks, E. E., Kalluri, A., Kunadi, N., & Tyler, B. M. (2022). Polymeric nanoparticles in brain cancer therapy: A review of current approaches. *Polymers*, *14*(14), 2963. doi:10.3390/polym14142963 PMID:35890738

Cartlidge, M. K., & Hill, A. T. (2017). Inhaled or nebulised ciprofloxacin for the maintenance treatment of bronchiectasis. *Expert Opinion on Investigational Drugs*, *26*(9), 1091–1097. doi:10.1080/13543784.2017.1364728 PMID:28778139

Cash, K. J., & Clark, H. A. (2010). Nanosensors and nanomaterials for monitoring glucose in diabetes. *Trends in Molecular Medicine*, *16*(12), 584–593. doi:10.1016/j.molmed.2010.08.002 PMID:20869318

Castro, K. C. D., Costa, J. M., & Campos, M. G. N. (2022). Drug-loaded polymeric nanoparticles: A review. *International Journal of Polymeric Materials*, *71*(1), 1–13. doi:10.1080/00914037.2020.1798436

Catalano, F., Accomasso, L., Alberto, G., Gallina, C., Raimondo, S., Geuna, S., Giachino, C., & Martra, G. (2015). Factors Ruling the Uptake of Silica Nanoparticles by Mesenchymal Stem Cells:Agglomeration Versus Dispersions, Absence Versus Presence of Serum Proteins. *Small*, *11*(24), 2919–2928. doi:10.1002mll.201400698 PMID:25689227

Catarina Pinto, R., Neufeld, R. J., Ribeiro, A. J., Francisco, V., & Nanoencapsulation, I. (2006). Methods for preparation of drug-loaded polymeric nanoparticles Nanomedicine. *Nanotechnol Biol Med*, *2*, 8–21. doi:10.1016/j.nano.2005.12.003

Cervantes, A., Alsina, M., Tabernero, J., Infante, J. R., LoRusso, P., Shapiro, G., Paz-Ares, L. G., Falzone, R., Hill, J., Cehelsky, J., White, A., Toudjarska, I., Bumcrot, D., Meyers, R., Hinkle, G., Svrzikapa, N., Sah, D. W., Vaishnaw, A., Gollob, J., & Burris, H. A. (2011). Phase I dose-escalation study of ALN-VSP02, a novel RNAi therapeutic for solid tumors with liver involvement. *Journal of Clinical Oncology*, *29*(15, suppl), 3025–3025. doi:10.1200/jco.2011.29.15_suppl.3025

Cha, C., Shin, S. R., Annabi, N., Dokmeci, M. R., & Khademhosseini, A. (2013). Carbon-Based Nanomaterials: Multi-functional Materials for Biomedical Engineering. *ACS Nano*, *7*(4), 2891–2897. doi:10.1021/nn401196a PMID:23560817

Chack, D., Agrawal, N., & Raghuwanshi, S. K. (2014). To analyse the performance of tapered and MMI assisted splitter on the basis of geographical parameters. *Optik (Stuttgart)*, *125*(11), 2568–2571. doi:10.1016/j.ijleo.2013.11.019

Chack, D., Raghuwanshi, S. K., Kumar, V., & Agrawal, N. (2013). Analyzing the Optimum Parameter of an 1x2 MMI Splitter. *2013 International Conference on Communication Systems and Network Technologies*. IEEE. 10.1109/CSNT.2013.41

Chacko, J. B., & Jose, S. (2023). PLGA-based nanoparticles for treatment of cerebral diseases. In P. Kesharwani (Ed.), *Poly(lactic-co-glycolic acid) (PLGA) Nanoparticles for Drug Delivery* (pp. 235–266). Elsevier. doi:10.1016/B978-0-323-91215-0.00018-2

Chahar, V., Sharma, B., Shukla, G., Srivastava, A., & Bhatnagar, A. (2018). Study of antimicrobial activity of silver nanoparticles synthesized using green and chemical approach. *Colloids and Surfaces. A, Physicochemical and Engineering Aspects*, *554*, 149–155. doi:10.1016/j.colsurfa.2018.06.012

Chairuangkitti, P., Lawanprasert, S., Roytrakul, S., Aueviriyavit, S., Phummiratch, D., Kulthong, K., Chanvorachote, P., & Maniratanachote, R. (2013). Silver nanoparticles induce toxicity in A549 cells via ROS-dependent and ROS-independent pathways. *Toxicology In Vitro*, *27*(1), 330–338. doi:10.1016/j.tiv.2012.08.021 PMID:22940466

Chakaya, J., Khan, M., Ntoumi, F., Aklillu, E., Fatima, R., Mwaba, P., Kapata, N., Mfinanga, S., Hasnain, S. E., Katoto, P. D. M. C., Bulabula, A. N. H., Sam-Agudu, N. A., Nachega, J. B., Tiberi, S., McHugh, T. D., Abubakar, I., & Zumla, A. (2021). Global Tuberculosis Report 2020–Reflections on the Global TB burden, treatment and prevention efforts. *International Journal of Infectious Diseases*, *113*, S7–S12. doi:10.1016/j.ijid.2021.02.107 PMID:33716195

Chakraborty, N., Lamba, M., Juglan, K. C., & Kumar, H. (2022). Temperature dependent thermodynamic studies of glycols in aqueous solutions of vitamin B3. In Journal of Physics: Conference Series, 2267(1), 012134). doi:10.1088/1742-6596/2267/1/012134

Chakraborty, N., Bhakri, K., Juglan, K. C., & Kumar, H. (2022). Physicochemical studies of polyethylene glycols in aqueous biotin solutions at different temperatures and constant pressure. *Journal of Physics: Conference Series*, *2267*(1), 012124. doi:10.1088/1742-6596/2267/1/012124

Chakraborty, N., Jha, D., Roy, I., Kumar, P., Gaurav, S. S., Marimuthu, K., Ng, O. T., Lakshminarayanan, R., Verma, N. K., & Gautam, H. K. (2022). Nanobiotics against antimicrobial resistance: Harnessing the power of nanoscale materials and technologies. *Journal of Nanobiotechnology*, *20*(1), 375. doi:10.118612951-022-01573-9 PMID:35953826

Chakraborty, N., Juglan, K. C., & Kumar, H. (2020). Study of thermodynamic and acoustic properties of niacin in aqueous hexylene glycol and propylene glycol at different temperatures. *ACS Omega*, *5*(50), 32357–32365. doi:10.1021/acsomega.0c04292 PMID:33376872

Chakraborty, N., Juglan, K. C., & Kumar, H. (2021). Volumetric and ultrasonic studies of molecular interactions of glycols in aqueous Niacin (vitamin B3) at different temperatures. *Journal of Molecular Liquids*, *332*, 115869. doi:10.1016/j.molliq.2021.115869

Chakraborty, N., Juglan, K. C., Kumar, H., & Singla, M. (2022). Measurement of the Density and Ultrasonic Speed of the Sound of Poly (ethylene glycols)(600 and 6000) in Aqueous Vitamin B5 Solutions at Different Temperatures. *Journal of Chemical & Engineering Data*, *67*(9), 2292–2306. doi:10.1021/acs.jced.2c00260

Chakraborty, N., Juglan, K. C., Kumar, H., & Singla, M. (2022). Study of thermodynamic parameters of ternary solutions of polyethylene glycols in aqueous biotin solutions at multiple temperatures. *The Journal of Chemical Thermodynamics*, *174*, 106876. doi:10.1016/j.jct.2022.106876

Chakraborty, N., Kaur, K., Juglan, K. C., & Kumar, H. (2020). Volumetric and ultrasonic studies on interactions of glycols in aqueous solutions of xylitol at different temperatures. *Journal of Chemical & Engineering Data*, *65*(4), 1435–1446. doi:10.1021/acs.jced.9b00869

Chakraborty, N., Kumar, H., Kaur, K., & Juglan, K. C. (2018). Acoustic and thermodynamic study of D-Panthenol in aqueous solutions of glycol at different temperatures. *The Journal of Chemical Thermodynamics*, *126*, 137–146. doi:10.1016/j.jct.2018.07.006

Chakraborty, N., Rani, M., & Juglan, K. C. (2020). Ultrasonic Investigation of Dichloromethane with Ethanolamine at Various Temperatures. *Plant Archives*, *20*, 2825–2829.

Chakravarty, M., & Vora, A. (2020). Nanotechnology-based antiviral therapeutics. *Drug Delivery and Translational Research 2020 11:3, 11*(3), 748–787. doi:10.1007/s13346-020-00818-0

Chalotra, R., Gupta, T., Chib, S., Amanat, M., Kumar, P., & Singh, R. (2023). Treatment of diabetic complications: Do flavonoids holds the keys? *Critical Reviews in Food Science and Nutrition*, 1–22. doi:10.1080/10408398.2023.2232868 PMID:37435788

Chaloupka, K., Malam, Y., & Seifalian, A. M. (2010). Nanosilver as a new generation of nanoproduct in biomedical applications. *Trends in Biotechnology*, *28*(11), 580–588. doi:10.1016/j.tibtech.2010.07.006 PMID:20724010

Chamcheu, J. C., Siddiqui, I. A., Adhami, V. M., Esnault, S., Bharali, D. J., Babatunde, A. S., Adame, S., Massey, R. J., Wood, G. S., Longley, B. J., Mousa, S. A., & Mukhtar, H. (2018). Chitosan-based nanoformulated (-)-epigallocatechin-3-gallate (EGCG) modulates human keratinocyte-induced responses and alleviates imiquimod-induced murine psoriasiform dermatitis. *International Journal of Nanomedicine*, *13*, 4189–4206. doi:10.2147/IJN.S165966 PMID:30057446

Chamundeeswari, M., Jeslin, J., & Verma, M. L. (2018). Nanocarriers for drug delivery applications. *Environmental Chemistry Letters 2018 17:2, 17*(2), 849–865. doi:10.1007/s10311-018-00841-1

Chan, W. C. W. (2017). *Nanomedicine 2.0.* ACS. doi:10.1021/acs.accounts.6b00629

Chandarana, M., Curtis, A., & Hoskins, C. (2018). The use of nanotechnology in cardiovascular disease. *Applied Nanoscience 2018 8:7, 8*(7), 1607–1619. doi:10.1007/s13204-018-0856-z

Chandra, S., Bharadwaj, R., & Mukherji, S. (2017). Label free ultrasensitive optical sensor decorated with polyaniline nanofibers: Characterization and immunosensing application. *Sensors and Actuators. B, Chemical*, *240*, 443–450. doi:10.1016/j.snb.2016.08.103

Chang, J., Jallouli, Y., Kroubi, M., Yuan, X. B., Feng, W., Kang, C. S., Pu, P., & Betbeder, D. (2009). Characterization of endocytosis of transferrin-coated PLGA nanoparticles by the blood–brain barrier. *International Journal of Pharmaceutics*, *379*(2), 285–292. doi:10.1016/j.ijpharm.2009.04.035 PMID:19416749

Chatterjee, K., Sarkar, S., Jagajjanani Rao, K., & Paria, S. (2014). Core/shell nanoparticles in biomedical applications. *Advances in Colloid and Interface Science*, *209*, 8–39. doi:10.1016/j.cis.2013.12.008 PMID:24491963

Chausali, N., Saxena, J., & Prasad, R. (2023). Nanotechnology as a sustainable approach for combating the environmental effects of climate change. *Journal of Agriculture and Food Research*, *12*, 100541. doi:10.1016/j.jafr.2023.100541

Chawla, D., Chakraborty, N., Juglan, K. C., & Kumar, H. (2021). Temperature-dependent physicochemical studies of some glycols in aqueous d-mannitol solution. *Chemical Papers*, *75*(4), 1497–1506. doi:10.100711696-020-01403-y

Chen, S., Zhang, Q., Hou, Y., Zhang, J., & Liang, X. (2013). Nanomaterials in medicine and pharmaceuticals: nanoscale materials developed with less toxicity and more efficacy. *EJNM*, *5*(2), 61-79. doi: . doi:10.1515/ejnm-2013-0003

Chen, C., Ma, Y. P., Du, S. Y., Wu, Y. Y., Shen, P. L., Yan, T., Li, X. Q., Song, Y. J., Zha, Z. B., & Han, X. (2021). Controlled CRISPR-Cas9 ribonucleoprotein delivery for sensitized photothermal therapy. *Small*, *2101155*(17), 2101155. doi:10.1002mll.202101155

Cheng, L., Zhang, X., Tang, J., Lv, Q., & Liu, J. (2021). Gene-engineered exosomes-thermosensitive liposomes hybrid nanovesicles by the blockade of CD47 signal for combined photothermal therapy and cancer immunotherapy. *Biomaterials*, *275*, 120964. doi:10.1016/j.biomaterials.2021.120964 PMID:34147721

Cheng, X., & Lee, R. J. (2016). The role of helper lipids in lipid nanoparticles (LNPs) designed for oligonucleotide delivery. *Advanced Drug Delivery Reviews*, *99*, 129–137. doi:10.1016/j.addr.2016.01.022

Cheng, X., Li, D., & Cui, R. (2023). Introducing a novel therapeutic supplement for osteoporosis: Remedial, cytotoxicity and antioxidant effects of plant extract green-formulated gold nanoparticles. *Journal of Engineering Research, 100151*. doi:10.1016/j.jer.2023.100151

Cheng, X., Xie, Q., & Sun, Y. (2023). Advances in nanomaterial-based targeted drug delivery systems. *Frontiers in Bioengineering and Biotechnology*, *11*, 1177151. doi:10.3389/fbioe.2023.1177151 PMID:37122851

Cheng, Z., Li, M., Dey, R., & Chen, Y. (2021). Nanomaterials for cancer therapy: Current progress and perspectives. *Journal of Hematology & Oncology*, *14*(1), 1–27. doi:10.118613045-021-01096-0

Chen, H., Gu, Z., An, H., Chen, C., Chen, J., Cui, R., Chen, S., Chen, W., Chen, X., Chen, X., Chen, Z., Ding, B., Dong, Q., Fan, Q., Fu, T., Hou, D., Jiang, Q., Ke, H., Jiang, X., ... Zhao, Y. (2018). Precise Nanomedicine for Intelligent Therapy of Cancer. *Science China. Chemistry*, *61*(12), 1503–1552. doi:10.100711426-018-9397-5

Chen, S., Du, K., & Zou, C. (2020). Current progress in stem cell therapy for type 1 diabetes mellitus. *Stem Cell Research & Therapy*, *11*(1), 1–13. doi:10.118613287-020-01793-6 PMID:32641151

Chen, T., Feng, X., Yin, Y., & Xu, Y. (2020). Investigation of the Effect of Alkyl Chain Length on Molecular Interactions Between Methyl Benzoate with Alcohols: A Study of Physicochemical Properties. *Journal of Solution Chemistry*, *49*(11), 1402–1418. doi:10.100710953-020-01029-4

Chen, W., Liu, K., & Zhang, J. (2022). Functional nanomaterials: From structures to biomedical applications. *Molecules (Basel, Switzerland)*, *27*(21), 7492. doi:10.3390/molecules27217492 PMID:36364319

Chen, X. Z., Tang, J.-H., Cui, Y.-N., Liu, M., & Mao, D. (2014). Phase equilibrium for ternary system NaH2PO4 + Na2SO4 + H2O in aqueous solution at 298.15 K. *Journal of Chemical & Engineering Data*, *59*(2), 481–484. doi:10.1021/je400932e

Chen, X., & Schluesener, H. J. (2008). Nanosilver: A nanoproduct in medical application. *Toxicology Letters*, *176*(1), 1–12. doi:10.1016/j.toxlet.2007.10.004 PMID:18022772

Chen, Y., Wang, M., Zhang, T., Du, E., Liu, Y., Qi, S., Xu, Y., & Zhang, Z. (2018). Autophagic effects and mechanisms of silver nanoparticles in renal cells under low dose exposure. *Ecotoxicology and Environmental Safety*, *166*, 71–77. doi:10.1016/j.ecoenv.2018.09.070 PMID:30248563

Chen, Y., Xiong, X., Chen, Y., Chen, L., Liu, G., Xiao, W., Shi, J., Chen, Z., & Luo, Y. (2023). MoS2-Nanoflower and Nanodiamond Co-Engineered Surface Plasmon Resonance for Biosensing. *Biosensors (Basel)*, *13*(5), 506. doi:10.3390/bios13050506 PMID:37232867

Chen, Y., Yang, T., Chen, S., Qi, S., Zhang, Z., & Xu, Y. (2020). Silver nanoparticles regulate autophagy through lysosome injury and cell hypoxia in prostate cancer cells. *Journal of Biochemical and Molecular Toxicology*, *34*(5), e22474. doi:10.1002/jbt.22474 PMID:32043710

Chen, Y., Zhong, H., Wang, J., Wan, X., Li, Y., Pan, W., Li, N., & Tang, B. (2019). Catalase-like metal-organic framework nanoparticles to enhance radiotherapy in hypoxic cancer and prevent cancer recurrence. *Chemical Science (Cambridge)*, *10*(22), 5773–5778. doi:10.1039/C9SC00747D

Chen, Z. P., Zhang, Y., Zhang, S., Xia, J. G., Liu, J. W., Xu, K., & Gu, N. (2008). Preparation and characterization of water-soluble monodisperse magnetic iron oxide nanoparticles via surface double-exchange with DMSA. *Colloids and Surfaces. A, Physicochemical and Engineering Aspects*, *316*(1–3), 210–216. doi:10.1016/j.colsurfa.2007.09.017

Chen, Z. Y., Wang, Y. X., Lin, Y., Zhang, J. S., Yang, F., Zhou, Q. L., & Liao, Y. Y. (2014). Advance of molecular imaging technology and targeted imaging agent in imaging and therapy. *BioMed Research International*, *2014*, 1–12. doi:10.1155/2014/819324 PMID:24689058

Chen, Z., Kang, L., Wang, Z., Xu, F., Gu, G., Cui, F., & Guo, Z. (2014). Recent progress in the research of biomaterials regulating cell behavior. *RSC Advances*, *4*(109), 63807–63816. doi:10.1039/C4RA05534A

Cherukuri, P., Glazer, E. S., & Curley, S. A. (2010). Targeted hyperthermia using metal nanoparticles. *Advanced Drug Delivery Reviews*, *62*(3), 339–345. doi:10.1016/j.addr.2009.11.006 PMID:19909777

Chevallet, M., Veronesi, G., Fuchs, A., Mintz, E., Michaud-Soret, I., & Deniaud, A. (2017). Impact of labile metal nanoparticles on cellular homeostasis. Current developments in imaging, synthesis and applications. *Biochimica et Biophysica Acta. G, General Subjects*, *1861*(6), 1566–1577. doi:10.1016/j.bbagen.2016.12.012 PMID:27993661

Chikan, V., & McLaurin, E. J. (2016). Rapid nanoparticle synthesis by magnetic and microwave heating. *Nanomaterials (Basel, Switzerland)*, *6*(85), 85. doi:10.3390/nano6050085 PMID:28335212

Chinnarao, D., Padmarao, C. V., Beena, C., Srilatha, M., Ramanjaneyulu, M. V. V., Choppara, P., Murali, N., & Rao, B. V. (2023). Acoustic, excess thermodynamical, molecular interaction and anti-microbial activity studies on binary liquid mixtures of geranyl acetate and benzyl benzoate in the temperature range of 303.15K–318.15K. *Journal of the Indian Chemical Society*, *100*(5), 100969. doi:10.1016/j.jics.2023.100969

Chis, A. A., Dobrea, C., Morgovan, C., Arseniu, A. M., Rus, L. L., Butuca, A., Juncan, A. M., Totan, M., Vonica-Tincu, A. L., Cormos, G., Muntean, A. C., Muresan, M. L., Gligor, F. G., & Frum, A. (2020). Applications and Limitations of Dendrimers in Biomedicine. *Molecules (Basel, Switzerland)*, *25*(17), 3982. doi:10.3390/molecules25173982 PMID:32882920

Choi, H. S., Ashitate, Y., Lee, J. H., Kim, S. H., Matsui, A., Insin, N., Bawendi, M. G., Semmler-Behnke, M., Frangioni, J. V., & Tsuda, A. (2010). Rapid translocation of nanoparticles from the lung airspaces to the body. *Nature Biotechnology*, *28*(12), 1300–1303. doi:10.1038/nbt.1696 PMID:21057497

Choi, J., Burns, A. A., Williams, R. M., Zhou, Z., Flesken-Nikitin, A., Zipfel, W. R., Wiesner, U., & Nikitin, A. Y. (2008). Core-shell silica nanoparticles as fluorescent labels for nanomedicine. *Journal of Biomedical Optics*, *12*(06), 1. doi:10.1117/1.2823149 PMID:18163823

Choi, Y. K. (2021). Emerging and re-emerging fatal viral diseases. *Experimental & Molecular Medicine*, *53*(5), 711–712. doi:10.103812276-021-00608-9 PMID:33953321

Choi, Y., Cho, B. K., Seok, S. H., Kim, C., Ryu, J. H., & Kwon, I. C. (2023). Controlled spatial characteristics of ligands on nanoparticles: Determinant of cellular functions. *Journal of Controlled Release*, *360*, 672–686. doi:10.1016/j.jconrel.2023.07.020 PMID:37437847

Chong, Y., Ge, C., Fang, G., Wu, R., Zhang, H., Chai, Z., Chen, C., & Yin, J. J. (2017). Light-Enhanced Antibacterial Activity of Graphene Oxide, Mainly via Accelerated Electron Transfer. *Environmental Science & Technology*, *51*(17), 10154–10161. doi:10.1021/acs.est.7b00663 PMID:28771330

Chopra, H., Bibi, S., Singh, I., Hasan, M. M., Khan, M. S., Yousafi, Q., Baig, A. A., Rahman, M. M., Islam, F., Emran, T. B., & Cavalu, S. (2022). Green Metallic Nanoparticles: Biosynthesis to Applications. *Frontiers in Bioengineering and Biotechnology*, *10*, 874742. doi:10.3389/fbioe.2022.874742 PMID:35464722

Chordiya, K., Patwa, H., Walode, S. G., & Chatur, V. M. (2021). Role of Nanoparticles in the Management of Diabetes. *Int. Journal of Pharmaceutical Sciences and Medicine*, *6*(4), 83–91. doi:10.47760/ijpsm.2021.v06i04.007

Chorny, M., Fishbein, I., Danenberg, H. D., & Golomb, G. (2002). Lipophilic drug loaded nanospheres prepared by nanoprecipitation: Effect of formulation variables on size, drug recovery and release kinetics. *Journal of Controlled Release*, *83*(3), 389–400. doi:10.1016/S0168-3659(02)00211-0 PMID:12387947

Choudhury, H., Pandey, M., Lim, Y. Q., Low, C. Y., Lee, C. T., Marilyn, T. C. L., Loh, H. S., Lim, Y. P., Lee, C. F., Bhattamishra, S. K., Kesharwani, P., & Gorain, B. (2020). Silver nanoparticles: Advanced and promising technology in diabetic wound therapy. *Materials Science and Engineering C*, *112*, 110925. doi:10.1016/j.msec.2020.110925 PMID:32409075

Chou, H., Lin, H., & Liu, J. M. (2015). A tale of the two PEGylated liposomal doxorubicins. *OncoTargets and Therapy*, *8*, 1719–1720. doi:10.2147/OTT.S79089

Chouhan, R., & Bajpai, A. K. (2010). Release dynamics of ciprofloxacin from swellable nanocarriers of poly (2-hydroxyethyl methacrylate): An in vitro study. *Nanomedicine; Nanotechnology, Biology, and Medicine*, *6*(3), 453–462. doi:10.1016/j.nano.2009.11.006 PMID:20044034

Chou, W.-C., Chen, Q., Yuan, L., Cheng, Y.-H., He, C., Monteiro-Riviere, N. A., Riviere, J. E., & Lin, Z. (2023). An artificial intelligence-assisted physiologically-based pharmacokinetic model to predict nanoparticle delivery to tumors in mice. *Journal of Controlled Release*, *361*, 53–63. doi:10.1016/j.jconrel.2023.07.040 PMID:37499908

Chow, J. C. (2022). Application of Nanomaterials in Biomedical Imaging and Cancer Therapy. *Nanomaterials (Basel, Switzerland)*, *12*(5), 726. doi:10.3390/nano12050726 PMID:35269214

Chung, C., Kim, Y. K., Shin, D., Ryoo, S. R., Hong, B. H., & Min, D. H. (2013). Biomedical applications of graphene and graphene oxide. *Accounts of Chemical Research*, *46*(10), 2211–2224. doi:10.1021/ar300159f

Chun, Y. W., Crowder, S. W., Mehl, S. C., Wang, X., Bae, H., & Sung, H.-J. (2013). THERAPEUTIC APPLICATION OF NANOTECHNOLOGY IN CARDIOVASCULAR AND PULMONARY REGENERATION. *Computational and Structural Biotechnology Journal*, *7*(8), e201304005. doi:10.5936/csbj.201304005 PMID:24688735

Cicha, I., Priefer, R., Severino, P., Souto, E. B., & Jain, S. (2022). Biosensor-Integrated Drug Delivery Systems as New Materials for Biomedical Applications. *Biomolecules*, *12*(9), 1198. doi:10.3390/biom12091198 PMID:36139035

Cicha, I., Singh, R., Garlichs, C. D., & Alexiou, C. (2016). Nano-biomaterials for cardiovascular applications: Clinical perspective. *Journal of Controlled Release*, *229*, 23–36. doi:10.1016/j.jconrel.2016.03.015 PMID:26988601

Cohen, J. D., Li, L., Wang, Y., Thoburn, C., Afsari, B., Danilova, L., Douville, C., Javed, A. A., Wong, F., Mattox, A., Hruban, R. H., Wolfgang, C. L., Goggins, M. G., Dal Molin, M., Wang, T.-L., Roden, R., Klein, A. P., Ptak, J., Dobbyn, L, & Papadopoulos, N. (2018). Detection and localization of surgically resectable cancers with a multi-analyte blood test. *Science*, *359*(6378), 926–930. doi:10.1126cience.aar3247

Colino, C. I., Lanao, J. M., & Gutierrez-Millan, C. (2021). Recent advances in functionalized nanomaterials for the diagnosis and treatment of bacterial infections. *Materials Science and Engineering C*, *121*, 111843. doi:10.1016/j.msec.2020.111843 PMID:33579480

Cordeiro, A. S., Patil-Sen, Y., Shivkumar, M., Patel, R., Khedr, A., & Elsawy, M. A. (2021). Nanovaccine delivery approaches and advanced delivery systems for the prevention of viral infections: From development to clinical application. *Pharmaceutics*, *13*(12), 2091. doi:10.3390/pharmaceutics13122091 PMID:34959372

Corrigan, O. I., & Li, X. (2009). Quantifying drug release from PLGA nanoparticulates. *European Journal of Pharmaceutical Sciences*, *37*(3-4), 477–485. doi:10.1016/j.ejps.2009.04.004 PMID:19379812

Coutinho, C., & Somoza, Á. (2019). MicroRNA sensors based on gold nanoparticles. *Analytical and Bioanalytical Chemistry*, *411*(9), 1807–1824. doi:10.100700216-018-1450-7 PMID:30390112

Couvreur, P., Barratt, G., Fattal, E., & Vauthier, C. (2002). Nanocapsule technology: a review. *Critical Reviews™ in Therapeutic Drug Carrier Systems, 19*(2).

Couvreur, P. (2013). Nanoparticles in drug delivery: Past, present and future. *Advanced Drug Delivery Reviews*, *65*(1), 21–23. doi:10.1016/j.addr.2012.04.010 PMID:22580334

Couvreur, P., Dubernet, C., & Puisieux, F. (1995). Controlled drug delivery with nanoparticles: Current possibilities and future trends. *European Journal of Pharmaceutics and Biopharmaceutics*, *41*(1), 2–13.

Craparo, E. F., & Bondì, M. L. (2012). Application of polymeric nanoparticles in immunotherapy. *Current Opinion in Allergy and Clinical Immunology*, *12*(6), 658–664. doi:10.1097/ACI.0b013e3283588c57 PMID:23095912

Crezee, J., Franken, N. A., & Oei, A. L. (2021). Hyperthermia-based anti-cancer treatments. *Cancers (Basel)*, *1240*(13), 1240. doi:10.3390/cancers13061240

Crinson, I., & Crinson, I. (2021). The Interdisciplinarity Field of Social Studies of Science and Technology (SSST). *The Biomedical Sciences in Society: An Interdisciplinary Analysis*, 1-16. doi:10.1007/978-981-15-9523-3_1

Crucho, C. I. (2015). Stimuli-responsive polymeric nanoparticles for nanomedicine. *ChemMedChem*, *10*(1), 24–38. doi:10.1002/cmdc.201402290 PMID:25319803

Crucho, C. I., & Barros, M. T. (2017). Polymeric nanoparticles: A study on the preparation variables and characterization methods. *Materials Science and Engineering C*, *80*, 771–784. doi:10.1016/j.msec.2017.06.004 PMID:28866227

Cruz-Hernández, C., López-Méndez, L. J., & Guadarrama, P. (2022). Dendronization: A practical strategy to improve the performance of molecular systems used in biomedical applications. *European Journal of Medicinal Chemistry*, *229*, 113988. doi:10.1016/j.ejmech.2021.113988 PMID:34801269

Cui, Z., & Mumper, R. J. (2002). Plasmid DNA-entrapped nanoparticles engineered from microemulsion precursors: In vitro and in vivo evaluation. *Bioconjugate Chemistry*, *13*(6), 1319–1327. doi:10.1021/bc0255586 PMID:12440869

Cun, D., Jensen, D. K., Maltesen, M. J., Bunker, M., Whiteside, P., Scurr, D., Foged, C., & Nielsen, H. M. (2011). High loading efficiency and sustained release of siRNA encapsulated in PLGA nanoparticles: Quality by design optimization and characterization. *European Journal of Pharmaceutics and Biopharmaceutics*, *77*(1), 26–35. doi:10.1016/j.ejpb.2010.11.008 PMID:21093589

D'Costa, G., Pisal, D.S., Rane, D.S.(2012). *Report on Synthesis of nanoparticles and functionalization: Co-precipitation method.*

da Silva, A. L., Silva, L. A., Cruz, F. F., Rocco, P. R. M., & Morales, M. M. (2020). Application of novel nanotechnologies in asthma. *Annals of Translational Medicine, 8*(5), 159. doi:10.21037/atm.2019.12.40 PMID:32309307

Dabla, P. K. (2010). Renal function in diabetic nephropathy. *World Journal of Diabetes, 1*(2), 48. doi:10.4239/wjd.v1.i2.48 PMID:21537427

Dadashpour, M., Firouzi-Amandi, A., Pourhassan-Moghaddam, M., Maleki, M. J., Soozangar, N., Jeddi, F., Nouri, M., Zarghami, N., & Pilehvar-Soltanahmadi, Y. (2018). Biomimetic synthesis of silver nanoparticles using Matricaria chamomilla extract and their potential anticancer activity against human lung cancer cells. *Materials Science and Engineering C, 92*, 902–912. doi:10.1016/j.msec.2018.07.053 PMID:30184820

Dadwal, M., Solan, D., & Pradesh, H. (2014). Polymeric nanoparticles as promising novel carriers for drug delivery: An overview. *Journal of Advanced Pharmacy Education & Research Jan-Mar, 4*(1).

Dai, M., & Ja, F. (2016). Engineered Protein Polymer-Gold Nanoparticle Hybrid Materials for Small Molecule Delivery. *Journal of Nanomedicine & Nanotechnology, 356*(7). doi:10.4172/2157-7439.1000356

Dai, Q., Wilhelm, S., Ding, D., Syed, A. M., Sindhwani, S., Zhang, Y., Chen, Y. Y., Macmillan, P., & Chan, W. C. W. (2018). Quantifying the Ligand-Coated Nanoparticle Delivery to Cancer Cells in Solid Tumours. *ACS Nano, 12*(8), 8423–8435. doi:10.1021/acsnano.8b03900 PMID:30016073

Daneman, R., & Prat, A. (2015). The Blood–Brain Barrier. *Cold Spring Harbor Perspectives in Biology, 7*(1), a020412. doi:10.1101/cshperspect.a020412 PMID:25561720

Dange, S. P., Chimankar, O. P., & Borkar, P. D. (2021). Physico-chemical analysis on binary liquid mixture of Nicotinic acid at different temperatures. *Indian Journal of Pure and Applied Physics, 59*(2), 132–137. doi:10.56042/ijpap.v59i2.33311

Danhier, F., Feron, O., & Préat, V. (2010). To exploit the tumor microenvironment: Passive and active tumor targeting of nanocarriers for anti-cancer drug delivery. *Journal of Controlled Release, 148*(2), 135–146. doi:10.1016/j.jconrel.2010.08.027 PMID:20797419

Darbasizadeh, B., Feyzi-barnaji, B., & Naderi, N. (2022). Chapter 19 - Toxicity and biocompatibility of nanomaterials: In vivo studies. In M. Saravanan, H. Barabadi, E. Mostafavi, & T. Webster (Eds.), Emerging Nanomaterials and Nano-Based Drug Delivery Approaches to Combat Antimicrobial Resistance (pp. 701-732): Elsevier. doi:10.1016/B978-0-323-90792-7.00014-2

Darville, N., van Heerden, M., Vynckier, A., De Meulder, M., Sterkens, P., Annaert, P., & Van den Mooter, G. (2014). Intramuscular Administration of Paliperidone Palmitate Extended-Release Injectable Microsuspension Induces a Subclinical Inflammatory Reaction Modulating the Pharmacokinetics in Rats. *Journal of Pharmaceutical Sciences, 103*(7), 2072–2087. doi:10.1002/jps.24014 PMID:24845884

Das, S., Kotcherlakota, R., & Patra, C. R. (2019). Noninvasive imaging techniques of metal nanoparticles and their future diagnostic applications. *Medical Imaging Methods: Recent Trends*, 119–141. https://doi.org/ doi:10.1007/978-981-13-9121-7_5/COVER

Das, B., Nayak, A. K., & Mallick, S. (2022). Lipid-based nanocarriers for ocular drug delivery: An updated review. *Journal of Drug Delivery Science and Technology, 76*, 103780. doi:10.1016/j.jddst.2022.103780

Das, S., Datta, S., Barman, A., & Barua, R. (2023). Smart Biodegradable and Bio-Based Polymeric Biomaterials for Biomedical Applications. In A. Kumar, P. Kumar, A. Srivastava, & V. Goyat (Eds.), *Modeling, Characterization, and Processing of Smart Materials* (pp. 56–82). IGI Global. doi:10.4018/978-1-6684-9224-6.ch003

Datta, S., & Barua, R. (2023). Fluorescent Nanomaterials and Its Application in Biomedical Engineering. In A. Rakha, A. Munawar, V. Khanna, & S. Bansal (Eds.), *Modeling and Simulation of Functional Nanomaterials for Forensic Investigation* (pp. 164–186). IGI Global. doi:10.4018/978-1-6684-8325-1.ch009

Davis, M. E., Zuckerman, J. E., Choi, C. H. J., Seligson, D., Tolcher, A., Alabi, C. A., Yen, Y., Heidel, J. D., & Ribas, A. (2010). Evidence of RNAi in humans from systemically administered siRNA via targeted nanoparticles. *Nature*, *464*(7291), 1067–1070. doi:10.1038/nature08956 PMID:20305636

de la Escosura-Muñiz, A., Parolo, C., & Merkoçi, A. (2010). Immunosensing using nanoparticles. *Materials Today*, *13*(7), 24–34. doi:10.1016/S1369-7021(10)70125-5

Debnath, S. K., & Srivastava, R. (2021). Drug Delivery With Carbon-Based Nanomaterials as Versatile Nanocarriers: Progress and Prospects. *Frontiers in Nanotechnology*, *3*, 644564. doi:10.3389/fnano.2021.644564

Deckers, R., & Moonen, C. T. (2010). Ultrasound triggered, image guided, local drug delivery. *Journal of Controlled Release*, *148*(1), 25–33. doi:10.1016/j.jconrel.2010.07.117 PMID:20709123

Deepika, G., Suresh, V., Rupula, K., Bantal, V., & Rb, S. (2023). Synthesis and evaluation of anti-inflammatory and anti-nociceptive potentials of biopolymer based curcumin nanoparticle construct: In silico, in vitro and in vivo studies. *Bioactive Carbohydrates and Dietary Fibre*, *30*, 100381. doi:10.1016/j.bcdf.2023.100381

Dehghani, P., Rad, M. E., Zarepour, A., Sivakumar, P. M., & Zarrabi, A. (2023). An insight into the polymeric nanoparticles applications in diabetes diagnosis and treatment. *Mini-Reviews in Medicinal Chemistry*, *23*(2), 192–216. doi:10.2174/1389557521666211116123002 PMID:34784864

Deitrich, R. A., & Erwin, V. G. (1971). Mechanism of the inhibition of aldehyde dehydrogenase in vivo by disulfiram and diethyldithiocarbamate. *Molecular Pharmacology*, *7*(3), 301–307. PMID:4328422

Delgado, J. A., Martin, S., Hare, J. I., Yates, J. W. T., & Barry, S. T. (2015). Tumour stromal morphology impacts nanomedicine cytotoxicity in patient-derived xenografts. *Nanomedicine; Nanotechnology, Biology, and Medicine*, *11*(5), 1247–1252. doi:10.1016/j.nano.2015.02.007 PMID:25752857

DeLong, R. K., Akhtar, U., Sallee, M., Parker, B., Barber, S., Zhang, J., Craig, M., Garrad, R., Hickey, A. J., & Engstrom, E. (2009). Characterization and performance of nucleic acid nanoparticles combined with protamine and gold. *Biomaterials*, *30*(32), 6451–6459. doi:10.1016/j.biomaterials.2009.07.067 PMID:19726081

Delplace, V., Couvreur, P., & Nicolas, J. (2014). Recent trends in the design of anticancer polymer prodrug nanocarriers. *Polymer Chemistry*, *5*(5), 1529–1544. doi:10.1039/C3PY01384G

Demirel, M., Parikh, A., Crespi, V., & Reed, S. (2007). *Biologically Inspired Nanomaterials: A Conference Report*. arXiv preprint arXiv:0708.0164.

Demolder, C., Molina, A., Hammond, F. L. III, & Yeo, W. H. (2021). Recent advances in wearable biosensing gloves and sensory feedback biosystems for enhancing rehabilitation, prostheses, healthcare, and virtual reality. *Biosensors & Bioelectronics*, *190*, 113443. doi:10.1016/j.bios.2021.113443 PMID:34171820

Deng, S., Gu, J., Jiang, Z., Cao, Y., Mao, F., Xue, Y., Wang, J., Dai, K., Qin, L., Wu, K., He, Q., & Cai, K. (2022). Application of nanotechnology in the early diagnosis and comprehensive treatment of gastrointestinal cancer. *Journal of Nanobiotechnology*, *20*(1), 415. doi:10.118612951-022-01613-4 PMID:36109734

Deng, W., Chen, W., Clement, S., Guller, A., Zhao, Z., Engel, A., & Goldys, E. M. (2018). Controlled Gene and Drug Release from a Liposomal Delivery Platform Triggered by X-Ray Radiation. *Nature Communications*, *2713*(9), 2713. doi:10.103841467-018-05118-3

Deng, Y., Zhang, X., Shen, H., He, Q., Wu, Z., Liao, W., & Yuan, M. (2020). Application of the nano-drug delivery system in treatment of cardiovascular diseases. *Frontiers in Bioengineering and Biotechnology*, *7*, 489. doi:10.3389/fbioe.2019.00489 PMID:32083068

Deng, Z. J., Morton, S. W., Ben-Akiva, E., Dreaden, E. C., Shopsowitz, K. E., & Hammond, P. T. (2013). Layer-by-layer nanoparticles for systemic codelivery of an anticancer drug and siRNA for potential triple-negative breast cancer treatment. *ACS Nano*, *7*(11), 9571–9584. doi:10.1021/nn4047925

Deol, P., & Khuller, G. K. (1997). Lung specific stealth liposomes: Stability, biodistribution and toxicity of liposomal antitubercular drugs in mice. *Biochimica et Biophysica Acta*, *1334*(2-3), 161–172. doi:10.1016/S0304-4165(96)00088-8 PMID:9101710

Desai, N., Momin, M., Khan, T., Gharat, S., Ningthoujam, R. S., & Omri, A. (2021). Metallic nanoparticles as drug delivery system for the treatment of cancer. *Expert Opinion on Drug Delivery*, *18*(9), 1261–1290. doi:10.1080/17425247.2021.1912008 PMID:33793359

Devaraj, P., Kumari, P., Aarti, C., & Renganathan, A. (2013). Synthesis and characterization of silver nanoparticles using cannonball leaves and their cytotoxic activity against MCF-7 cell line. *Journal of Nanotechnology*, *2013*, 2013. doi:10.1155/2013/598328

Devunuri, N., Kancherla, S., Chennuri, B. K., & Gardas, R. L. (2016). Apparent molar volume and isentropic compressibilities of antidepressant drugs (Citalopram HBr and Escitalopram oxalate) with water. *Journal of Molecular Liquids*, *216*, 347–353. doi:10.1016/j.molliq.2016.01.058

Dey, N., Kamatchi, C., Vickram, A. S., Anbarasu, K., Thanigaivel, S., Palanivelu, J., Pugazhendhi, A., & Ponnusamy, V. K. (2022). Role of Nanomaterials in Deactivating Multiple Drug Resistance Efflux Pumps - A Review. *Environmental Research*, *204*, 111968. doi:10.1016/j.envres.2021.111968

Dhal, K., Das, P., Singh, S., & Talukdar, M. (2023). Analysis of ultraacoustic behavior of l-aspartic acid in aqueous sodium benzoate and ammonium acetate media. *Journal of Molecular Liquids*, *376*, 121413. doi:10.1016/j.molliq.2023.121413

Dhal, K., Singh, S., & Talukdar, M. (2022). Ultraacoustic and conductometric studies on the interactions of l-glutamic acid with potassium sorbate and sodium benzoate in aqueous media. *Journal of Molecular Liquids*, *368*, 120761. doi:10.1016/j.molliq.2022.120761

Dhanya, C. S., Paul, W., Rekha, M. R., & Joseph, R. (2023). Solid lipid nanoparticles of lauric Acid: A prospective drug carrier for oral drug delivery. *Journal of Molecular Liquids*, *380*, 121738. doi:10.1016/j.molliq.2023.121738

Dhiman, M., Singh, K., Kaushal, J., Upmanyu, A., & Singh, D. P. (2019). Ultrasonic study of molecular interactions in polymeric solution of polypropylene glycol-400 and ethanol at 303 K. *Acta Acustica united with Acustica*, *105*(5), 743–752. doi:10.3813/AAA.919354

Dhull, A., Yu, C., Wilmoth, A. H., Chen, M., Sharma, A., & Yiu, S. (2023). Dendrimers in Corneal Drug Delivery: Recent Developments and Translational Opportunities. *Pharmaceutics*, *15*(6), 1591. doi:10.3390/pharmaceutics15061591 PMID:37376040

Di Trani, N., Liu, H.-C., Qi, R., Viswanath, D. I., Liu, X., Chua, C. Y. X., & Grattoni, A. (2021). Long-acting tunable release of amlodipine loaded PEG-PCL micelles for tailored treatment of chronic hypertension. *Nanomedicine; Nanotechnology, Biology, and Medicine*, *37*, 102417. doi:10.1016/j.nano.2021.102417 PMID:34171469

Diaconu, A., Chiriac, A.P., Neamtu, I., Nita, L.E. (2019). Magnetic Polymeric Nanocomposites. *Polymeric Nanomaterials in Nanotherapeutics*, 359–386. doi:10.1016/B978-0-12-813932-5.00010-8

Dianzani, C., Monge, C., Miglio, G., Serpe, L., Martina, K., Cangemi, L., Ferraris, C., Mioletti, S., Osella, S., Gigliotti, C. L., Boggio, E., Clemente, N., Dianzani, U., & Battaglia, L. (2020). Nanoemulsions as delivery systems for poly-chemotherapy aiming at melanoma treatment. *Cancers (Basel)*, *12*(5), 1198. doi:10.3390/cancers12051198

Diez-Pascual, A. M., & Rahdar, A. (2022). Functional Nanomaterials in Biomedicine: Current Uses and Potential Applications. *ChemMedChem*, *17*(16), e202200142. doi:10.1002/cmdc.202200142 PMID:35729066

Digiacomo, L., Renzi, S., Quagliarini, E., Pozzi, D., Amenitsch, H., Ferri, G., Pesce, L., Lorenzi, V. D., Matteoli, G., Cardarelli, F., & Caracciolo, G. (2023). Investigating the mechanism of action of DNA-loaded PEGylated lipid nanoparticles. *Nanomedicine; Nanotechnology, Biology, and Medicine*, *102697*, 102697. doi:10.1016/j.nano.2023.102697 PMID:37507061

Dilworth, L., Facey, A., & Omoruyi, F. (2021). Diabetes mellitus and its metabolic complications: The role of adipose tissues. *International Journal of Molecular Sciences*, *22*(14), 7644. doi:10.3390/ijms22147644 PMID:34299261

Dinakar, Y. H., Karole, A., Parvez, S., Jain, V., & Mudavath, S. L. (2023). Folate receptor targeted NIR cleavable liposomal delivery system augment penetration and therapeutic efficacy in breast cancer. *Biochimica et Biophysica Acta (BBA) -. Biochimica et Biophysica Acta. G, General Subjects*, *1867*(9), 130396. doi:10.1016/j.bbagen.2023.130396 PMID:37271407

Ding, S., Chen, L., Liao, J., Huo, Q., Wang, Q., Tian, G., & Yin, W. (2023). Harnessing Hafnium-Based Nanomaterials for Cancer Diagnosis and Therapy. *Small*, *19*(32), 2300341. doi:10.1002mll.202300341 PMID:37029564

Dipankar, C., & Murugan, S. (2012). The green synthesis, characterization and evaluation of the biological activities of silver nanoparticles synthesized from Iresine herbstii leaf aqueous extracts. *Colloids and Surfaces. B, Biointerfaces*, *98*, 112–119. doi:10.1016/j.colsurfb.2012.04.006 PMID:22705935

Dissanayake, T., Sun, X., Abbey, L., & Bandara, N. (2022). Recent advances in lipid-protein conjugate-based delivery systems in nutraceutical, drug, and gene delivery. *Food Hydrocolloids for Health*, *2*, 100054. doi:10.1016/j.fhfh.2022.100054

Dixit, A., & Juglan, K. C., Sharma. (2014). Acoustic parameter investigation of ternary mixture of n-butanol, water and acetic acid by using ultrasonic technique. *Journal of Chemical and Pharmaceutical Research*, *6*(10), 93–104.

Domingues, C., Santos, A., Alvarez-Lorenzo, C., Concheiro, A., Jarak, I., Veiga, F., Barbosa, I., Dourado, M., & Figueiras, A. (2022). Where is nano today and where is it headed? A review of nanomedicine and the dilemma of nanotoxicology. *ACS Nano*, *16*(7), 9994–10041. doi:10.1021/acsnano.2c00128 PMID:35729778

Domínguez-Aragón, A., Zaragoza-Contreras, E. A., Figueroa-Miranda, G., Offenhäusser, A., & Mayer, D. (2023). Electrochemical Immunosensor Using Electroactive Carbon Nanohorns for Signal Amplification for the Rapid Detection of Carcinoembryonic Antigen. *Biosensors (Basel)*, *13*(1), 63. doi:10.3390/bios13010063 PMID:36671898

Dong, C., Cao, C., Zhang, X., Zhan, Y., Wang, X., Yang, X., Zhou, K., Xiao, X., & Yuan, B. (2017). Wolfberry fruit (Lycium barbarum) extract mediated novel route for the green synthesis of silver nanoparticles. *Optik (Stuttgart)*, *130*, 162–170. doi:10.1016/j.ijleo.2016.11.010

Dong, X. (2018). Current Strategies for Brain Drug Delivery. *Theranostics*, *8*(6), 1481–1493. doi:10.7150/thno.21254 PMID:29556336

Dong, Y., Wu, X., Chen, X., Zhou, P., Xu, F., & Liang, W. (2021). Nanotechnology shaping stem cell therapy: Recent advances, application, challenges, and future outlook. *Biomedicine and Pharmacotherapy*, *137*, 111236. doi:10.1016/j.biopha.2021.111236 PMID:33486201

Donlan, R. M., & Costerton, J. W. (2002). Biofilms: Survival mechanisms of clinically relevant microorganisms. *Clinical Microbiology Reviews*, *15*(2), 167–193. doi:10.1128/CMR.15.2.167-193.2002 PMID:11932229

Đorđević, S., Gonzalez, M. M., Conejos-Sánchez, I., Carreira, B., Pozzi, S., Acúrcio, R. C., Satchi-Fainaro, R., Florindo, H. F., & Vicent, M. J. (2022). Current hurdles to the translation of nanomedicines from bench to the clinic. *Drug Delivery and Translational Research*, *12*(3), 1–26. doi:10.100713346-021-01024-2 PMID:34302274

Dorokhov, Y. L., Sheshukova, E. V., Kosobokova, E. N., Shindyapina, A. V., Kosorukov, V. S., & Komarova, T. V. (2016). Functional role of carbohydrate residues in human immunoglobulin G and therapeutic monoclonal antibodies. *Biochemistry (Moscow)*, *81*(8), 835–857. doi:10.1134/S0006297916080058 PMID:27677552

dos Santos, D. M. S., Pires, J. G., & Braga, A. S. (2019). Comparison between static and semi-dynamic models for microcosm biofilm formation on dentin. *Journal of Applied Oral Science*, *27*, 1–6. doi:10.1590/1678-7757-2018-0163 PMID:30624468

Dristant, U., Mukherjee, K., Saha, S., & Maity, D. (2023). An Overview of Polymeric Nanoparticles-Based Drug Delivery System in Cancer Treatment. *Technology in Cancer Research & Treatment*, *22*, 15330338231152083. doi:10.1177/15330338231152083 PMID:36718541

Duarte, A. A., Mohsin, S., & Golubnitschaja, O. (2018). Diabetes care in figures: Current pitfalls and future scenario. *The EPMA Journal*, *9*(2), 125–131. doi:10.100713167-018-0133-y PMID:29896313

Du, B., Jiang, X., Das, A., Zhou, Q., Yu, M., Jin, R., & Zheng, J. (2017). Glomerular barrier behaves as an atomically precise bandpass filter in a sub-nanometre regime. *Nature Nanotechnology*, *12*(11), 1096–1102. doi:10.1038/nnano.2017.170 PMID:28892099

Dubey, R., Prabhakar, P. K., & Gupta, J. (2022). Epigenetics: Key to improve delayed wound healing in type 2 diabetes. *Molecular and Cellular Biochemistry*, *477*(2), 371–383. doi:10.100711010-021-04285-0 PMID:34739665

Du, F., Ming, Y., Zeng, F., Yu, C., & Wu, S. (2013). A low cytotoxic and ratiometric fluorescent nanosensor based on carbon-dots for intracellular pH sensing and mapping. *Nanotechnology*, *24*(36), 365101. doi:10.1088/0957-4484/24/36/365101 PMID:23942146

Dufes, C., Uchegbu, I., & Schatzlein, A. (2005). Dendrimers in gene delivery. *Advanced Drug Delivery Reviews*, *57*(15), 2177–2202. doi:10.1016/j.addr.2005.09.017 PMID:16310284

Dugershaw, B. B., Aengenheister, L., Hansen, S. S. K., Hougaard, K. S., & Buerki-Thurnherr, T. (2020). Recent insights on indirect mechanisms in developmental toxicity of nanomaterials. *Particle and Fibre Toxicology*, *17*(1), 1–22. doi:10.118612989-020-00359-x PMID:32653006

Du, M., Yang, Z., Lu, W., Wang, B., Wang, Q., Chen, Z., Chen, L., Han, S., Cai, T., & Cai, Y. (2020). Design and development of spirulina polysaccharide-loaded nanoemulsions with improved the antitumor effects of paclitaxel. *Journal of Microencapsulation*, *37*(6), 403–412. doi:10.1080/02652048.2020.1767224

Duncan, R., & Gaspar, R. (2011). *Nanomedicine (s) under the Microscope*, 2101–2141. ACS. doi:10.1021/mp200394t

Duraivathi, C., Priya, J. J., Poongodi, J., & Jeyakumar, H. J. (2022). Ultrasonic study of molecular interactions in organic liquid with CCl4 at different temperature. *Materials Today: Proceedings*, *49*, 1968–1972. doi:10.1016/j.matpr.2021.08.140

Dutt, Y., Pandey, R. P., Dutt, M., Gupta, A., Vibhuti, A., Vidic, J., Raj, V. S., Chang, C.-M., & Priyadarshini, A. (2023). Therapeutic applications of nanobiotechnology. *Journal of Nanobiotechnology*, *21*(1), 148. doi:10.118612951-023-01909-z PMID:37149615

Duvic, M., & Talpur, R. (2008). Optimizing denileukin diftitox (Ontak) therapy. *Future Oncology (London, England)*, *4*(4), 457–469. doi:10.2217/14796694.4.4.457

Ealias, A. M., & Saravanakumar, M. P. (2017). A review on the classification, characterisation, synthesis of nanoparticles and their application. IOP Conf. Ser. *Materials Science and Engineering*, *263*, 032019.

Edgington-Mitchell, L. E., Barlow, N., Aurelio, L., Samha, A., Szabo, M., Graham, B., & Bunnett, N. (2017). Fluorescent diphenylphosphonate-based probes for detection of serine protease activity during inflammation. *Bioorganic & Medicinal Chemistry Letters*, *27*(2), 254–260. doi:10.1016/j.bmcl.2016.11.064

Ediz, E., Kurtay, G., Karaca, B., Büyük, İ., Gökdemir, F. Ş., & Aras, S. (2021). Green synthesis of silver nanoparticles from Phaseolus vulgaris L. extracts and investigation of their antifungal activities. *Hacettepe Journal of Biology and Chemistry*, *49*(1), 11–23. doi:10.15671/hjbc.680371

Efimov, A. A., Lizunova, A. A., Volkov, I. A., Mylnikov, D. A., Arsenov, P. V., & Ivanov, V. V. (2016). A new approach to the high-yield synthesis of nanoparticles by spark discharge. *Journal of Physics: Conference Series*, *741*, 741. doi:10.1088/1742-6596/741/1/012035

Egas, A. P., Talavera-Prieto, N. M., Ferreira, A. G., Santos, J. B., Santos, M. J., Almeida, Z. L., & Fonseca, I. M. (2021). Speed of sound and derived thermodynamic properties of glycerol. *The Journal of Chemical Thermodynamics*, *156*, 106367. doi:10.1016/j.jct.2020.106367

Egbuna, C., Parmar, V. K., Jeevanandam, J., Ezzat, S. M., Patrick-Iwuanyanwu, K. C., Adetunji, C. O., Khan, J., Onyeike, E. N., Uche, C. Z., Akram, M., Ibrahim, M. S., El Mahdy, N. M., Awuchi, C. G., Saravanan, K., Tijjani, H., Odoh, U. E., Messaoudi, M., Ifemeje, J. C., Olisah, M. C., & Ibeabuchi, C. G. (2021). Toxicity of Nanoparticles in Biomedical Application: Nanotoxicology. *Journal of Toxicology*, *9954443*, 1–21. doi:10.1155/2021/9954443

Eid, M. A., Lewis, R. W., Abdel-Mageed, A. B., & Kumar, M. V. (2002). Reduced response of prostate cancer cells to TRAIL is modulated by NFkappaB-mediated inhibition of caspases and bid activation. *International Journal of Oncology*. doi:10.3892/ijo.21.1.111 PMID:12063557

Elahi, N., Kamali, M., & Baghersad, M. H. (2018). Recent biomedical applications of gold nanoparticles: A review. *Talanta*, *184*, 537–556. doi:10.1016/j.talanta.2018.02.088 PMID:29674080

Elansary, M., Belaiche, M., Mouhib, Y., Lemine, O. M., Bentarhlia, N., & Bsoul, I. (2023). Novel biocompatible nanomaterial for biomedical application: Structural, morphological, magnetic, and in vivo toxicity investigations. *Ceramics International*, *49*(3), 4551–4570. doi:10.1016/j.ceramint.2022.09.341

Eldar-Boock, A., Polyak, D., Scomparin, A., & Satchi-Fainaro, R. (2013). Nano-sized polymers and liposomes designed to deliver combination therapy for cancer. *Current Opinion in Biotechnology*, *24*(4), 682–689. doi:10.1016/j.copbio.2013.04.014 PMID:23726153

Elkateb, H., Cauldbeck, H., Niezabitowska, E., Hogarth, C., Arnold, K., Rannard, S., & McDonald, T. O. (2023). High drug loading solid lipid nanoparticles, nanostructured lipid carriers and nanoemulsions for the dual drug delivery of the HIV drugs darunavir and ritonavir. *JCIS Open*, *11*, 100087. doi:10.1016/j.jciso.2023.100087

Elmehbad, N. Y., Mohamed, N. A., Abd El-Ghany, N. A., & Abdel-Aziz, M. M. (2023). Reinforcement of the antimicrobial activity and biofilm inhibition of novel chitosan-based hydrogels utilizing zinc oxide nanoparticles. *International Journal of Biological Macromolecules*, *246*, 125582. doi:10.1016/j.ijbiomac.2023.125582 PMID:37379952

El-Naggar, N. E., Hussein, M. H., & El-Sawah, A. A. (2017). Bio-fabrication of silver nanoparticles by phycocyanin, characterization, in vitro anticancer activity against breast cancer cell line and in vivo cytotxicity. *Scientific Reports*, *7*(1), 10844. doi:10.103841598-017-11121-3 PMID:28883419

Eloy, J. O., Petrilli, R., Topan, J. F., Antonio, H. M. R., Barcellos, J. P. A., Chesca, D. L., Serafini, L. N., Tiezzi, D. G., Lee, R. J., & Marchetti, J. M. (2016). Co-loaded paclitaxel/rapamycin liposomes: Development, characterization and in vitro and in vivo evaluation for breast cancer therapy. *Colloids and Surfaces. B, Biointerfaces*, *141*, 74–82. doi:10.1016/j.colsurfb.2016.01.032

Elsabahy, M., & Wooley, K. L. (2012). Design of polymeric nanoparticles for biomedical delivery applications. *Chemical Society Reviews*, *41*(7), 2545. doi:10.1039/c2cs15327k PMID:22334259

Elshahed, M. S., Bhupathiraju, V. K., Wofford, N. Q., Nanny, M. A., & McInerney, M. J. (2001). Metabolism of Benzoate, Cyclohex-1-ene Carboxylate, and Cyclohexane Carboxylate by "Syntrophus aciditrophicus" Strain SB in Syntrophic Association with H_2-Using Microorganisms. *Applied and Environmental Microbiology*, *67*(4), 1728–1738. doi:10.1128/AEM.67.4.1728-1738.2001 PMID:11282627

Emami, A., Ghafouri, H., & Sariri, R. (2023). Polyphyllin D-loaded solid lipid nanoparticles for breast cancer: Synthesis, characterization, in vitro, and in vivo studies. *International Journal of Pharmaceutics*, *639*, 122976. doi:10.1016/j.ijpharm.2023.122976 PMID:37088118

Erdem, İ., & Çakır, Ş. (2022). Green synthesis of silver nanoparticles using walnut shell powder and cynara sp. and their antibacterial activities. *Hacettepe Journal of Biology and Chemistry*, *50*(4), 335–347. doi:10.15671/hjbc.984727

Erdlenbruch, B., Jendrossek, V., Eibl, H., & Lakomek, M. (2000). Transient and controllable opening of the blood-brain barrier to cytostatic and antibiotic agents by alkylglycerols in rats. *Experimental Brain Research*, *135*(3), 417–422. doi:10.1007002210000553 PMID:11146820

Erdogan, O., Abbak, M., Demirbolat, G. M., Birtekocak, F., Aksel, M., Pasa, S., & Cevik, O. (2019). Green synthesis of silver nanoparticles via Cynara scolymus leaf extracts: The characterization, anticancer potential with photodynamic therapy in MCF7 cells. *PLoS One*, *14*(6), e0216496. doi:10.1371/journal.pone.0216496 PMID:31220110

Eslamian, M., & Shekarriz, M. (2009). Recent advances in nanoparticle preparation by spray and microemulsion methods. *Recent Patents on Nanotechnology*, *3*(2), 99–115. doi:10.2174/187221009788490068 PMID:19519594

Essien, E. N., Revi, N., Khatri, V., Liu, S., Van Thiel, G., & Bijukumar, D. (2023). Methotrexate and sulforaphane loaded PBA-G5-PAMAM dendrimers as a combination therapy for anti-inflammatory response in an intra-articular joint arthritic animal model. *International Journal of Pharmaceutics*, *642*, 123150. doi:10.1016/j.ijpharm.2023.123150 PMID:37336302

Estelrich, J., Sánchez-Martín, M. J., & Busquets, M. A. (2015). Nanoparticles in magnetic resonance imaging: From simple to dual contrast agents. *International Journal of Nanomedicine*, *10*, 1727–1741. doi:10.2147/IJN.S76501 PMID:25834422

Ethaib, S., Al-Qutaifia, S., Al-Ansari, N., & Zubaidi, S. L. (2022). Function of Nanomaterials in Removing Heavy Metals for Water and Wastewater Remediation: A Review. *Environments (Basel, Switzerland)*, *9*(10), 123. doi:10.3390/environments9100123

Etheridge, M. L., Campbell, S. A., Erdman, A. G., Haynes, C. L., Wolf, S. M., & Mccullough, J. (2013). The big picture on nanomedicine: The state of investigational and approved nanomedicine products. *Nanomedicine; Nanotechnology, Biology, and Medicine*, *9*(1), 1–14. doi:10.1016/j.nano.2012.05.013 PMID:22684017

Ettinger, A. R. (1995). Pegaspargase (Oncaspar). *Journal of Pediatric Oncology Nursing*, *12*(1), 46–48. doi:10.1177/104345429501200110

Fahmy, T.M., Fong, P.M., Goyal, A., & Saltzman, W.M. (2005). Targeted for drug delivery. Mater Today, 8, 18–26. doi: 71033-610. doi:10.1016/S1369-7021(05)

Falahati, M., Attar, F., Sharifi, M., Saboury, A. A., Salihi, A., Aziz, F. M., Kostova, I., Burda, C., Priecel, P., Lopez-Sanchez, J. A., Laurent, S., Hooshmand, N., & El-Sayed, M. A. (1864). 2020. Gold nanomaterials as key suppliers in biological and chemical sensing, catalysis, and medicine. *Biochimica et Biophysica Acta (BBA)-. Biochimica et Biophysica Acta. G, General Subjects*, *1864*(1), 129435. doi:10.1016/j.bbagen.2019.129435 PMID:31526869

Fan, R. Z., Fei, D., D'Aurelio, R., & Ge, Y. (2014). The Impact of Nanopharmaceuticals on Healthcare and Regulation. *Nanomedicine: Principles and Perspectives*, 355-364. doi:10.1007/978-1-4614-2140-5_17

Fang, R. H., Kroll, A. V., Gao, W., & Zhang, L. (2018). Cell Membrane Coating Nanotechnology. *Advanced Materials*, *30*(23), 1706759. doi:10.1002/adma.201706759 PMID:29582476

Fang, X., Wang, Y., Ma, X., Li, Y., Zhang, Z., Xiao, Z., Liu, L., Gao, X., & Liu, J. (2017). Mitochondria-targeting Au nanoclusters enhance radiosensitivity of cancer cells. *Journal of Materials Chemistry. B*, *5*(5), 4190–4197. doi:10.1039/C7TB00422B

Farah, M., Ali, M. A., Chen, S. M., Li, Y., Al-Hemaid, F. M., & Abou-Tarboush, F. M. (2016). Silver nanoparticle synthesized from Adenium obesum leaf extract: Anticancer, antimicrobial, antioxidant and catalytic activities. *Arabian Journal of Chemistry*, *9*(6), 970–975.

Fard, N. N., Noorbazargan, H., Mirzaie, A., Hedayati, Ch. M., Moghimiyan, Z., & Rahimi, A. (2018). Biogenic synthesis of Ag-NPs using Artemisia oliveriana extract and their biological activities for an effective treatment of lung cancer. *Artificial Cells, Nanomedicine, and Biotechnology*, *46*(sup3), 1047–1058. doi:10.1080/21691401.2018.1528983 PMID:30479160

Faria, M., Björnmalm, M., Thurecht, K. J., Kent, S. J., Parton, R. G., Kavallaris, M., Johnston, A. P. R., Gooding, J. J., Corrie, S. R., Boyd, B. J., Thordarson, P., Whittaker, A. K., Stevens, M. M., Prestidge, C. A., Porter, C. J. H., Parak, W. J., Davis, T. P., Crampin, E. J., & Caruso, F. (2018). Minimum information reporting in bio–nano experimental literature. *Nature Nanotechnology*, *13*(9), 777–785. doi:10.103841565-018-0246-4 PMID:30190620

Farina, E., Nabhen, J. J., Dacoregio, M. I., Batalini, F., & Moraes, F. Y. (2022). An overview of artificial intelligence in oncology. *Future Science OA*, *8*(8), FSO787. doi:10.2144/fsoa-2021-0074

Farjadian, F., Ghasemi, A., Gohari, O., Roointan, A., Karimi, M., & Hamblin, M. R. (2019). Nanopharmaceuticals and nanomedicines currently on the market: Challenges and opportunities. *Nanomedicine (London)*, *14*(1), 93–126. doi:10.2217/nnm-2018-0120 PMID:30451076

Fastier-Wooller, J. W., Dau, V. T., Dinh, T., Tran, C. D., & Dao, D. V. (2021). Pressure and Temperature Sensitive e-Skin for in situ Robotic Applications. *Materials & Design*, *208*, 109886. doi:10.1016/j.matdes.2021.109886

Fateh Basharzad, S., Hamidi, M., Maleki, A., Karami, Z., Mohamadpour, H., & Reza Saghatchi Zanjani, M. (2022). Polysorbate-coated mesoporous silica nanoparticles as an efficient carrier for improved rivastigmine brain delivery. *Brain Research*, *1781*, 147786. doi:10.1016/j.brainres.2022.147786 PMID:35041841

Fathi-Achachelouei, M., Knopf-Marques, H., Ribeiro da Silva, C. E., Barthès, J., Bat, E., Tezcaner, A., & Vrana, N. E. (2019). Use of nanoparticles in tissue engineering and regenerative medicine. *Frontiers in Bioengineering and Biotechnology*, *7*, 113. doi:10.3389/fbioe.2019.00113 PMID:31179276

Fatima, H., Charinpanitkul, T., & Kim, K. S. (2021). Fundamentals to Apply Magnetic Nanoparticles for Hyperthermia Therapy. *Nanomaterials*, *11*(5), 1203. doi:10.3390/nano11051203

Fessi, H. P. F. D., Puisieux, F., Devissaguet, J. P., Ammoury, N., & Benita, S. (1989). Nanocapsule formation by interfacial polymer deposition following solvent displacement. *International Journal of Pharmaceutics*, *55*(1), R1–R4. doi:10.1016/0378-5173(89)90281-0

Filoche, S. K., Zhu, M., & Wu, C. D. (2004). In situ biofilm formation by multi-species oral bacteria under flowing and anaerobic conditions. *Journal of Dental Research*, *83*(10), 802–806. doi:10.1177/154405910408301013 PMID:15381723

Finn, O. J., & Beatty, P. L. (2016). Cancer immunoprevention. *Current Opinion in Immunology*, *39*, 52–58. doi:10.1016/j.coi.2016.01.002

Firdhouse, M. J., & Lalitha, P. (2013). Biosynthesis of silver nanoparticles using the extract of Alternanthera sessilis-antiproliferative effect against prostate cancer cells. *Cancer Nanotechnology*, *4*(6), 137–143. doi:10.100712645-013-0045-4 PMID:26069509

Fischer, M., Appelhans, D., Schwarz, S., Klajnert, B., Bryszewska, M., Voit, B., & Rogers, M. (2010). Influence of surface functionality of poly(propylene imine) dendrimers on protease resistance and propagation of the scrapie prion protein. *Biomacromolecules*, *11*(5), 1314–1325. doi:10.1021/bm100101s PMID:20405854

Fisher, R. S., & Ho, J. (2002). Potential new methods for antiepileptic drug delivery. *CNS Drugs*, *16*(9), 579–593. doi:10.2165/00023210-200216090-00001 PMID:12153331

Fleige, E., Quadir, M. A., & Haag, R. (2012). Stimuli-responsive polymeric nanocarriers for the controlled transport of active compounds: Concepts and applications. *Advanced Drug Delivery Reviews*, *64*(9), 866–884. doi:10.1016/j.addr.2012.01.020 PMID:22349241

Fleischer, C. C., & Payne, C. K. (2014). Nanoparticle-cell interactions: Molecular structure of theprotein corona and cellular outcomes. *Accounts of Chemical Research*, *47*(8), 2651–2659. doi:10.1021/ar500190q PMID:25014679

Flemming, H. C., Neu, T. R., & Wozniak, D. J. (2007). The EPS matrix: The "House of Biofilm Cells.". *Journal of Bacteriology*, *189*(22), 7945–7947. doi:10.1128/JB.00858-07 PMID:17675377

Flühmann, B., Ntai, I., Brorchard, G., Simoens, S., & Mühlebach, S. (2018). SC. *European Journal of Pharmaceutical Sciences*. doi:10.1016/j.ejps.2018.11.019

Foged, C., Brodin, B., Frokjaer, S., & Sundblad, A. (2005). Particle size and surface charge affect particle uptake by human dendritic cells in an in vitro model. *International Journal of Pharmaceutics*, *298*(2), 315–322. doi:10.1016/j.ijpharm.2005.03.035

Fonseca-Santos, B., Gremião, M. P. D., & Chorilli, M. (2015). Nanotechnology-based drug delivery systems for the treatment of Alzheimer's disease. *International Journal of Nanomedicine*, *10*, 4981–5003. doi:10.2147/IJN.S87148

Fornaguera, C., Feiner-Gracia, N., Calderó, G., García-Celma, M. J., & Solans, C. (2015). Galantamine-loaded PLGA nanoparticles, from nano-emulsion templating, as novel advanced drug delivery systems to treat neurodegenerative diseases. *Nanoscale*, *7*(28), 12076–12084. doi:10.1039/C5NR03474D PMID:26118655

Foroozandeh, P., & Aziz, A. A. (2018). Insight into cellular uptake and intracellular trafficking of nanoparticles. *Nanoscale Research Letters*, *13*(1), 1–12. doi:10.118611671-018-2728-6 PMID:30361809

Foulkes, R., Man, E., Thind, J., Yeung, S., Joy, A., & Hoskins, C. (2020). The regulation of nanomaterials and nanomedicines for clinical application: Current and future perspectives. *Biomaterials Science*, *8*(17), 4653–4664. doi:10.1039/D0BM00558D PMID:32672255

Frampton, J. E. (2010). Mifamurtide. *Paediatric Drugs*, *12*(3), 141–153. doi:10.2165/11204910-000000000-00000

Freidus, L. G., Pradeep, P., Kumar, P., Choonara, Y. E., & Pillay, V. (2018). Alternative fluorophores designed for advanced molecular imaging. *Drug Discovery Today*, *23*(1), 115–133. doi:10.1016/j.drudis.2017.09.008 PMID:29111179

Freis, B., Ramírez, M. D. L. Á., Furgiuele, S., Journe, F., Cheignon, C., Charbonnière, L. J., Henoumont, C., Kiefer, C., Mertz, D., Affolter-Zbaraszczuk, C., Meyer, F., Saussez, S., Laurent, S., Tasso, M., & Bégin-Colin, S. (2023). Bioconjugation studies of an EGF-R targeting ligand on dendronized iron oxide nanoparticles to target head and neck cancer cells. *International Journal of Pharmaceutics*, *635*, 122654. doi:10.1016/j.ijpharm.2023.122654 PMID:36720449

Fresta, M., Puglisi, G., Giammona, G., Cavallaro, G., Micali, N., & Furneri, P. M. (1995). Pefloxacine mesylate-and ofloxacin-loaded polyethylcyanoacrylate nanoparticles: Characterization of the colloidal drug carrier formulation. *Journal of Pharmaceutical Sciences*, *84*(7), 895–902. doi:10.1002/jps.2600840721 PMID:7562444

Frigerio, B., Bizzoni, C., Jansen, G., Leamon, C. P., Peters, G. J., Low, P. S., Matherly, L. H., & Figini, M. (2019). Folate receptors and transporters: Biological role and diagnostic/therapeutic targets in cancer and other diseases. *Journal of Experimental & Clinical Cancer Research: Cr.* . doi:10.1186/s13046-019-1123-1

Fritea, L., Banica, F., Costea, T. O., Moldovan, L., Dobjanschi, L., Muresan, M., & Cavalu, S. (2021). Metal nanoparticles and carbon-based nanomaterials for improved performances of electrochemical (Bio) sensors with biomedical applications. *Materials (Basel)*, *14*(21), 6319. doi:10.3390/ma14216319 PMID:34771844

Fu, C., Liu, T., Li, L., Liu, H., Chen, D., & Tang, F. (2013). The absorption, distribution, excretion and toxicity of mesoporous silica nanoparticles in mice following different exposure routes. *Biomaterials*, *34*(10), 2565–2575. doi:10.1016/j.biomaterials.2012.12.043 PMID:23332175

Funda, G., Taschieri, S., Bruno, G. A., Grecchi, E., Paolo, S., Girolamo, D., & Del Fabbro, M. (2020). Nanotechnology Scaffolds for Alveolar Bone Regeneration. *Materials (Basel)*, *13*(1), 201. doi:10.3390/ma13010201 PMID:31947750

Fu, Q., Wang, J., & Liu, H. (2020). Chemo-immune synergetic therapy of esophageal carcinoma: Trastuzumab modified, cisplatin and fluorouracil co-delivered lipid–polymer hybrid nanoparticles. *Drug Delivery*, *27*(1), 1535–1543. doi:10.1080/10717544.2020.1837294

Gagliardi, A., Giuliano, E., Venkateswararao, E., Fresta, M., Bulotta, S., Awasthi, V., & Cosco, D. (2021). Biodegradable polymeric nanoparticles for drug delivery to solid tumors. *Frontiers in Pharmacology*, *12*, 601626. doi:10.3389/fphar.2021.601626 PMID:33613290

Gaikwad, S. S., Morade, Y. Y., Kothule, A. M., Kshirsagar, S. J., Laddha, U. D., & Salunkhe, K. S. (2023). Overview of phytosomes in treating cancer: Advancement, challenges, and future outlook. *Heliyon*, *9*(6), e16561. doi:10.1016/j.heliyon.2023.e16561 PMID:37260890

Gaikwad, S., Ingle, A., Gade, A., Rai, M., Falanga, A., Incoronato, N., Russo, L., Galdiero, S., & Galdiero, M. (2013, November 6). Antiviral activity of mycosynthesized silver nanoparticles against herpes simplex virus and human parainfluenza virus type 3. *International Journal of Nanomedicine*, 4303–4314. PMID:24235828

Ganachaud, F., & Katz, J. L. (2005). Nanoparticles and nanocapsules created using the ouzo effect: Spontaneous emulsification as an alternative to ultrasonic and high-shear devices. *ChemPhysChem*, *6*(2), 209–216. doi:10.1002/cphc.200400527 PMID:15751338

Ganesan, M., & Nagaraaj, P. (2020). Quantum dots as nanosensors for detection of toxics: A literature review. *Analytical Methods*, *12*(35), 4254–4275. doi:10.1039/D0AY01293A PMID:32940270

Ganta, S., Devalapally, H., Shahiwala, A., & Amiji, M. (2008). A review of stimuli-responsive nanocarriers for drug and genedelivery. *Journal of controlled release: official journal of the Controlled Release Society, 126*, 87-204.

Gao, C., Lyu, F., & Yin, Y. (2020). Encapsulated metal nanoparticles for catalysis. *Chemical Reviews*, *121*(2), 834–881. doi:10.1021/acs.chemrev.0c00237 PMID:32585087

Gao, D., Xu, H., Philbert, M. A., & Kopelman, R. (2008). Bioeliminable Nanohydrogels for Drug Delivery. *Nano Letters*, *8*(10), 3320–3324. doi:10.1021/nl8017274 PMID:18788823

Gao, J., Gu, H., & Xu, B. (2009). Multifunctional magnetic nanoparticles: Design, synthesis, and biomedical applications. *Accounts of Chemical Research*, *42*(8), 1097–1107. doi:10.1021/ar9000026 PMID:19476332

Gao, S., Yang, X., Xu, J., Qiu, N., & Zhai, G. (2021). Nanotechnology for boosting cancer immunotherapy and remodeling tumor microenvironment: The horizons in cancer treatment. *ACS Nano*, *15*(8), 12567–12603. doi:10.1021/acsnano.1c02103

García-García, G., Caro, C., Fernández-Álvarez, F., García-Martín, M. L., & Arias, J. L. (2023). Multi-stimuli-responsive chitosan-functionalized magnetite/poly(ε-caprolactone) nanoparticles as theranostic platforms for combined tumor magnetic resonance imaging and chemotherapy. *Nanomedicine; Nanotechnology, Biology, and Medicine*, *52*, 102695. doi:10.1016/j.nano.2023.102695 PMID:37394106

Garcia-Gonzalez, I., Mühleder, S., Fernández-Chacón, M., & Benedito, R. (2020). Genetic tools to study cardiovascular biology. *Frontiers in Physiology*, *11*, 1084. doi:10.3389/fphys.2020.01084 PMID:33071802

Garibyan, A., Delyagina, E., & Terekhova, I. (2023). Improving properties of baricitinib due to interaction with Pluronic micelles. *Journal of Molecular Liquids*, *382*, 121968. doi:10.1016/j.molliq.2023.121968

Gatti, T. H. H., Eloy, J. O., Ferreira, L. M. B., Silva, I. C. D., Pavan, F. R., Gremião, M. P. D., & Chorilli, M. (2018). Insulin-loaded polymeric mucoadhesive nanoparticles: Development, characterization and cytotoxicity evaluation. *Brazilian Journal of Pharmaceutical Sciences*, *54*(1), 54. doi:10.15902175-97902018000117314

Gaur, M., Misra, C., Yadav, A. B., Swaroop, S., Maolmhuaidh, F., Bechelany, M., & Barhoum, A. (2021). Biomedical applications of carbon nanomaterials: Fullerenes, quantum dots, nanotubes, nanofibers, and graphene. *Materials (Basel)*, *14*(20), 5978. doi:10.3390/ma14205978 PMID:34683568

Gautam, S., Das, D. K., Kaur, J., Kumar, A., Ubaidullah, M., Hasan, M., Yadav, K. K., & Gupta, R. K. (2023). Transition metal-based nanoparticles as potential antimicrobial agents: Recent advancements, mechanistic, challenges, and future prospects. *Discover Nano*, *18*(1), 84. Advance online publication. doi:10.118611671-023-03861-1 PMID:37382784

Gavas, S., Quazi, S., & Karpiński, T. M. (2021). Nanoparticles for Cancer Therapy: Current Progress and Challenges. *Nanoscale Research Letters*, *16*(1), 173. doi:10.118611671-021-03628-6 PMID:34866166

Ge, C., Du, J., Zhao, L., Wang, L., Liu, Y., Li, D., Yang, Y., Zhou, R., Zhao, Y., Chai, Z., & Chen, C. (2011). Binding of Blood Proteins to Carbon Nanotubes Reduces Cytotoxicity. *Proceedings of the National Academy of Sciences of the United States of America*, *108*(41), 16968–16973. doi:10.1073/pnas.1105270108 PMID:21969544

Geisow, M. J., & Evans, W. H. (1984). pH in the endosome: Measurements during pinocytosis and receptor-mediated endocytosis. *Experimental Cell Research*, *150*(1), 36–46. doi:10.1016/0014-4827(84)90699-2 PMID:6198190

Ge, J., Lei, J., & Zare, R. N. (2011). Bovine serum albumin–poly (methyl methacrylate) nanoparticles: An example of frustrated phase separation. *Nano Letters*, *11*(6), 2551–2554. doi:10.1021/nl201303q PMID:21553851

Ge, J., Zhang, Q., Zeng, J., Gu, Z., & Gao, M. (2020). Radiolabeling nanomaterials for multimodality imaging: New insights into nuclear medicine and cancer diagnosis. *Biomaterials*, *228*, 119553. doi:10.1016/j.biomaterials.2019.119553 PMID:31689672

Gerasimenko, A. Y., Ichkitidze, L. P., Podgaetsky, V. M., & Selishchev, S. V. (2015). Biomedical Applications of Promising Nanomaterials with Carbon Nanotubes. *Biomedical Engineering*, *48*(6), 310–314. doi:10.100710527-015-9476-z

Gertz, F., & Khitun, A. (2016). Biological cell manipulation by magnetic nanoparticles. *AIP Advances*, *6*(2), 025308. doi:10.1063/1.4942090

Ghaderi, S., Ramesh, B., & Seifalian, A. M. (2011). Fluorescence nanoparticles "quantum dots" as drug delivery system and their toxicity: A review. *Journal of Drug Targeting*, *19*(7), 475–486. doi:10.3109/1061186X.2010.526227 PMID:20964619

Ghaemi, F., Amiri, A., Bajuri, M. Y., Yuhana, N. Y., & Ferrara, M. (2021). Role of different types of nanomaterials against diagnosis, prevention and therapy of COVID-19. *Sustainable Cities and Society*, *72*, 103046. doi:10.1016/j.scs.2021.103046 PMID:34055576

Ghazanfar, H., Rizvi, S. W., Khurram, A., Orooj, F., & Qaiser, I. (2016). Impact of insulin pump on quality of life of diabetic patients. *Indian Journal of Endocrinology and Metabolism*, *20*(4), 506. doi:10.4103/2230-8210.183472 PMID:27366717

Gheibi Hayat, S. M., & Darroudi, M. (2019). Nanovaccine: A novel approach in immunization. *Journal of Cellular Physiology*, *234*(8), 12530–12536. doi:10.1002/jcp.28120 PMID:30633361

Gholami, A., Hashemi, S. A., Yousefi, K., Mousavi, S. M., Chiang, W.-H., Ramakrishna, S., Mazraedoost, S., Alizadeh, A., Omidifar, N., Behbudi, G., & Babapoor, A. (2020). 3D Nanostructures for Tissue Engineering, Cancer Therapy, and Gene Delivery. *Journal of Nanomaterials*, *1852946*, 1–24. doi:10.1155/2020/1852946

Gholami, A., Mousavi, S. M., Hashemi, S. A., Ghasemi, Y., Chiang, W.-H., & Parvin, N. (2020). Current trends in chemical modifications of magnetic nanoparticles for targeted drug delivery in cancer chemotherapy. *Drug Metabolism Reviews*, (52), 205–224. doi:10.1080/03602532.2020.1726943

Ghosh Tapash K. & Jasti Bhaskar R. (2009). *Oral controlled release Solid Dosage Forms; In theory and practice of contemporary Pharmaceutics*. CRC Press.

Ghosh, B., & Biswas, S. (2021). Polymeric micelles in cancer therapy: State of the art. *Journal of Controlled Release*, *332*, 127–147. doi:10.1016/j.jconrel.2021.02.016 PMID:33609621

Ghosh, S. (2004). Recent research and development in synthetic polymer-based drug delivery systems. *Journal of Chemical Research*, *2004*(4), 241–246. doi:10.3184/0308234041209158

Ghosh, S., Irvin, K., & Thayumanavan, S. (2007). Tunable disassembly of micelles using a redox trigger. *Langmuir*, *23*(15), 7916–7919. doi:10.1021/la700981z PMID:17567057

Giljohann, D. A., Seferos, D. S., Daniel, W. L., Massich, M. D., Patel, P. C., & Mirkin, C. A. (2010). Gold nanoparticles for biology and medicine. *Angewandte Chemie International Edition*, *49*(19), 3280–3294. doi:10.1002/anie.200904359 PMID:20401880

Gilligan, K. E., & Dwyer, R. M. (2017). Engineering exosomes for cancer therapy. *International Journal of Molecular Sciences*, *18*(6), 1122. doi:10.3390/ijms18061122

Gill, P. S., Wernz, J., Scadden, D. T., Cohen, P., Mukwaya, G. M., von Roenn, J. H., Jacobs, M., Kempin, S., Silverberg, I., Gonzales, G., Rarick, M. U., Myers, A. M., Shepherd, F., Sawka, C., Pike, M. C., & Ross, M. E. (1996). Randomized phase III trial of liposomal daunorubicin versus doxorubicin, bleomycin, and vincristine in AIDS-related Kaposi's sarcoma. *Journal of Clinical Oncology*, *14*(8), 2353–2364. doi:10.1200/JCO.1996.14.8.2353

Giustini, A. J., Petryk, A. A., Cassim, S. M., Tate, J. A., Baker, I., & Hoopes, P. J. (2010). Magnetic Nanoparticle Hyperthermia In Cancer Treatment. *Nano LIFE, 1*(1n02), . https://doi.org/ doi:10.1142/S1793984410000067

Goebel, J., Chmielewski, J., & Hrycyna, C. A. (2021). The roles of the human ATP-binding cassette transporters P-glycoprotein and ABCG2 in multidrug resistance in cancer and at endogenous sites: Future opportunities for structure-based drug design of inhibitors. *Cancer Drug Resistance (Alhambra, Calif.)*. doi:10.20517/cdr.2021.19 PMID:34993424

Goel, M., Mackeyev, Y., & Krishnan, S. (2023). Radiolabeled nanomaterial for cancer diagnostics and therapeutics: Principles and concepts. *Cancer Nanotechnology*, *14*(1), 1–36. doi:10.118612645-023-00165-y PMID:36865684

Golchin, A., Rekabgardan, M., Taheri, R. A., & Nourani, M. R. (2018). *Promotion of cell-based therapy: special focus on the cooperation of mesenchymal stem cell therapy and gene therapy for clinical trial studies. Cell Biology and Translational Medicine* (Vol. 4). Stem Cells and Cell Based Strategies in Regeneration. doi:10.1007/5584_2018_256

Goldberg, M. S. (2019). Improving cancer immunotherapy through nanotechnology. *Nature Reviews. Cancer*, *19*(10), 587–602. doi:10.103841568-019-0186-9

Gomathi, A. C., Xavier Rajarathinam, S. R., Mohammed Sadiq, A., & Rajeshkumar, S. (2020). Anticancer activity of silver nanoparticles synthesized using aqueous fruit shell extract of Tamarindus indica on MCF-7 human breast cancer cell line. *Journal of Drug Delivery Science and Technology*, *55*, 101376. doi:10.1016/j.jddst.2019.101376

Gong, H., Peng, R., & Liu, Z. (2013). Carbon nanotubes for biomedical imaging: The recent advances. *Advanced Drug Delivery Reviews*, *65*(15), 1951–1963. doi:10.1016/j.addr.2013.10.002 PMID:24184130

Gong, N., Sheppard, N. C., Billingsley, M. M., June, C. H., & Mitchell, M. J. (2021). Nanomaterials for T-cell cancer immunotherapy. *Nature Nanotechnology*, *16*(1), 25–36. doi:10.103841565-020-00822-y

González-Toro, D. C., Ryu, J. H., Chacko, R. T., Zhuang, J., & Thayumanavan, S. (2012). Concurrent binding and delivery of proteins and lipophilic small molecules using polymeric nanogels. *Journal of the American Chemical Society*, *134*(16), 6964–6967. doi:10.1021/ja3019143 PMID:22480205

Gopisetty, M. K., Kovács, D., Igaz, N., Rónavári, A., Bélteky, P., Rázga, Z., Venglovecz, V., Csoboz, B., Boros, I. M., Kónya, Z., & Kiricsi, M. (2019). Endoplasmic reticulum stress: Major player in size-dependent inhibition of P-glycoprotein by silver nanoparticles in multidrug-resistant breast cancer cells. *Journal of Nanobiotechnology*, *17*(1), 1–15. doi:10.118612951-019-0448-4 PMID:30670028

Govender, T., Stolnik, S., Garnett, M. C., Illum, L., & Davis, S. S. (1999). PLGA nanoparticles prepared by nanoprecipitation: Drug loading and release studies of a water soluble drug. *Journal of Controlled Release*, *57*(2), 171–185. doi:10.1016/S0168-3659(98)00116-3 PMID:9971898

Govindan, B., Sabri, M. A., Hai, A., Banat, F., & Haija, M. A. (2023). A Review of Advanced Multifunctional Magnetic Nanostructures for Cancer Diagnosis and Therapy Integrated into an Artificial Intelligence Approach. *Pharmaceutics*, *15*(3), 868. doi:10.3390/pharmaceutics15030868

Govindarajan, D. K., & Kandaswamy, K. (2022). Virulence factors of uropathogens and their role in host pathogen interactions. *Cell Surface (Amsterdam, Netherlands)*, *8*, 100075. doi:10.1016/j.tcsw.2022.100075 PMID:35198842

Govindarajan, D. K., & Kandaswamy, K. (2023). Antimicrobial peptides: A small molecule for sustainable healthcare applications. *Medicine in Microecology*, *18*, 100090. doi:10.1016/j.medmic.2023.100090

Govindarajan, D. K., Meghanathan, Y., Sivaramakrishnan, M., Kothandan, R., Muthusamy, A., Seviour, T. W., & Kandaswamy, K. (2022). Enterococcus faecalis thrives in dual-species biofilm models under iron-rich conditions. *Archives of Microbiology*, *204*(12), 710. doi:10.100700203-022-03309-7 PMID:36383258

Goyal, R., Macri, L. K., Kaplan, H. M., & Kohn, J. (2016). Nanoparticles and nanofibers for topical drug delivery. *Journal of Controlled Release*, *240*, 77–92. doi:10.1016/j.jconrel.2015.10.049 PMID:26518723

Grabowski, N., Hillaireau, H., Vergnaud, J., Tsapis, N., Pallardy, M., Kerdine-Römer, S., & Fattal, E. (2015). Surface coating mediates the toxicity of polymeric nanoparticles towards human-like macrophages. *International Journal of Pharmaceutics*, *482*(1-2), 75–83. doi:10.1016/j.ijpharm.2014.11.042 PMID:25448553

Grammatikopoulos, P., Steinhauer, S., Vernieres, J., Singh, V., & Sowwan, M. (2016). Nanoparticle design by gas-phase synthesis. *Advances in Physics: X*, *1*(1), 81–100. doi:10.1080/23746149.2016.1142829

Grana, A., Limpach, A., & Chauhan, H. (2013). Formulation considerations and applications of solid lipid nanoparticles. *American Pharmaceutical Review*, 16.

Greulich, C., Diendorf, J., Simon, T., Eggeler, G., Epple, M., & Köller, M. (2011). Uptake and intracellular distribution of silver nanoparticles in human mesenchymal stem cells. *Acta Biomaterialia*, *7*(1), 347–354. doi:10.1016/j.actbio.2010.08.003 PMID:20709196

Grislain, L., Couvreur, P., Lenaerts, V., Roland, M., Deprez-Decampeneere, D., & Speiser, P. (1983). Pharmacokinetics and distribution of a biodegradable drug carrier. *International Journal of Pharmaceutics*, *15*(3), 335–345. doi:10.1016/0378-5173(83)90166-7

Guerrini, L., Rodriguez-Loureiro, I., Correa-Duarte, M. A., Lee, Y. H., Ling, X. Y., García De Abajo, F. J., & Alvarez-Puebla, R. A. (2014). Chemical speciation of heavy metals by surface-enhanced Raman scattering spectroscopy: Identification and quantification of inorganic- and methyl-mercury in water. *Nanoscale*, *6*(14), 8368–8375. doi:10.1039/C4NR01464B PMID:24938410

Guimarães, D., Cavaco-Paulo, A., & Nogueira, E. (2021). Design of liposomes as drug delivery system for therapeutic applications. *International Journal of Pharmaceutics*, *601*, 120571. doi:10.1016/j.ijpharm.2021.120571 PMID:33812967

Guisbiers, G., Mejía-Rosales, S., & Deepak, F. L. (2012). Nanomaterial Properties: Size and Shape Dependencies. *Journal of Nanomaterials*, *180976*, 1–2. doi:10.1155/2012/180976

Gulumian, M., Andraos, C., Afantitis, A., Puzyn, T., & Coville, N. J. (2021). Importance of Surface Topography in Both Biological Activity and Catalysis of Nanomaterials: Can Catalysis by Design Guide Safe by Design? *International Journal of Molecular Sciences*, *22*(15), 8347. doi:10.3390/ijms22158347 PMID:34361117

Guo, J., Rahme, K., He, Y., Li, L. L., Holmes, J. D., & O'Driscoll, C. M. (2017). Gold nanoparticles enlighten the future of cancer theranostics. *International Journal of Nanomedicine*, *12*, 6131–6152. doi:10.2147/IJN.S140772 PMID:28883725

Guo, X., Shi, C., Yang, G., Wang, J., Cai, Z., & Zhou, S. (2014). Dual-responsive polymer micelles for target-cell-specific anticancer drug delivery. *Chemistry of Materials*, *26*(15), 4405–4418. doi:10.1021/cm5012718

Guo, Z., Zhang, P., Chakraborty, S., Chetwynd, A. J., Abdolahpur Monikh, F., Stark, C., Ali-Boucetta, H., Wilson, S., Lynch, I., & Valsami-Jones, E. (2021). Biotransformation modulates the penetration of metallic nanomaterials across an artificial blood–brain barrier model. *Proceedings of the National Academy of Sciences of the United States of America*, *118*(28), e2105245118. doi:10.1073/pnas.2105245118 PMID:34260400

Gu, P., Wusiman, A., Wang, S., Zhang, Y., Liu, Z., Hu, Y., Liu, J., & Wang, D. (2019). Polyethylenimine-coated PLGA nanoparticles-encapsulated Angelica sinensis polysaccharide as an adjuvant to enhance immune responses. *Carbohydrate Polymers*, *223*, 115128. doi:10.1016/j.carbpol.2019.115128 PMID:31427012

Gupta, R. (2017). Diabetes treatment by nanotechnology. *Journal of Biotechnology & Biomaterials*, *7*(3), 268. doi:10.4172/2155-952X.1000268

Gupta, V., Mohapatra, S., Mishra, H., Farooq, U., Kumar, K., Ansari, M. J., & Iqbal, Z. (2022). Nanotechnology in cosmetics and cosmeceuticals—A review of latest advancements. *Gels (Basel, Switzerland)*, *8*(3), 173. doi:10.3390/gels8030173 PMID:35323286

Gurav, D. D., Jia, Y. A., Ye, J., & Qian, K. (2019). Design of plasmonic nanomaterials for diagnostic spectrometry. *Nanoscale Advances*, *1*(2), 459–469. doi:10.1039/C8NA00319J PMID:36132258

Gürbüz, M. U., Ertürk, A. S., & Tülü, M. (2017). Synthesis of surface-modified TREN-cored PAMAM dendrimers and their effects on the solubility of sulfamethoxazole (SMZ) as an analog antibiotic drug. *Pharmaceutical Development and Technology*, *22*(5), 678–689. doi:10.1080/10837450.2016.1221425 PMID:27493125

Gurunathan, S., Jeong, J. K., Han, J. W., Zhang, X. F., Park, J. H., & Kim, J. H. (2015). Multidimensional effects of biologically synthesized silver NPs in Helicobacter pylori, Helicobacter felis, and human lung (L132) and lung carcinoma A549 cells. *Nanoscale Research Letters*, *10*(1), 35. doi:10.118611671-015-0747-0 PMID:25852332

Gurunathan, S., Qasim, M., Park, C., Yoo, H., Kim, J. H., & Hong, K. (2018). Cytotoxic Potential and Molecular Pathway Analysis of Silver Nanoparticles in Human Colon Cancer Cells HCT116. *International Journal of Molecular Sciences*, *19*(8), 2269. doi:10.3390/ijms19082269 PMID:30072642

Guterres, S. S., Alves, M. P., & Pohlmann, A. R. (2007). Polymeric nanoparticles, nanospheres and nanocapsules, for cutaneous applications. *Drug Target Insights*, *2*, 117739280700200002. doi:10.1177/117739280700200002 PMID:21901071

Gu, X., Zhou, J., Zhou, L., Xie, S., Petti, L., Wang, S., & Wang, F. (2018). Specific Binding of Antigen-Antibody in Physiological Environments: Measurement, Force Characteristics and Analysis. *Optics and Lasers in Engineering*, *104*, 252–258. doi:10.1016/j.optlaseng.2017.09.016

Gu, Z., Biswas, A., Zhao, M., & Tang, Y. (2011). Tailoring nanocarriers for intracellular protein delivery. *Chemical Society Reviews*, *40*(7), 3638–3655. doi:10.1039/c0cs00227e PMID:21566806

H. Sadegh;R. Shahryari-ghoshekandi. (2015). Functionalization of carbon nanotubes and its application in nanomedicine: A review. *Nanomedicine Journal, 2*(4), 231–248. https://doi.org/. 2015.04.001 doi:10.7508/nmj

Habumugisha, T., Zhang, Z., Fang, C., Yan, C., & Zhang, X. (2023). Uptake, bioaccumulation, biodistribution and depuration of polystyrene nanoplastics in zebrafish (Danio rerio). *The Science of the Total Environment*, *893*, 164840. doi:10.1016/j.scitotenv.2023.164840 PMID:37321508

Ha, H., Amicucci, C., Matteini, P., & Hwang, B. (2022). Mini review of synthesis strategies of silver nanowires and their applications. *Colloid and Interface Science Communications*, *50*, 100663. doi:10.1016/j.colcom.2022.100663

Hainfeld, J. F., Dilmanian, F. A., Zhong, Z., Slatkin, D. N., Kalef-Ezra, J. A., & Smilowitz, H. M. (2010). Gold Nanoparticles Enhance the Radiation Therapy of a Murine Squamous Cell Carcinoma. *Physics in Medicine and Biology*, *55*(11), 3045–3059. doi:10.1088/0031-9155/55/11/004

Hajifathali, A., Lasemi, M. V., Mehravar, M., Moshari, M. R., Alizadeh, A. M., & Roshandel, E. (2023). Novelty in improvement of CAR T cell-based immunotherapy with the aid of CRISPR system. *Hematology, Transfusion and Cell Therapy*. doi:10.1016/j.htct.2023.05.009 PMID:37451978

Haleem, A., Javaid, M., Singh, R. P., Rab, S., & Suman, R. (2023). Applications of nanotechnology in medical field: A brief review. *Global Health Journal (Amsterdam, Netherlands)*, *7*(2), 70–77. doi:10.1016/j.glohj.2023.02.008

Halkare, P., Punjabi, N., Wangchuk, J., Nair, A., Kondabagil, K., & Mukherji, S. (2019). Bacteria functionalized gold nanoparticle matrix based fiber-optic sensor for monitoring heavy metal pollution in water. *Sensors and Actuators. B, Chemical*, *281*, 643–651. doi:10.1016/j.snb.2018.10.119

Hall, J. B., Dobrovolskaia, M. A., Patri, A. K., & McNeil, S. E. (2007). *Characterization of nanoparticles for therapeutics*.

Hamilton, S. K., & Harth, E. (2009). Molecular dendritic transporter nanoparticle vectors provide efficient intracellular delivery of peptides. *ACS Nano*, *3*(2), 402–410. doi:10.1021/nn800679z PMID:19236078

Hamimed, S., Jabberi, M., & Chatti, A. (2022). Nanotechnology in drug and gene delivery. *Naunyn-Schmiedeberg's Archives of Pharmacology*, *395*(7), 769–787. doi:10.100700210-022-02245-z PMID:35505234

Han, F., Wang, J., Ding, L., Hu, Y., Li, W., Yuan, Z., Guo, Q., Zhu, C., Yu, L., Wang, H., Zhao, Z., Jia, L., Li, J., Yu, Y., Zhang, W., Chu, G., Chen, S., & Li, B. (2020). Tissue engineering and regenerative medicine: Achievements, future, and sustainability in Asia. *Frontiers in Bioengineering and Biotechnology*, *8*, 83. doi:10.3389/fbioe.2020.00083 PMID:32266221

Han, G., Noh, D., Lee, H., Lee, S., Kim, S., Yoon, H. Y., & Lee, S. H. (2023). Advances in mRNA therapeutics for cancer immunotherapy: From modification to delivery. *Advanced Drug Delivery Reviews*, *199*, 114973. doi:10.1016/j.addr.2023.114973 PMID:37369262

Hanna, E., Rémuzat, C., Auquier, P., & Toumi, M. (2017). Gene therapies development: Slow progress and promising prospect. *Journal of Market Access & Health Policy*, *5*(1), 1265293. doi:10.1080/20016689.2017.1265293 PMID:28265348

Hansen, S. F., & Baun, A. (2012). European regulation affecting nanomaterials-review of limitations and future recommendations. *Dose-Response*, *10*(3), dose-response.1. doi:10.2203/dose-response.10-029.Hansen PMID:22942870

Han, X., Xu, K., Taratula, O., & Farsad, K. (2019). Applications of nanoparticles in biomedical imaging. *Nanoscale*, *11*(3), 799–819. doi:10.1039/C8NR07769J PMID:30603750

Hare, J. I., Lammers, T., Ashford, M. B., Puri, S., Storm, G., & Barry, S. T. (2016). SC. *Advanced Drug Delivery Reviews*. doi:10.1016/j.addr.2016.04.025 PMID:27137110

Harish, V., Mohd, S., Tewari, D., Pandey, N. K., Vishwas, S., Babu, M. R., Salkini, M. A., Rehman, Z., Alotaibi, J. T., Alotaibi, R. F., Alrashed, F. A., Prasher, P., Sharma, N., Gupta, G., Jakhmola, V., Singh, Y., Pinto, T. J. A., Paudel, K. R., Mittal, N., & Singh, S. K. (2023). Unravelling the role of solid lipid nanoparticles in drug delivery: Journey from laboratory to clinical trial. *Journal of Drug Delivery Science and Technology*, *85*, 104616. doi:10.1016/j.jddst.2023.104616

Hartmann, P., Brezesinski, T., Sann, J., Lotnyk, A., Eufinger, J. P., Kienle, L., & Janek, J. (2013). Defect Chemistry of Oxide Nanomaterials with High Surface Area: Ordered Mesoporous Thin Films of the Oxygen Storage Catalyst CeO2-ZrO2. *ACS Nano*, *7*(4), 2999–3013. doi:10.1021/nn400255w PMID:23514447

Hasanzadeh, M., Shadjou, N., Lin, Y., & de la Guardia, M. (2017). Nanomaterials for use in immunosensing of carcinoembryonic antigen (CEA): Recent advances. *Trends in Analytical Chemistry*, *86*, 185–205. doi:10.1016/j.trac.2016.11.003

Hashimoto, S., Werner, D., & Uwada, T. (2012). Studies on the interaction of pulsed lasers with plasmonic gold nanoparticles toward light manipulation, heat management, and nanofabrication. *Journal of Photochemistry and Photobiology C, Photochemistry Reviews*, *13*(1), 28–54. doi:10.1016/j.jphotochemrev.2012.01.001

Hassani, S., Gharehaghaji, N., & Divband, B. (2022). Chitosan-coated iron oxide/graphene quantum dots as a potential multifunctional nanohybrid for bimodal magnetic resonance/fluorescence imaging and 5-fluorouracil delivery. *Materials Today. Communications*, *103589*(31), 103589. doi:10.1016/j.mtcomm.2022.103589

Hawkins, M. J., Soon-Shiong, P., & Desai, N. (2008). Protein nanoparticles as drug carriers in clinical medicine. *Advanced Drug Delivery Reviews*, *60*(8), 876–885. doi:10.1016/j.addr.2007.08.044 PMID:18423779

He, P., Yang, G., Zhu, D., Kong, H., Corrales- Ureña, Y. R., Ciacchi, L. C., Wei, G. (2022). *Journal of Nanobiotechnology,* (20), 483. doi:10.1186/s12951-022-01691-4

Healy, K. E., Harbers, G. M., Barber, T. A., & Sumner, D. R. (2000). Osteoblast Interactions with Engineered Surfaces. In J. E. Davies (Ed.), Bone engineering. em squared.

Heaton, L. L., López, E., Maini, P. K., Fricker, M. D., & Jones, N. S. (2012). Advection, diffusion, and delivery over a network. *Physical Review. E*, *86*(2), 021905. doi:10.1103/PhysRevE.86.021905 PMID:23005783

Hemlata, M., Meena, P. R., Singh, A. P., & Tejavath, K. K. (2020). Biosynthesis of Silver Nanoparticles Using Cucumis prophetarum Aqueous Leaf Extract and Their Antibacterial and Antiproliferative Activity Against Cancer Cell Lines. *ACS Omega*, *5*(10), 5520–5528. doi:10.1021/acsomega.0c00155 PMID:32201844

He, Q., Zhang, J., Chen, F., Guo, L., Zhu, Z., & Shi, J. (2010). An anti-ROS/hepatic fibrosis drug delivery system based on salvianolic acid B loaded mesoporous silica nanoparticles. *Biomaterials*, *31*(30), 7785–7796. doi:10.1016/j.biomaterials.2010.07.008 PMID:20674009

Heredia, K. L., Bontempo, D., Ly, T., Byers, J. T., Halstenberg, S., & Maynard, H. D. (2005). In situ preparation of protein–"smart" polymer conjugates with retention of bioactivity. *Journal of the American Chemical Society*, *127*(48), 16955–16960. doi:10.1021/ja054482w PMID:16316241

Herranz, F., Almarza, E., Rodríguez, I., Salinas, B., Rosell, Y., Desco, M., Bulte, J. W., & Ruiz-Cabello, J. (2011, July). The application of nanoparticles in gene therapy and magnetic resonance imaging. *Microscopy Research and Technique*, *74*(7), 577–591. doi:10.1002/jemt.20992 PMID:21484943

He, W., Zhou, Y. T., Wamer, W. G., Boudreau, M. D., & Yin, J. J. (2012). Mechanisms of the pH Dependent Generation of Hydroxyl Radicals and Oxygen Induced by Ag Nanoparticles. *Biomaterials*, *33*(30), 7547–7555. doi:10.1016/j.biomaterials.2012.06.076 PMID:22809647

He, Y., Du, Z., Ma, S., Cheng, S., Jiang, S., Liu, Y., Li, D., Huang, H., Zhang, K., & Zheng, X. (2016). Biosynthesis, Antibacterial Activity and Anticancer Effects against prostate Cancer (PC-3) cells of silver nanoparticles using Dimocarpus Longan Lour. Peel Extract. *Nanoscale Research Letters*, *11*(1), 300. doi:10.118611671-016-1511-9 PMID:27316741

He, Y., Du, Z., Ma, S., Liu, Y., Li, D., Huang, H., Jiang, S., Cheng, S., Wu, W., Zhang, K., & Zheng, X. (2016b). Effects of green-synthesized silver NPs on lung cancer cells in vitro and grown as xenograft tumors in vivo. *International Journal of Nanomedicine*, *11*, 1879. doi:10.2147/IJN.S103695 PMID:27217750

Heydari, R., & Rashidipour, M. (2015). Green synthesis of silver nanoparticles using extract of oak fruit hull (jaft): Synthesis and in vitro cytotoxic effect on mcf-7 cells. *International Journal of Breast Cancer*, *846743*, 1–6. doi:10.1155/2015/846743 PMID:25685560

Hilger, I., Hergt, R., & Kaiser, W. A. (2005). Use of magnetic nanoparticle heating in the treatment of breast cancer. *IEE Proceedings. Nanobiotechnology*, *152*(1), 33–39. doi:10.1049/ip-nbt:20055018 PMID:16441156

Hill, R. T. (2015). Plasmonic biosensors. *Wiley Interdisciplinary Reviews. Nanomedicine and Nanobiotechnology*, *7*(2), 152–168. doi:10.1002/wnan.1314 PMID:25377594

Holmes, H. F., Simonson, J. M., & Mesmer, R. E. (2000). Aqueous solutions of the mono-and di-hydrogenphosphate salts of sodium and potassium at elevated temperatures. Isopiestic results. *The Journal of Chemical Thermodynamics*, *32*(1), 77–96. doi:10.1006/jcht.1999.0571

Honary, S., & Zahir, F. (2013). Effect of zeta potential on the properties of nano-drug delivery systems-a review (Part 2). *Tropical Journal of Pharmaceutical Research*, *12*(2), 265–273.

Hong, H., Shi, J., Yang, Y., Zhang, Y., Engle, J. W., Nickles, R. J., Wang, X., & Cai, W. (2011). Cancer-targeted optical imaging with fluorescent zinc oxide nanowires. *Nano Letters*, *11*(9), 3744–3750. doi:10.1021/nl201782m PMID:21823599

Hong, R., Han, G., Fernández, J. M., Kim, B. J., Forbes, N. S., & Rotello, V. M. (2006). Glutathione-mediated delivery and release using monolayer protected nanoparticle carriers. *Journal of the American Chemical Society*, *128*(4), 1078–1079. doi:10.1021/ja056726i PMID:16433515

Hong, Y., Huh, Y.-M., Yoon, D. S., & Yang, J. (2012). Nanobiosensors Based on Localized Surface Plasmon Resonance for Biomarker Detection. *Journal of Nanomaterials, 759830*, 1–13. doi:10.1155/2012/759830

Horak, P., Leichsenring, J., Goldschmid, H., Kreutzfeldt, S., Kazdal, D., Teleanu, V., Endris, V., Gieldon, L., Allgaeuer, M., Volckmar, A. L., Dikow, N., Renner, M., Kirchner, M., Penzel, R., Ploeger, C., Brandt, R., Seker-Cin, H., Budczies, J., & Heilig, C. E. (2022). Assigning evidence to actionability: An introduction to variant interpretation in precision cancer medicine. *Genes, Chromosomes & Cancer, 61*(6), 303–313. doi:10.1002/gcc.22987

Horst, M. F., Coral, D. F., van Raap, M. B. F., Alvarez, M., & Lassalle, V. (2017). Hybrid nanomaterials based on gum Arabic and magnetite for hyperthermia treatments. *Materials Science and Engineering C, 74*, 443–450. doi:10.1016/j.msec.2016.12.035

Horvath, D., & Basler, M. (2023). PLGA Particles in Immunotherapy. *Pharmaceutics, 15*(2), 615. doi:10.3390/pharmaceutics15020615 PMID:36839937

Hoshyar, N., Gray, S., Han, H., & Bao, G. (2016). The effect of nanoparticle size on in vivo pharmacokinetics and cellular interaction. *Nanomedicine (London), 11*(6), 673–692. doi:10.2217/nnm.16.5 PMID:27003448

Hsu, J. C., Tang, Z., Eremina, O. E., Sofias, A. M., Lammers, T., Lovell, J. F., Zavaleta, C., Cai, W., & Cormode, D. P. (2023). Nanomaterial-based contrast agents. *Nature Reviews. Methods Primers, 3*(1), 30. doi:10.103843586-023-00211-4

Huang, B., Zhang, F., Cai, C., & Zhang, L. (2023). Toward understanding polymeric micelle stability regulated by diverse physico-chemical strategies and their stabilized mechanism. *Colloids and Surfaces. A, Physicochemical and Engineering Aspects, 674*, 131880. doi:10.1016/j.colsurfa.2023.131880

Huang, J., Wang, T., Zhu, P., & Xiao, J. (2013). Preparation, characterization, and thermal properties of the microencapsulation of a hydrated salt as phase change energy storage materials. *Thermochimica Acta, 557*, 1–6. doi:10.1016/j.tca.2013.01.019

Huang, Q., Wang, Y., Chen, X., Wang, Y., Li, Z., Du, S., Wang, L., & Chen, S. (2018). Nanotechnology-Based Strategies for Early Cancer Diagnosis Using Circulating Tumor Cells as a Liquid Biopsy. *Nanotheranostics, 2*(1), 21–41. doi:10.7150/ntno.22091 PMID:29291161

Huang, Q., Xu, S., Ouyang, Z., Yang, Y., & Liu, Y. (2021). Multi-scale nacre-inspired lamella-structured Ti-Ta composites with high strength and low modulus for load-bearing orthopedic and dental applications. *Materials Science and Engineering C, 118*, 111458. doi:10.1016/j.msec.2020.111458 PMID:33255043

Huang, Y., Li, X., Cao, J., Wei, X., Li, Y., Wang, Z., Cai, X., Li, R., & Chen, J. (2022). Use of dissociation degree in lysosomes to predict metal oxide nanoparticle toxicity in immune cells: Machine learning boosts nano-safety assessment. *Environment International, 164*, 107258. doi:10.1016/j.envint.2022.107258 PMID:35483183

Huang, Y., Yu, D., Qiu, Y., Chu, L., & Lin, Y. (2020). The Role of Nanomaterials in Modulating the Structure and Function of Biomimetic Catalysts. *Frontiers in Chemistry, 8*, 764. doi:10.3389/fchem.2020.00764 PMID:33134257

Hua, S., De Matos, M. B., Metselaar, J. M., & Storm, G. (2018). Current trends and challenges in the clinical translation of nanoparticulate nanomedicines: Pathways for translational development and commercialization. *Frontiers in Pharmacology, 9*, 790. doi:10.3389/fphar.2018.00790 PMID:30065653

Huo, Y., Singh, P., Kim, Y. J., Soshnikova, V., Kang, J., Markus, J., Ahn, S., Castro-Aceituno, V., Mathiyalagan, R., Chokkalingam, M., Bae, K. S., & Yang, D. C. (2018). Biological synthesis of gold and silver chloride nanoparticles by Glycyrrhiza uralensis and in vitro applications. *Artificial Cells, Nanomedicine, and Biotechnology, 46*(2), 303–312. doi:10.1080/21691401.2017.1307213 PMID:28375686

Husni, P., Lim, C., & Oh, K. T. (2023). Tumor microenvironment stimuli-responsive lipid-drug conjugates for cancer treatment. *International Journal of Pharmaceutics*, *639*, 122942. doi:10.1016/j.ijpharm.2023.122942 PMID:37037397

Hussain, S., Vanoirbeek, J. A., & Hoet, P. H. (2012). Interactions of nanomaterials with the immune system. *Wiley Interdisciplinary Reviews. Nanomedicine and Nanobiotechnology*, *4*(2), 169–183. doi:10.1002/wnan.166 PMID:22144008

Hu, X., & Liu, S. (2015). Recent advances towards the fabrication and biomedical applications of responsive polymeric assemblies and nanoparticle hybrid superstructures. *Dalton Transactions (Cambridge, England)*, *44*(9), 3904–3922. doi:10.1039/C4DT03609C

Iannazzo, D., Pistone, A., Salamò, M., Galvagno, S., Romeo, R., Giofré, S. V., Branca, C., Visalli, G., & Di Pietro, A. (2017). Graphene quantum dots for cancer targeted drug delivery. *International Journal of Pharmaceutics*, *518*(1–2), 185–192. doi:10.1016/j.ijpharm.2016.12.060 PMID:28057464

Ibrahim, H., Bindschaedler, C., Doelker, E., Buri, P., & Gurny, R. (1992). Aqueous nanodispersions prepared by a salting-out process. *International Journal of Pharmaceutics*, *87*(1-3), 239–246. doi:10.1016/0378-5173(92)90248-Z

Iglesias-Mayor, A., Amor-Gutiérrez, O., Costa-García, A., & de la Escosura-Muñiz, A. (2019). Nanoparticles as Emerging Labels in Electrochemical Immunosensors. *Sensors (Basel)*, *19*(23), 5137. doi:10.339019235137 PMID:31771201

Ijaz, S., Sultana, M., Shamim, R., & Bukhari, N. I. (2023). Development and DoE-ANN based optimization of novel swellable matrix-diffusible doxorubicin loaded zinc oxide nanoflowers using sonochemical-precipitation method. *International Journal of Pharmaceutics*, *633*, 122584. doi:10.1016/j.ijpharm.2023.122584 PMID:36621704

Ikezoe, T., Yang, Y., Bandobashi, K., Saito, T., Takemoto, S., Machida, H., Togitani, K., Koeffler, H. P., & Taguchi, H. (2005). Oridonin, a diterpenoid purified from Rabdosia rubescens, inhibits the proliferation of cells from lymphoid malignancies in association with blockade of the NF-κB signal pathways. *Molecular Cancer Therapeutics*, *4*(4), 578–586. doi:10.1158/1535-7163.MCT-04-0277 PMID:15827331

Imbuluzqueta, E., Gamazo, C., Lana, H., Campanero, M. Á., Salas, D., Gil, A. G., Elizondo, E., Ventosa, N., Veciana, J., & Blanco-Prieto, M. J. (2013). Hydrophobic gentamicin-loaded nanoparticles are effective against Brucella melitensis infection in mice. *Antimicrobial Agents and Chemotherapy*, *57*(7), 3326–3333. doi:10.1128/AAC.00378-13 PMID:23650167

Imig, J. D., & Ryan, M. J. (2013). Immune and inflammatory role in renal disease. *Comprehensive Physiology*, *3*(2), 957. doi:10.1002/cphy.c120028 PMID:23720336

Inamuddin. (2018). Applications of Nanocomposite Materials in Orthopedics. *Applications of Nanocomposite Materials in Orthopedics*, 1–328. doi:10.1016/C2016-0-05076-3

Indoria, S., Singh, V., & Hsieh, M. F. (2020). Recent advances in theranostic polymeric nanoparticles for cancer treatment: A review. *International Journal of Pharmaceutics*, *119314*(582), 119314. doi:10.1016/j.ijpharm.2020.119314

Iqbal, M. A., Md, S., Sahni, J. K., Baboota, S., Dang, S., & Ali, J. (2012). Nanostructured lipid carriers system: Recent advances in drug delivery. *Journal of Drug Targeting*, *20*(10), 813–830. doi:10.3109/1061186X.2012.716845

Islam, N. U., Amin, R., Shahid, M., Amin, M., Zaib, S., & Iqbal, J. (2017). A multi-target therapeutic potential of Prunus domestica gum stabilized nanoparticles exhibited prospective anticancer, antibacterial, urease-inhibition, anti-inflammatory and analgesic properties. *BMC Complementary and Alternative Medicine*, *17*(1), 276. doi:10.118612906-017-1791-3 PMID:28535789

Israel, L. L., Galstyan, A., Holler, E., & Ljubimova, J. Y. (2020). Magnetic iron oxide nanoparticles for imaging, targeting and treatment of primary and metastatic tumors of the brain. *Journal of Controlled Release*, *320*, 45–62. doi:10.1016/j.jconrel.2020.01.009

Israelsen, N. D., Hanson, C., & Vargis, E. (2015). Nanoparticle properties and synthesis effects on surface-enhanced Raman scattering enhancement factor: An introduction. *TheScientificWorldJournal, 124582*, 1–12. doi:10.1155/2015/124582 PMID:25884017

Itoo, A. M., Paul, M., Padaga, S. G., Ghosh, B., & Biswas, S. (2022). Nanotherapeutic Intervention in Photodynamic Therapy for Cancer. *ACS Omega*, *7*(7), 45882–45909. doi:10.1021/acsomega.2c05852

Ivone Vanessa Jurado-Davila, I. A. H. S. (2023). Phosphate removal using dolomite modified with ultrasound: Mathematical and experimental analysis. *Journal of Environmental Science and Health. Part A, Toxic/Hazardous Substances & Environmental Engineering*, *58*(5), 469–482. doi:10.1080/10934529.2023.2196928 PMID:37005870

Jabeen, S., Qureshi, R., Munazir, M., Maqsood, M., Munir, M., Shah, S. S. H., & Rahim, B. Z. (2021). Application of green synthesized silver nanoparticles in cancer treatment - A critical review. *Materials Research Express*, *8*(9), 092001. doi:10.1088/2053-1591/ac1de3

Jackson, J. K., Letchford, K., Wasserman, B. Z., Ye, L., Hamad, W. Y., & Burt, H. M. (2011). The use of nanocrystalline cellulose for the binding and controlled release of drugs. *International Journal of Nanomedicine*, *6*, 321. PMID:21383857

Jafernik, K., Ladniak, A., Blicharska, E., Czarnek, K., Ekiert, H., Wiącek, A. E., & Szopa, A. (2023). Chitosan-Based Nanoparticles as Effective Drug Delivery Systems—A review. *Molecules (Basel, Switzerland)*, *28*(4), 1963. doi:10.3390/molecules28041963 PMID:36838951

Jain, D., Hasan, N., Zafar, S., Thakur, J., Haider, K., Parvez, S., & Ahmad, F. J. (2023). Transferrin functionalized nanostructured lipid carriers for targeting Rivastigmine and Resveratrol to Alzheimer's disease: Synthesis, in vitro characterization and brain uptake analysis. *Journal of Drug Delivery Science and Technology*, *86*, 104555. doi:10.1016/j.jddst.2023.104555

Jain, K. K. (2010). Advances in the field of nanooncology. *BMC Medicine*, *8*(1), 83. doi:10.1186/1741-7015-8-83 PMID:21144040

Jain, K. K. (2020). An overview of drug delivery systems. *Drug Delivery System*, *2059*, 1–54. PMID:31435914

Jain, N., Jain, P., Rajput, D., & Patil, U. K. (2021). Green synthesized plant-based silver nanoparticles: Therapeutic prospective for anticancer and antiviral activity. *Micro and Nano Systems Letters*, *9*(1), 5. doi:10.118640486-021-00131-6

Jaiswal, M., Dudhe, R., & Sharma, P. K. (2015). Nanoemulsion: an advanced mode of drug delivery system. *3 Biotech, 5*, 123-127. doi:10.1007/s13205-014-0214-0

Jaiswal, J., Gupta, S. K., & Kreuter, J. (2004). Preparation of biodegradable cyclosporine nanoparticles by high-pressure emulsification-solvent evaporation process. *Journal of Controlled Release*, *96*(1), 169–178. doi:10.1016/j.jconrel.2004.01.017 PMID:15063039

Jakhmola, A., Anton, N., & Vandamme, T. F. (2012). Inorganic Nanoparticles Based Contrast Agents for X-ray Computed Tomography. *Advanced Healthcare Materials*, *1*(4), 413–431. doi:10.1002/adhm.201200032 PMID:23184772

Jalal, R. R., Ways, T. M. M., Abu Elella, M. H., Hassan, D. A., & Khutoryanskiy, V. V. (2023). Preparation of mucoadhesive methacrylated chitosan nanoparticles for delivery of ciprofloxacin. *International Journal of Biological Macromolecules*, *242*, 124980. doi:10.1016/j.ijbiomac.2023.124980 PMID:37236558

Jalil, A. T., Thabit, S. N., Hanan, Z. K., Alasheqi, M. Q., Al-Azzawi, A. K. J., Zabibah, R. S., & Fadhil, A. A. (2023). Modulating gut microbiota using nanotechnology to increase anticancer efficacy of the treatments. *Macromolecular Research*, *31*(8), 1–14. doi:10.100713233-023-00168-z

Jalota, S., Bhaduri, S. B., & Tas, A. C. (2007). Osteoblast proliferation on neat and apatite-like calcium phosphate-coated titanium foam scaffolds. *Materials Science and Engineering C*, *27*(3), 432–440. doi:10.1016/j.msec.2006.05.052

James, J. S. (1995). DOXIL approved for KS. *AIDS Treatment News*, (236), 6.

Jamkhande, P. G., Ghule, N. W., Bamer, A. H., & Kalaskar, M. G. (2019). Metal nanoparticles synthesis: An overview on methods of preparation, advantages and disadvantages, and applications. *Journal of Drug Delivery Science and Technology*, *53*, 101174. doi:10.1016/j.jddst.2019.101174

Jandt, K. D., & Watts, D. C. (2020). Nanotechnology in dentistry: Present and future perspectives on dental nanomaterials. *Dental Materials*, *36*(11), 1365–1378. doi:10.1016/j.dental.2020.08.006 PMID:32981749

Janež, A., Guja, C., Mitrakou, A., Lalic, N., Tankova, T., Czupryniak, L., Tabak, A. G., Prazny, M. P., & Smircic-Duvnjak, L. (2020). Insulin therapy in adults with type 1 diabetes mellitus: A narrative review. *Diabetes Therapy : Research, Treatment and Education of Diabetes and Related Disorders*, *11*(2), 387–409. doi:10.100713300-019-00743-7 PMID:31902063

Jangam, S. R., Hayter, G., & Dunn, T. C. (2013). Impact of glucose measurement processing delays on clinical accuracy and relevance. *Journal of Diabetes Science and Technology*, *7*(3), 660–668. doi:10.1177/193229681300700311 PMID:23759399

Jang, S. J., Yang, I. J., Tettey, C. O., Kim, K. M., & Shin, H. M. (2016). In-vitro anticancer activity of green synthesized silver nanoparticles on MCF-7 human breast cancer cells. *Materials Science and Engineering C*, *68*, 430–435. doi:10.1016/j.msec.2016.03.101 PMID:27524038

Janic, B., Brown, S. L., Neff, R., Liu, F., Mao, G., Chen, Y., Jackson, L., Chetty, I. J., Movsas, B., & Wen, N. (2021). Therapeutic enhancement of radiation and immunomodulation by gold nanoparticles in triple negative breast cancer. *Cancer Biology & Therapy*, *22*(2), 124–135. doi:10.1080/15384047.2020.1861923 PMID:33459132

Jarai, B. M., Kolewe, E. L., Stillman, Z. S., Raman, N., & Fromen, C. A. (2020). Polymeric nanoparticles. In *Nanoparticles for biomedical applications* (pp. 303–324). Elsevier. doi:10.1016/B978-0-12-816662-8.00018-7

Javed, R., Ahmad, M. A., & Ao, Q. (2019). Theranostic applications of nanobiotechnology in cancer. *Nanotheranostics: Applications and Limitations*, 277-295. doi:10.1007/978-3-030-29768-8_13

Jeanbart, L., & Swartz, M. A. (2015). Engineering opportunities in cancer immunotherapy. *Proceedings of the National Academy of Sciences of the United States of America*, *112*(47), 14467–14472. doi:10.1073/pnas.1508516112

Jeevanandam, J., Barhoum, A., Chan, Y. S., Dufresne, A., & Danquah, M. K. (2018). Review on nanoparticles and nanostructured materials: History, sources, toxicity and regulations. *Beilstein Journal of Nanotechnology*, *9*, 1050–1074. doi:10.3762/bjnano.9.98 PMID:29719757

Jengathe, S. P., Dhondge, S. S., Paliwal, L. J., Tangde, V. M., & Mondal, S. (2015). Effect of sodium chloride and myo-inositol on diphenhydramine hydrochloride drug in aqueous solution at different temperatures: Volumetric and acoustic approach. *The Journal of Chemical Thermodynamics*, *87*, 78–87. doi:10.1016/j.jct.2015.03.020

Jensen, T. L., Gøtzsche, C. R., & Woldbye, D. P. (2021). Current and future prospects for gene therapy for rare genetic diseases affecting the brain and spinal cord. *Frontiers in Molecular Neuroscience*, *14*, 695937. doi:10.3389/fnmol.2021.695937 PMID:34690692

Jeong, S. H., Lim, D., Kim, K., Kang, E., Lim, S., Ricci, J., Sung, S., & Kwon, M. (2016). A comprehensive evaluation of carboxylated nanodiamond as a topical drug delivery system. *International Journal of Nanomedicine*, *2381*, 2381. doi:10.2147/IJN.S104859

Jeong, Y. I., Cho, C. S., Kim, S. H., Ko, K. S., Kim, S. I., Shim, Y. H., & Nah, J. W. (2001). Preparation of poly (DL-lactide-co-glycolide) nanoparticles without surfactant. *Journal of Applied Polymer Science*, *80*(12), 2228–2236. doi:10.1002/app.1326

Jeon, H. J., Jeong, Y. I., Jang, M. K., Park, Y. H., & Nah, J. W. (2000). Effect of solvent on the preparation of surfactant-free poly (DL-lactide-co-glycolide) nanoparticles and norfloxacin release characteristics. *International Journal of Pharmaceutics*, *207*(1-2), 99–108. doi:10.1016/S0378-5173(00)00537-8 PMID:11036235

Jethara, S., Patel, M., & Patel, Al. (2014). Sustained Release Drug Delivery Systems: A Patent Overview. *Aperito Journal of Drug Designing and Pharmacology*, *1*, 1–14.

Jeyaraj, M., Sathishkumar, G., Sivanandhan, G., MubarakAli, D., Rajesh, M., Arun, R., Kapildev, G., Manickavasagam, M., Thajuddin, N., Premkumar, K., & Ganapathi, A. (2013). Biogenic silver nanoparticles for cancer treatment: An experimental report. *Colloids and Surfaces. B, Biointerfaces*, *106*, 86–92. doi:10.1016/j.colsurfb.2013.01.027 PMID:23434696

Jha, R., Singh, A., Sharma, P. K., & Fuloria, N. K. (2020). Smart carbon nanotubes for drug delivery system: A comprehensive study. *Journal of Drug Delivery Science and Technology*, *58*, 101811. doi:10.1016/j.jddst.2020.101811

Jha, S., Sharma, P. K., & Malviya, R. (2016). Hyperthermia: Role and risk factor for cancer treatment. *Achievements in the Life Sciences*, *10*(10), 161–167. doi:10.1016/j.als.2016.11.004

Jia, G., Hill, M. A., & Sowers, J. R. (2018). Diabetic cardiomyopathy: An update of mechanisms contributing to this clinical entity. *Circulation Research*, *122*(4), 624–638. doi:10.1161/CIRCRESAHA.117.311586 PMID:29449364

Jia, H. R., Zhu, Y. X., Duan, Q. Y., Chen, Z., & Wu, F. G. (2019). Nanomaterials meet zebrafish: Toxicity evaluation and drug delivery applications. *Journal of Controlled Release*, *311*, 301–318. doi:10.1016/j.jconrel.2019.08.022 PMID:31446084

Jiang, P. (2018). Dose Dependencies and Biocompatibility of Renal Clearable Gold Nanoparticles: From Mice to Non-human Primates. *Angewandte Chemie International Edition*, *57*(1), 266–271. doi:10.1002/anie.201710584 PMID:29160029

Jiang, X., Du, B., & Zheng, J. (2019). Glutathione-mediated biotransformation in the liver modulates nanoparticle transport. *Nature Nanotechnology*, *14*(9), 874–882. doi:10.103841565-019-0499-6 PMID:31308501

Jiang, X., Zhang, S., Ren, F., Chen, L., Zeng, J., Zhu, M., Cheng, Z., Gao, M., & Li, Z. (2017). Ultrasmall magnetic CuFeSe2 ternary nanocrystals for multimodal imaging guided photothermal therapy of cancer. *ACS Nano*, *11*(6), 5633–5645. doi:10.1021/acsnano.7b01032

Jiang, X., Zhu, C., & Ma, Y. (2013). Densities and viscosities of erythritol, xylitol, and mannitol in l-ascorbic acid aqueous solutions at T=(293.15 to 323.15) K. *Journal of Chemical & Engineering Data*, *58*(11), 2970–2978. doi:10.1021/je400395u

Jiang, Y., Wang, Z., & Dai, Z. (2016). Preparation of Silicon-Carbon-Based Dots@Dopamine and Its Application in Intracellular Ag+ Detection and Cell Imaging. *ACS Applied Materials & Interfaces*, *8*(6), 3644–3650. doi:10.1021/acsami.5b08089 PMID:26502274

Jiang, Z., Zhang, M., Li, P., Wang, Y., & Fu, Q. (2023). Nanomaterial-based CT contrast agents and their applications in image-guided therapy. *Theranostics*, *13*(2), 483–509. doi:10.7150/thno.79625 PMID:36632234

Jian, W. H., Wang, H. C., Kuan, C. H., Chen, M. H., Wu, H. C., Sun, J. S., & Wang, T. W. (2018). Glycosaminoglycan-based hybrid hydrogel encapsulated with polyelectrolyte complex nanoparticles for endogenous stem cell regulation in central nervous system regeneration. *Biomaterials*, *174*, 17–30. doi:10.1016/j.biomaterials.2018.05.009 PMID:29763775

Jia, S., Zhang, R., Li, Z., Li, J., Jia, S., Zhang, R., Li, Z., & Li, J. (2017). Clinical and biological significance of circulating tumor cells, circulating tumor DNA, and exosomes as biomarkers in colorectal cancer. *Oncotarget*, *8*(33), 55632–55645. doi:10.18632/oncotarget.17184 PMID:28903450

Jia, Y., Jiang, Y., He, Y., Zhang, W., Zou, J., Magar, K. T., Boucetta, H., Teng, C., & He, W. (2023). Approved Nanomedicine against Diseases. *Pharmaceutics*, *15*(3), 774. doi:10.3390/pharmaceutics15030774 PMID:36986635

Jiffrin, R., Razak, S. I. A., Jamaludin, M. I., Hamzah, A. S. A., Mazian, M. A., Jaya, M. A. T., Nasrullah, M. Z., Majrashi, M., Theyab, A., Aldarmahi, A. A., Aman, Z., Abdel-Daim, M. M., & Azad, A. K. (2022). Electrospun nanofiber composites for drug delivery: A review on current progresses. *Polymers*, *14*(18), 3725. doi:10.3390/polym14183725 PMID:36145871

Jin, B., Odongo, S., Radwanska, M., & Magez, S. (2023). Nanobodies: A Review of Generation, Diagnostics and Therapeutics. *International Journal of Molecular Sciences, 24*(6). . doi:10.3390/ijms24065994

Jin, C., Wang, K., Oppong-Gyebi, A., & Hu, J. (2020). Application of Nanotechnology in Cancer Diagnosis and Therapy - A Mini-Review. *International Journal of Medical Sciences*, *17*(18), 2964–2973. doi:10.7150/ijms.49801 PMID:33173417

Jin, L., Wang, Q., Chen, J., Wang, Z., Xin, H., & Zhang, D. (2019). Efficient delivery of therapeutic siRNA by Fe3O4 magnetic nanoparticles into oral cancer cells. *Pharmaceutics*, *11*(11), 615. doi:10.3390/pharmaceutics11110615

Jin, Y., Song, Y., Zhu, X., Zhou, D., Chen, C., Zhang, Z., & Huang, Y. (2012). Goblet cell-targeting nanoparticles for oral insulin delivery and the influence of mucus on insulin transport. *Biomaterials*, *33*(5), 1573–1582. doi:10.1016/j.biomaterials.2011.10.075 PMID:22093292

Jin, Z., Nguyen, K. T., Go, G., Kang, B., Min, H. K., Kim, S. J., Kim, Y., Li, H., Kim, C. S., Lee, S., Park, S., Kim, K. P., Huh, K. M., Song, J., Park, J. O., & Choi, E. (2019). Multifunctional Nanorobot System for Active Therapeutic Delivery and Synergistic Chemo-photothermal Therapy. *Nano Letters*, *19*(12), 8550–8564. doi:10.1021/acs.nanolett.9b03051

Ji, T., Zhao, Y., Wang, J., Zheng, X., Tian, Y., Zhao, Y., & Nie, G. (2013). Tumor Fibroblast Specific Activation of a Hybrid Ferritin Nanocage-Based Optical Probe for Tumor Microenvironment Imaging. *Small*, *9*(14), 2427–2431. doi:10.1002mll.201300600 PMID:23853124

Jomhori Baloch, M., Mosaddeghi, H., & Jamshidian-Mojaver, M. (2022). Structural view of insulin adsorption on the multiple sizes of Cu nanoparticles; molecular dynamics simulation study. *Archives of Biochemistry and Biophysics*, *722*, 109219. doi:10.1016/j.abb.2022.109219 PMID:35427577

Joseph, T. M., Mahapatra, D. K., Esmaeili, A., Piszczyk, Ł., Hasanin, M. S., Kattali, M., Haponiuk, J., & Thomas, S. (2023). Nanoparticles: Taking a Unique Position in Medicine. *Nanomaterials (Basel, Switzerland)*, *13*(3), 574. doi:10.3390/nano13030574 PMID:36770535

Joshi, A. S., Singh, P., & Mijakovic, I. (2020). Interactions of gold and silver nanoparticles with bacterial biofilms: Molecular interactions behind inhibition and resistance. *International Journal of Molecular Sciences*, *21*(20), 7658–7664. doi:10.3390/ijms21207658 PMID:33081366

Joubert, F., Munson, M. J., Sabirsh, A., England, R. M., Hemmerling, M., Alexander, C., & Ashford, M. B. (2023). Precise and systematic end group chemistry modifications on PAMAM and poly(l-lysine) dendrimers to improve cytosolic delivery of mRNA. *Journal of Controlled Release*, *356*, 580–594. doi:10.1016/j.jconrel.2023.03.011 PMID:36918085

Joudeh, N., & Linke, D. (2022). Nanoparticle classification, physicochemical properties, characterization, and applications: A comprehensive review for biologists. *Journal of Nanobiotechnology*, *20*(1), 262. doi:10.118612951-022-01477-8 PMID:35672712

Juglan, K. C., & Kumar, H. (2020). Volumetric and ultrasonic investigation of polyethylene glycols (PEG-200 and PEG-600) in aqueous solutions of sodium methylparaben at various temperatures. *The Journal of Chemical Thermodynamics*, *140*, 105916. doi:10.1016/j.jct.2019.105916

Juhairiyah, F., & de Lange, E. C. M. (2021). Understanding Drug Delivery to the Brain Using Liposome-Based Strategies: Studies that Provide Mechanistic Insights Are Essential. *The AAPS Journal*, *23*(6), 114. doi:10.120812248-021-00648-z PMID:34713363

Juneja, M., Suthar, T., Pardhi, V. P., Ahmad, J., & Jain, K. (2022). Emerging trends and promises of nanoemulsions in therapeutics of infectious diseases. *Nanomedicine (London)*, *17*(11), 793–812. doi:10.2217/nnm-2022-0006 PMID:35587031

Jung, J., & Perrut, M. (2001). Particle design using supercritical fluids: Literature and patent survey. *The Journal of Supercritical Fluids*, *20*(3), 179–219. doi:10.1016/S0896-8446(01)00064-X

Kalishwaralal, K., BarathManiKanth, S., Pandian, S. R. K., Deepak, V., & Gurunathan, S. (2010). Silver nanoparticles impede the biofilm formation by Pseudomonas aeruginosa and Staphylococcus epidermidis. *Colloids and Surfaces. B, Biointerfaces*, *79*(2), 340–344. doi:10.1016/j.colsurfb.2010.04.014 PMID:20493674

Kalombo, L., Lemmer, Y., Semete-Makokotlela, B., Ramalapa, B., Nkuna, P., Booysen, L. L., Naidoo, S., Hayeshi, R., Verschoor, J. A., & Swai, H. S. (2019). Spray-dried, nanoencapsulated, multi-drug anti-tuberculosis therapy aimed at once weekly administration for the duration of treatment. *Nanomaterials (Basel, Switzerland)*, *9*(8), 1167. doi:10.3390/nano9081167 PMID:31443150

Kamaly, N., Xiao, Z., Valencia, P. M., Radovic-Moreno, A. F., & Farokhzad, O. C. (2012). Targeted polymeric therapeutic nanoparticles: Design, development and clinical translation. *Chemical Society Reviews*, *41*(7), 2971–3010. doi:10.1039/c2cs15344k PMID:22388185

Kamaly, N., Yameen, B., Wu, J., & Farokhzad, O. C. (2016). Degradable controlled-release polymers and polymeric nanoparticles: Mechanisms of controlling drug release. *Chemical Reviews*, *116*(4), 2602–2663. doi:10.1021/acs.chemrev.5b00346 PMID:26854975

Kamau, S. W., Hassa, P. O., Steitz, B., Petri-fink, A., Hofmann, H., Hofmann-Amtenbrink, M., & Hottiger, M. O. (2006). Enhancement of the efficiency of non-viral gene delivery by application of pulsed magnetic field. *Nucleic Acids Research*, *34*(5), e40. doi:10.1093/nar/gkl035 PMID:16540591

Kambhampati, P. (2021). Nanoparticles, Nanocrystals, and Quantum Dots: What are the Implications of Size in Colloidal Nanoscale Materials? *The Journal of Physical Chemistry Letters*, *12*(20), 4769–4779. doi:10.1021/acs.jpclett.1c00754 PMID:33984241

Kamel, A. O., Awad, G. A., Geneidi, A. S., & Mortada, N. D. (2009, December). Preparation of intravenous stealthy acyclovir nanoparticles with increased mean residence time. *AAPS PharmSciTech*, *10*(4), 1427–1436. doi:10.120812249-009-9342-y PMID:19949904

Kanathasan, J. S., Swamy, V., Palanisamy, U. D., & Radhakrishnan, A. K. G. K. (2016). Legumain Targeting Peptide Conjugated Fluorescent Porous Silicon Nanoparticles for Breast Cancer Imaging. In P. Vincenzini (Ed.), *7th Forum on New Materials: Part F* (pp. 45-50). Trans Tech Publications. 10.4028/www.scientific.net/AST.102.45

Kanathasan, J. S., Gunasagaram, D., Khan, S. U., Palanisamy, U. D., Radhakrishnan, A. K., Ahemad, N., & Swamy, V. (2020). Linear versus branched peptide with same amino acid sequence for legumain-targeting in macrophages: Targeting efficiency and bioimaging potential. *ChemistrySelect*, *5*(32), 9911–9919. doi:10.1002lct.202002161

Kanathasan, J. S., Palanisamy, U. D., Radhakrishnan, A. K., Chakravarthi, S., Thong, T. B., & Swamy, V. (2022). Protease-targeting peptide-functionalized porous silicon nanoparticles for cancer fluorescence imaging. *Nanomedicine (London)*, *17*(21), 1511–1528. doi:10.2217/nnm-2022-0017

Kang, E. B., Lee, J. E., Mazrad, Z. A. I., In, I., Jeong, J. H., & Park, S. Y. (2018). pH-Responsible fluorescent carbon nanoparticles for tumor selective theranostics via pH-turn on/off fluorescence and photothermal effect in vivo and in vitro. *Nanoscale*, *10*(5), 2512–2523. doi:10.1039/C7NR07900A

Kang, M. S., Lee, S. Y., Kim, K. S., & Han, D. W. (2020). State of the Art Biocompatible Gold Nanoparticles for Cancer Theragnosis. *Pharmaceutics*, *12*(8), 701. doi:10.3390/pharmaceutics12080701 PMID:32722426

Kannan, R. M., Pitha, I., & Parikh, K. S. (2023). A new era in posterior segment ocular drug delivery: Translation of systemic, cell-targeted, dendrimer-based therapies. *Advanced Drug Delivery Reviews*, *200*, 115005. doi:10.1016/j.addr.2023.115005 PMID:37419213

Kansız, S., & Elçin, Y. M. (2023). Advanced liposome and polymersome-based drug delivery systems: Considerations for physicochemical properties, targeting strategies and stimuli-sensitive approaches. *Advances in Colloid and Interface Science*, *317*, 102930. doi:10.1016/j.cis.2023.102930 PMID:37290380

Karakatsanis, A., Christiansen, P. M., Fischer, L., Hedin, C., Pistioli, L., Sund, M., Rasmussen, N. R., Jørnsgård, H., Tegnelius, D., Eriksson, S., Daskalakis, K., Wärnberg, F., Markopoulos, C. J., & Bergkvist, L. (2016). The Nordic SentiMag trial: A comparison of super paramagnetic iron oxide (SPIO) nanoparticles versus Tc(99) and patent blue in the detection of sentinel node (SN) in patients with breast cancer and a meta-analysis of earlier studies. *Breast Cancer Research and Treatment*, *157*(2), 281–294. doi:10.100710549-016-3809-9 PMID:27117158

Karakuş, K. E., Sakarya, S., Yeşiltepe Mutlu, G., Berkkan, M., Muradoğlu, S., Can, E., Gökçe, T., Eviz, E., & Hatun, Ş. (2021). Benefits and drawbacks of Continuous Glucose Monitoring (CGM) use in young children with type 1 diabetes: A qualitative study from a country where the CGM is not reimbursed. *Journal of Patient Experience*, *8*, 23743735211056523. doi:10.1177/23743735211056523 PMID:34881352

Karayianni, M., Chroni, A., Chrysostomou, V., Giaouzi, D., Kafetzi, M., Selianitis, D., Sentoukas, T., & Pispas, S. (2023). Polymeric micelles for therapeutics and diagnosis. In M. S. Hasnain, A. K. Nayak, & T. M. Aminabhavi (Eds.), *Advanced Nanoformulations* (pp. 97–157). Academic Press. doi:10.1016/B978-0-323-85785-7.00019-X

Karimi, Z., Karimi, L., & Shokrollahi, H. (2013). Nano-magnetic particles used in biomedicine: Core and coating materials. *Materials Science and Engineering C*, *33*(5), 2465–2475. doi:10.1016/j.msec.2013.01.045 PMID:23623057

Karnwal, A., Kumar, G., Pant, G., Hossain, K., Ahmad, A., & Alshammari, M. B. (2023). Perspectives on Usage of Functional Nanomaterials in Antimicrobial Therapy for Antibiotic-Resistant Bacterial Infections. *ACS Omega*, *8*(15), 13492–13508. doi:10.1021/acsomega.3c00110 PMID:37091369

Karthikeyan, A., Senthil, N., & Min, T. (2020). Nanocurcumin: A promising candidate for therapeutic applications. *Frontiers in Pharmacology*, *11*, 487. doi:10.3389/fphar.2020.00487 PMID:32425772

Kasagana, V., Karumuri, S. S., & Margesan, M. T. (2011). Recent advances in smart drug delivery systems. *Int J Nov Drug Deliv Tech*, *1*(3), 201–207.

Kashyap, B. K., Singh, V. V., Solanki, M. K., Kumar, A., Ruokolainen, J., & Kesari, K. K. (2023). Smart Nanomaterials in Cancer Theranostics: Challenges and Opportunities. *ACS Omega*, *8*(16), 14290–14320. doi:10.1021/acsomega.2c07840 PMID:37125102

Kathiravan, V., Ravi, S., & Ashokkumar, S. (2014). Synthesis of silver nanoparticles from Melia dubia leaf extract and their in vitro anticancer activity. *Spectrochimica Acta. Part A: Molecular and Biomolecular Spectroscopy*, *130*, 116–121. doi:10.1016/j.saa.2014.03.107 PMID:24769382

Kaur, H., Chakraborty, N., Juglan, K. C., & Kumar, H. (2021). Volumetric and Acoustic Behavior of PEG-200 and PEG-600 in Aqueous D-Mannitol solutions at Different Temperatures. *Journal of Solution Chemistry*, *50*(8), 1079–1102. doi:10.100710953-021-01105-3

Kaur, H., Thakur, R. C., & Kumar, H. (2020). Effect of proteinogenic amino acids lserine/l-threonine on volumetric and acoustic behavior of aqueous 1-butyl-3-propyl imidazolium bromide at T=(288.15, 298.15, 308.15, 318.15) K. *The Journal of Chemical Thermodynamics*, *150*, 106211. doi:10.1016/j.jct.2020.106211

Kaur, I. P., Kakkar, V., Deol, P. K., Yadav, M., Singh, M., & Sharma, I. (2014). Issues and concerns in nanotech product development and its commercialization. *Journal of Controlled Release*, *193*, 51–62. doi:10.1016/j.jconrel.2014.06.005 PMID:24933600

Kaur, K., & Juglan, K. C. (2015). Studies of molecular interaction in the binary mixture of chloroform and methanol by using ultrasonic technique. *Der Pharma Chem*, *7*(2), 160–167.

Kaur, K., & Juglan, K. C. (2016). Ultrasonic velocity, density and viscosity studies of the binary mixtures of ethyl acetate with hexane. *Journal of Chemical and Pharmaceutical Research*, *87*, 49–53.

Kaur, K., Juglan, K. C., & Kumar, H. (2017). Investigation on temperature-dependent volumetric and acoustical properties of homologous series of glycols in aqueous sorbitol solutions. *Journal of Chemical & Engineering Data*, *62*(11), 3769–3782. doi:10.1021/acs.jced.7b00501

Kaur, K., Juglan, K. C., & Kumar, H. (2017, July). Thermo-acoustical molecular interaction study in binary mixtures of glycerol and ethylene glycol. *AIP Conference Proceedings*, *1860*(1), 020026. doi:10.1063/1.4990325

Keating, P., & Cambrosio, A. (2003). *Biomedical platforms: realigning the normal and the pathological in late-twentieth-century medicine*. Mit Press. doi:10.7551/mitpress/1622.001.0001

Ke, C. H., Sio, K. M., Wang, S. L., Kuo, Y., Huang, W. H., & Lin, C. S. (2022). The High Expression of Legumain in Canine Neoplasms: A Retrospective Analysis of 100 Cases. *Animals (Basel)*, *12*(4), 504. doi:10.3390/ani12040504

Ke, P. C., Lin, S., Parak, W. J., Davis, T. P., & Caruso, F. (2017). A Decade of the Protein Corona. *ACS Nano*, *11*(12), 11773–11776. doi:10.1021/acsnano.7b08008 PMID:29206030

Kerc, J., & Srcic, S. (1995). Thermal analysis of glassy pharmaceuticals. *Thermochimica Acta*, *248*, 81–95. doi:10.1016/0040-6031(94)01949-H

Keskinbora, K. H., & Jameel, M. A. (2018). Nanotechnology Applications and Approaches in Medicine: A Review. *J Nanosci Nanotechnol Res*, *2*(2), 6. www.imedpub.com

Kewal, K. (2014). Drug Delivery System. Methods in Molecular Biology. Springer. , doi:10.1007/978-1-4939-0363-4_1

Khaled, H. G. B., Khattech, I., & Jemal, M. (2011). Standard enthalpy of formation of disodium hydrogen phosphate hexahydrate and sodium diphosphate. *The Journal of Chemical Thermodynamics*, *43*(4), 521–526. doi:10.1016/j.jct.2010.11.008

Khaledian, M., Nourbakhsh, M. S., Saber, R., Hashemzadeh, H., & Darvishi, M. H. (2020). Preparation and evaluation of doxorubicin-loaded pla–peg–fa copolymer containing superparamagnetic iron oxide nanoparticles (Spions) for cancer treatment: Combination therapy with hyperthermia and chemotherapy. *International Journal of Nanomedicine*, *6167*(15), 6167–6182. doi:10.2147/IJN.S261638

Khalid, M., & El-Sawy, H. S. (2017). Polymeric nanoparticles: Promising platform for drug delivery. International journal of pharmaceutics, 528(1-2), 675-691.

Khalid, M. A. U., & Chang, S. H. (2022). Flexible strain sensors for wearable applications fabricated using novel functional nanocomposites: A review. *Composite Structures*, *284*, 115214. doi:10.1016/j.compstruct.2022.115214

Khalil, W. F., El-Sayyad, G. S., El Rouby, W. M. A., Sadek, M. A., Farghali, A. A., & El-Batal, A. I. (2020). Graphene oxide-based nanocomposites (GO-chitosan and GO-EDTA) for outstanding antimicrobial potential against some Candida species and pathogenic bacteria. *International Journal of Biological Macromolecules*, *164*, 1370–1383. doi:10.1016/j.ijbiomac.2020.07.205 PMID:32735925

Khan, I., Pandit, J., Ahmed, S., Zameer, S., Nikita, Ahmad, S., Bano, S., Ansari, M. D., Solanki, P., Jahan, R. N., Waheed, A., Aqil, M., & Sultana, Y. (2022). Development and evaluation of biodegradable polymeric lomustine nanofibres for the efficient tumor targeting: In vitro characterization, ex vivo permeation and degradation study. *Journal of Drug Delivery Science and Technology*, *75*, 103685. doi:10.1016/j.jddst.2022.103685

Khan, I., Saeed, K., & Khan, I. (2019). Nanoparticles: Properties, applications and toxicities. *Arabian Journal of Chemistry*, *12*(7), 908–931. doi:10.1016/j.arabjc.2017.05.011

Khan, M. A. (2021). Targeted Drug Delivery Using Tuftsin-bearing Liposomes: Implications in the Treatment of Infectious Diseases and Tumors. *Current Drug Targets*, *22*(7), 770–778. doi:10.2174/1389450121999201125200756 PMID:33243117

Khare, J. M., Dahiya, S., Gangil, B., & Ranakoti, L. (2021). Influence of different resins on Physico-Mechanical properties of hybrid fiber reinforced polymer composites used in human prosthetics. *Materials Today: Proceedings*, *38*, 345–349. doi:10.1016/j.matpr.2020.07.420

Kheiri, K., Sohrabi, N., Mohammadi, R., & Amini-Fazl, M. S. (2022). Preparation and characterization of magnetic nanohydrogel based on chitosan for 5-fluorouracil drug delivery and kinetic study. *International Journal of Biological Macromolecules*, *202*, 191–198. doi:10.1016/j.ijbiomac.2022.01.028 PMID:35033524

Kher, C., & Kumar, S. (2022). The application of nanotechnology and nanomaterials in cancer diagnosis and treatment: A review. *Cureus*, *14*(9), e29059. doi:10.7759/cureus.29059

Khorrami, S., Zarrabi, A., Khaleghi, M., Danaei, M., & Mozafari, M. R. (2018). Selective cytotoxicity of green synthesized silver nanoparticles against the MCF-7 tumor cell line and their enhanced antioxidant and antimicrobial properties. *International Journal of Nanomedicine*, *13*, 8013–8024. doi:10.2147/IJN.S189295 PMID:30568442

Khoshnoud, M. J., Siavashpour, A., Bakhshizadeh, M., & Rashedinia, M. (2018). Effects of sodium benzoate, a commonly used food preservative, on learning, memory, and oxidative stress in brain of mice. *Journal of Biochemical and Molecular Toxicology*, *32*(2), e22022. doi:10.1002/jbt.22022 PMID:29243862

Kiessling, F., Morgenstern, B., & Zhang, C. (2006). Contrast Agents and Applications to Assess Tumor Angiogenesis In Vivo by Magnetic Resonance Imaging. *Current Medicinal Chemistry*, *14*(1), 77–91. doi:10.2174/092986707779313516 PMID:17266569

Kiio, T. M., & Park, S. (2020). Nano-scientific Application of Atomic Force Microscopy in Pathology: From Molecules to Tissues. *International Journal of Medical Sciences*, *17*(7), 844–858. doi:10.7150/ijms.41805 PMID:32308537

Kim, T., Momin, E., Choi, J., Yuan, K., Zaidi, H., Kim, J., Park, M., Lee, N., Mcmahon, M. T., Quinones-hinojosa, A., Bulte, J. W. M., Hyeon, T., & Gilad, A. A. (2011). *116 jacs 2011 T Kim Mesoporous Silica-Coated Hollow Manganese Oxide Nanoparticles.pdf.* 2955–2961.

Kim, B. Y. S., Rutka, J. T., & Chan, W. C. W. (2010). Nanomedicine. *The New England Journal of Medicine*, *365*(25), 2434–2442. doi:10.1056/NEJMra0912273 PMID:21158659

Kim, C., Cho, E. C., Chen, J., Song, K. H., Au, L., Favazza, C., Zhang, Q., Cobley, C. M., Gao, F., Xia, Y., & Wang, L. V. (2010). In vivo molecular photoacoustic tomography of melanomas targeted by bioconjugated gold nanocages. *ACS Nano*, *4*(8), 4559–4564. doi:10.1021/nn100736c PMID:20731439

Kim, C., & Hong, J. H. (2009). Carbosilane and carbosiloxane dendrimers. *Molecules (Basel, Switzerland)*, *14*(9), 3719–3730. doi:10.3390/molecules14093719 PMID:19783954

Kim, D., Jeong, Y. Y., & Jon, S. (2010). A drug-loaded aptamer - Gold nanoparticle bioconjugate for combined ct imaging and therapy of prostate cancer. *ACS Nano*, *4*(7), 3689–3696. doi:10.1021/nn901877h PMID:20550178

Kim, H.-S., Kang, J.-H., Jang, J., Lee, E.-J., Kim, J. H., Byun, J., & Shin, U. S. (2023). Dual stimuli-responsive mesoporous silica nanoparticles for efficient loading and smart delivery of doxorubicin to cancer with RGD-integrin targeting. *European Journal of Pharmaceutical Sciences*, *188*, 106525. doi:10.1016/j.ejps.2023.106525 PMID:37437854

Kim, K.-R., Kim, D.-R., Lee, T., Yhee, J. Y., Kim, B.-S., Kwon, I. C., & Ahn, D.-R. (2013). Drug delivery by a self-assembled DNA tetrahedron for overcoming drug resistance in breast cancer cells. *Chemical Communications (Cambridge)*, *49*(20), 2010–2012. doi:10.1039/c3cc38693g

Kim, M., Kim, S.-B., Kim, J., Kim, K.-S., & Kim, D.-E. (2023). Co-delivery of curcumin and PTTG1 siRNA by galactose receptor-targeted liposomes for enhanced anti-tumor effects in hepatocellular carcinoma. *Journal of Drug Delivery Science and Technology*, *86*, 104692. doi:10.1016/j.jddst.2023.104692

Kim, Y. K., Zhang, M., Lu, J. J., Xu, F., Chen, B. A., Xing, L., & Jiang, H. L. (2016). PK11195-chitosan-graft-polyethylenimine-modified SPION as a mitochondria-targeting gene carrier. *Journal of Drug Targeting*, *24*(5), 457–467. doi: 10.3109/1061186X.2015.1087527

Kipper, M. J., Shen, E., Determan, A., & Narasimhan, B. (2002). Design of an injectable system based on bioerodible polyanhydride microspheres for sustained drug delivery. *Biomaterials*, *23*(22), 4405–4412. doi:10.1016/S0142-9612(02)00181-3 PMID:12219831

Kirtane, A. R., Verma, M., Karandikar, P., Furin, J., Langer, R., & Traverso, G. (2021). Nanotechnology approaches for global infectious diseases. *Nature Nanotechnology*, *16*(4), 369–384. doi:10.103841565-021-00866-8 PMID:33753915

Kishore, K., Pandey, A., Wagri, N. K., Saxena, A., Patel, J., & Al-Fakih, A. (2023). *Technological challenges in nanoparticle-modified geopolymer concrete: A comprehensive review on nanomaterial dispersion, characterization techniques and its mechanical properties*. Case Studies in Construction Materials.

Kitson, T. M. (1975). The effect of disulfiram on the aldehyde dehydrogenases of sheep liver. *The Biochemical Journal*, *151*(2), 407–412. doi:10.1042/bj1510407 PMID:3167

Kitson, T. M. (1983). Mechanism of inactivation of sheep liver cytoplasmic aldehyde dehydrogenase by disulfiram. *The Biochemical Journal*, *213*(2), 551–554. doi:10.1042/bj2130551 PMID:6615449

Klaine, S. J., Alvarez, P. J., Batley, G. E., Fernandes, T. F., Handy, R. D., Lyon, D. Y., Mahendra, S., McLaughlin, M. J., & Lead, J. R. (2008). Nanomaterials in the environment: Behavior, fate, bioavailability, and effects. *Environmental Toxicology and Chemistry*, *27*(9), 1825–1851. doi:10.1897/08-090.1 PMID:19086204

Kobayashi, H., Watanabe, R., & Choyke, P. L. (2014). Improving conventional enhanced permeability and retention (EPR) effects; what is the appropriate target? *Theranostics*, *4*(1), 81–89. doi:10.7150/thno.7193 PMID:24396516

Kodiha, M., Wang, Y. M., Hutter, E., Maysinger, D., & Stochaj, U. (2015). Off to the Organelles -Killing Cancer Cells with Targeted Gold Nanoparticles. *Theranostics*, *5*(4), 357–370. doi:10.7150/thno.10657 PMID:25699096

Kodsangma, A., Homsaard, N., Nadon, S., Rachtanapun, P., Leksawasdi, N., Phimolsiripol, Y., Insomphun, C., Seesuriyachan, P., Chaiyaso, T., Jantrawut, P., Inmutto, N., Ougizawa, T., & Jantanasakulwong, K. (2020). Effect of sodium benzoate and chlorhexidine gluconate on a bio-thermoplastic elastomer made from thermoplastic starch-chitosan blended with epoxidized natural rubber. *Carbohydrate Polymers*, *242*, 116421. doi:10.1016/j.carbpol.2020.116421 PMID:32564859

Komalla, V., & Haghi, M. (2020). Liposomes in the treatment of chronic respiratory conditions. In *Targeting chronic inflammatory lung diseases using advanced drug delivery systems* (pp. 375–392). Academic Press. doi:10.1016/B978-0-12-820658-4.00018-2

Konan, Y. N., Gurny, R., & Allémann, E. (2002). Preparation and characterization of sterile and freeze-dried sub-200 nm nanoparticles. *International Journal of Pharmaceutics*, *233*(1-2), 239–252. doi:10.1016/S0378-5173(01)00944-9 PMID:11897428

Kong, S. D., Lee, J., Ramachandran, S., Eliceiri, B. P., Shubayev, V. I., Lal, R., & Jin, S. (2012). Magnetic targeting of nanoparticles across the intact blood–brain barrier. *Journal of Controlled Release*, *164*(1), 49–57. doi:10.1016/j.jconrel.2012.09.021 PMID:23063548

Koo, O. M., Rubinstein, I., & Onyuksel, H. (2005). Role of nanotechnology in targeted drug delivery and imaging: A concise review. *Nanomedicine; Nanotechnology, Biology, and Medicine*, *1*(3), 193–212. doi:10.1016/j.nano.2005.06.004 PMID:17292079

Koo, Y. E. L., Cao, Y., Kopelman, R., Koo, S. M., Brasuel, M., & Philbert, M. A. (2004). Real-Time Measurements of Dissolved Oxygen Inside Live Cells by Organically Modified Silicate Fluorescent Nanosensors. *Analytical Chemistry*, *76*(9), 2498–2505. doi:10.1021/ac035493f PMID:15117189

Korake, S., Bothiraja, C., & Pawar, A. (2023). Design, development, and in-vitro/in-vivo evaluation of docetaxel-loaded PEGylated solid lipid nanoparticles in prostate cancer therapy. *European Journal of Pharmaceutics and Biopharmaceutics*, *189*, 15–27. doi:10.1016/j.ejpb.2023.05.020 PMID:37270157

Kościk, I., Jankowski, D., & Jagusiak, A. (2021). Carbon Nanomaterials for Theranostic Use. *C*, *8*(1), 3. doi:10.3390/c8010003

Kou, L., Hou, Y., Yao, Q., Guo, W., Wang, G., Wang, M., Fu, Q., He, Z., Ganapathy, V., & Sun, J. (2018). L-Carnitine-conjugated nanoparticles to promote permeation across blood–brain barrier and to target glioma cells for drug delivery via the novel organic cation/carnitine transporter OCTN2. *Artificial Cells, Nanomedicine, and Biotechnology*, *46*(8), 1605–1616. doi:10.1080/21691401.2017.1384385/SUPPL_FILE/IANB_A_1384385_SM9430.DOC PMID:28974108

Kourou, K., Exarchos, T. P., Exarchos, K. P., Karamouzis, M. V., & Fotiadis, D. I. (2015). Machine learning applications in cancer prognosis and prediction. *Computational and Structural Biotechnology Journal*, *13*, 8–17. doi:10.1016/j.csbj.2014.11.005

Kousar, K., Naseer, F., Abduh, M. S., Kakar, S., Gul, R., Anjum, S., & Ahmad, T. (2023). Green synthesis of hyaluronic acid coated, thiolated chitosan nanoparticles for CD44 targeted delivery and sustained release of Cisplatin in cervical carcinoma. *Frontiers in Pharmacology*, *13*, 1073004. doi:10.3389/fphar.2022.1073004 PMID:36712656

Kovács, D., Szoke, K., Igaz, N., Spengler, G., Molnár, J., Tóth, T., Madarász, D., Rázga, Z., Kónya, Z., Boros, I. M., & Kiricsi, M. (2016). Silver nanoparticles modulate ABC transporter activity and enhance chemotherapy in multidrug resistant cancer. *Nanomedicine; Nanotechnology, Biology, and Medicine*, *12*(3), 601–610. doi:10.1016/j.nano.2015.10.015 PMID:26656631

Kreuter, J., Ramge, P., Petrov, V., Hamm, S., Gelperina, S. E., Engelhardt, B., Alyautdin, R., von Briesen, H., & Begley, D. J. (2003). Direct evidence that polysorbate-80-coated poly(butyl cyanoacrylate) nanoparticles deliver drugs to the CNS via specific mechanisms requiring prior binding of the drug to the nanoparticles. *Pharmaceutical Research, 20*(3), 409–416. doi:10.1023/A:1022604120952 PMID:12669961

Krishna Bama, G., Anitha, R., & Ramachandran, K. (2010). On the thermal properties of aqueous solution of D-mannitol. *Nondestructive Testing and Evaluation, 25*(1), 67–75. doi:10.1080/10589750902994407

Ku, M. S. (2008). Use of the biopharmaceutical classification system in early drug development. *The AAPS Journal, 10*(1), 208–212. doi:10.120812248-008-9020-0 PMID:18446521

Kumar, S., Agrawal, N., Saha, C., & Jha, R. (2020). Optical Fiber-based Plasmonic Biosensors: Trends, Techniques and Applications.

Kumar, A., Chen, F., Mozhi, A., Zhang, X., Zhao, Y., Xue, X., Hao, Y., Zhang, X., Wang, P. C., & Liang, X.-J. (2013). Innovative pharmaceutical development based on unique properties of nanoscale delivery formulation. *Nanoscale, 5*(18), 8307–8325. doi:10.1039/c3nr01525d PMID:23860639

Kumar, A., Das, N., & Rayavarapu, R. G. (2023). Role of Tunable Gold Nanostructures in Cancer Nanotheranostics: Implications on Synthesis, Toxicity, Clinical Applications and Their Associated Opportunities and Challenges. *Journal of Nanotheranostics, 4*(1), 1–34. doi:10.3390/jnt4010001

Kumar, A., Singla, M. L., Kumar, A., & Rajput, J. K. (2019). Fabrication and linearisation of conformable POMANI-Mn3O4 nanocomposite based thermistor for temperature monitoring applications in prosthetic gloves. *Sensors and Actuators. A, Physical, 285*, 588–598. doi:10.1016/j.sna.2018.11.036

Kumar, H., & Behal, I. (2016). Volumetric and ultrasonic investigation of molecular interactions of l-serine and l-threonine in aqueous nicotinamide solutions at T= (288.15–318.15) K. *Journal of Molecular Liquids, 219*, 756–764. doi:10.1016/j.molliq.2016.04.019

Kumar, H., Kaur, K., Arti, S., & Singla, M. (2016). Study of thermodynamic properties of sodium dodecyl sulphate in aqueous solutions of alkoxyalkanols at different temperatures. *Journal of Molecular Liquids, 221*, 526–534. doi:10.1016/j.molliq.2016.06.027

Kumar, H., Kuča, K., Bhatia, S. K., Saini, K., Kaushal, A., Verma, R., Bhalla, T. C., & Kumar, D. (2020). Applications of Nanotechnology in Sensor-Based Detection of Foodborne Pathogens. *Sensors (Basel), 20*(7), 1966. doi:10.339020071966 PMID:32244581

Kumar, H., Singla, M., & Jindal, R. (2014). Investigations on solute–solvent interactions of amino acids in aqueous solutions of sodium dihydrogen phosphate at different temperatures. *Monatshefte für Chemie, 145*(7), 1063–1082. doi:10.100700706-014-1183-z

Kumar, H., Singla, M., & Mittal, H. (2016). Volumetric, acoustic and viscometric behaviour of dipotassium hydrogen phosphate and disodium hydrogen phosphate in aqueous solution of N-acetyl glycine at different temperatures. *The Journal of Chemical Thermodynamics, 94*, 204–220. doi:10.1016/j.jct.2015.10.017

Kumari, R., Saini, A. K., Kumar, A., & Saini, R. V. (2020). Apoptosis induction in lung and prostate cancer cells through silver nanoparticles synthesized from Pinus roxburghii bioactive fraction. *Journal of Biological Inorganic Chemistry, 25*(1), 23–37. doi:10.100700775-019-01729-3 PMID:31641851

Kumari, S., Juglan, K. C., & Sharma, A. (2014). Acoustic parameter investigation of tyrosine derivative in dimethyl sulpho oxide by ultrasonic technique. *Journal of Chemical and Pharmaceutical Research, 6*(11), 782–794.

Kumar, K. P. S., Bhowmik, D., Srivastava, S., Paswan, S., & Dutta, A. S. (2012). Sustained Release Drug Delivery System Potential. *The Pharma Innovation*, *1*(2), 48–60.

Kumar, M. (2013). Molecular Biology Application in Biomedicine and Toxicology. *Annals of the Romanian Society for Cell Biology*, 15–26. doi:10.3389/fgeed.2023.1200987

Kumar, M. R. (Ed.). (2008). *Handbook of particulate drug delivery*. American Scientific Publishers.

Kumar, M., Khan, M. A., Yadav, C. P., Pandey, D. K., & Singh, D. (2021). Ultrasonic characterization of binary mixture of 2, 3-dichloroaniline and polyethylene glycols. *The Journal of Chemical Thermodynamics*, *161*, 106557. doi:10.1016/j.jct.2021.106557

Kumar, S., Agrawal, N., Saha, C., & Jha, R. (2022). *Optical Fiber-Based Plasmonic Biosensors: Trends, Techniques, and Applications*. CRC Press. doi:10.3389/978-2-88974-680-4

Kumar, S., Fry, L. E., Wang, J.-H., Martin, K. R., Hewitt, A. W., Chen, F. K., & Liu, G.-S. (2023). RNA-targeting strategies as a platform for ocular gene therapy. *Progress in Retinal and Eye Research*, *92*, 101110. doi:10.1016/j.preteyeres.2022.101110 PMID:35840489

Kumar, Y., Koul, A., Singla, R., & Ijaz, M. F. (2023). Artificial intelligence in disease diagnosis: A systematic literature review, synthesizing framework and future research agenda. *Journal of Ambient Intelligence and Humanized Computing*, *14*(7), 8459–8486. doi:10.100712652-021-03612-z

Kumawat, T. K., Kumawat, V., Sharma, V., Pandit, A., & Biyani, M. (2023). *Applications of Nanomaterials in Diagnostics and Treatment of Cancer. Sustainable Nanomaterials for Biomedical Engineering: Impacts*. Challenges, and Future Prospects.

Kunzler, T. P., Drobek, T., Schuler, M., & Spencer, N. D. (2007). Systematic study of osteoblast and fibroblast response to roughness by means of surface-morphology gradients. *Biomaterials*, *28*(13), 2175–2182. doi:10.1016/j.biomaterials.2007.01.019 PMID:17275082

Kuppusamy, P., Ichwan, S. J., Al-Zikri, P. N., Suriyah, W. H., Soundharrajan, I., Govindan, N., Maniam, G. P., & Yusoff, M. M. (2016). In Vitro Anticancer Activity of Au, Ag Nanoparticles Synthesized Using Commelina nudiflora L. Aqueous Extract Against HCT-116 Colon Cancer Cells. *Biological Trace Element Research*, *173*(2), 297–305. doi:10.100712011-016-0666-7 PMID:26961292

Kurawattimath, V., Wilson, B., & Geetha, K. M. (2023). Nanoparticle-based drug delivery across the blood-brain barrier for treating malignant brain glioma. *OpenNano*, *10*, 100128. doi:10.1016/j.onano.2023.100128

Kurzin, A. V., Evdokimov, A. N., Golikova, V. S., & Fedorov, V. A. (2012). Solubility of potassium and sodium orthophosphates in ethylene glycol. *Russian Journal of Applied Chemistry*, *85*(5), 841–842. doi:10.1134/S1070427212050278

Kwiatkowska, A., Drabik, M., Lipko, A., Grzeczkowicz, A., Stachowiak, R., Marszalik, A., & Granicka, L. H. (2022). Composite Membrane Dressings System with Metallic Nanoparticles as an Antibacterial Factor in Wound Healing. *Membranes*, *12*(2), 215. doi:10.3390/membranes12020215 PMID:35207136

Kwon, H. Y., Lee, J. Y., Choi, S. W., Jang, Y., & Kim, J. H. (2001). Preparation of PLGA nanoparticles containing estrogen by emulsification–diffusion method. *Colloids and Surfaces. A, Physicochemical and Engineering Aspects*, *182*(1-3), 123–130. doi:10.1016/S0927-7757(00)00825-6

La Zerda, A. D., Liu, Z., Bodapati, S., Teed, R., Vaithilingam, S., Khuri-Yakub, B. T., Chen, X., Dai, H., & Gambhir, S. S. (2010). Ultrahigh sensitivity carbon nanotube agents for photoacoustic molecular imaging in living mice. *Nano Letters*, *10*(6), 2168–2172. doi:10.1021/nl100890d PMID:20499887

Labieniec-Watala, M., Karolczak, K., Siewiera, K., & Watala, C. (2013). The Janus face of PAMAM dendrimers used to potentially cure nonenzymatic modifications of biomacromolecules in metabolic disorders—A critical review of the pros and cons. *Molecules (Basel, Switzerland)*, *18*(11), 13769–13811. doi:10.3390/molecules181113769 PMID:24213655

Lamba M., Chakraborty, N., Juglan, K. C., & Kumar, H. (2022). Thermodynamic-Acoustic Studies of Mixture Vitamin B7 Glycols at Different Temperatures. *Lett. Appl. NanoBioScience*, *12*(4).

Lammers, T. (2018). PT NU SC. *Journal of Controlled Release#*. doi:10.1016/j.jconrel.2018.11.031

Lammers, T., & Ferrari, M. (2020). The success of nanomedicine. *Nano Today*, *31*, 100853. doi:10.1016/j.nantod.2020.100853 PMID:34707725

Lamprecht, A. L. F., Ubrich, N., Yamamoto, H., Schäfer, U., Takeuchi, H., Maincent, P., & Lehr, C. M. (2001). Biodegradable nanoparticles for targeted drug delivery in the treatment of inflammatory bowel disease. *The Journal of Pharmacology and Experimental Therapeutics*, *299*(2), 775–781. PMID:11602694

Langer, R. (1990). New methods of drug delivery. *Science*, *249*(4976), 1527–1533. doi:10.1126cience.2218494 PMID:2218494

Langer, R. (1998). Drug delivery and targeting. *Nature*, *392*, 5–10. PMID:9579855

Leal-Junior, A., & Frizera-Neto, A. (n.d.). *Optical Fiber Sensors for the Next Generation of Rehabilitation Robotics*. Science Direct. http://www.sciencedirect.com:5070/book/9780323859523/optical-fiber-sensors-for-the-next-generation-of-rehabilitation-rob
otics

Leary, S. P., Liu, C. Y., & Apuzzo, M. L. (2006). Toward the emergence of nanoneurosurgery: part III—nanomedicine: targeted nanotherapy, nanosurgery, and progress toward the realization of nanoneurosurgery. *Neurosurgery*, *58*(6), 1009–1026. doi:10.1227/01.NEU.0000217016.79256.16 PMID:16723880

Lebeaux, D., Chauhan, A., Rendueles, O., & Beloin, C. (2013). From in vitro to in vivo models of bacterial biofilm-related infections. *Pathogens (Basel, Switzerland)*, *2*(2), 288–356. doi:10.3390/pathogens2020288 PMID:25437038

Lee, J. H., & Yeo, Y. (2015). Controlled drug release from pharmaceutical nanocarriers. *Chemical Engineering Science*, *125*, 75–84. doi:10.1016/j.ces.2014.08.046 PMID:25684779

Lee, K. W. K., Periasamy, S., Mukherjee, M., Xie, C., Kjelleberg, S., & Rice, S. A. (2014). Biofilm development and enhanced stress resistance of a model, mixed-species community biofilm. *The ISME Journal*, *8*(4), 894–907. doi:10.1038/ismej.2013.194 PMID:24152718

Lee, K., Conboy, M., Park, H. M., Jiang, F., Kim, H. J., Dewitt, M. A., Mackley, V. A., Chang, K., Rao, A., Skinner, C., Shobha, T., Mehdipour, M., Liu, H., Huang, W. C., Lan, F., Bray, N. L., Li, S., Corn, J. E., Kataoka, K., & Murthy, N. (2017). Nanoparticle delivery of Cas9 ribonucleoprotein and donor DNA in vivo induces homology-directed DNA repair. *Nature Biomedical Engineering*, *1*(11), 889–901. doi:10.103841551-017-0137-2 PMID:29805845

Lee, M. J., Lee, S. J., Yun, S. J., Jang, J. Y., Kang, H., Kim, K., Choi, I. H., & Park, S. (2015). Silver nanoparticles affect glucose metabolism in hepatoma cells through production of reactive oxygen species. *International Journal of Nanomedicine*, 55. doi:10.2147/IJN.S94907 PMID:26730190

Lee, S. H., & Jun, B. H. (2019). Silver nanoparticles: Synthesis and application for nanomedicine. *International Journal of Molecular Sciences*, *20*(4), 865. Advance online publication. doi:10.3390/ijms20040865 PMID:30781560

Lee, S. H., Kim, B. S., Kim, S. H., Choi, S. W., Jeong, S. I., Kwon, I. K., Kang, S. W., Nikolovski, J., Mooney, D. J., Han, Y.-K., & Kim, Y. H. (2003). Elastic biodegradable poly (glycolide-co-caprolactone) scaffold for tissue engineering. *Journal of Biomedical Materials Research. Part A*, *66*(1), 29–37. doi:10.1002/jbm.a.10497 PMID:12833428

Lee, S. Y., Hong, E., Jeong, J. Y., Cho, J., Seo, J., Ko, H., & Cho, H.-J. (2019). Esterase-sensitive cleavable histone deacetylase inhibitor-coupled hyaluronic acid nanoparticles for boosting anticancer activities against lung adenocarcinoma. *Biomaterials Science*, *7*(11), 4624–4635. doi:10.1039/C9BM00895K PMID:31451819

Lee, S.-Y., Yang, C.-Y., Peng, C.-L., Wei, M.-F., Chen, K.-C., Yao, C.-J., & Shieh, M.-J. (2016). A theranostic micelleplex co-delivering SN-38 and VEGF siRNA for colorectal cancer therapy. *Biomaterials*, *86*, 92–105. doi:10.1016/j.biomaterials.2016.01.068

Lee, Y., El Andaloussi, S., & Wood, M. J. (2012). Exosomes and microvesicles: Extracellular vesicles for genetic information transfer and gene therapy. *Human Molecular Genetics*, *21*(R1), R125–R134. doi:10.1093/hmg/dds317

Lee, Y., Kamada, N., & Moon, J. J. (2021). Oral nanomedicine for modulating immunity, intestinal barrier functions, and gut microbiome. *Advanced Drug Delivery Reviews*, *179*, 114021. doi:10.1016/j.addr.2021.114021 PMID:34710529

Lemarchand, C., Gref, R., Passirani, C., Garcion, E., Petri, B., Müller, R., Costantini, D., & Couvreur, P. (2006). Influence of polysaccharide coating on the interactions of nanoparticles with biological systems. *Biomaterials*, *27*(1), 108–118. doi:10.1016/j.biomaterials.2005.04.041 PMID:16118015

Lembo, D., Donalisio, M., Civra, A., Argenziano, M., & Cavalli, R. (2018, January 2). Nanomedicine formulations for the delivery of antiviral drugs: A promising solution for the treatment of viral infections. *Expert Opinion on Drug Delivery*, *15*(1), 93–114. doi:10.1080/17425247.2017.1360863 PMID:28749739

Leo, E., Brina, B., Forni, F., & Vandelli, M. A. (2004). In vitro evaluation of PLA nanoparticles containing a lipophilic drug in water-soluble or insoluble form. *International Journal of Pharmaceutics*, *278*(1), 133–141. doi:10.1016/j.ijpharm.2004.03.002 PMID:15158956

Leroux, J. C., Allemann, E., Doelker, E., & Gurny, R. (1995). New approach for the preparation of nanoparticles by an emulsification-diffusion method. *European Journal of Pharmaceutics and Biopharmaceutics*, *41*(1), 14–18.

Li, C., Zhou, L., & Yang, H. (2017). *Self-assembled Exopolysaccharide Nanoparticles for Bioremediation and Green Synthesis of Noble Metal Nanoparticles*.

Liang, K., Xie, Q., Nie, J., & Deng, J. (2021). Study on the effect of education for insulin injection in diabetic patients with new simulation tools. *Medicine*, *100*(14), e25424. doi:10.1097/MD.0000000000025424 PMID:33832143

Liang, S., Sun, M., Lu, Y., Shi, S., Yang, Y., Lin, Y., Feng, C., Liu, J., & Dong, C. (2020). Cytokine-induced killer cells-assisted tumor-targeting delivery of Her-2 monoclonal antibody-conjugated gold nanostars with NIR photosensitizer for enhanced therapy of cancer. *Journal of Materials Chemistry. B*, *8*(36), 8368–8382. doi:10.1039/D0TB01391A

Liao, H., Nehl, C. L., & Hafner, J. H. (2006). Biomedical applications of plasmon resonant metal nanoparticles. *Nanomedicine (London)*, *1*(2), 201–208. doi:10.2217/17435889.1.2.201 PMID:17716109

Liao, S. H., Liu, C. H., Bastakoti, B. P., Suzuki, N., Chang, Y., Yamauchi, Y., Lin, F. H., & Wu, K. C. W. (2015). Functionalized magnetic iron oxide/alginate core-shell nanoparticles for targeting hyperthermia. *International Journal of Nanomedicine*, *10*, 3315. doi:10.2147/IJN.S68719 PMID:26005343

Liao, X., Song, W., Zhang, X., Zhan, H., Liu, Y., Wang, Y., & Zheng, Y. (2019). Hetero-contact microstructure to program discerning tactile interactions for virtual reality. *Nano Energy*, *60*, 127–136. doi:10.1016/j.nanoen.2019.03.048

Liao, X., Wang, W., Wang, L., Jin, H., Shu, L., Xu, X., & Zheng, Y. (2021). A highly stretchable and deformation-insensitive bionic electronic exteroceptive neural sensor for human-machine interfaces. *Nano Energy*, *80*, 105548. doi:10.1016/j.nanoen.2020.105548

Li, B., Zhang, T., & Tang, M. (2022). Toxicity mechanism of nanomaterials: Focus on endoplasmic reticulum stress. *The Science of the Total Environment*, *834*, 155417. doi:10.1016/j.scitotenv.2022.155417 PMID:35472346

Libby, P., & Ridker, P. M. (2004). Inflammation and atherosclerosis: Role of C-Reactive protein in risk assessment. *The American Journal of Medicine*, *116*(6), 9–16. doi:10.1016/j.amjmed.2004.02.006 PMID:15050187

Li, D. W., Qin, L. X., Li, Y., Nia, R. P., Long, Y. T., & Chen, H. Y. (2011). CdSe/ZnS quantum dot–Cytochrome c bioconjugates for selective intracellular O2˙– sensing. *Chemical Communications*, *47*(30), 8539–8541. doi:10.1039/c1cc13160e PMID:21709927

Li, F., You, M., Li, S., Hu, J., Liu, C., Gong, Y., Yang, H., & Xu, F. (2020). Paper-based point-of-care immunoassays: Recent advances and emerging trends. *Biotechnology Advances*, *39*, 107442. doi:10.1016/j.biotechadv.2019.107442 PMID:31470046

Li, H., Wei, W., & Xu, H. (2022). Drug discovery is an eternal challenge for the biomedical sciences. *Acta Materia Medica*, *1*(1), 1–3. doi:10.15212/AMM-2022-1001

Li, J., Zhang, L., Tao, Y., Sun, Z., Ge, Y., & Hu, S. (2023). Combination of transcatheter arterial chemoembolization and anti-PD-L1 liposomes therapy suppressed hepatocellular carcinoma progression in mice. *European Journal of Pharmaceutical Sciences*, *106549*, 106549. doi:10.1016/j.ejps.2023.106549 PMID:37524271

Li, J., Zhang, W., Chung, T. F., Slipchenko, M. N., Chen, Y. P., Cheng, J. X., & Yang, C. (2015). Highly sensitive transient absorption imaging of graphene and graphene oxide in living cells and circulating blood. *Scientific Reports*, *5*(June), 1–9. doi:10.1038rep12394 PMID:26202216

Li, L., Guo, Q., Liu, Y., Lu, M., Yang, J., Ge, Y., Zhang, Q., Sun, B., Wang, X., Liang-cheng, L., & Ren, L. (2021). Targeted combination therapy for glioblastoma by co-delivery of doxorubicin, YAP-siRNA and gold nanorods. *Journal of Materials Science and Technology*, *63*, 81–90. doi:10.1016/j.jmst.2020.03.009

Lin, P. C., Lin, S., Wang, P. C., & Sridhar, R. (2014). Techniques for physicochemical characterization of nanomaterials. *Biotechnology advances, 32*(4), 711-726.99.

Lin, J., Chen, X., & Huang, P. (2016). Graphene-Based Nanomaterials for Bioimaging Graphical abstract HHS Public Access. *Advanced Drug Delivery Reviews*, *105*, 242–254. doi:10.1016/j.addr.2016.05.013 PMID:27233213

Lipsky, J. J., Shen, M. L., & Naylor, S. (2001). In vivo inhibition of aldehyde dehydrogenase by disulfiram. *Chemico-Biological Interactions*, *130-132*(1-3), 93–102. doi:10.1016/S0009-2797(00)00225-8 PMID:11306034

Li, Q., Liu, Y., Huang, Z., Guo, Y., & Li, Q. (2022). Triggering Immune System with Nanomaterials for Cancer Immunotherapy. *Frontiers in Bioengineering and Biotechnology*, *10*, 878524. doi:10.3389/fbioe.2022.878524

Li, Q., Tang, Z., Zhang, Y., Yuan, T., Yuan, B., Du, L., & Jin, Y. (2023). Application of low-intensity ultrasound by opening blood–brain barrier for enhanced brain-targeted drug delivery. *International Journal of Pharmaceutics*, *642*, 123191. doi:10.1016/j.ijpharm.2023.123191 PMID:37391108

Li, R., Liu, B., & Gao, J. (2017). The application of nanoparticles in diagnosis and theranostics of gastric cancer. *Cancer Letters*, *386*, 123–130. doi:10.1016/j.canlet.2016.10.032 PMID:27845158

Li, S., Chen, L., & Fu, Y. (2023). Nanotechnology-based ocular drug delivery systems: Recent advances and future prospects. *Journal of Nanobiotechnology*, *21*(1), 1–39. doi:10.118612951-023-01992-2 PMID:37480102

Li, S., Li, W., & Khashab, N. (2012). Stimuli-responsive nanomaterials for controlled release applications. *Nanotechnology Reviews*, *1*(6), 493–513. doi:10.1515/ntrev-2012-0033

Li, S., Meng Lin, M., Toprak, M. S., Kim, D. K., & Muhammed, M. (2010). Nanocomposites of polymer and inorganic nanoparticles for optical and magnetic applications. *Nano Reviews*, *1*(1), 5214. doi:10.3402/nano.v1i0.5214 PMID:22110855

Liu, A., Chai, X., Zhu, S., Chin, P., He, M., Xu, Y.-J., & Liu, Y. (2023). Effects of N-succinyl-chitosan coating on properties of astaxanthin-loaded PEG-liposomes: Environmental stability, antioxidant/antibacterial activities, and in vitro release. *International Journal of Biological Macromolecules*, *244*, 125311. doi:10.1016/j.ijbiomac.2023.125311 PMID:37302627

Liu, C., Han, D., Liang, P., Li, Y., & Cao, F. (2021). The current dilemma and breakthrough of stem cell therapy in ischemic heart disease. *Frontiers in Cell and Developmental Biology*, *9*, 636136. doi:10.3389/fcell.2021.636136 PMID:33968924

Liu, G. W., Guzman, E. B., Menon, N., & Langer, R. S. (2023). Lipid Nanoparticles for Nucleic Acid Delivery to Endothelial Cells. *Pharmaceutical Research*, *40*(1), 3–25. doi:10.100711095-023-03471-7 PMID:36735106

Liu, H., Zhang, J., Chen, X., Du, X. S., Zhang, J. L., Liu, G., & Zhang, W. G. (2016). Application of iron oxide nanoparticles in glioma imaging and therapy: From bench to bedside. *Nanoscale*, *8*(15), 7808–7826. doi:10.1039/C6NR00147E PMID:27029509

Liu, J., Huang, Y., Kumar, A., Tan, A., Jin, S., Mozhi, A., & Liang, X.-J. (2014). pH-Sensitive nano-systems for drug delivery in cancer therapy. *Biotechnology Advances*, *32*(4), 693–710. doi:10.1016/j.biotechadv.2013.11.009 PMID:24309541

Liu, J., Miao, L., Sui, J., Hao, Y., & Huang, G. (2019). Nanoparticle cancer vaccines: Design considerations and recent advances. *Asian Journal of Pharmaceutical Sciences*, *15*(5), 576–590. doi:10.1016/j.ajps.2019.10.006 PMID:33193861

Liu, M., Wei, X., Zheng, Z., Li, Y., Li, M., Lin, J., & Yang, L. (2023). Recent Advances in Nano-Drug Delivery Systems for the Treatment of Diabetic Wound Healing. *International Journal of Nanomedicine*, *18*, 1537–1560. doi:10.2147/IJN.S395438 PMID:37007988

Liu, Q., Wang, S., & Cai, L. (2014). Diabetic cardiomyopathy and its mechanisms: Role of oxidative stress and damage. *Journal of Diabetes Investigation*, *5*(6), 623–634. doi:10.1111/jdi.12250 PMID:25422760

Liu, S., Liang, H., Sun, T., Yang, D., & Cao, M. (2018). A recoverable dendritic polyamidoamine immobilized TEMPO for efficient catalytic oxidation of cellulose. *Carbohydrate Polymers*, *202*, 563–570. doi:10.1016/j.carbpol.2018.09.016 PMID:30287037

Liu, T., Lu, Y., Zhan, R., Qian, W., & Luo, G. (2023). Nanomaterials and nanomaterials-based drug delivery to promote cutaneous wound healing. *Advanced Drug Delivery Reviews*, *193*, 114670. doi:10.1016/j.addr.2022.114670 PMID:36538990

Liu, T., Zou, H., Mu, J., Zhang, X., Liu, G., Yu, N., Yuan, B., Yuan, X., Liang, X., & Guo, S. (2023). PDLLA length on anti-breast cancer efficacy of acid-responsive self-assembling mPEG-PDLLA–docetaxel conjugates. *Chinese Chemical Letters*, *34*(9), 108135. doi:10.1016/j.cclet.2023.108135

Liu, W., Wei, J., Chen, Y., Huo, P., & Wei, Y. (2013). Electrospinning of poly(L-lactide) nanofibers encapsulated with water-soluble fullerenes for bioimaging application. *ACS Applied Materials & Interfaces*, *5*(3), 680–685. doi:10.1021/am400037s PMID:23327807

Liu, X. L., & Fan, H. M. (2014). Innovative magnetic nanoparticle platform for magnetic resonance imaging and magnetic fluid hyperthermia applications. *Current Opinion in Chemical Engineering*, *4*, 38–46. doi:10.1016/j.coche.2013.12.010

Liu, X., Li, C., Lv, J., Huang, F., An, Y., Shi, L., & Ma, R. (2020). Glucose and H_2O_2 dual-responsive polymeric micelles for the self-regulated release of insulin. *ACS Applied Bio Materials*, *3*(3), 1598–1606. doi:10.1021/acsabm.9b01185

Liu, Y., Li, S., Ding, C., Ge, Z., Aierken, A., Li, J., Qin, L., Liu, J., Guo, X., Wang, Y., Xing, Z., Yuan, F., & Zhou, P. (2023). Dual-responsive and controlled-release paclitaxel-loaded mesoporous silicon nanoparticles with cell membrane coating for homologous targeted therapy of tongue squamous cell carcinoma. *Materials & Design*, *229*, 111886. doi:10.1016/j.matdes.2023.111886

Liu, Y., Zeng, S., Ji, W., Yao, H., Lin, L., Cui, H., Santos, H. A., & Pan, G. (2022). Emerging theranostic nanomaterials in diabetes and its complications. *Advancement of Science*, *9*(3), 2102466. doi:10.1002/advs.202102466 PMID:34825525

Liu, Y., Zhu, S., Gu, Z., & Chen, C. (2023). Toxicology of nanomaterials: From toxicokinetics to toxicity mechanisms. In Y. Yin, Y. Lu, & Y. Xia (Eds.), *Encyclopedia of Nanomaterials* (1st ed., pp. 718–732). Elsevier. doi:10.1016/B978-0-12-822425-0.00025-7

Li, Y., Ma, Z., Ren, Y., Lu, D., Li, T., Li, W., Wang, J., Ma, H. M., & Zhao, J. (2021). Tissue engineering strategies for peripheral nerve regeneration. *Frontiers in Neurology*, *12*, 768267. doi:10.3389/fneur.2021.768267 PMID:34867754

Li, Y., Wang, X., Zhang, Y., Nie, G., Nie, G., & Nie, G. (2020). Recent Advances in Nanomaterials with Inherent Optical and Magnetic Properties for Bioimaging and Imaging-Guided Nucleic Acid Therapy. *Bioconjugate Chemistry*, *31*(5), 1234–1246. doi:10.1021/acs.bioconjchem.0c00126 PMID:32302478

Li, Y., Xu, R., & Zuo, Y. (2022). Effects and Detection Methods of Potential Toxic Chemicals in Cosmetics: Metals, Phenoxyethanol and Aloe Vera. *Highlights in Science. Engineering and Technology*, *6*, 9–17.

Li, Z., Xu, K., Qin, L., Zhao, D., Yang, N., Wang, D., & Yang, Y. (2023). Hollow Nanomaterials in Advanced Drug Delivery Systems: From Single-to Multiple Shells. *Advanced Materials*, *35*(12), 2203890. doi:10.1002/adma.202203890 PMID:35998336

Llop, J., & Lammers, T. (2021). Nanoparticles for Cancer Diagnosis, Radionuclide Therapy and Theranostics. *ACS Nano*, *15*(11), 16974–16981. doi:10.1021/acsnano.1c09139 PMID:34748314

Lockman, P. R., Mumper, R. J., Khan, M. A., & Allen, D. D. (2002). Nanoparticle technology for drug delivery across the blood-brain barrier. *Drug Development and Industrial Pharmacy*, *28*(1), 1–13. doi:10.1081/DDC-120001481 PMID:11858519

Lohcharoenkal, W., Wang, L., Chen, Y. C., & Rojanasakul, Y. (2014). Protein nanoparticles as drug delivery carriers for cancer therapy. *BioMed Research International*, *2014*, 1–12. doi:10.1155/2014/180549 PMID:24772414

Lokendra, S., Niteshkumar, A., Himnashu, B., Bhupal, A., & Taresh, S. (2021). Application of Fiber Optics in Bio-Sensing. In H.-C. Guillermo (Ed.), *Fiber Optics*. IntechOpen.

Lombardi, G., Del Bianco, P., Brandes, A. A., Eoli, M., Rudà, R., Ibrahim, T., Lolli, I., Rizzato, S., Daniele, B., Pace, A., Pasqualetti, F., Caccesse, M., Bergo, E., Magni, G., Salvo, G. L. D., & Zagonel, V. (2021). Patient-reported outcomes in a phase II randomised study of regorafenib compared with lomustine in patients with relapsed glioblastoma (the REGOMA trial). *European Journal of Cancer*, *155*, 179–190. doi:10.1016/j.ejca.2021.06.055 PMID:34388515

Longinotti, M. P., & Corti, H. R. (2004). Electrical conductivity and complexation of sodium borate in trehalose and sucrose aqueous solutions. *Journal of Solution Chemistry*, *33*(8), 1029–1040. doi:10.1023/B:JOSL.0000048053.92048.7b

Longmire, M., Choyke, P. L., & Kobayashi, H. (2008). Clearance properties of nano-sized particles and molecules as imaging agents: Considerations and caveats. *Nanomedicine (London)*, *3*(5), 703–717. doi:10.2217/17435889.3.5.703 PMID:18817471

López-Lorente, Á. I. (2021). Recent developments on gold nanostructures for surface enhanced Raman spectroscopy: Particle shape, substrates and analytical applications. A review. *Analytica Chimica Acta*, *1168*, 338474. doi:10.1016/j.aca.2021.338474 PMID:34051992

Lo, S. T., Kumar, A., Hsieh, J. T., & Sun, X. (2013). Dendrimer nanoscaffolds for potential theranostics of prostate cancer with a focus on radiochemistry. *Molecular Pharmaceutics*, *10*(3), 793–812. doi:10.1021/mp3005325

Lou, F., Dong, S., Zhu, K., Chen, X., & Ma, Y. (2023). Thermal Insulation Performance of Aerogel Nano Porous Materials: Characterization and Test Methods. *Gels (Basel, Switzerland)*, *9*(3), 220. doi:10.3390/gels9030220 PMID:36975669

Lou, H. Y., Zhao, W., Zeng, Y., & Cui, B. (2018). The Role of Membrane Curvature in Nanoscale Topography-Induced Intracellular Signaling. *Accounts of Chemical Research*, *51*(5), 1046–1053. doi:10.1021/acs.accounts.7b00594 PMID:29648779

Lou, Z., Wang, L., Jiang, K., Wei, Z., & Shen, G. (2020). Reviews of wearable healthcare systems: Materials, devices and system integration. *Materials Science and Engineering R Reports*, *140*, 100523. doi:10.1016/j.mser.2019.100523

Lu, C. H., & Hsiao, J. K. (2023). Diagnostic and therapeutic roles of iron oxide nanoparticles in biomedicine. *Tzu-Chi Medical Journal*, *35*(1), 11. doi:10.4103/tcmj.tcmj_65_22 PMID:36866343

Lu, C., & Urban, M. W. (2018). Stimuli-responsive polymer nano-science: Shape anisotropy, responsiveness, applications. *Progress in Polymer Science*, *78*, 24–46. doi:10.1016/j.progpolymsci.2017.07.005

Lu, M., Yang, X., Yang, Y., Qin, P., Wu, X., & Cai, Z. (2017). Nanomaterials as assisted matrix of laser desorption/ionization time-of-flight mass spectrometry for the analysis of small molecules. *Nanomaterials (Basel, Switzerland)*, *7*(4), 87. doi:10.3390/nano7040087 PMID:28430138

Lundstrom, K. (2023). Viral vectors engineered for gene therapy. In *International Review of Cell and Molecular Biology*. Academic Press.

Lungwitz, U., Breunig, M., Blunk, T., & Göpferich, A. (2005). Polyethylenimine-based non-viral gene delivery systems. *European Journal of Pharmaceutics and Biopharmaceutics*, *60*(2), 247–266. doi:10.1016/j.ejpb.2004.11.011 PMID:15939236

Lu, S., Hao, D., Xiang, X., Pei, Q., & Xie, Z. (2023). Carboxylated paclitaxel prodrug nanofibers for enhanced chemotherapy. *Journal of Controlled Release*, *355*, 528–537. doi:10.1016/j.jconrel.2023.02.013 PMID:36787820

Maatouk, B., Jaffa, M. A., Karam, M., Fahs, D., Nour-Eldine, W., Hasan, A., Jaffa, A. A., & Mhanna, R. (2021). Sulfated alginate/polycaprolactone double-emulsion nanoparticles for enhanced delivery of heparin-binding growth factors in wound healing applications. *Colloids and Surfaces. B, Biointerfaces*, *208*, 112105. doi:10.1016/j.colsurfb.2021.112105 PMID:34536674

Mabrouk, A. A., El-Mezayen, N. S., Awaad, A. K., Tadros, M. I., El-Gazayerly, O. N., & El-Refaie, W. M. (2023). Novel celecoxib-loaded chitosan-fucoidan nanoparticles as potential immunotherapy for oral squamous cell carcinoma: Mechanistic insights. *Journal of Drug Delivery Science and Technology*, *81*, 104228. doi:10.1016/j.jddst.2023.104228

Macêdo, D. C. D. S., Cavalcanti, I. D. L., Medeiros, S. M., Souza, J. B., Lira Nogueira, M. C. B., & Cavalcanti, I. M. F. (2022). Nanotechnology and tuberculosis: An old disease with new treatment strategies. *Tuberculosis (Edinburgh, Scotland)*, *135*, 102208. doi:10.1016/j.tube.2022.102208 PMID:35567896

Machtakova, M., Thérien-Aubin, H., & Landfester, K. (2022). Polymer nano-systems for the encapsulation and delivery of active biomacromolecular therapeutic agents. *Chemical Society Reviews*, *51*(1), 128–152. doi:10.1039/D1CS00686J PMID:34762084

Magenheim, B., Levy, M. Y., & Benita, S. (1993). A new in vitro technique for evaluating drug release profile from colloidal carriers-ultrafiltration technique at low pressure. *International Journal of Pharmaceutics*, *94*(1-3), 115–123. doi:10.1016/0378-5173(93)90015-8

Ma, H., & Xue, M. A. Q. (2021). Recent advances in the photothermal applications of two-dimensional nanomaterials: Photothermal therapy and beyond. *Journal of Materials Chemistry. A, Materials for Energy and Sustainability*, *9*(9), 17569–17591. doi:10.1039/D1TA04134G

Mahamuni-Badiger, P., & Dhanavade, M. J. (2023). Challenges and toxicity assessment of inorganic nanomaterials in biomedical applications: Current status and future roadmaps. *Journal of Drug Delivery Science and Technology*, *104806*, 104806. doi:10.1016/j.jddst.2023.104806

Maharjan, R., Hada, S., Lee, J. E., Han, H.-K., Kim, K. H., Seo, H. J., Foged, C., & Jeong, S. H. (2023). Comparative study of lipid nanoparticle-based mRNA vaccine bioprocess with machine learning and combinatorial artificial neural network-design of experiment approach. *International Journal of Pharmaceutics*, *640*, 123012. doi:10.1016/j.ijpharm.2023.123012 PMID:37142140

Mahendran, G., & Kumari, B. R. (2016). Biological activities of silver nanoparticles from Nothapodytes nimmoniana (Graham) Mabb. fruit extracts. *Food Science and Human Wellness*, *5*(4), 207–218. doi:10.1016/j.fshw.2016.10.001

Maiti, D., Tong, X., Mou, X., & Yang, K. (2019). Carbon-Based Nanomaterials for Biomedical Applications: A Recent Study. *Frontiers in Pharmacology*, *9*, 1401. doi:10.3389/fphar.2018.01401 PMID:30914959

Ma, J., Liu, R., Wang, X., Liu, Q., Chen, Y., Valle, R. P., Zuo, Y. Y., Xia, T., & Liu, S. (2015). Crucial role of lateral size for graphene oxide in activating macrophages and stimulating pro-inflammatory responses in cells and animals. *ACS Nano*, *9*(10), 10498–10515. doi:10.1021/acsnano.5b04751

Majeed, S., Bakhtiar, N. F. B., Danish, M., Ibrahim, M. M., & Hashim, R. (2019). Green approach for the biosynthesis of silver nanoparticles and its antibacterial and antitumor effect against osteoblast MG-63 and breast MCF-7 cancer cell lines. *Sustainable Chemistry and Pharmacy*, *12*, 100138. doi:10.1016/j.scp.2019.100138

Majka, J., Babiński, L., & Olek, W. (2017). Sorption isotherms of waterlogged subfossil Scots pine wood impregnated with a lactitol and trehalose mixture. *Holzforschung*, *71*(10), 813–819. doi:10.1515/hf-2017-0006

Majumder, N., Das, N. G., & Das, S. K. (2020). Polymeric micelles for anticancer drug delivery. *Therapeutic Delivery*, *11*(10), 613–635. doi:10.4155/tde-2020-0008

Makabenta, J. M. V., Nabawy, A., Li, C. H., Schmidt-Malan, S., Patel, R., & Rotello, V. M. (2021). Nanomaterial-based therapeutics for antibiotic-resistant bacterial infections. *Nature Reviews. Microbiology*, *19*(1), 23–36. doi:10.103841579-020-0420-1 PMID:32814862

Makarov, V. V., Love, A. J., Sinitsyna, O. V., Makarova, S. S., Yaminsky, I. V., Taliansky, M. E., & Kalinina, N. O. (2014). "Green" nanotechnologies: Synthesis of metal nanoparticles using plants. [англоязычная версия]. *Acta Naturae (English Ed.)*, *6*(1 (20)), 35–44. doi:10.32607/20758251-2014-6-1-35-44 PMID:24772325

Makvandi, P., Song, H., Yiu, C. K., Sartorius, R., Zare, E. N., Rabiee, N., Wu, W. X., Paiva-Santos, A. C., Wang, X. D., Yu, C. Z., & Tay, F. R. (2023). Bioengineered materials with selective antimicrobial toxicity in biomedicine. *Military Medical Research*, *10*(1), 8. doi:10.118640779-023-00443-1 PMID:36829246

Malekghasemi, S., Mokhtarani, B., Hamzehzadeh, S., Sharifi, A., & Mirzaei, M. (2016). Liquid–liquid equilibria of aqueous biphasic systems of ionic liquids and dipotassium hydrogen phosphate at different temperatures: Experimental study and thermodynamic modeling. *Journal of Molecular Liquids*, *219*, 95–103. doi:10.1016/j.molliq.2016.03.026

Maleki, M., Pourhassan-Moghaddam, M., Karimi, A., Akbarzadeh, A., Zarghami, N., & Mohammadi, S. (2019). Synthesis, characterisation, and application of chamomile gold nanoparticles in molecular diagnostics: A new component for PCR kits. *Biointerface Research in Applied Chemistry*, *9*(6), 4635–4641. doi:10.33263/BRIAC96.635641

Mali, S. (2013). Delivery systems for gene therapy. *Indian Journal of Human Genetics*, *19*(1), 3. doi:10.4103/0971-6866.112870 PMID:23901186

Mallakpour, S., & Behranvand, V. (2016). Polymeric nanoparticles: Recent development in synthesis and application. *Express Polymer Letters*, *10*(11), 895–913. doi:10.3144/expresspolymlett.2016.84

Malviya, N., Malviya, S., Saxena, R., Chauhan, V., & Dhere, M. (2022). Smart Biodegradable Polymeric Nanoparticles: Synthesis, Characterization, and Applications. In Advancements in Controlled Drug Delivery Systems (pp. 257-280). IGI Global.

Malviya, R., Fuloria, S., Verma, S., Subramaniyan, V., Sathasivam, K. V., Kumarasamy, V., Hari Kumar, D., Vellasamy, S., Meenakshi, D. U., Yadav, S., Sharma, A., Fuloria, N. K. (2021). Commercial utilities and future perspective of nanomedicines. *PeerJ,* 9e12392. doi:10.7717/peerj.12392

Mandal, D., Anand, K., & Prabhakar, P. K. (2023). Biomedical Applications of Nanofluids in Drug Delivery. In *Novel Technologies in Biosystems, Biomedical & Drug Delivery* (pp. 105–124). Springer Nature Singapore. doi:10.1007/978-981-99-5281-6_5

Manhas, P., Sharma, R., Wangoo, N., Saini, R., Saima, Agrewala, J. N., & Sharma, R. K. (2023). Dox-loaded TPU-PLGA nanoparticles embedded chitosan hydrogel formulation as an effective anti-cancer therapy. *Journal of Molecular Liquids*, *383*, 122170. doi:10.1016/j.molliq.2023.122170

Manimaran, V., Sivakumar, P. M., Narayanan, J., Parthasarathi, S., & Prabhakar, P. K. (2021). Nanoemulsions: A Better Approach for Antidiabetic Drug Delivery. *Current Diabetes Reviews*, *17*(4), 486–495. doi:10.2174/1573399817666201209095205 PMID:33297917

Mansoori, G. A., & Soelaiman, T. A. F. (2005). Nanotechnology—An introduction for the standards community. *Journal of ASTM International*, *2*(6), 1–22.

Mansoor, S., Kondiah, P. P., Choonara, Y. E., & Pillay, V. (2019). Polymer-based nanoparticle strategies for insulin delivery. *Polymers*, *11*(9), 1380. doi:10.3390/polym11091380 PMID:31443473

Mao, F. X., Wen, L., Sun, C. X., Zhang, S. H., Wang, G. L., Zeng, J. F., Wang, Y., Ma, J., Gao, M., & Li, Z. (2016). Ultrasmall Biocompatible Bi_2Se_3 Nanodots for Multimodal Imaging-Guided Synergistic Radiophotothermal Therapy Against Cancer. *ACS Nano*, *10*(12), 11145–11155. doi:10.1021/acsnano.6b06067

Markman, J. L., Rekechenetskiy, A., Holler, E., & Ljubimova, J. Y. (2013). Nanomedicine therapeutic approaches to overcome cancer drug resistance. *Advanced Drug Delivery Reviews*, *65*(13-14), 1866–1879. doi:10.1016/j.addr.2013.09.019 PMID:24120656

Markowicz-Piasecka, M., Sikora, J., Szymański, P., Kozak, O., Studniarek, M., & Mikiciuk-Olasik, E. (2015). PAMAM dendrimers as potential carriers of gadolinium complexes of iminodiacetic acid derivatives for magnetic resonance imaging. *Journal of Nanomaterials*, *2015*, 2015. doi:10.1155/2015/394827

Mark, S. W. (2011). *Torchilin., Vladimir P., Drug delivery systems*. Access Science, McGraw-Hill Companies.

Martínez, G., Merinero, M., Pérez-Aranda, M., Pérez-Soriano, E. M., Ortiz, T., Villamor, E., Begines, B., & Alcudia, A. (2020). Environmental impact of nanoparticles' application as an emerging technology: A review. *Materials (Basel)*, *14*(1), 166. doi:10.3390/ma14010166 PMID:33396469

Marzi, M., Osanloo, M., Vakil, M. K., Mansoori, Y., Ghasemian, A., Dehghan, A., & Zarenezhad, E. (2022). Applications of metallic nanoparticles in the skin cancer treatment. *BioMed Research International*, *2022*, 1–20. doi:10.1155/2022/2346941 PMID:36420097

Mascolo, M. C., Pei, Y., & Ring, T. A. (2013). Room temperature co-precipitation synthesis of magnetite nanoparticles in a large pH window with different bases. *Materials (Basel)*, *6*(12), 5549–5567. doi:10.3390/ma6125549 PMID:28788408

Mason, T. G., Wilking, J. N., Meleson, K., Chang, C. B., & Graves, S. M. (2006). Nanoemulsions: Formation, structure, and physical properties. *Journal of Physics Condensed Matter*, *18*(41), R635–R666. doi:10.1088/0953-8984/18/41/R01

Mata, R., Nakkala, J. R., & Sadras, S. R. (2015). Biogenic silver NPs from Abutilon indicum: Their antioxidant, antibacterial and cytotoxic effects in vitro. *Colloids and Surfaces. B, Biointerfaces*, *128*, 76–86. doi:10.1016/j.colsurfb.2015.01.052 PMID:25701118

Matea, C. T., Mocan, T., Tabaran, F., Pop, T., Mosteanu, O., Puia, C., Iancu, C., & Mocan, L. (2017). Quantum dots in imaging, drug delivery and sensor applications. *International Journal of Nanomedicine*, *12*, 5421–5431. doi:10.2147/IJN.S138624 PMID:28814860

Mathurin, J., Pancani, E., Deniset-Besseau, A., Kjoller, K., Prater, C. B., Gref, R., & Dazzi, A. (2018). How to unravel the chemical structure and component localization of individual drug-loaded polymeric nanoparticles by using tapping AFM-IR. *Analyst*, *143*(24), 5940–5949. doi:10.1039/C8AN01239C PMID:30345433

Matiyani, M., Rana, A., Karki, N., Garwal, K., Pal, M., & Sahoo, N. G. (2023). Development of multi-functionalized graphene oxide based nanocarrier for the delivery of poorly water soluble anticancer drugs. *Journal of Drug Delivery Science and Technology*, *83*, 104412. doi:10.1016/j.jddst.2023.104412

Maurer, M. S., Fontana, M., Berk, J., Gustafsson, F., Simoes, M., Grogan, M., Fernandes, F., Gottlieb, R. L., Kubanek, M., Poulsen, S., Damy, T., Diemberger, I., Tahara, N., Yu, W.-C., Tang, W. H. W., Obic, L., Gonzalez-Duarte, A., Sekijima, Y., White, M. T., & Gillmore, J. D. (2023). Primary results from apollo-B, a phase 3 study of patisiran in patients with transthyretin-mediated amyloidosis with cardiomyopathy. *Journal of Cardiac Failure*, *29*(4), 550. doi:10.1016/j.cardfail.2022.10.013

Maus, A., Strait, L., & Zhu, D. (2021). Nanoparticles as delivery vehicles for antiviral therapeutic drugs. *Engineered Regeneration*, *2*, 31–46. doi:10.1016/j.engreg.2021.03.001

Ma, W., Zhan, Y., Zhang, Y., Mao, C., Xie, X., & Lin, Y. (2021). The biological applications of DNA nanomaterials: Current challenges and future directions. *Signal Transduction and Targeted Therapy*, *6*(1), 351. doi:10.103841392-021-00727-9 PMID:34620843

Ma, W., Zhan, Y., Zhang, Y., Shao, X., Xie, X., Mao, C., Cui, W., Li, Q., Shi, J., Li, J., Fan, C., & Lin, Y. (2019). An intelligent DNA nanorobot with in vitro enhanced protein lysosomal degradation of HER2. *Nano Letters*, *19*(7), 4505–4517. doi:10.1021/acs.nanolett.9b01320

Mayer, K. M., & Hafner, J. H. (2011). Localized Surface Plasmon Resonance Sensors. *Chemical Reviews*, *111*(6), 3828–3857. doi:10.1021/cr100313v PMID:21648956

McClements, D., & Xiao, H. (2017). Is nano safe in foods? Establishing the factors impacting the gastrointestinal fate and toxicity of organic and inorganic food-grade nanoparticles. *npj Science of Food*, *1*(1), 6. . doi:10.1038/s41538-017-0005-1

McDougald, D., Rice, S. A., Barraud, N., Steinberg, P. D., & Kjelleberg, S. (2012). Should we stay or should we go: Mechanisms and ecological consequences for biofilm dispersal. *Nature Reviews. Microbiology*, *10*(1), 39–50. doi:10.1038/nrmicro2695 PMID:22120588

McNamara, K., & Tofail, S. A. M. (2013). Biomedical applications of nanoalloys. *Nanoalloys. From Fundamentals to Emergent Applications*, 345–371. doi:10.1016/B978-0-12-394401-6.00010-2

McNamara, K., & Tofail, S. A. M. (2016). Nanoparticles in biomedical applications. *Advances in Physics: X*, *2*(1), 54–88. doi:10.1080/23746149.2016.1254570

Md Anwar Nawaz, R., Darul Raiyaan, G. I., Sivakumar, K., & Arunachalam, K. D. (2023). Nanomedicine Regulation and Future Prospects. *Advances in Novel Formulations for Drug Delivery*, 67-80. doi:10.1002/9781394167708.ch4

Medintz, I. L., Stewart, M. H., Trammell, S. A., Susumu, K., Delehanty, J. B., Mei, B. C., Melinger, J. S., Blanco-Canosa, J. B., Dawson, P. E., & Mattoussi, H. (2010). Quantum-dot/dopamine bioconjugates function as redox coupled assemblies for in vitro and intracellular pH sensing. *Nature Materials*, *9*(8), 676–684. doi:10.1038/nmat2811

Meglioli, M., Mergoni, G., Artioli, F., Ghezzi, B., Manfredi, M., Macaluso, G. M., & Lumetti, S. (2023). A Novel Self-Assessment Method for Training Access Cavity on 3D Printed Endodontic Models. *Dentistry Journal*, *11*(6), 152. doi:10.3390/dj11060152 PMID:37366675

Mendes, R., Fernandes, A. R., & Baptista, P. V. (2017). Gold nanoparticle approach to the selective delivery of gene silencing in cancer—The case for combined delivery? *Genes*, *8*(3), 94. doi:10.3390/genes8030094

Meng, L., Xia, X., Yang, Y., Ye, J., Dong, W., Ma, P., Jin, Y., & Liu, Y. (2016). Co-encapsulation of paclitaxel and baicalein in nanoemulsions to overcome multidrug resistance via oxidative stress augmentation and P-glycoprotein inhibition. *International Journal of Pharmaceutics*, *513*(1-2), 8–16. doi:10.1016/j.ijpharm.2016.09.001

Mertdinç-Ülküseven, S., Khakzad, F., Aslan, C., Onbasli, K., Çevik, Ç., İşçi, S., Balcı-Çağıran, Ö., Acar, H. Y., Öveçoğlu, M. L., & Ağaoğulları, D. (2023). Fe_2B magnetic nanoparticles: Synthesis, optimization and cytotoxicity for potential biomedical applications. *Journal of Science. Advanced Materials and Devices*, *8*(3), 100602. doi:10.1016/j.jsamd.2023.100602

Metawea, O. R. M., Teleb, M., Haiba, N. S., Elzoghby, A. O., Khafaga, A. F., Noreldin, A. E., Khattab, S. N., & Khalil, H. H. (2023). Folic acid-poly(N-isopropylacrylamide-maltodextrin) nanohydrogels as novel thermo-/pH-responsive polymer for resveratrol breast cancer targeted therapy. *European Polymer Journal*, *182*, 111721. doi:10.1016/j.eurpolymj.2022.111721

Mhlwatika, Z., & Aderibigbe, B. A. (2018). Application of Dendrimers for the Treatment of Infectious Diseases. *Molecules (Basel, Switzerland)*, *23*(9), 2205. doi:10.3390/molecules23092205 PMID:30200314

Michlewska, S., Garaiova, Z., Šubjakova, V., Hołota, M., Kubczak, M., Grodzicka, M., Okła, E., Naziris, N., Balcerzak, Ł., Ortega, P., de la Mata, F. J., Hianik, T., Waczulikova, I., Bryszewska, M., & Ionov, M. (2023). Lipid-coated ruthenium dendrimer conjugated with doxorubicin in anti-cancer drug delivery: Introducing protocols. *Colloids and Surfaces. B, Biointerfaces*, *227*, 113371. doi:10.1016/j.colsurfb.2023.113371 PMID:37244201

Mickolajczyk, K. J., Geyer, E. A., Kim, T., Rice, L. M., & Hancock, W. O. (2019). Direct observation of individual tubulin dimers binding to growing microtubules. *Proceedings of the National Academy of Sciences of the United States of America*, *116*(15), 7314–7322. doi:10.1073/pnas.1815823116 PMID:30804205

Miclăuş, T., Beer, C., Chevallier, J., Scavenius, C., Bochenkov, V. E., Enghild, J. J., & Sutherland, D. S. (2016). Dynamic Protein Coronas Revealed as a Modulator of Silver Nanoparticle Sulphidation In Vitro. *Nature Communications*, *7*(1), 11770. doi:10.1038/ncomms11770 PMID:27278102

Miethling-Graff, R., Rumpker, R., Richter, M., Verano-Braga, T., Kjeldsen, F., Brewer, J., Hoyland, J., Rubahn, H. G., & Erdmann, H. (2014). Exposure to silver nanoparticles induces size- and dose-dependent oxidative stress and cytotoxicity in human colon carcinoma cells. *Toxicology In Vitro*, *28*(7), 1280–1289. doi:10.1016/j.tiv.2014.06.005 PMID:24997297

Mihai, M. M., Dima, M. B., Dima, B., & Holban, A. M. (2019). Nanomaterials for wound healing and infection control. *Materials (Basel), 12*(13), 2176. doi:10.3390/ma12132176 PMID:31284587

Mihranyan, A., Ferraz, N., & Stromme, M. (2012). Current status and prospects of nanotechnology in cosmetics. *Progress in Materials Science, 57*(5), 875–910. doi:10.1016/j.pmatsci.2011.10.001

Milano, G., Innocenti, F., & Minami, H. (2022). Liposomal irinotecan (Onivyde): Exemplifying the benefits of nanotherapeutic drugs. *Cancer Science, 113*(7), 2224–2231. doi:10.1111/cas.15377

Miranda, R. R., Gorshkov, V., Korzeniowska, B., Kempf, S. J., Neto, F. F., & Kjeldsen, F. (2018). Co-exposure to silver nanoparticles and cadmium induce metabolic adaptation in HepG2 cells. *Nanotoxicology, 12*(7), 781–795. doi:10.1080/17435390.2018.1489987 PMID:29996704

Miranda, R. R., Sampaio, I., & Zucolotto, V. (2022). Exploring silver nanoparticles for cancer therapy and diagnosis. *Colloids and Surfaces. B, Biointerfaces, 210*, 112254. doi:10.1016/j.colsurfb.2021.112254 PMID:34896692

Mirazi, N., Shoaei, J., Khazaei, A., & Hosseini, A. (2015). A comparative study on effect of metformin and metformin-conjugated nanotubes on blood glucose homeostasis in diabetic rats. *European Journal of Drug Metabolism and Pharmacokinetics, 40*(3), 343–348. doi:10.100713318-014-0213-x PMID:24969688

Mirón-Barroso, S., Domènech, E. B., & Trigueros, S. (2021). Nanotechnology-Based Strategies to Overcome Current Barriers in Gene Delivery. *International Journal of Molecular Sciences, 22*(16), 8537. doi:10.3390/ijms22168537 PMID:34445243

Mirrahimi, M., Khateri, M., Beik, J., Ghoreishi, F. S., Dezfuli, A. S., Ghaznavi, H., & Shakeri-Zadeh, A. (2019). Enhancement of Chemoradiation by Co-incorporation of Gold Nanoparticles and Cisplatin into Alginate Hydrogel. *Journal of Biomedical Materials Research. Part B, Applied Biomaterials, 107*(8), 2658–2663. doi:10.1002/jbm.b.34356

Mirza, Z., & Karim, S. (2021, February). Nanoparticles-based drug delivery and gene therapy for breast cancer: Recent advancements and future challenges. *Seminars in cancer biology*, (69), 226-237. Academic Press. doi:10.1016/j.semcancer.2019.10.020

Mirzaali, F., Dizaj, S. M., Shahi, S., Memar, M. Y., & Parnia, F. (2023). The Antibacterial Effect of Tetracycline-loaded Mesoporous Silica Nanoparticles in the Gingival Fluid at Implant-abutment Junction: A Randomized Clinical Trial Study. *Pharmaceutical Nanotechnology, 11*(2), 208–216. doi:10.2174/2211738511666230106151403 PMID:36617708

Mirza, S., Ahmad, M. S., Shah, M. I. A., & Ateeq, M. (2019). Magnetic nanoparticles: Drug delivery and bioimaging applications. In *Metal Nanoparticles for Drug Delivery and Diagnostic Applications*. Elsevier Inc., doi:10.1016/B978-0-12-816960-5.00011-2

Mishra, A., Kumar, R., Mishra, J., Dutta, K., Ahlawat, P., Kumar, A., Dhanasekaran, S., Gupta, A. K., Sinha, S., Bishi, D. K., Gupta, P. K., & Nayak, S. (2023). Strategies facilitating the permeation of nanoparticles through blood-brain barrier: An insight towards the development of brain-targeted drug delivery system. *Journal of Drug Delivery Science and Technology, 86*, 104694. doi:10.1016/j.jddst.2023.104694

Mishra, A., Pradhan, D., Halder, J., Biswasroy, P., Rai, V. K., Dubey, D., Kar, B., Ghosh, G., & Rath, G. (2022). Metal nanoparticles against multi-drug-resistance bacteria. *Journal of Inorganic Biochemistry, 237*, 111938. doi:10.1016/j.jinorgbio.2022.111938 PMID:36122430

Mishra, M., Gupta, A. D., Dadhich, R., Ahmad, M. N., Dasgupta, A., Chopra, S., & Kapoor, S. (2023). Mycobacterial lipid-derived immunomodulatory drug- liposome conjugate eradicates endosome-localized mycobacteria. *Journal of Controlled Release, 360*, 578–590. doi:10.1016/j.jconrel.2023.07.013 PMID:37442202

Missaoui, W. N., Arnold, R. D., & Cummings, B. S. (2018). Toxicological status of nanoparticles: What we know and what we don't know. *Chemico-Biological Interactions*, *295*, 1–12. doi:10.1016/j.cbi.2018.07.015 PMID:30048623

Mistry, N., Bandyopadhyaya, R., & Mehra, S. (2022). Enhancement of Antimycobacterial Activity of Rifampicin Using Mannose-Anchored Lipid Nanoparticles against Intramacrophage Mycobacteria. *ACS Applied Bio Materials*, *5*(12), 5779–5789. doi:10.1021/acsabm.2c00796 PMID:36441965

Mitchell, M. J., Billingsley, M. M., Haley, R. M., Wechsler, M. E., Peppas, N. A., & Langer, R. (2021). Engineering precision nanoparticles for drug delivery. *Nature Reviews. Drug Discovery*, *20*(2), 101–124. doi:10.103841573-020-0090-8

Mitchell, S. L., & Carlson, E. E. (2018). Tiny things with enormous impact: Nanotechnology in the fight against infectious disease. *ACS Infectious Diseases*, *4*(10), 1432–1435. doi:10.1021/acsinfecdis.8b00138 PMID:30070819

Miyata, K., Christie, R. J., & Kataoka, K. (2011). Polymeric micelles for nano-scale drug delivery. *Reactive & Functional Polymers*, *71*(3), 227–234. doi:10.1016/j.reactfunctpolym.2010.10.009

Moasses Ghafary, S., Rahimjazi, E., Hamzehil, H., Modarres Mousavi, S. M., Nikkhah, M., & Hosseinkhani, S. (2022). Design and preparation of a theranostic peptideticle for targeted cancer therapy: Peptide-based codelivery of doxorubicin/curcumin and graphene quantum dots. *Nanomedicine; Nanotechnology, Biology, and Medicine*, *42*, 102544. doi:10.1016/j.nano.2022.102544 PMID:35192939

Mohammed, H. A., Khan, R. A., Singh, V., Yusuf, M., Akhtar, N., Sulaiman, G. M., & Al-Subaiyel, A. M. (2023). Solid lipid nanoparticles for targeted natural and synthetic drugs delivery in high-incidence cancers, and other diseases: Roles of preparation methods, lipid composition, transitional stability, and release profiles in nanocarriers' development. *Nanotechnology Reviews*, *12*(1), 20220517 doi:10.1515/ntrev-2022-0517

Mohan, T. M., Sastry, S. S., & Murthy, V. R. K. (2011). Thermodynamic, Dielectric and Conformational Studies on Hydrogen Bonded Binary Mixtures of Propan-1-ol with Methyl Benzoate and Ethyl Benzoate. *Journal of Solution Chemistry*, *40*(1), 131–146. doi:10.100710953-010-9634-6

Mohanty, S., Mishra, S., Jena, P., Jacob, B., Sarkar, B., & Sonawane, A. (2012). An investigation on the antibacterial, cytotoxic, and antibiofilm efficacy of starch-stabilized silver nanoparticles. *Nanomedicine (London)*, *8*(6), 916–924. doi:10.1016/j.nano.2011.11.007 PMID:22115597

Moinard-Chécot, D., Chevalier, Y., Briançon, S., Beney, L., & Fessi, H. (2008). Mechanism of nanocapsules formation by the emulsion–diffusion process. *Journal of Colloid and Interface Science*, *317*(2), 458–468. doi:10.1016/j.jcis.2007.09.081 PMID:17936772

Mokhtar, N., Fouda, F., Zaazaa, A. M., & Mahmoud, M. H. (2023). Nano-Encapsulation of Doxorubicin Using Pectin: Safety an Activity on Chemotherapy-Induced Cardiotoxicity in Carcinoma Mice. *Letters in Applied NanoBioScience*, *12*(4), 107. doi:10.33263/LIANBS124.107

Molaei, M. J. (2023). Carbon quantum dots-based fluorescent layered double hydroxide for targeted drug delivery application. *Diamond and Related Materials*, *137*, 110135. doi:10.1016/j.diamond.2023.110135

Molaei, M. J., & Salimi, E. (2022). Magneto-fluorescent superparamagnetic Fe_3O_4@ SiO_2@ alginate/carbon quantum dots nanohybrid for drug delivery. *Materials Chemistry and Physics*, *126361*(288), 126361. doi:10.1016/j.matchemphys.2022.126361

Mondal, R. (2021). Nanotechnology in Microbiology. *Nanotechnology for Advances in Medical Microbiology*, 269-293. doi:10.1007/978-981-15-9916-3_11

Mongin, C., Garakyaraghi, S., Razgoniaeva, N., Zamkov, M., & Castellano, F. N. (2016). Direct observation of triplet energy transfer from semiconductor nanocrystals. *Science*, *351*(6271), 369–372. doi:10.1126cience.aad6378 PMID:26798011

Monopoli, M. P., Åberg, C., Salvati, A., & Dawson, K. A. (2012). Biomolecular coronas provide the biological identity of nanosized materials. *Nature Nanotechnology*, *7*(12), 779–786. doi:10.1038/nnano.2012.207 PMID:23212421

Montalti, M., Cantelli, A., & Battistelli, G. (2015). Nanodiamonds and silicon quantum dots: Ultrastable and biocompatible luminescent nanoprobes for long-term bioimaging. *Chemical Society Reviews*, *44*(14), 4853–4921. doi:10.1039/C4CS00486H PMID:26051500

Monte, J. P., Fontes, A., Santos, B. S., Pereira, G. A., & Pereira, G. (2023). Recent advances in hydroxyapatite/polymer/silver nanoparticles scaffolds with antimicrobial activity for bone regeneration. *Materials Letters*, *134027*, 134027. doi:10.1016/j.matlet.2023.134027

Mosleh-Shirazi, S., Abbasi, M., Moaddeli, M. R., Vaez, A., Shafiee, M., Kasaee, S. R., Amani, A. M., & Hatam, S. (2022). Nanotechnology Advances in the Detection and Treatment of Cancer: An Overview. In Nanotheranostics (Vol. 6, Issue 4, pp. 400–423). Ivyspring International Publisher. doi:10.7150/ntno.74613

Mourdikoudis, S., Pallares, R. M., & Thanh, N. T. (2018). Characterization techniques for nanoparticles: Comparison and complementarity upon studying nanoparticle properties. *Nanoscale*, *10*(27), 12871–12934. doi:10.1039/C8NR02278J PMID:29926865

Mrugacz, M., Bryl, A., & Zorena, K. (2021). Retinal vascular endothelial cell dysfunction and neuroretinal degeneration in diabetic patients. *Journal of Clinical Medicine*, *10*(3), 458. doi:10.3390/jcm10030458 PMID:33504108

Mujawar, M. A., Gohel, H., Bhardwaj, S. K., Srinivasan, S., Hickman, N., & Kaushik, A. (2020). Nano-enabled biosensing systems for intelligent healthcare: Towards COVID-19 management. *Materials Today. Chemistry*, *17*, 100306. doi:10.1016/j.mtchem.2020.100306 PMID:32835155

Mukherjee, S., Ray, S., & Thakur, R. S. (2009). Solid lipid nanoparticles: A modern formulation approach in drug delivery system. *Indian Journal of Pharmaceutical Sciences*, *71*(4), 349–358. doi:10.4103/0250-474X.57282 PMID:20502539

Mukhtar, M., Bilal, M., Rahdar, A., Barani, M., Arshad, R., Behl, T., Brisc, C., Banica, F., & Bungau, S. (2020). Nanomaterials for diagnosis and treatment of brain cancer: Recent updates. *Chemosensors (Basel, Switzerland)*, *8*(4), 117. doi:10.3390/chemosensors8040117

Mukundan, D., Mohankumar, R., & Vasanthakumari, R. (2015). Green synthesis of silver nanoparticles using leaves extract of Bauhinia tomentosa linn and its invitro anticancer potential. *Materials Today: Proceedings*, *2*(9), 4309–4316. doi:10.1016/j.matpr.2015.10.014

Müller, R., Maaben, S., Weyhers, H., & Mehnert, W. (1996). Phagocytic uptake and cytotoxicity of solid lipid nanoparticles (SLN) sterically stabilized with poloxamine 908 and poloxamer 407. *Journal of Drug Targeting*, *4*(3), 161–170. doi:10.3109/10611869609015973 PMID:8959488

Mundekkad, D., & Cho, W. C. (2022). Nanoparticles in Clinical Translation for Cancer Therapy. *International Journal of Molecular Sciences*, *23*(3), 1685. doi:10.3390/ijms23031685 PMID:35163607

Murakami, T., Hiroshima, Y., Matsuyama, R., Homma, Y., Hoffman, R. M., & Endo, I. (2019). Role of the tumor microenvironment in pancreatic cancer. *Annals of Gastroenterological Surgery*, *3*(2), 130–137. doi:10.1002/ags3.12225

Mura, S., Nicolas, J., & Couvreur, P. (2013). Stimuli-responsive nanocarriers for drug delivery. *Nature Materials*, *12*(11), 991–1003. doi:10.1038/nmat3776 PMID:24150417

Mushtaq, G., Khan, J. A., Joseph, E., & Kamal, M. A. (2015). Nanoparticles, Neurotoxicity and Neurodegenerative Diseases. *Current Drug Metabolism*, *16*(8), 676–684. doi:10.2174/1389200216666150812122302 PMID:26264205

Mussa Farkhani, S., Asoudeh Fard, A., Zakeri-Milani, P., Shahbazi Mojarrad, J., & Valizadeh, H. (2017). Enhancing antitumor activity of silver nanoparticles by modification with cell-penetrating peptides. *Artificial Cells, Nanomedicine, and Biotechnology*, *45*(5), 1029–1035. doi:10.1080/21691401.2016.1200059 PMID:27357085

Mustfa, S. A., Maurizi, E., McGrath, J., & Chiappini, C. (2021). Nanomedicine approaches to negotiate local biobarriers for topical drug delivery. *Advanced Therapeutics*, *4*(1), 2000160. doi:10.1002/adtp.202000160

Muthoosamy, K., & Manickam, S. (2023). Nanomaterials for disease diagnostics. *Mikrochimica Acta*, *190*(4), 143. doi:10.100700604-023-05724-z PMID:36933103

Muthukrishnan, G., Roberts, C. A., Chen, Y. C., Zahn, J. D., & Hancock, W. O. (2004). Patterning surface-bound microtubules through reversible DNA hybridization. *Nano Letters*, *4*(11), 2127–2132. doi:10.1021/nl048816b

Nafee, N., Schneider, M., Schaefer, U. F., & Lehr, C. M. (2009). Relevance of the colloidal stability of chitosan/PLGA nanoparticles on their cytotoxicity profile. *International Journal of Pharmaceutics*, *381*(2), 130–139. doi:10.1016/j.ijpharm.2009.04.049 PMID:19450671

Nagarjuna, A., Raju, K., Kotilingaiah, N., & Praveen, B. (2023). Comparitive study of Binary liquid mixtures containing P-methoxy Benzoate Acid and Amides. *European Chemical Bulletin*, *12*, 3395–3407. doi:10.31838/ecb/2023.12.si6.3022023.06/06/2023

Nagarjun, B., Sarma, A. V., Rao, G. V. R., & Rambabu, C. (2013). Thermodynamic and Acoustic Study on Molecular Interactions in Certain Binary Liquid Systems Involving Ethyl Benzoate. *Journal of Thermodynamics*, *2013*, 1–9. doi:10.1155/2013/285796

Nain, A. K., Pal, R., & Neetu. (2014). Physicochemical study of solute–solute and solute–solvent interactions of l-phenylalanine in (water+ arabinose/glucose/sucrose) solutions at different temperatures. *The Journal of Chemical Thermodynamics*, *68*, 169–182. doi:10.1016/j.jct.2013.09.008

Nair, H. A. S., Periasamy, S., Yang, L., Kjelleberg, S., & Rice, S. A. (2017). Real Time, Spatial, and Temporal Mapping of the Distribution of c-di-GMP during Biofilm Development. *The Journal of Biological Chemistry*, *292*(2), 477–487. doi:10.1074/jbc.M116.746743 PMID:27899451

NajafiKhoshnoo, S., Kim, T., Tavares-Negrete, J. A., Pei, X., Das, P., Lee, S. W., Rajendran, J., & Esfandyarpour, R. (2023). A 3D Nanomaterials-Printed Wearable, Battery-Free, Biocompatible, Flexible, and Wireless pH Sensor System for Real-Time Health Monitoring. *Advanced Materials Technologies*, *8*(8), 2201655. doi:10.1002/admt.202201655

Nakkala, J. R., Mata, R., Raja, K., Khub Chandra, V., & Sadras, S. R. (2018). Green synthesized silver nanoparticles: Catalytic dye degradation, in vitro anticancer activity and in vivo toxicity in rats. *Materials Science and Engineering C*, *91*, 372–381. doi:10.1016/j.msec.2018.05.048 PMID:30033267

Nakkala, J. R., Mata, R., & Sadras, S. R. (2017). Green synthesized nano silver: Synthesis, physicochemical profiling, antibacterial, anticancer activities and biological in vivo toxicity. *Journal of Colloid and Interface Science*, *499*, 33–45. doi:10.1016/j.jcis.2017.03.090 PMID:28363102

Nana, A. B. A., Marimuthu, T., Kondiah, P. P. D., Choonara, Y. E., Du Toit, L. C., & Pillay, V. (2019). Multifunctional Magnetic Nanowires: Design, Fabrication, and Future Prospects as Cancer Therapeutics. *Cancers (Basel)*, *11*(12), 1956. doi:10.3390/cancers11121956 PMID:31817598

Nankar, R., Prabhakar, P. K., & Doble, M. (2017). Hybrid drug combination: Combination of ferulic acid and metformin as anti-diabetic therapy. *Phytomedicine*, *37*, 10–13. doi:10.1016/j.phymed.2017.10.015 PMID:29126698

Narayanaswamy, R., & Torchilin, V. P. (2019). Hydrogels and Their Applications in Targeted Drug Delivery. *Molecules (Basel, Switzerland)*, *24*(3), 603. doi:10.3390/molecules24030603 PMID:30744011

Naresh, V., & Lee, N. (2021a). A Review on Biosensors and Recent Development of Nanostructured Materials-Enabled Biosensors. *Sensors (Basel)*, *21*(4), 1109. doi:10.339021041109 PMID:33562639

Naseem, B., Khan, M., & Jamal, M. A. (2016). Acoustical studies of pharmaceutical excipients in binary solvent mixtures. *Journal of Molecular Liquids*, *220*, 581–591. doi:10.1016/j.molliq.2016.04.091

Naser, R., Abu-Huwaij, R., Al-khateeb, I., Abbas, M. M., & Atoom, A. M. (2021, May). Green synthesis of zinc oxide nanoparticles using the root hair extract of Phoenix dactylifera: Antimicrobial and anticancer activity. *Applied Nanoscience*, *11*(5), 1747–1757. doi:10.100713204-021-01837-0

Nassiri Koopaei, N., & Abdollahi, M. (2016). Opportunities and obstacles to the development of nanopharmaceuticals for human use. *Daru : Journal of Faculty of Pharmacy, Tehran University of Medical Sciences*, *24*, 1–6. 10.1186%2Fs40199-016-0163-8 PMID:27716350

National Research Council. (2003). *Large-scale biomedical science: exploring strategies for future research.* National Academies Press. doi:10.17226/10718

Navabhatra, A., Brantner, A., & Yingngam, B. (2022). Artificial neural network modeling of nanostructured lipid carriers containing 5-*O*-caffeoylquinic acid-rich *Cratoxylum formosum* leaf extract for skin application. *Advanced Pharmaceutical Bulletin*, *12*(4), 801–817. doi:10.34172/apb.2022.082 PMID:36415630

Naveen, E., Ramnath, B. V., Elanchezhian, C., & Nazirudeen, S. S. M. (2017). Influence of organic corrosion inhibitors on pickling corrosion behaviour of sinter-forged C45 steel and 2% Cu alloyed C45 steel. *Journal of Alloys and Compounds*, *695*, 3299–3309. doi:10.1016/j.jallcom.2016.11.133

Nayaka, S., Chakraborty, B., Pallavi, S. S., Bhat, M. P., Shashiraj, K. N., & Ghasti, B. (2020). Synthesis of biogenic silver nanoparticles using Zanthoxylum rhetsa (Roxb.) DC seed coat extract as reducing agent and in-vitro assessment of anticancer effect on A549 lung cancer cell line. *International Journal of Pharmaceutical Research*, *12*(3), 302–314.

Nayak, D., Ashe, S., Rauta, P. R., Kumari, M., & Nayak, B. (2016). Bark extract mediated green synthesis of silver nanoparticles: Evaluation of antimicrobial activity and antiproliferative response against osteosarcoma. *Materials Science and Engineering C*, *58*, 44–52. doi:10.1016/j.msec.2015.08.022 PMID:26478285

Nayak, D., & Tippavajhala, V. K. (2021). A comprehensive review on preparation, evaluation and applications of deformable liposomes. *Iranian Journal of Pharmaceutical Research*, *20*(1), 186–205. doi:10.22037/ijpr.2020.112878.13997 PMID:34400952

Neamatallah, T. (2023). Delayed inflammatory reaction to hyaluronic acid lip filler after the Pfizer-BioNTech COVID-19 vaccine: A case report. *Heliyon*, *9*(7), e18274. doi:10.1016/j.heliyon.2023.e18274 PMID:37539264

Nel, A. E., Madler, L., Velegol, D., Xia, T., Hoek, E. M., Somasundaran, P., Klaessig, F., Castranova, V., & Thompson, M. (2009). Understanding Biophysicochemical Interactions at the Nano-Bio Interface. *Nature Materials*, *8*(7), 543–557. doi:10.1038/nmat2442 PMID:19525947

Nel, A., Xia, T., Mädler, L., & Li, N. (2006). Toxic Potential of Materials at the Nanolevel. *Science*, *311*(5761), 622–627. doi:10.1126cience.1114397 PMID:16456071

Netrusov, A. I., Liyaskina, E. V., Kurgaeva, I. V., Liyaskina, A. U., Yang, G., & Revin, V. V. (2023). Exopolysaccharides Producing Bacteria: A Review. *Microorganisms*, *11*(6), 1541. doi:10.3390/microorganisms11061541 PMID:37375041

Nezhadi, S., Norouzi, P., Rasouli, A., Akbari Javar, H., Ostad, S. N., & Dorkoosh, F. (2023). Co-delivery of paclitaxel and regorafenib by F127/TPGS mixed micelles for triple negative breast cancer treatment. *Journal of Drug Delivery Science and Technology*, *86*, 104673. doi:10.1016/j.jddst.2023.104673

Ng, E. Y., & Etehadtavakol, M. (Eds.). (2017). *Application of infrared to biomedical sciences*. Springer., doi:10.1007/978-981-10-3147-2

Nguyen, C.-H., Banh, K.-S., An, T. N. M., Anh, N. T. H., Dang, C.-H., Doan, V.-D., Chi, T. T. K., Vu-Quang, H., & Nguyen, T.-D. (2023). Cyclodextrin modified with different groups to enhance the drug delivery efficiency of gold nanoparticles to treat cancer. *Arabian Journal of Chemistry*, *16*(9), 105079. doi:10.1016/j.arabjc.2023.105079

Nguyen, P. H. D., Jayasinghe, M. K., Le, A. H., Peng, B., & Le, M. T. (2023). Advances in drug delivery systems based on red blood cells and their membrane-derived nanoparticles. *ACS Nano*, *17*(6), 5187–5210. doi:10.1021/acsnano.2c11965 PMID:36896898

Nguyen, T. T., Chuang, E.-Y., Chen, Y.-P., Tseng, P.-C., Jhan, M.-K., Lai, C.-Y., Wang, Y.-T., Hung, Y.-P., Changou, C. A., Lee, C.-M., Chen, C.-L., & Lin, C.-F. (2023). Anticancer polypyrrole-polyethylenimine drug-free nanozyme for precise B-cell lymphoma therapy. *Biomedicine and Pharmacotherapy*, *160*, 114397. doi:10.1016/j.biopha.2023.114397 PMID:36796279

Nguyen, V. H., Thuy, V. N., Van, T. V., Dao, A. H., & Lee, B.-J. (2022). Nanostructured lipid carriers and their potential applications for versatile drug delivery via oral administration. *OpenNano*, *8*, 100064. doi:10.1016/j.onano.2022.100064

Nicolle, L. E. (2014). Catheter associated urinary tract infections. *Antimicrobial Resistance and Infection Control*, *3*(1), 1–8. doi:10.1186/2047-2994-3-23 PMID:25075308

Nii-Trebi, N. I. (2017). Emerging and Neglected Infectious Diseases: Insights, Advances, and Challenges. *BioMed Research International*, *5245021*, 1–15. doi:10.1155/2017/5245021 PMID:28286767

Ni, K., Lan, G., Song, Y., Hao, Z., & Lin, W. (2020). Biomimetic nanoscale metal-organic framework harnesses hypoxia for effective cancer radiotherapy and immunotherapy. *Chemical Science (Cambridge)*, *11*(29), 7641–7653. doi:10.1039/D0SC01949F

Ni, K., Lan, G., Veroneau, S. S., Duan, X., Song, Y., & Lin, W. (2018). Nanoscale metal-organic frameworks for mitochondria-targeted radiotherapy-radiodynamic therapy. *Nature Communications*, *4321*(9), 4321. doi:10.103841467-018-06655-7

Nilavukkarasi, M., Vijayakumar, S., & Kumar, S. P. (2020). Biological synthesis and characterization of silver nanoparticles with Capparis zeylanica L. leaf extract for potent antimicrobial and anti proliferation efficiency. *Materials Science for Energy Technologies*, *3*, 371–376. doi:10.1016/j.mset.2020.02.008

Niwa, T., Takeuchi, H., Hino, T., Kunou, N., & Kawashima, Y. (1993). Preparations of biodegradable nanospheres of water-soluble and insoluble drugs with D, L-lactide/glycolide copolymer by a novel spontaneous emulsification solvent diffusion method, and the drug release behavior. *Journal of Controlled Release*, *25*(1-2), 89–98. doi:10.1016/0168-3659(93)90097-O

Norizan, M. N., Moklis, M. H., Demon, S. Z. N., Halim, N. A., Samsuri, A., Mohamad, I. S., Knight, V. F., & Abdullah, N. (2020). Carbon nanotubes: Functionalisation and their application in chemical sensors. *RSC Advances*, *10*(71), 43704–43732. doi:10.1039/D0RA09438B PMID:35519676

Nune, S. K., Gunda, P., Thallapally, P. K., Lin, Y. Y., Forrest, M. L., & Berkland, C. J. (2009). Nanoparticles for biomedical imaging. *Expert Opinion on Drug Delivery*, *6*(11), 1175–1194. doi:10.1517/17425240903229031 PMID:19743894

Oerlemans, C., Bult, W., Bos, M., Storm, G., Nijsen, J. F., & Hennink, W. E. (2010). Polymeric micelles in anticancer therapy: Targeting, imaging and triggered release. *Pharmaceutical Research*, *27*(12), 2569–2589. doi:10.100711095-010-0233-4

Oh, J., Feldman, M. D., Kim, J., Condit, C., Emelianov, S., & Milner, T. E. (2006). Detection of magnetic nanoparticles in tissue using magneto-motive ultrasound. *Nanotechnology*, *17*(16), 4183–4190. doi:10.1088/0957-4484/17/16/031 PMID:21727557

Oh, S. Y., Lee, M. J., Heo, N. S., Kim, S., Oh, J. S., Lee, Y., Jeon, E. J., Moon, H., Kim, H. S., Park, T. J., Moon, G., Chun, H. S., & Huh, Y. S. (2019). Cuvette-Type LSPR Sensor for Highly Sensitive Detection of Melamine in Infant Formulas. *Sensors (Basel)*, *19*(18), 3839. doi:10.339019183839 PMID:31491964

Oladipo, A. O., Lebelo, S. L., & Msagati, T. A. M. (2023). Nanocarrier design–function relationship: The prodigious role of properties in regulating biocompatibility for drug delivery applications. *Chemico-Biological Interactions*, *377*, 110466. doi:10.1016/j.cbi.2023.110466 PMID:37004951

Oldfrey, B., Tchorzewska, A., Jackson, R., Croysdale, M., Loureiro, R., Holloway, C., & Miodownik, M. (2021). Additive manufacturing techniques for smart prosthetic liners. *Medical Engineering & Physics*, *87*, 45–55. doi:10.1016/j.medengphy.2020.11.006 PMID:33461673

Oleiwi, J. K., Hamad, Q. A., & Abdulrahman, S. A. (2022). Flexural, impact and max. shear stress properties of fibers composite for prosthetic socket. *Materials Today: Proceedings*, *56*, 3121–3128. doi:10.1016/j.matpr.2021.12.368

Omanović-Mikličanin, E., Badnjević, A., Kazlagić, A., & Hajlovac, M. (2020). Nanocomposites: A brief review. *Health and Technology*, *10*(1), 51–59. doi:10.100712553-019-00380-x

Omrani, M., Naimi-Jamal, M. R., & Far, B. F. (2022). The design of multi-responsive nanohydrogel networks of chitosan for controlled drug delivery. *Carbohydrate Polymers*, *298*, 120143. doi:10.1016/j.carbpol.2022.120143 PMID:36241333

Osial, M., & Pregowska, A. (2022). The Application of Artificial Intelligence in Magnetic Hyperthermia Based Research. *Future Internet*, *356*(14), 356. doi:10.3390/fi14120356

Othman, A. K., El Kurdi, R., Badran, A., Mesmar, J., Baydoun, E., & Patra, D. (2022). Liposome-based nanocapsules for the controlled release of dietary curcumin: PDDA and silica nanoparticle-coated DMPC liposomes enhance the fluorescence efficiency and anticancer activity of curcumin. *RSC Advances*, *12*(18), 11282–11292. doi:10.1039/D2RA00071G PMID:35425076

Othman, N., Masarudin, M. J., Kuen, C. Y., Dasuan, N. A., Abdullah, L. C., & Md. Jamil, S. N. A. (2018). Synthesis and optimization of chitosan nanoparticles loaded with L-ascorbic acid and thymoquinone. *Nanomaterials (Basel, Switzerland)*, *8*(11), 920. doi:10.3390/nano8110920 PMID:30405074

Otsuka, H., Nagasaki, Y., & Kataoka, K. (2003). PEGylated nanoparticles for biological and pharmaceutical applications. *Advanced Drug Delivery Reviews*, *55*(3), 403–419. doi:10.1016/S0169-409X(02)00226-0 PMID:12628324

Ouyang, Z., Gao, Y., Shen, M., & Shi, X. (2021). Dendrimer-based nanohybrids in cancer photomedicine. *Materials Today. Bio*, *10*, 100111. doi:10.1016/j.mtbio.2021.100111 PMID:34027382

Padhi, S., Nayak, A. K., & Behera, A. (2020). Type II diabetes mellitus: A review on recent drug based therapeutics. *Biomedicine and Pharmacotherapy*, *131*, 110708. doi:10.1016/j.biopha.2020.110708 PMID:32927252

Padinjarathil, H., Joseph, M. M., Unnikrishnan, B. S., Preethi, G. U., Shiji, R., Archana, M. G., Maya, S., Syama, H. P., & Sreelekha, T. T. (2018). Galactomannan endowed biogenic silver NPs exposed enhanced cancer cytotoxicity with excellent biocompatibility. *International Journal of Biological Macromolecules*, *118*, 1174–1182. doi:10.1016/j.ijbiomac.2018.06.194 PMID:30001604

Pahle, J., & Walther, W. (2016). Vectors and strategies for nonviral cancer gene therapy. *Expert Opinion on Biological Therapy*, *16*(4), 443–461. doi:10.1517/14712598.2016.1134480 PMID:26761200

Palaiologou, M. M., Arianas, G. K., & Tsierkezos, N. G. (2006). Thermodynamic investigation of dimethyl sulfoxide binary mixtures at 293.15 and 313.15 K. *Journal of Solution Chemistry*, *35*(11), 1551–1565. doi:10.100710953-006-9082-5

Palaniappan, P., Sathishkumar, G., & Sankar, R. (2015). Fabrication of nano-silver particles using Cymodocea serrulata and its cytotoxicity effect against human lung cancer A549 cells line. *Spectrochimica Acta. Part A: Molecular and Biomolecular Spectroscopy*, *138*, 885–890. doi:10.1016/j.saa.2014.10.072 PMID:25467657

Palanikumar, L., Al-Hosani, S., Kalmouni, M., Nguyen, V. P., Ali, L., Pasricha, R., Barrera, F. N., & Magzoub, M. (2020). pH-responsive high stability polymeric nanoparticles for targeted delivery of anticancer therapeutics. *Communications Biology*, *3*(1), 1–17. doi:10.103842003-020-0817-4 PMID:32127636

Palani, R., & Geetha, A. (2009). Acoustical and excess thermodynamic studies of molecular interaction in aqueous mixed solvent systems at 303, 308 and 313 K. *Physics and Chemistry of Liquids*, *47*(5), 542–552. doi:10.1080/00319100802562862

Palit, S., & Hussain, C. M. (2020). Functionalization of nanomaterials for industrial applications: recent and future perspectives. In *Handbook of functionalized nanomaterials for industrial applications* (pp. 3–14). Elsevier. doi:10.1016/B978-0-12-816787-8.00001-6

Pal, J., Singh, K. M., Aditya, S., Ganesh, P., Hwa, C. K., & Sangsul, L. (2020). Bottom-Up and Top-Down Approaches for MgO. In K. Selcan (Ed.), *Sonochemical Reactions*. IntechOpen.

Palmerston Mendes, L., Pan, J., & Torchilin, V. P. (2017). Dendrimers as Nanocarriers for Nucleic Acid and Drug Delivery in Cancer Therapy. *Molecules (Basel, Switzerland)*, *22*(9), 1401. doi:10.3390/molecules22091401 PMID:28832535

Panda, P. K., & Jain, S. K. (2023). Doxorubicin bearing peptide anchored PEGylated PLGA nanoparticles for the effective delivery to prostate cancer cells. *Journal of Drug Delivery Science and Technology*, *86*, 104667. doi:10.1016/j.jddst.2023.104667

Pandey, S., & Bodas, D. (2020). High-quality quantum dots for multiplexed bioimaging: A critical review. *Advances in Colloid and Interface Science*, *278*, 102137. doi:10.1016/j.cis.2020.102137 PMID:32171116

Pan, F., Khan, M., Ragab, A. H., Javed, E., Alsalmah, H. A., Khan, I., Lei, T., Hussain, A., Mohamed, A., Zada, A., & Ansari, M. Z. (2023). Recent advances in the structure and biomedical applications of nanodiamonds and their future perspectives. *Materials & Design*, *233*, 112179. doi:10.1016/j.matdes.2023.112179

Pankhurst, Q. A., Connolly, J., Jones, S. K., & Dobson, J. (2003). Applications of magnetic nanoparticles in biomedicine. *Journal of Physics. D, Applied Physics*, *36*(13), R167–R181. doi:10.1088/0022-3727/36/13/201

Pantidos, N., & Horsfall, L. E. (2014). Biological synthesis of metallic nanoparticles by bacteria, fungi, and plants. *Journal of Nanomedicine & Nanotechnology*, *5*(233). Advance online publication. doi:10.4172/2157-7439.1000233

Pan, X., Wang, Q., He, P., Liu, K., Ni, Y., Chen, L., Ouyang, X., Huang, L., Wang, H., & Xu, S. (2020). A bionic tactile plastic hydrogel-based electronic skin constructed by a nerve-like nanonetwork combining stretchable, compliant, and self-healing properties. *Chemical Engineering Journal*, *379*, 122271. doi:10.1016/j.cej.2019.122271

Pan, Y., Guan, J., Gao, Y., Zhu, Y., Li, H., Guo, H., He, Q., Guan, Z., & Yang, Z. (2023). Modified ASO conjugates encapsulated with cytidinyl/cationic lipids exhibit more potent and longer-lasting anti-HCC effects. *Molecular Therapy. Nucleic Acids*, *32*, 807–821. doi:10.1016/j.omtn.2023.04.028 PMID:37251692

Panyam, J., & Labhasetwar, V. (2003). Biodegradable nanoparticles for drug and gene delivery to cells and tissue. *Advanced Drug Delivery Reviews*, *55*(3), 329–347. doi:10.1016/S0169-409X(02)00228-4 PMID:12628320

Pardridge, W. M. (2023). Brain gene therapy with Trojan horse lipid nanoparticles. *Trends in Molecular Medicine*, *29*(5), 343–353. doi:10.1016/j.molmed.2023.02.004 PMID:36907687

Parenti, C. C., Binelli, A., Caccia, S., Della Torre, C., Magni, S., Pirovano, G., & Casartelli, M. (2020). Ingestion and effects of polystyrene nanoparticles in the silkworm Bombyx mori. *Chemosphere*, *257*, 127203. doi:10.1016/j.chemosphere.2020.127203 PMID:32480083

Park, E. J., Brasuel, M., Behrend, C., Philbert, M. A., & Kopelman, R. (2003). Ratiometric optical PEBBLE nanosensors for real-time magnesium ion concentrations inside viable cells. *Analytical Chemistry*, *75*(15), 3784–3791. doi:10.1021/ac0342323 PMID:14572044

Park, J. H., Gu, L., Von Maltzahn, G., Ruoslahti, E., Bhatia, S. N., & Sailor, M. J. (2009). Biodegradable luminescent porous silicon nanoparticles for in vivo applications. *Nature Materials*, *8*(4), 331–336. doi:10.1038/nmat2398

Park, W., Heo, Y. J., & Han, D. K. (2018). New opportunities for nanoparticles in cancer immunotherapy. *Biomaterials Research*, *22*(1), 1–10. doi:10.118640824-018-0133-y

Park, Y. C., Oh, E. J., Jo, J. H., Jin, Y. S., & Seo, J. H. (2016). Recent advances in biological production of sugar alcohols. *Current Opinion in Biotechnology*, *37*, 105–113. doi:10.1016/j.copbio.2015.11.006 PMID:26723007

Parsamanesh, N., Moossavi, M., Bahrami, A., Butler, A. E., & Sahebkar, A. (2018). Therapeutic potential of curcumin in diabetic complications. *Pharmacological Research*, *136*, 181–193. doi:10.1016/j.phrs.2018.09.012 PMID:30219581

Parthasarathy, L. K., Ratnam, L., Seelan, S., Tobias, C., Casanova, M. F., & Parthasarathy, R. N. (2006). Mammalian inositol 3-phosphate synthase: Its role in the biosynthesis of brain inositol and its clinical use as a psychoactive agent. Biology of Inositols and Phosphoinositides. *Sub-Cellular Biochemistry*, *39*, 293–314. doi:10.1007/0-387-27600-9_12 PMID:17121280

Patel, H. S., Shaikh, S. J., Ray, D., Aswal, V. K., Vaidya, F., Pathak, C., Varade, D., Rahdar, A., & Sharma, R. K. (2022). Structural transitions in mixed Phosphatidylcholine/Pluronic micellar systems and their in vitro therapeutic evaluation for poorly water-soluble drug. *Journal of Molecular Liquids*, *364*, 120003. doi:10.1016/j.molliq.2022.120003

Patel, M. P., Patel, R. R., & Patel, J. K. (2010). Chitosan mediated targeted drug delivery system: A review. *Journal of Pharmacy & Pharmaceutical Sciences*, *13*(4), 536–557. doi:10.18433/J3JC7C PMID:21486530

Patel, P., Hanini, A., Shah, A., Patel, D., Patel, S., Bhatt, P., & Pathak, Y. V. (2019). Surface Modification of Nanoparticles for Targeted Drug Delivery. In *Surface Modification of Nanoparticles for Targeted Drug Delivery* (pp. 19–31). Springer International Publishing. doi:10.1007/978-3-030-06115-9_2

Patel, P., & Shah, J. (2017). Safety and Toxicological Considerations of Nanomedicines: The Future Directions. *Current Clinical Pharmacology*, *12*(2), 73–82. doi:10.2174/1574884712666170509161252 PMID:28486906

Pathomthongtaweechai, N., & Muanprasat, C. (2021). Potential applications of chitosan-based nanomaterials to surpass the gastrointestinal physiological obstacles and enhance the intestinal drug absorption. *Pharmaceutics*, *13*(6), 887. doi:10.3390/pharmaceutics13060887 PMID:34203816

Patil, P. P., Bohara, R. A., Meshram, J. V., Nanaware, S. G., & Pawar, S. H. (2019, February 1). Hybrid chitosan-ZnO nanoparticles coated with a sonochemical technique on silk fibroin-PVA composite film: A synergistic antibacterial activity. *International Journal of Biological Macromolecules*, *122*, 1305–1312. doi:10.1016/j.ijbiomac.2018.09.090 PMID:30227212

Patil, S., Gao, Y. G., Lin, X., Li, Y., Dang, K., Tian, Y., Zhnag, W. J., Jiang, S. F., Qadir, A., & Qian, A. R. (2019). The development of functional non-viral vectors for gene delivery. *International Journal of Molecular Sciences*, *20*(21), 5491. doi:10.3390/ijms20215491 PMID:31690044

Patnaik, P., Chakraborty, N., Kaur, P., Juglan, K. C., & Kumar, H. (2021). Thermodynamic and Acoustic Investigation of D-Panthenol in Homologous Series of Polyethylene Glycol at Different Temperatures. *Advances in fundamental and smart material: Select proceedings of ICFMMP*.

Patra, J. K., Das, G., Fraceto, L. F., Estefania, V. R. C., Maria del Pilar, R.-T., Acosta-Torres, L. S., Diaz-Torres, L. A., Grillo, R., Swamy, M. K., Sharma, S., Habtemariam, S., & Shin, H.-S. (2018). Nano based drug delivery systems: Recent developments and future prospects. *Journal of Nanobiotechnology*, *16*(1), 71. doi:10.118612951-018-0392-8 PMID:30231877

Paunovska, K., Loughrey, D., Sago, C. D., Langer, R., & Dahlman, J. E. (2019). Using large datasets to understand nanotechnology. *Advanced Materials*, *31*(43), 1902798. doi:10.1002/adma.201902798 PMID:31429126

Pautler, M., & Brenner, S. (2022). *Nanomedicine: Promises and challenges for the future of public health*. Dove Press. doi:10.2147/IJN.S13816

Pearce, J. (2011). Mathematical models of laser-induced tissue thermal damage. *International journal of hyperthermia: The official journal of European Society for Hyperthermic Oncology. International Journal of Hyperthermia*, *27*(8), 741–750. doi:10.3109/02656736.2011.580822 PMID:22098359

Pecot, C. V., Calin, G. A., Coleman, R. L., Lopez-Berestein, G., & Sood, A. K. (2011). RNA interference in the clinic: Challenges and future directions. *Nature Reviews. Cancer*, *11*(1), 59–67. doi:10.1038/nrc2966 PMID:21160526

Peer, D., Karp, J. M., Hong, S., Farokhzad, O. C., Margalit, R., & Langer, R. (2007). Nanocarriers as an emerging platform forcancer therapy. *Nature Nanotechnology*, *2*(12), 751–760. doi:10.1038/nnano.2007.387 PMID:18654426

Peer, D., & Lieberman, J. (2011). Special delivery: Targeted therapy with small RNAs. *Gene Therapy*, *18*(12), 1127–1133. doi:10.1038/gt.2011.56 PMID:21490679

Pei, J., Fu, B., Jiang, L., & Sun, T. (2019). Biosynthesis, characterization, and anticancer effect of plant-mediated silver nanoparticles using Coptis chinensis. *International Journal of Nanomedicine*, *14*, 1969–1978. doi:10.2147/IJN.S188235 PMID:30936697

Pei, Z., Lei, H., & Cheng, L. (2023). Bioactive inorganic nanomaterials for cancer theranostics. *Chemical Society Reviews*, *52*(6), 2031–2081. doi:10.1039/D2CS00352J PMID:36633202

Pelaz, B., Alexiou, C., Alvarez-Puebla, R. A., Alves, F., Andrews, A. M., Ashraf, S., Balogh, L. P., Ballerini, L., Bestetti, A., Brendel, C., Bosi, S., Carril, M., Chan, W. C. W., Chen, C., Chen, X., Chen, X., Cheng, Z., Cui, D., Du, J., & Parak, W. J. (2017). Diverse Applications of Nanomedicine. *ACS Nano*, *11*(3), 2313–2381. doi:10.1021/acsnano.6b06040 PMID:28290206

Pelaz, B., Del Pino, P., Maffre, P., Hartmann, R., Gallego, M., Rivera-Fernández, S., De La Fuente, J. M., Nienhaus, G. U., & Parak, W. J. (2015). Surface Functionalization of Nanoparticles with Polyethylene Glycol: Effects on Protein Adsorption and Cellular Uptake. *ACS Nano*, *9*(7), 6996–7008. doi:10.1021/acsnano.5b01326 PMID:26079146

Pellico, J., Gawne, P. J., & de Rosales, R. T. (2021). Radiolabelling of nanomaterials for medical imaging and therapy. *Chemical Society Reviews*, *50*(5), 3355–3423. doi:10.1039/D0CS00384K PMID:33491714

Peng, F., Setyawati, M. I., Tee, J. K., Ding, X., Wang, J., Nga, M. E., Ho, H. K., & Leong, D. T. (2019). Nanoparticles Promote In Vivo Breast Cancer Cell Intravasation and Extravasation by Inducing Endothelial Leakiness. *Nature Nanotechnology*, *14*(3), 279–286. doi:10.103841565-018-0356-z PMID:30692675

Peng, T., Xu, W., Li, Q., Ding, Y., & Huang, Y. (2023). Pharmaceutical liposomal delivery—Specific considerations of innovation and challenges. *Biomaterials Science*, *11*(1), 62–75. doi:10.1039/D2BM01252A PMID:36373563

Peracchia, M. T., Gref, R., Minamitake, Y., Domb, A., Lotan, N., & Langer, R. (1997). PEG-coated nanospheres from amphiphilic diblock and multiblock copolymers: Investigation of their drug encapsulation and release characteristics. *Journal of Controlled Release*, *46*(3), 223–231. doi:10.1016/S0168-3659(96)01597-0

Perevedentseva, E., Lin, Y.-C., & Cheng, C.-L. (2021). A review of recent advances in nanodiamond-mediated drug delivery in cancer. *Expert Opinion on Drug Delivery*, *18*(3), 369–382. doi:10.1080/17425247.2021.1832988 PMID:33047984

Peserico, A., Di Berardino, C., Russo, V., Capacchietti, G., Di Giacinto, O., Canciello, A., Rapini, C. C. S., & Barboni, B. (2022). Nanotechnology-Assisted Cell Tracking. *Nanomaterials (Basel, Switzerland)*, *12*(9), 1414. doi:10.3390/nano12091414 PMID:35564123

Petanovska-Ilievska, B., Velkoska-Markovska, L., & Jankulovska, M. S. (2017). Development of reverse-phase high-performance liquid chromatography method for simultaneous determination of sodium benzoate and potassium sorbate in beverages. *Acta Chromatographica*, *29*(3), 345–358. doi:10.1556/1326.2017.29.3.05

Petersen, L. K., Sackett, C. K., & Narasimhan, B. (2010). High-throughput analysis of protein stability in polyanhydride nanoparticles. *Acta Biomaterialia*, *6*(10), 3873–3881. doi:10.1016/j.actbio.2010.04.004 PMID:20388561

Piccolo, O., Lincoln, J. D., Melong, N., Orr, B. C., Fernandez, N. R., Borsavage, J., Berman, J. N., Robar, J., & Ha, M. N. (2022). Radiation Dose Enhancement Using Gold Nanoparticles with a Diamond Linear Accelerator Target: A Multiple Cell Type Analysis. *Scientific Reports*, *1559*(12), 1559. doi:10.103841598-022-05339-z

Pierobon, M., & Akyildiz, I. F. (2012). Capacity of a diffusion-based molecular communication system with channel memory and molecular noise. *IEEE Transactions on Information Theory*, *59*(2), 942–954. doi:10.1109/TIT.2012.2219496

Pillai, C. K. S., & Sharma, C. P. (2010). Absorbable polymeric surgical sutures: Chemistry, production, properties, biodegradability, and performance. *Journal of Biomaterials Applications*, *25*(4), 291–366. doi:10.1177/0885328210384890 PMID:20971780

Pimentel, R. G. C., Robles Botero, V., Martínez, E. S. M., Gómez García, C., & Hinestroza, J. P. (2016). Soybean agglutinin-conjugated silver nanoparticles nanocarriers in the treatment of breast cancer cells. *Journal of Biomaterials Science. Polymer Edition*, *27*(3), 218–234. doi:10.1080/09205063.2015.1116892 PMID:26540350

Pinheiro, R. G. R., Coutinho, A. J., Pinheiro, M., & Neves, A. R. (2021). Nanoparticles for Targeted Brain Drug Delivery: What Do We Know? *International Journal of Molecular Sciences*, *22*(21), 11654. doi:10.3390/ijms222111654 PMID:34769082

Pino, P., Bosco, F., Mollea, C., & Onida, B. (2023). Antimicrobial Nano-Zinc Oxide Biocomposites for Wound Healing Applications: A Review. *Pharmaceutics*, *15*(3), 970. doi:10.3390/pharmaceutics15030970 PMID:36986831

Pires, D., Mandal, M., Matos, A. I., Peres, C., Catalão, M. J., Azevedo Pereira, J. M., Satchi-Fainaro, R., Florindo, H. F., & Anes, E. (2023). Development of Chitosan Particles Loaded with siRNA for Cystatin C to Control Intracellular Drug-Resistant Mycobacterium tuberculosis. *Antibiotics (Basel, Switzerland)*, *12*(4), 729. doi:10.3390/antibiotics12040729 PMID:37107091

Pishavar, E., Ramezani, M., & Hashemi, M. (2019). Co-delivery of doxorubicin and TRAIL plasmid by modified PAMAM dendrimer in colon cancer cells, in vitro and in vivo evaluation. *Drug Development and Industrial Pharmacy*, *45*(12), 1931–1939. doi:10.1080/03639045.2019.1680995

Pitt, C. G., Gratzl, M. M., Kimmel, G. L., Surles, J., & Schindler, A. (1981). Aliphatic polyesters II. The degradation of poly (DL-lactide), poly (epsilon-caprolactone), and their copolymers in vivo. *Biomaterials*, *2*(4), 215–220. doi:10.1016/0142-9612(81)90060-0 PMID:7326315

Plackal Adimuriyil George, B., Kumar, N., Abrahamse, H., & Ray, S. S. (2018). Apoptotic efficacy of multifaceted biosynthesized silver nanoparticles on human adenocarcinoma cells. *Scientific Reports*, *8*(1), 14368. doi:10.103841598-018-32480-5 PMID:30254325

Pondman, K. M., Bunt, N. D., Maijenburg, A. W., van Wezel, R. J. A., Kishore, U., Abelmann, L., ten Elshof, J. E., & ten Haken, B. (2015). Magnetic drug delivery with FePd nanowires. *Journal of Magnetism and Magnetic Materials*, *380*, 299–306. doi:10.1016/j.jmmm.2014.10.101

Poon, W., Kingston, B. R., Ouyang, B., Ngo, W., & Chan, W. C. W. (2020). A framework for designing delivery systems. *Nature Nanotechnology*, *15*(10), 819–829. doi:10.103841565-020-0759-5

Popova, V., Poletaeva, Y., Chubarov, A., & Dmitrienko, E. (2023). pH-Responsible Doxorubicin-Loaded Fe_3O_4@$CaCO_3$ Nanocomposites for Cancer Treatment. *Pharmaceutics*, *15*(3), 771. doi:10.3390/pharmaceutics15030771 PMID:36986632

Porfiryeva, N. N., Semina, I. I., Salakhov, I. A., Moustafine, R. I., & Khutoryanskiy, V. V. (2021). Mucoadhesive and mucus-penetrating interpolyelectrolyte complexes for nose-to-brain drug delivery. *Nanomedicine (London)*, *37*, 102432. doi:10.1016/j.nano.2021.102432 PMID:34186258

Pourmadadi, M., Ahmadi, M., & Yazdian, F. (2023). Synthesis of a novel pH-responsive Fe3O4/chitosan/agarose double nanoemulsion as a promising Nanocarrier with sustained release of curcumin to treat MCF-7 cell line. *International Journal of Biological Macromolecules*, *235*, 123786. doi:10.1016/j.ijbiomac.2023.123786 PMID:36828092

Pourmadadi, M., Eshaghi, M. M., Ostovar, S., Mohammadi, Z., Sharma, R. K., Paiva-Santos, A. C., Rahmani, E., Rahdar, A., & Pandey, S. (2023). Innovative nanomaterials for cancer diagnosis, imaging, and therapy: Drug deliveryapplications. *Journal of Drug Delivery Science and Technology*, *82*, 104357. doi:10.1016/j.jddst.2023.104357

Pourmadadi, M., Yazdian, F., Koulivand, A., & Rahmani, E. (2023). Green synthesized polyvinylpyrrolidone/titanium dioxide hydrogel nanocomposite modified with agarose macromolecules for sustained and pH-responsive anticancer drug release. *International Journal of Biological Macromolecules*, *240*, 124345. doi:10.1016/j.ijbiomac.2023.124345 PMID:37054860

Prabhakar, P. K. (2016). Pathophysiology of secondary complications of diabetes mellitus. *Pathophysiology*, *9*(1), 32–36.

Prabhakar, P. K., & Sivakumar, P. M. (2019). Protein tyrosine phosphatase 1B inhibitors: A novel therapeutic strategy for the management of type 2 diabetes mellitus. *Current Pharmaceutical Design*, *25*(23), 2526–2539. doi:10.2174/1381612825666190716102901 PMID:31333090

Prabha, S., Durgalakshmi, D., Rajendran, S., & Lichtfouse, E. (2021). Plant-derived silica nanoparticles and composites for biosensors, bioimaging, drug delivery and supercapacitors: A review. *Environmental Chemistry Letters*, *19*(2), 1667–1691. doi:10.100710311-020-01123-5 PMID:33199978

Prabhu, D., Arulvasu, C., Babu, G., Manikandan, R., & Srinivasan, P. (2013). Biologically synthesized green silver nanoparticles from leaf extract of Vitex negundo L. induce growth-inhibitory effect on human colon cancer cell line HCT15. *Process Biochemistry (Barking, London, England)*, *48*(2), 317–324. doi:10.1016/j.procbio.2012.12.013

Prajapati, B. G., Prajapati, B., & Khunt, D. (2023). In-vivo pharmacokinetics study of exemestane hydrochloride self-nanoemulsifying drug delivery systems via oral route. *Letters in Applied NanoBioScience*, *12*(4), 98. doi:10.33263/LIANBS124.098

Praphawatvet, T., Peters, J. I., & Williams, R. O. III. (2020). Inhaled nanoparticles–An updated review. *International Journal of Pharmaceutics*, *587*, 119671. doi:10.1016/j.ijpharm.2020.119671 PMID:32702456

Prasad, D & Harsh Chauhan, (2013, October 25). *Key targeting approaches for Pharmaceutical Drug Delivery*. American Pharmaceutical Review. https://www.americanpharmaceuticalreview.com/Featured-Articles/148744-Key-Targeting-Approaches-for-Pharmaceutical-Drug-Delivery/

Proniewicz, E. (2023). Metallic nanoparticles as effective sensors of bio-molecules. *Spectrochimica Acta. Part A: Molecular and Biomolecular Spectroscopy*, *288*, 122207. doi:10.1016/j.saa.2022.122207 PMID:36502763

Puleo, D. A., & Nanci, A. (1999). Understanding and controlling the bone-implant interface. *Biomaterials*, *20*(23–24), 2311–2321. doi:10.1016/S0142-9612(99)00160-X PMID:10614937

Pursel, S., Horn, M. W., Demirel, M. C., & Lakhtakia, A. (2005). Growth of sculptured polymer submicronwire assemblies by vapor deposition. *Polymer*, *46*(23), 9544–9548. doi:10.1016/j.polymer.2005.07.092

Pushpalatha, R., Selvamuthukumar, S., & Kilimozhi, D. (2017). Nanocarrier mediated combination drug delivery for chemotherapy–A review. *Journal of Drug Delivery Science and Technology*, *39*, 362–371. doi:10.1016/j.jddst.2017.04.019

Qamar, S. A., Asgher, M., Khalid, N., & Sadaf, M. (2019). Nanobiotechnology in health sciences: Current applications and future perspectives. *Biocatalysis and Agricultural Biotechnology*, *22*, 101388. doi:10.1016/j.bcab.2019.101388

Qian, W., Xu, S., Zhang, X., Li, C., Yang, W., Bowen, C. R., & Yang, Y. (2021). Differences and similarities of photocatalysis and electrocatalysis in two-dimensional nanomaterials: Strategies, traps, applications and challenges. *Nano-Micro Letters*, *13*(1), 1–38. doi:10.100740820-021-00681-9 PMID:34264418

Qi, K., Xing, X., Zada, A., Li, M., Wang, Q., Liu, S. Y., Lin, H., & Wang, G. (2020, February 1). Transition metal doped ZnO nanoparticles with enhanced photocatalytic and antibacterial performances: Experimental and DFT studies. *Ceramics International*, *46*(2), 1494–1502. doi:10.1016/j.ceramint.2019.09.116

Qin, L., Cui, Z., Wu, Y., Wang, H., Zhang, X., Guan, J., & Mao, S. (2022). Challenges and strategies to enhance the systemic absorption of inhaled peptides and proteins. *Pharmaceutical Research*, 1–19. doi:10.100711095-022-03435-3 PMID:36385216

Quintana, A., Raczka, E., Piehler, L., Lee, I., Myc, A., Majoros, I., Patri, A. K., Thomas, T., Mulé, J., & Baker, J. R. Jr. (2002). Design and function of a dendrimer-based therapeutic nanodevice targeted to tumor cells through the folate receptor. *Pharmaceutical Research*, *19*(9), 1310–1316. doi:10.1023/A:1020398624602 PMID:12403067

Quintanar-Guerrero, D., Allémann, E., Doelker, E., & Fessi, H. (1997). A mechanistic study of the formation of polymer nanoparticles by the emulsification-diffusion technique. *Colloid & Polymer Science*, *275*(7), 640–647. doi:10.1007003960050130

Rack, H. J., & Qazi, J. I. (2006). Titanium alloys for biomedical applications. *Materials Science and Engineering C*, *26*(8), 1269–1277. doi:10.1016/j.msec.2005.08.032

Radovic-Moreno, A. F., Lu, T. K., Puscasu, V. A., Yoon, C. J., Langer, R., & Farokhzad, O. C. (2012). Surface charge-switching polymeric nanoparticles for bacterial cell wall-targeted delivery of antibiotics. *ACS Nano*, *6*(5), 4279–4287. doi:10.1021/nn3008383 PMID:22471841

Raffi, M., Rumaiz, A. K., Hasan, M. M., & Shah, S. I. (2007). Studies of the growth parameters for silver nanoparticle synthesis by inert gas condensation. *Journal of Materials Research*, *22*(12), 3378–3384. doi:10.1557/JMR.2007.0420

Rahdar Abbas, K. S. A. F. (2018). Pluronic as nano-carrier platform for drug delivery systems. *Nanomed Res J*, *3*(4), 174–179.

Rahmani, D., Torbat, N. A., & Boddohi, S. (2023). Synthesis and characterization of pH-responsive PCL-PVA polymersome for dual delivery to breast cancer cells. *European Polymer Journal*, *191*, 112032. doi:10.1016/j.eurpolymj.2023.112032

Rahmani, P., & Shojaei, A. (2021). A review on the features, performance and potential applications of hydrogel-based wearable strain/pressure sensors. *Advances in Colloid and Interface Science*, *298*, 102553. doi:10.1016/j.cis.2021.102553 PMID:34768136

Rahman, M. M., Islam, M. R., Islam, M. T., Harun-Or-Rashid, M., Islam, M., Abdullah, S., Uddin, M. B., Das, S., Rahaman, M. S., Ahmed, M., Alhumaydhi, F. A., Emran, T. B., Mohamed, A. A. R., Faruque, M. R. I., Khandaker, M. U., & Mostafa-Hedeab, G. (2022). Stem cell transplantation therapy and neurological disorders: Current status and future perspectives. *Biology (Basel)*, *11*(1), 147. doi:10.3390/biology11010147 PMID:35053145

Rahman, M. S., Hossain, K. S., Das, S., Kundu, S., Adegoke, E. O., Rahman, M. A., Hannan, M. A., Uddin, M. J., & Pang, M. G. (2021). Role of insulin in health and disease: An update. *International Journal of Molecular Sciences*, *22*(12), 6403. doi:10.3390/ijms22126403 PMID:34203830

Rai, M., Yadav, A., & Gade, A. (2009). Silver nanoparticles as a new generation of antimicrobials. *Biotechnology Advances*, *27*(1), 76–83. doi:10.1016/j.biotechadv.2008.09.002 PMID:18854209

Rai, R., Alwani, S., & Badea, I. (2019). Polymeric nanoparticles in gene therapy: New avenues of design and optimization for delivery applications. *Polymers*, *11*(4), 745. doi:10.3390/polym11040745 PMID:31027272

Raja, G., Jang, Y. K., Suh, J. S., Kim, H. S., Ahn, S. H., & Kim, T. J. (2020). Microcellular environmental regulation of silver nanoparticles in cancer therapy: *A critical review, cancers (Basel)*. . doi:10.3390/cancers12030664

Rajaei, M., Rashedi, H., Yazdian, F., Navaei-Nigjeh, M., Rahdar, A., & Díez-Pascual, A. M. (2023). Chitosan/agarose/graphene oxide nanohydrogel as drug delivery system of 5-fluorouracil in breast cancer therapy. *Journal of Drug Delivery Science and Technology*, *82*, 104307. doi:10.1016/j.jddst.2023.104307

Rajendran, A. K., Kim, H. D., Kim, J. W., Bae, J. W., & Hwang, N. S. (2023). Nanotechnology in tissue engineering and regenerative medicine. *Korean Journal of Chemical Engineering*, *40*(2), 286–301. doi:10.100711814-022-1363-1

Ramezani Farani, M., Azarian, M., Heydari Sheikh Hossein, H., Abdolvahabi, Z., Mohammadi Abgarmi, Z., Moradi, A., Mousavi, S. M., Ashrafizadeh, M., Makvandi, P., Saeb, M. R., & Rabiee, N. (2022). Folic acid-adorned curcumin-loaded iron oxide nanoparticles for cervical cancer. *ACS Applied Bio Materials*, *5*(5), 1305–1318. doi:10.1021/acsabm.1c01311

Ramos, A. P., Cruz, M. A. E., Tovani, C. B., & Ciancaglini, P. (2017). Biomedical applications of nanotechnology. *Biophysical Reviews*, *9*(2), 79–89. doi:10.100712551-016-0246-2 PMID:28510082

Rane, A. V., Kanny, K., Abitha, V. K., & Thomas, S. (2018). Methods for synthesis of nanoparticles and fabrication of nanocomposites. In *Synthesis of inorganic nanomaterials* (pp. 121–139). Woodhead Publishing. doi:10.1016/B978-0-08-101975-7.00005-1

Rani, R., Sethi, K., & Singh, G. (2019). Nanomaterials and Their Applications in Bioimaging. *Nanotechnology in the Life Sciences*, (October), 429–450. doi:10.1007/978-3-030-16379-2_15

Ranjan, S., Dasgupta, N., Singh, S., & Gandhi, M. (2019). Toxicity and regulations of food nanomaterials. *Environmental Chemistry Letters*, *17*(2), 929–944. doi:10.100710311-018-00851-z

Rank Miranda, R., Pereira da Fonseca, M., Korzeniowska, B., Skytte, L., Lund Rasmussen, K., & Kjeldsen, F. (2020). Elucidating the cellular response of silver nanoparticles as a potential combinatorial agent for cisplatin chemotherapy. *Journal of Nanobiotechnology*, *18*(1), 164. doi:10.118612951-020-00719-x PMID:33168016

Ranson, M. R., Cheeseman, S., White, S., & Margison, J. (2001). Caelyx (stealth liposomal doxorubicin) in the treatment of advanced breast cancer. *Critical Reviews in Oncology/Hematology*, *37*(2), 115–120. doi:10.1016/S1040-8428(00)00107-4

Rao,, B.P. (2013). Characterization of Exopolysaccharide from Bacillus amyloliquefaciens BPRGS for its Bioflocculant Activity. *International Journal of Scientific and Engineering Research*, *4*, 1696–1704.

Rao, J. P., & Geckeler, K. E. (2011). Polymer nanoparticles: Preparation techniques and size-control parameters. *Progress in Polymer Science*, *36*(7), 887–913. doi:10.1016/j.progpolymsci.2011.01.001

Rarokar, N., Agrawal, R., Yadav, S., Khedekar, P., Ravikumar, C., Telange, D., & Gurav, S. (2023). Pteroyl-γ-l-glutamate/ Pluronic® F68 modified polymeric micelles loaded with docetaxel for targeted delivery and reduced toxicity. *Journal of Molecular Liquids*, *369*, 120842. doi:10.1016/j.molliq.2022.120842

Rasheed, M., Ali, A., Kanwal, S., Ismail, M., Sabir, N., & Amin, F. (2019). Synergy of green tea reduced tamoxifen-loaded silver nanoparticles exhibit OGT downregulation in breast cancer cell line. *Digest Journal of Nanomaterials and Biostructures*, *14*(3), 695–704.

Rashid, R., Naqash, A., Bader, G. N., & Sheikh, F. A. (2020). Nanotechnology and diabetes management: Recent advances and future perspectives. *Application of Nanotechnology in Biomedical Sciences*, 99-117. doi:10.1007/978-981-15-5622-7_6

Rauf, A., Abu-Izneid, T., Khalil, A. A., Hafeez, N., Olatunde, A., Rahman, M., Semwal, P., Al-Awthan, Y. S., Bahattab, O. S., Khan, I. N., Khan, M. A., & Sharma, R. (2022). Nanoparticles in clinical trials of COVID-19: An update. *International Journal of Surgery*, *104*, 106818. doi:10.1016/j.ijsu.2022.106818 PMID:35953020

Raula, J., Eerikäinen, H., Lähde, A., & Kauppinen, E. I. (2007). Aerosol flow reactor method for the synthesis of multicomponent drug nano-and microparticles. In *Nanoparticulate Drug Delivery Systems* (pp. 111–128). CRC Press.

Rawat, P., & Gupta, S. (2021). Dual engineered gold nanoparticle based synergistic prophylaxis delivery system for HIV/ AIDS. *Medical Hypotheses*, *150*, 110576. doi:10.1016/j.mehy.2021.110576 PMID:33799160

Ray, S. S., & Bandyopadhyay, J. (2021). Nanotechnology-enabled biomedical engineering: Current trends, future scopes, and perspectives. *Nanotechnology Reviews*, *10*(1), 728–743. doi:10.1515/ntrev-2021-0052

Razavi, M. S., Abdollahi, A., Malek-Khatabi, A., Ejarestaghi, N. M., Atashi, A., Yousefi, N., Ebrahimnejad, P., Elsawy, M. A., & Dinarvand, R. (2023). Recent advances in PLGA-based nanofibers as anticancer drug delivery systems. *Journal of Drug Delivery Science and Technology*, *85*, 104587. doi:10.1016/j.jddst.2023.104587

Redhead, H. M., Davis, S. S., & Illum, L. (2001). Drug delivery in poly (lactide-co-glycolide) nanoparticles surface modified with poloxamer 407 and poloxamine 908: In vitro characterisation and in vivo evaluation. *Journal of Controlled Release*, *70*(3), 353–363. doi:10.1016/S0168-3659(00)00367-9 PMID:11182205

Reed, S. M., Clegg, R. S., & Hutchison, J. E. (2003). *Tuning the electrical properties of monolayers by using internal peptide bonds.*

Reis, C. P., Neufeld, R. J., Ribeiro, A. J., & Veiga, F. (2006). Nanoencapsulation II. Biomedical applications and current status of peptide and protein nanoparticulate delivery systems. *Nanomedicine; Nanotechnology, Biology, and Medicine, 2*(2), 53–65. doi:10.1016/j.nano.2006.04.009 PMID:17292116

Ren, Q., Liang, Z., Jiang, X., Gong, P., Zhou, L., Sun, Z., Xiang, J., Xu, Z., Peng, X., Li, S., Li, W., Cai, L., & Tang, J. (2019). Enzyme and pH dual-responsive hyaluronic acid nanoparticles mediated combination of photodynamic therapy and chemotherapy. *International Journal of Biological Macromolecules, 130*, 845–852. doi:10.1016/j.ijbiomac.2019.03.030 PMID:30844454

Ren, R., Lim, C., Li, S., Wang, Y., Song, J., Lin, T. W., Muir, B. W., Hsu, H. Y., & Shen, H. H. (2022). Recent advances in the development of lipid-, metal-, carbon-, and polymer-based nanomaterials for antibacterial applications. *Nanomaterials (Basel, Switzerland), 12*(21), 3855. doi:10.3390/nano12213855 PMID:36364631

Revia, R. A., & Zhang, M. (2016). Magnetite nanoparticles for cancer diagnosis, treatment, and treatment monitoring: Recent advances. *Materials Today, 19*(3), 157–168. doi:10.1016/j.mattod.2015.08.022

Rezaei, N., Kazem Arki, M., Miri-Lavasani, Z., Solhi, R., Khoramipour, M., Rashedi, H., Aghdaei, H. A., Hossein-Khannazer, N., Mostafavi, E., & Vosough, M. (2023). Co-delivery of doxorubicin and paclitaxel via niosome nanocarriers attenuates cancerous phenotypes in gastric cancer cells. *European Journal of Pharmaceutics and Biopharmaceutics, 188*, 33–47. doi:10.1016/j.ejpb.2023.04.016 PMID:37105361

Rhodes, C. J. (2011). Electron Spin Resonance.: Part One: A Diagnostic Method in the Biomedical Sciences. *Science Progress, 94*(1), 16–96. doi:10.3184/003685011X12982218769939 PMID:21548528

Ribeiro, E. B., de Marchi, P. G., Honorio-França, A. C., França, E. L., & Soler, M. A. (2020). Interferon-gamma carrying nanoemulsion with immunomodulatory and anti-tumor activities. *Journal of Biomedical Materials Research. Part A, 108*(2), 234–245. doi:10.1002/jbm.a.36808

Rice, M. K., & Ruder, W. C. (2013). Creating biological nanomaterials using synthetic biology. *Science and Technology of Advanced Materials*. PMID:27877637

Rideau, E., Dimova, R., Schwille, P., Wurm, F. R., & Landfester, K. (2018). Liposomes and polymersomes: A comparative review towards cell mimicking. *Chemical Society Reviews, 47*(23), 8572–8610. doi:10.1039/C8CS00162F

Riley, M. K. II, & Vermerris, W. (2017). Recent advances in nanomaterials for gene delivery—A review. *Nanomaterials (Basel, Switzerland), 7*(5), 94. doi:10.3390/nano7050094 PMID:28452950

Ritz, S., Schöttler, S., Kotman, N., Baier, G., Musyanovych, A., Kuharev, J., Landfester, K., Schild, H., Jahn, O., Tenzer, S., & Mailänder, V. (2015). Protein Corona of Nanoparticles: Distinct Proteins Regulate the Cellular Uptake. *Biomacromolecules, 16*(4), 1311–1321. doi:10.1021/acs.biomac.5b00108 PMID:25794196

Rizvi, S. B., Ghaderi, S., Keshtgar, M., & Seifalian, A. M. (2010). Semiconductor quantum dots as fluorescent probes for in vitro and in vivo bio-molecular and cellular imaging. *Nano Reviews, 1*(1), 5161. doi:10.3402/nano.v1i0.5161 PMID:22110865

Robert, H., & Pierce, X. G. (2019). Applications of Quantum Dots in Bioimaging and Bioassays. *Material Matters : Chemistry Driving Performance*.

Roco, M. C. (2011). The long view of nanotechnology development: The National Nanotechnology Initiative at 10 years. *Journal of Nanoparticle Research, 13*(2), 427–445. doi:10.100711051-010-0192-z

Rojo, M. C., Arroyo López, F. N., Lerena, M. C., Mercado, L., Torres, A., & Combina, M. (2015). Evaluation of different chemical preservatives to control Zygosaccharomyces rouxii growth in high sugar culture media. *Food Control, 50*, 349–355. doi:10.1016/j.foodcont.2014.09.014

Roma-Rodrigues, C., Rivas-García, L., Baptista, P. V., & Fernandes, A. R. (2020). Gene therapy in cancer treatment: Why go nano? *Pharmaceutics*, *12*(3), 233. doi:10.3390/pharmaceutics12030233 PMID:32151052

Romero, C. M., & Negrete, F. (2004). Effect of temperature on partial molar volumes and viscosities of aqueous solutions of α-dl-Amino butyric acid, dl-Norvaline and dl-Norleucine. *Physics and Chemistry of Liquids*, *42*(3), 261–267. doi:10.1080/00319100410001659596

Rosenblum, D., Joshi, N., Tao, W., Karp, J. M., & Peer, D. (2018). Progress and challenges towards targeted delivery of cancer therapeutics. *Nature Communications*, *9*(1), 1410. doi:10.103841467-018-03705-y PMID:29650952

Rosen, J. E., Yoffe, S., Meerasa, A., Verma, M., & Gu, F. X. (2011). Nanotechnology and Diagnostic Imaging: New Advances in Contrast Agent Technology. *Journal of Nanomedicine & Nanotechnology*, *2*(5). doi:10.4172/2157-7439.1000115

Rouge, J. (2023). RNA and nanocarriers: Next generation drug and delivery platform take center stage. *Trends in Biotechnology*, *41*(3), 281–282. doi:10.1016/j.tibtech.2022.12.019 PMID:36609034

Roy, H., Panda, S. P., Panda, S. K., Tripathi, A. K., Srivastava, S. K., Nayak, B. S., Singh, P. K., & Singh, G. D. (2023). N-trimethyl chitosan and tripalmitin loaded solid lipid nanoparticles of tofacitinib citrate: Characterization and in-vivo anti-inflammatory assessment. *Journal of Drug Delivery Science and Technology*, *87*, 104789. doi:10.1016/j.jddst.2023.104789

Roy, I., Ohulchanskyy, T. Y., Pudavar, H. E., Bergey, E. J., Oseroff, A. R., Morgan, J., Dougherty, T. J., & Prasad, P. N. (2003). Ceramic-based nanoparticles entrapping water-insoluble photosensitizing anticancer drugs: A novel drug-carrier system for photodynamic therapy. *Journal of the American Chemical Society*, *125*(26), 7860–7865. doi:10.1021/ja0343095 PMID:12823004

Rudramurthy, G. R., Swamy, M. K., Sinniah, U. R., & Ghasemzadeh, A. (2016). Nanoparticles: Alternatives against drug-resistant pathogenic microbes. *Molecules (Basel, Switzerland)*, *21*(7), 836. doi:10.3390/molecules21070836 PMID:27355939

Rümenapp, C., Gleich, B., & Haase, A. (2012). Magnetic nanoparticles in magnetic resonance imaging and diagnostics. *Pharmaceutical Research*, *29*(5), 1165–1179. doi:10.100711095-012-0711-y PMID:22392330

Sá, A. G. A., de Meneses, A. C., de Araújo, P. H. H., & de Oliveira, D. (2017). A review on enzymatic synthesis of aromatic esters used as flavor ingredients for food, cosmetics and pharmaceuticals industries. *Trends in Food Science & Technology*, *69*, 95–105. doi:10.1016/j.tifs.2017.09.004

Sadeghi, R., Hosseini, R., & Jamehbozorg, B. (2008). Effect of sodium phosphate salts on the thermodynamic properties of aqueous solutions of poly (ethylene oxide) 6000 at different temperatures. *The Journal of Chemical Thermodynamics*, *40*(9), 1364–1377. doi:10.1016/j.jct.2008.05.007

Safi, I. (2000). Recent aspects concerning DC reactive magnetron sputtering of thin films: A review. *Surface and Coatings Technology*, *127*(2-3), 203–218. doi:10.1016/S0257-8972(00)00566-1

Sahoo, S. K., Parveen, S., & Panda, J. J. (2007). The present and future of nanotechnology in human health care. *Nanomedicine, 3*, 20–31. doi:10.1016/j.nano.2006.11.008

Sahoo, S. K., & Labhasetwar, V. (2003). Nanotech approaches to drug delivery and imaging. *Drug Discovery Today*, *8*(24), 1112–1120. doi:10.1016/S1359-6446(03)02903-9 PMID:14678737

Sahu, T., Ratre, Y. K., Chauhan, S., Bhaskar, L. V. K. S., Nair, M. P., & Verma, H. K. (2021). Nanotechnology based drug delivery system: Current strategies and emerging therapeutic potential for medical science. *Journal of Drug Delivery Science and Technology*, *63*, 102487. doi:10.1016/j.jddst.2021.102487

Saini, R. K., Bagri, L. P., Bajpai, A. K., & Mishra, A. (2018). Responsive polymer nanoparticles for drug delivery applications. In *Stimuli Responsive Polymeric Nanocarriers for Drug Delivery Applications* (Vol. 1, pp. 289–320). Woodhead Publishing. doi:10.1016/B978-0-08-101997-9.00015-1

Sakthi Devi, R., Girigoswami, A., Siddharth, M., & Girigoswami, K. (2022). Applications of gold and silver nanoparticles in theranostics. *Applied Biochemistry and Biotechnology*, *194*(9), 4187–4219. doi:10.100712010-022-03963-z PMID:35551613

Sakuri, S., Surojo, E., Ariawan, D., & Prabowo, A. R. (2020). Investigation of Agave cantala-based composite fibers as prosthetic socket materials accounting for a variety of alkali and microcrystalline cellulose treatments. *Theoretical & Applied Mechanics Letters*, *10*(6), 405–411. doi:10.1016/j.taml.2020.01.052

Saleh, T. A. (2020a). Nanomaterials: Classification, properties, and environmental toxicities. *Environmental Technology & Innovation*, *20*, 101067. doi:10.1016/j.eti.2020.101067

Saleh, T. A. (2020b). Trends in the sample preparation and analysis of nanomaterials as environmental contaminants. *Trends in Environmental Analytical Chemistry*, *28*, e00101. doi:10.1016/j.teac.2020.e00101

Salesa, B., Ferrús-Manzano, P., Tuñón-Molina, A., Cano-Vicent, A., Assis, M., Andrés, J., & Serrano-Aroca, Á. (2023). Study of biological properties of gold nanoparticles: Low toxicity, no proliferative activity, no ability to induce cell gene expression and no antiviral activity. *Chemico-Biological Interactions*, *382*, 110646. doi:10.1016/j.cbi.2023.110646 PMID:37506996

Salhi, B., Hossain, M. K., Mukhaimer, A. W., & Al-Sulaiman, F. A. (2016). Nanowires: A new pathway to nanotechnology-based applications. *Journal of Electroceramics*, *37*(1), 34–49. doi:10.100710832-016-0037-y PMID:32214875

Saltzman, M. W., & Torchilin, V. P. (2021, April). *Drug delivery system*. AccessScience. . https://www.accessscience.com/content/article/a757275 doi:10.1036/1097-8542.757275

Salvetti, A., Gambino, G., Rossi, L., De Pasquale, D., Pucci, C., Linsalata, S., Innocenti, A. D., Nitti, S., Prato, M., Ippolito, C., & Ciofani, G. (2020). Stem cell and tissue regeneration analysis in low-dose irradiated planarians treated with cerium oxide nanoparticles. *Materials Science and Engineering C*, *115*, 111113. doi:10.1016/j.msec.2020.111113 PMID:32600713

Samad, A., Sultana, Y., & Aqil, M. (2007). Liposomal drug delivery systems: An update review. *Current Drug Delivery*, *4*(4), 297–305. doi:10.2174/156720107782151269

Samanta, B., Yan, H., Fischer, N. O., Shi, J., Jerry, D. J., & Rotello, V. M. (2008). Protein-passivated Fe(3)O(4) nanoparticles: Low toxicity and rapid heating for thermal therapy. *Journal of Materials Chemistry*, *18*(11), 1204–1208. doi:10.1039/b718745a PMID:19122852

Samavati, S. S., Kashanian, S., Derakhshankhah, H., & Rabiei, M. (2022). Nanoparticle application in diabetes drug delivery. *Journal of Nanoparticle Research*, *24*(9), 178. doi:10.100711051-022-05547-8

Samiei, M., Farjami, A., Dizaj, S. M., & Lotfipour, F. (2016). Nanoparticles for antimicrobial purposes in Endodontics: A systematic review of in vitro studies. *Materials Science and Engineering C*, *58*, 1269–1278. doi:10.1016/j.msec.2015.08.070 PMID:26478430

Samuel, P., Sundarraj, S., & Sudarmani, D. N. P. (2023). *Nanotechnology-Based Stem Cell Therapy: Current Status and Perspectives*. IntechOpen. doi:10.5772/intechopen.109275

Sanchez-Gaytan, B. L., Fay, F., Lobatto, M. E., Tang, J., Ouimet, M., Kim, Y., van der Staay, S. E. M., van Rijs, S. M., Priem, B., Zhang, L., Fisher, E. A., Moore, K. J., Langer, R., Fayad, Z. A., & Mulder, W. J. (2015). HDL-mimetic PLGA nanoparticle to target atherosclerosis plaque macrophages. *Bioconjugate Chemistry*, *26*(3), 443–451. doi:10.1021/bc500517k PMID:25650634

Sánchez-López, E., Guerra, M., Dias-Ferreira, J., Lopez-Machado, A., Ettcheto, M., Cano, A., Espina, M., Camins, A., Garcia, M. L., & Souto, E. B. (2019). Current applications of nanoemulsions in cancer therapeutics. *Nanomaterials (Basel, Switzerland)*, *9*(6), 821. doi:10.3390/nano9060821

Sands, I., Lee, J., & Chen, Y. (2023). Nanotechnology for DNA and RNA delivery. In T. J. Webster (Ed.), *Nanomedicine* (2nd ed., pp. 81–111). Woodhead Publishing. doi:10.1016/B978-0-12-818627-5.00008-7

Saneja, A., Kumar, R., Mintoo, M. J., Dubey, R. D., Sangwan, P. L., Mondhe, D. M., Panda, A. K., & Gupta, P. N. (2019). Gemcitabine and betulinic acid co-encapsulated PLGA-PEG polymer nanoparticles for improved efficacy of cancer chemotherapy. *Materials Science and Engineering C*, *98*, 764–771. doi:10.1016/j.msec.2019.01.026

Sani, A., Cao, C., & Cui, D. (2021). Toxicity of gold nanoparticles (AuNPs): A review. *Biochemistry and Biophysics Reports*, *26*, 100991. doi:10.1016/j.bbrep.2021.100991 PMID:33912692

Sanles-Sobrido, M., Rodríguez-Lorenzo, L., Lorenzo-Abalde, S., González-Fernández, Á., Correa-Duarte, M. A., Alvarez-Puebla, R. A., & Liz-Marzán, L. M. (2009). Label-free SERS detection of relevant bioanalytes on silver-coated carbon nanotubes: The case of cocaine. *Nanoscale*, *1*(1), 153–158. doi:10.1039/b9nr00059c PMID:20644874

San-Martin, C. R., Zhang, Y., Hamoh, T., Berendse, L., Klijn, C., Li, R., Sigaeva, A., Kawałko, J., Li, H. T., Tehrani, J., Mzyk, A., & Schirhagl, R. (2023). Fluorescent nanodiamond labels: Size and concentration matters for sperm cell viability. *Materials Today. Bio*, *20*, 100629. doi:10.1016/j.mtbio.2023.100629 PMID:37441134

Santagneli, S. H., de Araujo, C. C., Strojek, W., Eckert, H., Poirier, G., Ribeiro, S. J. L., & Messaddeq, Y. (2007). Structural studies of NaPO3– MoO3 glasses by solid-state nuclear magnetic resonance and Raman spectroscopy. *The Journal of Physical Chemistry B*, *111*(34), 10109–10117. doi:10.1021/jp072883n PMID:17683136

Santo, D., Mendonça, P. V., Lima, M. S., Cordeiro, R. A., Cabanas, L., Serra, A., Coelho, J. F. J., & Faneca, H. (2019). Poly (ethylene glycol)-block-poly (2-aminoethyl methacrylate hydrochloride)-Based Polyplexes as Serum-Tolerant Nanosystems for Enhanced Gene Delivery. *Molecular Pharmaceutics*, *16*(5), 2129–2141. doi:10.1021/acs.molpharmaceut.9b00101

Sapsford, K. E., Pons, T., Medintz, I. L., & Mattoussi, H. (2006). Biosensing with Luminescent Semiconductor Quantum Dots. *Sensors (Basel)*, *6*(8), 925–953. doi:10.33906080925

Saramago, S., Magalhães, J., & Pinheiro, M. (2021). Tuberculosis vaccines: An update of recent and ongoing clinical trials. *Applied Sciences (Basel, Switzerland)*, *11*(19), 9250. doi:10.3390/app11199250

Sarkar, S., & Kotteeswaran, V. (2018). Green synthesis of silver nanoparticles from aqueous leaf extract of Pomegranate (Punica granatum) and their anticancer activity on human cervical cancer cells. *Advances in Natural Sciences: Nanoscience and Nanotechnology*, *9*(2), 025014. doi:10.1088/2043-6254/aac590

Satsangi, N. (2020). Synthesis and characterization of biocompatible silver nanoparticles for anticancer application. *Journal of Inorganic and Organometallic Polymers and Materials*, *30*(6), 1907–1914. doi:10.100710904-019-01372-0

Sau, S., Alsaab, H. O., Bhise, K., Alzhrani, R., Nabil, G., & Iyer, A. K. (2018). Multifunctional nanoparticles for cancer immunotherapy: A groundbreaking approach for reprogramming malfunctioned tumor environment. *Journal of Controlled Release, 274*, 24–34. doi:10.1016/j.jconrel.2018.01.028 PMID:29391232

Sawai, J,, Yamamoto, O., Hotta, M., Kojima, H., & Sasamoto, T. (1998). Antibacterial characteristics of heated zinc oxide powders on Escherichia coli and Staphylococcus aureus; Kanetsu shori sareta sanka aen funmatsu no daichokin oyobi oshoku budoukyukin ni taisuru kokin tokusei. *Nippon Kagaku Kaishi (Journal of the Chemical Society of Japan, Chemistry and Industrial Chemistry).*

Saxena, R., Sharma, P., Kumar, S., Agrawal, N., Sharma, S. K., & Awasthi, A. (2023). Modulation of mitochondria by viral proteins. *Life Sciences, 313*, 121271. doi:10.1016/j.lfs.2022.121271 PMID:36526048

Scaffaro, R., Maio, A., & Citarrella, M. C. (2021). Ionic tactile sensors as promising biomaterials for artificial skin: Review of latest advances and future perspectives. *European Polymer Journal, 151*, 110421. doi:10.1016/j.eurpolymj.2021.110421

Scatena, R. (2012). Mitochondria and cancer: A growing role in apoptosis, Cancer cell metabolism and dedifferentiation. *Advances in Experimental Medicine and Biology, 942*, 287–308. doi:10.1007/978-94-007-2869-1_13 PMID:22399428

Schmidt, H. H., Wixner, J., Planté-Bordeneuve, V., Muñoz-Beamud, F., Lladó, L., Gillmore, J. D., Mazzeo, A., Li, X., Arum, S., Jay, P. Y., & Adams, D. (2022). Patisiran treatment in patients with hereditary transthyretin-mediated amyloidosis with polyneuropathy after liver transplantation. *American Journal of Transplantation, 22*(6), 1646–1657. doi:10.1111/ajt.17009 PMID:35213769

Schuemann, J., Bagley, A. F., Berbeco, R., Bromma, K., Butterworth, K. T., Byrne, H. L., Chithrani, B. D., Cho, S. H., Cook, J. R., Favaudon, V., Gholami, Y. H., Gargioni, E., Hainfeld, J. F., Hespeels, F., Heuskin, A.-C., Ibeh, U. M., Kuncic, Z., Kunjachan, S., Lacombe, S., & Krishnan, S. (2020). Roadmap for metal nanoparticles in radiation therapy: Current status, translational challenges, and future directions. *Physics in Medicine and Biology, 65*(21), 21RM02. doi:10.1088/1361-6560/ab9159 PMID:32380492

Schulte, P. A., & Salamanca-Buentello, F. (2007). Ethical and scientific issues of nanotechnology in the workplace. *Environmental Health Perspectives, 115*(1), 5–12. doi:10.1289/ehp.9456 PMID:17366812

Scott, R. P., & Quaggin, S. E. (2015). The cell biology of renal filtration. *The Journal of Cell Biology, 209*(2), 199–210. doi:10.1083/jcb.201410017 PMID:25918223

Sebestyen, Z., Prinz, I., Déchanet-Merville, J., Silva-Santos, B., & Kuball, J. (2020). Translating gammadelta (γδ) T cells and their receptors into cancer cell therapies. *Nature Reviews. Drug Discovery, 19*(3), 169–184. doi:10.103841573-019-0038-z

Seib, F. P., Jones, G. T., Rnjak-Kovacina, J., Lin, Y., & Kaplan, D. L. (2013). pH-dependent anticancer drug release from silk nanoparticles. *Advanced Healthcare Materials, 2*(12), 1606–1611. doi:10.1002/adhm.201300034 PMID:23625825

Sekar, R., Basavegowda, N., Thathapudi, J. J., Sekhar, M. R., Joshi, P., Somu, P., & Baek, K.-H. (2023). Recent Progress of Gold-Based Nanostructures towards Future Emblem of Photo-Triggered Cancer Theranostics: A Special Focus on Combinatorial Phototherapies. *Pharmaceutics, 433*(15), 433. doi:10.3390/pharmaceutics15020433

Selvamuthukumar, S., & Velmurugan, R. (2012). Nanostructured lipid carriers: A potential drug carrier for cancer chemotherapy. *Lipids in Health and Disease, 11*(1), 1–8. doi:10.1186/1476-511X-11-159

Semaltianos, N. G. (2010). Nanoparticles by laser ablation. *Critical Reviews in Solid State and Material Sciences, 35*(2), 105–124. doi:10.1080/10408431003788233

Sengupta, S., Pal, S., Pal, A., Maity, S., Sarkar, K., & Das, M. (2023). A review on synthesis, toxicity profile and biomedical applications of graphene quantum dots (GQDs). *Inorganica Chimica Acta*, *557*, 121677. doi:10.1016/j.ica.2023.121677

Şen, Ö., Emanet, M., Marino, A., Belenli Gümüş, M., Bartolucci, M., Doccini, S., Catalano, F., Genchi, G. G., Santorelli, F. M., Petretto, A., & Ciofani, G. (2021). Evaluation of the therapeutic potential of resveratrol-loaded nanostructured lipid carriers on autosomal recessive spastic ataxia of Charlevoix-Saguenay patient-derived fibroblasts. *Materials & Design*, *209*, 110012. doi:10.1016/j.matdes.2021.110012

Seo, B., Lim, K., Kim, S. S., Oh, K. T., Lee, E. S., Choi, H. G., Shin, B. S., & Youn, Y. S. (2019). Small gold nanorods-loaded hybrid albumin nanoparticles with high photothermal efficacy for tumor ablation. *Colloids and Surfaces. B, Biointerfaces*, *1*(179), 340–351. doi:10.1016/j.colsurfb.2019.03.068

Serafinelli, C., Fantoni, A., Alegria, E. C. B. A., & Vieira, M. (2023). Recent Progresses in Plasmonic Biosensors for Point-of-Care (POC) Devices: A Critical Review. *Chemosensors (Basel, Switzerland)*, *11*(5), 303. doi:10.3390/chemosensors11050303

Sercombe, L., Veerati, T., Moheimani, F., Wu, S. Y., Sood, A. K., & Hua, S. (2015). Advances and challenges of liposome assisted drug delivery. *Frontiers in Pharmacology*, *286*(6). doi:10.3389/fphar.2015.00286

Serrano-Aroca, Á., Cano-Vicent, A., Sabater i Serra, R., El-Tanani, M., Aljabali, A. A. A., Tambuwala, M. M., & Mishra, Y. K. (2022). Scaffolds in the microbial resistant era: Fabrication, materials, properties and tissue engineering applications. *Materials Today. Bio*, *100412*, 100412. Advance online publication. doi:10.1016/j.mtbio.2022.100412 PMID:36097597

Sethi, A. K., Samal, R., Lahiri, B., Das, A., Kumar, G., & Behera, S. (2018). Awareness, attitude and practice regarding disinfection and handling of extracted teeth among the students in a dental college in India. *Journal of International Society of Preventive & Community Dentistry*, *8*(6), 488–494. doi:10.4103/jispcd.JISPCD_314_18 PMID:30596038

Shahazidy, U., Jamal, M. A., Muneer, M., Naseem, B., & Qureshi, A. K. (2022). Elucidation of molecular interactions between sugar alcohol and dimethyl sulfoxide in aqueous system: Volumetric and acoustic study. *Journal of Molecular Liquids*, *350*, 118543. doi:10.1016/j.molliq.2022.118543

Shan, S., Li, Q., Criswell, T., Atala, A., & Zhang, Y. (2023). Stem cell therapy combined with controlled release of growth factors for the treatment of sphincter dysfunction. *Cell & Bioscience*, *13*(1), 1–23. doi:10.118613578-023-01009-3 PMID:36927578

Shan, X., Gong, X., Li, J., Wen, J., Li, Y., & Zhang, Z. (2022). Current approaches of nanomedicines in the market and various stage of clinical translation. *Acta Pharmaceutica Sinica. B*, *12*(7), 3028–3048. doi:10.1016/j.apsb.2022.02.025

Shao, L., Gao, Y., & Yan, F. (2011). Semiconductor quantum dots for biomedicial applications. *Sensors (Basel)*, *11*(12), 11736–11751. doi:10.3390111211736 PMID:22247690

Shao, L., Kahraman, N., Yan, G., Wang, J., Ozpolat, B., & Ittmann, M. (2020). Targeting the TMPRSS2/ERG fusion mRNA using liposomal nanovectors enhances docetaxel treatment in prostate cancer. *The Prostate*, *80*(1), 65–73. doi:10.1002/pros.23918

Sharma, G., Dhankar, G., Thakur, K., Raza, K., & Katare, O. P. (2016). Benzyl Benzoate-Loaded Microemulsion for Topical Applications: Enhanced Dermatokinetic Profile and Better Delivery Promises. *AAPS PharmSciTech*, *17*(5), 1221–1231. doi:10.120812249-015-0464-0 PMID:26669889

Sharma, G., Sharma, A. R., Nam, J. S., Doss, G. P. C., Lee, S. S., & Chakraborty, C. (2015). Nanoparticle based insulin delivery system: The next generation efficient therapy for Type 1 diabetes. *Journal of Nanobiotechnology*, *13*(1), 1–13. doi:10.118612951-015-0136-y PMID:26498972

Sharma, P., Rana, S., Barick, K. C., Kumar, C., Salunke, H. G., & Hassan, P. A. (2014). Biocompatible phosphate anchored Fe3O4 nanocarriers for drug delivery and hyperthermia. *New Journal of Chemistry*, *38*(11), 5500–5508. doi:10.1039/C4NJ01431F

Sharoyko, V. V., Berdichevsky, G. M., Vasina, L. V., Shemchuk, O. S., Maystrenko, D. N., Molchanov, O. E., Abdelhalim, A. O. E., Nashchekin, A. V., Nerukh, D. A., Tochilnikov, G. V., Murin, I. V., & Semenov, K. N. (2023). Covalent conjugates based on nanodiamonds with doxorubicin and a cytostatic drug from the group of 1,3,5-triazines: Synthesis, biocompatibility and biological activity. *Biochimica et Biophysica Acta (BBA) -. Biochimica et Biophysica Acta. G, General Subjects*, *1867*(9), 130384. doi:10.1016/j.bbagen.2023.130384 PMID:37209777

Shedrack, R. K., Peter, K., Judith, S., Dominic, O., Peter, M., & Naomi, M. (2022). Biogenic synthesis of silver nanoparticles using Azadirachta indica methanolic bark extract and their anti-proliferative activities against DU-145 human prostate cancer cells. *African Journal of Biotechnology*, *21*, 64–72.

Shelma, R. (2022). Polymeric Nanoparticles for Drug Delivery. In *A Holistic and Integrated Approach to Lifestyle Diseases* (pp. 319–332). Apple Academic Press.

Shen, C., Xue, Y., Li, Y., Wei, M., Wen, M., Zhang, L., & Shang, L. (2023). Kinetically regulated one-pot synthesis of cationic gold nanoparticles and their size-dependent antibacterial mechanism. *Journal of Materials Science and Technology*, *162*, 145–156. doi:10.1016/j.jmst.2023.03.061

Shen, X., Cui, Z., Wei, Y., Huo, Y., Yu, D., Zhang, X., & Mao, S. (2023). Exploring the potential to enhance drug distribution in the brain subregion via intranasal delivery of nanoemulsion in combination with borneol as a guider. *Asian Journal of Pharmaceutical Sciences*, *100778*(6), 100778. Advance online publication. doi:10.1016/j.ajps.2023.100778 PMID:38089837

Shen, Z., Chen, T., Ma, X., Ren, W., Zhou, Z., Zhu, G., Zhang, A., Liu, Y., Song, J., Li, Z., Ruan, H., Fan, W., Lin, L., Munasinghe, J., Chen, X., & Wu, A. (2017). Multifunctional Theranostic Nanoparticles Based on Exceedingly Small Magnetic Iron Oxide Nanoparticles for T_1-Weighted Magnetic Resonance Imaging and Chemotherapy. *ACS Nano*, *11*(11), 10992–11004. doi:10.1021/acsnano.7b04924

Sheoran, R., Khokra, S. L., Chawla, V., & Dureja, H. (2019). Recent patents, formulation techniques, classification and characterization of liposomes. *Recent Patents on Nanotechnology*, *13*(1), 17–27. doi:10.2174/1872210513666181127110413

Sherje, A. P., Jadhav, M., Dravyakar, B. R., & Kadam, D. (2018). Dendrimers: A versatile nanocarrier for drug delivery and targeting. *International Journal of Pharmaceutics*, *548*(1), 707–720. doi:10.1016/j.ijpharm.2018.07.030 PMID:30012508

Shete, H. K., Prabhu, R. H., & Patravale, V. B. (2014). Endosomal Escape: A Bottleneck in Intracellular Delivery. *Journal of Nanoscience and Nanotechnology*, *14*(1), 460–474. doi:10.1166/jnn.2014.9082 PMID:24730275

Shi, J., Votruba, A. R., Farokhzad, O. C., & Langer, R. (2010). Nanotechnology in drug delivery and tissue engineering: From discovery to applications. *Nano Letters*, *10*(9), 3223–3230. doi:10.1021/nl102184c PMID:20726522

Shi, M., Shen, K., Yang, B., Zhang, P., Lv, K., Qi, H., Wang, Y., Li, M., Yuan, Q., & Zhang, Y. (2021). An electroporation strategy to synthesize the membrane-coated nanoparticles for enhanced anti-inflammation therapy in bone infection. *Theranostics*, *11*(5), 2349–2363. doi:10.7150/thno.48407 PMID:33500729

Shim, M., Shi Kam, N. W., Chen, R. J., Li, Y., & Dai, H. (2002). Functionalization of carbon nanotubes for biocompatibility and biomolecular recognition. *Nano Letters*, *2*(4), 285–288. doi:10.1021/nl015692j

Shinde, S. B., Fernandes, C. B., & Patravale, V. B. (2012, April 30). Recent trends in in-vitro nanodiagnostics for detection of pathogens. *Journal of Controlled Release*, *159*(2), 164–180. doi:10.1016/j.jconrel.2011.11.033 PMID:22192572

Shin, J., Anisur, R. M., Ko, M. K., Im, G. H., Lee, J. H., & Lee, I. S. (2009). Hollow manganese oxide nanoparticles as multifunctional agents for magnetic resonance imaging and drug delivery. *Angewandte Chemie International Edition*, *48*(2), 321–324. doi:10.1002/anie.200802323 PMID:19040234

Shi, X., Tian, Y., Liu, Y., Xiong, Z., Zhai, S., Chu, S., & Gao, F. (2022). Research Progress of Photothermal Nanomaterials in Multimodal Tumor Therapy. *Frontiers in Oncology*, *939365*(12), 939365. doi:10.3389/fonc.2022.939365

Shi, Y., Zhu, C., Fu, T., Gao, X., & Ma, Y. (2020). Volumetric and Viscometric Properties of Maltitol in Glycylglycine Aqueous Solutions at T= 293.15–333.15 K. *Journal of Chemical & Engineering Data*, *66*(1), 360–367. doi:10.1021/acs.jced.0c00731

Shkodra-Pula, B., Vollrath, A., Schubert, U. S., & Schubert, S. (2020). Polymer-based nanoparticles for biomedical applications. *Frontiers of Nanoscience*, *16*, 233–252. doi:10.1016/B978-0-08-102828-5.00009-7

Shoaib, A., Azmi, L., Pal, S., Alqahtani, S. S., Rahamathulla, M., Hani, U., Alshehri, S., Ghoneim, M. M., & Shakeel, F. (2022). Integrating nanotechnology with naturally occurring phytochemicals in neuropathy induced by diabetes. *Journal of Molecular Liquids*, *350*, 118189. doi:10.1016/j.molliq.2021.118189

Shrestha, N., Araujo, F., Shahbazi, M. A., Mäkilä, E., Gomes, M. J., Airavaara, M., Kauppinen, E. I., Raula, J., Salonen, J., Hirvonen, J., Sarmento, B., & Santos, H. A. (2016). Oral hypoglycaemic effect of GLP-1 and DPP4 inhibitor based nanocomposites in a diabetic animal model. *Journal of Controlled Release*, *232*, 113–119. doi:10.1016/j.jconrel.2016.04.024 PMID:27091697

Shruti, A., Bage, N., & Kar, P. (2023). Nanomaterials based sensors for analysis of food safety. *Food Chemistry*, 137284. PMID:37703589

Siafaka, P. I., Okur, N. Ü., Karantas, I. D., Okur, M. E., & Gündoğdu, E. A. (2021). Current update on nanoplatforms as therapeutic and diagnostic tools: A review for the materials used as nanotheranostics and imaging modalities. *Asian Journal of Pharmaceutical Sciences*, *16*(1), 24–46. doi:10.1016/j.ajps.2020.03.003 PMID:33613728

Sibuyi, N. R. S., Thipe, V. C., Panjtan-Amiri, K., Meyer, M., & Katti, K. V. (2021). Green synthesis of gold nanoparticles using Acai berry and elderberry extracts and investigation of their effect on prostate and pancreatic Cancer cells. *BJGP Open*, *8*. doi:10.1177/1849543521995310 PMID:33643450

Siddique, S., & Chow, J. C. (2020). Application of nanomaterials in biomedical imaging and cancer therapy. *Nanomaterials (Basel, Switzerland)*, *10*(9), 1700. doi:10.3390/nano10091700 PMID:32872399

Siegel, R., Ma, J., Zou, Z., & Jemal, A. (2014). Cancer statistics. *CA: a Cancer Journal for Clinicians*, *64*(1), 9–29. doi:10.3322/caac.21208 PMID:24399786

Silva, N. P., M. F. P., & C. M. (2012). Dendrimers as potential platforms in nanotechnology-based drug delivery systems. *IOSR Journal of Pharmacy*, *2*(5), 23–30. doi:10.9790/3013-25602330

Silva, P., Bonifácio, B., Ramos, M., Negri, K., Maria Bauab, T., & Chorilli, M. (2013). Nanotechnology-based drug delivery systems and herbal medicines: A review. *International Journal of Nanomedicine*, *1*, 1. doi:10.2147/IJN.S52634

Silverman, J. A., & Deitcher, S. R. (2013). Marqibo® (vincristine sulfate liposome injection) improves the pharmacokinetics and pharmacodynamics of vincristine. *Cancer Chemotherapy and Pharmacology*, *71*(3), 555–564. doi:10.100700280-012-2042-4

Sim, S., & Wong, N. K. (2021). Nanotechnology and its use in imaging and drug delivery (Review). *Biomedical Reports*, *14*(5), 42. doi:10.3892/br.2021.1418 PMID:33728048

Singh, P. K., & Bhatt, S. C. (2010). Investigation of acoustical parameters of polyvinyl acetate. *Applied physics research*, *2*(1)

Singh, R. (2019). Nanotechnology based therapeutic application in cancer diagnosis and therapy. *3 Biotech 9*(11), 415. . doi:10.1007/s13205-019-1940-0

Singh, B. N., & Kim, K. H. (2000). Floating drug delivery systems: An approach to oral controlled drug delivery via gastric retention. *Journal of Controlled Release*, *63*(3), 235–259. doi:10.1016/S0168-3659(99)00204-7 PMID:10601721

Singh, D., Yadav, E., Falls, N., Kumar, V., Singh, M., & Verma, A. (2019). RETRACTED ARTICLE: Phytofabricated silver nanoparticles of Phyllanthus emblica attenuated diethylnitrosamine-induced hepatic cancer via knock-down oxidative stress and inflammation. *Inflammopharmacology*, *27*(5), 1037–1054. doi:10.100710787-018-0525-6 PMID:30219979

Singh, L., Agrawal, N., Gola, K. K., Saha, C., & Pareek, P. (2022). Numerical investigation of all optical SR flip-flop using plasmonic metal–insulator-metal (MIM) waveguides. *Optical and Quantum Electronics*, *54*(6), 381. doi:10.100711082-022-03666-z

Singh, L., Agrawal, N., & Saha, C. (2021). Investigation of Glucose Sensor by using Plasmonic MIM Waveguide Based M. *2021 IEEE MTT-S International Microwave and RF Conference (IMARC)*. IEEE. 10.1109/IMaRC49196.2021.9714533

Singh, L., Agrawal, N., Saha, C., & Kaushik, B. K. (2022). A Plus Shaped Cavity in Optical Fiber Based Refractive Index Sensor. *IEEE Transactions on Nanobioscience*, *21*(2), 199–205. doi:10.1109/TNB.2021.3121779 PMID:34673494

Singh, L., Agrawal, N., Saha, C., Singh, B. M., & Singh, T. (2022). Highly Sensitive Plus Shaped Cavity in Silicon Fiber for RI Detection of Water Samples. *Silicon*, *14*(13), 7819–7828. doi:10.100712633-021-01519-0

Singh, L., Iadicicco, A., Agrawal, N., Saha, C., & Chauhan, R. (2022). A compact formulation of all optical signal router by using plasmonic waveguides. *Optical and Quantum Electronics*, *54*(8), 478. doi:10.100711082-022-03878-3

Singh, L., Kruger, H. G., Maguire, G. E. M., Govender, T., & Parboosing, R. (2017). The role of nanotechnology in the treatment of viral infections. *Therapeutic Advances in Infectious Disease*, *4*(4), 105–131. doi:10.1177/2049936117713593 PMID:28748089

Singh, M., & Singh, N. (2017). Nanotechnology in sports medicine: A perspective on latest developments. *International Journal of Nanomedicine*, *12*, 871–881.

Singh, R., & Lillard, J. W. Jr. (2009). Nanoparticle-based targeted drug delivery. *Experimental and Molecular Pathology*, *86*(3), 215–223. doi:10.1016/j.yexmp.2008.12.004 PMID:19186176

Singh, S., Shauloff, N., Sharma, C. P., Shimoni, R., Arnusch, C. J., & Jelinek, R. (2021). Carbon dot-polymer nanoporous membrane for recyclable sunlight-sterilized facemasks. *Journal of Colloid and Interface Science*, *592*, 342–348. doi:10.1016/j.jcis.2021.02.049 PMID:33677194

Si, P., Razmi, N., Nur, O., Solanki, S., Pandey, C. M., Gupta, R. K., Malhotra, B. D., Willander, M., & De La Zerda, A. (2021). Gold nanomaterials for optical biosensing and bioimaging. *Nanoscale Advances*, *3*(10), 2679–2698. doi:10.1039/D0NA00961J PMID:36134176

Siqueira, G., Bras, J., & Dufresne, A. (2010). Cellulosic bionanocomposites: A review of preparation, properties and applications. *Polymers*, *2*(4), 728–765. doi:10.3390/polym2040728

Skonieczny, M., Królikowska, M., & Królikowski, M. (2023). Investigation of thermodynamic properties of dimethyl phosphate-based ILs for use as working fluids in absorption refrigeration technology. *Molecules (Basel, Switzerland)*, *28*(4), 1940. doi:10.3390/molecules28041940 PMID:36838928

Slowing, I. I., Trewyn, B. G., & Lin, V. S. (2007). Mesoporous silica nanoparticles for intracellular delivery of membrane-impermeable proteins. *Journal of the American Chemical Society*, *129*(28), 8845–8849. doi:10.1021/ja0719780 PMID:17589996

Snow, A., Lin, L., Hunsucker, S. A., Wang, Y., Liu, R., & Armistead, P. M. (2022). Development of a mRNA lipid nanoparticle (mRNA-LNP) cancer vaccine to prevent leukemia relapse after stem cell transplant. *Blood, 140*(Supplement 1), 7382–7383. doi:10.1182/blood-2022-160218

Soares, S., Sousa, J., Pais, A., & Vitorino, C. (2018). Nanomedicine: Principles, properties, and regulatory issues. *Frontiers in Chemistry*, *360*, 360. doi:10.3389/fchem.2018.00360 PMID:30177965

Sobhanan, J., Anas, A., & Biju, V. (2023). Nanomaterials for Fluorescence and Multimodal Bioimaging. *Chemical Record (New York, N.Y.)*, *23*(3), e202200253. doi:10.1002/tcr.202200253 PMID:36789795

Sofi, M. A., Sunitha, S., Sofi, M. A., Pasha, S. K., & Choi, D. (2022). An overview of antimicrobial and anticancer potential of silver nanoparticles. *Journal of King Saud University. Science*, *34*(2), 101791. doi:10.1016/j.jksus.2021.101791

Soisuwan, S., Teeranachaideekul, V., Wongrakpanich, A., Langguth, P., & Junyaprasert, V. B. (2019). Impact of uncharged and charged stabilizers on in vitro drug performances of clarithromycin nanocrystals. *European Journal of Pharmaceutics and Biopharmaceutics : Official Journal of Arbeitsgemeinschaft Fur Pharmazeutische Verfahrenstechnik e.V*, *137*, 68–76. doi:10.1016/j.ejpb.2019.02.004

Soleimani, M., Zaabi, A., Merheb, M., & Matar, R. (2016). Nanoparticles in Gene Therapy. *International Journal of Integrative Biology*, *17*, 7–16.

Soliman, N. M., Shakeel, F., Haq, N., Alanazi, F. K., Alshehri, S., Bayomi, M., Alenazi, A. S. M., & Alsarra, I. A. (2022). Development and Optimization of Ciprofloxacin HCl-Loaded Chitosan Nanoparticles Using Box–Behnken Experimental Design. *Molecules (Basel, Switzerland)*, *27*(14), 4468. doi:10.3390/molecules27144468

Song, J., Yang, X., Jacobson, O., Lin, L., Huang, P., Niu, G., Ma, Q., & Chen, X. (2015). Sequential Drug Release and Enhanced Photothermal and Photoacoustic Effect of Hybrid Reduced Graphene Oxide-Loaded Ultrasmall Gold Nanorod Vesicles for Cancer Therapy. *ACS Nano*, *9*(9), 9199–9209. doi:10.1021/acsnano.5b03804

Song, K. C., Lee, H. S., Choung, I. Y., Cho, K. I., Ahn, Y., & Choi, E. J. (2006). The effect of type of organic phase solvents on the particle size of poly (d, l-lactide-co-glycolide) nanoparticles. *Colloids and Surfaces. A, Physicochemical and Engineering Aspects*, *276*(1-3), 162–167. doi:10.1016/j.colsurfa.2005.10.064

Song, N., Guo, H., Ren, J., Hao, S., & Wang, X. (2018). Synergistic anti-tumor effects of dasatinib and dendritic cell vaccine on metastatic breast cancer in a mouse model. *Oncology Letters*, *15*(5), 6831–6838. 10.3892%2Fol.2018.8188

Song, S., Shim, M. K., Yang, S., Lee, J., Yun, W. S., Cho, H., Moon, Y., Min, J. Y., Han, E. H., Yoon, H. Y., & Kim, K. (2023). All-in-one glycol chitosan nanoparticles for co-delivery of doxorubicin and anti-PD-L1 peptide in cancer immunotherapy. *Bioactive Materials*, *28*, 358–375. doi:10.1016/j.bioactmat.2023.05.016 PMID:37334068

Song, X., Zhao, Y., Wu, W., Bi, Y., Cai, Z., Chen, Q., Li, Y., & Hou, S. (2008). PLGA nanoparticles simultaneously loaded with vincristine sulfate and verapamil hydrochloride: Systematic study of particle size and drug entrapment efficiency. *International Journal of Pharmaceutics*, *350*(1-2), 320–329. doi:10.1016/j.ijpharm.2007.08.034 PMID:17913411

Soni, S., Ruhela, R. K., & Medhi, B. (2016). Nanomedicine in Central Nervous System (CNS) Disorders: A Present and Future Prospective. *Advanced Pharmaceutical Bulletin*, *6*(3), 319–335. doi:10.15171/apb.2016.044 PMID:27766216

Soppimath, K. S., Aminabhavi, T. M., Kulkarni, A. R., & Rudzinski, W. E. (2001). Biodegradable polymeric nanoparticles as drug delivery devices. *Journal of Controlled Release*, *70*(1-2), 1–20. doi:10.1016/S0168-3659(00)00339-4 PMID:11166403

Soufi, G. J., & Iravani, S. (2020). Eco-friendly and sustainable synthesis of biocompatible nanomaterials for diagnostic imaging: Current challenges and future perspectives. *Green Chemistry*, *22*(9), 2662–2687. doi:10.1039/D0GC00734J

Soundararajan, D., Ramana, L. N., Shankaran, P., & Krishnan, U. M. (2022). Nanoparticle-based strategies to target HIV-infected cells. *Colloids and Surfaces. B, Biointerfaces*, *213*, 112405. doi:10.1016/j.colsurfb.2022.112405 PMID:35255375

Souri, M., Soltani, M., Kashkooli, F. M., Shahvandi, M. K., Chiani, M., Shariati, F. S., Mehrabi, M. R., & Munn, L. L. (2022). Towards principled design of cancer nanomedicine to accelerate clinical translation. *Materials Today. Bio*, *13*, 100208. doi:10.1016/j.mtbio.2022.100208 PMID:35198957

Souto, E. B., Souto, S. B., Campos, J. R., Severino, P., Pashirova, T. N., Zakharova, L. Y., Silva, A. M., Durazzo, A., Lucarini, M., Izzo, A. A., & Santini, A. (2019). Nanoparticle delivery systems in the treatment of diabetes complications. *Molecules (Basel, Switzerland)*, *24*(23), 4209. doi:10.3390/molecules24234209 PMID:31756981

Sowmiya, P., Dhas, T. S., Inbakandan, D., Anandakumar, N., Nalini, S., Suganya, K. U., Remya, R. R., Karthick, V., & Kumar, C. V. (2023). Optically active organic and inorganic nanomaterials for biological imaging applications: A review. *Micron (Oxford, England)*, *172*, 103486. doi:10.1016/j.micron.2023.103486 PMID:37262930

Spadari, C. C., Lanser, D. M., Araújo, M. V., De Jesus, D. F., Lopes, L. B., Gelli, A., & Ishida, K. (2023). Oral delivery of brain-targeted miltefosine-loaded alginate nanoparticles functionalized with polysorbate 80 to treat cryptococcal meningitis. *The Journal of Antimicrobial Chemotherapy*, *78*(4), 1092–1101. doi:10.1093/jac/dkad053 PMID:36881722

Speranza, G. (2021). Carbon nanomaterials: Synthesis, functionalization and sen[1] Speranza, G., Carbon nanomaterials: Synthesis, functionalization and sensing applications, Nanomaterials 11 (2021).sing applications. *Nanomaterials (Basel, Switzerland)*, *11*(4). PMID:33918769

Spirescu, V. A., Chircov, C., Grumezescu, A. M., & Andronescu, E. (2021). Polymeric nanoparticles for antimicrobial therapies: An up-to-date overview. *Polymers*, *13*(5), 724. doi:10.3390/polym13050724 PMID:33673451

Sriraman, S. K., Geraldo, V., Luther, E., Degterev, A., & Torchilin, V. (2015). Cytotoxicity of PEGylated liposomes co-loaded with novel pro-apoptotic drug NCL-240 and the MEK inhibitor cobimetinib against colon carcinoma in vitro. *Journal of Controlled Release*, *220*, 160–168. doi:10.1016/j.jconrel.2015.10.037

Sriram, M., Zong, K., Vivekchand, S., & Gooding, J. (2015). Single Nanoparticle Plasmonic Sensors. *Sensors (Basel)*, *15*(10), 25774–25792. doi:10.3390151025774 PMID:26473866

Srivastav, A. K., Karpathak, S., Rai, M. K., Kumar, D., Misra, D. P., & Agarwal, V. (2023). Lipid based drug delivery systems for oral, transdermal and parenteral delivery: Recent strategies for targeted delivery consistent with different clinical application. *Journal of Drug Delivery Science and Technology*, *85*, 104526. doi:10.1016/j.jddst.2023.104526

Sternling, C. A., & Scriven, L. E. (1959). Interfacial turbulence: Hydrodynamic instability and the Marangoni effect. *AIChE Journal. American Institute of Chemical Engineers*, *5*(4), 514–523. doi:10.1002/aic.690050421

Su, C., Liu, Y., Li, R., Wu, W., Fawcett, J.P., & Gu, J. (2019). Absorption, distribution, metabolism and excretion of the biomaterials used in Nanocarrier drug delivery systems. *Adv Drug Deliv. Rev*, *143*, 97-114. undefined. doi:10.1016/j.addr.2019.06.008

Subhan, M. A., & Subhan, T. (2022). Safety and global regulations for application of nanomaterials. In *Nanomaterials Recycling* (pp. 83–107). Elsevier. doi:10.1016/B978-0-323-90982-2.00005-6

Subhra, T., Loganathan, S., Nanomaterials, M. E., & Applications, T. B. (2021). *Springer Series in Biomaterials Science and Engineering, 16*. Springer. https://www.springer.com/series/10955

Subramaniam, B., Rajewski, R. A., & Snavely, K. (1997). Pharmaceutical processing with supercritical carbon dioxide. *Journal of Pharmaceutical Sciences*, *86*(8), 885–890. doi:10.1021/js9700661 PMID:9269864

Suen, M. S., Lin, Y. C., & Chen, R. (2018). A flexible multifunctional tactile sensor using interlocked zinc oxide nanorod arrays for artificial electronic skin. *Sensors and Actuators. A, Physical*, *269*, 574–584. doi:10.1016/j.sna.2017.11.053

Suhaimi, N. A. A., Ahmad, S., Husna, S. M. N., Elena Sarmiento, M., Acosta, A., Norazmi, M. N., Ibrahim, J., Mohamud, R., & Kadir, R. (2022). Application of liposomes in the treatment of infectious diseases. *Life Sciences*, *305*, 120734. doi:10.1016/j.lfs.2022.120734 PMID:35760094

Suhre, K., McCarthy, M. I., & Schwenk, J. M. (2021). Genetics meets proteomics: Perspectives for large population-based studies. *Nature Reviews. Genetics*, *22*(1), 19–37. doi:10.103841576-020-0268-2 PMID:32860016

Sung, D., Sanchez, A., & Tward, J. D. (2023). Successful salvage brachytherapy after infusion of gold auroshell nanoshells for localized prostate cancer in a human patient. *Advances in Radiation Oncology*, *8*(4), 101202. doi:10.1016/j.adro.2023.101202 PMID:37082724

Sun, J., Russell, C. C., Scarlett, C. J., & McCluskey, A. (2020). Small molecule inhibitors in pancreatic cancer. *RSC Medicinal Chemistry*, *11*(2), 164–183. doi:10.1039/C9MD00447E

Sun, Q., Sun, X., Ma, X., Zhou, Z., Jin, E., Zhang, B., Shen, Y., Van Kirk, E. A., Murdoch, W. J., Lott, J. R., Lodge, T. P., Radosz, M., & Zhao, Y. (2014). Integration of Nanoassembly Functions for an Effective Delivery Cascade for Cancer Drugs. *Advanced Materials*, *26*(45), 7615–7621. doi:10.1002/adma.201401554 PMID:25328159

Sun, X., Huang, X., Yan, X., Wang, Y., Guo, J., Jacobson, O., Liu, D., Szajek, L. P., Zhu, W., Niu, G., Kiesewetter, D. O., Sun, S., & Chen, X. (2014). Chelator-Free 64CuIntegrated Gold Nanomaterials for Positron Emission Tomography Imaging Guided Photothermal Cancer Therapy. *ACS Nano*, *8*(8), 8438–8446. doi:10.1021/nn502950t

Sun, Y. P., Zhou, B., Lin, Y., Wang, W., Fernando, K. A. S., Pathak, P., Meziani, M. J., Harruff, B. A., Wang, X., Wang, H., Luo, P. G., Yang, H., Kose, M. E., Chen, B., Veca, L. M., & Xie, S.-Y. (2006). Quantum-sized carbon dots for bright and colorful photoluminescence. *Journal of the American Chemical Society*, *128*(24), 7756–7757. doi:10.1021/ja062677d PMID:16771487

Sun, Y., Lu, Y., Yin, L., & Liu, Z. (2020). The roles of nanoparticles in stem cell-based therapy for cardiovascular disease. *Frontiers in Bioengineering and Biotechnology*, *8*, 947. doi:10.3389/fbioe.2020.00947 PMID:32923434

Sun, Y., Zhang, Y., Liu, X., Tingting, Y., Shen, L., Ye, D., Kong, X., Su, Y., & Tian, Q. (2023). The preparation of high minoxidil loaded transfersomes and its gel for effective topical treatment of alopecia. *Journal of Drug Delivery Science and Technology*, *84*, 104458. doi:10.1016/j.jddst.2023.104458

Surana, H., Agarwal, N., Udaykumar, A., & Darekar, R. (2019). *Blackbox-Based Night Vision Camouflage Robot for Defence Applications*. Computing, Communication and Signal Processing. doi:10.1007/978-981-13-1513-8_64

Surmenev, R. A., Surmeneva, M. A., & Ivanova, A. A. (2014). Significance of calcium phosphate coatings for the enhancement of new bone osteogenesis—A review. *Acta Biomaterialia*, *10*(2), 557–579. doi:10.1016/j.actbio.2013.10.036 PMID:24211734

Suryanarayana, C., & Prabhu, B. (2007). Synthesis of nanostructured materials by inert-gas condensation methods. In *Nanostructured materials* (pp. 47–90). William Andrew Publishing. doi:10.1016/B978-081551534-0.50004-X

Su, Y., Xie, Z., Kim, G. B., Dong, C., & Yang, J. (2015). Design strategies and applications of circulating cell-mediated drug delivery systems. *ACS Biomaterials Science & Engineering*, *1*(4), 201–217. doi:10.1021/ab500179h PMID:25984572

Syeda, U. A., Battillo, D., Visaria, A., & Malin, S. K. (2023). The importance of exercise for glycemic control in type 2 diabetes. *American Journal of Medicine Open*, *9*, 100031. doi:10.1016/j.ajmo.2023.100031

Taher, M., Susanti, D., Haris, M. S., Rushdan, A. A., Widodo, R. T., Syukri, Y., & Khotib, J. (2023). PEGylated liposomes enhance the effect of cytotoxic drug: A review. *Heliyon*, *9*(3), e13823. doi:10.1016/j.heliyon.2023.e13823 PMID:36873538

Taiwo, B. O., Romdhani, H., Lafeuille, M. H., Bhojwani, R., Milbers, K., & Donga, P. (2023). Treatment and comorbidity burden among people living with HIV: A review of systematic literature reviews. *Journal of Drug Assessment*, *12*(1), 1–11. doi:10.1080/21556660.2022.2149963 PMID:36582675

Takeuchi, I., Suzuki, T., & Makino, K. (2021). Iontophoretic transdermal delivery using chitosan-coated PLGA nanoparticles for transcutaneous immunization. *Colloids and Surfaces. A, Physicochemical and Engineering Aspects*, *608*, 125607. doi:10.1016/j.colsurfa.2020.125607

Tang, G. P., Zeng, J. M., Gao, S. J., Ma, Y. X., Shi, L., Li, Y., Too, H.-P., & Wang, S. (2003). Polyethylene glycol modified polyethylenimine for improved CNS gene transfer: Effects of PEGylation extent. *Biomaterials*, *24*(13), 2351–2362. doi:10.1016/S0142-9612(03)00029-2 PMID:12699673

Tang, L., Li, J., Zhao, Q., Pan, T., Zhong, H., & Wang, W. (2021). Advanced and innovative nano-systems for anticancer targeted drug delivery. *Pharmaceutics*, *1151*(13), 1151. doi:10.3390/pharmaceutics13081151

Tang, X., Fu, J., & Qin, H. (2023). Microwave-induced thermoacoustic imaging with functional nanoparticles. *Journal of Innovative Optical Health Sciences*, *16*(02), 2230014. doi:10.1142/S1793545822300142

Tan, P., Li, H. S., Wang, J., & Gopinath, S. C. B. (2021). Silver nanoparticle in biosensor and bioimaging: Clinical perspectives. *Biotechnology and Applied Biochemistry*, *68*(6), 1236–1242. doi:10.1002/bab.2045 PMID:33043496

Tan, Q., Wu, C., Li, L., Shao, W., & Luo, M. (2022). Nanomaterial-Based Prosthetic Limbs for Disability Mobility Assistance: A Review of Recent Advances. *Journal of Nanomaterials*, *2022*, 1–10. doi:10.1155/2022/3425297

Tantra, R., Schulze, P., & Quincey, P. (2010). Effect of nanoparticle concentration on zeta-potential measurement results and reproducibility. *Particuology*, *8*(3), 279–285. doi:10.1016/j.partic.2010.01.003

Tao, Y., Li, M., Kim, B., & Auguste, D. T. (2017). Incorporating gold nanoclusters and target-directed liposomes as a synergistic amplified colorimetric sensor for HER2-positive breast cancer cell detection. *Theranostics*, *7*(4), 899–911. doi:10.7150/thno.17927 PMID:28382162

Taruno, K., Kurita, T., Kuwahata, A., Yanagihara, K., Enokido, K., Katayose, Y., Nakamura, S., Takei, H., Sekino, M., & Kusakabe, M. (2019). Multicenter clinical trial on sentinel lymph node biopsy using superparamagnetic iron oxide nanoparticles and a novel handheld magnetic probe. *Journal of Surgical Oncology*, *120*(8), 1391–1396. doi:10.1002/jso.25747 PMID:31667855

Tashakori-Miyanroudi, M., Janzadeh, A., Seifalian, A., Aboutaleb, N., Azizi, Y., & Ramezani, F. (2022). Will carbon nanotube/nanofiber bring new hope for the treatment of heart damage? A systematic review. *Nanomedicine (London)*, *17*(29), 2189–2205. doi:10.2217/nnm-2022-0113 PMID:36896892

Teixeira, M. I., Lopes, C. M., Amaral, M. H., & Costa, P. C. (2023). Surface-modified lipid nanocarriers for crossing the blood-brain barrier (BBB): A current overview of active targeting in brain diseases. *Colloids and Surfaces. B, Biointerfaces*, *221*, 112999. doi:10.1016/j.colsurfb.2022.112999 PMID:36368148

Tenchov, R., Sasso, J. M., & Zhou, Q. A. (2023). PEGylated Lipid Nanoparticle Formulations: Immunological Safety and Efficiency Perspective. *Bioconjugate Chemistry*, *34*(6), 941–960. doi:10.1021/acs.bioconjchem.3c00174 PMID:37162501

Teo, G., Suzuki, Y., Uratsu, S. L., Lampinen, B., Ormonde, N., Hu, W. K., DeJong, T. M., & Dandekar, A. M. (2006). Silencing leaf sorbitol synthesis alters long-distance partitioning and apple fruit quality. *Proceedings of the National Academy of Sciences of the United States of America*, *103*(49), 18842–18847. doi:10.1073/pnas.0605873103 PMID:17132742

Thakur, A., Juglan, K. C., Kumar, H., & Kaur, K. (2019). Investigation on molecular interaction of glycols in methanol solutions of methylparaben (methyl 4–hydroxybenzoate) at different temperatures through thermo-acoustical analysis. *Journal of Molecular Liquids*, *288*, 111014. doi:10.1016/j.molliq.2019.111014

Thakur, A., & Kathpalia, R. (2022). Engineered nanoparticles (ENPs): Unexplored potential and limitations. [IJBB]. *Indian Journal of Biochemistry & Biophysics*, *59*(12), 1163–1170. doi:10.56042/ijbb.v59i12.67304

Thankappan, B., Thomas, A., Sakthivadivel, A., Shanmuganathan, N., & Angayarkanni, J. (2023). In vitro and in vivo antimicrobial activity of self-assembled melittin nanoparticles: A comparative study with melittin peptide. *Colloids and Surfaces. B, Biointerfaces*, *226*, 113331. doi:10.1016/j.colsurfb.2023.113331 PMID:37150105

Thapa, R. K., & Kim, J. O. (2023). Nanomedicine-based commercial formulations: Current developments and future prospects. *Journal of Pharmaceutical Investigation*, *53*(1), 19–33. doi:10.100740005-022-00607-6

Tharkar, P., Varanasi, R., Wong, W. S. F., Jin, C. T., & Chrzanowski, W. (2019). Nano-enhanced drug delivery and therapeutic ultrasound for cancer treatment and beyond. *Frontiers in Bioengineering and Biotechnology*, *7*, 324. doi:10.3389/fbioe.2019.00324

Thirumaran, S., Suguna, M., & Selvi, S. R. (2009). Acoustic and Thermodynamic Studies of Ternary Liquid Mixtures at Different Temperatures. *Research Journal of Chemistry and Environment*, *13*(3), 81–89.

Thi, T. T. H., Suys, E. J., Lee, J. S., Nguyen, D. H., Park, K. D., & Truong, N. P. (2021). Lipid-based nanoparticles in the clinic and clinical trials: From cancer nanomedicine to COVID-19 vaccines. *Vaccines*, *9*(4), 359. doi:10.3390/vaccines9040359 PMID:33918072

Thomas, F. (2022, May). An Evolving Approach to Drug Delivery, Published on: May 3, 2022, Pharmaceutical Technology. *Pharmaceutical Technology*, *46*(5), 26–27.

Tian, H., He, Z., Sun, C., Yang, C., Zhao, P., Liu, L., Leong, K. W., Mao, H. Q., Liu, Z., & Chen, Y. (2018). Uniform core-shell nanoparticles with thiolated hyaluronic acid coating to enhance oral delivery of insulin. *Advanced Healthcare Materials*, *7*(7), 1–12. doi:10.1002/adhm.201800285

Tian, N., Duan, H., Cao, T., Dai, G., Sheng, G., Chu, H., & Sun, Z. (2023). Macrophage-targeted nanoparticles mediate synergistic photodynamic therapy and immunotherapy of tuberculosis. *RSC Advances*, *13*(3), 1727–1737. doi:10.1039/D2RA06334D PMID:36712647

Tojo, C., de Dios, M., & Barroso, F. (2010). Surfactant effects on microemulsion-based nanoparticle synthesis. *Materials (Basel)*, *4*(1), 55–72. doi:10.3390/ma4010055 PMID:28879976

Tomsia, A. P., Launey, M. E., Lee, J. S., Mankani, M. H., Wegst, U. G. K., & Saiz, E. (2011). Nanotechnology Approaches for Better Dental Implants. *The International Journal of Oral & Maxillofacial Implants, 26*(Suppl), 25. /pmc/articles/PMC3087979/

Tong, L., Liu, D., Cao, Z., Zheng, N., Mao, C., Liu, S., He, L., & Liu, S. (2023). Research status and Prospect of non-viral vectors based on siRNA: A review. *International Journal of Molecular Sciences*, *24*(4), 3375. doi:10.3390/ijms24043375 PMID:36834783

Tong, R., & Langer, R. (2015). Nanomedicines Targeting the Tumor Microenvironment. *Cancer Journal (Sudbury, Mass.)*, *21*(4), 314–321. doi:10.1097/PPO.0000000000000123 PMID:26222084

Torchilin, V. (2000). Drug targeting. *European journal of pharmaceutical sciences: official journal of the European Federation for Pharmaceutical Sciences.*

Torchilin, V. P. (2006). Multifunctional nanocarriers. *Advanced Drug Delivery Reviews*, *58*(14), 1532–1555. doi:10.1016/j.addr.2006.09.009 PMID:17092599

Tran, K. A., Kondrashova, O., Bradley, A., Williams, E. D., Pearson, J. V., & Waddell, N. (2021). Deep learning in cancer diagnosis, prognosis and treatment selection. *Genome Medicine*, *152*(13), 152. doi:10.118613073-021-00968-x

Tran, V. N., Strnad, O., Šuman, J., Veverková, T., Sukupová, A., Cejnar, P., Hynek, R., Kronusová, O., Šach, J., Kaštánek, P., & Viktorová, J. (2023). Cannabidiol nanoemulsion for eye treatment – Anti-inflammatory, wound healing activity and its bioavailability using in vitro human corneal substitute. *International Journal of Pharmaceutics*, *643*, 123202. doi:10.1016/j.ijpharm.2023.123202 PMID:37406946

Trimaille, T., Pichot, C., Elaissari, A., Fessi, H., Briançon, S., & Delair, T. (2003). Poly (D, L-lactic acid) nanoparticle preparation and colloidal characterization. *Colloid & Polymer Science*, *281*(12), 1184–1190. doi:10.100700396-003-0894-1

Trivedi, M., & Dahryn Trivedi, A. B. (2015). Spectroscopic characterization of disodium hydrogen orthophosphate and sodium nitrate after biofield treatment. *Journal of Chromatography & Separation Techniques*, *5*(6). doi:10.4172/2157-7064.1000282

Trüeb, R. M. (2016). Serum Biotin Levels in Women Complaining of Hair Loss. *International Journal of Trichology*, *8*(2), 73–77. doi:10.4103/0974-7753.188040 PMID:27601860

Tsai, H., Chang, K., Lee, W., & Fuh, C. B. (2022). Rapid Preparation of Fluorescent Carbon Dots from Pine Needles for Chemical Analysis. *Nanomaterials (Basel, Switzerland)*, *12*(1), 66. doi:10.3390/nano12010066 PMID:35010016

Tsoi, K. M., Macparland, S. A., Ma, X. Z., Spetzler, V. N., Echeverri, J., Ouyang, B., Fadel, S. M., Sykes, E. A., Goldaracena, N., Kaths, J. M., Conneely, J. B., Alman, B. A., Selzner, M., Ostrowski, M. A., Adeyi, O. A., Zilman, A., McGilvray, I. D., & Chan, W. C. W. (2016). Mechanism of hard-nanomaterial clearance by the liver. *Nature Materials*, *15*(11), 1212–1221. doi:10.1038/nmat4718 PMID:27525571

Turan, O., Bielecki, P., Perera, V., Lorkowski, M., Covarrubias, G., Tong, K., Yun, A., Rahmy, A., Ouyang, T., Raghunathan, S., Gopalakrishnan, R., Griswold, M. A., Ghaghada, K. B., Peiris, P. M., & Karathanasis, E. (2019). Delivery of drugs into brain tumors using multicomponent silica nanoparticles. *Nanoscale*, *11*(24), 11910–11921. doi:10.1039/C9NR02876E

Turney, D. J. (2009). *Nanomaterials*. EC. https://ec.europa.eu/health/scientific_committees/opinions_layman/nanomaterials/en/l-2/1.htm

Turos, E., Reddy, G. S. K., Greenhalgh, K., Ramaraju, P., Abeylath, S. C., Jang, S., Dickey, S., & Lim, D. V. (2007). Penicillin-bound polyacrylate nanoparticles: Restoring the activity of β-lactam antibiotics against MRSA. *Bioorganic & Medicinal Chemistry Letters*, *17*(12), 3468–3472. doi:10.1016/j.bmcl.2007.03.077 PMID:17420125

Turrina, C., Schoenen, M., Milani, D., Klassen, A., Rojas Gonzaléz, D. M., Cvirn, G., Mela, P., Berensmeier, S., Slabu, I., & Schwaminger, S. P. (2023). Application of magnetic iron oxide nanoparticles: Thrombotic activity, imaging and cytocompatibility of silica-coated and carboxymethyl dextrane-coated particles. *Colloids and Surfaces. B, Biointerfaces*, *228*, 113428. doi:10.1016/j.colsurfb.2023.113428 PMID:37379701

Ulery, B. D., Nair, L. S., & Laurencin, C. T. (2011). Biomedical applications of biodegradable polymers. *Journal of Polymer Science. Part B, Polymer Physics*, *49*(12), 832–864. doi:10.1002/polb.22259 PMID:21769165

Umpierrez, G. E., & Klonoff, D. C. (2018). Diabetes technology update: Use of insulin pumps and continuous glucose monitoring in the hospital. *Diabetes Care*, *41*(8), 1579–1589. doi:10.2337/dci18-0002 PMID:29936424

Unal, N., Bakirhan, N., Yucel, C., & Savluk, M. (2022). Antimicrobial effective nanoparticles: Mechanisms and recent achievements. Medicine Science I. *Medicine Science*, *11*(2), 905. doi:10.5455/medscience.2021.12.401

Unser, S., Bruzas, I., He, J., & Sagle, L. (2015). Localized Surface Plasmon Resonance Biosensing: Current Challenges and Approaches. *Sensors (Basel)*, *15*(7), 15684–15716. doi:10.3390150715684 PMID:26147727

Upadhyay, R. K. (2014). Drug Delivery Systems, CNS Protection, and the Blood Brain Barrier. *BioMed Research International*, *2014*, 1–37. doi:10.1155/2014/869269 PMID:25136634

Upmanyu, A., Dhiman, M., Singh, D. P., & Kumar, H. (2021). Thermo-viscous investigations of molecular interactions for the binary mixtures of polyethylene glycol-400 and polyethylene glycol-600 with dimethyl sulfoxide and water at different temperatures. *Journal of Molecular Liquids*, *334*, 115939. doi:10.1016/j.molliq.2021.115939

Upmanyu, A., & Singh, D. P. (2014). Ultrasonic studies of molecular interactions in polymer solution of the Polyisobutylene (PIB) and Benzene. *Acta Acustica united with Acustica*, *100*(3), 434–439. doi:10.3813/AAA.918723

Usmani, A., Mishra, A., Jafri, A., Arshad, M., & Siddiqui, M. A. (2019). Green synthesis of silver nanocomposites of Nigella sativa seeds extract for hepatocellular carcinoma. *Current Nanomaterials*, *4*(3), 191–200. doi:10.2174/2468187309666190906130115

Utembe, W., Tlotleng, N., & Kamng'ona, A. W. (2022). A systematic review on the effects of nanomaterials on gut microbiota. *Current Research in Microbial Sciences*, *3*, 100118. doi:10.1016/j.crmicr.2022.100118 PMID:35909630

Vaid, P., Raizada, P., Saini, A. K., & Saini, R. V. (2020). Biogenic silver, gold and copper nanoparticles-A sustainable green chemistry approach for cancer therapy. *Sustainable Chemistry and Pharmacy*, *16*, 100247. doi:10.1016/j.scp.2020.100247

Valent, P., Groner, B., Schumacher, U., Superti-Furga, G., Busslinger, M., Kralovics, R., Zielinski, C., Penninger, J. M., Kerjaschki, D., Stingl, G., Smolen, J. S., Valenta, R., Lassmann, H., Kovar, H., Jäger, U., Kornek, G., Müller, M., & Sörgel, F. (2016). Paul Ehrlich (1854–1915) and his contributions to the foundation and birth of translational medicine. *Journal of Innate Immunity*, *8*(2), 111–120. doi:10.1159/000443526 PMID:26845587

Vallari, R. C., & Pietruszko, R. (1982). Human aldehyde dehydrogenase: Mechanism of inhibition of disulfiram. *Science*, *216*(4546), 637–639. doi:10.1126cience.7071604 PMID:7071604

van Eck, N. J., & Waltman, L. (2010). Software survey: VOSviewer, a computer program for bibliometric mapping. *Scientometrics*, *84*(2), 523–538. doi:10.100711192-009-0146-3 PMID:20585380

Van Teunenbroek, T., Baker, J., & Dijkzeul, A. (2017). Towards a more effective and efficient governance and regulation of nanomaterials. *Particle and Fibre Toxicology*, *14*(1), 54. doi:10.118612989-017-0235-z PMID:29258600

van Vliet, E. F., Knol, M. J., Schiffelers, R. M., Caiazzo, M., & Fens, M. H. A. M. (2023). Levodopa-loaded nanoparticles for the treatment of Parkinson's disease. *Journal of Controlled Release*, *360*, 212–224. doi:10.1016/j.jconrel.2023.06.026 PMID:37343725

Vargas-Molinero, H. Y., Serrano-Medina, A., Palomino-Vizcaino, K., López-Maldonado, E. A., Villarreal-Gómez, L. J., Pérez-González, G. L., & Cornejo-Bravo, J. M. (2023). Hybrid Systems of Nanofibers and Polymeric Nanoparticles for Biological Application and Delivery Systems. *Micromachines*, *14*(1), 208. doi:10.3390/mi14010208 PMID:36677269

Varo, R., Chaccour, C., & Bassat, Q. (2020). Update on malaria. *Medicina Clínica (English Ed.)*, *155*(9), 395–402. doi:10.1016/j.medcle.2020.05.024 PMID:32620355

Vasanth, K., Ilango, K., MohanKumar, R., Agrawal, A., & Dubey, G. P. (2014). Anticancer activity of Moringa oleifera mediated silver nanoparticles on human cervical carcinoma cells by apoptosis induction. *Colloids and Surfaces. B, Biointerfaces*, *117*, 354–359. doi:10.1016/j.colsurfb.2014.02.052 PMID:24681047

Vashist, A., Vashist, A., Gupta, Y. K., & Ahmad, S. (2014). Recent advances in hydrogel based drug delivery systems for the human body. *Journal of Materials Chemistry. B*, *2*(2), 147–166. doi:10.1039/C3TB21016B PMID:32261602

Vasir, J., & Labhasetwar, V. (2007). Biodegradable nanoparticles for cytosolic delivery of therapeutics☆. *Advanced Drug Delivery Reviews*, *59*(8), 718–728. doi:10.1016/j.addr.2007.06.003 PMID:17683826

Vaudagna, M. V., Aiassa, V., Marcotti, A., Pince Beti, M. F., Constantín, M. F., & Pérez, M. F., & Silvero C., M. J. (2023). Titanium Dioxide Nanoparticles in sunscreens and skin photo-damage. Development, synthesis and characterization of a novel biocompatible alternative based on their in vitro and in vivo study. *Journal of Photochemistry and Photobiology*, *15*, 100173. doi:10.1016/j.jpap.2023.100173

Vazquez-Prada, K. X., Moonshi, S. S., Wu, Y., Akther, F., Tse, B. W., Sokolowski, K. A., Peter, K., Wang, X., Xu, G., & Ta, H. T. (2023). A Spiky Silver-Iron Oxide Nanoparticle for Highly Efficient Targeted Photothermal Therapy and Multimodal Imaging of Thrombosis. *Small*, *19*(11), 2205744. doi:10.1002mll.202205744 PMID:36634995

Vazquez-Rodriguez, A., Vasto-Anzaldo, X. G., Leon-Buitimea, A., Zarate, X., & Morones-Ramirez, J. R. (2020). Antibacterial and Antibiofilm Activity of Biosynthesized Silver Nanoparticles Coated with Exopolysaccharides Obtained from Rhodotorula mucilaginosa. *IEEE Transactions on Nanobioscience*, *19*(3), 498–503. doi:10.1109/TNB.2020.2985101 PMID:32248119

Vega, D. M., Di Meglio, M., del Valle Alonso, S., Alvira, F., & Montanari, J. (2023). *Nanomaterials for Diagnosis, Treatment, and Prevention of Human Cutaneous Leishmaniasis: A Review*. OpenNano.

Veiseh, O., & Langer, R. (2015). A smart insulin patch. *Nature*, *524*(7563), 39–40. doi:10.1038/524039a PMID:26245577

Veiseh, O., Tang, B. C., Whitehead, K. A., Anderson, D. G., & Langer, R. (2015). Managing diabetes with nanomedicine: Challenges and opportunities. *Nature Reviews. Drug Discovery*, *14*(1), 45–57. doi:10.1038/nrd4477 PMID:25430866

Veith, A. P., Henderson, K., Spencer, A., Sligar, A. D., & Baker, A. B. (2019). Therapeutic strategies for enhancing angiogenesis in wound healing. *Advanced Drug Delivery Reviews*, *146*, 97–125. doi:10.1016/j.addr.2018.09.010 PMID:30267742

Venkateshaiah, A., Padil, V. V. T., Nagalakshmaiah, M., Waclawek, S., Černík, M., & Varma, R. S. (2020). Microscopic Techniques for the Analysis of Micro and Nanostructures of Biopolymers and Their Derivatives. *Polymers*, *12*(3), 512. doi:10.3390/polym12030512 PMID:32120773

Ventura, J. A. (2015). Design and Synthesis of Polymeric Nanoparticles for Drug and Protein Delivery.

Verastegui, Y., Cheng, J., & Kolczynski, D. (2014). Multisubstrate Isotope Labeling and Metagenomic Analysis of Active. *mBio*, *5*(4), e01157-14. Advance online publication. doi:10.1128/mBio.01157-14 PMID:25028422

Verma, I. M., & Weitzman, M. D. (2005). GENE THERAPY: Twenty-First Century Medicine. *Annual Review of Biochemistry*, *74*(1), 711–738. doi:10.1146/annurev.biochem.74.050304.091637 PMID:15952901

Vijayan, R., Joseph, S., & Mathew, B. (2018). Indigofera tinctoria leaf extract mediated green synthesis of silver and gold nanoparticles and assessment of their anticancer, antimicrobial, antioxidant and catalytic properties. *Artificial Cells, Nanomedicine, and Biotechnology*, *46*(4), 861–871. doi:10.1080/21691401.2017.1345930 PMID:28681622

Vijayaram, S., Razafindralambo, H., Sun, Y.-Z., Vasantharaj, S., Ghafarifarsani, H., Hoseinifar, S. H., & Raeeszadeh, M. (2023). Applications of green synthesized metal nanoparticles – a review. *Biological Trace Element Research*. doi:10.100712011-023-03645-9 PMID:37046039

Vimaladevi, M., Divya, K. C., & Girigoswami, A. (2016). Liposomal nanoformulations of rhodamine for targeted photodynamic inactivation of multidrug resistant gram negative bacteria in sewage treatment plant. *Journal of Photochemistry and Photobiology. B, Biology*, *162*, 146–152. doi:10.1016/j.jphotobiol.2016.06.034 PMID:27371913

Vinhas, R., Mendes, R., Fernandes, A. R., & Baptista, P. V. (2017). Nanoparticles—Emerging potential for managing leukemia and lymphoma. *Frontiers in Bioengineering and Biotechnology*, *5*, 79. doi:10.3389/fbioe.2017.00079

Virupannanavar, D., Shah, M. A., & Assad, R. (2023). Harnessing biomedical applications of bionanomaterials through omics approach. In *Synthesis of Bionanomaterials for Biomedical Applications* (pp. 379–394). Elsevier. doi:10.1016/B978-0-323-91195-5.00003-9

Vivanco-Benavides, L. E., Martínez-González, C. L., Mercado-Zúñiga, C., & Torres-Torres, C. (2022). Machine learning and materials informatics approaches in the analysis of physical properties of carbon nanotubes: A review. *Computational Materials Science*, *201*, 110939. doi:10.1016/j.commatsci.2021.110939

Vivek, R., Thangam, R., Muthuchelian, K., Gunasekaran, P., Kaveri, K., & Kannan, S. (2012). Green biosynthesis of silver nanoparticles from Annona squamosa leaf extract and its in vitro cytotoxic effect on MCF-7 cells. *Process Biochemistry (Barking, London, England)*, *47*(12), 2405–2410. doi:10.1016/j.procbio.2012.09.025

Vojdani, S., Ghaderian, S. M. H., Zali, A., Rakhshan, A., Oraee Yazdani, S., Poursheikhani, A., Zerehpoush, F. B., & Sharifi, G. (2021). Altered expression of EGFR and miR-34a derived from serum and tumoral tissue was associated with glioblastoma multiform. *Experimental and Molecular Pathology*, *121*, 104655. doi:10.1016/j.yexmp.2021.104655 PMID:34062187

von Roemeling, C., Jiang, W., Chan, C. K., Weissman, I. L., & Kim, B. Y. S. (2017). Breaking Down the Barriers to Precision Cancer Nanomedicine. *Trends in Biotechnology*, *35*(2), 159–171. doi:10.1016/j.tibtech.2016.07.006 PMID:27492049

Vyas, S. P., & Khar, R. K. (2004). *Targeted & controlled drug delivery: novel carrier systems*. CBS publishers & distributors.

Wabler, M., Zhu, W., Hedayati, M., Attaluri, A., Zhou, H., Mihalic, J., Geyh, A., Deweese, T. L., Ivkov, R., & Artemov, D. (2014). Magnetic resonance imaging contrast of iron oxide nanoparticles developed for hyperthermia is dominated by iron content. *International Journal of Hyperthermia*, *30*(3), 192–200. doi:10.3109/02656736.2014.913321 PMID:24773041

Waidi, Y. O., Barua, R., & Datta, S. (2023). Metals, Polymers, Ceramics, Composites Biomaterials Used in Additive Manufacturing for Biomedical Applications. In A. Kumar, P. Kumar, A. Srivastava, & V. Goyat (Eds.), *Modeling, Characterization, and Processing of Smart Materials* (pp. 165–184). IGI Global. doi:10.4018/978-1-6684-9224-6.ch008

Walia, N., Dasgupta, N., Ranjan, S., Ramalingam, C., & Gandhi, M. (2019). Food-grade nanoencapsulation of vitamins. *Environmental Chemistry Letters*, *17*(2), 991–1002. doi:10.100710311-018-00855-9

Walia, S. S., & Prasad, D. N. (2022). Silver sulfadiazine: Action on burn wound sepsis and infections. *Journal of Drug Delivery and Therapeutics*, *12*(4), 154–161. doi:10.22270/jddt.v12i4.5419

Walkey, C. D., & Chan, W. C. W. (2012). Understanding and controlling the interaction of nanomaterials with proteins in a physiological environment. *Chemical Society Reviews*, *41*(7), 2780–2799. doi:10.1039/C1CS15233E PMID:22086677

Walkey, C. D., Olsen, J. B., Guo, H., Emili, A., & Chan, W. C. W. (2012). Nanoparticle size and surface chemistry determine serum protein adsorption and macrophage uptake. *Journal of the American Chemical Society*, *134*(4), 2139–2147. doi:10.1021/ja2084338 PMID:22191645

Walkey, C. D., Olsen, J. B., Song, F., Liu, R., Guo, H., Olsen, D. W. H., Cohen, Y., Emili, A., & Chan, W. C. W. (2014). Protein corona fingerprinting predicts the cellular interaction of gold and silver nanoparticles. *ACS Nano*, *8*(3), 2439–2455. doi:10.1021/nn406018q PMID:24517450

Wang, A. Z., Langer, R., & Farokhzad, O. C. (2012). Nanoparticle Delivery of Cancer Drugs. *Annual Review of Medicine*, *63*(1), 185–198. doi:10.1146/annurev-med-040210-162544 PMID:21888516

Wang, C., Ravi, S., Martinez, G. V., Chinnasamy, V., Raulji, P., Howell, M., Davis, Y., Mallela, J., Seehra, M. S., & Mohapatra, S. (2012). Dual-purpose magnetic micelles for MRI and gene delivery. *Journal of Controlled Release*, *163*(1), 82–92. doi:10.1016/j.jconrel.2012.04.030 PMID:22561339

Wang, H., Gu, W., Xiao, N., Ye, L., & Xu, Q. (2014). Chlorotoxin-conjugated graphene oxide for targeted delivery of an anticancer drug. *International Journal of Nanomedicine*, *9*(1), 1433–1442. doi:10.2147/IJN.S58783

Wang, H., Huff, T. B., Zweifel, D. A., He, W., Low, P. S., Wei, A., & Cheng, J. X. (2005). In vitro and in vivo two-photon luminescence imaging of single gold nanorods. *Proceedings of the National Academy of Sciences of the United States of America*, *102*(44), 15752–15756. doi:10.1073/pnas.0504892102 PMID:16239346

Wang, H., Qin, L., Zhang, X., Guan, J., & Mao, S. (2022). Mechanisms and challenges of nanocarriers as non-viral vectors of therapeutic genes for enhanced pulmonary delivery. *Journal of Controlled Release*, *352*, 970–993. doi:10.1016/j.jconrel.2022.10.061 PMID:36372386

Wang, J., Zhang, L., Peng, F., Shi, X., & Leong, D. T. (2018). Targeting Endothelial Cell Junctions with Negatively Charged Gold Nanoparticles. *Chemistry of Materials*, *30*(11), 3759–3767. doi:10.1021/acs.chemmater.8b00840

Wang, L., Sun, Q., Wang, X., Wen, T., Yin, J. J., Wang, P., Bai, R., Zhang, X. Q., Zhang, L. H., Lu, A. H., & Chen, C. (2015). Using Hollow Carbon Nanospheres as a Light-Induced Free Radical Generator to Overcome Chemotherapy Resistance. *Journal of the American Chemical Society*, *137*(5), 1947–1955. doi:10.1021/ja511560b PMID:25597855

Wang, L., Yuan, Y., Lin, S., Huang, J., Dai, J., Jiang, Q., Cheng, D., & Shuai, X. (2016). Photothermo-chemotherapy of cancer employing drug leakage-free gold nanoshells. *Biomaterials*, *78*, 40–49. doi:10.1016/j.biomaterials.2015.11.024

Wang, M., Zhang, M., Hu, X., Wang, W., Zhang, Y., Zhang, L., & Wang, J. (2023). Lipid-functionalized gold nanorods with plug-to-direct mitochondria targeting ligand for synergetic photothermal-chemotherapy of tumor therapy. *European Journal of Pharmaceutics and Biopharmaceutics*, *185*, 71–81. doi:10.1016/j.ejpb.2023.02.010 PMID:36828240

Wang, Q., Du, J., Ouyang, R., Liu, B., Miao, Y., & Li, Y. (2023). Recent advances in functional bismuth chalcogenide nanomaterials: Cancer theranostics, antibacterial and biosensing. *Coordination Chemistry Reviews*, *492*, 215281. doi:10.1016/j.ccr.2023.215281

Wang, S.-Y., Shi, X.-C., Zhu, G.-Y., Zhang, Y.-J., Jin, D.-Y., Zhou, Y.-D., Liu, F.-Q., & Laborda, P. (2021). Application of surface-enhanced Raman spectroscopy using silver and gold nanoparticles for the detection of pesticides in fruit and fruit juice. *Trends in Food Science & Technology*, *116*, 583–602. doi:10.1016/j.tifs.2021.08.006

Wang, W., Tasset, A., Pyatnitskiy, I., Mohamed, H. G., Taniguchi, R., Zhou, R., & Wang, H. (2022). Ultrasound triggered organic mechanoluminescence materials. *Advanced Drug Delivery Reviews*, *186*, 114343. doi:10.1016/j.addr.2022.114343 PMID:35580814

Wang, X., Fan, Y., Yan, J., & Yang, M. (2022). Engineering polyphenol-based polymeric nanoparticles for drug delivery and bioimaging. *Chemical Engineering Journal*, *439*, 135661. doi:10.1016/j.cej.2022.135661

Wang, X., Meng, X., Mao, K., Chen, H., Cong, X., Liu, F., Wang, J., Liu, S., Xin, Y., Zhu, G., Tan, H., Yang, Y.-G., & Sun, T. (2023). Maleimide as the PEG end-group promotes macrophage-targeted drug delivery of PEGylated nanoparticles in vivo by enhancing interaction with circulating erythrocytes. *Biomaterials*, *300*, 122187. doi:10.1016/j.biomaterials.2023.122187 PMID:37302279

Wang, X., Wang, X., Wang, M., Zhang, D., Yang, Q., Liu, T., Lei, R., Zhu, S., Zhao, Y., & Chen, C. (2018). Probing Adsorption Behaviors of BSA onto Chiral Surfaces of Nanoparticles. *Small*, *14*(1703982), 1703982. doi:10.1002mll.201703982 PMID:29573549

Wang, X., Zhong, X., Li, J., Liu, Z., & Cheng, L. (2021). Inorganic nanomaterials with rapid clearance for biomedical applications. *Chemical Society Reviews*, *50*(15), 8669–8742. doi:10.1039/D0CS00461H PMID:34156040

Wang, Y., Cai, R., & Chen, C. (2019). The Nano–Bio Interactions of Nanomedicines: Understanding the Biochemical Driving Forces and Redox Reactions. *Accounts of Chemical Research*, *52*(6), 1507–1518. doi:10.1021/acs.accounts.9b00126 PMID:31149804

Wang, Y., Ji, J.-Y., Guo, K., Zhang, T., Zhong, X.-C., Zhuang, Z.-M., Zhong, Y.-F., Lin, X.-F., Du, Y.-Z., Chen, J., & Tan, W.-Q. (2023). Gene liposome nanocomplex-loaded dermal substitute promotes diabetic chronic wound healing and angiogenesis in rat. *Biomedicine and Pharmacotherapy*, *163*, 114794. doi:10.1016/j.biopha.2023.114794 PMID:37121150

Wang, Y., Qin, Z., Buehler, M. J., & Xu, Z. (2016). Intercalated Water Layers Promote Thermal Dissipation at Bio-Nano Interfaces. *Nature Communications*, *7*(1), 12854. doi:10.1038/ncomms12854 PMID:27659484

Wang, Y., Wang, H., Zhu, X. X., Guan, Y., & Zhang, Y. (2020). Smart microneedle patches for rapid, and painless transdermal insulin delivery. *Journal of Materials Chemistry. B*, *8*(40), 9335–9342. doi:10.1039/D0TB01822H PMID:32969458

Wang, Y., Yuan, K., Shang, Z., Tan, G., Zhong, Q., He, Y., Miao, G., Lai, K., Li, Y., & Wang, X. (2023). Construction of nanohydrogels for enhanced delivery of hydrophilic and hydrophobic drugs and improving chemotherapy efficacy. *European Polymer Journal*, *186*, 111838. doi:10.1016/j.eurpolymj.2023.111838

Wang, Z., Deng, X., Ding, J., Zhou, W., Zheng, X., & Tang, G. (2018). Mechanisms of drug release in pH-sensitive micelles for tumor-targeted drug delivery system: A review. *International Journal of Pharmaceutics*, *535*(1–2), 253–260. doi:10.1016/j.ijpharm.2017.11.003 PMID:29113804

Wang, Z., Ma, W., Fu, X., Qi, Y., Zhao, Y., & Zhang, S. (2023). Development and applications of mRNA treatment based on lipid nanoparticles. *Biotechnology Advances*, *65*, 108130. doi:10.1016/j.biotechadv.2023.108130 PMID:36933868

Wang, Z., Qiao, R., Tang, N., Lu, Z., Wang, H., Zhang, Z., Xue, X., Huang, Z., Zhang, S., Zhang, G., & Li, Y. (2017). Active targeting theranostic iron oxide nanoparticles for MRI and magnetic resonance-guided focused ultrasound ablation of lung cancer. *Biomaterials*, *127*, 25–35. doi:10.1016/j.biomaterials.2017.02.037 PMID:28279919

Wan, X., Song, Y., Song, N., Li, J., Yang, L., Li, Y., & Tan, H. (2016). The preliminary study of immune superparamagnetic iron oxide nanoparticles for the detection of lung cancer in magnetic resonance imaging. *Carbohydrate Research*, *419*, 33–40. doi:10.1016/j.carres.2015.11.003 PMID:26649917

Warmińska, D. (2012). Volumetric and acoustic properties of D-mannitol in aqueous sodium or magnesium chloride solutions over the temperature range of 293.15–313.15 K. *Carbohydrate Research*, *349*, 44–51. doi:10.1016/j.carres.2011.12.004 PMID:22221791

Weber, C. F., Beahm, E. C., & Watson, J. S. (1999). Modeling thermodynamics and phase equilibria for aqueous solutions of trisodium phosphate. *Journal of Solution Chemistry*, *28*(11), 1207–1238. doi:10.1023/A:1021784515522

Wei, C., Xu, Y., Shen, Q., Li, R., Xiao, X., Saw, P. E., & Xu, X. (2023). Role of long non-coding RNAs (lncRNAs) in cancer: From subcellular localization to nanoparticles (NPs)-mediated targeted regulation. *Molecular Therapy. Nucleic Acids*, *33*, 774–793. doi:10.1016/j.omtn.2023.07.009 PMID:37655045

Weissleder, R., & Pittet, M. J. (2008). Imaging in the era of molecular oncology. *Nature 2008 452:7187*, *452*(7187), 580–589. doi:10.1038/nature06917

Wei, X., Han, Y., Quan, L., Liu, C., Liao, Y., & Eur, J. (2013). Oily nanosuspension for long-acting intramuscular delivery of curcumin didecanoate prodrug: Preparation, characterization and in vivo evaluation. *Pharmaceutical Sciences*, *49*(2), 286–293. doi:10.1016/j.ejps.2013.03.010 PMID:23542494

Wilhelm, S., Tavares, A. J., Dai, Q., Ohta, S., Audet, J., Dvorak, H. F., & Chan, W. C. W. (2016). Analysis of nanoparticle delivery to tumours. *Nature Reviews. Materials*, *1*(5), 16014. doi:10.1038/natrevmats.2016.14

Windell, D. L., Mourabit, S., Moger, J., Owen, S. F., Winter, M. J., & Tyler, C. R. (2023). The influence of size and surface chemistry on the bioavailability, tissue distribution and toxicity of gold nanoparticles in zebrafish (*Danio rerio*). *Ecotoxicology and Environmental Safety*, *260*, 115019. doi:10.1016/j.ecoenv.2023.115019 PMID:37269610

Woiski, C., Dobslaw, D., & Engesser, K. H. (2020). Isolation and characterization of 2-butoxyethanol degrading bacterial strains. *Biodegradation*, *31*(3), 153–169. doi:10.100710532-020-09900-3 PMID:32356147

Wolfram, J., Zhu, M., Yang, Y., Shen, J., Gentile, E., Paolino, D., Fresta, M., Nie, G., Chen, C., Shen, H., Ferrari, M., & Zhao, Y. (2015). Safety of Nanoparticles in Medicine. *Current Drug Targets*, *16*(14), 1671–1681. doi:10.2174/1389450115666140804124808 PMID:26601723

Wong, C. Y., Al-Salami, H., & Dass, C. R. (2018). Microparticles, microcapsules and microspheres: A review of recent developments and prospects for oral delivery of insulin. *International Journal of Pharmaceutics*, *537*(1-2), 223–244. doi:10.1016/j.ijpharm.2017.12.036 PMID:29288095

Wong, C. Y., Martinez, J., & Dass, C. R. (2016). Oral delivery of insulin for treatment of diabetes: Status quo, challenges and opportunities. *The Journal of Pharmacy and Pharmacology*, *68*(9), 1093–1108. doi:10.1111/jphp.12607 PMID:27364922

Wong, J. K., Mohseni, R., Hamidieh, A. A., MacLaren, R. E., Habib, N., & Seifalian, A. M. (2017). Will nanotechnology bring new hope for gene delivery? *Trends in Biotechnology*, *35*(5), 434–451. doi:10.1016/j.tibtech.2016.12.009 PMID:28108036

Wong, K. H., Lu, A., Chen, X., & Yang, Z. (2020). Natural ingredient-based polymeric nanoparticles for cancer treatment. *Molecules (Basel, Switzerland)*, *25*(16), 3620. doi:10.3390/molecules25163620 PMID:32784890

Wong, P. T., & Choi, S. K. (2015, May 13). Mechanisms of drug release in nanotherapeutic delivery systems. *Chemical Reviews*, *115*(9), 3388–3432. doi:10.1021/cr5004634 PMID:25914945

Wong, W. F., Ang, K. P., Sethi, G., & Looi, C. Y. (2023). Recent Advancement of Medical Patch for Transdermal Drug Delivery. *Medicina*, *59*(4), 778. doi:10.3390/medicina59040778 PMID:37109736

Wong, X. Y., Sena-Torralba, A., Álvarez-Diduk, R., Muthoosamy, K., & Merkoçi, A. (2020). Nanomaterials for Nanotheranostics: Tuning Their Properties According to Disease Needs. *ACS Nano*, *14*(3), 2585–2627. doi:10.1021/acsnano.9b08133 PMID:32031781

Wu, B., Feng, J., Zeng, T., Guo, Q., Zhang, Z., Ding, C., Tian, B., & Sai, S. (2022). Flurbiprofen loaded thermosensitive nanohydrogel for ophthalmic anti-inflammatory therapy. *Journal of Drug Delivery Science and Technology*, *70*, 103253. doi:10.1016/j.jddst.2022.103253

Wu, B., Wang, Y., Lee, Y. H., Horst, A., Wang, Z., Chen, D. R., Sureshkumar, R., & Tang, Y. J. (2010, February 15). Comparative eco-toxicities of nano-ZnO particles under aquatic and aerosol exposure modes. *Environmental Science & Technology*, *44*(4), 1484–1489. doi:10.1021/es9030497 PMID:20102184

Wu, D., Sedgwick, A. C., Gunnlaugsson, T., Akkaya, E. U., Yoon, J., & James, T. D. (2017). Fluorescent chemosensors: The past, present and future. *Chemical Society Reviews*, *46*(23), 7097–7472. doi:10.1039/C7CS00240H PMID:29019488

Wu, H., Nan, J., Yang, L., Park, H. J., & Li, J. (2023). Insulin-loaded liposomes packaged in alginate hydrogels promote the oral bioavailability of insulin. *Journal of Controlled Release*, *353*, 51–62. doi:10.1016/j.jconrel.2022.11.032 PMID:36410613

Wu, J., Du, X., Zhang, D., Cui, J., Zhang, X., Duan, X., Trant, J. F., & Li, Y. (2023). A nanodiamond chemotherapeutic folate receptor-targeting prodrug with triggerable drug release. *International Journal of Pharmaceutics*, *630*, 122432. doi:10.1016/j.ijpharm.2022.122432 PMID:36435503

Wu, J., Liu, H., Chen, W., Ma, B., & Ju, H. (2023). Device integration of electrochemical biosensors. *Nature Reviews Bioengineering*, *1*(5), 346–360. doi:10.103844222-023-00032-w PMID:37168735

Wu, M., Zhang, Z., Yong, J., Schenk, P. M., Tian, D., Xu, Z. P., & Zhang, R. (2022). Determination and Imaging of Small Biomolecules and Ions Using Ruthenium (II) Complex-Based Chemosensors. *Topics in Current Chemistry (Cham)*, *380*(5), 29. doi:10.100741061-022-00392-8 PMID:35695976

Wu, Q., Miao, W. S., Zhang, Y. D., Gao, H. J., & Hui, D. (2020). Mechanical properties of nanomaterials: A review. *Nanotechnology Reviews*, *9*(1), 259–273. doi:10.1515/ntrev-2020-0021

Wu, S., Gan, T., Xie, L., Deng, S., Liu, Y., Zhang, H., Hu, X., & Lei, L. (2022). Antibacterial performance of graphene oxide/alginate-based antisense hydrogel for potential therapeutic application in *Staphylococcus aureus* infection. *Biomaterials Advances*, *141*, 213121. doi:10.1016/j.bioadv.2022.213121 PMID:36162343

Wu, S., Li, Z., Han, J., & Han, S. (2011). Dual colored mesoporous silica nanoparticles with pH activable rhodamine-lactam for ratiometric sensing of lysosomal acidity. *Chemical Communications*, *47*(40), 11276–11278. doi:10.1039/c1cc14627k PMID:21931895

Wust, P., Hildebrandt, B., Sreenivasa, G., Rau, B., Gellermann, J., Riess, H., Felix, R., & Schlag, P. M. (2002). Hyperthermia in combined treatment of cancer. *The Lancet. Oncology*, *3*(8), 487–497. doi:10.1016/S1470-2045(02)00818-5 PMID:12147435

Wu, X., Tan, S., Xing, Y., Pu, Q., Wu, M., & Zhao, J. X. (2017). Graphene oxide as an efficient antimicrobial nanomaterial for eradicating multi-drug resistant bacteria in vitro and in vivo. *Colloids and Surfaces. B, Biointerfaces*, *157*, 1–9. doi:10.1016/j.colsurfb.2017.05.024 PMID:28554055

Wu, Y., Ali, M. R. K., Chen, K., Fang, N., & El-Sayed, M. A. (2019). Gold nanoparticles in biological optical imaging. *Nano Today*, *24*, 120–140. doi:10.1016/j.nantod.2018.12.006

Xie, H., & Smith, J. W. (2010). Fabrication of PLGA nanoparticles with a fluidic nanoprecipitation system. *Journal of Nanobiotechnology*, *8*(1), 1–7. doi:10.1186/1477-3155-8-18 PMID:20707919

Xie, J., Li, A., & Li, J. (2017). Advances in pH-sensitive polymers for smart insulin delivery. *Macromolecular Rapid Communications*, *38*(23), 1700413. doi:10.1002/marc.201700413 PMID:28976043

Xie, L., Jin, W., Chen, H., & Zhang, Q. (2019). Superparamagnetic iron oxide nanoparticles for cancer diagnosis and therapy. *Journal of Biomedical Nanotechnology*, *15*(2), 215–416. doi:10.1166/jbn.2019.2678

Xie, S., Ai, L., Cui, C., Fu, T., Cheng, X., Qu, F., & Tan, W. (2021). Functional aptamer-embedded nanomaterials for diagnostics and therapeutics. *ACS Applied Materials & Interfaces*, *13*(8), 9542–9560. doi:10.1021/acsami.0c19562 PMID:33595277

Xiong, J., Dong, X., Li, S., Jiang, F., Chen, J., Yu, S., Dong, B., & Su, Q. (2021). Effects of (Pro) renin receptor on diabetic cardiomyopathy pathological processes in rats via the PRR-AMPK-YAP pathway. *Frontiers in Physiology*, *12*, 657378. doi:10.3389/fphys.2021.657378 PMID:34122131

Xu, C., Dobson, H. E., Yu, M., Gong, W., Sun, X., Park, K. S., Kennedy, A., Zhou, X., Xu, J., Xu, Y., Tai, A. W., Lei, Y. L., & Moon, J. J. (2023). STING agonist-loaded mesoporous manganese-silica nanoparticles for vaccine applications. *Journal of Controlled Release*, *357*, 84–93. doi:10.1016/j.jconrel.2023.03.036 PMID:36948420

Xu, C., Li, S., Chen, J., Wang, H., Li, Z., Deng, Q., Li, J., Wang, X., Xiong, Y., Zhang, Z., Yang, X., & Li, Z. (2023). Doxorubicin and erastin co-loaded hydroxyethyl starch-polycaprolactone nanoparticles for synergistic cancer therapy. *Journal of Controlled Release*, *356*, 256–271. doi:10.1016/j.jconrel.2023.03.001 PMID:36871643

Xue, N., Ding, X., Huang, R., Jiang, R., Huang, H., Pan, X., Min, W., Chen, J., Duan, J. A., Liu, P., & Wang, Y. (2022). Bone tissue engineering in the treatment of bone defects. *Pharmaceuticals (Basel, Switzerland)*, *15*(7), 879. doi:10.3390/ph15070879 PMID:35890177

Xu, J., & Chow, E. K.-H. (2023). Biomedical applications of nanodiamonds: From drug-delivery to diagnostics. *SLAS Technology*, *28*(4), 214–222. doi:10.1016/j.slast.2023.03.007 PMID:37004790

Xu, J., Xiang, L., Liu, Q., Gilmore, H., Wu, J., Tang, J., & Madabhushi, A. (2016). Stacked sparse autoencoder (SSAE) for nuclei detection on breast cancer histopathology images. *IEEE Transactions on Medical Imaging*, *35*(1), 119–130. doi:10.1109/TMI.2015.2458702 PMID:26208307

Xu, L., Wang, J., Wang, J., Lu, S.-Y., Yang, Q., Chen, C., Yang, H., Hong, F., Wu, C., Zhao, Q., Cao, Y., & Liu, H. (2022). Polypyrrole-iron phosphate-glucose oxidase-based nanocomposite with cascade catalytic capacity for tumor synergistic apoptosis-ferroptosis therapy. *Chemical Engineering Journal*, *131671*(427), 131671. doi:10.1016/j.cej.2021.131671

Xu, L., Wang, X., Wang, W., Sun, M., Choi, W. J., Kim, J. Y., Hao, C., Li, S., Qu, A., Lu, M., Wu, X., Colombari, F. M., Gomes, W. R., Blanco, A. L., de Moura, A. F., Guo, X., Kuang, H., Kotov, N. A., & Xu, C. (2022). Enantiomer-dependent immunological response to chiral nanoparticles. *Nature*, *601*(7893), 366–373. doi:10.103841586-021-04243-2 PMID:35046606

Xu, Q., Akkurt, N., Zou, Z., Liu, Y., Feng, J., Yu, C., Ding, Y., Xiong, Y., Zhou, J., Zang, Y., & Ding, Y. (2020). Synthesis and characterization of disodium hydrogen phosphate dodecahydrate-lauric-palmitic acid used for indoor energy storage floor units. *Journal of Thermal Science*, *29*(2), 477–485. doi:10.100711630-020-1273-7

Xu, Y., & Schoonen, M. A. A. (2000). The Absolute Energy Positions of Conduction and Valence Bands of Selected Semiconducting Minerals. *The American Mineralogist*, *85*(3-4), 543–556. doi:10.2138/am-2000-0416

Xu, Y., Wang, X., Zhang, W. L., Lv, F., & Guo, S. (2018). Recent progress in two-dimensional inorganic quantum dots. *Chemical Society Reviews*, *47*(2), 586–625. doi:10.1039/C7CS00500H PMID:29115355

Yadav, D., Amini, F., & Ehrmann, A. (2020). Recent advances in carbon nanofibers and their applications–a review. *European Polymer Journal*, *138*, 109963. doi:10.1016/j.eurpolymj.2020.109963

Yadav, D., Anwar, M. F., Garg, V., Kardam, H., Beg, M. N., Suri, S., Gaur, S., & Asif, M. (2014). Development of polymeric nanopaclitaxel and comparison with free paclitaxel for effects on cell proliferation of MCF-7 and B16F0 carcinoma cells. *Asian Pacific Journal of Cancer Prevention*, *15*(5), 2335–2340. doi:10.7314/APJCP.2014.15.5.2335 PMID:24716980

Yang, W., Liang, H., Ma, S., Wang, D., & Huang, J. (2019). Gold nanoparticle based photothermal therapy: Development and application for effective cancer treatment. *Sustainable Materials and Technologies*, (22), e00109. doi:10.1016/j.susmat.2019.e00109

Yang, F., Xue, J., Wang, G., & Diao, Q. (2022). Nanoparticle-based drug delivery systems for the treatment of cardiovascular diseases. *Frontiers in Pharmacology*, *13*, 999404. doi:10.3389/fphar.2022.999404 PMID:36172197

Yang, H. W., Hua, M. Y., Liu, H. L., Huang, C. Y., Tsai, R. Y., Lu, Y. J., Chen, J.-Y., Tang, H.-J., Hsien, H.-Y., Chang, Y.-S., Yen, T.-C., Chen, P.-Y., & Wei, K. C. (2011). Self-protecting core-shell magnetic nanoparticles for targeted, traceable, long half-life delivery of BCNU to gliomas. *Biomaterials*, *32*(27), 6523–6532. doi:10.1016/j.biomaterials.2011.05.047 PMID:21645920

Yang, H. Y., Jang, M. S., Li, Y., Lee, J. H., & Lee, D. S. (2017). Multifunctional and Redox-Responsive Self-Assembled Magnetic Nanovectors for Protein Delivery and Dual-Modal Imaging. *ACS Applied Materials & Interfaces*, *9*(22), 19184–19192. doi:10.1021/acsami.7b03747

Yang, J., Dai, D., Lou, X., Ma, L., Wang, B., & Yang, Y. W. (2020). Supramolecular nanomaterials based on hollow mesoporous drug carriers and macrocycle-capped CuS nanogates for synergistic chemo-photothermal therapy. *Theranostics*, *10*(2), 615–629. doi:10.7150/thno.40066 PMID:31903141

Yang, T., Yao, Q., Cao, F., Liu, Q., Liu, B., & Wang, X. H. (2016). Silver nanoparticles inhibit the function of hypoxia-inducible factor-1 and target genes: Insight into the cytotoxicity and antiangiogenesis. *International Journal of Nanomedicine*, *11*, 6679–6692. doi:10.2147/IJN.S109695 PMID:27994464

Yang, X., Mo, W., Shi, Y., Fang, X., Xu, Y., He, X., & Xu, Y. (2023). Fumaria officinalis-loaded chitosan nanoparticles dispersed in an alginate hydrogel promote diabetic wounds healing by upregulating VEGF, TGF-β, and b-FGF genes: A preclinical investigation. *Heliyon*, *9*(7), e17704. doi:10.1016/j.heliyon.2023.e17704 PMID:37519642

Yang, Y., Jiang, Y., Xu, J., & Yu, J. (2007). Conducting polymeric nanoparticles synthesized in reverse micelles and their gas sensitivity based on quartz crystal microbalance. *Polymer*, *48*(15), 4459–4465. doi:10.1016/j.polymer.2007.06.005

Yan, Q., Yuan, W., Sun, X., Zhang, M.-J., Cen, F., Zhou, S.-Y., Wu, W.-B., Xu, Y.-C., Tong, L.-H., & Ma, Z.-H. (2018). Asparaginyl endopeptidase enhances pancreatic ductal adenocarcinoma cell invasion in an exosome-dependent manner and correlates with poor prognosis. *International Journal of Oncology*, *52*(5), 1651–1660. doi:10.3892/ijo.2018.4318

Yan, T., Su, M., Wang, Z., & Zhang, J. (2023). Second Near-Infrared Plasmonic Nanomaterials for Photoacoustic Imaging and Photothermal Therapy. *Small*, *19*(30), 2300539. doi:10.1002mll.202300539 PMID:37060228

Yao, D., Liu, N. N., & Mo, B. W. (2020). Assessment of proliferation, migration and differentiation potentials of bone marrow mesenchymal stem cells labeling with silica-coated and amine-modified superparamagnetic iron oxide nanoparticles. *Cytotechnology*, *72*(4), 513–525. doi:10.100710616-020-00397-5 PMID:32394163

Yao, D., Wu, L. A. S., Zhang, M., Fang, H., Li, D., Sun, Y., Gao, X., & Lu, C. (2022). Stretchable vertical graphene arrays for electronic skin with multifunctional sensing capabilities. *Chemical Engineering Journal*, *431*, 134038. doi:10.1016/j.cej.2021.134038

Yao, Y., Su, Z., Liang, Y., & Zhang, N. (2015). pH-Sensitive carboxymethyl chitosan-modified cationic liposomes for sorafenib and siRNA co-delivery. *International Journal of Nanomedicine*, 6185–6198. doi:10.2147/IJN.S90524

Yaqoob, A. A., Ahmad, H., Parveen, T., Ahmad, A., Oves, M., Ismail, I. M., Qari, H. A., Umar, K., & Mohamad Ibrahim, M. N. (2020). Recent advances in metal decorated nanomaterials and their various biological applications: A review. *Frontiers in Chemistry*, *8*, 341. doi:10.3389/fchem.2020.00341 PMID:32509720

Yasmin Begum, M. (2023). Co-loading of doxorubicin and gemcitabine on folic acid functionalized carbon nanotubes; a molecular dynamics simulation study. *Journal of Molecular Liquids*, *384*, 122244. doi:10.1016/j.molliq.2023.122244

Yeh, Y. C., Huang, T. H., Yang, S. C., Chen, C. C., & Fang, J. Y. (2020). Nano-based drug delivery or targeting to eradicate bacteria for infection mitigation: A review of recent advances. *Frontiers in Chemistry*, *8*, 286. doi:10.3389/fchem.2020.00286 PMID:32391321

Ye, L., Cao, Z., Liu, X., Cui, Z., Li, Z., Liang, Y., Zhu, S., & Wu, S. (2022). Noble metal-based nanomaterials as antibacterial agents. *Journal of Alloys and Compounds*, *164091*, 164091. doi:10.1016/j.jallcom.2022.164091

Yeom, J.-H., Shin, E., Jin, H., Liu, H., Luo, Y., Nam, Y., Ryu, M., Song, W., Chi, H., Kim, J., Lee, K., & Bae, J. (2023). Aptamer-conjugated gold nanoparticles platform as the intracellular delivery of antibodies for cancer therapy. *Journal of Industrial and Engineering Chemistry*, *126*, 480–491. doi:10.1016/j.jiec.2023.06.036

Yetisgin, A. A., Cetinel, S., Zuvin, M., Kosar, A., & Kutlu, O. (2020). Therapeutic Nanoparticles and Their Targeted Delivery Applications. *Molecules (Basel, Switzerland)*, *25*(9), 2193. doi:10.3390/molecules25092193 PMID:32397080

Ying, N., Lin, X., Xie, M., & Zeng, D. (2022). Effect of surface ligand modification on the properties of anti-tumor nanocarrier. *Colloids and Surfaces. B, Biointerfaces*, *220*, 112944. doi:10.1016/j.colsurfb.2022.112944 PMID:36274398

Yingngam, B. (2023a). Chapter 11 - Modern solvent-free microwave extraction with essential oil optimization and structure-activity relationships. In R. Atta ur (Ed.), Studies in Natural Products Chemistry (Vol. 77, pp. 365-420): Elsevier. doi:10.1016/B978-0-323-91294-5.00011-7

Yingngam, B. (2023b). New Drug Discovery. In M. S. Aslam & M. A. Ahmad (Eds.), *Multidisciplinary Applications of Natural Science for Drug Discovery and Integrative Medicine* (pp. 134–184). IGI Global. doi:10.4018/978-1-6684-9463-9.ch005

Yingngam, B., Chiangsom, A., Pharikarn, P., Vonganakasame, K., Kanoknitthiran, V., Rungseevijitprapa, W., & Prasitpuriprecha, C. (2019). Optimization of menthol-loaded nanocapsules for skin application using the response surface methodology. *Journal of Drug Delivery Science and Technology*, *53*, 101138. doi:10.1016/j.jddst.2019.101138

Yin, H., Kanasty, R. L., Eltoukhy, A. A., Vegas, A. J., Dorkin, J. R., & Anderson, D. G. (2014). Non-viral vectors for gene-based therapy. *Nature Reviews. Genetics*, *15*(8), 541–555. doi:10.1038/nrg3763 PMID:25022906

Yin, N., Wang, X., Yang, T., Ding, Y., Li, L., Zhao, S., Li, P., Xu, X., & Zhu, L. (2021). Multifunctional Fe_3O_4 cluster@ quantum dot-embedded mesoporous SiO_2 nanoplatform probe for cancer cell fluorescence-labelling detection and photothermal therapy. *Ceramics International*, *47*(6), 8271–8278. doi:10.1016/j.ceramint.2020.11.188

Yi, Z., Ye, J., Kikugawa, N., Kako, T., Ouyang, S., Stuart-Williams, H., Yang, H., Cao, J., Luo, W., Li, Z., Liu, Y., & Withers, R. L. (2010). An Orthophosphate Semiconductor with Photooxidation Properties under Visible-Light Irradiation. *Nature Materials*, *9*(7), 559–564. doi:10.1038/nmat2780 PMID:20526323

You, C. C., De, M., & Rotello, V. M. (2005). Monolayer-protected nanoparticle–protein interactions. *Current Opinion in Chemical Biology*, *9*(6), 639–646. doi:10.1016/j.cbpa.2005.09.012 PMID:16226485

Younas, A., Dong, Z., Hou, Z., Asad, M., Li, M., & Zhang, N. (2023). A chitosan/fucoidan nanoparticle-loaded pullulan microneedle patch for differential drug release to promote wound healing. *Carbohydrate Polymers*, *306*, 120593. doi:10.1016/j.carbpol.2023.120593 PMID:36746584

Yuan, H., Zhou, L., Qi, Z., Zhang, C., & Wang, C. (2022). Preparation of pH-responsive solanesol-based poly (glutamic acid) micellar carrier for doxorubicin delivery. *Materials Today. Communications*, *33*, 104800. doi:10.1016/j.mtcomm.2022.104800

Yuan, J., Zhang, Y., Zhang, Y., Mo, Y., & Zhang, Q. (2021). Effects of metal nanoparticles on tight junction-associated proteins via HIF-1α/miR-29b/MMPs pathway in human epidermal keratinocytes. *Particle and Fibre Toxicology*, *18*(1), 1–22. doi:10.118612989-021-00405-2 PMID:33407654

Yuan, L., Chen, Q., Riviere, J. E., & Lin, Z. (2023). Pharmacokinetics and tumor delivery of nanoparticles. *Journal of Drug Delivery Science and Technology*, *83*, 104404. doi:10.1016/j.jddst.2023.104404 PMID:38037664

Yue, N. N., Xu, H. M., Xu, J., Zhu, M. Z., Zhang, Y., Tian, C. M., Nie, Y. Q., Yao, J., Liang, Y. J., Li, D. F., & Wang, L. S. (2023). Application of Nanoparticles in the Diagnosis of Gastrointestinal Diseases: A Complete Future Perspective. *International Journal of Nanomedicine*, *18*, 4143–4170. doi:10.2147/IJN.S413141 PMID:37525691

Yu, G., He, X., Li, X., & Wu, Y. (2022). Driving neoantigen-based cancer vaccines for personalized immunotherapy into clinic: A burdensome journey to promising land. *Biomedicine and Pharmacotherapy*, *153*, 113464. doi:10.1016/j.biopha.2022.113464 PMID:36076493

Yu, L. (2001). Amorphous pharmaceutical solids: Preparation, characterization and stabilization. *Advanced Drug Delivery Reviews*, *48*(1), 27–42. doi:10.1016/S0169-409X(01)00098-9 PMID:11325475

Yu, M., Wu, J., Shi, J., & Farokhzad, O. C. (2016). Nanotechnology for protein delivery: Overview and perspectives. *Journal of Controlled Release*, *240*, 24–37. doi:10.1016/j.jconrel.2015.10.012 PMID:26458789

Yusuf, A., Almotairy, A. R. Z., Henidi, H., Alshehri, O. Y., & Aldughaim, M. S. (2023). Nanoparticles as Drug Delivery Systems: A Review of the implication of nanoparticles' physicochemical properties on responses in biological systems. *Polymers*, *15*(7), 1596. doi:10.3390/polym15071596 PMID:37050210

Zahid, M., Kim, B., Hussain, R., Amin, R., & Park, S. H. (2013). DNA nanotechnology: A future perspective. *Nanoscale Research Letters*, *8*(1), 1–13. doi:10.1186/1556-276X-8-119 PMID:23497147

Zamani, P., Mashreghi, M., Rezazade Bazaz, M., Zargari, S., Alizadeh, F., Dorrigiv, M., Abdoli, A., Aminianfar, H., Hatamipour, M., Zarqui, J., Behboodiar, S., Samsami, Y., Sokhangouy, S. K., Sefidbakht, Y., Uskoković, V., Rezayat, S. M., Jaafari, M. R., & Mozaffari-Jovin, S. (2023). Characterization of stability, safety and immunogenicity of the mRNA lipid nanoparticle vaccine Iribovax® against COVID-19 in nonhuman primates. *Journal of Controlled Release*, *360*, 316–334. doi:10.1016/j.jconrel.2023.06.025 PMID:37355212

Zaman, M., Ahmad, E., Qadeer, A., Rabbani, G., & Khan, R. H. (2014). Nanoparticles in relation to peptide and protein aggregation. *International Journal of Nanomedicine*, *9*, 899–912. PMID:24611007

Zarrintaj, P., Saeb, M. R., Ramakrishna, S., & Mozafari, M. (2018). Biomaterials selection for neuroprosthetics. *Current Opinion in Biomedical Engineering*, *6*, 99–109. doi:10.1016/j.cobme.2018.05.003

Zeghoud, S., Chandran, D., Amor, I. B., Hemmami, H., Mohankumar, P., & Emran, T. B. (2023). Nanotechnology and nanomaterials in the treatment and diagnosis of cancer: Correspondence. *Annals of Medicine and Surgery (London)*, *85*(5), 2258–2260. doi:10.1097/MS9.0000000000000677

Zeng, Q., Qi, X., Shi, G., Zhang, M., & Haick, H. (2022). Wound dressing: From nanomaterials to diagnostic dressings and healing evaluations. *ACS Nano*, *16*(2), 1708–1733. doi:10.1021/acsnano.1c08411 PMID:35050565

Zhang, L., Pornpattananangkul, D., Hu, C.-M.J., & Huang, C.-M. (2010) *Development of Nanoparticles for Antimicrobial Drug Delivery*. Research Gate.

Zhang, H., Gu, Z., Li, W., Guo, L., Wang, L., Guo, L., Wang, L., Guo, L., Ma, S., Han, B., & Chang, J. (2022). pH-sensitive O-carboxymethyl chitosan/sodium alginate nanohydrogel for enhanced oral delivery of insulin. *International Journal of Biological Macromolecules*, *223*, 433–445. doi:10.1016/j.ijbiomac.2022.10.274 PMID:36347366

Zhang, H., Ji, Z., Xia, T., Meng, H., Low-Kam, C., Liu, R., Pokhrel, S., Lin, S., Wang, X., Liao, Y.-P., Wang, M., Li, L., Rallo, R., Damoiseaux, R., Telesca, D., Mädler, L., Cohen, Y., Zink, J. I., & Nel, A. E. (2012). Nel, A. E. Use of Metal Oxide Nanoparticle Band Gap To Develop a Predictive Paradigm for Oxidative Stress and Acute Pulmonary Inflammation. *ACS Nano*, *6*(5), 4349–4368. doi:10.1021/nn3010087 PMID:22502734

Zhang, H., Wang, T., He, W., Wang, J., & Li, X. (2022). Irinotecan loaded ROS-responsive liposomes containing thioether phosphatidylcholine for improving anticancer activity. *Journal of Drug Delivery Science and Technology*, *71*, 103321. doi:10.1016/j.jddst.2022.103321

Zhang, J., Mou, L., & Jiang, X. (2020). Surface chemistry of gold nanoparticles for health-related applications. *Chemical Science (Cambridge)*, *11*(4), 923–936. doi:10.1039/C9SC06497D PMID:34084347

Zhang, J., Pan, Y., Shi, Q., Zhang, G., Jiang, L., Dong, X., Gu, K., Wang, H., Zhang, X., Yang, N., Li, Y., Xiong, J., Yi, T., Peng, M., Song, Y., Fan, Y., Cui, J., Chen, G., Tan, W., & Zhou, C. (2022). Paclitaxel liposome for injection (Lipusu) plus cisplatin versus gemcitabine plus cisplatin in the frst-line treatment of locally advanced or metastatic lung squamous cell carcinoma: A multicenter, randomized, open-label, parallel controlled clinical study. *Cancer Communications (London, England)*, *42*(1), 3–16. doi:10.1002/cac2.12225

Zhang, J., Yue, X., Zeng, Y., Hua, E., Wang, M., & Sun, Y. (2018). Bacillus amyloliquefaciens levan and its silver nanoparticles with antimicrobial properties. *Biotechnology, Biotechnological Equipment*, *32*(6), 1583–1589. doi:10.1080/13102818.2018.1523690

Zhang, K., Liu, X., Samuel Ravi, S. O. A., Ramachandran, A., Aziz Ibrahim, I. A., Nassir, A. M., & Yao, J. (2019). Synthesis of silver nanoparticles (Ag-NPs) from leaf extract of Salvia miltiorrhiza and its anticancer potential in human prostate cancer LNCaP cell lines. *Artificial Cells, Nanomedicine, and Biotechnology*. doi:10.1080/21691401.2019.1638792 PMID:31299869

Zhang, L. X., Xie, X. X., Liu, D. Q., Xu, Z. P., & Liu, R. T. (2018). Efficient co-delivery of neo-epitopes using dispersion-stable layered double hydroxide nanoparticles for enhanced melanoma immunotherapy. *Biomaterials*, *174*, 54–66. doi:10.1016/j.biomaterials.2018.05.015

Zhang, L., Beatty, A., Lu, L., Abdalrahman, A., Makris, T. M., Wang, G., & Wang, Q. (2020). Microfluidic-assisted polymer-protein assembly to fabricate homogeneous functional nanoparticles. *Materials Science and Engineering C*, *110768*(111), 110768. doi:10.1016/j.msec.2020.110768

Zhang, L., Gu, F. X., Chan, J. M., Wang, A. Z., Langer, R. S., & Farokhzad, O. C. (2008). Nanoparticles in medicine: Therapeutic applications and developments. *Clinical Pharmacology and Therapeutics*, *83*(5), 761–769. doi:10.1038j.clpt.6100400

Zhang, L., Jiang, Y., Ding, Y., Povey, M., & York, D. (2007, June). Investigation into the antibacterial behaviour of suspensions of ZnO nanoparticles (ZnO nanofluids). *Journal of Nanoparticle Research*, *9*(3), 479–489. doi:10.100711051-006-9150-1

Zhang, L., Ji, X., Su, Y., Zhai, X., Xu, H., Song, B., Jiang, A., Guo, D., & He, Y. (2021). Fluorescent silicon nanoparticles-based nanotheranostic agents for rapid diagnosis and treatment of bacteria-induced keratitis. *Nano Research*, *14*(1), 52–58. doi:10.100712274-020-3039-7

Zhang, M., Li, X. H., Gong, Y. D., Zhao, N. M., & Zhang, X. F. (2002). Properties and biocompatibility of chitosan films modified by blending with PEG. *Biomaterials*, *23*(13), 2641–2648. doi:10.1016/S0142-9612(01)00403-3 PMID:12059013

Zhang, M., Wang, W., Cui, Y., Zhou, N., & Shen, J. (2018). Magnetofluorescent Carbon Quantum Dot Decorated Multiwalled Carbon Nanotubes for Dual-Modal Targeted Imaging in Chemo-Photothermal Synergistic Therapy. *ACS Biomaterials Science & Engineering*, *4*(1), 151–162. doi:10.1021/acsbiomaterials.7b00531

Zhang, R., & James, T. D. (2023). Responsive probes and molecular bioimaging. *Chemistry, an Asian Journal*, *18*(5), e202300058. doi:10.1002/asia.202300058 PMID:36722771

Zhang, W. (2016). Application of Fe 3 O 4 nanoparticles functionalized carbon nanotubes for electrochemical sensing of DNA hybridization. *Journal of Applied Electrochemistry*, *46*(5), 559–566. doi:10.100710800-016-0952-2

Zhang, W., Singh, R., Wang, Z., Li, G., Xie, Y., Jha, R., Marques, C., Zhang, B., & Kumar, S. (2023). Humanoid shaped optical fiber plasmon biosensor functionalized with graphene oxide/multi-walled carbon nanotubes for histamine detection. *Optics Express*, *31*(7), 11788–11803. doi:10.1364/OE.486844 PMID:37155805

Zhang, W., Yang, Y., & Cui, B. (2021). New perspectives on the roles of nanoscale surface topography in modulating intracellular signaling. *Current Opinion in Solid State and Materials Science*, *25*(1), 100873. doi:10.1016/j.cossms.2020.100873 PMID:33364912

Zhang, X. Q., Xu, X., Bertrand, N., Pridgen, E., Swami, A., & Farokhzad, O. C. (2012). Interactions of nanomaterials and biological systems: Implications to personalized nanomedicine. *Advanced Drug Delivery Reviews*, *64*(13), 1363–1384. doi:10.1016/j.addr.2012.08.005 PMID:22917779

Zhang, X., Meng, L., Lu, Q., Fei, Z., & Dyson, P. J. (2009). Targeted delivery and controlled release of doxorubicin to cancer cells using modified single-wall carbon nanotubes. *Biomaterials*, *30*(30), 6041–6047. doi:10.1016/j.biomaterials.2009.07.025 PMID:19643474

Zhang, X., Wei, Z., Ding, Z., Lv, W., Li, J., Li, X., Liu, H., Yu, P., Yang, X., & Gan, L. (2023). Boosting doxil-based chemoimmunotherapy via reprogramming tumor-associated macrophages. *Chemical Engineering Journal*, *451*, 138971. doi:10.1016/j.cej.2022.138971

Zhang, Y., Li, M., Gao, X., Chen, Y., & Liu, T. (2019). Nanotechnology in cancer diagnosis: Progress, challenges and opportunities. *Journal of Hematology & Oncology*, *12*(1), 1–13. doi:10.118613045-019-0833-3 PMID:31847897

Zhang, Y., & Liu, H. (2019). Nanowires for High-Efficiency, Low-Cost Solar Photovoltaics. *Crystals*, *9*(2), 87. doi:10.3390/cryst9020087

Zhang, Y., Wang, P., Wang, Y., Li, J., Qiao, D., Chen, R., Yang, W., & Yan, F. (2021). Gold nanoparticles promote the bone regeneration of periodontal ligament stem cell sheets through activation of autophagy. *International Journal of Nanomedicine*, *16*, 61–73. doi:10.2147/IJN.S282246 PMID:33442250

Zhang, Y., Wang, R., Dong, Y., Huang, G., Ji, B., & Wang, Q. (2020). Assessment of biotin interference in thyroid function tests. *Medicine*, *99*(9), e19232. doi:10.1097/MD.0000000000019232 PMID:32118725

Zhang, Z., Fu, X., Wang, Y., Wang, J., Feng, S., Zhao, Z., Zheng, L., Zhang, J., Zhang, X., & Peng, Y. (2023). In vivo anti-hepatitis B activity of Artemisia argyi essential oil-loaded nanostructured lipid carriers. Study of its mechanism of action by network pharmacology and molecular docking. *Phytomedicine*, *116*, 154848. doi:10.1016/j.phymed.2023.154848 PMID:37163901

Zhang, Z., Gao, F., Bu, H., Xiao, J., & Li, Y. (2012). Solid lipid nanoparticles loading candesartan cilexetil enhance oral bioavailability: In vitro characteristics and absorption mechanism in rats. *Nanomedicine (London)*, *8*(5), 740–744. doi:10.1016/j.nano.2011.08.016 PMID:21930110

Zhao, L., Xiao, C., Ding, J., He, P., Tang, Z., Pang, X., Zhuang, X., & Chen, X. (2013). Facile one-pot synthesis of glucose-sensitive nanogel via thiol-ene click chemistry for self-regulated drug delivery. *Acta Biomaterialia*, *9*(5), 6535–6543. doi:10.1016/j.actbio.2013.01.040 PMID:23403168

Zhao, M. X., & Zeng, E. Z. (2015). Application of functional quantum dot nanoparticles as fluorescence probes in cell labeling and tumor diagnostic imaging. *Nanoscale Research Letters*, *10*(1), 1–9. doi:10.118611671-015-0873-8 PMID:25897311

Zhao, R., & Sun, Y. (2018). Polymeric Flexible Immunosensor Based on Piezoresistive Micro-Cantilever with PEDOT/PSS Conductive Layer. *Sensors (Basel)*, *18*(2), 451. doi:10.339018020451 PMID:29401669

Zhao, W., Cao, H., Wan, C. S., & Zhang, W. B. (2002). Application of nanotechnology in biomedical sciences. *Di Yi Jun Yi Da Xue Xue Bao*, *22*(5), 461–463. PMID:12390718

Zhao, W., Hanson, L., Lou, H. Y., Akamatsu, M., Chowdary, P. D., Santoro, F., Marks, J. R., Grassart, A., Drubin, D. G., Cui, Y., & Cui, B. (2017). Nanoscale manipulation of membrane curvature for probing endocytosis in live cells. *Nature Nanotechnology*, *12*(8), 750–756. doi:10.1038/nnano.2017.98 PMID:28581510

Zhao, Y., Pang, B., Detering, L., Luehmann, H., Yang, M., Black, K., Sultan, D., Xia, Y., & Liu, Y. (2018). Melanocortin 1 Receptor Targeted Imaging of Melanoma With Gold Nanocages and Positron Emission Tomography. *Molecular Imaging*, *17*. Advance online publication. doi:10.1177/1536012118775827 PMID:29873290

Zhao, Y., Wang, C., Wang, L., Yang, Q., Tang, W., She, Z., & Deng, Y. (2012). A frustrating problem: Accelerated blood clearance of PEGylated solid lipid nanoparticles following subcutaneous injection in rats. *European Journal of Pharmaceutics and Biopharmaceutics*, *81*(3), 506–513. doi:10.1016/j.ejpb.2012.04.023 PMID:22580209

Zhao, Z., Anselmo, A. C., & Mitragotri, S. (2022). Viral vector-based gene therapies in the clinic. *Bioengineering & Translational Medicine*, *7*(1), e10258. doi:10.1002/btm2.10258 PMID:35079633

Zhao, Z., Ukidve, A., Kim, J., & Mitragotri, S. (2020). Targeting Strategies for Tissue-Specific Drug Delivery. *Cell*, *181*(1), 151–167. doi:10.1016/j.cell.2020.02.001 PMID:32243788

Zheng, X., Zhang, P., Fu, Z., Meng, S., Dai, L., & Yang, H. (2021). Applications of nanomaterials in tissue engineering. *RSC Advances*, *11*(31), 19041–19058. doi:10.1039/D1RA01849C PMID:35478636

Zheng, Y., Hong, X., Wang, J., Feng, L., Fan, T., Guo, R., & Zhang, H. (2021). 2D Nanomaterials for Tissue Engineering and Regenerative Nanomedicines: Recent Advances and Future Challenges. *Advanced Healthcare Materials*, *10*(7), 2001743. doi:10.1002/adhm.202001743 PMID:33511775

Zhong, Y., Peng, F., Wei, X., Zhou, Y., Wang, J., Jiang, X., Su, Y., Su, S., Lee, T., & He, Y. (2012). Microwave-assisted synthesis of biofunctional and fluorescent silicon nanoparticles using proteins as hydrophilic ligands. *Angewandte Chemie International Edition*, *51*(34), 8485–8489. doi:10.1002/anie.201202085

Zhou, G., Lu, Y., Zhang, H., Chen, Y., Yu, Y., Gao, J., & Zhong, Y. (2013). A novel pulsed drug-delivery system: Polyelectrolyte layer-by-layer coating of chitosan–alginate microgels. *International Journal of Nanomedicine*, *8*, 877. PMID:23486565

Zhou, H., Hernandez, C., Goss, M., Gawlik, A., & Exner, A. A. (2015). Biomedical Imaging in Implantable Drug Delivery Systems. *Current Drug Targets*, *16*(6), 672–682. doi:10.2174/1389450115666141122211920 PMID:25418857

Zhou, H., Zhang, B., Zheng, J., Yu, M., Zhou, T., Zhao, K., Jia, Y., Gao, X., Chen, C., & Wei, T. (2014). The Inhibition of Migration and Invasion of Cancer Cells by Graphene via the Impairment of Mitochondrial Respiration. *Biomaterials*, *35*(5), 1597–1607. doi:10.1016/j.biomaterials.2013.11.020 PMID:24290441

Zhou, J., Hu, Z., Zabihi, F., Chen, Z., & Zhu, M. (2020). Progress and Perspective of Antiviral Protective Material. *Advanced Fiber Materials*, *2*(3), 123–139. doi:10.100742765-020-00047-7

Zhou, Z., Song, J., Nie, L., & Chen, X. (2016). Reactive oxygen species generating systems meeting challenges of photodynamic cancer therapy. *Chemical Society Reviews*, *45*(23), 6597–6626. doi:10.1039/C6CS00271D

Zhu, G., Agrawal, N., Singh, R., Kumar, S., Zhang, B., Saha, C., & Kumar, C. (2020). A novel periodically tapered structure-based gold nanoparticles and graphene oxide – Immobilized optical fiber sensor to detect ascorbic acid. *Optics & Laser Technology*, *127*, 106156. doi:10.1016/j.optlastec.2020.106156

Zhu, H., Yang, C., & Ma, K. (2022). Nanovesicles for transdermal drug delivery. In A. K. Nayak, M. S. Hasnain, T. M. Aminabhavi, & V. P. Torchilin (Eds.), *Applications of Nanovesicular Drug Delivery* (pp. 103–114). Academic Press., doi:10.1016/B978-0-323-91865-7.00012-2

Zhu, H., Zhang, L., Kou, F., Zhao, J., Lei, J., & He, J. (2024). Targeted therapeutic effects of oral magnetically driven pectin nanoparticles containing chlorogenic acid on colon cancer. *Particuology*, *84*, 53–59. doi:10.1016/j.partic.2023.02.021

Zhu, Q., Chen, Z., Paul, P. K., Lu, Y., Wu, W., & Qi, J. (2021). Oral delivery of proteins and peptides: Challenges, status quo and future perspectives. *Acta Pharmaceutica Sinica. B*, *11*(8), 2416–2448. doi:10.1016/j.apsb.2021.04.001 PMID:34522593

Zhu, R., Zhang, F., Peng, Y., Xie, T., Wang, Y., & Lan, Y. (2022). Current progress in cancer treatment using nanomaterials. *Frontiers in Oncology*, *930125*(12), 930125. doi:10.3389/fonc.2022.930125

Zhu, X., Radovic-Moreno, A. F., Wu, J., Langer, R., & Shi, J. (2014). Nanomedicine in the management of microbial infection–overview and perspectives. *Nano Today*, *9*(4), 478–498. doi:10.1016/j.nantod.2014.06.003 PMID:25267927

Zhu, Y. G., Gillings, M., & Penuelas, J. (2020). Integrating biomedical, ecological, and sustainability sciences to manage emerging infectious diseases. *One Earth*, *3*(1), 23–26. doi:10.1016/j.oneear.2020.06.004 PMID:34173527

Zhu, Y. Y., Li, W., Zhao, X., Zhou, Z. J., Wang, Y. T., Cheng, Y. Y., Huang, Q., & Zhang, Q. (2017). Hyaluronic Acid-Encapsulated Platinum Nanoparticles for Targeted Photothermal Therapy of Breast Cancer. *Journal of Biomedical Nanotechnology*, *13*(11), 1457–1467. doi:10.1166/jbn.2017.2446

Zhu, Y., Li, J., Li, W., Zhang, Y., Yang, X., Chen, N., Sun, Y., Zhao, Y., Fan, C., & Huang, Q. (2012). The Biocompatibility of Nanodiamonds and Their Application in Drug Delivery Systems. *Theranostics*, *2*(3), 302–312. doi:10.7150/thno.3627 PMID:22509196

Zhu, Y., Tang, R., Yu, Y., Yu, Z., Wang, K., Wang, Y., & Han, D. (2023). Efficient co-production of xylooligosaccharides and glucose from vinegar residue by biphasic phenoxyethanol-maleic acid pretreatment. *Fermentation (Basel, Switzerland)*, *9*(1), 61. doi:10.3390/fermentation9010061

Zhu, Y., Wang, B., Chen, J., He, J., & Qiu, X. (2023). Facile Synthesis of Three Types of Mesoporous Silica Microspheres as Drug Delivery Carriers and their Sustained-Release Properties. *Current Drug Delivery*, *20*(9), 1337–1350. doi:10.2174/1567201819666220616121602 PMID:35713141

Ziebarth, J., & Mainardes, R. M. (2023). Preparation, characterization and in vitro evaluation of chitosan nanoparticles for the oral delivery of GLP-1 analog liraglutide. *Journal of Thermal Analysis and Calorimetry*, *148*(6), 2443–2455. doi:10.100710973-022-11909-0

Zielińska, A., Carreiró, F., Oliveira, A. M., Neves, A., Pires, B., Venkatesh, D. N., Durazzo, A., Lucarini, M., Eder, P., Silva, A. M., Santini, A., & Souto, E. B. (2020). Polymeric nanoparticles: Production, characterization, toxicology and ecotoxicology. *Molecules (Basel, Switzerland)*, *25*(16), 3731. doi:10.3390/molecules25163731 PMID:32824172

Zielińska, A., Costa, B., Ferreira, M. V., Miguéis, D., Louros, J. M. S., Durazzo, A., Lucarini, M., Eder, P., Chaud, M. V., Morsink, M., Willemen, N., Severino, P., Santini, A., & Souto, E. B. (2020). Nanotoxicology and Nanosafety: Safety-By-Design and Testing at a Glance. *International Journal of Environmental Research and Public Health*, *17*(13). doi:10.3390/ijerph17134657 PMID:32605255

Zielińska, A., Ferreira, N. R., Durazzo, A., Lucarini, M., Cicero, N., Mamouni, S. E., Silva, A. M., Nowak, I., Santini, A., & Souto, E. B. (2019). Development and optimization of alpha-pinene-loaded solid lipid nanoparticles (SLN) using experimental factorial design and dispersion analysis. *Molecules (Basel, Switzerland)*, *24*(15), 2683. doi:10.3390/molecules24152683 PMID:31344802

Zingg, R., & Fischer, M. (2019). The consolidation of nanomedicine. *Wiley Interdisciplinary Reviews. Nanomedicine and Nanobiotechnology*, *11*(6), e1569. doi:10.1002/wnan.1569 PMID:31240855

Ziobro, D., Dąbrowski, R., Tykarska, M., Drzewiński, W., Filipowicz, M., Rejmer, W., Kuśmierek, K., Morawiak, P., & Piecek, W. (2012). Synthesis and properties of new ferroelectric and antiferroelectric liquid crystals with a biphenylyl benzoate rigid core. *Liquid Crystals*, *39*(8), 1011–1032. doi:10.1080/02678292.2012.691560

Zishan, M., Zeeshan, A., & Faisal, S. (2017). Vesicular drug delivery system used for liver diseases. *World J Pharm Sci.*, *5*(4), 28–35.

Zolkepli, H., Widodo, R. T., Mahmood, S., Salim, N., Awang, K., Ahmad, N., & Othman, R. (2022). A Review on the Delivery of Plant-Based Antidiabetic Agents Using Nanocarriers: Current Status and Their Role in Combatting Hyperglycaemia. *Polymers*, *14*(15), 2991. doi:10.3390/polym14152991 PMID:35893954

Zong, Q., Dong, N., Yang, X., Ling, G., & Zhang, P. (2021). Development of gold nanorods for cancer treatment. *Journal of Inorganic Biochemistry*, *220*, 111458. doi:10.1016/j.jinorgbio.2021.111458 PMID:33857697

Zou, Z., Iwata, M., Yamanishi, Y., & Oki, S. (2022). Epigenetic landscape of drug responses revealed through large-scale ChIP-seq data analyses. *BMC Bioinformatics*, *23*(1), 51. doi:10.118612859-022-04571-8 PMID:35073843

Zweers, M. L., Grijpma, D. W., Engbers, G. H., & Feijen, J. (2003). The preparation of monodisperse biodegradable polyester nanoparticles with a controlled size. *Journal of Biomedical Materials Research. Part B, Applied Biomaterials*, *66*(2), 559–566. doi:10.1002/jbm.b.10046 PMID:12861608

About the Contributors

Pranav Kumar Prabhakar has received his PhD in Biotechnology from Indian Institute of Technology (IIT) Madras, India during the period of 2011 and he has completed his master in biochemistry from Patna University Bihar, India in 2003. Currently, he is working as Assistant Professor in Lovely Professional University Punjab, India. He has successfully completed his Administrative responsibilities as research coordinator of the school. His research has included synergy, Phytomedicine, metabolic disorders. He is serving as an editorial member of several reputed journals & expert Reviewers for journals. He has authored 85+ research articles, 5 books, 15 book chapters. He has been listed in World's top 2% scientist (a list prepared by Stanford University, USA) in 2021, 2022, and 2023. He is a member of Royal Society of Chemistry and Asia-Pacific Chemical, Biological& Environmental Engineering Society (APCBEES).

Ajit Prakash is a postdoc in UNC, Chapel Hill. I did my B.Sc and M.Sc. from India and complete PhD in 2016 from Nanyang Technological University, Singapore. He works on drug development for Ras protein and also study the properties of G alpha protein. His research work involves protein expression, purification followed by NMR and X-ray crystallization and also cell culture work.

***

Niteshkumar Agrawal (S'19, M'22, SM'23) received his Ph.D. Degree from IIST/URSC, ISRO Thiruvananthapuram, and M.Tech. Degree from IIT (ISM) Dhanbad. He is currently working as an Associate Professor at Pillai College of Engineering (Autonomous), Mumbai University. He is an Ex. Project Researcher at IIST/URSC, ISRO Thiruvananthapuram during 2018-21 and Ex. Visiting Researcher at Liaocheng University (LCU), China during Mar-Nov 2019. He has more than 13 years of Research & Development, Teaching & Training, Industry, and, Administration Experience. He has authored 02 scientific books (with CRC Press, Traylor & Francis Publications, and Namya Publications) and 02 book contributions, 15 articles in scientific journals, and 05 international conferences. He has 03 completed/ongoing research projects and contracts financed by the ICSSR, Govt. of India (5 Lacs), Mumbai University, Govt. of Maharashtra (0.25 Lacs), and Siemens India Ltd, Kalwa Mumbai (5 Lacs). There is one Copyright, Government of India registered under his name. He has delivered more than 20 Invited Talks/Technical Sessions/Training Sessions at various institutions and organizations. He has guided 03 postgraduate students and is currently guiding 02 Ph.D. scholars. He is also the recipient of an AICTE-INAE/ Department of Space (DoS)-TRF Fellowship and a Chinese Government Scholarship for International Students. He is an IEEE Senior Member, and an active member of OSA, & SPIE. Currently serves as Industry Liasoning Officer, IRE Committee at IEEE Bombay Section (Since May 23).

He is Ex. Industry Coordinator for IEEE EMBS Chapter Kerala State (2021-22), Track Chair, ESST, IEEE INDICON-2022 Conference, Kochi, India, Meta Reviewer of IEEE Biosensors Conference-2023 London, UK, Meta-Reviewer/TPC Member, IEEE Sensors Conference-2022, Dallas, Texas USA, and Meta-Reviewer, IEEE I4Tech 2022 International Conference, Pune, India. His current research interests include Optics, Nanomaterials, Plasmonics, Sensors, Avionics, and Nanotechnology.

Mayank Bahuguna is a Ph.D. student working in a field of Environmental Biotechnology and its application for diverse problems.

Ranjit Barua is a Senior Researchers at Centre for Healthcare Science and Technology, IIEST-SHIBPUR. Core research area Bio-Mechanical System, 3D Bioprinting, Tissue Engineering.

Swati Bhathley is doing Masters in Physics in Lovely Professional University.

Nabaparna Chakraborty is working as Assistant Professor in Lovely professional University and published 30 research papers in Indexed journals.

Purva Chandorkar is a PhD Scholar from MIT-WPU in the department of Pharmaceutics. She has completed her Masters in Pharmaceutics from MIT-WPU. She has three publications in journals like "International Journal of Pharmacy, Biology and Applied Sciences" and "Research Journal of Biotechnology." She has successfully filed a design patent along with her colleagues. She has presented two posters in International e-poster presentation conferences held by "SNJB" and "BNCP" College of Pharmacy.

Sachin Chavan is a Professor at Bharati Vidhyapeeth (Deemed to be University), College of Engineering, Pune, Maharashtra, India. His research area of interest is nanotechology, Nano fibers synthesis and their various applications.

Babita Deka is currently working as assistant professor at NETES institute of Pharmaceutical science. Also persuing PhD at Srimanta Sankaradeva University of Health Sciences, Guwahati.

Sunita Devi did a Masters of Sciences from Panjab University, Chandigarh, India and doing Ph. D. from Lovely Professional University, Punjab, India

İlker Erdem graduated from Ege University Food Engineering Department in 1999. He had his MSc degree at İzmir Institute of Technology (IZTECH) from Biotechnology and Bioengineering MSc Program (2002) and his PhD degree at IZTECH from Chemical Engineering PhD Program (2009). He has been working on ceramic nano materials and their applications (e.g. ceramic membranes, photocatalytic nano ceramics) and different applications of various materials, currently at Abdullah Gül University Nanotechnology Engineering Department as an assistant professor.

Ashpinder Kaur Gill is M. Sc. in Physics from Panjab University Chandigarh and doing Ph. D. from Lovely Professional University, Phagwara Punjab, India.

Sanjay Gupta is a Senior Professor and Principal of the institution (Himalayan School of Biosciences) with an interest in Bioprocess Engineering, Environmental Biotechnology. A tremendous experience of more than 27 years in teaching and 109 publications, with many more to come.

Swati Jagdale is a highly accomplished academic and researcher in the field of pharmaceutics. She earned her B.Pharm. (1998), M.Pharm. (2000) from Pune University, and Ph.D. (2009) from Shivaji University Kolhapur. Currently, she holds the prestigious position of Professor in the Department of Pharmaceutics at the School of Health Sciences and Technology in Pune. Dr. Jagdale's significant contributions to the field of pharmaceutics are widely recognized, with more than 80 research articles published in reputed national and international journals, along with five authored books and ten book chapters. She holds one Indian patent and two patents from the Republic of South Africa, with an additional five Indian patents currently in process. She has also received funding for her research projects from the Council of Scientific and Industrial Research (CSIR) (Amount 21.36 Lakh) and AICTE-MODROB grant (Rs. 17.22 Lacs), in addition to completing two minor research projects at Savitribai Phule Pune University (4.9 Lakhs). As an experienced guide, Dr. Jagdale has successfully mentored 75 M. Pharm. students and 06 Ph.D. students, with four M. Pharm. and three Ph.D. students currently working on their projects under her guidance. Dr. Jagdale has presented her research work at various national and international conferences and also serves as a member of the Board of Studies under Science and Technology for Faculty of Pharmaceutics at Savitribai Phule Pune University. Her research article on ""Formulation and Evaluation of Gastroretentive Drug Delivery System of Propranolol Hydrochloride"" was one of the top five downloaded articles in AAPS PharmSciTech in 2012. She had also previously served as a member of the Board of Studies for Faculty of Pharmaceutics at the University of Pune.

Kailash Chandra Juglan is working as Professor and Associate Dean in Department of Physics, Lovely Professional University University, He has supervised 7 PhD and 30 masters thesis. He has published 75 research papers in indexed journals.

Jayasree S Kanathasan is Program Coordinator in Biomedical Science Department at the Faculty of Applied Sciences, Lincoln University. Dr Jayasree completed her undergraduate degree in Biomedical Science from University Tunku Abdul Rahman. She pursued her postgraduate studies in Master of Engineering Science (Research) and Doctor of Philosophy in Biomedical Engineering at Monash University Malaysia sponsored by Ministry of Higher Education (MOHE) and Monash University scholarship. She designed her PhD project on peptide functionalized fluorescent porous silicon and carbon dot nanoparticles for breast cancer imaging which was awarded with FRGS grant and known as one of the outstanding projects in the round of application for the year 2016. Her work was presented in International Conference on Advances in Functional Materials, University of California, Los Angeles.

Minhaj A. Khan working as Associate Professor in Department of Biochemistry under School of Bioengineering and Biosciences LPU

Shreedevi Kulkarni has completed BE (Instrumentation Technology), MTech (Biomedical Instrumentation) and PhD (Electrical and Electronic Engineering and Sciences). The research area relates to development of a method for the analysis of drug in low concentration and this relates to microsystem. The project was accepted and completed under INUP (Indian Nanotechnology User Program) at IITB,

Mumbai. The research interest are in sensors, biomedical instruments, microsystems, rehabilitative and assistive devices. She also completed bootcamp on virtual labs development, IITB. Have been a mentor for the development of the virtual labs in association with IITB. Worked as the regional and nodal coordinator for virtual lab. Have handled projects related to a number of biomedical instruments.

Devi Nallappan is a lecturer at the Department of Biomedical Science, Lincoln University College. Dr. Devi earned a Bachelor of Applied Science (Hons) in Bioindustrial Technology with first-class honors from University of Malaysia Kelantan in 2016. She went on to complete her PhD in Biomedical Science, with a focus on Biochemistry, at Universiti Malaya in 2022. Dr Devi's research during her PhD investigated the use of natural compounds to prevent and treat high-fat diet-induced obesity and its associated complications. She also worked on nano biomedicine-related projects, concentrating on the green synthesis of nanoparticles and their potential biological effects. Dr Devi has published numerous ISI-indexed reviews and research articles and has been awarded best oral and poster presenter in symposiums and conferences.

Kajal Parashar is working as PhD scholar in School of Bioengineering and Biosciences LPU

Pooja Patowary is currently working as an Assistant Professor in the Department of Pharmaceutical Chemistry at NETES Institute of Pharmaceutical Science, Shantipur, Mirza since 2018. Pursuing PhD in the Department of Pharmaceutical Sciences, Dibrugarh University. Graduation and post graduation were completed in 2017 from Departments of Pharmaceutical Sciences, Dibrugarh University.

Sandeep Poddar, Deputy Vice Chancellor (Research & Innovation), Member of Board of Studies, Lincoln University College, Malaysia, has been graduated from University of Calcutta in 1993 with Honours in Zoology, he has obtained Post Graduate Diploma in Dietetics from All India Institute of Hygiene and Public Health 1995, Master of Science in Zoology with specialization in Biochemical Genetics from Dayalbagh Educational Institute 1998 with distinction. He has completed PhD in Zoology from Vivekananda Institute of Medical Sciences on Cytotoxicity in 2004. After completing PhD he pursued Post Doctoral Research in different projects on Hemoglobinopathies and Oral Cancer mutation. He has published several research papers, filed patent and organized international conferences, and also edited books in Malaysia, Australia and India. Dr Sandeep obtained his MBA from Lincoln University College, Malaysia as well. Dr Sandeep is Fellow member of World Researchers Associations and Life members of Different associations including Indian Science Congress Association. Dr Sandeep is founder Assistant Secretary of Dr Tarak Nath Podder Memorial Foundation, Kolkata, India

Akash Podutwar is a PhD scholar in the department of pharmaceutics at MIT-World Peace university, Pune. He has received his Master of Pharmacy in Pharmaceutics from MIT-World Peace university, Pune itself. He has several publications in well known journals like "Journal of Pharmaceutical Research International" and "International Journal of Recent Scientific Research". Also he has one design patent titled "Novel integrated dissolution-disintegration apparatus" which is successfully filed in 2022.

Satish Polshettiwar is working as HoD and Asst Professor at School of Health Sciences and Technology MIT-WPU Pune. Published more than 50 research and review article in peer review journal. Filed 7 Indian patent and 2 patent has been granted. Published 3 textbook on Pharm Microbiology and Pharm Engineering.

Suyash Saxena, as a young researcher and Assistant Professor, has served and contributed significantly in the field of medical science and education more than 14 years. He is actively involved in the area of Advance surgical instrumentation, Clinical Biochemistry and oxidative stress etc. He has received various awards including Best Teacher Award (2022). He has significantly contributed in the novel invention not only in the field of medical science but also in enhancing women empowerment as, evidenced by published more than 25 patents. He has contributed significantly as author of several chapters in National book related to the effect of COVID 19 in organ system. H has organized several conferences/seminars in the field of medical sciences, research methodology and IPR.

Rahul Saxena is a dynamic and enthusiastic young researcher and academician. He has served and contributed significantly in the field of medical science and education as a Professor and researcher more than 17 years. His research concentrates on identification of various sorts of preventive measures of infection during surgical process, facilitating surgeons and patients of sub urbs and lower economic group. Apart from that free radicals mediated biomolecular deterioration and their role in the etiology of diseases have been focused by him. By means of several invention, evidenced by published more than 30 patents, he has contributed significantly not only in the field of medical science but also in enhancing women empowerment, and helping the geriatric population and students of rural areas. In the post COVID era, he has published two research books in relation to the effect of COVID 19 in various field of medical sciences. He has organized several conferences/seminars in the field of medical sciences, research methodology and IPR to impart the knowledge and motivate the young researchers. In addition, he has received several prestigious awards from various Research & Academic Bodies as Young scientist award, best teacher award etc. He has served as a Reviewer of various National and International journals in the field of medical sciences.

Demet Saylan is currently a Lecturer at Abdullah Gul University. She earned her Bachelor degree in biology in Turkiye. Later, she finished her Master's and PhD in cancer research in the UK. She is interested in bioactive compounds in food and their role in human cancers.

Garima Shandilya is a Phd (Nanotechnology) Scholar, Bharati Vidhyapeeth (Deemed to be University), College of Engineering, Pune, Maharashtra, India. She is working in the field of Nanotechnology and its applications in nanomedicine, nanoagronomics and nanobiotechnology.

Charu Sharma is a Ph.D. Student working in the field of Bioremediation in wastewater.

Vandana Singh, an Assistant Professor in the Department of Microbiology at School of Allied Health Sciences of Sharda University, holds a Ph.D. in Microbiology. She earned her M.Sc. in Microbiology from the University of Pune, Pune(India) and then She completed her Ph.D. in Microbiology from Noida International University, Noida (India). With over 12 years of teaching and research experience, her areas of expertise include Medical Microbiology, Environmental microbiology, Food microbiology, Microbial nanotechnology, Nano-materials, and microbial biotechnology. Her passion for microbiology is evident in her dedication to producing good-quality research, leading to numerous publications in the form of research articles, review papers and book chapters, in peer-reviewed and reputed journals. Her research interests focus on Medical Microbiology, Nanotechnology, Toxicity, Microbial Fuel cells, Wastewater Treatment, Biological Wastewater Treatment, Environmental Biotechnology, Bioremediation of Water and Wastewater Treatment, Biodegradation, Biofilms production, Biosurfactant production, remediation of pollutants etc.

Ajit Pal Singh, as a young researcher and Assistant Professor, has served and contributed significantly in the field of medical science and education more than 5 years. He is actively involved in the area of Medical Laboratory Technology. He has received various awards including Best Teacher Award (2022). He has significantly contributed in the novel invention not only in the field of medical science but also in enhancing women empowerment as, evidenced by published more than 25 patents. He has contributed significantly as author of several chapters in National book related to the effect of COVID 19 in organ system. H has organized several conferences/seminars in the field of medical sciences, research methodology and IPR.

Kirtan Tarwadi is a Professor, Bharati Vidhyapeeth (Deemed to be University), College of Engineering, Pune, Maharashtra, India. Her research areas are biotechnology, biochemistry and nanotechnology.

S. K. Tripathy is working as Associate Professor in Department of Electronics and Communication Engineering of National Institute of Technology Silchar, Assam. He obtained Ph.D. (Engg.) degree in optoelectronics materials from Indian Institute of Technology (ISM) Dhanbad, India, M. Tech. degree in Digital Systems from Motilal Nehru National Institute of Technology Allahabad, India and B.E. in Electronics and Communication Engineering from BPUT, Odisha, India in the year 2014, 2009 and 2003, respectively. His teaching interests are Microelectronics, VLSI Design and Physics of Semiconductor Devices. His research interests include Modeling of Semiconductor Devices, Photonics sensors, Renewable Energy and Materials for Optoelectronics applications.

Bancha Yingngam, an Associate Professor at Ubon Ratchathani University in Thailand, brings a wealth of knowledge and experience in Pharmaceutical Sciences and Technology. His academic path started in 2005, when he graduated with a bachelor's degree in pharmacy, receiving second-class honors. Driven by his passion for green chemistry and the pharmacy and pharmaceutical industry, he furthered his studies, obtaining a Ph.D. in 2011 from the same university. Between 2013 and 2021, during his postdoctoral fellowship at Karl-Franzens-Universität Graz, Austria, he extended his research focus to include optimization and machine learning algorithms. This focus has significantly influenced his field, as exemplified by his Scopus H-index of 10. Throughout his career, Dr. Yingngam has written over twenty scholarly articles, book chapters, and conference papers. His research largely explores optimization algorithms and the integration of machine learning in the pharmaceutical sciences. He is currently authoring book chapters that delve into artificial intelligence applications for green chemistry and pharmacy. His research has been acknowledged and published in various esteemed journals, and his contributions have enriched several key publications in his field. His exceptional work has twice earned him the "Outstanding Research Award in Health Science" from Ubon Ratchathani University in 2020 and 2022. Beyond his extensive research, Dr. Yingngam excels as an educator and mentor, having guided 1 Ph.D. student and 10 master's students in Austria toward achieving their academic and professional aspirations. Furthermore, his dedication to his field is showcased in his review of more than 100 articles listed in the Scopus database. Through his work in research and education, Dr. Yingngam continues to advance pharmaceutical sciences and technology.

Index

D

E

F

G

H

I

M

N

P

Q

www.ingramcontent.com/pod-product-compliance
Lightning Source LLC
LaVergne TN
LVHW060251011026
849161LV00011B/2693
* 9 7 9 8 3 6 9 3 0 4 4 8 8 *